INTEGRATED OBSTETRICS
AND GYNAECOLOGY
FOR POSTGRADUATES

INTEGRATED OBSTETRICS
AND GYNAECOLOGY
FOR POSTGRADUATES

EDITED BY

C. J. DEWHURST

M.B. Ch.B. F.R.C.S.(Ed.) F.R.C.O.G.

Professor of Obstetrics and Gynaecology
Institute of Obstetrics and Gynaecology at
Queen Charlotte's Hospital and
Chelsea Hospital for Women
University of London

BLACKWELL SCIENTIFIC PUBLICATIONS
OXFORD LONDON EDINBURGH
MELBOURNE

© 1972 by Blackwell Scientific Publications
Osney Mead, Oxford
3 Nottingham Street, London, W1
9 Forrest Road, Edinburgh
P.O. Box 9, North Balwyn, Victoria, Australia

ISBN 0 632 06660 1

First published 1972

Distributed in the USA by
F. A. Davis Company, 1915 Arch Street,
Philadelphia, Pennsylvania

Printed and bound in
Great Britain by
William Clowes & Sons Limited
London, Colchester and Beccles

CONTENTS

LIST OF CONTRIBUTORS

J.M.BRUDENELL M.B. B.S. F.R.C.S. M.R.C.O.G.
Consultant Obstetrician and Gynaecologist, King's College Hospital, London &
Queen Victoria Hospital, East Grinstead
Diabetes, thyroid diseases and adrenal diseases complicating pregnancy
General surgical procedures
Urinary tract injuries

G.V.P.CHAMBERLAIN M.D. B.S. F.R.C.S. F.R.C.O.G.
Consultant Obstetrician, Queen Charlotte's Hospital, London;
Consultant Gynaecologist, Chelsea Hospital for Women, London
The foetus

D.A.DAVEY Ph.D. M.B. B.S. M.R.C.S. F.R.C.O.G.
Professor of Obstetrics and Gynaecology, University of
Cape Town, South Africa
Normal pregnancy: physiology and management
Dysfunctional uterine bleeding

C.J.DEWHURST M.B. ch.B. F.R.C.S.(ED.) F.R.C.O.G.
Professor of Obstetrics and Gynaecology, Institute of Obstetrics and
Gynaecology, Queen Charlotte's Hospital and Chelsea Hospital for
Women, University of London
Normal and abnormal development of the genital organs
Gynaecological Disorders in Childhood and Adolescence
The normal puerperium
Pre-eclampsia, eclampsia, hypertension and chronic renal disease
Miscellaneous disorders complicating pregnancy
Abnormalities of the puerperium

Obstetric operations and procedures
Maternal and perinatal mortality
The menopause and climacteric
Benign and pre-malignant lesions of the vulva, vagina and cervix

R.M.FEROZE M.D. B.S. F.R.C.S. F.R.C.O.G.
Consultant Obstetrician and Gynaecologist, King's College
Hospital, London; Consultant Obstetrician, Queen Charlotte's
Maternity Hospital, London
Tumours of the female genital tract
Tumours of the vulva and vagina
Benign tumours of the uterus
Malignant disease of the cervix
Malignant disease of the uterine body
Tumours of the ovary

J.M.HOLMES M.D. B.S. F.R.C.O.G.
Consultant Obstetrician and Gynaecologist, University College
Hospital, London
Abnormal uterine action and prolonged labour
Contracted pelvis, disproportion and obstructed labour
Maternal injuries and complications
Resuscitation of the newborn

E.D.MORRIS M.D. B.ch. F.R.C.S. M.R.C.O.G.
Consultant Obstetrician and Gynaecologist, Guy's Hospital, London;
Consultant Obstetrician, Queen Charlotte's Maternity Hospital, London
Fertilization, implantation, placental function, early development
Contraception and sterilization
Malpositions of the occiput, malpresentations, multiple pregnancy, hydramnios,
oligohydramnios and post maturity

G.D.PINKER M.B. B.S. F.R.C.S. F.R.C.O.G.
Consultant Gynaecologist and Obstetrician, St. Mary's Hospital, London;
Consultant Gynaecologist, Middlesex, Samaritan and Bolingbroke Hospitals
Infertility and dyspareunia

J.D.ROBERTSON M.D. F.R.C.S.(Ed) M.R.C.O.G.
Complications of the third stage of labour
Heart disease in pregnancy

Blood disorders in pregnancy
Endometriosis
Pelvic infection

J.S.SCOTT M.D. Ch.B. F.R.C.S. F.R.C.O.G.
Professor of Obstetrics and Gynaecology, University of Leeds
Abortion, ectopic pregnancy and trophoblastic growths
Antepartum haemorrhage
Prolapse and stress incontinence of urine

R.P.SHEARMAN M.D. D.G.O. F.R.C.O.G.
Professor Obstetrics and Gynaecology, University of Sydney, Australia
Control of ovarian function
The intersexes
Primary amenorrhoea
Secondary amenorrhoea
Hirsutism and virilism
Endocrine changes during pregnancy
Induction of ovulation

PREFACE

Our purpose in writing this book has been to produce a comprehensive account of what the specialist in training in obstetrics and gynaecology must know. Unfortunately for him, he must now know a great deal, not only about his own subject, but about certain aspects of closely allied specialities such as endocrinology, biochemistry, cytogenetics, psychiatry, etc. Accordingly we have tried to offer the postgraduate student not only an advanced textbook in obstetrics and gynaecology but one which integrates the relevant aspects of other subjects which nowadays impinge more and more on the clinical field.

To achieve this aim within, we hope, a reasonable compass we have assumed some basic knowledge which the reader will have assimilated throughout his medical training, and we have taken matters on from there. Fundamental facts not in question are stated as briefly as is compatible with accuracy and clarity, and discussion is then deveoted to more advanced aspects. We acknowledge that it is not possible even in this way to provide all the detail some readers may wish, so an appropriate bibliography is provided with each chapter. Wherever possible we have tried to give a positive opinion and our reasons for holding it, but to discuss nonetheless other important views; this we believe to be more helpful than a complete account of all possible opinions which may be held. We have chosen moreover to lay emphasis on fundamental aspects of the natural and the disease processes which are discussed; we believe concentration on these basic physiological and pathological features to be important to the proper training of a specialist.

Clinical matters are, of course, dealt with in detail too, whenever theoretical discussion of them is rewarding. There are, however, some clinical aspects which cannot, at specialist level, be considered in theory with real benefit; examples of these are *how* to palpate a pregnant woman's abdomen and *how* to apply obstetric forceps. In general these matters are considered very briefly or perhaps not at all; this is not a book on *how* things are done, but on how correct treatment is chosen, what advantages one choice has over another, what complications are to be expected, etc. Practical matters, we believe, are better learnt in practice and with occasional reference to specialised textbooks devoted solely to them.

A word may be helpful about the manner in which the book is set out. We would willingly have followed the advice given to Alice when about to testify at the trial of the Knave of Hearts in Wonderland, 'Begin at the beginning, keep on until you come to the end and then stop'. But this advice is difficult to follow when attempting to find the beginning of complex subjects such as those to which this book is devoted. Does the beginning lie with fertilization; or with the events which lead up to it; or with the genital organs upon the correct function of which any pregnancy must depend; or does it lie somewhere else? And which direction must we follow then? The disorders of reproduction do not lie in a separate compartment from genital tract diseases, but each is clearly associated with the other for at least part of a woman's life. Although we have attempted to integrate obstetrics with gynaecology and with their associated specialities, some separation is essential in writing about them, and the plan we have followed is broadly this—we begin with the female child in utero, follow her through childhood to puberty, through adolescence to maturity, through pregnancy to motherhood, through her reproductive years to the climacteric and into old age. Some events have had to be taken out of order however, although reiteration has been avoided by indicating to the reader where in the book are to be found other sections dealing with different aspects of any subject under consideration.

We hope that our efforts will provide a coherent, integrated account of the field we have attempted to cover which will be to the satisfaction of our readers.

ACKNOWLEDGMENTS

In the presentation of this book, we have received assistance from numerous sources, and we wish to record our gratitude to all who have helped. We would specially like to indicate our indebtedness to those authors, publishers and editors listed below who have allowed us to reproduce material previously published elsewhere. To: Mr David Currie, Mr T. M. Coltart, Dr W. J. Garrett, Professor Sir Norman Jeffcoate, Dr Henry Roberts, Dr George Craig, Dr P. P. Franklyn, Professor W. J. Hamilton, Professor Llewellyn-Jones, Dr M. N. Grumbach, Dr J. B. Brown, Dr M. G. Coyle, Professor F. E. Hytten, Dr I. Leitch, Dr J. P. Gusdon Jr, Dr P. M. Elliott, Dr C. G. Paine, Dr S. Leon Israel, Dr E. C. Gillespie, Dr H. Steven, Professor R. W. Beard, Dr J. D. N. Nabarro, Dr N. W. Oakley, Dr R. C. Turner, Sir George Godber, Professor Harvey Carey, Professor J. P. Greenhill, Dr C. A. Salvatore, Dr J. A. Loraine, Dr E. T. Bell, Dr H. F. Traut, Dr A. Kuder, Dr A. L. Southam, Dr R. M. Richart, Dr A. M. Sutherland, Dr N. Vorys, Dr A. S. Neri, Dr Goerttler, Dr D. N. Danforth, and Dr E. E. Philipp; to Messrs: C. C. Thomas & Co, Baillière, Tindall and Cassell, Butterworth Medical Publications, Faber and Faber, Blackwell Scientific Publications, E. & S. Livingstone, The Surgical Publishing Co of Chicago, C. V. Mosby & Co., Gillmore and Lawrence, Harper & Rowe, Butterworth & Co., W. B. Saunders & Co., John Sherratt & Son, Controller of Her Majesty's Stationery Office, W. Heffer & Sons, and W. Heinemann Medical Books; and to the Editors of: *Australia and New Zealand Journal of Obstetrics and Gynaecology, Hoeber Medical Journals, The Lancet, British Medical Journal, Journal of Obstetrics and Gynaecology of the British Commonwealth, Proceedings of the New York Academy of Sciences, Journal of Pathology and Bacteriology, Bulletin of The Johns Hopkins Hospital, American Journal of Obstetrics and Gynaecology, Journal of the International College of Surgeons, Proceedings of the Royal Medico-Chirurgical Society of Glasgow.*

We would like to offer our most grateful thanks also to: Mr Stuart Campbell, Dr Magnus Haines, Dr H. P. Ferreira, Dr J. Smitham, Dr Peter Renou, Dr P. N. Cowan, Dr J. Pryse-Davies, Mr A. Gillespie, Professor J. M. Beazley, Dr Mary Lucas, Miss Baker, Miss Lumby, Mrs Apsey, Miss Platt, Miss Collins, Miss Miller and Miss Brodie, all of whom have given direct and most valuable assistance with the preparation of this book by supplying many of its illustrations or typing the manscript.

It has been a great pleasure for us all to co-operate in this venture with Blackwell Scientific Publications to whom we are grateful for their help, understanding and forebearance.

CHAPTER 1

NORMAL AND ABNORMAL DEVELOPMENT OF THE GENITAL ORGANS

Any account of the development of the genital organs should contain not only the details of how they are formed but also why they form as they do in the two sexes. The determinants of sex are more fully considered in Chapter 4. At this point it will be sufficient to state briefly the relationship between the sex chromosomes, the gonads and the other genital organs.

Sexual development depends initially on the arrangement of the sex chromosomes. Normal men have an XY sex chromosome arrangement

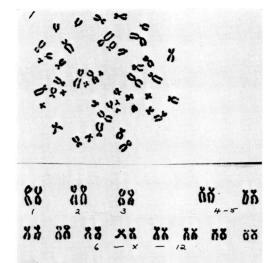

Fig. 1.1(b). Normal female karyotype. The Y chromosome resembles the small acrocentric ones of groups 21 and 22 but is usually distinguishable from them. The X chromosome resembles those of the largest group—6 to 12—and cannot be separately distinguished except by special techniques.

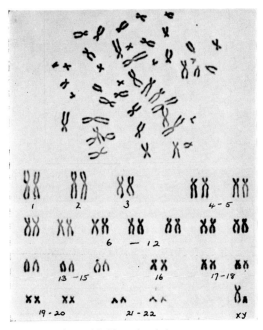

Fig. 1.1(a). Normal male karyotype.

and normal women an XX one (Fig. 1.1). Sometimes, however, individuals are born with additional sex chromosomes and are XXY, XYY, XXYY, XXX, XXXX, etc., and others with a single X only; still others have different arrangements which need not concern us here.

If a Y chromosome is present, however, with one or more X chromosomes testes will form in the early embryo; if two or more X chromosomes are present without a Y ovaries form. If a single X chromosome is present alone normal definitive gonadal tissue does not form and the gonads are represented by whitish streaks of tissue.

The relationship between the gonad and the development of the other genital organs is, in summary, this. If testes form in the early embryo that individual will develop male genital organs. If testes do not form the individual will develop female genital organs whether ovaries are present or not. It may be concluded that the arrangement of the sex chromosomes determines the nature of the gonad, which in turn determines the differentiation of the other genital organs.

We will now turn our attention to how the genital organs develop.

THE DEVELOPMENT OF THE GENITAL ORGANS

Most embryological accounts agree on the principles of genital tract development as a whole, although different views are held on the development of the gonad and vagina.

The genital organs and those of the urinary tract arise in the intermediate mesoderm on either side of the root of the mesentery, beneath the epithelium of the coelom. The pronephros, a few transient excretory tubules in the cervical region, appears first but quickly degenerates. The duct which begins in association with the pronephros persists and extends caudally to open at the cloaca, connecting as it does so with some of the tubules of the mesonephros shortly to appear. The duct is called the mesonephric (Wolffian) duct. The mesonephros itself, the second primitive kidney, develops as a swelling bulging into the dorsal wall of the coelom of the thoracic and upper lumbar regions. The mesonephros in the male persists in part as the excretory portion of the male genital system; in the female a few vestiges only survive (Fig. 1.2). The genital ridge in which the gonad of each sex is to develop is visible as a swelling on the medial aspect

of the mesonephros; the paramesonephric (Mullerian) duct, from which much of the female genital tract will develop, forms as an ingrowth of coelomic epithilium on its lateral aspect (10 mm C.R. length; 5–6 weeks). The ingrowth forms a groove and then a tube and sinks below the surface.

DEVELOPMENT OF THE UTERUS AND FALLOPIAN TUBES

The two paramesonephric (Mullerian) ducts then extend caudally until they reach the urogenital sinus, about 9 weeks; the blind ends project into the posterior wall of the sinus as the Mullerian tubercle. At the beginning of the third month the Mullerian and Wolffian ducts and mesonephric tubules are all present and capable of development [Fig. 1.2(a)]. From this point onwards in the female there is degeneration of the Wolffian system and marked growth of the Mullerian system [Fig. 1.2(b)]. In the male the opposite occurs [Fig. 1.2(c)]. The lower ends of the Mullerian ducts come together in the mid-line and fuse and develop into the uterus and cervix; the cephalic ends of the duct remain separate to form the fallopian tubes. The thick muscular walls of the uterus and cervix develop from proliferation of mesenchyme around the fused portions of the ducts.

DEVELOPMENT OF THE VAGINA

There is difference of opinion about the precise events in vaginal development. At the point where the mesonephric ducts protrude their solid tips into the dorsal wall of the urogenital sinus as the Mullerian tubercle (30 mm stage; 9 weeks) there is a marked growth of tissue from which the vagina will ultimately form. Koff (1933) describes the formation of paired sinovaginal bulbs as posterior evaginations of the urogenital sinus; there is also stratification of the cells lining that part of the sinus, and this obliterates the Mullerian tubercle. The sinovaginal bulbs, which become solidified by further epithilial proliferation, fuse with the lower end of the Mullerian ducts to form the vaginal plate. This plate quickly grows in all dimensions, greatly increasing the distance between the cervix

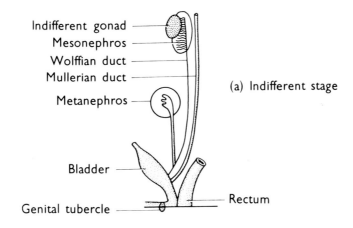

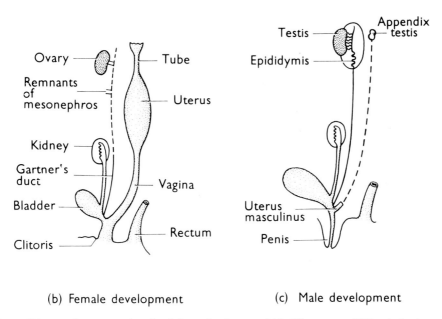

Fig. 1.2. Diagramatic representation of genital tract development. (a) Indifferent stage. (b) Female development. (c) Male development (By courtesy of Baillière, Tindall and Cassell.)

and the urogenital sinus. Later, the central cells of this plate break down to form the vaginal lumen.

According to Koff, approximately the upper four-fifths of the vagina is formed by the Mullerian ducts and the lower fifth from the urogenital sinus by the growth of the sino-

vaginal bulbs. He regards the hymen as being totally derived from the sinus epithilium. Vilas (1932) and Bulmer (1957) and others hold a different view. They believe that the sinus up-growth extends up to the cervix, displacing the Mullerian component completely, the vagina

(a) Indifferent stage

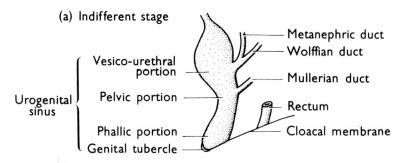

Urogenital sinus
- Vesico-urethral portion
- Pelvic portion
- Phallic portion
- Genital tubercle

- Metanephric duct
- Wolffian duct
- Mullerian duct
- Rectum
- Cloacal membrane

(b) Female development

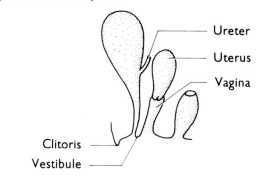

- Ureter
- Uterus
- Vagina
- Clitoris
- Vestibule

(c) Male development

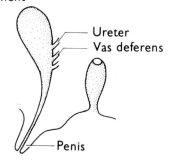

- Ureter
- Vas deferens
- Penis

Fig. 1.3. Diagramatic representation of lower genital tract development. (a) Indifferent stage. (b) Female development. (c) Male development. (By courtesy of Baillière, Tindall and Cassell.)

being thus derived wholly from the endoderm of the urogenital sinus. It seems certain that some of the vagina is formed from the urogenital sinus, but it is not certain whether the Mullerian component is involved or not.

THE DEVELOPMENT OF THE EXTERNAL GENITALIA

The primitive cloaca becomes divided by a transverse septum into an anterior urogenital portion and a posterior rectal portion. The urogenital portion of the cloacal membrane breaks down shortly after division is complete (15 mm C.R. length). The urogenital sinus develops further into three portions (Fig. 1.3). There is an external, expanded, phallic part, a deeper, narrow, pelvic part between it and the region of the Mullerian tubercle, and a vesico-urethral part connected superiorly to the allantois. Externally in this region the genital tubercle forms a conical projection around the anterior part of the cloacal membrane. Two pairs of swellings, a medial pair (the genital folds) and a lateral pair (genital swellings) are then formed by proliferation of mesoderm round the end of the urogenital sinus. Development up to this time (50 mm C.R. length; 10 weeks) is the same in the male and the female. Differentiation then occurs. The bladder and urethra form from the vesico-urethral portion of the urogenital sinus and the vestibule from the pelvic and phallic portions (Fig. 1.3). The genital tubercle enlarges only slightly and becomes the clitoris. The genital folds become the labia minora and the genital swellings enlarge to become the labia majora. In the male greater enlargement of the genital tubercle forms the penis. The genital folds fuse over a deep groove formed between them to become the penile part of the male urethra. The genital swellings enlarge, fuse and form the scrotum.

The final stage of the development of the clitoris or penis and the formation of the anterior surface of the bladder and the anterior abdominal wall up to the umbilicus is the result of growth of mesoderm extending ventrally round the body wall on each side to unite in the midline anteriorly.

DEVELOPMENT OF THE GONADS

The primitive gonad is first evident in embryos of 5·5–7·5 mm C.R. length (5 weeks). According to Gillman (1948) the gonad is of triple origin from the coelomic epithilium of the genital ridge, the underlying mesoderm and the primitive germ cells which come from an extragenital source (see below).

The gonad forms as a bulge on the medial aspect of the mesonephric ridge. Its histological appearances are alike in the early stages, whether it is to be testis or ovary. There is a proliferation of cells in and beneath the coelomic epithilium of the genital ridge. By 5 or 6 weeks these cells are seen spreading as ill-defined cords (sex cords) into the ridge, breaking up the mesenchyme into loose strands. Primitive germ cells are distinguishable as much larger structures, lying at first between the cords and then within them.

The differentiation of the testes is evident about 7 weeks by the disappearance of germ cells from the peripheral zone and gradual differentiation of remaining cells in fibroblasts and later into the tunica albuginea. The deeper parts of the sex cords give rise to the rete testis, the seminiferous and straight tubules. The first indication that the gonad will become an ovary is failure of these testicular changes to appear. The primitive ovary passes first into the stage of differentiation and growth, and later into that of follicle formation. The sex cords below the coelomic epithelium develop extensively, with many primitive germ cells evident in this active cellular zone (Fig. 1.4). The epithelial cells in this area are known as pregranulosa cells. The active growth phase then follows, involving the pregranulosa cells and the germ cells, which are now much reduced in size (14–16 weeks). This proliferation greatly enlarges the bulk of the

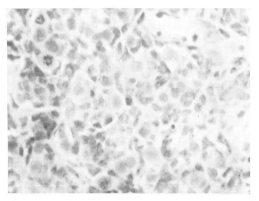

Fig. 1.4. Detail of immature ovary showing small epithelial cells (pregranulosa cells) and larger germ cells, two of which (top left) show mitotic figures. (By courtesy of the Editor of *Journal of Pathology and Bacteriology*.)

gonad. The next stage (20 weeks onwards) shows the primitive germ cells (now known as oöcytes) becoming surrounded by a ring of pregranulosa cells; stromal cells developed from the ovarian mesenchyme later surround the pregranulosa cells, now known as granulosa cells, and follicle formation is complete (Fig. 1.5). An interesting

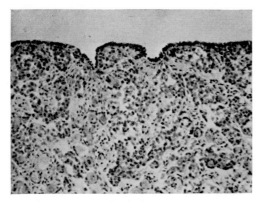

Fig. 1.5. A later ovary (31 weeks) showing, at the cortex, remaining islands of pregranulosa cells and numerous formed primary follicles. (By courtesy of the Editor of *Journal of Pathology and Bacteriology*.)

feature of the formation of follicles and the development of stroma is the disintegration of those oöcytes which do not succeed in encircling themselves with a capsule of pregranulosa cells.

The interpretation of changes of this kind in early embryos is highly specialized, and other workers, although observing similar appearances, have interpreted them differently. Willis (1962) summarizes these different views.

The origin of the germ cells is another subject about which conflicting views have been expressed. It is now generally accepted that they arise in the endoderm before the formation of the mesoderm of the lateral plate and somite formation (Pinkerton *et al.* 1961). Pinkerton and his colleagues described germ cells as migrating along the endoderm of the yolk sac, into the gut, through the mesenchyme at the route of the mesentery and into the primitive gonad. It seems probable that the presence of the germ cells is essential for subsequent development of the gonad. Rapid proliferation of germ cells

follows, until they become surrounded by granulosa cells as described above and become oöcytes. Mitotic division, by which the germ cells have been increasing in numbers, then ceases and they enter the first stage of meiosis.

The number of oöcytes is greatest sometime during pregnancy, and thereafter declines. Baker (1963) found that the total population of germ cells rose from some 600,000 at 2 months to a peak of almost 7,000,000 at 5 months. At birth the number had fallen to 2,000,000, of which half were atretic. After 28 weeks or so of intra-uterine life an increasing degree of follicle development is evident in the ovary. Follicles

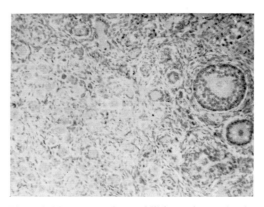

Fig. 1.6. Numerous primary follicles and two showing early development in the ovary of a child stillborn at 39 weeks. (By courtesy of the Editor of *Journal of Pathology and Bacteriology*.)

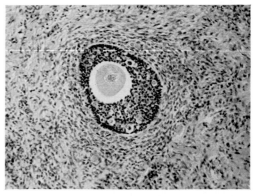

Fig. 1.7. More mature follicles in a child stillborn at 40 weeks. (By courtesy of the Editor of *Journal of Pathology and Bacteriology*.)

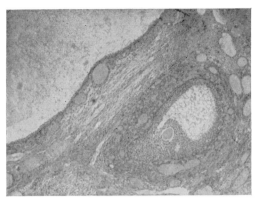

Fig. 1.8. Ovary from a child stillborn at 36 weeks showing a maturing Graafian follicle, to the right, and the edge of a large cystic follicle to the left. (By courtesy of the Editor of *Journal of Pathology and Bacteriology*.)

at various stages of development, and of various sizes, are seen (Pryse-Davies & Dewhurst 1970) (Figs. 1.6, 1.7 and 1.8).

GENITAL TRACT MALFORMATIONS

Numerous malformations of the genital tract have been described, some of little clinical significance, others of considerable importance.

Uterine anomalies

ABSENCE OF THE UTERUS

The uterus may be absent or of such rudimentary development as to be incapable of function of any kind. This type of anomaly is usually found when the vagina is absent also, the case presenting is one of primary amenorrhoea (see Chapter 5). Absence of the uterus may be associated with the development of the lower part of the vagina, which then ends blindly. This combination of features should suggest a diagnosis of testicular feminization (see Chapter 4); however, similar development of the lower vagina only, and absence of the uterus, may occasionally be found in XX patients with ovaries. No treatment is of course possible for the uterine abnormality as such; it must be

stressed however, that if the diagnosis is testicular feminization, testicular removal may be indicated on account of the increased risk of malignant change in the testes. Whether the patient be XY or XX, however, attention to psychological aspects of the case may be almost the most important facet of management.

FUSION ANOMALIES

Fusion anomalies of various kinds are not uncommon (Fig. 1.9) and may present clinically either in association with pregnancy or in other ways. The lesser degrees of fusion defects are quite common, the cornual parts of the uterus remaining separate, giving the organ a heart-shaped appearance. It is doubtful if such a minor degree of fusion defect *per se* gives rise to clinical symptoms or signs. The presence of a septum extending over some or all of the uterine cavity, however, is likely to give rise to clinical features. Such a septate or subseptate uterus may be of normal external appearance or of arcuate outline. Clinically, this state of affairs may come to light as a case of repeated unsuccessful pregnancy, when it is often suggested that the implantation of the conceptus is on the thin septum, giving rise to consistent early interruption of the pregnancy (see Chapter 4); a second likely method of presentation is as repeated transverse lie of the foetus in late pregnancy, since it tends to lie with the head in one cornu and the breech in the other (see Chapter 22).

In more extreme forms of failure of fusion the clinical features may be less, rather than more, marked. Two almost separate uterine bodies with one cervix are probably less likely to be associated with repeated abnormal lies than the lesser degrees of fusion defect mentioned above. Complete duplication of the uterus and cervix (uterus didelphys) if associated with any clinical fault at all might present as obstruction, or partial obstruction, to descent of the head in late pregnancy or labour by the non-pregnant horn.

Rudimentary development of one horn may give rise to a very serious situation if a pregnancy is implanted there. Rupture of the horn with profound bleeding may occur as the pregnancy

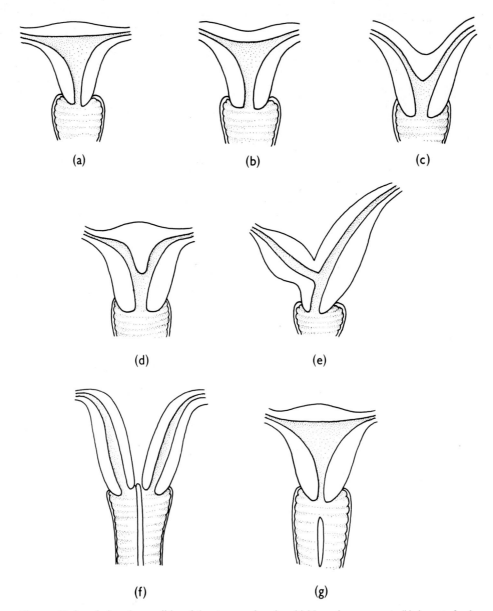

Fig. 1.9. Various fusion abnormalities of the uterus and vagina. (a) Normal appearances. (b) Arcuate fundus with little effect on the shape of the cavity. (c) Bicornuate uterus. (d) Subseptate uterus with normal outline. (e) Rudimentary horn. (f) Uterus didelphys. (g) Normal uterus with partial vaginal septum.

increases in size. The clinical picture will, in some ways, resemble that of a ruptured ectopic pregnancy, with the difference that the amenorrhoea would probably be measured in months rather than weeks; shock may be profound. A poorly developed or rudimentary horn may give rise to dysmenorrhoea and pelvic pain if there is any obstruction to communication between the horn and the main uterine cavity or the vagina. Surgical removal would then be indicated.

Vaginal anomalies

ABSENCE OF THE VAGINA

Absence of the vagina is generally associated with absence of the uterus, as indicated above. Rarely, the uterus may be present and the vagina, or at any rate a large part of it, absent.

In the more common circumstances of absence of both vagina and uterus the patient will probably present about 16 years or so of age with primary amenorrhoea. Secondary sexual characteristics should be present, since the ovaries are normally developed. This combination of normal secondary sexual development and primary amenorrhoea should suggest an anatomical cause, such as an imperforate or absent vagina, for the failure to menstruate. Inspection of the vulva, abdominal examination and rectal examination will be required to exclude the presence of any retained blood in a part of the upper genital tract.

Vulval development should be normal apart from the absence of the vaginal introitus (Fig. 1.10).

The presumptive diagnosis of absence of the vagina can generally be made without difficulty at the first examination. A very short vagina arising in the testicular feminizing syndrome may be mistaken for simple absence, so in every case of apparent vaginal absence a buccal smear, at least, should be performed and, if possible, a chromosome analysis. If the buccal smear is chromatin negative and the chromosome analysis confirms XY sex chromosomes, the case takes on an entirely different aspect (see Chapter 4).

An intravenus pyelogram is desirable in view of the frequent association of the renal tract

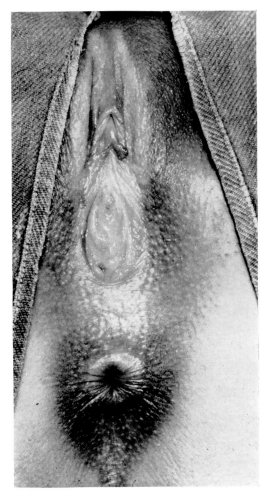

Fig. 1.10. Vulval appearances in a case of absence of the vagina.

anomalies which may have a bearing on treatment (Fig. 1.11). If there is any suggestion that there is a functioning uterus present laparoscopy is indicated to confirm or refute this, indeed, laparoscopy may be employed in any apparent case of vaginal absence to avoid the possibility of error, since the technique is simple and the upset to the patient comparatively small.

Once the diagnosis is certain, consideration must be given to the construction of an artificial vagina. Rarely, one sees patients in whom this is unnecessary, since attempted intercourse has so

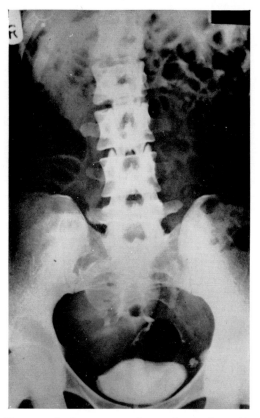

Fig. 1.11. An intravenous pyelogram in a patient with absence of the vagina, showing a single pelvic kidney.

indented the perineal area that enjoyable coitus for both wife and husband has been experienced. Such cases are, of course, exceptional. The timing and nature of surgical procedure required to construct an artificial vagina require some discussion. The technique introduced by McIndoe and Read (McIndoe & Bannister 1958) has, until recently, been the one most commonly used. In this procedure a cavity is created between the bladder and bowel at the site which the natural vagina would occupy; this cavity is then lined by a split-skin graft taken from the thigh and applied on a plastic mould. The anatomical result in successful cases can be remarkably good.

There are, none the less, difficulties and disadvantages to this technique (Jackson 1965).

The postoperative period is painful and sometimes protracted; the graft does not always take well and granulations can form over part of the cavity, giving rise to some discharge; pressure necrosis between the mould and the urethra, bladder or rectum can lead to fistula formation. A further, and greater, disadvantage is the tendency for the vagina to contract unless a dilator is worn or the vagina is used for intercourse regularly. The ideal timing of the procedure, therefore, is some 6 months or so before marriage, so that the woman can wear a dilator throughout this time to prevent contraction, which thereafter can be prevented through natural intercourse; a longer interval may lead to irregular use of a dilator, when contraction can occur very rapidly. It is, moreover, a great psychological disadvantage for a girl who knows she has such an abnormality and requires such an operation to have to wait until she finds someone who wishes to marry her before it can be done. Her relationship with young men is certain to be influenced.

The operation of vulvovaginoplasty introduced by Williams (1964) has obvious psychological advantages in this respect, since it appears that it can be performed on 17 or 18 year-old unmarried girls without the risk of significant contraction when regular intercourse is not indulged in for some time. Williams's account should be consulted for the details of this unusual technique, when it will be evident that the operative procedure is simple, quick and relatively comfortable for the patient. Functionally, the results seem good. The only apparent disadvantage is the unusual angle of the vagina (Fig. 1.12), which may displease a purist surgeon. The angle may, however, lead to a maximum of clitoral stimulation at intercourse and may account for good functional results.

The combination of absence of most of the lower vagina in association with a functioning uterus presents a difficult problem. The upper fragment of vagina will collect menstrual blood and a clinical picture, similar in many ways to haematocolpos (see below) will be seen. Diagnosis, however, would be more difficult and it may not be at all certain how much of the vagina is absent, and thus how extensive the dissection

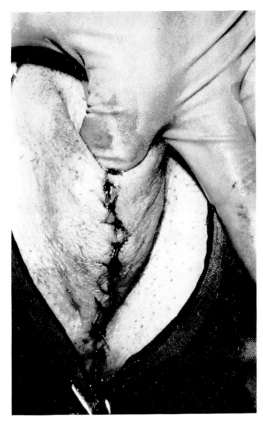

Fig. 1.12. A vagina constructed by the Williams vulvo-vaginoplasty method.

requires to be to release the retained fluid. Rectal examination may reveal a bulging swelling at a high level, which may give the initial clue to the nature of the abnormality. Laparoscopy will be helpful by confirming the presence of the uterus and indicating if the tubes contain retained blood also. If doubt remains the abdomen should be opened to establish for certain the precise state of affairs.

The problem of treatment is a difficult one. If a dissection upwards is made as in the McIndoe–Read technique the blood can be released, but its discharge for some time later may interfere with the application of the mould and the 'take' of the skin graft in the artificial vagina. The approach advocated by Jeffcoate (1969) may provide the solution. He suggests that after the

dissection has been made to open into the fragment of upper vagina, the walls of this portion, now stretched and greatly extended, should be brought down and stitched to the introital area, so lining the new vagina with its own skin and obviating the risk of contraction. Jeffcoate calls this 'the advancement of the vagina'.

HAEMATOCOLPOS

An imperforate membrane may exist at the lower end of the vagina; this is loosely referred to as an imperforate hymen, although the hymen can usually be distinguished separately (Fig. 1.13). The condition is seldom recognized clinically until puberty, when retention of menstrual flow gives rise to the clinical features of haematocolpos; rarely, the case may present in the newborn as hydrocolpos (see Chapter 2). The features of haematocolpos are, predominantly, three: ab-

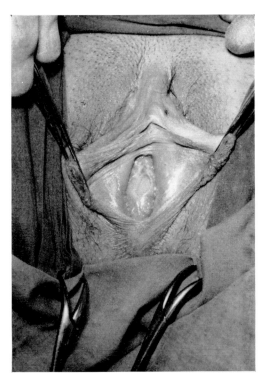

Fig. 1.13. An imperforate membrane occluding the vaginal introitus in a case of haematocolpos. Note the hymen clearly visible immediately distal to the membrane

dominal pain, amenorrhoea, and interference
with micturition. The patient is usually aged
about 14 or 15 years, but may be much older.
A clear history may be given of regular lower
abdominal pain for some months past, but a less
clear-cut history is not uncommon. The patient
may be brought to hospital as an acute emergency
if urinary retention develops. The examination
will reveal a lower abdominal swelling if there is
urinary retention; per rectum a large, bulging
mass in the vagina may be appreciated (Fig. 1.14).

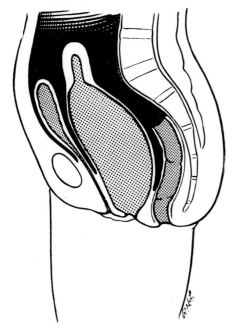

Fig. 1.14. Drawing of the pelvis contents in a case of
haematocolpos.

Vulval inspection will reveal the imperforate
membrane, which may or may not be blueish in
colour depending upon its thickness. Diagnosis
may be more difficult if the vagina is imperforate
over some distance in its lower part or if there
is obstruction in one half of a septate vagina
(Macdonald 1960).

Treatment is usually very simple, since all
that is required is incision of the membrane and
the release of the retained blood. Redundant
portions of the membrane may then be snipped

away, but nothing more should be done at that
time. Fluid will drain away naturally over some
days. Examination a few weeks later is desirable
to ensure that no pelvic mass remains which
might suggest the condition of haematosalpinx.
In fact, haematosalpinx is most uncommon
except in cases of very long-standing, or in
association with retention of blood in a fragment
of upper vagina. On those rare occasions when a
haematosalpinx is discovered, laparotomy is
desirable, the distended tube being removed or
preserved, as seems best. Haematometra scarcely
seems to be a realistic clinical entity, the thick
uterine walls permitting very little blood to
collect therein. The subsequent menstrual
history and fertility of patients who are successfully treated for haematocolpos is probably
not significantly different from that of normal
women.

A vaginal septum extending throughout all or
part of the vagina is not uncommonly encountered. Such a septum lies in the sagittal
plane in the mid-line, although if one side of the
vagina has been habitually used for coitus the
septum may have become displaced laterally
to such an extent that it may not be obvious that
one is present. The condition may be found in
association with a completely double uterus and
cervix, or with a single uterus only. In obstetrics
the septum may be important if a foetus presenting by the breech enters the vagina astride it,
when serious tearing may occur. For this reason
it is wise to arrange division of the vaginal
septum as a formal surgical procedure whenever
one is discovered during pregnancy. There is
then no risk of a serious situation arising acutely
during labour. The septum may occasionally
appear to be associated with dyspareunia,
when similar management will be indicated.

Vulval anomalies

Doubt about the sex of a child due to faults in
the development of the external genitalia may
arise in various circumstances. These are discussed fully in Chapter 4. Rarely, anomalies
in the development of bowel or bladder may give
rise to considerable abnormality in the appearance of the vulva. The anus may open

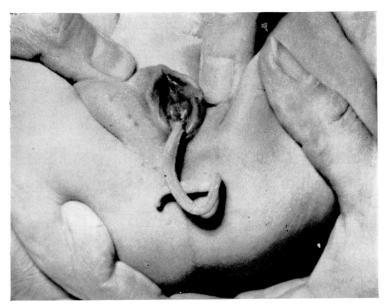

Fig. 1.15. Ectopic opening of the anus at the fourchette.

immediately adjacent to the vagina or just within it (Fig. 1.15). Bladder exstrophy will give rise to a bifid clitoris and anterior displacement of the vagina, in addition to the bladder deformity itself. These unusual cases are more fully discussed by Stephens (1963), Dewhurst (1963), and others.

Gonadal anomalies

Gonadal development may be markedly interfered with in certain patients with sex chromosome abnormalities (XO, XX/XO, XY/XO etc.). In these patients who present in clinical practise as examples of gonadal dysgenesis the gonads are represented by whitish streaks of tissue without the characteristic histological features of ovary or testis. In other patients with pure gonadal dysgenesis similar gonadal appearances may be observed, although the sex chromosomes are either XX or XY.

Testes may be discovered in phenotypic females with testicular feminization and other varieties of male intersex. Both testicular and ovarian tissue may be present together in the rare condition of hermaphroditism.

All these conditions are discussed in detail in Chapter 4.

Wolffian duct anomalies

Remnants of the lower part of the Wolffian duct system may be evident as vaginal cysts, or remnants of the upper part as thin-walled cysts lying within the layers of the broad ligament (parovarian cysts). It is doubtful whether the vaginal cyst *per se* calls for surgical removal, although removal is usually undertaken. Cysts situated at the upper end of the vagina may be found to burrow deeply into the region of the broad ligament and base of the bladder, and should be approached surgically with considerable caution. A palpable, and probably parovarian, cyst will require surgical exploration, since its precise nature will be unknown until the abdomen is opened. Such cysts normally shell out easily from the broad ligament.

Renal tract anomalies

The association between congenital malformations of the genital tract and those of the renal tract has already been mentioned. Whenever a malformation of the genital organs of any significant degree presents in clinical practice some investigation to confirm or refute a renal tract anomaly will be wise. An intravenous pyelogram can be arranged without great upset to the patient and will probably be sufficient in the first instance. Lesions such as absence of one kidney, a double renal element on one or both sides, a double ureter, a pelvic kidney (Fig. 1.11), etc., may not call for immediate treatment but may do so later; moreover, it is as well to be aware of such anomalies if the abdomen is to be opened for exploration or treatment of the genital tract lesion itself.

ECTOPIC URETER

One abnormality which can apparently present with gynaecological symptoms is the ectopic

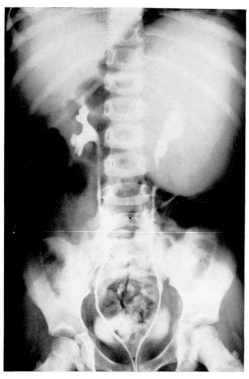

Fig. 1.16. An intravenous pyelogram in a child with an imperforate vagina. Both ureters open ectopically into the posterior urethra.

ureter (Fig. 1.16). A ureter opening abnormally is usually an additional one, although sometimes a single one may be ectopic. The commonest site of the opening is the vestibule, followed closely by the urethra and then the vagina; other sites are less common. The main symptom is uncontrollable wetness. The amount of moisture appearing at the vulva may, however, be small and is sometimes mistaken for a vaginal discharge. This confusion, together with difficulties in confirming the diagnosis of an ectopic ureter even when this is suspected, may lead to many patients being investigated for years before the condition is recognized. Mitchell (1961) reported a case in which the diagnosis was made for the first time at the age of 43 years!

Diagnosis can sometimes be easy, but is usually not so. The orifice at the vestibule may be clearly visible, but more often careful search is necessary to locate it, if it can be seen at all. Cystoscopy and urethroscopy may be necessary to establish, if nothing else, whether normal ureteric openings exist in the bladder. Radiological study is often helpful by indicating a double element on one side or both sides. The intravenous injection of indigocarmine, although theoretically likely to be useful, is often of little value, since concentration in the affected part of the kidney is often too poor to show up the opening well. Treatment will generally involve the urological surgeon rather than the gynaecologist. Partial nephrectomy and ureterectomy are likely to be the most satisfactory treatment, but it should be remembered that the tract of the ureter can be tortuous, and surgery may be difficult.

REFERENCES

BAKER T.G. (1963) *Proc. R. Soc.* **158**, 417.
BULMER D. (1957) *J. Anat.* **91**, 490.
DEWHURST C.J. (1963) *The Gynaecological Disorders of Infants and Children*, London, Cassell, p. 39.
GILLMAN J. (1948) *Contributions to Embryology, No.* 210, Vol. 32. Carnegie Institute of Washington Publication 575, p. 83.
JACKSON I. (1965) *J. Obstet. Gynaec. Br. Commonw.* **72**, 336.

Jeffcoate T.N.A. (1969) *J. Obstet. Gynaec. Br. Commonw.* **76**, 961.

Koff A.K. (1933) *Contributions to Embryology, No. 140*, Vol. 24. Carnegie Institute of Washington Publication 443, p. 61.

Macdonald C.R. (1960) *J. Obstet. Gynaec. Br. Commonw.* **67**, 848.

McIndoe A.H. & Bannister J.B. (1938) *J. Obstet. Gynaec. Br. Emp.* **45**, 490.

Mitchell R.J. (1961) *J. Obstet. Gynaec. Br. Commonw.* **68**, 299.

Pinkerton J.H.M., McKay D.G., Adams E.C. & Hertig A.H. (1961) *Obstet. & Gynaec., N.Y.* **18**, 152.

Pryse-Davies J. & Dewhurst C.J. (1971) *J. Path.* **103**, 5.

Stephens F. Douglas (1963) *Congenital Malformations of the Rectum, Anus and Genito-urinary Tracts*. Edinburgh and London, Livingstone, p. 4.

Vilas E. (1932) *Z. Anat. EntwGesch.* **98**, 263.

Williams E.A. (1964) *J. Obstet. Gynaec. Br. Commonw.* **71**, 511.

Willis R.A. (1962) *The Borderland of Embryology and Pathology*, 2nd edn. London, Butterworths, p. 47.

CHAPTER 2

GYNAECOLOGICAL DISORDERS IN
CHILDHOOD AND ADOLESCENCE

Happily, children are seldom afflicted by diseases of the genital organs, but when they are the problems concerned are not the same in miniature as those which occur in later life; these little patients present particular gynaecological problems of their own which are worthy of our attention. During adolescence important physiological and emotional changes occur, to which greater attention is now being paid by gynaecologists. Genital tract disease may then be seen more often than during childhood itself.

Endocrinology, anatomy and physiology

The endocrinology of the childhood years will first be discussed briefly so that some of the disorders encountered may be understood more fully. The subject has recently been reviewed by Pennington *et al.* (1969). During the first week or two of life, a child enjoys a certain amount of passive oestrogenic stimulation which has passed across the placenta from the mother. This time is characterized by transient, but distinct, clinical features. Some growth of the breasts occurs then in most babies born at term, and the enlargement can sometimes be quite considerable and may be accompanied by a discharge of fluid from the nipple. A clear vaginal discharge is evident in most female babies also; moistening of the genitalia is noticeable which will not be evident for most of the rest of childhood. This discharge may be blood-stained— a form of withdrawal bleeding occurring because oestrogen levels in the baby gradually fall and are no longer able to sustain the endometrium.

The amount of bleeding is seldom sufficient to cause concern, but may alarm the attendants if they are unaware of its nature. Ten to fifteen per cent of babies may have a blood-stained loss of this kind during the first few weeks or so of life. After this neonatal period of passive hormone stimulation there follows a number of years when the genital organs receive little stimulus from the sex hormones. Oestrogens, gonadotrophins and adrenal hormones may be found in the child's urine during this time, but in small amounts only. The pelvic organs suffer from an oestrogen deficiency which is responsible for some of the clinical conditions shortly to be described. Gradual increase in hormone secretion during childhood leads ultimately to the commencement of secondary sexual development, growth spurt and menstruation.

A child's genital organs reflect this hormone background. The uterus at birth is somewhat larger than it will be for some years. Uterine hypertrophy has taken place under the influence of maternal oestrogens, but very soon the uterus becomes smaller and shows the characteristics of the unstimulated uterus of the child. It is straight in form, without fundal hypertrophy and the cervix is relatively longer than in the adult; the ratio of cervix to body of the uterus in the first week of life may be 1:1; later, when this hypertrophy has disappeared, the ratio of cervix to body becomes 2:1; at puberty, when the uterus has developed as a result of the child's own oestrogenic stimulation, this ratio will be 1:2. The changes in the ovary during intrauterine life are dealt with in Chapter 1. At

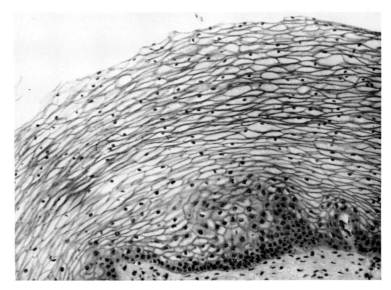

Fig. 2.1. Section of the vaginal epithelium of a newborn baby (compare Fig. 2.2).

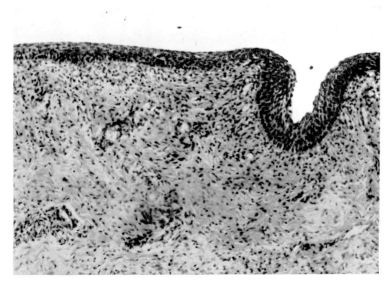

Fig. 2.2 Section of vaginal wall of an infant dying after the neonatal period.

birth, and during the first few weeks of life, more cystic follicles may be seen than is the case later. Limited follicle development continues throughout childhood, however, reducing still further the number of ova present at puberty.

The changes which occur in the vagina have the most significance so far as clinical disorders are concerned. The vagina at birth is lined by squamous epithelium which is many layers thick (Fig. 2.1), the cells being rich in glycogen.

Within 2 or 3 weeks, however, most of the superficial layers become exfoliated and the vagina is lined by stratified squamous epithelium a few cells thick only (Fig. 2.2). The reaction of the vagina, which in the newborn child is acid, with a pH of less than 5, soon becomes alkaline (pH 7) due to oestrogen deprivation. It is lack of this protective acid secretion which makes the vagina of the child so susceptible to infections by low-grade organisms that cause the vaginitis shortly to be described.

CLINICAL DISORDERS

Most of the gynaecological disorders of childhood may conveniently be discussed in three groups. Group I, disorders of the newborn period. Group II, disorders of the years of oestrogen deficiency between this time and puberty. Group III, pubertal disorders.

Group I
Neonatal disorders

Some of the transient clinical manifestations of the early neonatal period have already been described. In addition to these, however, various congenital malformations involving the genital tract may call for investigation and treatment. These have recently been reviewed by Dewhurst (1968). The intersexual disorders form one important group which is discussed in Chapter 4. Another group of congenital malformations is that in which the bowel opens into the upper or lower genital tract. Surgical treatment of some kind is generally necessary at a comparatively early stage and a surgical opinion should always be requested quickly. Consultation between gynaecologist and a paediatric surgeon will be an advantage in such cases. In one malformation—that of a congenital imperforate membrane occluding the lower vagina—mistakes in diagnosis may arise if the doctor is unaware of the disorder or does not elicit the physical signs correctly. This condition is called hydrocolpos.

HYDROCOLPOS

The lower part of the vagina is occluded by an imperforate membrane usually situated immediately above the hymen (Fig. 2.3). Above this obstruction the vagina becomes distended to a varying amount by watery or, usually, milky, fluid, which probably collects there as a result of the passive hormone stimulation already mentioned, to which the foetus *in utero* in late pregnancy is always subjected. The quantity of fluid which collects may vary from a few millilitres to many ounces, so modifying the

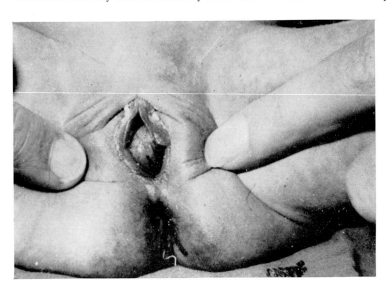

Fig. 2.3. Bulging vaginal membrane in a child with hydrocolpos.

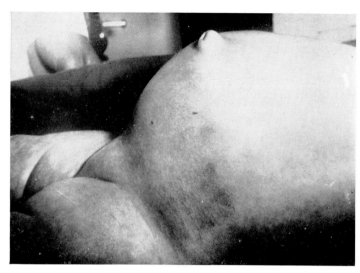

Fig. 2.4. Enormous abdominal swelling in an 8-day-old child with hydrocolpos.

clinical features of the condition. If a large quantity of fluid is present there may be retention of urine, abdominal pain and a lower abdominal swelling which sometimes assumes large proportions. Inspection of the vulva usually reveals a bulging membrane, and the diagnosis can readily be made. Difficulties in diagnosis may occur if the abdominal swelling is thought so large that hydrocolpos is not seriously considered (Fig. 2.4); or if the obstruction at the lower end of the vagina is more extensive than a simple membrane. In the latter case no bulge will be evident, but rectal examination should disclose a swelling at a higher level. Correct diagnosis permits the condition to be treated properly by simple incision of the membrane and release of the retained fluid. It must be emphasized, however, that there are several cases on record in which laparotomy, or even hysterectomy, has been performed without the correct diagnosis being made; in one such case the child died (Joseph *et al.* 1966).

An interesting aspect of this condition is the origin of the fluid. It has already been suggested that the fluid accumulates as a result of passive hormone stimulation. Study of histological sections of the vagina and cervix from children stillborn or dying in the neonatal period indicates that considerable desquamation and outpouring

of the fluid may be seen (Pryse-Davies & Dewhurst 1971). If there is vaginal obstruction but only a small volume of fluid collects, symptoms may not arise until the amount is increased by the menstrual flow about puberty; the case then presents as haemotocolpos (see p. 1). If a much greater quantity of fluid collects in the vagina at birth, clinical features will be evident very soon and treatment will be called for. Most cases of hydrocolpos become manifest during the first week or so of life, or not until they present as haemotocolpos at puberty. A further interesting aspect of the condition, as with genital tract malformations in general, is the association with anomalies of the renal tract. The condition may be associated with imperforate anus and congenital abnormalities of the colon, bladder and ureter, and urinary tract investigation will usually be wise.

Group II
Disorders of the low oestrogen years

The commonest gynaecological disorder of childhood—vulvovaginitis—occurs during these years. There are several possible aetiological factors concerned but the most important are the ease with which infection may be introduced into the child's vagina and the lack of protective acid secretion during this time. Many cases of childhood vulvovaginitis are due to infection with organisms of low virulence rather than to specific pathogenic ones. Gonorrhoea was, at one time, a common cause of this condition, but is now fortunately seen much less often. The usual bacteriological finding in a case of vulvo-vaginitis is a mixed bacterial flora, no specific organism preponderating; specific organisms are sometimes found, but this is seldom the case by the time the patient is seen by the gynae-cologist, although it may be more common at an earlier stage in the illness. Sore throats, scarlet fever and other exanthemata have some-times been noted in cases of vulvovaginitis, and in some of these, haemolytic streptococci have been isolated. *Trichomonas vaginalis* infestations in children are not common, although they may be seen more frequently in the child near to puberty. Similarly, infestations with *Candida albicans* are rare and when they are found pre-disposing factors are present, such as diabetes or treatment with a broad-spectrum antibiotic. A foreign body in the vagina of a little girl will undoubtedly give rise to discharge and vulval soreness. In these circumstances the discharge is usually blood-stained and foul-smelling. In the presence of these features examination under anaesthesia is necessary to exclude a foreign body, but in the absence of them it is unlikely to be indicated; foreign bodies are comparatively rare findings in children presenting with vaginal discharge, and vulval soreness and examination under anaesthesia has been undertaken too often in the past. A further cause worthy of mention is a threadworm infestation which sometimes gives rise to this condition.

Although the presence of a vaginal discharge and vulval soreness is common to all cases, the degree of annoyance or discomfort caused is variable. If the vulva is sore the child is likely to complain of pain on micturition. It is important to establish if a vaginal discharge is a prominent feature or whether the soreness is the main one, discharge being only slight or absent (see lichen sclerosus). Inquiry as to how often, and in what manner, the vulva is cleansed will also be help-ful; imperfect vulval hygiene is sometimes evident and is certain to aggravate the irritation.

Examination can usually be performed with-out upset to the parent or child. Simple inspection of the vulva will show whether there is consider-able soreness or not (Fig. 2.5). The vulva is usually reddened and may be swollen, and gentle separation of the labia will reveal a small amount of discharge present. If none can be seen, a rectal examination may permit a small amount of

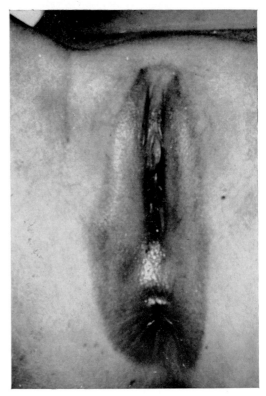

Fig. 2.5. Vulval soreness secondary to a vaginal discharge.

the discharge to be 'milked down' to the in-troitus. Bacteriological studies are not always helpful in cases of vulvovaginitis in childhood. If useful results are to be obtained, however, it is necessary to provide suitable samples for examination; a swab hastily taken from the region of the introitus will not give reliable in-formation. With gentleness, however, a small amount of discharge may be taken with a platinum loop from within the lower vagina itself, and a smear made on a slide, which can then be examined. It should be possible to obtain a small amount of discharge also with a pipette, and some of this discharge may be added at once to Stewart's medium, to permit culture, and the remainder put directly onto a slide for examination for *Trichomonas vaginalis* or *Candida albicans*. Threadworm ova may also be recognized in this way.

Treatment with an appropriate antibiotic will be helpful if a specific organism has been isolated, but as has already been said, such cases are uncommon. For non-specific vaginitis the application of Dienoestrol cream to the vulva each night for about 2 weeks is often most helpful, since it increases the natural vaginal protection and allows the infection to be overcome; because the soreness is relieved, the morale of the patient and parents is greatly improved. It is wise also to give some instruction to parents and child in elementary hygiene of the vulva. The vulva should be bathed daily at least, perhaps more often. Antiseptics should not be added to the water used, since they usually make matters worse. After cleansing, drying with a soft towel should be undertaken. If soap or detergent used to wash the child's underclothes is not completely removed by rinsing, this may maintain a vulval irritation. Clothing the child unwisely in unsuitable thick undergarments in warm weather may increase vulval moisture and, again, aggrevate the symptoms.

If the discharge is gonococcal, advice from a venereologist should be sought, since other members of the family may need examination and treatment as well. *Trichomonas* and *Candida* infestations in children respond well to oral therapy; Metronidozole may be used against *trichomonas* in doses of 200 mg three times daily for 10 days; a smaller dose for a younger child— say 100 mg for a child under 12 years—may be necessary. For *Candida albicans*, nystatin may be given as an oral suspension or as a tablet; one tablet (500,000 units) three times daily for a week may be taken by an older child; for a younger one a suspension in doses of 2–4 ml (200,000–400,000 units) three times daily may be preferable. Threadworm infestations usually respond well to a piperazine preparation such as Antepar.

LICHEN SCLEROSUS

Vulval soreness is not always secondary to a vaginal discharge. A generalized skin disease such as eczema or lichen sclerosus may be to blame. Lichen sclerosus can be present anywhere on the body surface, but has a special tendency to affect the genital area. Discreet, white, flattened papules may be seen in the early stages; later, these colase to form larger plaques (Fig. 2.6). The histological appearances are hyperkeratosis of the epidermis itself, flattening of the rete pegs and disappearance of elastic

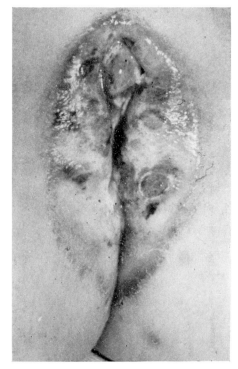

Fig. 2.6. Lichen sclerosus of the vulva with some secondary infection in a 4 year-old child.

fibres from the superficial layers of the dermis, where the collagen shows a hyaline change; in the deeper layers a zone of round-cell infiltration is seen. In many cases the degree of irritation is less severe than would be expected from the appearance of the skin, but itching can be marked, especially if any secondary infection is present. For treatment of acute cases, careful

attention to vulval hygiene is desirable in all
cases. Cleansing with 1% cetrimide may be
helpful and is less painful than soap and water.
Aureomycin cream may be useful if the lesion
is infected. Ditkowsky *et al.* (1956) reported an
improvement in all their cases beyond puberty,
but Kindler (1953) found that most of her cases
were unaffected at this time. Barclay *et al.*
(1966), reporting five cases and reviewing recent
literature, concluded that spontaneous resolution may occur at puberty, but does not always
do so.

LABIAL ADHESIONS

This is a simple condition not uncommon in
young girls, and is sometimes seen even in older
ones, in which the labial minora become adherent to each other, usually from behind,
forwards, leaving a tiny opening through which
urine is passed. The line of adhesion is quite
thin and almost translucent in early cases
but becomes firmer and thicker as time goes by
(Fig. 2.7). The importance of the condition is
not intrinsic to the disease itself but is concerned
with the fact that it may be mistaken for absence
of the vagina; this may result in inaccurate and
disturbing advice being given to the parents,
who already may be greatly distressed by the
condition. The aetiology is unknown but is
thought to be concerned with the low oestrogen
values of early childhood or with poor hygiene.
It seems likely that it is concerned with oestrogen
lack, as the adhesions seldom persist after the
pubertal period and can be encouraged to separate
spontaneously by local oestrogen therapy (see
below); moreover, a similar condition sometimes
occurs in very old ladies. Imperfect vulval
hygiene is less convincing as an aetiological
factor, since children with the disorder seldom
appear neglected in this way. Some authorities
consider that some cases of labial adhesions may
be congenital in origin (Campbell 1940; Stephens
1966) but others do not agree; however, adhesions may develop quite soon after the neonatal period.

Simple treatment is all that is required. The
adhesions can be separated with a fine probe,
although a general anesthetic may be necessary

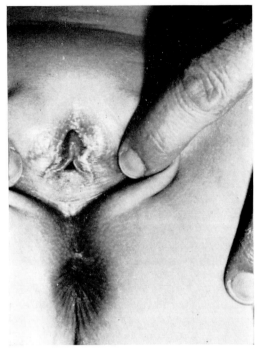

Fig. 2.7. Labial adhesions simulating absence of the
vagina.

for this if they are firm. Alternatively, oestrogen
cream may be applied by the child's mother to the
line of the adhesions each night; the adhesions
then usually separate spontaneously in some
10–14 days (Huffman 1958; Dewhurst 1963,
1968). They may re-form, however, and it may
be advisable to warn the mother of this, suggesting
that she looks for early signs of it from time
to time; if they seem to be re-forming they
can easily be drawn apart and simple cream
applied.

Group III
Puberty and its disorders

PHYSIOLOGICAL CONSIDERATIONS

A general account only of the physiology of
puberty and menstruation will be given here,
the endocrine control of menstruation under
normal and abnormal conditions being examined
in greater detail in Chapters 3 and 35.

Hormonal changes

In the hormonal sense the control of the menstruation begins with the pituitary gland and its secretion of the gonadotrophic hormones, follicle-stimulating hormone (FSH) and luteinizing hormone (LH). Pituitary activity is, however, under the control of higher centres, as Harris *et al.* (1952) established by implanting the pituitary of immature animals into mature ones and demonstrating the immature pituitary capable of function when stimulated by a mature hypothalamus. This hypothalamic control of pituitary activity is a complex process involving various releasing factors (RF) and will be considered in detail in Chapter 3. Briefly, FSH stimulates the development of a Graafian follicle in the ovary. Ovulation results from the combined action of FSH and LH. During any single cycle one Graafian follicle alone achieves full development and ovulates; rarely, two and, more rarely still, more than two follicles ovulate. For the production of the meagre return of one ovum per month, however, many follicles commence development and undergo follicle atresia once an ovum is shed by one of them. This abortive development clearly occurs to a considerable extent even during childhood, evidence of it being visible in the ovaries at any age before the menarche. Such development can be explained by the recognition of gonadotrophic excretion throughout childhood indicating gonadotrophic production be the pituitary even during these early days (Pennington & Dewhurst 1969). Nothing is known, however, of the FSH/LH ratio during this time—a ratio which must be critical so far as complete Graafian follicle formation is concerned. The degree of ovarian activity in childhood, however, probably accounts for the gradual increase in oestrogen production and excretion as the child grows older, resulting first in secondary sexual development and later in a uterine response and menstruation.

The developing Graafian follicle produces oestrogens; after ovulation the corpus luteum produces oestrogens and progesterone. These hormones have an important interrelationship with hypothalamic releasing factors, and so indirectly with FSH and LH. This relationship to is considered much more closely later (Chapter 3), but may be summarized as follows. At the time of menstruation, in response to falling levels of oestrogen and progesterone there is a surge of FSH/RF which causes a peak of FSH production. This, together with a continuing low level of LH secretion, causes follicle maturation. Oestrogen production accordingly rises again; this rise inhibits FSH/RF and shuts down FSH production but frees LH/RF, so stimulating the ovulation peak of LH secretion. Oestrogen and progesterone secreted by the corpus luteum then quickly inhibit further LH/RF, and so further LH, secretion. As the steroidal output from the corpus luteum falls, menstruation occurs, and the cycle begins again.

Ovarian changes

As a result of stimulation by the pituitary gonadotrophins many follicles in the ovary commence maturation each month. In the primary follicle the ovum is surrounded by a single layer of granulosa cells. These cells multiply quickly, many layers of granulosa cells being produced. During multiplication the cells secrete a fluid—liquor folliculi—which gradually distends the developing follicle to form a central, fluid-filled cavity. The layers of granulosa cells surrounding the cavity are then called the membrana granulosa. There is a localized proliferation of granulosa cells at one point—the discus proligerus, or cumulus oöphorus—which contains the ovum within its depths. The stromal cells outside the granulosa layer become formed into a layer of spindle cells—the theca interna—whilst outside this, in turn, is a zone of flattened cells—the theca externa (Fig. 2.8).

Gradual increase in the size of the Graafian follicle occurs. At the same time, the follicle makes its way towards the periphery of the ovary, the discus proligerus always facing the surface; this progress is evidently facilitated by the formation of a cone-shaped development of theca interna cells which form at the same point.

Ovulation occurs at full follicle maturation, the ovum being discharged into, or very close

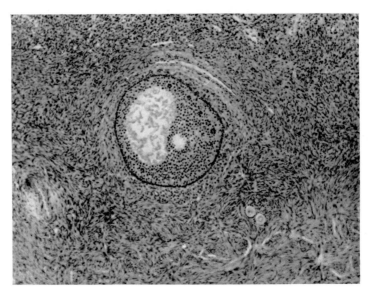

Fig. 2.8. Histological appearances of a developing Graafian follicle.

to, the ostium of the fallopian tube, which by normal tubal motility has been approximated to the ovary at the appropriate time. At ovulation the ovum has undergone the first stage of meiotic division (maturation division) reducing the number of chromosomes from 46 to 23 and casting off the first polar body. The second maturation division occurs after fertilization. At the time the ovum is surrounded by a pale-staining zone—the zona pellucida—and outside this area is a ring of granulosa cells—the corona radiata.

The ruptured follicle collapses over a small quantity of blood and fluid left within and is transformed into the corpus luteum. The granulosa cells and the theca interna cells increase in size and take on a swollen appearance as a result of the process of luteinization; during this process, fluid, rich in carotene, is deposited within the cell cytoplasm, giving the corpus luteum an increasingly yellow colour as development proceeds. The cells of the corpus luteum become thrown into folds as they collapse into the empty cavity, giving it a characteristic appearance histologically (Fig. 2.9).

Activity of the corpus luteum continues for some 9–10 days, when degenerative changes commence if there has not been fertilization of the ovum. This coincides with a fall in oestrogen and progesterone production, until the endometrium cannot be maintained and menstruation occurs.

It is probable that many early menstrual cycles are anovulatory, the developing follicles producing oestrogens which bring about the proliferation changes in the endometrium shortly to be described; when the follicle finally degenerates, oestrogen levels fall and anovular withdrawal haemorrhage results; early cycles are therefore frequently irregular both in interval and duration of flow (see below). At a still earlier stage in the pubertal years the slow rise in the secretion of oestrogen by increasing follicular activity produces the secondary sexual development shortly to be described.

Uterine changes

The changes occurring in the uterus as a result of the ovarian activity described above are most important ones. Immediately following the menstruation the endometrium is thin; glands are narrow and straight and are lined by cuboidal epithelium; the stroma is compact. The action of oestrogen on this thin uterine lining is to

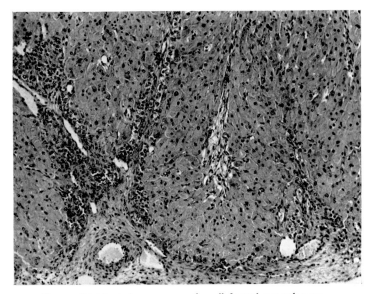

Fig. 2.9. Histological appearances of a well-formed corpus luteum.

produce growth of all the elements present. Glands become longer but remain straight; the epithelial lining becomes tall and columnar, the nuclei occupying a basal position (Fig. 2.10). The stromal cells increase in number and become more loosely packed together, the whole stroma being vascular and abundant. This is the stage of proliferation.

Following ovulation and the addition of progesterone activity to the oestrogen effect described, the secretory phase of development occurs. The glands become more tortuous and

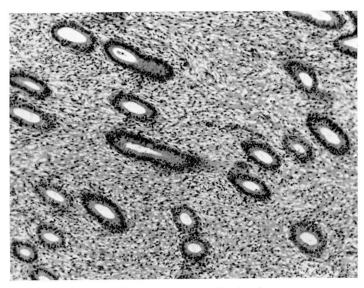

Fig. 2.10. Endometrium in the proliferative phase.

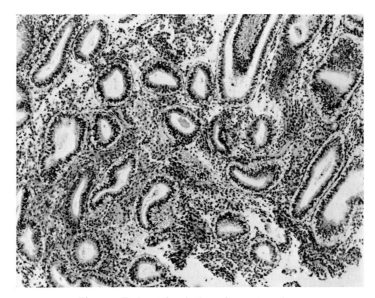

Fig. 2.11. Endometrium in the early secretory phase.

corkscrew-like. The epithelial lining demonstrates a series of changes during which the nuclei become displaced from their basal position towards the centre of the cell by the formation of subnuclear vacuoles (Fig. 2.11). These are usually readily recognizable as clear areas deep to the nucleus. The gland lumina are seen to contain more secretion as the days go by, until maximum secretion is achieved about day 25 of a 28 day cycle; this secretion is rich in glycogen (Fig. 2.12). Stromal cells become further increased in size and are loosely arranged,

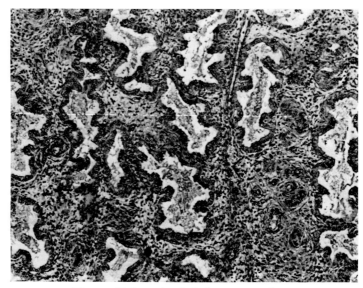

Fig. 2.12. Endometrium in the late secretory phase.

giving the stroma an oedematous appearance which may begin to resemble the decidua of early pregnancy. The arterioles of the endometrium, which are spiralling outwards towards the cavity from the arteries in the basal area, become more and more coiled.

With regression in the corpus luteum the levels of oestrogen and progesterone in the blood fall, and the maintenance of the endometrium is withdrawn. Shrinkage occurs and there is constriction of the spiral arteries, stasis, necrosis and bleeding. The endometrium, with the exception of the deeper basal zone which retains an effective blood supply, breaks down and is cast off as menstrual flow.

The changes in cervical mucus during the ovarian cycle are equally important to the occurrence of a pregnancy. The cervical mucus in the days immediately following menstruation is thick, opaque and of small amount only. Increased secretion of mucus occurs during the proliferative phase, the peak corresponding with that of oestrogen production shortly before ovulation. At this point the cervical mucus is not only much greater in amount but is thin and watery and allows the passage of spermatozoa with great facility. A property of the mucus demonstrable with increasing oestrogen secretion and maximal about the time of ovulation is that of spinnbarkeit; this refers to the property of being able to be drawn out in long threads. A further property exhibited to its greatest extent at the time of ovulation is arborization; that is, fern-like formation visible when a drop of mucus is placed on a glass-slide, allowed to dry and examined under a microscope.

During the secretory phase of the cycle there is a return to the viscid, thicker mucus of the time immediately following the end of menstruation.

Hormone cytology of the vagina

The vaginal epithelium is the most accessible end-organ reflecting the hormonal turmoil of the menstrual cycle. Provided that they are interpreted with care by an experienced cytologist, smears from the vaginal fornix will help to form a general impression of hormonal activity.

Clear changes in cytology are to be seen throughout the normal menstrual cycle, so that for maximum information serial smears are needed.

The vaginal epithelium during reproductive life is made up of four discernible types of cell (Fig. 2.13). Basal cells are firmly attached to the

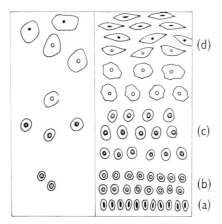

(a) Basal layer (not seen in smears).
(b) Parabasal layer.
(c) Intermediate squames.
(d) Superficial squames.

Fig. 2.13. Diagram of vaginal epithelial cell types. On the right the cells are represented in their normal orientation; on the left they are as seen in vaginal smears.

basement membrane and do not exfoliate, but parabasal cells, intermediate cells and superficial cells may be seen in different circumstances. When oestrogen levels are low there will be preponderance of parabasal cells staining blue with Papanicolau's stain. With greater oestrogen activity there is increase in the number of superficial cells, which stain pink at high oestrogen levels. The nucleus of these cells is pyknotic. Progesterone dominance gives a smear containing a large percentage of intermediate cells which may stain either pink or blue with Papanicolau's stain.

In essence, therefore, throughout one menstrual cycle postmenstrual smears show a relatively high proportion of intermediate cells; with progressive follicular maturation there is a rapid increase in cornified superficial cells. At the time of ovulation the smear shows few leucocytes, whilst the squames are large, separate and have small pyknotic nuclei. After ovulation the leucocyte population increases rapidly, the squames become folded and grouped in clumps, while the number of intermediate cells increases. Later in the luteal phase there is progressive cytolysis.

To attempt more objective assessment the maturation index, eosinophilic index and cornification index have been evolved by various workers. The maturation index relates to the percentage of parabasal, intermediate and superficial cells present, the eosinophilic index to the percentage of pink-staining cells, and the cornification index to the percentage of squamous cells with pyknotic nuclei, omitting from the count, in this instance, parabasal cells.

Androgen activity is believed by some workers in this field to be reflected in the vaginal smear; others refute this view, regarding so-called androgen appearances as identical with those of oestrogen deficiency.

CLINICAL FEATURES

During the pubertal years many important changes occur, in which gynaecologists are now taking a greater interest. The first sign of pubertal development is usually breast growth (Tanner 1962). Growth in height occurs about the same time. Breast growth is usually seen first between the ages of 8 and 13 years, with an average around 11 years. Pubic hair development usually follows next, and later the appearance of axillary hair; this in turn is followed by the first menstrual period. Variations in this pattern are frequent, however, and anxiety on this account alone is needless (Dewhurst 1969; Marshall & Tanner 1969). The most common variation is the appearance of menstruation before axillary hair, and this event may sometimes precede the appearance of pubic hair. Less commonly, pubic hair growth may occur before breast growth. It is worthy of mention that breast growth is not uncommonly unequal during the early stages, the breasts becoming equal in size as growth proceeds.

The age of the menarche has been investigated in great detail by workers in most countries and different results have been obtained, since the onset of menstruation is influenced by factors such as nutrition and environment. In the United States of America, Fluhmann (1956) has examined all preceding work in detail. In Britain several studies have been carried out over the last two decades and have been reviewed by Roberts & Dann (1967). Despite work of this kind it must be emphasized that there is considerable variation in the age of the menarche from one girl to another; to expect a girl to conform too rigidly to a pattern is a mistake that may result in unnecessary investigation and treatment. A generalization which still gives a reliable working rule is that of Wilson & Sutherland (1950), that we can expect a girl in Britain to have her first period between the ages of 10 and 16 years, about half the girls menstruating by the time they are 13 to $13\frac{1}{2}$ years old. The problems concerned with the investigation of primary amenorrhea are dealt with in Chapter 5.

PRECOCIOUS SEXUAL DEVELOPMENT

Sexual development must be considered precocious if there is breast and pubic hair growth before the age of 8 years or menstrual periods before the age of 10 years (Fig. 2.14).

The most common cause of this finding is the premature release of the gonadotrophins from the anterior pituitary without any organic lesion being present—the so-called constitutional precocious puberty (Jolly 1955; Eberline et al. 1960). Here, the signs of puberty usually appear in their correct order and the bone-age and the child's height are several years in advance of the chronological age. Gonadotrophins should be present in the urine, although absence from a single 24 hr specimen should not be regarded as significant. There should, of course, be no abdominal or pelvic swelling palpable, although in some cases retention cysts of follicular type may form in the ovaries and may reach a considerable size. These, however, are the result of the premature ovarian stimulation and are not the cause of the abnormality. The next most

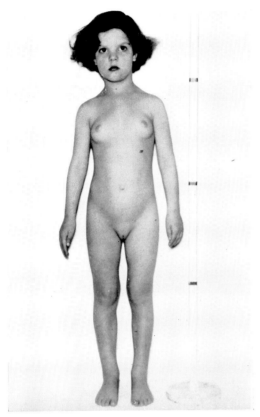

Fig. 2.14. A child aged 5 years with constitutional precocious puberty. (By permission of Baillière, Tindall and Cassell.)

this diagnosis and will call for laparotomy; what has been said already, however, about the possibility of a large follicular cyst in a case of constitutional precocious puberty should be remembered, and if such a lesion be found at operation ovarian tissue must be conserved. A feminizing tumour if present is best treated by oöphorectomy, as most are benign.

Two other examples of premature sexual development must be mentioned. Premature thelarche (Fig. 2.16) is a condition in which breast growth is the only sign of precocious development, and premature pubarche a condition in which pubic hair growth is the only sign of sexual development. The conditions may represent unusual sensitivity of end-organs to the usual low level of hormones in the blood during childhood. In neither case is treatment required beyond simple explanation once careful examination and appropriate investigation have been carried out. The breast enlargement may be unilateral and is sometimes transient, as it

common cause of precocious sexual development is, again, the premature release of gonadotrophin by the pituitary, this time stimulated by the presence of some intracranial lesion, such as meningitis, encephalitis, a cerebral tumour, etc. The example shown in Fig. 2.15. is due to Albright's syndrome.

Less common than either of these lesions is premature sexual development due to a feminizing tumour of the ovary (see Chapter 44). Here, the various landmarks of puberty may not appear in their usual order and vaginal bleeding may be out of all proportion to the degree of breast development. Gonadotrophin is often said to be absent from the urine, but this is not always the case. The presence of a pelvic tumour will be the most significant feature pointing to

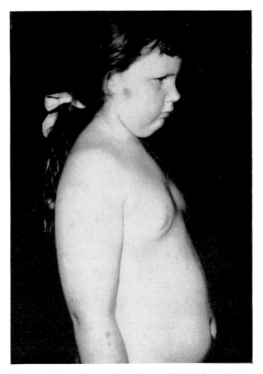

Fig. 2.15. Precocious puberty due to Albright's syndrome.

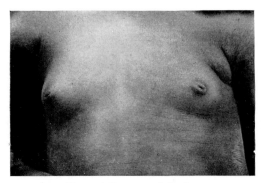

Fig. 2.16. Premature thelarche.

was in the case shown in Fig. 2.16. The breasts began to decrease in size again after 6 months.

EXCESSIVE MENSTRUAL BLEEDING

In considering this symptom it must again be emphasized that early menstrual cycles seldom occur so regularly as in later life. The interval between periods, their duration and the amount of loss are often variable for some months or longer in most girls. Such variation is within physiological limits, and investigation and treatment are unnecessary. Occasionally, however, periods occur more frequently or are more heavy, the parents are alarmed and take their daughter to see a doctor.

The mother and child should then be questioned closely to determine the amount of loss, in order to decide if there is real cause for anxiety or not. A general examination is necessary to exclude any important associated abnormality but a pelvic examination can seldom be carried out in full. Inspection of the vulva, and bimanual rectal examination are nearly always possible and are often helpful in excluding a gross lesion. Examination of the blood should be undertaken in case any significant anaemia is present.

In the treatment of mild cases it may be sufficient to give firm reassurance to mother and child that such episodes are not uncommon and are usually transient. The patient may be given a small calendar on which to keep a record of the days of future bleeding which may help to indicate that little is, in fact, wrong. Iron and dietary advice may be useful. In more severe cases admission to hospital may be necessary. This allows the severity of the condition to be assessed more accurately, and permits more intensive treatment of anaemia, should this be necessary. Heavy bleeding can generally be controlled by a progestogen such as norethisterone (Primolut N) 5 mg three times a day, or norethynodrel (Enavid) 10 mg twice a day, which should stop the bleeding within a few days. The drug should be continued for a further 3 weeks and then stopped to permit withdrawal haemorrhage to occur. Two or three courses are advisable, after which the treatment may be stopped to see if regularity will be resumed. Curettage may be required in protracted cases (Sutherland 1953) and more complete blood studies called for in view of the unlikely, but possible, association of a blood-coagulation defect. Only in very exceptional cases indeed is more surgery to be contemplated. Excessive puberty bleeding is usually a self-limiting disease; any delaying tactics are therefore likely to be helpful by allowing spontaneous recovery to take place.

DYSMENORRHOEA

Not only are early menstrual cycles irregular, but they are frequently anovular. Anovular menstruation seldom causes pain, so that a girl's first few periods will probably be pain-free. Dysmenorrhoea becomes more common later when regular ovulation is established. Dysmenorrhoea during the first few cycles may suggest it to be due more to the incorrect attitude of the girl and her parents towards menstruation than to painful contraction of the uterine muscle. In such cases it may be manifest when interviewing the parents that the girl has been influenced by hearing graphic accounts of her mother's suffering, which not surprisingly may affect her own. It may not be easy to undo the harm done in this kind of case, but a simple explanation of the physiology of menstruation given sympathetically should help. Exercise should be encouraged and the patient should join in games at school whenever she can. Codeine or aspirin may be helpful in providing a more traditional remedy as well. Simple measures of this kind should be used for a while. In more severe cases, in older girls, the use of the 'Pill' to inhibit ovulation and to allow painless menstruation has obvious advantages. Simple dilatation of the cervix under general anaesthesia may be effective, at least for a time, if a progestogen is not favoured.

Other childhood disorders

GENITAL TRACT TUMOURS

Sarcoma botryoides

Tumours during childhood are fortunately uncommon. The most serious is the botryoid sarcoma, which is often grape-like (as its name suggests) but at other times consists of a large, fleshy mass—as we see it in Fig. 2.17. The con-

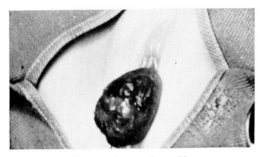

Fig. 2.17. Sarcoma botryoides.

dition probably belongs to the group of mesodermal mixed tumours of the genital tract. Histological features are varied; the stroma is myxomatous and contains fusiform cells singly or in groups; pleomorphism is usually marked; two distinguishing features are the presence of rhabdomyoblasts—large cells with vacuolated eosinophilic cytoplasm—and muscle fibres showing cross-striations.

In the early stages the tumour spreads extensively in the subepithelial tissues of the vagina or cervix whilst retaining a covering of epithelium, giving it a polyp-like appearance. Progress of the disease may be so rapid that the patient is overwhelmed by it and treatment is hardly

possible; in other cases, however, there may be time for curative treatment, provided this is started soon enough and is sufficiently radical. Delay may arise because of the similarity of early lesions to simple polypi, and only when they have been removed and have recurred and then removed again is their nature apparent. It must be emphasized that, rare though botryoid sarcoma is, simple polypi in childhood are rarer still.

It is probable that only radical surgical treatment is likely to be effective. This may involve removing the uterus appendages and vagina or even the bladder or rectum, or both as well. The position of the tumour may influence the extent of the surgical treatment necessary to cure it. If the growth is early and confined to the cervix alone, then hysterectomy and partial vaginectomy may be sufficient. If extension to the posterior fornix has occurred this treatment may still suffice, but if the anterior wall of the vagina is involved the proximity of the bladder base makes anterior exenteration necessary if the patient's life is to be saved. Some authorities feel that this treatment is too radical for children, but many such children go to school, play games and lead very full lives with an ileal bladder or colostomy, or both.

Carcinoma of cervix

This is very rare indeed during childhood and nearly all examples reported have been adenocarcinomata. The presenting feature has always been vaginal bleeding, subsequent investigation leading to the discovery of a tumour. As might be expected, treatment has been mostly ineffective, but some children have survived for 5 years or more.

Ovarian cysts and tumours

These have been reported not infrequently during childhood. The types of tumour found in the child do not differ markedly from those seen in the adult, but certain tumours tend to be seen more often than in later life. The commonest ovarian tumour of the child and adolescent is the teratoma, which is usually found in the form of the well-known dermoid cyst. Half the tumours in the combined series reviewed by Dewhurst (1963) were cystic, or solid, benign teratomata. Simple cysts of follicular type may be found especially in the new-born and very young baby; dysgerminomata appear to be relatively more common than in the adult.

Clinically, the presenting feature is more often torsion than is the case in older patients; sometimes, operation for undiagnosed abdominal pain has led to the tumour's discovery. In the differential diagnosis Wilms's tumour, mesenteric cysts, enlarged spleen, distended bladder and hydrocolpos may need to be considered. Operation is required and the tumour must be dealt with in the most appropriate manner. Cysts which are clearly benign must be removed by ovarian cystectomy, and not by oöphorectomy. It should be recalled that the common cyst—the dermoid—is often bilateral, and ovarian conservation is most important.

Solid ovarian tumours may be benign (fibroma) or malignant (teratoma, carcinoma or dysgerminoma). A solid, well-defined tumour likely to be benign should be dealt with by salpingo-oöphorectomy in the first instance; subsequent treatment may be considered in the light of the histological report. The dysgerminomata are not of a high degree of malignancy and are relatively radio-sensitive, two characteristics which suggest that unilateral removal may be sufficient here too. The child may then be left with a chance of fertility; if a recurrence were detected later, radiotherapy could be employed.

REFERENCES

BARCLAY D.L., MACEY H.B. & REED R.J. (1966) *Obstet. Gynec., N.Y.* **27**, 637.

CAMPBELL J.F. (1940) *J. Am. Ass.* **115**, 513.

DEWHURST C.J. (1963) *Gynaecological Disorders of Infants and Children.* Cassell, London, p. 24.

DEWHURST C.J. (1968) *J. Obstet. Gynaec. Br. Commonw.* **75**, 377.

DITKOWSKY S.P., FALK A.B., BAKER N. & SCHAFFNER M. (1956) *Am. J. Dis. Child.* **91**, 52.

EBERLEIN W.R., BONGIOVANNI A.M., JONES I.T. & YAKOVAC W.C. (1960) *J. Pediat.* **57**, 484.

FLUHMANN C.J. (1956) *The Management of Menstrual Disorders.* Philadelphia, Saunders, p. 69.

HARRIS G.W. & JACOBSOHN D. (1952) *Proc. R. Soc. B.* **139**, 263.

HUFFMAN J.W. (1958) *Pediat. Clins N. Am.* Feb., p. 38.

JOLLY H. (1955) *Sexual Precocity.* Oxford, Blackwell.

JOSEPH M.K., NAYAR B.G. & KANNANKUTTY M. (1966) *Br. med. J.* i, 89.

KINDLER T. (1953) *Br. J. Derm.* **65**, 269.

MARSHALL W.A. & TANNER J.M. (1969) *Archs Dis. Childh.* **44**, 291.

PENNINGTON G.W. & DEWHURST C.J. (1969) *Archs Dis. Childh.* **44**, 629.

PRYSE-DAVIES J. & DEWHURST C.J. (1971) *J. Path.* **103**, 5.

ROBERTS D.A. & DANN T.C. (1967) *Br. J. prev. soc. Med.* **21**, 170.

STEPHENS F.D. (1966) *Aust. N.Z. J. Obstet. Gynec.* **5**, 64.

SUTHERLAND A.M. (1953) *Glasg. med. J.* **34**, 496.

TANNER J.M. (1962) *Growth at Adolescence.* Oxford, Blackwell.

WILSON D.C. & SUTHERLAND I. (1950) *Br. med. J.* ii, 862.

CHAPTER 3

CONTROL OF OVARIAN FUNCTION

Rapid progress has been made in understanding the mechanisms of ovarian control and the subject has been reviewed recently (Shearman 1969). New knowledge is accumulating with such speed, however, that any review of the subject must be read with a retrospective glance to the time it was written, rather than when it is published.

The concept of neural control of anterior pituitary function is sufficiently well established not to need detailed discussion here, the classical hypothesis of Harris having been amply confirmed. More recently, attention has focused on hypothalamic releasing factors controlling pituitary trophic hormone release, and most recently on those areas within the hypothalamus controlling these releasing factors and those factors which in turn control these areas.

Two hypothalamic factors controlling gonadotrophin release have been described in animals and the human (Schally et al. 1967), luteinizing hormone release factor (LRF) and follicle-stimulating hormone release factor (FSH-RF).

LUTEINIZING HORMONE RELEASE
FACTOR (LRF)

This factor has been the subject of extensive reviews (Harris 1961; Guillemin 1964; Schally et al. 1968). Current evidence suggests that there are two different areas synthesizing LRF—one in the suprachiasmatic region and another in the arcuateventromedial region. While these areas secrete the hormones, they are stored in the median eminence (Martini et al. 1968). Thence

they pass, via the hypothalamopituitary portal circulation, to the anterior pituitary. While earlier work suggested that LRF was a polypeptide with a molecular weight of about 1,200–2,000 (Ratner et al. 1967), recent evidence suggests that it may be much smaller (Schally et al. 1968).

LRF is inactive when given to hypophysectomized animals, but when administered to intact animals will stimulate LH release from the anterior pituitary, even to the point of inducing ovulation (Arimura et al. 1967; Schally et al. 1968). LRF does not appear to be species specific.

As more is learned, the controlling mechanisms of the releasing factors become more complex. Barraclough (1966) suggested that of the two hypothalamic areas controlling LRF, one would stimulate basal secretion, the other—effective only in the female—causing cyclic release. It is now suggested (Martini et al. 1968) that the male and female hypothalamus are closer together in this respect than previously believed.

The comparatively simple 'negative feedback control' of gonadal steroids on the hypothalamus and pituitary is no longer really tenable. Now, 'long', 'short', 'negative' and 'positive' feedback mechanisms must be considered (Martini et al. 1968). Either locally or systemically in large amounts, oestrogens will act on the hypothalamus to reduce hypothalamic stores of LRF in the median eminence—a 'long negative' feedback. Small amounts of oestrogens will deplete LH stores and increase plasma LH—a 'long positive' feedback. It is thought that the receptor site for this control is in the median eminence, not the pituitary.

The concept of 'short feedback' control is more recent. These are controls 'independent from the hormones secreted by the peripheral target gland and in which the signal is provided by pituitary hormones themselves' (Martini et al. 1968). It has been shown that implantation of LH into the median eminence will cause a decrease in pituitary LH stores ('short negative' feedback), while the administration of LH to hypophysectomized animals will reduce plasma levels of LRF.

FOLLICLE-STIMULATING HORMONE
RELEASE FACTOR (FSH-RF)

Clearly established by Igarashi & McCann (1964) as a separate factor from LRF and previously believed to be a polypeptide, it is now thought that FSH-RF is a much smaller molecule—probably a polyamine (Schally et al. 1968). Some single amines have been shown to deplete pituitary FSH in vivo.

Purified FSH-RF has no effect in the hypophysectomized animal, but will increase plasma FSH in the intact animal and deplete pituitary FSH. FSH-RF administered to anovulatory women has induced ovulation (Igarashi et al. 1967). It is not species specific.

FSH-RF is synthesized in a single area in the hypothalamus (the paraventricular area)—unlike LRF—but like the latter is stored in the median eminence.

Oestrogens, either given systemically or implanted into the median eminence, reduce pituitary FSH levels, while systemic oestradiol will reduce FSH-RF stores in the median eminence ('long negative' feedback). Progesterone will inhibit both FSH and FSH-RF in the female animal, but not the male. There is also evidence for a 'long positive' feedback of oestrogens on the hypothalamus.

As with LRF, a 'short negative' feedback for FSH-RF has been demonstrated (Martini et al. 1968). Exogenous FSH will cause a fall in both pituitary FSH and median eminence FSH-RF, the primary action being an inhibition of synthesis and storage of FSH-RF. The receptors for these protein hormones are highly specific.

There is no cross-over reaction at this level with LH, FSH or ACTH.

The long dormant discussion of the effect of the pineal gland on gonadal function has been revived with the demonstration of the effect of indoles on gonadotrophic function. A specific pineal-produced neuro humour affecting this system has been postulated and named 'melatonin' (Wurtman 1967). It may add to one's sense of universal order to reflect that pinealectomy will delay sexual maturation in the Japanese quail (Sayler & Wolfson 1968). The systemic administration of melatonin to rats suggests that the secretion of LH, but not FSH, is inhibited (Martini et al. 1968).

These findings relate to laboratory animals and their relevance to human reproduction remain to be determined. It is, however, a consistent source of Darwinian delight that findings in laboratory animals so frequently apply, with little change, to the human scene.

THE GONADOTROPHINS

Fortunately, there is no need to complicate further an already difficult picture by postulating the existence of three gonadotrophins in the human, as has frequently been done in the recent past. Savard et al. (1965) review their own evidence in the human and evidence from other species (monkey, sow, ewe, guinea-pig and rabbit) that prolactin (LTH) is not luteotrophic. In the human, prolactin has yet to be demonstrated as an entity separate from growth hormone, although on clinical grounds there are good reasons to believe it must exist.

The two proven human gonadotrophins are FSH and LH, also called interstitial cell-stimulating hormone (ICSH) because of its action in the male. The two hormones are produced by different pituitary cells.

Follicle-stimulating hormone (FSH)

The isolation of pure FSH from either the pituitary or postmenopausal urine has presented many problems. Steelman et al. (1956) published preliminary data on a highly purified FSH which they claimed to be homogenous. In 1959,

Steelman and Segaloff gave data on porcine, ovine and human pituitary and urinary FSH, indicating a molecular weight of between 29,000 and 30,000. In 1961, Greep pointed out that no product so far obtained would satisfy all modern criteria of purity. In 1964, Roos and Gemzell described a method of preparation from the pituitary giving an extremely potent preparation of FSH 'homogenous in both the ultracentrifuge and in the free zone-electrophoresis apparatus'. More recently, Butt (1967) has given more detailed characterization of FSH extracted from human pituitaries. He noted a carbohydrate content of just over 24%. Since it is possible that the specificity of trophic action is dependent on carbohydrate sequences, this is of considerable importance.

For many years some workers suggested that in urine there were not two distinct hormones, but rather one, with both FSH and LH activity (Loraine 1958). Improvements in extraction procedures have yielded urinary extracts with increasingly high FSH/LH ratios (Donini et al. 1964b; Reichert & Parlow 1964) with adequate separation of FSH and LH (Blatt et al. 1966). This has culminated in the preparation from postmenopausal urine by Donini et al. (1966a, b) of 'biologically pure' FSH.

Probably the most graphic description of the action of pure FSH is Greep's (1959), ' . . . it will not lead to stimulation of the uterus: the ovaries will exhibit many mature but not cystic follicles and no follicles that are in preovulatory swelling; the preparation will not produce any trace of luteinization or thecal swelling in the hypophysectomized female rat nor any enlargement of the prostate in males'.

Greep (1961) reviews evidence from the rat, rabbit, sheep and cow that excessive stimulation with FSH, while not effecting the growth of individual follicles, brings more and more follicles to maturity. This artificial production of a state of readiness for superovulation is very relevant to the problem of dosage control in human therapeutics (Chapter 34). It should be reiterated that pure FSH, although capable of producing follicular maturation, is not by itself capable of inducing ovulation or initiating ovarian steroidogenesis. For this LH is needed as well.

Luteinizing hormone (LH)

Like FSH, LH is a glycoprotein and its structure, partially clarified by Li (1961), has been documented further by the Birmingham group (Butt 1967). It is thought that LH consists of two non-identical sub-units, different from each other in amino-acid composition, carbohydrate content and electrophoretic mobility (Holcomb et al. 1968).

Greep (1961) has pointed out that while LH administered alone has no detectable effect in the immature animal, in the adult animal many of its effects can be seen with the naked eye—superovulation, luteinization and the effects of promoted steroidogenesis on the genital tract. For all of these effects prior priming with FSH is essential. The receptor cell for the steroidogenic ferment created by LH is quite unmoved by FSH alone.

For obvious reasons there is little known of the effect of LH on human ovarian steroidogenesis in vivo. Even the somewhat coarse index of its effect on the lifespan of the corpus luteum is uncertain. Short (1964) reviews the evidence of others, and provides much of his own, that the lifespan of the ovine corpus luteum is unaffected by either LH or HCG. Moor & Rowson (1964) provide evidence that hysterectomy in the sheep before the thirteenth day of a 16 day cycle will prolong the life of the corpus luteum, and because of this a uterine 'luteolysin' has been postulated. The weight of evidence suggests that the endometrium produces this 'luteolysin' in the sheep, cow and some small laboratory animals. The human uterus does not seem to be effective in this way, but the problem in the human warrants re-examination. There is no evidence in the human that LH has either trophic or lytic qualities with regard to the corpus luteum (Neill et al. 1967).

There is evidence that HCG can prolong the life of the human corpus luteum in the non pregnant human female (Browne & Venning 1938; Brown & Bradbury 1947). This may, however, merely demonstrate one of the differences between HCG and LH.

Although it is not clear just how closely in vitro studies can be applied to in vivo behaviour,

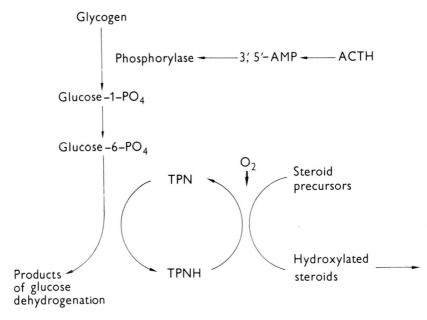

Fig. 3.1. Haynes's concept of the mechanism of action of ACTH. (From Haynes *et al.* (1960), by courtesy of the Editor of *Recent Progress in Hormone Research*.)

they do at least provide useful information about the synthetic potential of the tissues studied. Savard *et al.* (1965) have shown that HCG and human LH will increase the synthesis of all steroids, including progesterone and oestrogens, in human corpus luteum preparations.

The mechanism(s) by which LH increased steroidogenesis is not yet clear. Savard *et al.* (1965) suggest that the Haynes concept (Haynes *et al.* 1960) of the action of corticotrophin on the adrenal cortex (Fig. 3.1) may not be directly applicable to the action of LH. After reviewing evidence relating to the effect of gonadotrophins on 20-hydroxylation and side-chain cleavage of cholesterol, Savard concludes that in addition, an important role of LH is in the added stimulation of 'steroidogenic' cholesterol from earlier precursors. Savard's later work (1967) indicates that LH has a site specific effect on the concentration of cyclic AMP (adenosine $3',5'$-monophosphate) in luteal tissue. In tissue slices of corpus luteum exposed to LH, increased concentration of cyclic AMP precedes by 15–20 min any significant increase in steroid synthesis.

The effect of LH at a synthetic site prior to cholesterol production remains controversial. Savard's evidence suggests such a role in bovine corpus luteum but not in human tissue (Savard 1967), while Armstrong (1967) concludes that in the rabbit 'LH does not stimulate progesterone synthesis as a result of an action prior to cholesterol production', not could he find evidence in the bovine ovary to support Savard.

OVARIAN STEROIDOGENESIS

Accepting that LH promotes ovarian steroidogenesis, exclusive attention should not be focused on the follicle and corpus luteum as the sole sites of response. Savard *et al.* (1965) on the basis of *in vitro* findings discuss three separate steroidogenic compartments in the ovary, all of which are responsive to LH stimulation after prior or concurrent exposure to FSH. These are as follows:

(1) The stroma, which may synthesize androstenedione, dehydro-*epi*androsterone,

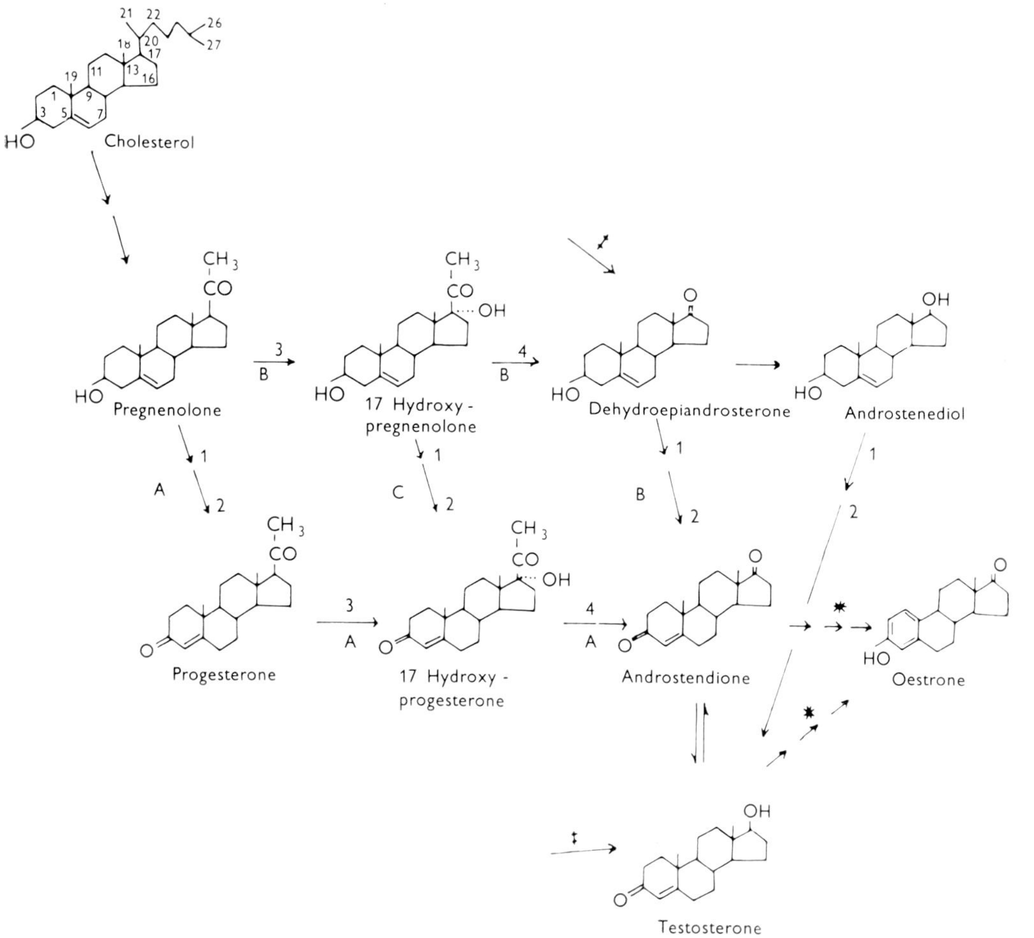

Fig. 3.2. Some pathways of ovarian steroidogenesis. (From Shearman & Cox (1966), by courtesy of the Editor of *Obstetrual and Gynecological Surveys*.)

testosterone and small quantities of oestradiol and progesterone. This role of the stroma has been amplified by Mattingy & Huang (1969).

(2) The follicle, synthesizing mainly oestradiol with trace amounts of progesterone and androgens.

(3) The corpus luteum, producing progesterone as the dominant hormone, but significant quantities of oestradiol also.

There are very few data on the changes in steroidogenesis coincidental with cellular changes during the human menstrual cycle. Short (1962, 1964) has taken advantage of the large amount of follicular and luteal fluid present in the mare ovary to study steroid production *in vivo*. On the basis of his results he puts forward the 'two cell theory' which 'postulates that the theca interna cells have all the enzyme systems necessary for the synthesis of oestradiol-17β from cholesterol, whereas the granulosal cells have only a weak 17-hydroxylase ability and little or no 17-desmolase activity'. Short suggests that the synthetic potential of the granulosal cells is not evident in the follicular phase because of its avascularity. After ovulation with a rapid ingrowth of blood vessels, the capacity of the lutein-transformed granulosa becomes dominant. He concludes that in the mare, changes in steroid secretion so clearly evident after ovulation are 'a direct result of the change in cell type', the thecal cells of the follicle producing oestrogens and androstenedione, the granulosal-derived luteal cells producing predominantly progesterone.

Savard (1964) and Pearlman (1964) emphasize the species variability in production of steroids by the corpus luteum. *In vitro*, the human corpus luteum produces significant quantities of oestrogen, and the urinary excretion pattern of oestrogens in the luteal phase of the cycle indicates that this also occurs *in vivo*. It may be relevant that whereas in the mare—studied by Short—the thecal cells almost entirely disappear after ovulation, in the human they remain prominent as the theca lutein cells.

Ryan & Petro (1966) have studied the steroidal potential of human granulosal and thecal cells *in vitro*. They conclude that in the human the differences are quantitative rather than qualitative. Both cells convert precursor pregnenolone to oestrogens, but this is of much greater degree in thecal cells. Granulosal cells showed a striking preference for the conversion of pregnenolone to progesterone.

There are many adequate recent reviews of ovarian steroid biogenesis and metabolism (Brooksbank 1964; Dorfman 1963; Dorfman *et al.* 1963; Engel & Langer 1961; Goldzieher 1964; Ryan & Smith 1965) and these have been summarized by Shearman & Cox (1966).

The main pathways are shown in Fig. 3.2. The Δ^4 (A) pathway hitherto considered dominant has ample support from the Δ^5 (B) steps, (Ryan & Smith 1961; Smith & Ryan 1962). Kase (1964) has suggested that the Δ^5 pathway may be characteristic of all non-luteinized tissue.

While it should be noted that all oestrogens appear to be produced from androgenic precursors (Chapter 7), it must be emphasized that steroids occurring as part of a biosynthetic pathway may not be secreted in appreciable amounts.

SECRETION AND EXCRETION PATTERNS OF GONADOTROPHINS AND OVARIAN STEROIDS IN OVULATORY CYCLES

Gonadotrophins

For obvious reasons there are virtually no data on the pituitary content of gonadotrophins in the human during the menstrual cycle. Using prostatic weight in the hypophysectomized rat as the end-point, McArthur (1965) has long held that there is a peak of LH excretion at midcycle and that it is detectable at all other times of the cycle. Using the more sensitive ovarian ascorbic-acid depletion test, Fukushima *et al.* (1964), and Rosemberg & Keller (1965) have also found a midcycle peak in LH excretion. Similar results have been reported by Wide & Gemzell (1962) and Mishell (1966) using an immunological method. In plasma, Yokata *et al.* (1965) have found clear evidence of a midcycle increase in LH levels. Using a radio-immunoassay for LH, which is more sensitive than methods hitherto developed, Bagshawe *et al.* (1966) described midcycle peaks of LH in both serum and urine (Fig. 3.3) and their findings in plasma have been confirmed by Odell *et al.* (1967) and Neill *et al.* (1967).

The physiological pattern of FSH excretion remains in dispute. Relatively non-specific assays have yielded little useful information despite a vast amount of work. Even using the more specific and sensitive method of ovarian augmentation, differing results have been obtained. Brown (1959) in a study of four women, found the highest levels in urine during the first part of the cycle in three of them, but in the fourth there was a peak just after midcycle. Fukushima *et al.* (1964) found high levels during menstruation and low or undetectable levels in the rest of the cycle, whereas Rosemberg & Keller (1965) found FSH throughout the cycle with a tendency to a midcycle peak. The need for vertical pooling of urine to obtain measurable levels is a very real problem with this method. If methods for radio-immune assay of FSH such as that developed by Faiman & Ryan (1967a) prove to satisfy reliability criteria, much more information

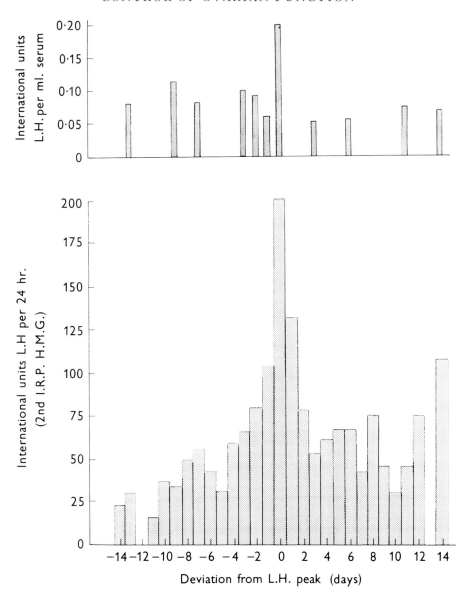

Fig. 3.3. Urinary and serum levels of luteinizing hormone during the normal menstrual cycle. (From Bagshawe *et al.* (1966), by courtesy of the Editor of *Lancet*.)

should be forthcoming soon. Using this technique they (Faiman & Ryan 1967b) found two peaks of FSH, one early in the proliferative phase and a second at or near the time of ovulation.

OVARIAN STEROIDS

If there remains uncertainty about the physiological relationship of FSH and LH during the normal cycle there is, fortunately, a little more certainty and uniformity of opinion about the ovarian steroidal response to this stimulus, at least in terms of urinary excretion.

Using a double isotope method, Svendson & Sorensen (1964) found levels of unconjugated oestrone and oestradiol of between 0·1 and 0·3 μg/l throughout most of the cycle. Only around the time of ovulation was there a significant increase. Shutt (1969), using a method based on competitive protein binding, has shown oestradiol levels of 18 ng/100 ml in the follicular phase and 47 ng/100 ml in the luteal phase.

There is reliable information about the levels of plasma progesterone during the cycle. The studies of Woolever (1963) show the expected

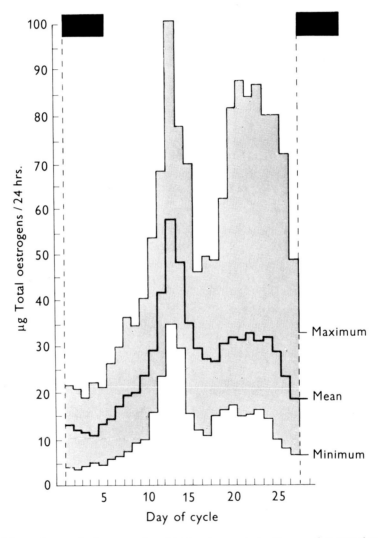

Fig. 3.4. Mean and range of urinary excretion of total oestrogens during the normal menstrual cycle. (From Brown *et al.* (1959), by the courtesy of the Editor of *Journal of Obstetrics and Gynaecology of the British* Commonwealth.)

rise in the luteal phase with a sharp fall before the onset of menstruation.

In a study using the extremely sensitive, precise and specific method of competitive protein binding, Neill *et al.* (1967) have shown low levels of plasma progesterone (< 0·2–1·8 m μg/ml) in the follicular phase. It is only after the midcycle peak of LH that an increase in plasma progesterone is seen, reaching 10–19 m μg/ml 3–5 days later with a sharp fall before the onset of menstruation. The excretion patterns of the three classical oestrogens and pregnanediol are fully documented following the early work of Brown (1955a, b) and Klopper (1957). Oestrogen excretion patterns have been fully reviewed by Brown *et al.* (1959) and Brown & Matthew (1962). The mean and normal range values for oestrogens (oestrone, oestradiol and oestriol) obtained from a study of sixteen women are shown in Fig. 3.4. Typically, the pattern is biphasic. During the first 2 or 3 days of menstruation oestrogen excretion is low. In a 28-day cycle there is then a fairly rapid rise to a well-defined peak at midcycle, usually termed the *ovulation peak*. This is followed by a fall in oestrogen excretion and then a second, broader, rise—the luteal maximum. In the last few days of the cycle there is a decrease in oestrogen excretion, and menstruation follows.

It has been believed that in the non-pregnant individual, urinary oestriol is derived only from secreted oestrone and/or oestradiol, although it is now well established that oestriol in pregnancy is predominantly derived from non-oestrogenic precursors produced by the foetus. More recently, work by Barlow & Logan (1967) suggests that at least in the luteal phase, precursors of urinary oestriol other than oestrone and/or oestradiol may be involved.

In contrast, the excretion pattern of pregnanediol is uniphasic. During the follicular phase excretion is usually less than 1 mg 24 hr. Shortly after ovulation the levels increase, reaching a maximum midway through the luteal phase and then declining before menstruation. The results in Fig. 3.5 are typical of those seen in a spontaneous ovulatory cycle.

The pattern in conceptual cycles is different. Brown (1956) produced data on the pattern of

oestrogen excretion in the conceptual cycle of a woman ovulating spontaneously. A further increase beyond the luteal maximum is already obvious before the first missed period. If ovulation is physiologically induced in anovulatory

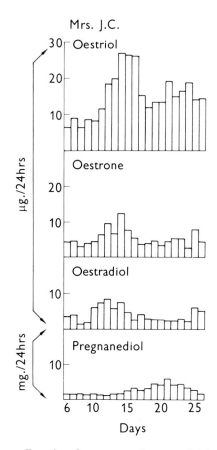

Fig. 3.5. Excretion of oestrogens and pregnanediol during the normal menstrual cycle. (From Shearman (1969), by courtesy of Charles C. Thomas, Publisher.)

females an identical pattern can be produced (Fig. 3.6).

It should be emphasized that although there is a qualitative similarity in excretion patterns from one woman to another, quantitatively there are large interpersonal differences. A clear picture may only be obtained by serial assays.

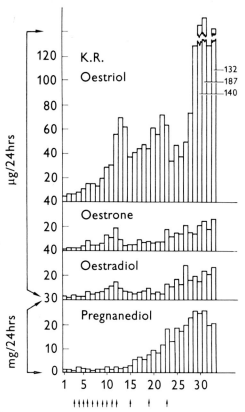

Fig. 3.6. Urinary steroid excretion during a conceptual cycle.

Days 3–9 –75 i.u. F.S.H. (Pergonal)

Days 10–11 –150 i.u. F.S.H. (Pergonal)

Day 12 –75 i.u. F.S.H. (Pergonal) + 2,000 units H.C.G.

Days 15,19 and 23 –500 units H.C.G.

REFERENCES

ARIMURA A., SCHALLY A.V., SAITO T., MULLER E.E. & BOWERS C.Y. (1967) *Endocrinology,* **80,** 515.

ARMSTRONG D.T. (1967) In *Recent Research on Gonadotrophic Hormones* (edited by E.T. Bell & J.A. Loraine). Edinburgh and London, Livingstone, p. 188.

BAGSHAWE K.D., WILDE C.E. & ORR A.H. (1966) *Lancet,* i, 1118.

BARLOW J.J. & LOGAN C.M. (1967) *Am. J. Obstet. Gynec.* 98, 687.

BARRACLOUGH C.A. (1966) *Recent Prog. Horm. Res.* **22,** 503.

BLATT W.R., PARK M.Y., TAYMOR M.L. & TODD R. (1966) *J. clin. Endocr. Metab.* 26, 189.

BROOKSBANK B.W.L. (1964) *Clin. Obstet. Gynec.* 7, (No. 4), 1120.

BROWN J.B. (1955a) *Lancet,* **ii,** 320.

BROWN J.B. (1955b) *Mem. Soc. Endocr.* 3, 1.

BROWN J.B. (1956) *Lancet,* i, 704.

BROWN J.B., KELLAR R. & MATTHEW G.D. (1959) *J. Obstet. Gynaec. Br. Commonw.* **66,** 177.

BROWN J.B. & MATTHEW G.D. (1962) *Recent Prog. Horm. Res.* **18,** 337.

BROWN P.S. (1959) *J. Endocr.* 18, 46.

BROWN W.E. & BRADBURY J.T. (1947) *Am. J. Obstet. Gynec.* **53,** 749.

BROWNE J.S.L. & VENNING E.H. (1938) *Am. J. Physiol.* **123,** 26.

BUTT W.R. (1967) In *Recent Research on Gonadotrophic Hormones* (edited by E.T. Bell & J.A. Loraine). Edinburgh and London, Livingstone, p. 129.

DONINI P., PUZZUOLI D. & MONTEZEMELO R. (1964a) *Acta endocr. Kbh.* 45, 321.

DONINI P., PUZZUOLI D. & D'ALESSIO I. (1964b) *Acta endocr. Kbh.* 45, 329.

DONINI P., PUZZUOLI D., D'ALESSIO I., LUNENFELD B., ESHKOL A. & PARLOW A.F. (1966a) *Acta endocr.* 52, 169.

DONINI P., PUZZUOLI D., D'ALESSIO I., LUNENFELD B., ESHKOL A. & PARLOW A.F. (1966b) *Acta endocr.* 52, 186.

DORFMAN R.I. (1963) *Obstetl gynec. Surv.* 18, 65.

DORFMAN R.K., FORCHIELLI E. & GUT M. (1963) *Recent Progr. Horm. Res.* 19, 251.

ENGEL L.L. & LANGER L.J. (1961) *A. Rev. Biochem.* 30, 499.

FAIMAN C. & RYAN R.J. (1967a) *J. clin. Endocr. Metab.* 27, 444.

FAIMAN C. & RYAN R.J. (1967b) *J. clin. Endocr. Metab.* 27, 1711.

FUKUSHIMA M., STEVENS V.C., GANTT C.L. & VORYS N. (1964) *J. clin. Endocr. Metab.* 24, 205.

GOLDZIEHER J.W. (1964) *Clin. Obstet. Gynec.* 7 (No. 4), 1160.

GREEP R.O. (1959) *Recent Prog. Horm. Res.* 15, 139.

GREEP R.O. (1961) In *Sex and Internal Secretions* (edited by W.C. Young). Baltimore, Williams and Wilkins, p. 240.

GUILLEMIN R. (1964) *Recent Prog. Horm. Res.* 20, 89.

HARRIS G.W. (1961) In *Control of Ovulation* (edited by C.A. Villee). Oxford, Pergamon Press, p. 56.

HAYNES R.C., SUTHERLAND E.W. & RALL T.W. (1960) *Recent Prog. Horm. Res.* 16, 121.

HOLCOMB G.N., LAMKIN W.M., JAMES S.A., WADE J. & WARD D.N. (1968) *Endocrinology*, 83, 1293.

IGARASHI M. & McCANN S.M. (1964) *Endocrinology*, 74, 446.

IGARASHI M., YOKOTA N. EHARA Y., MAYUZUMI R. & MATSUMOTO S. (1967) In *Proceedings of Vth World Congress of Gynaecology and Obstetrics* (edited by C. Wood). Sydney, Butterworths, p. 349.

KASE N. (1964) *Am. J. Obstet. Gynec.* 90, 1268.

KLOPPER A.K. (1957) *J. Obstet. Gynaec. Br. Commonw.* 64, 504.

LI C.H. (1961) In *Human Pituitary Gonadotropins* (edited by A. Albert). Springfield, Thomas, p. 364.

LORAINE J.A. (1958) *Clinical Application of Hormone Assay.* Edinburgh and London, Livingstone, p. 15.

MARTINI L., FRASCHINI F. & MOTTA M. (1968) *Recent Prog. Horm. Res.* 24, 439.

MATTINGLY R.F. & HUANG W.Y. (1969) *Am. J. Obstet. Gynec.* 103, 679.

MISHELL D.R. (1966) *Am. J. Obstet. Gynec.* 95, 747.

MOOR R.M. & ROWSON L.E.A. (1964)*Nature, Lond.* 201, 522.

McARTHUR J.W. (1965) In *Human Ovulation* (edited by C.S. Keefer). London, Churchill, p. 94.

NEILL J.D., JOHANSSON E.D.B., DATTA J.K. & KNOBIL E. (1967) *J. clin. Endocr. Metab.* 27, 1167.

ODELL W.D., ROSS G.T. & PLAYFORD P.L. (1967) *J. clin. Invest.* 46, 248.

PEARLMAN W.H. (1964) *Recent Prog. Horm. Res.* 20, 338.

RATNER A., DHARIWAL A.P.S. & McCANN S.M. (1967) *Clin. Obstet. Gynec.* 10, 106.

REICHERT L.W. & PARLOW A.F. (1964) *J. clin. Endocr. Metab.* 24, 1040.

ROOS P. & GEMZELL C.A. (1964) *Biochim. biophys. Acta,* 82, 218.

ROSEMBERG E. & KELLER P.J. (1965) *J. clin. Endocr. Metab.* 25, 1262.

RYAN K.J. & PETRO Z. (1966) *J. clin. Endocr. Metab.* 26, 46.

RYAN K.J. & SMITH O.W. (1961) *J. biol. Chem.* 236, 2207.

RYAN K.J. & SMITH O.W. (1965) *Recent Prog. Horm. Res.* 21, 367.

SAVARD K. (1964) *Recent Prog. Horm. Res.* 20, 334.

SAVARD K. (1967) In *Recent Research on Gonadotrophic Hormones* (edited by E.T. Bell & J. A. Loraine). Edinburgh and London, Livingstone, p. 170.

SAVARD K., MARSH J.M. & RICE B.F. (1965) *Recent Prog. Horm. Res.* 21, 285.

SAYLER A. & WOLFSON A. (1968) *Endocrinology* 83, 1237.

SCHALLY A.V., ARIMURA A., BOWERS C.Y., KASTIN A.M., SAWANO S. & REDDING T.W. (1968) *Recent Prog. Horm. Res.* 24, 497.

SCHALLY A.V., MULLER E.E., ARIMURA A., BOWERS C.Y., SAITO T., REDDING T.W., SAWANO S. & PIZZOLATO F. (1967) *J. clin. Endocr. Metab.* 27, 755.

SHEARMAN R.P. (1969) *Induction of Ovulation.* Springfield, Thomas.

SHEARMAN R.P. & COX R.I. (1966) *Obstetl gynec. Surv.* 21, 1.

SHORT, R.V. (1962) *J. Endocr.* 24, 59.

SHORT R.V. (1964) *Recent Prog. Horm. Res.* 20, 303.

SHUTT D.A. (1969) *Steroids,* 13, 69.

SMITH O.W. & RYAN K.J. (1962) *Am. J. Obstet. Gynec.* 84, 141.

STEELMAN S.L., KELLY T.L., SEGALOFF A. & WEBER G.F. (1956) *Endocrinology,* 59, 156.

STEELMAN S.L. & SEGALOFF A. (1959) *Recent Prog. Horm. Res.* 15, 115.

SVENDSON R. & SORENSEN B. (1964) *Acta endocr.* 47, 235.

WIDE L. & GEMZELL C. (1962) *Acta endocr.* 39, 539.

WOOLEVER C.A. (1963) *Am. J. Obstet. Gynec.* 85, 981.

WURTMAN R.J. (1967) In *Neuroendocrinology* (edited by L. Martini & W.F. Ganong), Vol. 11. New York, Academic Press, p. 19.

YOKOTA N., IGARASHI M. & MATSUMOTO S. (1965) *Endocr. jap.* 12, 92.

CHAPTER 4

THE INTERSEXES

It is more than usually difficult to compress this subject into a brief chapter. Extensive publications have been edited by Jones & Scott (1958), Overzier (1963), Dewhurst & Gordon (1969) and more briefly, written by Dewhurst (1963), Federman (1967) and Money (1968a). This section will deal only with intersexes determined predominantly by aberration in intra-uterine development. Virilism arising *de novo* in older children and adults is discussed in Chapter 7.

Before it is possible to discuss intersexuality at a rational level, it is necessary to establish just what is meant by sex.

In normal individuals the sex at birth is assigned after inspection of the external genitals: the sex of rearing will be decided on this inspection. Since this frequently made, but nevertheless important, decision is effected so rapidly and superficially, it is worthwhile looking further back to sexual differentiation in an attempt to determine what factors are responsible for sex assignment.

NORMAL SEXUAL DIFFERENTIATION

At fertilization the ovum and the sperm contain the haploid number of chromosomes—in the human ovum 22 autosomes plus one X chromosome, in the sperm 22 autosomes with either an X or Y chromosome. This union will normally result in a conceptus with 46 chromosomes; a female with 44 autosomes and XX sex chromosomes (46/XX) or a male with a similar number of autosomes and XY sex chromosomes (46/XY). Thus will be determined *chromosomal* sex.

Despite this initial chromosome directive the early embryo is morphologically sexually indifferent, with Wolffian and Mullerian ducts and an undifferentiated gonadal ridge. The first objective sign of sexual differentiation is the development from the gonadal ridge of the embryonic testis or ovary, the former evoked by an XY, the latter by an XX, sex chromosome complement. Thus will be determined *gonadal* sex.

In the normal female foetus, Wolffian structures will atrophy, the Mullerian ducts will develop into uterus, tubes and upper vagina, while the cloaca assumes normal female characteristics. In the normal male, the Mullerian structures will regress and the Wolffian ducts will develop into vas deferens, seminal vessels and epididymis. Concurrently, the cloaca will masculinize, with the development of penis, penile urethra and scrotum. Thus will be determined *internal genital* and *external genital* sex.

From simple inspection will be determined the *sex of rearing*, and it is on this, more than anything else, that the psychosexual orientation of the individual will depend (Money 1968a).

We have then, to deal with five sorts of sex—chromosomal, gonadal, internal genital, external genital or body sex (phenotype) and, finally, sex of rearing.

The simplest explanation of all of this would be to say that beyond the chromosome level the ovary is responsible for female differentiation and the testes for masculine development. The sequences are, however, more fascinating and capable of almost infinite variety. Jost (1958) has shown in a series of elegant experiments that if the gonads are removed from a foetus before the stage of gonadal differentiation, then, irrespective of chromosomal sex, development will be along female lines. That is, whether the embryo is chromosomally male or female, without a gonad Mullerian structures will develop into uterus, tubes and upper vagina and the cloaca will develop into a vulva and lower vagina. Female development may, therefore, be regarded as the neutral or asexual norm (Jones & Wilkins 1961) the ovary itself playing no part in this development. At the foetal level female organogenesis does not depend on the presence of an ovary, but male development is very dependent on the presence of a testis.

For masculine differentiation to occur it is then necessary to postulate that the foetal testis does three, and possibly four, things:

First, that the testis will produce a Mullerian inhibitor which will halt the otherwise inexorably neutral development of uterus, tubes and upper vagina.

Secondly, that it possesses a Wolffian evocator which will cause positive development of the Wolffian apparatus.

Thirdly, that it will induce the cloaca to develop into a penis with penile urethra and scrotum.

Fourthly, perhaps, that it will imprint on the hypothalamus a potential for male type of non-cyclic release of luteinizing hormone, instead of the cyclic female patterns (Pfeiffer 1936; Smith & Peng 1967). This sexually exclusive imprinting mechanism on the hypothalamus appears less certain because of the findings of Martini *et al.* (1968) (see Chapter 3).

It would be easier if one substance from the testis was responsible for this remarkable transformation, but because of experimental and clinical evidence it is necessary to postulate that the intra-uterine testis produces at least two (Jones & Wilkins 1961), and possibly three, substances during embryonic induction.

The transformation of the Wolffian ducts and concurrent inhibition of Mullerian structures appears to be the consequence of a local evocating action of the testis on the same side of the body, and is seen to be effective in a centripetal fashion. Masculine differentiation of the external genitals, on the other hand, though still depending on the presence of a testis, appears to be mediated through the action of a circulating substance— a true hormone, probably testosterone. Whereas the circulating substance may modify profoundly the external genitals, it has no effect itself on Mullerian or Wolffian structures. Excessive androgens circulating in the blood of a female foetus—as in the adrenogenital syndrome— may cause complete masculinization of the external genitals, but will never affect internal genital sex.

ABNORMAL SEXUAL DIFFERENTIATION AND CLASSIFICATION OF INTERSEX

Taken in sequence then, intersexuality may occur because of abnormality in the sex chromosomes; because of gonadal defects in the presence of normal chromosomes—a gonadal mixture as in true hermaphroditism, or absence of gonads as in true gonadal agenesis; further in the presence of a testis, intersex may occur because the gonad is defective in one or other of its inducor roles; or to complicate matters further there may be end-organ resistance—partial or complete— to normally competent foetal testes; given normal chromosomes and gonads the external genitals of a female infant may be modified by the effect of a circulating androgen; and finally, all of the foregoing may be normal, but a degree of behavioural intersexuality, such as homosexuality or transvestism, may be superimposed by aberrations in the sex of rearing.

It is probably now reasonable to attempt a definition, and then a classification, of intersex. An intersex may be defined as an individual where there is conflict at any level between chromosomal sex, gonadal sex, internal genital sex, external genital (phenotypical) sex or the sex of rearing.

No classification will suit every student. The classification here suits the writer, but at the

same time he is fully conscious of its imper-
fections.

(1) Chromosomal level
    (i) True Turner's syndrome and
        Turner's mosaic
    (ii) Triplo X female
    (iii) Klinefelter's syndrome
    (iv) Mixed gonadal dysgenesis
    (v) XYY male
(2) Gonadal level
    (i) True hermaphroditism
    (ii) True gonadal agenesis
    (iii) Virilizing male intersex
(3) End-organ resistance
    (i) Complete: testicular feminization
    (ii) Partial: cryptorchid hypospadiac
        male intersex
    (iii) Familial male intersex (Lubs,
        Gilbert-Dreyfus, Reifenstein)
(4) Female intersexuality
    (i) Progressive: congenital adrenal
        hyperplasia (adrenogenital syn-
        drome)
    (ii) Non-progressive: due to:
        (a) Maternal androgen
        (b) Exogenous synthetic pro-
            gestogen
        (c) Spontaneous

Overlap here is unavoidable. Some true
hermaphrodites have chromosomal abnormality,
but since their claim to uniqueness lies in their
dual gonads they are classified here at that level.
Similarly, although the virilizing male intersex
lacks a Mullerian inhibitor and is, therefore,
included in the gonadal level, these children also
have partial end-organ resistance.

Chromosomal level

Although it had been postulated in 1923 by
Painter that karyotypic disturbance in the human
might lead to some types of intersex, it took 25
years of technical progress for this proposition
to move beyond the realm of theory. The ex-
plosion that cleared the pathway to this exciting
territory was the discovery of the sex chromatin
body in 1949. This strikingly original observation

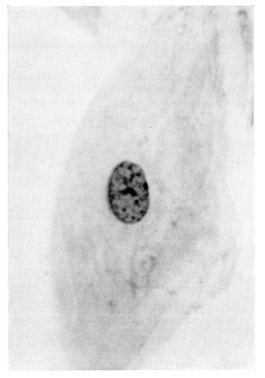

Fig. 4.1. Chromatin-positive buccal smear.

was made by Barr when studying the neuronal
cells of cats and has since been extended to other
interphase cells in most animal species, including
man (Fig. 4.1). Between 20 and 30% of cells from
the female will show a dense mass of hetero-
chromatin beneath the nuclear membrane—
the Barr body (Barr 1963). With the charming
exception of the Virginia opossum, sex chromatin
is not found in the male. Cells for study are most
conveniently obtained from buccal smears,
although leucocyte 'drumsticks' have the same
significance. The work of Lyon (1962) has indicated that the Barr body is one of the two X
chromosomes, and that it is largely a matter of
chance whether the maternal or paternal X is
sent to the wall. The number of Barr bodies is
one less than the number of X chromosomes: no
sex chromatin (chromatin negative) indicates
that the cells are XO or XY, one Barr body means
XX or XXY, two Barr bodies XXX or XXXY and
so on. In some chromosome mosaics (see p. 56)

the percentage of chromatin-positive cells may lie between 2 and 15%.

Abnormalities of sex chromosomes may consist of sex chromosome deletion or addition. This chromosomal polymorphy may arise during meiosis, when each cell of the conceptus will be similarly affected, or after conception during mitosis, when two or more stem lines will arise, giving chromosomal mosaicism. The arguments for the more common mechanism of meiotic or somatic (mitotic) non-disjunction and the less common mechanisms of anaphase lagging or translocation are dealt with fully by Ford (1963).

TURNER'S SYNDROME

First described by Turner (1938) the syndrome included short stature, sexual infantilism, cubitus valgus and webbing of the neck. The nipples are widely spaced and *pectus cavum* is commonly present. Congenital cardiac lesions—particularly coarctation of the aorta—may be present. The diagnosis may rarely be made in the neonatal period by the presence of peripheral oedema.

Most patients are chromatin negative and their karyotype 45/XO. Some will have partial deletion of the second X and others 45/XO, 46/XX mosaicism. Buccal smears in mosaics will usually show between 5 and 15% of cells as chromatin positive, while those with partial X deletion may have small Barr bodies. They are phenotypic females with normal but infantile vulva, uterus, vagina and tubes. No gonads are present, the gonadal area being represented characteristically by 'streaks' of fibrous tissue which may resemble ovarian stroma. Some of the XO/XX mosaics may have primordial follicles. Since this problem more commonly presents with primary amenorrhoea, it is discussed more fully in Chapter 5.

The majority of 45/XO embryos will abort. It is of more than passing interest that an early 45/XO abortus *does* have primordial follicles, but these have disappeared by the time of birth in the non-aborted conceptus.

TRIPLE X FEMALE

Presumably the result of the fertilization of a non-disjunctional XX ovum by an X-carrying sperm, this syndrome described by Jacobs *et al.* (1959) may never reach the level of clinical consciousness. They may have oligomenorrhoea, premature menopause or be of normal fertility. Mental retardation is common. Two Barr bodies are seen in buccal smears.

KLINEFELTER'S SYNDROME

The original syndrome described by Klinefelter *et al.* (1942) included atrophy of the seminiferous tubules, azoospermia, gynaecomastia and eunuchoidism; the last two features are by no means constant, while mental retardation is common. Assumed, in its most common form, to be the results of fertilization of an XX nondisjunctional ovum by a Y sperm, the usual buccal smear is chromatin positive and the karyotype XXY. Less frequently, more exotic sex chromosome patterns such as XXXY, XY/XXY are present. The gynaecologist will meet this problem more frequently in the azoospermic male partner of an infertile marriage. The subject is exhaustively reviewed by Paulsen *et al.* (1968).

MIXED GONADAL DYSGENESIS

This syndrome may present at birth with an infant displaying equivocal external genitals— usually clitoral hypertrophy and variable degrees of labioscrotal fusion. Less frequently, the infant may be phenotypically female and develop slight clitoral hypertrophy at puberty. Least often, it will be an accidental diagnosis when investigating what is clinically a 'typical' case of Turner's syndrome or true gonadal agenesis (Shearman 1968). First described by Greenblatt (1958) and delineated more clearly by Sohval (1964), this subject has been fully reviewed by Federman (1967).

Buccal smears from these individuals are usually chromatin negative, while the karyotype usually shows evidence of mosaicism—most frequently XO/XY. Internal genital sex is feminine, while, as mentioned above, external genital sex is equivocal, with sufficient feminine characteristics to dictate a feminine sex of rearing. The gonadal area shows wide variability;

there may be a unilateral testis with a contralateral 'streak' gonad, or gonad plus tumour, or gonadal tumour only. The frequency of these tumours—variably classified as dysgerminoma, seminoma, gonadoma and gonadoblastoma—found in 10 of 23 patients in one series (Federman 1967) and 8 of 26 patients in another series (Teter & Boczkowski 1967) has considerable influence in the management of these patients. This is discussed more fully in Chapter 44.

XYY MALE

The first descriptions of this syndrome by the Edinburgh group have been amply confirmed. Significantly taller than average, with variable intelligence, the clinical feature that has dominated most reports to date is of violent antisocial behaviour. Demonstration of a defendent's XYY karyotype has already been accepted as grounds for acquittal, because of diminished responsibility, in one murder trial in Australia. The full clinical spectrum of this karyotype is yet to be determined, however, as most publications relate to findings in inmates of gaols or psychiatric institutions. Its prevalence in 'normal' individuals is not yet known but there have been reports of this chromosome pattern in males showing no evidence of antisocial behaviour.

Gonadal level

TRUE HERMAPHRODITISM

For this diagnosis to be reached, true testicular and ovarian tissue must be present—not just stroma, but both primordial follicles and seminiferous tubules. External genital sex and internal genital sex vary widely, the former as a rule being predominantly male, while a uterus is usually present. Gonadal elements may be lateral, a testis on one side and ovary on the other, unilateral, with a testis or ovary and an ovotestis on the other; or bilateral, with an ovotestis on each side.

The chromosomal structure of these individuals is usually 46/XX, but mosaics of 46/XX, 47/XXY or 46/XX, 48/XXYY have been recorded.

The rarest karyotype is 46/XY. One of our own patients (Shearman et al. 1964) had this karyotype in leucocytes, skin and testis, while the ovarian tissue was chromatin negative. Since karyotypes from the ovary were not prepared, a 46/XX, 45/XO mosaic cannot be excluded completely.

There is no satisfactory explanation for the fascinating embryological problem of the true hermaphrodite. The interested reader may refer to the reviews of Jones & Scott (1958), Overzier (1963) and Federman (1967).

TRUE GONADAL AGENESIS

Also called pure gonadal dysgenesis, this syndrome is characterized by the complete absence of germinal tissue, female external and internal

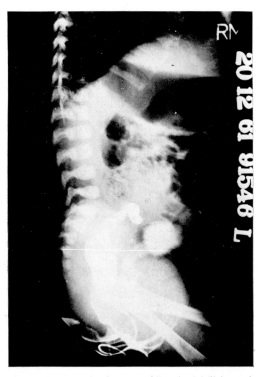

Fig. 4.2. X-ray study of a neonatal intersex (virilizing male intersex) showing bladder anteriorly and vagina and uterus posteriorly. (From Shearman (1968), by courtesy of the Editor of *Journal of Obstetrics and Gynaecology of the British Commonwealth.*)

genital sex, and absence of other congenital malformation. Buccal smears may be positive or negative and karyotype 46/XX or 46/XY.

The individuals are a perfect justification for the translation of Jost's finding in rabbits to the human. Irrespective of chromosomal sex, for reasons that remain obscure (? auto-immune) no gonad develops. Female differentiation therefore occurs as the neutral or asexual norm, but of course in the absence of gonadal tissue, sexual infantilism is the rule.

Since the usual presentation is that of primary amenorrhoea and sexual infantilism in an individual of normal—or slightly increased—height, this condition will be discussed more fully in Chapter 5.

VIRILIZING MALE INTERSEX

These children are an eloquent testimony to the multi-faceted inducor role of the foetal testis. At birth the clitoris is enlarged with variable degrees of labioscrotal fusion and a urogenital sinus. Identical external genitals may be seen in the various forms of female pseudo-hermaphroditism and in cryptorchid hypospadiac male intersex. Radiological studies show a normal vagina, uterus and fallopian tubes (Fig. 4.2).

Bilateral testes are apparent, usually in the 'ovarian' fossa, sometimes in the inguinal regions, buccal smears are chromatin negative and karyotype 46/XY. The testicular tissue is identical to that of a normal male of the same age (Fig. 4.3). Left untreated, a virilizing puberty is inevitable.

This syndrome is explicable by the presence of testes lacking the normal Muellerian inhibitor and partial cloacal resistance to normal intra-uterine androgen production.

End-organ resistance

TESTICULAR FEMINISM

This syndrome was first properly documented by Morris in 1953. It is unusual for the condition to be diagnosed in the neonate, as on routine examination the baby appears completely feminine. Occasionally, the presence of an inguinal hernia in childhood containing a testis will suggest the diagnosis, but the majority of cases present at puberty with primary amenorrhoea. The characteristic clinical picture is that of a female of normal height with well-developed breasts, but scanty or absent axillary and pubic hair (Fig. 4.4). The vulva is completely feminine but

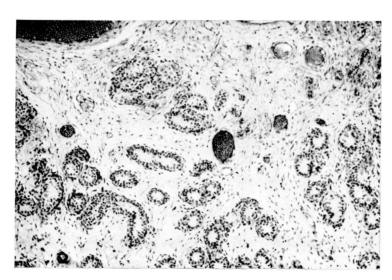

Fig. 4.3. Testicular tissue removed from the abdomen of the patient shown in Fig. 4.2. at the age of 3½ years.

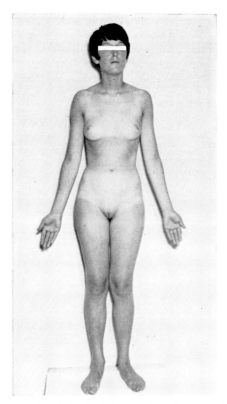

Fig. 4.4. Testicular feminism (patient of the late Dr. Keith Harrison).

It is clear that these testes are hormonally competent both *in utero* and after puberty. Mullerian inhibition is complete, the feature being one of end-organ resistance to testosterone. Enormous doses of exogenous testosterone produce no virilization in these patients. Even the very sensitive test of intradermal administration of testosterone produces no effect on the local hair follicles. Breast development at puberty is thought to be due to normal adrenal and testicular oestrogen levels acting on an end-organ resistant to androgen.

CRYPTORCHID HYPOSPADIAC MALE INTERSEX

These infants will present at birth with clitoral hypertrophy, a urethral sinus at the base of the

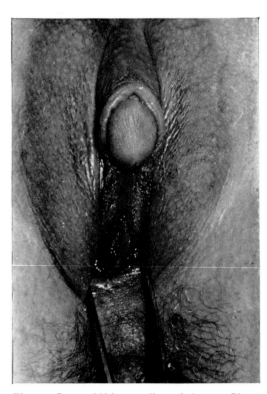

Fig. 4.5. Cryptorchid hypospadiac male intersex. Picture taken at the age of 14 years when the patient was undergoing a masculinizing puberty. Enlarged clitoris and normal urethral opening are visible. There was no vagina or uterus.

the vagina is short and 'blind', the uterus and tubes absent. Bilateral testes may be in the inguinal canal or near the 'ovarian fossa'.

Testicular tissue removed from the postpuberal patient shows tubules lined with immature germ cells and Sertoli cells, while Leydig cells are prominent.

Buccal smears are chromatin negative and the karyotype 46/XY. Since the condition is familial, it is not uncommon to see 'sisters' with the same condition.

Although there is evidence for oestrogen synthesis by these gonads in some patients (Stitch & Oakey 1967), the overwhelming bulk of data show normal male testosterone production in these patients with levels of plasma testosterone identical to those seen in postpuberal males (Federman 1967; Jeffcoate *et al.* 1968).

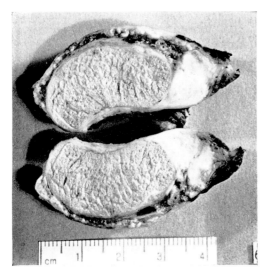

Fig. 4.6. Section of the abdominal testis removed from the patient shown in Fig. 4.5 .

by Wilkins of the role of corticosteroids in treatment. A full review of this extensive subject is not relevant to a section dealing with intersex, and the reader is referred to Wilkins (1965) and Chapter 7. Jones & Scott (1958) give a beautiful historical review of this condition. In essence there is congenital deficiency in enzymes essential for the transformation of progesterone to cortisol (see Chapter 7) most frequently in 21-hydroxylase (with or without salt loss) less frequently 11-hydroxylase (hypertensive form) and least frequently 3-β-ol-dehydrogenase (invariable and severe salt loss). In an effort to produce sufficient cortisol, the hypothalamic thermostat for corticotrophin release is 'turned up', with excessive production of steroidal intermediaries—17-hydroxyprogesterone, androstenedione, dehydro*epi*androsterone and 11-hydroxy-21-deoxycortisol. The excess androgen will produce variable masculinization of the external genitals of an affected female foetus (the male equivalent, *macrogenitosoma praecox*, is not an intersex and

shaft and variable degrees of labioscrotal fusion. In extreme cases the vulva on simple inspection will appear to be quite normal except for clitoral enlargement (Fig. 4.5). However, unlike the virilizing male intersex there is no uterus, vagina or fallopian tubes. Buccal smears are chromatin negative, karyotype 46/XY and the gonads testes, with no significant features to distinguish them from other intra-abdominal or inguinal testes (Fig. 4.6). If left untreated a male-type puberty is inevitable.

FAMILIAL MALE INTERSEX

The familial types of male intersex (apart from the testicular feminization) associated with the eponyms of Lubs, Gilbert-Dreyfus and Reifenstein are excessively rare and have been reviewed by Federman (1967).

Female intersexuality

CONGENITAL ADRENAL HYPERPLASIA
(ADRENOGENITAL SYNDROME)

The pathogenesis of this condition has become fully documented since the original observations

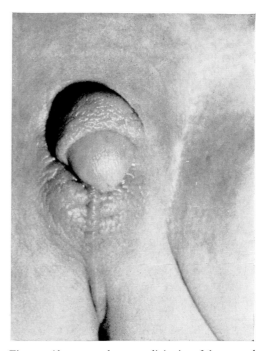

Fig. 4.7. Almost complete masculinization of the external genitals in a female with congenital adrenal hyperplasia. The tip of the completely penile urethra is visible.

will not be discussed here) and metabolities of these intermediaries will be reflected by an increased urinary secretion of 17-oxosteroids, pregnanetriol and pregnanetriolone.

The syndrome may present in the newborn with clitoral hypertrophy, variable labioscrotal fusion and urogenital sinus, or in extreme cases virtually complete masculinization of the external genitals with apparent cryptorchidism (Fig. 4.7). Internal genital, gonadal and chromosomal sex are never affected, representing once more a beautiful clinical confirmation of Jost's postulates. In children less severely affected in an anatomical sense, the diagnosis may become apparent by salt loss soon after birth, or present with the development of precocious heterosexual puberty. In the least severe form, the condition may not declare itself until puberty, and is described in the sections dealing with hirsutism and virilism (Chapter 7) and primary amenorrhoea (Chapter 5).

NON-PROGRESSIVE FEMALE INTERSEX

It may come as something of a relief to find a syndrome whose title—with a little thought—is self-explanatory. These individuals are female at chromosomal, gonadal and internal genital level. At birth the external genital sex is equivocal, resembling the sex in common forms of congenital adrenal hyperplasia, and there is no further progression of the virilism. As might be expected, this condition is related to exposure of an otherwise normal female foetus to an abnormal androgenic stimulus *in utero*. Overzier (1963) gives an excellent review of the subject.

The stimulus for this type of intersex may be endogenous or exogenous. The classic example of the former is the case described by Brentnall (1945) of a woman who developed virilism during pregnancy from what ultimately proved to be an arrhenoblastoma. The female infant had labioscrotal fusion, clitoral hypertrophy and a urogenital sinus.

The exogenous stimulus may be testosterone given to the mother or certain synthetic progestins given early in pregnancy in the treatment of habitual or threatened abortion (Grumbach *et al.* 1959). Much less frequently the condition

may arise spontaneously or in women given stilboestrol during pregnancy (Wilkins 1960).

As in the external genital virilism of congenital adrenal hyperplasia, internal genital sex is never affected.

DIFFERENTIAL DIAGNOSIS AND TREATMENT

Any obstetrician, at any time, may be confronted with a newborn baby whose sex cannot be assigned with certainty on simple inspection. The management of the problem begins at this point, when the mother asks, 'Is it a boy or a girl?'

It is clinically indefensible to say, 'I *think* it's a boy—or a girl'. Both immediately and in long-term management, it is far better to indicate that ambiguity exists that will be rapidly resolved by further study. The problems inherent in this unfortunate clinical situation have been nicely discussed by Money (1965, 1968b).

It is of paramount importance to make a proper assignment of the sex of rearing as rapidly as is possible. The assistance of a paediatrician experienced in these problems is invaluable—in fact, mandatory.

'There are two good sex assignment rules to follow. The first is: do not assign a newborn hermaphrodite to the sex for which it cannot by surgery be made coitally adequate. This rule applies regardless of genetic or gonadal sex and also of hormonal sex, which can be controlled pharmacologically. The rule applies chiefly to male hermaphrodites with a clitoropenis which cannot be properly masculinized but in whom an artificial vagina can be successfully constructed.

The second rule is: do not impose a sex reassignment on older hermaphrodite children and adults if psychologically it would be equivalent to an announcement that you yourself should be reassigned'. (Money 1968b).

Briefly, the requisite investigation will be buccal smears, chromosome studies, urinary steroids, radiography and, occasionally, explanatory laparotomy. It should be remembered that in the first 48 hr of life urinary steroids may be normal even in severe adrenal hyperplasia,

THE INTERSEXES

DIAGNOSIS	EXTERNAL GENITAL SEX	INTERNAL GENITAL SEX	GONADAL SEX	SEX CHROMATIN	SEX CHROMOSOMES	URINARY STEROIDS AT BIRTH	SEX OF REARING	TREATMENT HORMONAL	SURGICAL
CHROMOSOMAL LEVEL									
Turner's Syndrome	♀	♀	Nil or ♀	−ve or 5–15% +ve mosaic	XO XO/XX etc.	Not relevant.	♀	Oestrogens at age of normal puberty.	Nil.
Triplo X Female	♀	♀	♀	2 Barr bodies	XXX	Not relevant.	♀	Nil.	Nil.
Klinefelter's Syndrome	♂	♂	♂	+ve or 2 or more Barr bodies	XXY XXXY etc.	Not relevant.	♂	May need testosterone.	Nil.
XYY Male	♂	♂	♂	−ve	XYY	Not relevant.	♂	Nil.	Nil.
Mixed Gonadal Dysgenesis	Equivocal	♀	Nil or ♂	−ve or mosaic	XY, XO/XXXY XX/XY etc.	17 OS normal pregnanetriol normal pregnanetriolone not found.	♀	Oestrogens at age of normal puberty.	Clitoridectomy and vulval correction. Removal of gonad or gonadal 'streak'.
GONADAL LEVEL									
True Hermaphrodite	Equivocal leaning to ♂	♀ and ♂ variable	♀ and ♂ invariable	Usually +ve Sometimes −ve	XX,XO/XY XY etc.	17OS normal pregnanetriol normal pregnanetriolone not found.	Usually ♂ Sometimes ♀	Dependent on sex of rearing.	Exploratory laparotomy; excision of inappropriate organs.
True Gonadal Agenesis	♀	♀	Nil	−ve or +ve	XX or XY	Not relevant.	♀	Oestrogens at age of normal puberty.	Excision of gonadal 'streaks' in XY patients.
Virilising Male Intersex	Equivocal	♀	♂	−ve	XY	As for mixed gonadal dysgenesis	♀	Oestrogens at age of normal puberty	Clitoridectomy and vulval correction. Bilateral orchidectomy.
END ORGAN RESISTANCE									
Testicular Feminism	♀	Nil to ♂	♂	−ve	XY	Not relevant.	♀	Nil except ?testosterone after orchidectomy	?Orchidectomy as prophylaxis against seminoma.
Cryptorchid Hypospadiac Male Intersex	Equivocal	Nil to ♂	♂	−ve	XY	As for mixed gonadal dysgenesis	Usually ♀	Oestrogens at age of normal puberty.	Clitoridectomy and vulval correction and orchidectomy in infancy. Artificial vagina 17–20.
FEMALE INTERSEX									
Congenital Adrenal Hyperplasia	♀ to equivocal to ♂	♀	♀	+ve	XX	17OS ++ Pregnanetriol ++ Pregnanetriolone ++	♀	Corticosteroids from time of diagnosis.	Clitoridectomy and vulval correction in infancy.
Non-progressive Female Intersex	Equivocal	♀	♀	+ve	XX	As for mixed gonadal dysgenesis	♀	Nil.	Clitoridectomy and vulval correction in infancy.

Table 4.1. Clinical and cytogenetic findings in intersexuality.

and that evidence of salt loss may make treatment mandatory before hormonal confirmation of the diagnosis is reached. Reports on buccal smears may not be reliable in the first week of life. Instillation of gastrografin into the urosinus will be invaluable in determining the internal genital sex. Corrective surgery of the external genitals—particularly clitoridectomy—should be undertaken before the child is old enough to notice her difference from other girls—usually between the age of 2 and 3 years. Exploratory laparotomy will usually only be indicated in male intersexes or where true hermaphroditism is suspected. A good working rule is that a male intersex showing virilism at birth will virilize at puberty. If the assigned sex is female, the testes should be excised long before puberty. It is invaluable at laparotomies of this type to have available facilities for frozen section of biopsied gonads.

The construction of an artificial vagina where indicated, and the use of exogenous gonadal steroids to induce feminization, is discussed in Chapters 1 and 5.

A summary of the complex problem of intersexuality is shown in Table 4.1.

It requires tact, experience and more than a little dissimulation to deal adequately with the parents. Very few parents are able to understand the problems of inappropriate chromosomes or gonads without some permanent doubt about the gender role of their child. Although, perhaps, intellectually dishonest, it is better to come down firmly on the side of sex of rearing with appropriate explanation and diagrams regarding operative and hormonal treatment. It is the height of folly to tell parents that a child to be reared as a little girl has testicular tissue; the problem can usually be resolved by explanations involving potentially abnormal hormone production and the need for corrective surgery.

REFERENCES

BARR M.L. (1963) In *Intersexuality* (edited by C. Overzier), London and New York, Academic Press, p. 48.

BRENTNALL C.P. (1945) *J. Obstet. Gynaec. Br. Commonw.* **52**, 235.

DEWHURST C.J. (1963) *Gynaecological Disorders of Infants and Children.* London, Cassell.

DEWHURST C.J. & GORDON R.R. (1969) *The Intersexual Disorders.* London, Baillière, Tindall & Cassell.

FEDERMAN D.D. (1967) *Abnormal Sexual Development.* Philadelphia, Saunders.

FORD C.E. (1963) In *Intersexuality* (edited by C. Overzier). London and New York, Academic Press, p. 86.

GREENBLATT R.B. (1958) *Recent Prog. Horm. Res.* **14**, 335.

GRUMBACH M.M., DU CHARME J.R. & MOLOSHOK R.E. (1959) *J. clin. Endocr. Metab.* **19**, 1369.

JACOBS P.A., BAIKIE A.G., COURT BROWN W.M., MACGREGOR T.N., MACLEAN N. & HARNDEN D.G. (1959) *Lancet*, ii, 423.

JEFFCOATE S.L., BROOKS R.V. & PRUNTY F.T.G. (1968) *Br. med. J.* i, 208.

JONES H.W. & SCOTT W.W. (editors) (1958) *Hermaphroditism, Genital Anomalies and Related Disorders.* Baltimore, Williams and Wilkins.

JONES H.W. & WILKINS L. (1961) *Amr. J. Obstet. Gynec.* **82**, 1142.

JOST A. (1958) In *Hermaphroditism, Genital Anomalies and Related Endocrine Disorders* (edited by H. W. Jones & W.W. Scott). Baltimore, Williams and Wilkins.

KLINEFELTER H.F., REIFENSTEIN E.C. & ALBRIGHT F.J. (1942) *Clin. Endocr.* **2**, 615.

LYON M.F. (1962) *Am. J. hum. Genet.* **14**, 135.

MARTINI L., FRASCHINI F. & MOTTA M. (1968) *Recent Prog. Horm. Res.* **24**, 439.

MONEY J. (1965) *Pediatrics, Springfield, Illinois*, **36**, 51.

MONEY J. (1968a) *Sex Errors of the Body.* Baltimore, Johns Hopkins Press.

MONEY J. (1968b) In *Gynecologic Endocrinology* (edited by J.J. Gold). New York, Hoeber, p. 449.

MORRIS J. McL. (1953) *Am. J. Obstet. Gynec.* **65**, 1192.

OVERZIER C. (1963) *Intersexuality.* London, Academic Press.

PAINTER T.S. (1923) *J. exp. Zool.* **37**, 291.

PAULSEN C.A., GORDON D.L. & CARPENTER R.W. (1968) *Recent Prog. Horm. Res.* **24**, 321.

PFEIFFER C.A. (1936) *Am. J. Anat.* **58**, 195.

SHEARMAN R.P. (1968) *J. Obstet. Gynaec. Br. Commonw.* **75**, 1013.

SHEARMAN R.P., SINGH S., LEE C.W.G., HUDSON B. & ILBERY P.L.T. (1964) *J. Obstet. Gynaec. Br. Commonw.* **71**, 627.

SMITH W.N.A. & PENG M.T. (1967) *J. Embryol. exp. Morph.* **17**, 171.

SOHVAL A.R. (1964) *Am. J. Med.* **36**, 281.

STITCH S.R. & OAKLEY R.E. (1967) *J. Endocr.* **38**, xviii.

TETER J. & BOCZKOWSKI K. (1967) *Cancer, N.Y.* **20**, 1301.

TURNER H.H. (1938) *Endocrinology*, **23**, 566.

WILKINS L. (1960) *Acta endocr., Copenh.* **35** (supplement 51), 671.

WILKINS L. (1965) *Diagnosis and Treatment of Endocrine Disorders in Childhood and Adolescence*, 3rd edition. Springfield, Thomas.

CHAPTER 5

PRIMARY AMENORRHOEA

The differential diagnosis of primary amenorrhoea has long been an interesting intellectual exercise, an exercise that has become more fascinating with the unfolding knowledge of genetic and hormonal influences on phenotypic development. With proper management it should be possible for all of these patients to lead a normal life, although many will be infertile.

The normal menarche requires a nice integration of hypothalamus, pituitary, ovary and uterus, and a patent effluent canal for menstrual bleeding. Abberations in any of these may result in failure of sexual maturation or absence of menarche. It is now apparent that many, if not the majority, of abnormalities responsible for primary amenorrhoea are determined *in utero*, some of them prior to conception. It is very rarely indeed that a precise reason cannot be found for primary amenorrhoea, although the cause of the condition is, in some cases, obscure at present. This subject has been dealt with briefly elsewhere (Shearman 1968).

There is considerable overlap between the problems of intersexuality and primary amenorrhoea. To save repetition it is assumed that the various factors—genetic, gonadal and hormonal—involved in intra-uterine sexual differentiation will have been read in Chapter 4.

THE CLINICAL PROBLEM

There is difference of opinion about the age at which primary amenorrhoea should be investigated. Eighteen years is an age often advanced, and this may be reasonable in the patient who has developed normal secondary sexual characteristics and in whom cryptomenorrhoea has been excluded. But those with primary amenorrhoea and sexual infantilism should be investigated at the age of 15 or 16, or even earlier if there are stigmata suggestive of Turner's syndrome or virilism.

A working classification of the causes of primary amenorrhoea is shown in Table 5.1.

CLASSIFICATION OF PRIMARY AMENORRHOEA

A. CHROMOSOMAL
    Turner's syndrome.
    Mixed gonadal dysgenesis.

B. GONADAL
    True Hermaphrodite.
    True gonadal agenesis.
    Virilising male intersex.

C. END ORGAN RESISTANCE
    Testicular feminization.
    Cryptorchid Hypospadiac male intersex.

D. HYPOTHALMUS-PITUITARY
    Pan hypopituitarism.
    Asexual ateliotic dwarfism.
    Lawrence-Moon-Beidl syndrome.
    Olfacto genital syndrome.
    Hypogonadotrophic eunuchoidism.
    Pre-pubertal polycystic ovaries.

E. ADRENAL HYPERPLASIA

F. GYNAETRESIA
    Congenital absence of uterus and vagina.
    Cryptomenorrhoea.

G. DELAYED MENARCHE

Table 5.1. Classification: primary amenorrhoea.

In the majority of individuals with primary amenorrhoea, it is possible to arrive at a fairly firm provisional diagnosis from the history and the results of physical examination. It is only in a minority that there is a need to go beyond fairly simple outpatient investigations.

The most important initial distinction is whether the patient is sexually infantile or whether there is evidence of secondary sexual characteristics. The importance of this distinction should be clear. A girl of 15 or 16 who has no secondary sexual characteristics obviously has not been exposed to any form of stimulation from gonadal hormones. Individuals with sexual infantilism can be further divided into those in whom there is idiopathic delay of sexual development and those in whom there is pathological sexual infantilism, the cause of which may lie in the hypothalamic pituitary area or in the gonad.

Idiopathic delay and precocious puberty are two ends of a fairly wide frequency distribution curve. Girls with idiopathic delay may not commence sexual maturation until the age of 15 or 16. Differentiation of this condition from pathological sexual infantilism may require observation for a year or more. Closely related is the obese young girl with delayed menstruation and puberty, frequently mislabelled Fröhlich's syndrome. Most young girls who show this triad have no detectable pathological lesion, and spontaneous remission will occur in the majority.

The majority of patients with sexual infantilism due to congenital hypothalamic pituitary disturbances, such as Lorain-Lévi syndrome or Laurence-Moon-Biedl syndrome, will have been recognized clinically before the age of puberty, and its absence is only another incident in a long history. Lorain-type dwarfism is usually manifest by the third or fourth year with growth retardation and unfolds with evidence of persistently juvenile features, hypogonadism, hypothyroidism and sometimes hypo-adrenocorticism. Although there is no doubt about the homogeneity of the Laurence-Moon-Biedl syndrome, the classical features of retinitis pigmentosa, polydactylism or syndactylism and mental retardation will be evident in infancy.

Most girls with sexual infantilism who are seen by the gynaecologist appear to be quite well in every way except for the infantilism. The patient's height is important. If she is less than 4 ft 10 in (147 cm) tall it is very likely that one or other of the chromosomal abnormalities leading to gonadal dysgenesis will be present. Much less frequently, the diagnosis will be panhypopituitarism.

Less frequently still, a diagnosis of ateliotic dwarfism may be reached. This may be asexual (with permanent sexual infantilism) or sexual (with spontaneous puberty). The latter group undergo spontaneous puberty at a relatively late age, so that asexual forms of ateliosis cannot be distinguished with certainty until the age of about 25, although there is usually a strong family history. Unlike sexual ateliosis, the asexual form is usually non-familial, except for the well-documented Hutterites (Rimion et al. 1968).

If, in addition to being short the patient has a web neck, increased carrying angle or perhaps even a congenital cardiac lesion, then it requires only modest clinical skill to suspect a diagnosis of Turner's syndrome (Fig. 5.1). This may usually be confirmed by finding chromatin-negative buccal smears. The majority of these short, chromatin-negative individuals prove on further investigation to be cases of true Turner's syndrome with a karyotype of 45/XO. Somewhat less frequently, mosaics such as XO/XX will be found. Under these circumstances between 5 and 15% of cells may be chromatin positive. Rarely, buccal smears may be normal. Although most mosaics are sexually infantile with a female phenotype, some may have menstruated, while others (XO/XY) may show variable degrees of virilism. This last group is probably better classified under the heading of mixed gonadal dysgenesis. As a rule, knowledge of the exact karyotype is interesting, but is not essential for proper clinical management. Laparotomy or laparoscopy should only be considered when there is disparity between clinical findings, especially phenotype, and laboratory investigations.

For the taller patient with sexual infantilism the diagnosis usually lies between true gonadal

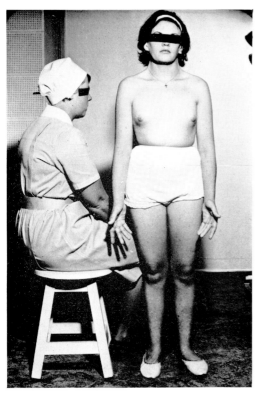

Fig. 5.1. Turner's syndrome—height 4 ft 10 in. Note webbed neck and widely spaced nipples. Oestrogens have caused breast growth.

agenesis and hypogonadotrophic eunuchoidism. Examination of the buccal smear may be helpful. Very rarely in this group the smear will be chromatin negative with a 46/XY karyotype (Ford 1963; Philip *et al.* 1965). If a chromatin-positive buccal smear is present, as a rule the karyotype is 46/XX. Clinically there is no way of distinguishing this picture due to hypo-gonadotrophic eunuchoidism from the less frequent instance of true gonadal agenesis. Demonstration of primordial follicles will establish the former diagnosis and absence the latter. The same information can, however, be obtained without recourse to surgery, by serial assay of gonadotrophins or by studying the effect of exogenous gonadotrophins on urinary oestrogen excretion (Shearman 1964; Shearman & Cox 1965; Swyer *et al.* 1968). The patient with hypogonadotrophic eunuchoidism will have undetectable levels of urinary gonadotrophins and show a satisfactory increase of urinary oestrogens after gonadotrophin stimulation. The reverse is true of the patient with true gonadal agenesis.

This group of patients should always have the sense of smell tested, as some may belong to the currently obscure 'olfacto genital' syndrome (Belaisch *et al.* 1965; Teter 1967; Mroueh & Kase 1968). This potentially fascinating syndrome requires further documentation, and at the moment is only distinguishable from hypo-gonadotrophic eunuchoidism by the anosmia.

Three cases of our own have shown sexual infantilism, normal or above normal height and absent or scanty sexual hair. The response to clomiphene is interesting. In normal individuals there is an immediate increase in serum LH. The results from one of our patients are shown in Fig. 5.2. It will be noted that clomiphene had no significant impact on serum LH but that exogenous gonadotrophins cause a satisfactory increase in urinary oestrogen excretion, indicating the presence of primordial follicles.

Delay in menstruation in a patient who has reached puberty is a different problem. An initial and simple distinction is to note whether the changes of puberty have been feminizing or masculinizing. If the patient has some female secondary sexual characteristics then obviously she has been exposed to some endogenous sex steroid stimulation. This statement is only valid if one can be certain that this sexual maturation has not been induced by the prolonged administration of exogenous steroids in an unwise attempt to induce vaginal bleeding before a proper diagnosis has been made. Far too frequently a patient in her late teens or early twenties will present with 'secondary amenorrhoea'. On careful questioning it is found that all of the patient's periods have been induced by hormone therapy given intermittently over many years, and that neither the patient, nor her mother, can recall whether the secondary sexual characteristics preceded or followed this treatment.

In a patient with normal female habitus, some local abnormality within the genital tract

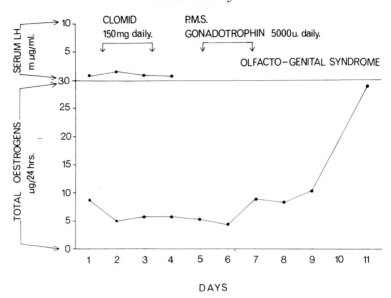

Fig. 5.2 Response of serum LH to clomiphene and of urinary oestrogens to clomiphene and gonadotrophins in the olfactogenital syndrome.

should be excluded forthwith. There may be an imperforate hymen or undeveloped vagina with cryptomenorrhoea. The uterus and vagina may be congenitally absent, in which case ovarian function is usually normal (Brown *et al.* 1959). If it is found that the patient has a blind vagina without any evidence of a uterus, even though she may otherwise be quite feminine, the most likely diagnosis is the syndrome of testicular feminization. The testes may be palpable in the inguinal region, while axillary and pubic hair is usually scanty. Buccal smears are chromatin negative and the karyotype 46/XY. Since the condition is familial, 'sisters' with the same problem may present.

If the patient has no local genital abnormality, and if some female secondary sexual characteristics have developed spontaneously, it is possible to await, with some degree of confidence, the onset of spontaneous menstruation. This may be delayed until the age of 19 or 20.

Primary amenorrhoea may occur in an apparent female who shows virilizing changes at puberty. This may be due to mild congenital adrenal hyperplasia that has not been detected

previously, or the postpuberal form of adrenal hyperplasia. The steroidal aberrations are the same as those found in congenital adrenal hyperplasia presenting in children (Brooks *et al.* 1960). Such a diagnosis may be confirmed by finding chromatin-positive buccal smears, and increased urinary excretion of 17-ketosteroids, pregnanetriol and pregnanetriolone. An adrenal tumour may be excluded by the ability of dexamethasone to suppress these levels (see Chapter 7).

If the buccal smears are chromatin negative, virilizing male intersexuality or cryptorchid hypospadiac male intersexuality should be considered. Today, these conditions should be diagnosed and treated long before the age of puberty. Figure 4.5 (p. 50) shows the genitalia of a child born with an enlarged clitoris and a 'urogenital sinus'. The initial, and statistically more likely, diagnosis of congenital adrenal hyperplasia was excluded by finding chromatin-negative buccal smears and normal urinary steroids. One testis was found in an inguinal hernia at the age of 3 years and removed. Despite the enlarged clitoris the other gonad was not explored, and when first seen at the age of 14 this girl was having a masculinizing puberty. The residual testis in the left 'ovarian' fossa was removed, followed by clitoridectomy. The patient has no uterus, fallopian tubes or vagina and represents a classic example of cryptorchid hypospadiac male intersex. Buccal smears were chromatin negative and karyotype 46/XY.

While both true hermaphroditism and virilizing ovarian tumour are excessively rare, each must nevertheless be considered as a possible diagnosis in any apparent female who presents at puberty with virilism. Figures 5.3 and 5.4 show biopsies from the gonads of a patient known to be a true hermaphrodite at the age of 4 years. The testis was left *in situ* and at the age of 13 the patient suddenly developed a masculinizing puberty, having been brought up as a female. The abdominal testis was removed and the early virilism regressed rapidly.

Sections of the testis removed after the masculinizing puberty are shown in Fig. 4.6 (p. 51).

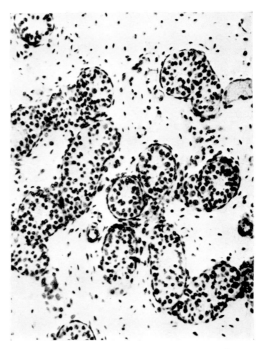

Fig. 5.4. Biopsy from testis removed from a true hermaphrodite during infancy. (From Shearman *et al.* (1964), by courtesy of the Editor of *Journal of Obstetrics and Gynaecology of the British Commonwealth.*)

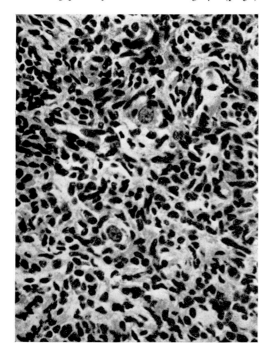

Fig. 5.3. Biopsy of ovarian tissue from true hermaphrodite. (From Shearman *et al.* (1964), by courtesy of the Editor of *Journal of Obstetrics and Gynaecology of the British Commonwealth.*)

Short of virilism, primary amenorrhoea may be the presenting symptom in some girls who, having had a female type of onset of puberty, develop severe acne and hirsutism. Mild postpuberal adrenal hyperplasia should be considered in this instance. Rarely the diagnosis will prove to be prepuberal polycystic ovaries (Teter 1967). These patients show the expected hyperresponsiveness to diagnostic gonadotrophin stimulation (see Chapter 6) and the inverted relationship of urinary 17-oxosteroids and oestrogens after dexamethasone suppression (Netter 1961; Crooke *et al.* 1963).

Treatment

The aim of treatment should be to attain the maximum physiological function of which the individual patient is capable. This may be complete fertility; it may be the prospect of fertility; often it will end with attainment of functional sexual maturation but irrevocable infertility. Only very rarely—if ever—will it be necessary to settle for anything less. No attempt should ever be made to treat those patients until a firm diagnosis is reached.

TURNER'S SYNDROME AND GONADAL AGENESIS

The only treatment for these patients is to achieve sexual maturation with exogenous steroids. An initial dose of 0·01 mg of ethinyl oestradiol twice daily for 3 weeks in every month will cause primary breast-bud development if it is given for several months, but only rarely will withdrawal bleeding occur. Then definitive treatment with a larger amount of oestrogen and an added progestin is started and continued cyclically for an indefinite time. The easiest and

cheapest way to do this is to use an oral contraceptive of the sequential type. The writer's preference of this purpose is one containing not more than 80 μg of ethinyloestradiol or mestranol. Many people use oestrogens alone, but the addition of a progestin for 6 or 10 days each month gives much better cycle control and appears to cause better breast development. Laparotomy should only be considered when there is discrepancy between the clinical findings and the laboratory data. If virilism is present, as it may be in XO/XY mosaics, the area of the gonadal streaks should be excised to prevent the risk of development of a malignant tumour (Teter & Boczkowski 1967).

Although virilism is usual, a similar problem may arise in the non-virilized chromosomal intersex. Figure 5.5 shows a dysgerminoma removed from a non-virilized but sexually in-

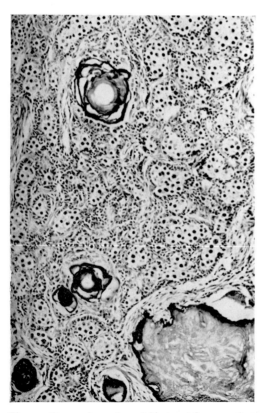

Fig. 5.5. Dysgerminoma (gonadoblastoma) from a patient with a mixed gonadal dysgenesis.

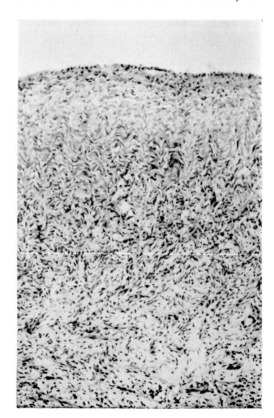

Fig. 5.6. Section from streak gonad on the contralateral side to that shown in Fig. 5.5.

fantile patient of normal height whose chromosomes showed XO/XY mosaicism. The gonadal streak from the contralateral side is shown in Fig. 5.6. Because of the frequency of this complication (see Chapter 4) it is the writer's preference to perform laparotomy on all XY or XO/XY mosaics and perform bilateral adnexectomy.

GONADAL CAUSES WITH OR WITHOUT VIRILISM

Definitive treatment aims to achieve transformation to a potentially sexually competent adult; this means the surgical removal of sources of inappropriate hormonal stimulus (usually testicular tissue) and reconstruction of the external genitals along female lines. This should be done before the age of 4 years.

The testes should be removed from patients with the testicular feminizing syndrome because of the risk of development of a malignant gonadal tumour. The degree of risk is not known with certainty, but Jones (1958) states that the incidence of malignant degeneration is 'not above 5%'. Most evidence suggests that these testes do not produce oestrogens; there are recent data that the failure of target organ response is related to a deficiency of enzymes in the peripheral metabolism and utilization of testosterone. If the testes are removed before puberty, breast development will not occur, but surgery should be considered after sexual maturation.

DISORDERS OF HYPOTHALAMUS AND PITUITARY GLAND

Pituitary dwarfs with an isolated deficiency in human growth hormone (HGH) will undergo spontaneous puberty. Those who have panhypopituitarism from a craniopharyngioma or other causes should be treated initially with HGH, made sexually mature with gonadal steroids, and then treated with human pituitary or human menopausal gonadotrophin to induce ovulation when pregnancy is desired. The ateliotic asexual dwarf will require the same treatment.

With the exception of the need for HGH, the same treatment is used for those with hypogonadotrophic eunuchoidism with or without anosmia. In the writer's experience, clomiphene is not useful in these cases (Shearman 1968, and Fig. 5.2).

ADRENAL HYPERPLASIA

If this condition presents at the time of puberty it is treated specifically with corticosteroids. In the rare event that ovulation does not follow, clomiphene is the additional treatment of choice. Unlike those cases diagnosed in infancy, the external genitals of the patients discussed here are usually normal.

GYNAETRESIA

Cryptomenorrhoea obviously requires treatment as soon as the diagnosis is made. This presents no difficulty in patients with a simple imperforate 'hymen', but when there is total absence of the vagina with haematometra above it, there may be great difficulty in retaining reproductive potential.

Complete gynaetresia is rarely diagnosed until several years after puberty, which is normal in these patients. The definitive treatment is to construct an artificial vagina at a suitable age.

DELAYED MENARCHE

Clearly, this diagnosis may only be made in retrospect. The onset of puberty in these patients is usually late, but providing that some secondary female characteristics have developed spontaneously and progressively, and providing that all other causes have been excluded, no treatment should be offered. Spontaneous resolution will occur, but sometimes not until the age of 20.

Conclusions

Abnormalities in the normal progression of factors responsible for sexual differentiation *in utero* are the commonest causes of primary amenorrhoea; the factors responsible for normal differentiation should be understood for a rational approach to the clinical problem of primary amenorrhoea, and are discussed fully in Chapter 4.

With suitable investigation a precise diagnosis can usually be reached, and it is possible to treat these patients on rational and physiological principles. All should be able to lead normal, sexually mature lives, but the prospect of fertility may be possible for a minority only.

REFERENCES

BELAISCH J., MUSSET R. & NETTER A. (1965) *Annls Endocr.* **26**, 267.

BROOKS R.V., MATTINGLY D., MILLS I.H. & PRUNTY F.T.G. (1960) *Br. med. J.* **i**, 1294.

BROWN J.B., KELLAR R. & MATTHEW G.D. (1959) *J. Obstet. Gynaec. Br. Commonw.* **66**, 177.

CROOKE A.C., BUTT W.R., PALMER R., MORRIS R., EDWARDS R.L., TAYLOR C.W. & SHORT R.V. (1963) *Br. med. J.* **i**, 1119.

FORD C.E. (1963) In *Intersexuality* (edited by C. Overzier). London and New York, Academic Press, p. 86.

JONES H.W. (1958) In *Hermaphroditism, Genital Anomalies and Related Disorders* (edited by H.W. Jones & W.W. Scott). Baltimore, Williams and Wilkins, p. 172.

MROUEH A. & KASE N. (1968) *Am. J. Obstet. Gynec.* **100**, 525.

NETTER A. (1961) *Proc. R. Soc. Med.* **54**, 1006.

PHILIP J., SELE V., TROLLE D. & MOLLER B. (1965) *Fert. Steril.* **17**, 795.

RIMION D.C., MERIMEE T.J., RABINOWITZ D. & McKUSICK V.A. (1968) *Recent Prog. Horm. Res.* **24**, 365.

SHEARMAN R.P. (1964) *Br. med. J.* **ii**, 1115.

SHEARMAN R.P. (1968) *J. Obstet. Gynaec. Br. Commonw.* **75**, 1101.

SHEARMAN R.P. (1969) *Induction of Ovulation.* Springfield, Thomas.

SHEARMAN R.P. & COX R.I. (1965) *Am. J. Obstet. Gynec.* **92**, 747.

SHEARMAN R.P., SINGH S., LEE C.W.G., HUDSON B. & ILBERY P.L.T. (1964) *J. Obstet. Gynaec. Br. Commonw.* **71**, 627.

SWYER G.I.M., LITTLE V., LAWRENCE D. & COLLINS J. (1968) *Br. med. J.* **i**, 349.

TETER J. (1967) In *Proceedings of Vth World Congress of Gynaecology and Obstetrics* (edited by E.C. Wood). Sydney, Butterworth, p. 272.

TETER J. & BOCZKOWSKI K. (1967) *Cancer, N.Y.* **20**, 1301.

CHAPTER 6

SECONDARY AMENORRHOEA

Definitions of secondary amenorrhoea vary; while some things are capable of objective, precise definition, categorization here, like so much else in medicine, must be arbitrary. It is defined here as the secondary absence of menstruation for more than 12 months, excluding physiological causes such as pregnancy, lactation and normal menopause. Premature menopause is equally difficult to define. The average age of the menopause in Australia is 51. A premature menopause is defined here as secondary ovarian failure before the age of 35.

Custom usually dictates that any writing on secondary amenorrhoea should be accompanied by a list of causes. Since secondary amenorrhoea is a symptom and not a specific disease, it would be possible, given a sufficiently obsessive mind, to fill several pages with such a list. As this approach has never seemed to produce a real understanding of this complex problem the traditional practice will not be followed.

It should be stressed again that secondary amenorrhoea is a symptom, and that it may be due to a multitude of causes. The gynaecologist working in this area must have a high index of clinical suspicion for systemic disease. If he does not, these fascinating diagnostic and therapeutic problems will be annexed by the physician, as has already occurred in many centres. The gynaecologist will be left holding the baby—literally—as his only contribution. This subject has been fully reviewed elsewhere (Shearman 1969b).

In its simplest terms, normal menstrual function requires a uterus that will respond to appropriate hormonal stimulus, an ovary that combines the dual functions of ovulation and normal steroidogenesis, and an hypothalamo-pituitary axis that will give the gonad the stimulus to do both of these things.

Secondary amenorrhoea may result from faults in any of these. The uterus, which may be considered the end organ, may be unresponsive to ovaries that are functioning normally. This may be due to *amenorrhoea traumatica*, while in some countries endometrial tuberculosis is a common cause of secondary amenorrhoea. The ovary may be unresponsive because of a premature menopause. Alternatively, its hormonal function may be excessive and abnormal, as with functioning ovarian tumours, cystic glandular hyperplasia or the Stein-Leventhal syndrome. Finally, and most frequently, the fault may lie in the pituitary and/or hypothalamus.

For reasons that remain obscure, an isolated deficiency in gonadotrophin secretion as a secondary phenomenon occurs far more commonly than deficiency of other pituitary trophic hormones. This may frequently be emotionally determined, and the spontaneous cure rate in short-term amenorrhoea of this type is high. There may be reflex inhibition of the hypothalamic gonadotrophin release centres by drugs such as reserpine, phenothiazines or oral contraceptives, or by general diseases such as depressive states, *anorexia nervosa*, diabetes, thyrotoxicosis or any severe debilitating illness. There may be specific inhibition of gonadotrophin secretion by abnormal ectopic steroid synthesis, as is seen in virilizing adrenal hyperplasia, Cushing's syndrome or adrenal tumour. Finally, there may be a destructive lesion in the area such as tumour or Sheehan's syndrome—pituitary infarction following severe postpartum haemorrhage (Sheehan 1937).

In each patient a comprehensive history is mandatory. Any factors operative at the time of onset must be elicited specifically. If the amenorrhoea follows pregnancy the patient should be asked whether curettage was undertaken for secondary postpartum haemorrhage or abortion. If there is such a history, then *amenorrhoea traumatica* (Asherman 1950; Foix *et al.* 1966) is a far more likely diagnosis than pituitary failure. Here the problem is obliteration of the endometrial cavity by intra-uterine adhesions, pituitary and ovarian function being quite normal.

If following delivery there was a large postpartum haemorrhage and failure of lactation, Sheehan's syndrome should be considered, remembering that some pituitary trophic function may be left intact, gonadotrophins usually being the first affected.

Weight change at or near the time of onset of secondary amenorrhoea is common and important. Obesity may be related. Far more frequently the patient gives a history of weight loss. The commonest history given is that of a mildly overweight teenager who goes on a 'crash diet'. The onset of amenorrhoea is abrupt, preceding significant weight loss and persisting even when the lost weight is regained. It is doubtful if this condition should be regarded as a mild form of *anorexia nervosa*. Typically, the patient with the latter condition will insist that her food intake is adequate, while the group of girls discussed here have no such reticence in describing in detail the rigorous diet they have followed.

Secondary amenorrhoea will often occur abruptly with a major environmental change. Short-term secondary amenorrhoea is common in nurses commencing training and women entering the armed services. Short- and long-term amenorrhoea is seen frequently in migrants.

A syndrome which appears to be more common recently is the development of amenorrhoea after treatment with oral contraceptives (Shearman 1966c; Shearman 1968).

Every patient with secondary amenorrhoea should be asked whether hot flushes are present or not. If so, this may produce the only clinical evidence of premature menopause, as they are never present in 'idiopathic' amenorrhoea.

The patient should be asked specifically about galactorrhoea. If this has developed after childbirth but persists after breast-feeding ceases and is associated with amenorrhoea, a diagnosis of Chiari-Frommel syndrome will be reached. If the galactorrhoea and amenorrhoea have developed with no temporal relationship to pregnancy, the syndrome described by Forbes *et al.* (1954) and Argonz & del Castillo (1953) should be considered. In either case an otherwise asymptomatic pituitary tumour may be present (Shearman & Turtle 1969).

Any change in hair-growth patterns should be elicited. Progressive hirsutes associated with amenorrhoea would suggest adrenal hyperplasia or tumour, virilizing ovarian tumour, polycystic ovaries or, rarely, acromegaly.

As stated earlier, not all patients who menstruate ovulate. Very rarely a patient with a relatively regular menstrual cycle will prove to be persistently anovulatory. More frequently, there is associated gross menstrual irregularity. Variable amenorrhoea interspersed with heavy vaginal bleeding would suggest, but by no means prove, a diagnosis of endometrial hyperplasia. Progressively scanty and irregular periods, particularly if associated with hirsutism, should suggest the possibility of polycystic ovaries. When the patient does have some menstrual bleeding, the incidence and degree of premenstrual symptoms will give a rough clinical clue to the frequency of ovulatory cycles. Most ovulatory cycles are preceded by some subjective disturbances—breast soreness, abdominal bloating, mild depression or tension, lower abdominal discomfort—while anovulatory periods often appear without warning. These subjective symptoms, however, should be interpreted with caution and a degree of scepticism.

Physical examination should be meticulous. Signs of thyroid dysfunction should be sought and the distribution of scalp and body hair noted carefully. The association of amenorrhoea, hypertension and hirsutes should suggest the possibility of *Cushing's syndrome*, while pigmentation will indicate the need to exclude Addison's disease. Virilism—that is, deepening of the voice, male-type baldness, clitoral enlargement and breast atrophy—if present in addition to hirsutes and amenorrhoea would suggest a virilizing tumour or adrenal hyperplasia. Impressive hirsutes and some clitoral enlargement may, however, be present in patients with polycystic ovaries (Chapter 7).

Whether or not the patient has given a history of galactorrhoea, attempts should be made to demonstrate its presence or absence during physical examination. Adequate vaginal examination is essential. In many unmarried women it is better to perform this under anaesthesia.

Further investigations

It is sometimes difficult to decide just how far investigation should be carried in any particular patient. If there is even the slightest suspicion of organic disease in a patient with secondary amenorrhoea the fullest investigation necessary to reach a diagnosis is mandatory. If from the history and physical examination there is no suggestion of organic disease, clinical enthusiasm should be tempered by judgement.

In general terms, secondary amenorrhoea of less than 12 months' duration in a patient who is otherwise well and who has no abnormal physical findings is not an indication for immediate investigation. The spontaneous cure rate with amenorrhoea of short duration is high. In this group the only justification for earlier investigation may be the pressing one of infertility.

When secondary amenorrhoea has been present for more than a year further investigation is necessary, but the type of investigations carried out will depend on the clinical problem. If the patient is not concerned by current or potential infertility, investigations should be limited to those necessary to exclude clinically undetectable organic disease. These would include X-ray of the chest, skull and pituitary fossa, dilatation and curettage, assay of urinary 17-ketosteroids and hydroxysteroids, and thyroid-function studies. Amenorrhoea may be the only symptom in a patient with pulmonary tuber-

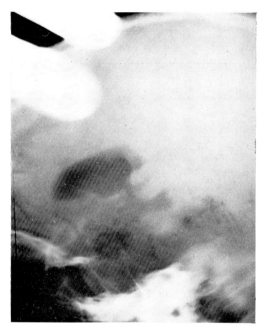

Fig. 6.1. Air studies showing a pituitary adenoma in a patient with secondary amenorrhoea. There were no other symptoms or signs. (From Shearman (1969), by courtesy of Charles C. Thomas, Publisher). The tumour is seen extending beyond the sella turcica elevating the floor of the third ventricle.

culosis or pituitary tumour (Fig. 6.1), while endometrial tuberculosis is a relatively frequent cause in some countries (Jeffcoate 1967). Not all patients with major adrenal disease are significantly hirsute.

It is uncommon for secondary amenorrhoea to be the presenting symptom in patients with thyroid dysfunction. In our own series only two women, one hyperthyroid the other hypothyroid, had amenorrhoea as their dominant symptom. Both are now euthyroid, but only the thyrotoxic patient has had restoration of normal menstrual function. Determination of the basal metabolic rate is of little assistance in assessing thyroid function in patients where the disease is not obvious clinically. Much more useful information will be obtained by measuring protein-bound iodine (PBI), tri-iodothyronine resin and ^{131}I uptakes. Of these three investigations, only the last is unaffected by the administration of gonadal steroids. If the patient is taking, or has taken in the previous 6 weeks, any oestrogenic preparation, the results of PBI and ^{131}I resin uptake may be quite misleading (Winnikoff & Taylor 1966).

If the patient is concerned by actual or potential infertility, then investigations additional to those already mentioned are necessary. The only purpose of these is to decide whether

For the married patient, the husband's seminal analysis should be normal. At the time of curettage, tubal patency should be established, and if this is in doubt after a Rubin's test, hysterosalpingography is indicated. If any endometrium is present, the histological pattern will give some idea of endogenous oestrogen production (Fig. 6.2). As already mentioned, in

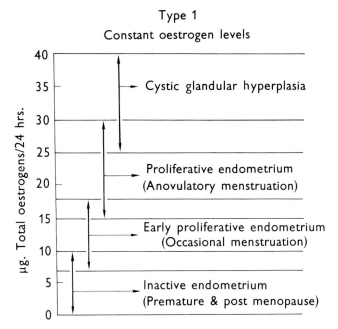

Fig. 6.2. Relationship of urinary oestrogens to endometrial pattern. (From Brown *et al.* (1959), by courtesy of the Editor of *Journal of Obstetrics and Gynaecology of the British Commonwealth.*)

or not the patient is suitable for definitive treatment; that is, induction of ovulation.

In the married patient with actual infertility the decision to make these further investigations rests with the husband and wife. Many unmarried women—and their mothers—are, however, worried by potential fertility, and it is completely reasonable to assess the possibilities of inducing ovulation so that a prognosis can be given. Under these circumstances the complete investigation of anovulation in an unmarried women is fully justifiable. Treatment, however, should not be contemplated until after marriage.

countries where genital tuberculosis is found, part of the endometrium should be cultured or inoculated into guinea-pigs for acid-fast bacilli.

Steroidal substitution therapy has a very limited place in the investigation of amenorrhoea. If *amenorrhoea traumatica* is suspected from the history, one or two courses—most conveniently and cheaply given as an oral contraceptive of the sequential type—might be given. If the uterus can be made to bleed, then the fault clearly lies elsewhere. The prolonged use of this type of treatment in amenorrhoeic women before a diagnosis is reached is to be deplored.

After these preliminary investigations have been completed, patients may be divided into several groups. Those in whom anovulation is secondary to organic disease such as thyrotoxicosis, Cushing's syndrome or virilizing adrenal hyperplasia, will have treatment directed to their primary disease.

The majority of patients will appear quite well in every way except for their anovulation, and it is in this group that final selection for treatment with one or other of the therapeutic substances discussed in Chapter 34 must be made. Most of these women will have absent or disordered gonadotrophin release as their primary problem. Some, clinically indistinguishable, may have a premature menopause.

In these apparently well women the following groups must be distinguished.

(1) Premature menopause
(2) Polycystic ovaries
(3) Cystic glandular hyperplasia
(4) 'Idiopathic' amenorrhoea with or without galactorrhoea
(5) Persistent anovulatory cycles

There is no way to detect, on clinical grounds alone, the patients with premature menopause.

This may occur even in teenagers (Baramki & Jones 1966), and attempts to treat such patients are bound to fail.

The clinical vagaries of patients with polycystic ovaries have been fully reviewed by Jeffcoate (1964) and Goldzieher (Goldzieher & Axelrod 1963; Goldzieher & Green 1962) and are discussed more fully in Chapter 7. Not all are obese or hirsute and the enlarged ovaries may escape detection on physical examination. Gynaecography may be of assistance but offers no real advantage over culdoscopy or laparoscopy. Assay of urinary pregnanetriolene and Δ^5-pregnenetriol may assist in the diagnosis (Cox & Shearman 1961; Shearman & Cox 1965; Shearman & Cox 1966; Shearman *et al.* 1961).

Cystic glandular hyperplasia is an unsatisfactory name for a well-recognized syndrome. The endometrium is not constantly hyperplastic nor are urinary oestrogens constantly grossly increased (Brown & Matthew 1962). Serial study over several months may be necessary to establish the diagnosis.

True galactorrhoea should be distinguished from the serous discharge often obtained from parous patients (Fig. 6.3). The presence of galactorrhoea in patients with 'idiopathic' amenorrhoea excludes a premature menopause,

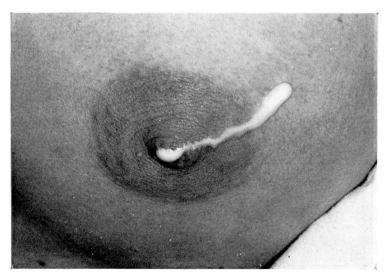

Fig. 6.3. True galactorrhoea in a nulliparous patient.

but may, on the other hand, indicate the presence of pituitary tumour.

The various syndromes of secondary amenorrhoea associated with unphysiological lactation have attracted interest for a long time. First described by Hippocrates, then by Chiari and Frommel and later by Ahumada, Argonz and del Castillo, and Forbes *et al.* these conditions have become an eponymic jungle. Whether the condition occurs *postpartum*, spontaneously, in relationship to drug therapy (phenothiazines, oral contraceptives, digoxin, reserpine) or is associated with a pituitary adenoma, the clinical presentation is identical. It seems better to use the term 'secondary amenorrhoea with inappropriate lactation'. The hormonal environment of these patients has been discussed by Shearman & Turtle (1970). Urinary oestrogens are usually in the postmenopausal range and, as expected from a dependent target organ, the uterus is small and endometrium absent or proliferative. Levels of serum LH are in the low–normal range and, acromegalics apart, growth-hormone studies are usually quantitatively and qualitatively normal. The response to clomiphene is usually good, indicating that the physiological disturbance is hypothalamic, rather than in the pituitary.

It is of the greatest importance to realize that one normal X-ray of the pituitary fossa does not exclude for all time the presence of a pituitary tumour. Follow-up X-rays and screening of visual fields should be undertaken at yearly intervals.

A valuable follow-up by Rankin *et al.* (1969) has indicated that the outlook for spontaneous cure in cases presenting *postpartum* may be better than previously believed. In nine patients followed for 10 or more years, seven resumed spontaneous periods. In the group where the syndrome was unrelated to previous pregnancy no spontaneous remissions were observed.

Patients without galactorrhoea who have a history of weight loss and/or environmental change related to the onset of amenorrhoea will probably prove to have hypothalamic amenorrhoea, as will those where amenorrhoea developed after treatment with oral contraceptives (Shearman 1966c; Shearman 1968). But in none of these people can one confidently exclude a premature menopause on history or clinical examination.

Patients with repeated anovulatory cycles have a variable oestrogen excretion and no evidence of a luteal phase rise in urinary pregnanediol, while endometrium obtained at any stage in their usually irregular cycles is proliferative in pattern.

Once a diagnosis of anovulatory bleeding has been established—whether this is associated with proliferative or hyperplastic endometrium—it is reasonable to embark on treatment without added investigations. The other groups may only be differentiated by further study. The most useful tools here are study of endogenous gonadotrophins or the response to exogenous gonadotrophins.

Considerable assistance may accrue from knowledge of endogenous gonadotrophin production, providing this is studied correctly. Radio-immunoassay of LH has not yet been employed sufficiently widely, nor is radio-immune assay of FSH sufficiently well developed, to be certain of their role in clinical investigation. It is probable, however, that in the future these assays will be of great value.

At the moment bio-assay of gonadotrophins is used most widely, and of the methods available the 'mouse uterus test' for total gonadotrophins in urine is in widespread use. This has the disadvantages of being time-consuming and relatively non-specific, since an undefined mixture of LH and FSH is assayed. However, if it is correctly employed (and as long as its lack of specificity is remembered), information of some assistance may be obtained. Single, isolated assays may be quite misleading. Loraine & Bell (1966) have shown the great daily variation that may occur in postmenopausal women. In 'idiopathic' amenorrhoea total gonadotrophins are usually low (Kistner 1966) but may be well within the normal range (Shearman 1966b). Three of our own patients who have had single estimations well above the postmenopausal range have subsequently been shown to respond to exogenous gonadotrophins, and two have conceived. The assay is not sufficiently specific to detect the increased LH levels usually present in patients with polycystic ovaries. For this reason serial assay of total gonadotrophins is necessary for really meaningful information, and this has the obvious disadvantage of time and cost. Because of these problems, it is difficult to accept such classifications as hypogonadotrophic, normogonadotrophic or hypergonadotrophic amenorrhoea that are currently in widespread clinical use.

Ideally, final assessment should be based on a knowledge of both endogenous gonadotrophin production and the ovarian response to exogenous gonadotrophins. We have developed (Shearman 1964b; Shearman 1966a; Shearman & Box 1966) a standardized gonadotrophin-stimulation test which will screen the differential response of patients with polycystic ovaries, cystic glandular hyperplasia, 'idiopathic' secondary amenorrhoea, or those with ovarian failure. These results have been confirmed by Swyer et al. (1968). Pregnant Mares Serum (PMS) gonadotrophin in a dose of 5,000 units is given intramuscularly for 3 days. Twenty-four hour urine collections continued for 8 days and either oestrone alone (Brown 1963) or total oestrogens (Brown et al. 1968) are measured daily. We have also shown that homologous preparations may be used for the same purpose (Shearman & Cox 1966). Cox et al. (1966) have used Pergonal® equivalent to 225 I.U. FSH daily for 3 days. In this department we have continued to use heterologous gonadotrophins, as HMG is expensive and HPG is, and probably will remain, in relatively short supply. In this way we have been able to keep homologous preparations for therapeutic rather than diagnostic work. PMS gonadotrophin has now been given to more than 200 women for diagnostic purposes. There have been no adverse subjective reactions. All patients subsequently proven to have polycystic ovaries had palpable ovarian enlargement which regressed. One patient developed bilateral ovarian enlargement, palpable abdominally. There was no evidence of ascites, but there was for 2 days some mild malaise. This short exposure is insufficient to create antibodies. Of these women, none who have had responsive ovaries, and have been subsequently treated, have failed to respond to clomiphene and/or HMG.

Four patterns of oestrogen excretion are seen in response to this stimulus (Shearman 1964a; Shearman 1966a; Shearman 1969a) and these results have been confirmed using HMG (Cox et al. 1966).

PATIENTS WITH NO OBSERVED INCREASE IN URINARY OESTROGENS

This pattern is seen most frequently in patients lacking ovarian follicles, whether this lack is primary (gonadal agenesis or dysgenesis) or secondary (premature menopause). Basal oestrogen excretion is less than 10 μg /24 hr, and there is no increase following gonadotrophin stimulation (Fig. 6.4.).

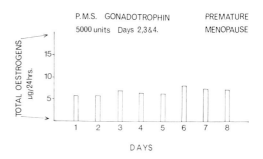

Fig. 6.4. Response to gonadotrophin stimulation in a patient with premature menopause.

Occasionally (Shearman 1968) the stimulus of 5,000 units PMS daily for 3 days may be below the threshold of response in an individual with secondary amenorrhoea who does have responsive ovaries at a higher dose level. This is more common in patients with primary amenorrhoea due to hypogonadotrophic eunuchoidism. It has been our practice to assay endogenous gonadotrophin excretion in those patients showing no increase in oestrogen excretion following stimulation. Of those stimulated, twelve have shown no increase. Two of these were patients with Turner's syndrome, stimulated to exclude any adrenal oestrogen response to PMS. Of the other ten, four have had total gonadotrophins in the postmenopausal range, while in six they were undetectable or at the lower limit of normal. It is a source of some surprise—and anxiety when attempting to assess prognosis—that one patient with no increase of urinary oestrogens and urinary gonadotrophins well above the post-menopausal range re-presented 2 years after investigation. There had been no periods but she complained of sore breasts and nausea. On examination she was 3 months pregnant. More recently we have found serum LH—assayed by radio-immunoassay—in the 'postmenopausal range' in several patients with responsive ovaries.

PATIENTS WITH POLYCYSTIC OVARIES

These patients show a considerable increase in urinary oestrogens, the levels rising to at least 100 μg/24 hr after stimulation and often exceeding 300 μg/24 hr (Fig. 6.5). This same type of

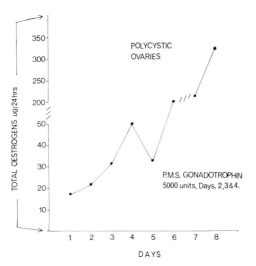

Fig. 6.5. Response to gonadotrophin stimulation in a patient with polycystic ovaries.

excessive response has been found by all workers (Cox *et al.* 1966; Crooke *et al.* 1963; Gemzell *et al.* 1960; Shearman 1964a; Shearman & Cox 1966) except Mahesh & Greenblatt (1964a, b). The increased urinary excretion of oestrogens is accompanied by a rise in urinary 17-keto-steroids (Gemzell *et al.* 1960; Keettel *et al.* 1957).

CYSTIC GLANDULAR HYPERPLASIA

Basal oestrogen excretion is at least equal to that found in the mid-follicular phase of the normal cycle, and frequently much higher. The initial high level of oestrogen excretion is not increased further by exogenous gonadotrophins (Shearman 1966a). For clinical purposes, however, it is as a rule unnecessary to stimulate these patients diagnostically, as careful clinical study will usually make the diagnosis apparent.

PATIENTS WITH 'IDIOPATHIC' AMENORRHOEA

Basal oestrogen excretion is usually less than 15 μg/24 hr. With these levels of oestrogens it is unusual to obtain any endometrium at curettage. A minority of patients, clinically indistinguishable, will have proliferative endometrium and basal total oestrogens of between 15 and 20 μg/24 hr.

After stimulation there is a modest increase in oestrogen excretion. A positive response is defined as an increase in total oestrogen excretion of at least 15 μg/24 hr above the basal level. A characteristic response is shown in Fig. 6.6.

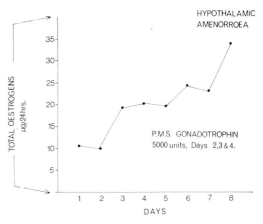

Fig. 6.6. Response to gonadotrophin stimulation in a patient with hypothalamic amenorrhoea.

Prognosis

As mentioned previously, the prospect of spontaneous cure in secondary amenorrhoea of short duration is good. In long-term amenor-rhoea—arbitrarily assessed as 12 months—it is not possible to give accurate figures. Where it is due to organic disease, the prognosis will depend on the primary cause and its amena-bility to treatment. In otherwise well women it has been stated that the spontaneous cure rate approaches 60%. The writer's experience suggests that this figure is far too high, only about 15% of women experiencing spontaneous restoration of menstruation.

Treatment

Treatment must never be undertaken until a diagnosis has been reached. As mentioned above, those patients who have organic disease causing the amenorrhoea will have their treat-ment directed at this cause. Those with no organic disease will fall into two groups: (i) those who wish to conceive; (ii) those who do not wish to conceive.

The treatment for the first group is to induce ovulation, and this is discussed in Chapter 34. For those in Group ii decisions regarding treat-ment are in some ways, more difficult. It should be stated quite clearly that absence of men-struation itself does no harm, but the gynaecolo-gist may only reassure his patient about this if he has excluded underlying organic disease. In this group of otherwise well women, treatment would only be undertaken for one of two reasons; either that for the particular patient concerned, the act of menstrual bleeding is of significant emotional importance; or that there is a valid reason to replace or modify the existing en-dogenous hormonal pattern.

The majority of women are prepared to accept amenorrhoea if they can be persuaded that lack of menstrual bleeding is, in itself, harmless. For some women, amenorrhoea appears to present a threat to their body image, menstrual bleeding being a visible red badge of femininity. This group may properly be treated with exogenous hormones, conveniently and cheaply given as an oral contraceptive of the sequential type.

Hormonal replacement elsewhere is con-troversial. The theoretical basis of this therapy rests on the assumption—which is yet to be proven with certainty—that absence of ovarian hormones is harmful. Treatment should logically be based on a knowledge of each patient's hor-monal environment.

(i) Those with high oestrogen production. It is unusual to find a patient with more than 12 months' secondary amenorrhoea who has hyperplastic endometrium. In this small group urinary oestrogens fluctuate, but for much of the time are above the levels found in the follicular phase of a normal cycle. The possible hazard of endometrial carcinoma should not be ignored. Treatment with norethisterone 5 mg twice daily for 7 days each month will ensure secretory transformation and cause regular withdrawal bleeds.

(ii) Some patients will have a urinary oestro-gen excretion fluctuating between 10 and 30 μg/24 hr and proliferative endometrium. Emotional reasons apart, there seems no reason to treat these women with hormones.

(iii) Some women will be hormonal castrates with urinary oestrogens in the postmenopausal range—less than 15 μg/24 hr. As a rule, no endometrium is obtained on curettage. This steroidal environment is shared by those with a premature menopause and most women with hypothalamic amenorrhoea. Uterine and vaginal atrophy is common and readily explicable; far less certain are the postulated results of oesteo-porosis and coronary atherosclerosis. The value of treatment, certain in terms of uterine and vaginal response, conjectural for bone and blood vessel, must be weighed against the venous thrombo-embolic risks of substitution treatment. A patient with a premature menopause may demand treatment for her hot flushes. Paren-thetically, it is interesting that a clinically similar patient with an identical steroidal pattern due to hypothalamic amenorrhoea will not com-plain of hot flushes. On balance it is probably better to treat these women symptomatically, using a sequential-type oral contraceptive as in the first group. A disadvantage of this therapeutic approach in those with hypothalamic amenor-rhoea, is that possible spontaneous cure will be masked.

It should once more be stressed that even in

the absence of visual symptoms, serial X-rays of the pituitary fossa at yearly intervals are mandatory in women with apparent hypothalamic amenorrhoea, whether galactorrhoea is present or not.

ASHERMAN'S SYNDROME

Treatment aimed at breaking down intra-uterine adhesions will sometimes cure this condition. After this has been done the end-result may be improved by leaving *in situ* an intra-uterine device such as a Lippes loop. Pregnancy may occur, but the risk of *placenta accreta* should be stressed to both the woman and her husband before treatment and pregnancy are attempted.

REFERENCES

AHUMADA J.C. & DEL CASTILLO E.B. (1932) quoted by Argonz J. & Del Castillo E.B. (1953).
ARGONZ J. & DEL CASTILLO E.B. (1953) *J. clin. Endocr. Metab.* **13**, 79.
ASHERMAN J.G. (1950) *J. Obstet. Gynaec. Br. Commonw.* **57**, 892.
BARAMKI T.A. & JONES H.W. (1966) *Am. J. Obstet. Gynec.* **96**, 990.
BROWN J.B. (1963) Personal communication.
BROWN J.B., KELLAR R. & MATTHEW G.D. (1959) *J. Obstet. Gynaec. Br. Commonw.* **66**, 177.
BROWN J.B., MACLEOD S.O., MACNAUGHTON C., SMITH M.A. & SMYTH B. (1968) *J. Endocr.* **42**, 5.
BROWN J.B. & MATTHEW G.D. (1962) *Recent Prog. Horm. Res.* **18**, 337.
CHIARI J., BRAUN C. & SPAETH J. (1855) Cited by Greenblatt *et al.* (1966).
COX R.I., COX L.W. & BLACK T.L. (1966) *Lancet*, ii, 888.
COX R.I. & SHEARMAN R.P. (1961) *J. clin. Endocr. Metab.* **21**, 586.
CROOKE A.C., BUTT W.R., PALMER R.F., MORRIS R., EDWARDS R.L. & ANSON C.J. (1963) *J. Obstet. Gynaec. Br. Commonw.* **70**, 604.
FOIX A., BRUNO R.O., DAVISON T. & LEMA B. (1966) *Am. J. Obstet Gynec.* **96**, 1027.
FORBES A.P., HENNEMAN D.H., GRISWOLD G.C. & ALBRIGHT F. (1951) *J. clin. Endocr. Metab.* **11**, 749.
FROMMEL J.T. (1882) Cited by Greenblatt *et al.* (1966).
GEMZELL C.A., DICZFALUSY E. & TILLINGER K.G. (1960) *Ciba Foundation Colloquia on Endocrinology* **13**, 191.
GOLDZIEHER J.W. & AXELROD L.R. (1963) *Fert. Steril.* **14**, 631.
GOLDZIEHER J.W. & GREEN J.A. (1962) *J. clin. Endocr. Metab.* **22**, 325.
HIPPOCRATES, Genuine works of. Translated by F. Adams. Baltimore, Williams and Wilkins, p. 310 (1939).
JEFFCOATE T.N.A. (1964) *Am. J. Obstet. Gynec.* 88, 143.
JEFFCOATE T.N.A. (1967) *Principles of Gynaecology*, 3rd edn. London, Butterworths, p. 651.
KEETTEL W.C., BRADBURY J.T. & STODDARD F.J. (1957) *Am. J. Obstet. Gynec.* **73**, 954.
KISTNER R.W. (1966) *Fert. Steril* **17**, 569.
LORAINE J.A. & BELL E.T. (1966) *Hormone assays and their clinical application*, 2nd edn. Edinburgh and London, Livingstone, p. 38.
MAHESH V.B. & GREENBLATT R.B. (1964a) *J. clin. Endocr. Metab.* **24**, 1293.
MAHESH V.B. & GREENBLATT R.B. (1964b) *Recent Prog. Horm. Res.* **20**, 341.
RANKIN J.S., GOLDFARB A.F. & RAKOFF A.E. (1969) *Obstet. Gynec. N.Y.* **33**, 1.
SHEARMAN R.P. (1964a) *Br. med. J.* ii, 1115.
SHEARMAN R.P. (1964b) *Med. Res.* **1**, 115.
SHEARMAN R.P. (1966a) *Australas. Ann. Med.* **15**, 266.
SHEARMAN R.P. (1966b) *The clinical uses of human gonadotrophins.* Proceedings of a private scientific meeting sponsored by G.D. Searle. London, Royal Society of Medicine, p. 75.
SHEARMAN R.P. (1966c) *Lancet*, ii, 1110.
SHEARMAN R.P. (1968) *Lancet*, i, 325.
SHEARMAN R.P. (1969a) In *Modern Trends in Gynaecology*, *Series 4* (edited by R.J. Kellar). London, Butterworths, p. 28.
SHEARMAN R.P. (1969b) *Induction of Ovulation.* Springfield, Thomas.
SHEARMAN R.P., COX R.I. & GANNON A. (1961) *Lancet*, i, 260.
SHEARMAN R.P. & COX R.I. (1965) *Am. J. Obstet. Gynec.* **92**, 747.
SHEARMAN R.P. & COX R.I. (1966) *Obstet. Gynec. Surv.* **21**, 1.
SHEARMAN R.P. & TURTLE J. (1970) *Am. J. Obstet. Gynec.* **106**, 818.
SHEEHAN H.L. (1937) *J. Path. Bact.* **45**, 189.
SWYER G.I.M., LITTLE V., LAWRENCE D. & COLLINS J. (1968) *Br. med. J.* i, 349.
WINNIKOFF D. & TAYLOR K. (1966) *Med. J. Aust.* ii, 108.

CHAPTER 7

HIRSUTISM AND VIRILISM

It is easier to define virilism than hirsutism. Although one may define *hirsutism* as 'excessive growth of hair on the body in an abnormal position' there are immediate difficulties in trying to quantitate the word excessive. Initially, it appears reasonable to apply the word excessive, in this context, to a degree of hairgrowth that worries the patient. It must be admitted that some women will become obsessed with a degree of hirsutism that would escape all but the most careful scrutiny; but if the patient is worried she is not to be dismissed lightly.

Hirsutism is very commonly present without any evidence of virilism; virilism is very rarely, if ever, present—apart from the neonate—without evidence of hirsutism. *Virilism* is defined here as one or more of the following: clitoral hypertrophy, breast atrophy, male-type baldness and deepening of the voice. It is usual to include amenorrhoea in this spectrum but it has been deliberately excluded here, both because amenorrhoea unassociated with actual or potential virilism is common, and because some grave causes of virilism may present with ovulatory or menstrual function still intact (see p. 79).

Because of rapid advances in techniques of steroid chemistry, there has been a correspondingly rapid advance in clinical knowledge of these vexing problems. Many short and long reviews of the subject have appeared (Brooksbank 1961; Shearman 1961; Goldzieher 1964; Shearman & Cox 1966; Prunty 1967a, b).

Unfortunately, the extraordinary change in biochemical and clinical knowledge has not made possible universal therapeutic triumph.

THE BIOCHEMISTRY OF HIRSUTISM AND VIRILISM

Hirsutism may be the outcome of excessive androgen production or excessive end-organ response. Virilism is invariably due to excessive androgenic stimulation. Although the prime mover may be as disparate as the hypothalamus, the pituitary, or even bronchogenic carcinoma, the final source of production in the non-pregnant individual will always be steroidogenic tissue—either the adrenal cortex or the gonad. It is fortunate, and embryologically understandable, that the ovary and the adrenal cortex share many common steps in biosynthesis.

Figure 7.1. shows a skeletal outline of some of the more important pathways of adrenocortical biosynthesis. Aldosterone is excluded as it is not relevant to the present topic. It will be noted:

(i) that in the synthesis of cortisol from progesterone, sequential hydroxylation at C_{17}, C_{21} and C_{11} occurs, steps of considerable importance in the genesis of congenital adrenal hyperplasia,
(ii) that androstenedione is produced from 17-hydroxyprogesterone; and
(iii) that oestrogens are produced from androgenic precursors.

The last two statements are equally valid for the ovary, but as the ovary possesses neither 21- nor 11-hydroxylases, the first is not applicable.

It should also be noted that alternate pathways may occur both physiologically and pathologically. An important alternate pathway may

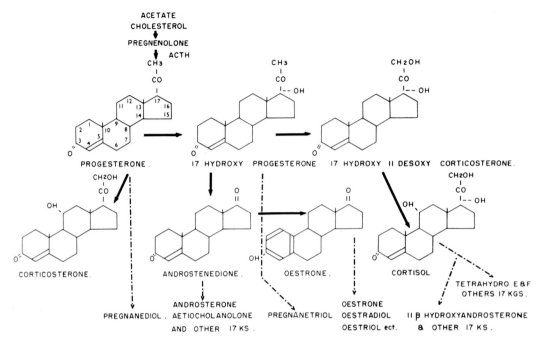

Fig. 7.1. Outline of some steps in adrenocortical biosynthesis.

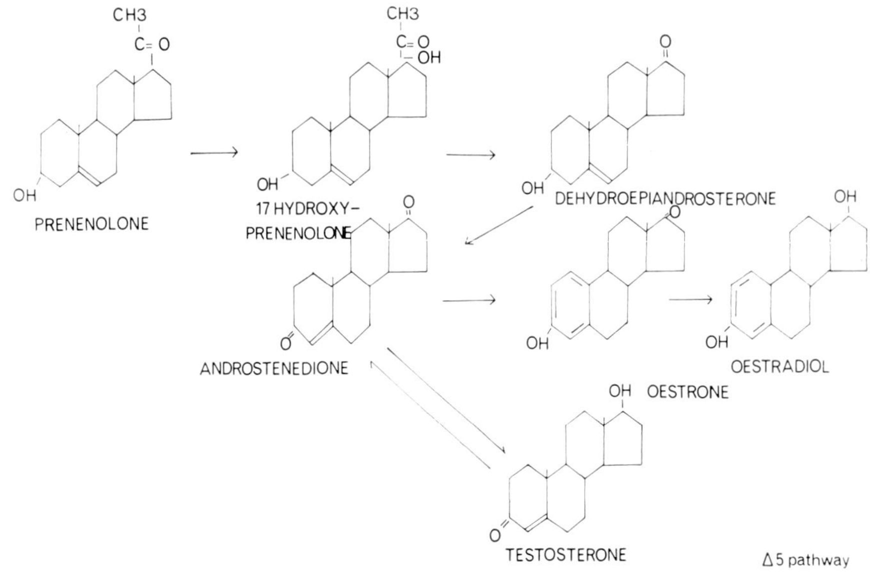

Fig. 7.2. An alternate pathway of steroid biosynthesis.

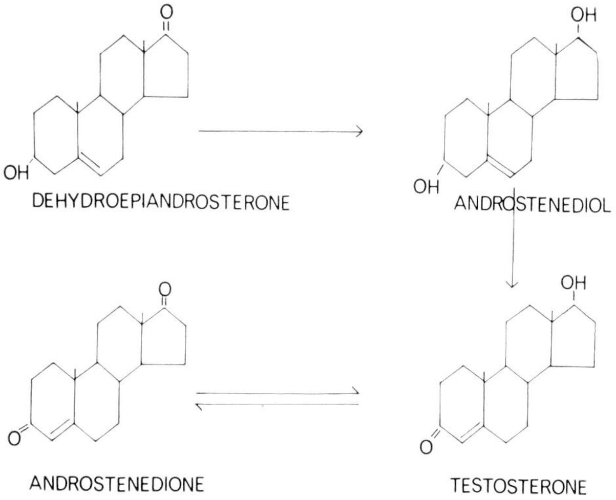

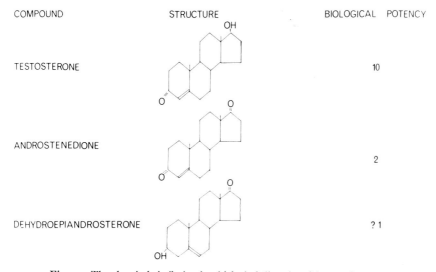

Fig. 7.3. Interconversion of some androgens.

occur in ovary and/or adrenal in either circumstance (Fig. 7.2). Conversion of androgens of weak biological activity—such as androstenedione or dehydro-epiandrostene (DHEA)—to the strongest androgen, testosterone, may occur either in abnormal ovarian or adrenal tissue—particularly the former, or by conversion elsewhere in the body (Fig. 7.3). The chemical similarity but different biological potency of three of these androgens should be stressed (Fig. 7.4).

Other metabolic pathways that are of particular relevance in discussing congenital adrenal hyperplasia and the Stein-Leventhal syndrome (polycystic ovaries) are shown in Fig. 7.5.

It is necessary to have a grasp of the significance of some of the steroidal estimations that are used in assessing the clinical problems to be

COMPOUND	STRUCTURE	BIOLOGICAL POTENCY
TESTOSTERONE		10
ANDROSTENEDIONE		2
DEHYDROEPIANDROSTERONE		? 1

Fig. 7.4. The chemical similarity, but biological disparity of three androgens.

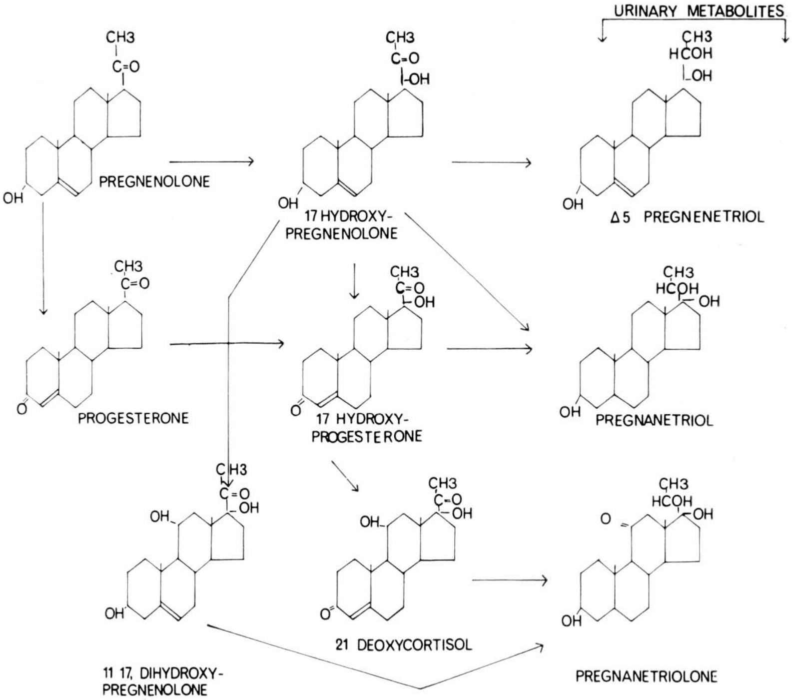

Fig. 7.5. Abnormal pathways of adrenocortical biosynthesis.

discussed in this chapter. Some, or all, of the following may be employed.

   (i) 17-Oxosteroids (17-ketosteroids).
   (ii) 17-Hydroxycorticosteroids.
   (iii) Cortisol.
   (iv) Testosterone.
   (v) Pregnanetriol, Δ^5-pregnenetriol and pregnanetriolone.

With the exception of the final steps in the formation of the characteristic steroids cortisol and aldosterone, most pathways of adrenocortical steroidogenesis are common to both adrenal and ovary. Unfortunately, because of shared precursors and common metabolites it is often difficult to establish whether the ovary or adrenal cortex is the source of the measured steroid, or whether both may be involved.

17-Oxosteroids

Strictly speaking, the term should be neutral 17-oxosteroids. It will include any neutral steroid (therefore excluding oestrogens) with an oxo grouping in the C_{17} position (Fig. 7.6).

It will be noted from a glance at the bottom line of Fig. 7.1 that the 17-oxosteroids are a heterogeneous group, derived from precursors of differing chemical and *biological* potencies. They may derive from C_{17} precursors of weak, or no, biological androgenic activity, such as androstenedione or DHEA, C_{21} precursors of no androgenic activity, such as cortisol; or C_{17} precursors with strong androgenic activity, such as testosterone. Testosterone itself is not a 17-oxosteroid but contributes to the level of these steroids in normal women. The problem of biological potency of precursors is seen clearly here (Fig. 7.7). *The urinary 17-oxosteroids bear some chemical resemblance to their secreted precursors but give no indication of either their biological potency or the site of origin.* Small amounts (chemically) of secreted testosterone will produce profound biological effects, but will have little effect on the total neutral 17-oxosteroids.

17 OXOSTEROID.

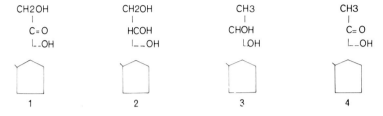

1,2 & 3 = 17 OXOGENIC STEROIDS.

123 & 4 = 17 HYDROXYCORTICOSTEROIDS.

Fig. 7.6. 17-Oxosteroids and 17-hydroxycorticosteroids.

In general terms ovarian tissue—either normal or pathological—is better at producing testosterone than the adrenal cortex. The latter preferentially secretes androstenedione and DHEA. The reasons for this difference are not clear.

17-hydroxysteroids

This term is often used interchangeably with 17-ketogenic steroids (17-oxogenic steroids).

The difference is shown in Fig. 7.6. For most clinical purposes the interchange is reasonable. A 17-hydroxysteroid is any steroid with an hydroxyl group in the C_{17} position. A 17-oxogenic (ketogenic) steroid is a steroid that on suitable treatment will loose its side-chain and become a 17-oxo (keto) steroid. The first of these side-chains shown in Fig. 7.6 is common to cortisol, cortisone, tetrahydrocortisone and

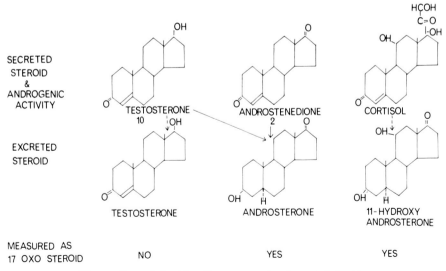

Fig. 7.7. Interrelationships of some secreted and excreted steroids.

tetrahydrocortisol, and under normal circumstances these would make up the bulk of 17-oxogenic steroids. The third side-chain, shown as a 17-oxogenic steroid, normally contributes a negligible amount of the total quantity of these steroids in urine. This is the side-chain of steroids such as pregnanetriol, pregnanetriolone and Δ^5-pregnenetriol. These can be considerably increased in congenital adrenal hyperplasia. Generally speaking, an increase in the 17-oxogenic steroids will indicate increased cortisol secretion, but this is not always true, and as with 17-oxosteroids the limitations of this investigation need to be realized.

Cortisol

Currently the most useful estimations of this steroid are to be done from plasma, rather than urine. Cortisol may be measured non-specifically as 'Porter-Silber chromogens', rather more sensitively by fluorescence, and with the greatest specificity, accuracy and precision by competitive protein binding. Normally there is a significant circadian rhythym—high levels in the morning, low levels at night. The diurnal variation is lost in Cushing's syndrome and depressive states.

Testosterone

This may be measured in urine or blood and methods may include, exclude, or measure separately, epitestosterone. Measurements in plasma or urine at the moment are technically difficult, but may be very helpful in static studies of the hirsute female, and particularly in dynamic studies aimed at differentiating ovarian or adrenal sources of hirsutism.

Pregnanetriol, pregnanetriolone and Δ^5-pregnenetriol

There are, as yet, no easy methods of measuring these steroids in urine; however, where facilities are available their assay may facilitate considerably the diagnosis of adrenal hyperplasia or polycystic ovaries.

THE CLINICAL PROBLEMS

The individual syndromes producing hirsutes or virilism will be discussed initially; a clinical approach to the investigation and differential diagnosis of the hirsute patient will then be presented.

The features of the various syndromes are most conveniently considered under the following headings:

  (i) Congenital causes.
 (ii) Iatrogenic virilization.
(iii) Masculinizing tumours of the ovary.
 (iv) Adrenal hyperplasia.
  (v) Adrenal tumour.
 (vi) Cushing's syndrome.
(vii) Stein-Leventhal syndrome (polycystic ovaries).
(viii) 'Idiopathic' hirsutism.
 (ix) Acromegaly.
  (x) Hirsutism during pregnancy.

(i) CONGENITAL CAUSES

For the most part, these have been considered in Chapter 4. Congenital adrenal hyperplasia has been discussed briefly in that chapter and will be further considered in (iv) below.

(ii) IATROGENIC VIRILIZATION

This may occur during treatment with androgens. There are no absolute indications to use androgens in women, and in most women virilized in this way this unfortunate complication is unecessary and avoidable. With the exception of its use in some women with disseminated breast carcinoma, testosterone has little valid place in the treatment of women. If used for any of the more arguable reasons—endometriosis, frigidity, premenstrual tension—the dose should not exceed 150–200 mg of methyltestosterone by mouth in any one month. In susceptible women even this amount will cause acne, or even early hirsutes.

(iii) MASCULINIZING TUMOURS OF THE OVARY

The pathology of ovarian tumours has long been a field of conflict among morbid anatomists.

With functioning tumours of the ovary it may be impossible to correlate structure with function. Although the classical arrhenoblastoma is clearly masculinizing, virilism may also occur with granulosal tumours, thecomas, luteomas, hilus-cell tumours or adrenal-rest tumours. Although usually endocrinologically inert, pseudomucinous cystadenomata, Brenner and Krukenberg tumours may rarely cause virilism. The problem is fully discussed by Prunty (1967a).

It is doubtful if the endocrine changes attributable to the dysgerminoma or gonadoblastoma are truly causal. Where virilism does occur it is more reasonably explained on chromosomal and other intra-uterine influences (Chapter 4).

Virilizing ovarian tumours may present at any age. The clinical picture is usually one of initial defeminization (amenorrhoea and breast atrophy) with concurrent, or rapidly following, hirsutism

and virilism (Fig. 7.8). The changes in personality may be striking, and have been well documented by Elliott & Heseltine (1967).

Clinically, the presence of palpable ovarian pathology would suggest such a diagnosis. In its absence—and these tumours, particularly hilus-cell tumours, are often so small that they are not palpable—hormonal investigations are of considerable assistance.

Because of the prediliction of ovarian tissues to produce testosterone (Prunty 1967a) urinary 17-oxosteroids are usually normal. In clinical practice the abrupt onset of virilism in the absence of elevated urinary 17-oxosteroids points very strongly to a gonadal cause. Occasionally, the levels may be increased. In these patients, differentiation from adrenal hyperplasia should be clear after dexamethasone suppression (see p. 80) and from adrenal tumour after perirenal air studies or laparotomy.

(iv) ADRENAL HYPERPLASIA

The most familiar form of adrenal hyperplasia is the adrenogenital syndrome, which is usually manifest at birth. The condition should be suspected in any infant born with abnormal external genitals. If the condition is unrecognized and untreated, and provided that the infant does not die from electrolyte disturbance, progressive virilization will occur. In one infant seen recently at this unit, pubic hair began to grow at the age of 18 months, but usually it does not appear until later in life. Body, axillary and facial hair develops progressively. It is usually accepted that without treatment menstruation does not occur, but that this is not invariable is demonstrated by the following clinical details.

The patient, aged 32 years, attended the endocrine clinic of King George V Memorial Hospital complaining of hirsutism, infertility and progressive male-type baldness. Abnormal genitals had been noticed in childhood, and growth of pubic and axillary hair had commenced at the age of 5 years. Somatic growth ceased when the patient was aged 12, and this was followed by the development of facial hirsutism and later of temporal recession of hair (Fig. 7.9). Menstruation commenced when the patient was aged 9,

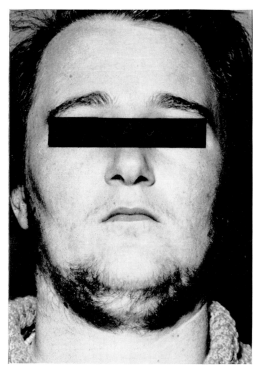

Fig. 7.8. Patient with arrhenoblastoma. (From Elliott & Heseltine (1967), by courtesy of the Editor of *Australian and New Zealand Journal of Obstetrics and Gynaecology*.)

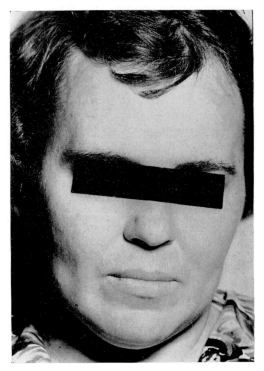

Fig. 7.9. Temporal recession of hair in untreated adrenal hyperplasia. (From Shearman (1969), by courtesy of Charles C. Thomas, Publisher.)

and had continued regularly since then. When she was aged 19, the external genitals had been corrected surgically. Endometrial biopsy on two occasions elsewhere had shown secretory endometrium, but the patient had not succeeded in becoming pregnant. The clitoris was 2·5 cm long and the blood pressure was 240/130 mmHg.

During a dexamethasone-suppression test, the 17-oxosteroid excretion fell from 25–30 mg to 2 mg in 24 hr, and on maintenance therapy with prednisone it has remained between 5 and 8 mg in 24 hr. At the same time the blood pressure has fallen to 130/80–90 mmHg. Eight months after the initiation of therapy the patient became pregnant, but had a spontaneous abortion during the tenth week. She became pregnant again, and has been delivered of a normal male infant (Shearman 1961).

Occasionally, adrenal hyperplasia may not become obvious until after puberty. In these cases, hirsutism and oligomenorrhoea progressing to amenorrhoea are usual, but normal ovulatory menstruation may persist. The biochemical disturbance in these patients is essentially similar to that seen in infants with congenital hyperplasia (Brooks *et al.* 1960).

In this syndrome, the 17-oxosteroid excretion is invariably elevated. In infants, amounts in excess of 1 mg/day must be regarded as abnormal; in adults, 17-oxosteroid excretion in excess of 25 mg/day is usual. Urinary 17-oxogenic steroid excretion in the resting state may be normal, but if large quantities of pregnanetriol and pregnanetriolone are being excreted the 17-oxogenic steroid excretion may be increased.

Urinary pregnanetriol excretion is usually increased (Bongiovanni 1953) and in the normotensive type pregnanetriolone has been detected in the urine on all occasions when it has been sought (Finkelstein 1959; Cox 1960). If elevated 17-oxosteroid excretion is found and pregnanetriolone is detected in the urine, the diagnosis of adrenal hyperplasia is virtually assured. Further confirmation can be obtained by suppressing endogenous production of adrenal androgen with corticosteroids. If a virilizing tumour is present, complete suppression will not follow. Suppression tests should be done—and interpreted properly. After 2 days for basal study, dexamethasone is given in a dose of 0·5 mg four times daily for 2 days and then 2 mg four times daily for 4 days. Urinary 17-oxosteroids should fall below 6 mg/24 hr. With adrenal tumour a decrease to 20, or even 10–15, mg/24 hr may occur, but suppression to the degree seen in adrenal hyperplasia will occur very rarely.

The pathogenesis of this condition has become clearer since the observation by Wilkins *et al.* (1950) that cortisone would arrest the virilization. In 1951, Bartter *et al.* suggested that the primary disorder was in the synthesis of cortisol. It will be recalled that 17-hydroxyprogesterone is converted into cortisol by hydroxylation at C_{21} and then C_{11}. In the more common form of this syndrome there is a defect in hydroxylation at C_{21}. The resulting low levels of cortisol cause an increase in ACTH secretion, which stimulates both the reticular and fasciculate zones of the adrenal cortex to produce excessive amounts of oestrogen, androgen and 17-hydroxyprogesterone. The increase in circulating androgen and oestrogen inhibits secretion of pituitary gonadotrophin, so that ovarian function does not become established.

The excessive amounts of 17-hydroxyprogesterone will cause an increase in the excretion of pregnanetriol, and since 11-hydroxylation is unimpaired, the production of 21-desoxycortisol (Jailer *et al.* 1955) will be reflected by the excretion of pregnanetriolone (Fukushima *et al.* 1959) (Fig. 7.5). Administration of cortisone inhibits the production of corticotrophin-release factor (CRF) and the stimulus to production of excessive androgen is removed. This in turn is followed by increased secretion of gonadotrophins, with restoration of ovarian function in most cases.

In the less common hypertensive form of adrenal hyperplasia, Bongiovanni & Eberlein (1958) demonstrated the presence of compound S and excessive quantities of desoxycorticosterone, which appeared to be due to a defect in 11-hydroxylation. This postulate is supported by the production of similar steroid abnormalities in subjects treated with a substance specifically inhibiting 11-β-hydroxylation — metapyrone (Liddle *et al.* 1958, 1959). However, it has been pointed out (Cox 1960) that simple defects in either C_{21} or C_{11} hydroxylation will not explain all the complexities of abnormal steroid excretion in these patients. Very rarely, in clinically very severe disease, the defect may be in 3-β-ol-dehydrogenase.

(v) TUMOURS OF THE ADRENAL CORTEX

These tumours may produce a wide variety of clinical features—primary aldosteronism, Cushing's syndrome, virilization in women or gynaecomastia in men. The endocrine disturbances may be related to the area of the cortex from which the tumour arises; aldosterone is secreted by the glomerulosa, and tumours of this area will cause hypertension and potassium loss (Conn & Louis 1956). Pure tumours of the fascicular zone will secrete excessive amounts of cortisol and corticosterone, causing Cushing's syndrome. Neoplasia of the reticularis will

produce a clinical picture that varies with the age and sex of the patient and the relative amounts of androgen and oestrogen secreted. Very frequently there is considerable overlap in the clinical picture produced, particularly in the two last-mentioned groups. Some patients with Cushing's syndrome will present with virilization, whereas in others it may be minimal.

Virilizing tumours may occur at any age. In children the onset is usually with growth of axillary and pubic hair, development of acne, clitoral enlargement and deepening voice. In the adult the clinical picture may be identical with that of virilizing ovarian tumours or adrenal hyperplasia. Occasionally, ovulatory menstruation may persist, but amenorrhoea is the general rule.

Urinary 17-oxosteroid excretion is usually considerably increased. Levels of over 50 mg/day are common, and with adrenal carcinoma excretion may exceed 100 mg/day. These levels are considerably higher than those seen in adrenal hyperplasia, but clinically these tumours cannot be distinguished from hyperplasia or ovarian tumour. As mentioned previously, patients with virilizing ovarian tumours *usually* have normal urinary 17-oxosteroids. Dexamethasone suppression is very helpful in differentiating adrenal tumour from hyperplasia. It is important to realize that some suppression of urinary steroids may be seen during dexamethasone suppression, but that the levels do not fall as low as those seen in adrenal hyperplasia. Perirenal air studies may demonstrate the lesion.

(vi) CUSHING'S SYNDROME

When this syndrome was first described in 1932, Cushing ascribed it to pituitary dysfunction. In 1943 Albright pointed out that overactivity of the adrenal cortex, whether from hyperplasia or tumour, was an invariable feature of this syndrome. It is now known that the pituitary may be of clinical importance in those cases due to adrenal hyperplasia (Salassa *et al.* 1959), and follow-up for evidence of pituitary tumour is mandatory.

The symptoms and signs of Cushing's syndrome in its classical form are well known. But the spectacular combination of obesity, moon face, cutaneous striae, subcutaneous ecchymoses,

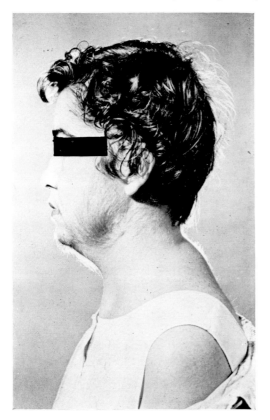

Fig. 7.10. Hirsutism in Cushing's syndrome due to adrenal carcinoma.

osteoporosis, hyperglycaemia, hirsutism and amenorrhoea is rarely seen in any one patient, and often some of the 'classical' manifestations may be absent. The disease is more common in women, and may be difficult to recognize in its early states.

The essence of Cushing's syndrome is overproduction of cortisol, and final diagnosis may depend on demonstration of this. The urinary 17-oxogenic steroids and 17-hydroxysteroids excretion will be increased as a rule, while urinary 17-oxosteroids are usually moderately increased. When the syndrome is due to adrenal carcinoma (Fig. 7.10) enormous levels of urinary steroids may be reached. Plasma cortisol levels are of great value in screening these patients.

A useful routine is to take plasma for cortisol estimation at 8 a.m. and 9 p.m., then at midnight to give 2 mg of dexamethasone and repeat the estimation the following morning. Characteristically, the normal diurnal variation is lost and there is no suppression after the midnight dose of dexamethasone. Typical results from a normal patient and another with Cushing's syndrome due to adrenal hyperplasia are seen in Table 7.1.

(vii) STEIN-LEVENTHAL SYNDROME

It is now 35 years since Stein and Leventhal first described this baffling syndrome. The results of an immense amount of work have since been published dealing with the chemical and clinical

PLASMA CORTISOL
µg/100 ml

	NORMAL	CUSHINGS
DAY 1 -8 A.M.	21.2	28.3
9 P.M.	14.2	22.6
12 midnight	2mg. DEXAMETHASONE	
DAY 2 - 8 A.M.	1.8	25.5

TABLE 1

Table 7.1. Plasma cortisol in a normal patient and another with Cushing's syndrome from adrenal hyperplasia.

vagaries of this condition, and many adequate reviews are available (Goldzieher & Green 1962; Goldzieher & Axelrod 1963; Jeffcoate 1964; Shearman & Cox 1966; Prunty 1967a).

The classical picture is of an obese, hirsute, infertile female with oligomenorrhoea and bilaterally enlarged polycystic ovaries. It is now apparent that obesity is not common, and that while hirsutism is customary, it is by no means

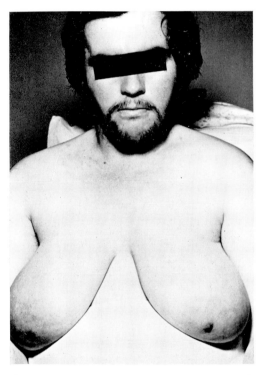

Fig. 7.11. Extensive hirsutism associated with polycystic ovaries. (From Shearman (1969), by courtesy of Charles C. Thomas, Publisher.)

universal. It may, however, be impressive (Fig. 7.11). Clitoral enlargement is uncommon, but may occur.

The enlarged ovaries may be difficult to feel on examination, even under anaesthesia, and additional help by gynaecography, culdoscopy or laparoscopy is frequently needed. Occasionally, the ovaries, although polycystic, may not be enlarged. The macroscopic appearance is typical,

but microscopic examination of the ovarian tissue reveals no unique feature.

The biochemical literature on this subject is now enormous. In essence, although these ovaries can produce oestrogens—occasionally to excess—they do so at the expense of excessive androgen production. Plasma testosterone is frequently elevated. Although there is ample evidence of enzymic deficiency *in vitro* in the ovarian tissue from many of these patients, there is equally valid evidence incriminating involvement of the adrenal cortex (Shearman 1961; Shearman & Cox 1965; Barlow 1969). The basic disturbance lies, almost certainly, in the hypothalamus.

Of hormone assays that may be employed routinely, the following are relevant. 17-oxosteroids are usually normal or at the upper limit of normal, oestrogens are usually within the range found in the follicular phase of the cycle before the rise to the midcycle peak. Pregnanetriolone is found in the urine of almost all patients—a distinction shared only by those with adrenal hyperplasia—and as discussed in Chapter 6 there is invariably an excessive oestrogen response to a standardized gonadotrophin stimulation test (Shearman & Cox 1966; Shearman 1969).

(viii) 'IDIOPATHIC' HIRSUTISM

This classification—a monument to medical ignorance—remains a convenient, if increasingly untidy, categorization of these women with hirsutism who are completely lacking in evidence of organic disease. It seems indisputable that there are some women whose hair follicles are excessively responsive to a normal androgenic stimulus, often racial and/or familial. The unknown frontiers of this group have been pushed further back by technical advances. There is now very valid evidence that many women cast into this clinical mould, while having normal urinary ketosteroids and normal reproductive function, do have levels of plasma testosterone significantly above the normal range (Casey *et al.* 1966). Although the source is sometimes the adrenal, more frequently the 'normal' ovary is to blame. This is, again, a reminder that oestrogens are produced from androgenic precursors.

(ix) ACROMEGALY

This is an uncommon disease, and it is even less common for hirsutism to be the presenting, or even the main, symptom. However, it may be, and the alert clinician will suspect the condition if there is associated atypical arthropathy, carpal-tunnel syndrome and growth of extremities. Urinary 17-oxosteroids and 17-hydroxysteroids may be slightly increased; glucose tolerance may be diabetic but the final court of appeal, even in the absence of radiological evidence of pituitary tumour, is study of plasma growth hormone (HGH). Basal levels are increased and the normal response to hyper- and hypoglycaemia is lost.

(x) HIRSUTISM IN PREGNANCY

It is unusual for hirsutes to develop for the first time during pregnancy, but there are many well-documented cases (Sohval 1965). Very rarely this may be due to the first manifestation of a genuinely coincidental cause such as an arrhenoblastoma (Brentnall 1945). More commonly, no such intercurrent pathology is found.

Clinical approach to differential diagnosis

Two popular misconceptions should be dismissed forthwith. It is often stated that provided there is no interference with menstrual function, hirsutism must be either familial or idiopathic. Although it is usually correct, this belief is wrong sufficiently often to make it essential to look further into the problem of the woman with excessive hair growth, even in the presence of normal ovulatory menstruation, or even in those with a history of recent pregnancy.

Figure 7.10 shows a florid example of this problem. This woman's presenting symptom was hirsutism. She had, when first seen, completely normal ovulatory cycles. She also had

carcinomatosis from an adrenal carcinoma producing Cushing's syndrome.

It is also sometimes stated, that provided the woman has normal urinary 17-oxosteroids, no further investigations are needed. Because of the ubiquitous role of testosterone and its lack of impact on 17-oxosteroids, stressed throughout this chapter, this belief is untenable. Figure 7.12

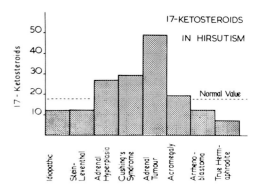

Fig. 7.12. Histogram of 17-oxosteroid (labelled Ketosteroids here) excretion in some patients with hirsutism.

shows a histogram of 17-oxosteroids excretion in a group of our own hirsute patients. The most severely virilized patients in the group—a true hermaphrodite and one with an arrhenoblastoma —had normal oxosteroids.

It is not meant as a placebo to say that a full history and examination are mandatory. The gynaecologist who restricts his field of vision to the subumbilical area will flounder—and deserve to.

The history itself may suggest adrenal hyperplasia (Fig. 7.9), the appearance Cushing's syndrome (Figs. 7.10 and 7.14), or even acromegaly. Often, in fact usually, clinical suspicion may be directed along a certain line, but confirmation will require extensive assessment of the patient's hormonal environment which may be beyond the capacity of many hospitals. An attempt has been made to compress into a flow-sheet (Fig. 7.13) what would otherwise be a long and garrulous discussion.

It should be re-emphasized that hirsutism *must* be investigated, irrespective of the patient's menstrual cycle.

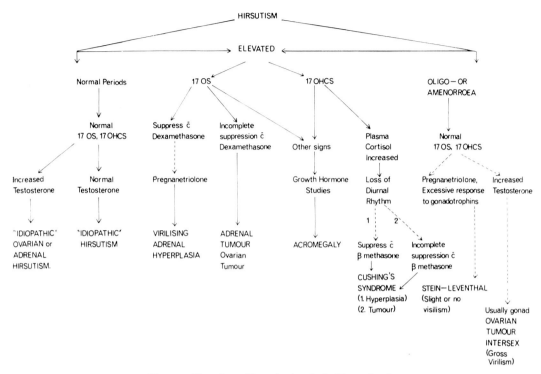

Fig. 7.13. Flow-sheet of investigations in the hirsute female.

In the majority of hirsute women seen with normal periods, 17-oxosteroids and 17-hydroxysteroids will be normal, and one will reach a diagnosis, by exclusion, of 'idiopathic' hirsutism. If facilities for assay are available, plasma testosterone is frequently increased, and dynamic studies of the adrenal and ovary involving ACTH, HMG/HPG stimulation and oestrogen/corticosteroid suppression may isolate the origin of the disturbance. This may have relevance to treatment (see p. 86).

If, on the other hand, the patient has oligomenorrhoea or amenorrhoea, and the 17-oxosteroids are found to be normal (not just once, but on several occasions), the Stein-Leventhal syndrome should be considered. The presence of urinary pregnanetriolone and an increasing response to exogenous gonadotrophins will confirm the diagnosis.

If, in the presence of gross virilism, the urinary 17-oxosteroids are normal, it would be an intelligent guess that there was a gonadal

basis for the problem—an inappropriate gonad or a tumour of the appropriate gland. Testosterone levels will be always increased.

If urinary 17-oxosteroids are increased, whether the periods are normal or not, further investigation is mandatory. In this group the adrenal is usually—but not always—at fault. In the purely virilizing group, dexamethasone suppression (see p. 80) will distinguish tumour from hyperplasia. In the Cushingoid group, plasma cortisol estimations will usually confirm or deny the diagnosis, but differentiation between tumour and hyperplasia may rest with the final court of appeal—exploratory surgery.

Acromegaly should be a constant phantom in the mind of the clinician who sees this type of patient. Like most phantoms, proof of existence is more difficult than initial suspicion, but without the latter, proof will never be forthcoming. Because of the very serious therapeutic implications involved, absolute proof is needed before the necessary radical treatment is invoked.

TREATMENT

Treatment here, as in any other branch of medicine, if it is to be rational, must be based on a proper diagnosis of cause, and an equally proper knowledge of the natural history of the causal condition. Where there is serious underlying pathology, treatment must be directed at this cause, and the results may be singularly rewarding both for the patient and her medical advisors (Figs. 7.14 and 7.15).

This treatment may involve bilateral adrenalectomy for hyperplastic Cushing's syndrome, removal of adrenal or ovarian tumours, hypophysectomy for acromegaly or prednisone for virilizing adrenal hyperplasia. Here the treatment is life-saving and a cure of hirsutism and associated infertility a bonus issue.

More difficult in some respects is the important majority where there is no life-threatening

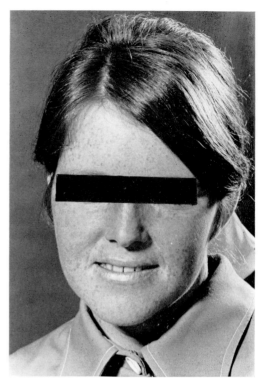

Fig. 7.15. The same patient as shown in Fig. 7.14, 6 months after bilateral adrenalectomy, maintained on cortisone acetate, 25 mg twice daily and 9-α-fluoro-hydrocortisone, 0·1 mg daily.

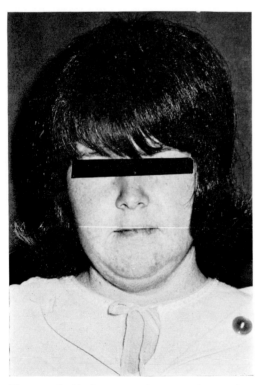

Fig. 7.14. Cushing's syndrome from adrenal hyperplasia before treatment.

cause for the clinical dilemma. The potential risks of treatment must be weighed against the therapeutic result. It should be realized that even with specific treatment, fully mature hair follicles acquire a degree of autonomy which is not readily reversed. In this majority group the patient's hopes should be distinguished from Salinger's roof beams, and not raised too high.

Numerically, the largest group will be those lacking serious pathology—those with the Stein-Leventhal syndrome or 'idiopathic' hirsutism.

The simultaneous treatment of hirsutism and infertility in patients with polycystic ovaries is mutually incompatible. In the writer's experience, wedge resection has no effect on any hirsutism present, a failing shared by clomiphene, although either approach has a place in the treatment of infertility (Chapter 34). The hirsutism may be controlled, and may sometimes remit, after long-term ovarian inhibition. This is most conveniently achieved by an orthodox oral contraceptive, but it is usually necessary to persevere with treatment for at least 6 months before initial results can be assessed. This treatment does not interfere with later specific treatment aimed at infertility.

Medical treatment in the 'idiopathic' group is generally unrewarding. Where dynamic studies of the adrenal and ovary are possible appropriate suppressive therapy may be indicated, but in general, corticosteroids give disappointing results and ovarian suppression only a little better. It should be borne in mind that long-term therapy with corticosteroids may produce complications worse than the original condition, and this cannot be regarded as trivial treatment.

Treatment with anti-androgens has, so far, been a great disappointment. Local cosmetic management can give better results than is often appreciated. If the patient can be persuaded to do so, shaving is a better approach than the use of depilatory waxes or creams, and the frequency of removal may be reduced by judicious bleaching.

REFERENCES

ALBRIGHT F. (1943) *Harvey Lect.* **38**, 123. Thomas, Springfield, Illinois.

BARLOW J.J. (1969) *Am. J. Obstet. Gynec.* **103**, 585.

BARRTTER F.C., ALBRIGHT F., FORBES A.P., LEAF A., DEMPSEY E. & CARROLL E. (1951) *J. clin. Invest.* **30**, 237.

BONGIOVANNI A.M. (1953) *Bull. Johns. Hopkins Hosp.* **92**, 244.

BONGIOVANNI A.M. & EBERLEIN W.R. (1958) *J. clin. Invest.* **35**, 693.

BRENTNALL C.P. (1945) *J. Obstet. Gynaec. Br. Commonw.* **52**, 235.

BROOKS R.V., MATTINGLY D., MILLS I.H. & PRUNTY F.T.G. (1960) *Br. med. J.* i, 1294.

BROOKSBANK B.W.L. (1961) *Physiol. Rev.* **41**, 623.

CASEY J.H., BURGER H.G., KENT J.R., KELLIE A.G., MOXHAM A., NABARRO J. & NABARRO J.D.N. (1966) *J. clin. Endocr. Metab.* **26**, 1370.

CONN J.W. & LOUIS L.H. (1956) *Ann. intern. Med.* **44**, 1.

COX R.I. (1960) *Acta endocr. Kbh.* **33**, 477.

CUSHING H. (1932) *Bull. Johns Hopkins Hosp.* **50**, 137.

ELLIOTT P. & HESELTINE M. (1967) *Aust. N.Z. J. Obstet. Gynaec.* **7**, 194.

FINKELSTEIN M. (1959) *Acta endocr. Kbh.* **30**, 489.

FUKUSHIMA D.K., BRADLOW H.L., HELLMAN L. & GALLAGHER T.F. (1959) *J. clin. Endocr. Metab.* **19**, 393.

GOLDZIEHER J.W. (1964) *Clin. Obstet. Gynec.* **7**, 1136.

GOLDZIEHER J.W. & AXELROD L.R. (1963) *Fert. Steril.* **14**, 631.

GOLDZIEHER J.W. & GREEN J.A. (1962) *J. clin. Endocr. Metab.* **22**, 325.

JAILER J.W., GOLD J.J., WIELE R.V. & LIEBERMAN S. (1955) *J. clin. Invest.* **34**, 1639.

JEFFCOATE T.N.A. (1964) *Am. J. Obstet. Gynec.* **88**, 143.

LIDDLE G.W., ESTEP H.L., KENDALL J.W., WILLIAMS W.C. & TOWNES A.W. (1959) *J. clin. Endocr. Metab.* **19**, 875.

LIDDLE G.W., ISLAND D., LACE E.M. & HARRIS A.P. (1958) *J. clin. Endocr. Metab.* **18**, 906.

PRUNTY F.T.G. (1967a) *J. Endocr.* **38**, 85.

PRUNTY F.T.G. (1967b) *J. Endocr.* **38**, 203.

SALASSA R.M., KEARNS T.P., KERNOHAN J.W., SPRAGUE R.G. & MACCARTY C.S. (1959) *J. clin. Endocr. Metab.* **19**, 1523.

SALINGER J.D. (1963) *Raise High the Roof Beams, Carpenters; and Seymour, An Introduction.* London, Heinemann.

SHEARMAN R.P. (1961) *Med. J. Aust.* i, 921.

SHEARMAN R.P. (1961) *Aust. N.Z. J. Obstet. Gynaec.* **1**, 24.

SHEARMAN R.P. (1969) *Induction of Ovulation.* Springfield, Thomas.

SHEARMAN R.P. & COX R.I. (1965) *Am. J. Obstet. Gynec.* **92**, 747.

SHEARMAN R.P. & COX R.I. (1966) *Obstet. Gynec. Surv.* **21**, 1.

SOHVAL A.R. (1965) In *Medical, Surgical and Gynaecological Complications of Pregnancy*, 2nd edn. (edited by Rovinsky & Guttmacher). Baltimore, Williams and Wilkins.

WILKINS L., LEWIS R.A., KLEIN R. & ROSEMBERG E. (1950) *Bull. Johns Hopkins Hosp.* **86**, 249.

CHAPTER 8

FERTILIZATION, IMPLANTATION, PLACENTAL FUNCTION, EARLY DEVELOPMENT

In this chapter a number of very important events will be examined in some detail. These are fertilization, implantation of the zygote, formation of the placenta and a consideration of some of its important functions; the early development of the embryo will be more briefly considered, with special reference to the importance of early embryonic development in obstetric practice.

Germ-Cell Maturation

Primordial germ cells appear in the yolk sac about 25 days' gestation and migrate via the ventral duct mesentery to the primary gonadal folds. At the end of the month there may be over a thousand in the area of the future gonad.

At $7\frac{1}{2}$ weeks the testis is recognizable, at which time multiplication by mitosis ends and the germ cells enter upon a long-resting premeiotic phase. The central cells of tubules degenerate. Much later the attached cells will divide to form spermatogonia, whose successive redivisions produce the primary spermatocyte, the secondary spermatocyte and spermatids. The latter mature to spermatozoa by a series of at least six recognizable stages (Clermont 1963). In man the division of spermatogonia to mature spermatozoa (Fig. 8.1) occupies a period of not less than 64 days. The process of spermatogenesis occupies a longer time than mitosis and is under the control of local factors which are as yet ill-understood. These stimulate maturation in waves of activity. The tubules are apparently controlled by FSH and the Leydig cells by ICSH.

In the future female, mitosis continues during migration of germ cells to the primary gonadal folds and up to 2 months' gestational age. At

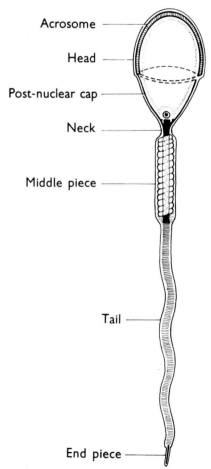

Fig. 8.1. Drawing of a spermatozoon.

Acrosome

Head

Post-nuclear cap

Neck

Middle piece

Tail

End piece

this time the first, or leptotene, stage appears with polarization of chromosomes which are clumped at one edge of the nucleus; then follows the zygotene stage with homologous pairs of chromosomes lying parallel to each other; by 4 months the first pachytene oöcytes can be detected (Baker 1963). In the human female at 5 months there are nearly seven million eggs present. Many of these have entered the diplotene stage, the pairs beginning to split but remaining together at various points (chiasma) where genetic exchange is thought to occur; here they rest until just before ovulation, though 'rest' does in fact include both metabolic and mechanical activity.

In pre-ovulation, which is controlled by FSH and LH, the cell passes from rest to the first metaphase, remaining there for 12 hr before passing through the first anaphase with elimination of the first polar body [Fig. 8.2(a)]. It then enters the second metaphase, which is followed after some time by fertilization. With fertilization is associated the production of the second polar body, and the ovum—now having reached its final stages—joins the male gamete to form the zygote.

Fertilization

The process of capacitation of spermatozoa involves changes in the acrosome and also the accumulation of hyaluronidase. Penetration of the cumulus oöphorus may be assisted by these changes, but it is not thought that hyaluronidase is involved in passage of the sperm through the zona pellucida. Following entry of a sperm into the egg, there begins at the site of contact, and thence passing over the surface of the zona pellucida, a reaction which prevents the passage of further sperms. This prevents polyspermia and the risk of polyploidy.

Following entry of the sperm, its postnuclear cap disappears and the head detaches from the tail. The head, possibly with the midpiece still attached, reorganizes in the centre of the ovum and becomes larger, exhibiting many nucleoli and showing distinct chromatin material. Entry of the sperm, as noted, triggers off the second maturation division of the ovum

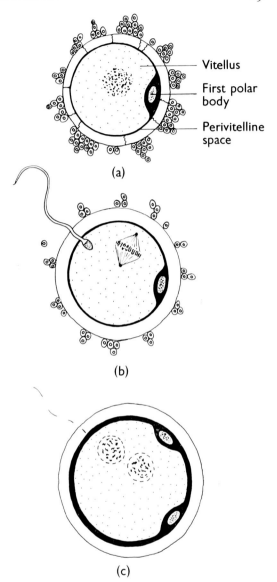

Vitellus

First polar body

Perivitelline space

(a)

(b)

(c)

Fig. 8.2. (a) Secondary oöcyte and first polar body formation following the first stage of meiosis. (b) Penetration of the sperm stimulating the second meiotic division of the oöcyte. (c) The second polar body has formed; male and female pronuclei have formed prior to fusion. (Redrawn from Llewellyn-Jones, *Fundamentals of Obstetrics and Gynaecology*. London, Faber & Faber.)

[Fig. 8.2(b) and (c)], following which the chromosomes of ovum and sperm fuse.

Following fusion the nucleoli disappear and

there ensues a brief period of rest, which is succeeded by much chemical activity. A first cleavage division occurs within 24 hr of fertilization and divisions follow roughly every 22 hr, successive ones occurring at right-angles. Divisions are normally into equal halves.

Implantation

During this time the fertilized ovum is being transported along the fallopian tube by a mixture

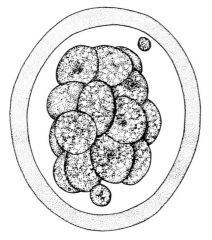

Fig. 8.3. Diagrammatic representation of the morula stage.

of ciliary action and peristalsis, passing the isthmus at 96–120 hr when of the 16–50-cell size. Until this time there has been little alteration in overall size, and the cell mass—likened to a mulberry—is known as a morula (Fig. 8.3). Within the centre of this mass there soon develops a space filled with fluid—the blastocyst cavity [Fig. 8.4(a)]. The surrounding sphere of cells forms the trophoblast. The inner aspect of the trophoblast is at one pole thickened by the inner cell mass. The size of the ovum now rapidly increases to about 300 μm and the zona pellucida becomes extremely thin.

The inner cell mass will form the embryo, yolk sac and amniotic cavity, whilst the trophoblast forms the placenta, chorion and extra embryonic mesoderm. The change from morula to blastocyst is seen in the first 24 hr after entry of the fertilized ovum into the uterus, which normally occurs at $3\frac{1}{2}$–5 days after fertilization. Shortly thereafter the amniotic cavity appears in the inner cell mass [Fig. 8.4(b)] and erosion of the endometrium by the trophoblast usually begins in an area between the mouths of two decidual glands. Decidual glycogen is concentrated in the area of implantation, possibly in response to the presence of trophoblast. Maternal cells and glycogen are both absorbed as embryotrophe. Regeneration of maternal epithelium at the implantation site is rapid and the tropho-

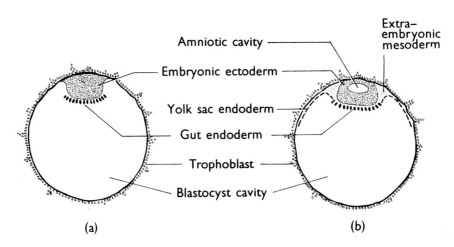

Fig. 8.4. Drawing of the formation of the inner cell mass and amniotic cavity.

blast is fully embedded by the eighth or ninth day after ovulation. The embryonic pole with the inner cell mass penetrates first, and most deeply, into the decidua.

Early Chorionic development

When the blastocyst imbeds at 7 days syncytiotrophoblast and cytotrophoblast are defined, and lacunar spaces appear in the syncytium in the next 48 hr. Two or three days after this there advance into the surrounding tissues early villi, each of which consists of cytotrophoblast surrounded by syncytium. The lacunar clefts soon become filled with maternal blood from eroded maternal capillaries, and a slow circulation of this is evident by 12 days (Fig. 8.5).

Mesodermal cores become evident in the villi by the thirteenth day (Fig. 8.6), foetal blood vessels appearing subsequently and a foetal placental circulation being established when the heart starts to beat at 21–22 days. At 16–17 days the surface of the blastocyst is covered by branching villi which are best developed at the embryonic pole where the placenta will finally be established; the chorion here is known as chorion frondosum, in contrast to the smooth chorion (chorion laeve) covering the remainder of the embryonic sphere. At 4 weeks spiral arteries of the endometrium, which in the progestational phase exhibit to-and-fro looping and marked dilatation, become eroded, with an increased rate of flow in the intervillous space.

The definitive number of stem villi is apparently established by 12 weeks' gestation. Placental growth thereafter continues until term, and possibly beyond, by a continuing increase in size of stem villi with sprouting and

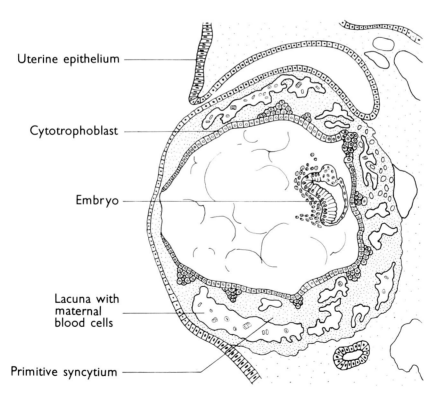

Uterine epithelium

Cytotrophoblast

Embryo

Lacuna with maternal blood cells

Primitive syncytium

Fig. 8.5. Drawing of the early development of the trophoblast. (Redrawn from Hamilton-Boyd & Mossman, *Human Embryology*.)

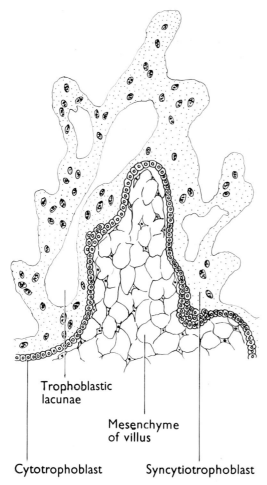

Fig. 8.6. More definitive development of chorionic villi with entry of mesodermal cores.

branching of their growing ends. This branching and rebranching causes the villi to fill the expanding lacunar space, which itself expands by virtue of coincident uterine growth in the area of placental attachment. We can now speak of this as the intervillous space, in which a brisk circulation has been established by about 5–6 weeks.

FOETAL VESSELS IN THE PLACENTA

Main branches of the umbilical arteries and veins can be seen running together on the foetal surface of the placental chorion outside the transparent amnion. From these main branches

at the chorionic surface paired branches are given off at intervals which enter the stalk of a primary villus, following its ramifications to reach the terminal villi. Up to 200 of these foetal units have been described in the mature placenta, though more recent writers suggest that between 60 and 80 may be a more usual number. Each primary stem villus, with all its ramifications, forms one foetal unit, but these foetal units are grouped together by incomplete septa which, arising from maternal tissues, divide the maternal aspect of the placenta into the somewhat indistinct lobulations known as cotyledons. Each cotyledon must include more than one foetal unit, as there are normally some 30 cotyledons.

THE INTERVILLOUS SPACE

This develops as the lacunar spaces of the early trophoblast expand and fuse, an arterial in-flow to the spaces being developed after the fourth week of gestation by erosion of spiral arteries. From the way in which the space develops it is unlikely that preformed and static channels exist for maternal blood flow. On the maternal aspect the intervillous space is enclosed by a layer of basal cytotrophoblast fused with decidua and interrupted by ridges and septa, the largest of which separate the placental cotyledons. Maternal spiral artery in-flow and venous out-flow openings are distributed throughout the basal plate. The circulation within the space must be comparatively brisk, though variable, whilst the nature of the flow would lead one to expect that the composition of intervillous blood would not be uniform. Intervillous circulation has been studied by Indian ink injection studies in monkeys and in isolated human uteri, and by angiography. Some 60–80 spiral arterial in-flows are evident in the mature placenta, which are fewer than the number of arterial openings which can be demonstrated histologically. Thus, even when the uterus is at rest, some arterial in-flow sites may be temporarily out of action. This will be referred to later when discussing alteration in flow during uterine activity.

Though the quantitative aspects of the inter-villous circulation are still speculative, and even the size of the space is uncertain, it is known that maternal arterial blood enters through the spiral arteries in the basal plate as forceful jets, each about 1 mm in diameter, and that venous drainage also occurs through openings scattered haphazardly in this plate. Crawford (1962) emphasized that the area immediately above an arterial in-flow is relatively free of villi, forming an intracotyledonary space, a concept confirmed by Freese (1966). The latter suggested that such an arrangement would permit a constant unobstructed in-flow of maternal blood at sufficient hydrostatic pressure to facilitate exchange of substances between maternal and foetal blood. An increase in size of the functioning vessels in the last trimester has been described. The entering blood jet (Borell jet) enters at a pressure 60–70 mmHg above the resting intervillous space pressure (9 and 15 mmHg) and is directed towards the chorionic plate.

Losing momentum, the blood is further impeded by the villi and is displaced from the centre of the cotyledon by the entry of the succeeding jet, so producing a doughnut shape on injection studies. As it spreads laterally the blood percolates progressively more slowly between villi, and finally leaves the intervillous space by the venous openings in the basal plate. Villi near these outflows will be surrounded by poorly-oxygenated blood and those near the chorionic plate by well-oxygenated blood. This has been termed a multivillous flow system. The mixed flow in the intervillous space accounts for the variable results which have been obtained in analysing that blood. During uterine relaxation the pressure in the space approximates to the intra-amniotic pressure (Martin 1965), while the pressure in the pelvic veins is slightly, but significantly, lower. Earlier authors demonstrated considerable variations in intro-amniotic resting pressure and found that the intervillous space pressure could actually be lower (Hellman *et al.* 1957). Injection studies have demonstrated that as uterine contractions become stronger the amount of contrast medium entering the intervillous space is reduced proportionally. In monkeys the in-flow will cease when contractions exceed 35 mmHg. It will be recalled that individual spiral arteries can be shut off from time to time even during uterine relaxation.

The volume of the space is important in considering the speed of blood flow, but it may not be constant. Moreover, in the normal full-term placenta the parenchymatous tissues which are involved in exchange of gases or metabolites are thought to account for 79% of its volume, and the intervillous space occupies between 37·5 and 42·5% of the parenchyma from the twenty-eighth week to term (Aherne & Dunnill 1966).

THE PLACENTA

The placenta, defined as an apposition or fusion of the foetal membranes to the uterine mucosa for physiological exchange, has been investigated by gross anatomy, injection techniques, large-tissue sections, histochemistry, histology, electron-microscopy and enzyme digestion, as well as by placental perfusion. Some confusion has arisen because each different approach may involve its own vocabulary. Even with a single method of study there are revealed wide discrepancies between different areas and even between contiguous areas of the same placenta. Finally, it may be difficult to distinguish between normal ageing processes and pathological change. Indeed, no pathological change has been described which has not also been reported in 'normal' placentas (Benirschke & Driscoll 1967). It is probable that the composition of the placenta, as well as its size, could alter during development (Dancis 1962). Whilst the well-being of the foetus must, of course, demand sufficient healthy placental tissue to allow transfer or synthesis of substances needed for foetal homeostasis, growth and differentiation, one cannot insist that every functional change must be associated with convincing morphological change. The Grosser (1927) classification of placental types was based upon the number of tissue layers which intervened between foetal and maternal blood in different species. In the haemochorial placentas of man and monkey all the layers are of foetal origin. They comprise syncytiotrophoblast, the connective tissue of the villi and the foetal capillary wall. This classification does not tell us how efficient is a given placental type. Efficiency can vary from one area to another and can be modified by such diverse factors as high altitude, anoxia, hypertension, endotoxin and ageing. Placental growth continues until term, and perhaps beyond, with the formation of new villi and with no general senescence or decrease in efficiency (Crawford 1962; Villee 1962). In a normal mature placenta dilated capillaries occupy most of the cross-sectional area of villi, less than 5% of villi being small with contracted vessels and a fibrous stroma. Light- and electron-microscopy reveal that in the normal human placenta cytotrophoblast cells persist to term, though they may be so flattened between the triple-layered basement membrane and the syncytiotrophoblast that they do not necessarily form a complete layer. Nuclei of the syncytium are smaller and more electron-dense than those of the cytotrophoblast. The cytoplasm is also more highly differentiated and the surface of the syncytium is covered with microvilli. At term the number of these falls, evidence of pinocytosis (see p. 95), lessens and foetal vessels approach the villous surface. Thinning of syncytium, reduction in the number of cytotrophoblast cells, increased stromal fibrosis, fibrin deposition, infarction and foetal endarteritus have been described as normal ageing processes in villi (Wilkin 1965). It was stressed by Amoroso (1961) that foetal capillaries are always covered with a layer of cytotrophoblast as well as by syncytium, however thin the former may become. In areas where the capillary lies close to the surface of the villa and the syncytium has become very thin, passive filtration is possibly facilitated. Such areas are known as vasculosyncytial membranes, but are not common in the normal placenta (Fox 1967). In other areas the syncytium is relatively thick, contains many nuclei and a considerable amount of alkaline phosphatase, which suggests involvement in active transfer. These are known as syncytial knots.

A close relation has been demonstrated between placental and birth weights and chorionic villous area (Aherne & Dunnill 1966). Gross changes (e.g. accessory lobes, circumvallate placenta, and even placenta accreta) are comparatively unimportant. The overall size or weight of a placenta is at best a crude guide to its functional capacity, except for the very small placenta, which often proves inadequate, possibly because it produces a high foetal peripheral vascular resistance. Even placenta–foetal weight ratios are a crude measurement and, moreover, depend on a meticulous, reproducible method of preparation of the placenta before it is weighed. Infarcts have been quantitated by Little (1960), who found a significant correlation with foetal mortality. Calcification of the placenta on the other hand, seems comparatively unimportant (Tindall & Scott 1965). A reduction of villous surface area in pre-eclampsia has been confirmed by Aherne & Dunnill (1966). However, it is probable that reduction of inter-villous blood flow will not only decrease concentration gradients from maternal to foetal blood but might also interfere with the function of placental tissue itself, as this depends for its nourishment upon maternal, and not foetal, blood. This, of course, need not produce structural changes, though there is experimental evidence that placental size can be limited by uterine blood supply.

Experiments involving high-altitude sheep suggested that chronic hypoxia can result in a placenta which permits oxygen to diffuse more easily. This could result from an increased functional area or involve alterations in thickness and composition of trophoblast, or be caused by opening-up and formation of extra capillaries. The experiments of Metcalfe et al. (1962) showed that the placenta became larger in relation to foetal size, whilst the incidence of twinning in high altitudes lessens (Lichty et al. 1957).

Amnion and Chorion

These have been described at length by Bourne (1962). Amnion varies in thickness from one-fiftieth to one-half of a millimetre and is devoid of nerves and blood vessels. It consists of five layers, though the function of each is uncertain.

The extraplacental chorion is from 0·2 to 0·02 mm thick and comprises four layers, the outermost of which, two to ten cells in depth, is formed of trophoblast with ghost villi.

PLACENTAL FUNCTIONS

Four functions have been attributed to the placenta:

(1) Respiratory function.
(2) Nutrient function.
(3) Hormone function.
(4) The so-called 'barrier' function.

These functions cannot be discussed without reference first being made to placental transport mechanisms.

Transport mechanisms

Various mechanisms are involved in the transport of substances across the placenta:

(1) Simple diffusion.
(2) Facilitated diffusion.
(3) Active transport.
(4) Special processes.

SIMPLE DIFFUSION

Molecules of a substance pass from a region of higher to one of lower concentration until the concentrations in the two areas become equal. The driving force is the thermal agitation of the molecules and no additional energy is needed. Two main groups of substances are involved:

(a) Substances concerned with the maintenance of biochemical homeostasis (water, electrolytes, oxygen, carbon dioxide).
(b) The majority of foreign substances (with the important exception of antimetabolites).

The quantity of a substance transferred in unit time follows Fick's equation. This will be considered in more detail when oxygen transfer is discussed (p. 96); it will suffice here to say that the constant K for a substance other than oxygen is determined by its molecular size (compounds of molecular weight below 600 passing easily whilst those of molecular weight above 1,000 pass hardly at all), its spatial configuration (the L isomer passing more readily than the D isomer), the degree of ionization (unionized molecules passing more freely), its lipid solubility (lipid-soluble drugs being favoured) and the partition coefficient for the substance between maternal and foetal blood.

FACILITATED DIFFUSION

Transfer between compartments occurs more quickly than in simple diffusion, though there is no difference in the equilibrium eventually attained. Carrier systems are thought to be involved. The process is concerned mainly with substances involved in foetal nutrition such as natural sugars and most water-soluble vitamins.

ACTIVE TRANSPORT

Here it is postulated that placental work is involved, because the concentrations reached on the foetal side cannot be explained by the physical laws of diffusion. Antimetabolites, inorganic ions, endogenous substrates and amino acids where selective transfer of the L isomer is most marked are substances which make up this group.

SPECIAL PROCESSES

These involve substances of immunologic, but not pharmacologic, importance. Two mechanisms are included under this heading:

(a) *Pinocytosis*. This is a process whereby tiny droplets of plasma are engulfed by a villus and discharged into the foetal circulation at a relatively slow rate.
(b) *Leakage*. Minute breaks in a placental villus have been implicated as a route of transfer of intact blood cells to the foetus from the maternal circulation. It has been demonstrated by the injection into the mother of red blood cells of abnormal shape and their subsequent recovery from the foetus.

Respiratory function

OXYGEN TRANSFER

An adequate supply of oxygen can be thought of as the transfer to the foetus of a sufficient quantity of oxygen, at a sufficient tension to enable the interior of foetal cells to receive an amount of oxygen adequate for their metabolic needs. It has been suggested that the critical oxygen tension in capillary blood which would allow adequate penetration of cells must be 15 mmHg or above. Oxygen is rapidly utilized and there are minimal stores, so that oxygen supply is a function which cannot be disturbed, even temporarily, without serious metabolic consequences to the foetus.

As oxygen is a substance which is transferred by diffusion, its passage through the placenta will occur according to a modified form of Fick's equation. The quantity of oxygen transferred in unit time (Qt) will be proportional to the effective area available for gas exchange (A), and will depend on the size of the gradient between the mean oxygen tension of maternal blood in the intervillous space and the mean oxygen tension in foetal placental blood: $PO_2(m) - PO_2(f)$. Transfer of the gas will be inversely related to the distance which separates foetal and maternal blood (d). The equation is completed by inclusion of the constant K which relates to the physical properties of the intervening tissues and the nature of the substance being transferred. In the case of oxygen it is a comparatively small figure. The equation may now be written $Qt = [PO_2(m) - PO_2(f)]K$. Oxygen transfer is facilitated by a high-pressure gradient, a small diffusion distance, freely-permeable intervening tissues and a large available area of exchange.

To understand the quantitative aspects of oxygen transfer more would need to be known about the extent to which trophoblast acted as a barrier to diffusion. We would also have to measure oxygen tension and saturation in umbilical venous, umbilical arterial, uterine arterial and uterine venous blood, as well as knowing the umbilical and uterine blood flows. It is obvious that many of these facts are not obtainable at present. During life the area of exchange cannot be measured, and measurement of villous surface area even *in vitro* is difficult and time-consuming. The area available for diffusion could be greater than the villous surface, if the additional surface provided by microvilli is included, or, alter-

natively could be less than the villous surface area if the limiting factor is the surface area of the foetal capillary bed. The distance will vary in different regions of the same placenta. It could be increased by local fibrin deposition, by formation of syncytial knots and possibly by the presence near the villi of a layer of relatively stagnant blood. The distance would lessen in areas of temporary or permanent thinning of trophoblast or where dilated foetal capillaries bulge the villus surface. Evidence has been adduced of reversible thinning in response to hypoxia. The average distance involved has been estimated as 3·5–6·5 mm, which is five to ten times that in the lung. Despite this, Adamson (1965) has presented evidence suggesting that the efficiency of the placenta is very similar to that of the lung, though its reserve of function is less.

It has been suggested that Qt, $PO_2(m)$ and $PO_2(f)$ are measurable or calculable. Were this so, then the expression could be rewritten $KA/d = Qt/[PO_2(m) - PO_2(f)] = D$ a value which has been named the diffusing capacity of a given placenta. Diffusing capacity has been shown to increase under high-altitude conditions (Metcalfe *et al.* 1962).

Maternal oxygen tension : $PO_2(m)$

Despite the hyperventilation of pregnancy, maternal arterial blood has a mean oxygen tension of only 97·1 mmHg (88·8–109·6) during pregnancy, which is similar to the range in the non-pregnant state, though PCO_2 has fallen from 40mm Hg to between 31 and 33 mmHg. This represents a pH change of 0·06 pH unit.

Arterial blood reaching the uterus has three functions.

One portion supplies the needs of the myometrium; estimates suggest that 25% of the blood may be so utilized. The remaining blood, which enters the intervillous space, subserves two functions. Firstly it supplies the oxygen needs of the placenta itself. At term the oxygen requirements of this very active organ have been estimated as 10 ml/kg/min, compared with 5 ml/kg/min for the foetus itself. Up to a third of the intervillous space flow could, therefore, be taken up in supplying placental needs. Secondly, the remaining intervillous blood supplies the foetal needs.

During pregnancy it is probable that the relative needs of myometrium, placenta and foetus will vary, and consequently the proportions of uterine blood supply involved in each function will also vary.

The anatomy of the intervillous space makes it obvious that the blood within it is not likely to be of uniform composition and it is therefore unlikely that sampling will produce consistent readings or ones from which $PO_2(m)$ would be calculated.

If over a given short time foetal and placental oxygen needs remain steady, then a quicker flow through the intervillous space would result in decreased maternal arteriovenous oxygen difference. This would in turn produce a higher $PO_2(m)$ so favouring materno-foetal transfer. Although it has been calculated that the intervillous space occupies 37·5–42·5% of the parenchymatous volume of the placenta (which is 79% of its total volume), it is not known whether this is the size in life nor is it certain that the size is constant.

There is evidence that maternal anaemia can be compensated for by an increased rate of flow, as can the chronic hypoxia of high-altitude conditions.

Foetal oxygen tension: $PO_2(f)$

The defects of studying cord-blood oxygen levels have already been stressed. As on the maternal side, alterations of foetal blood flow in the placenta will have a profound effect upon $PO_2(f)$. It was shown by Dawes (1962) that the placenta provides the maximum peripheral resistance in the foetus, and that the steadily increasing foetal blood-flow rates of pregnancy are initially the result of the opening-up of new vessels, but during later pregnancy are related to an increasing foetal blood pressure; the larger the foetus the higher the blood pressure which has to be maintained. For a foetus of 3·3 kg requiring 5 ml of oxygen/kg/min, cord blood flows of between 165 and 330 ml/min would be necessary (Bartels *et al.* 1962). These in turn demand a cardiac output of about 118 ml/kg/min. It was shown by Metcalfe *et al.* in 1962 that up to a fifth of the foetal blood reaching the placenta is shunted from arterial to venous side without entering into gaseous exchange. It has been claimed that arteriovenous communications occur at all levels in villi, and it is known that foetal blood can continue to flow in cotyledons which are temporarily deprived of maternal arterial in-flow. Hypoxia can in part be countered by an increase of foetal blood pressure and of foetal placental flow. The placental perfusion experiments of Panigel (1962) suggest that foetal placental vessels dilate in response to carbon dioxide and constrict in response to oxygen so that part of the control of flow, and hence $PO_2(f)$, may be peripheral. During hypoxia the umbilical blood flow is maintained by the response of foetal pulmonary blood vessels to asphyxia. This causes intense constriction, so diminishing the already small pulmonary blood flow and diverting the blood to the aorta and umbilical circulation.

Consideration of $PO_2(m) - PO_2(f)$ gradient demands close examination of foetal and maternal perfusion ratios. In long-term sheep catheterization experiments Battaglia (1967) found a PO_2 gradient of 40 mmHg between maternal arterial blood entering the intervillous space and foetal reduced blood entering the villi. Further, the blood in the uterine vein and that in the umbilical vein had an identical PO_2. Umbilical venous blood has an oxygen saturation of between 70 and 80% at a PO_2 of 30–40 mmHg. It must be remembered, however, that umbilical arterial blood is more representative of the arterial supply to foetal tissue, and this is normally 50–60% saturated with a PO_2 of 20–25 mmHg. Despite this low PO_2 the oxygen supply to tissues is usually adequate.

BLOOD PROPERTIES INVOLVED IN GAS EXCHANGE

Oxygen is slightly soluble in plasma, but the amount carried in solution is normally small, being of the order of 0·3 ml/100 ml of blood.

The quantity so carried will depend on oxygen tension and upon the solubility coefficients of oxygen in plasma and in the substance of the red blood cell, respectively. The bulk of oxygen is transported as oxyhaemoglobin. The quantity carried will depend on the number of grams of haemoglobin per 100 ml of blood. Each gram when fully saturated carries 1·34 ml of oxygen at standard temperature and pressure, a conversion factor being necessary for other temperatures and pressures. If the percentage saturation of a given blood is plotted against oxygen tension, the result is the oxygen dissociation curve for that blood. For haemoglobin F and haemoglobin A this is an S-shaped curve. Its shape and position will be altered by changes in PCO_2 and pH (the Bohr effect). As the blood becomes more acid it gives up oxygen.

Maternal blood in the intervillous space acquires fixed acid and carbon dioxide from the foetus. These liberate oxygen, which is the more avidly taken up by foetal blood because it has surrendered both fixed and volatile acid. This double effect is probably extremely important in oxygen transfer, and may increase the effective PO_2 difference by at least 12 mmHg.

In vitro, foetal and maternal blood exhibit different dissociation curves, the PO_2 required to produce half saturation being much lower in foetal than in maternal blood. The difference is closely related to the percentage of haemoglobin F in the foetal whole blood, yet it is known that in concentrated solution haemoglobin A and haemoglobin F produce identical curves. Further, when blood was tested which contained 69% haemoglobin F as a congenital abnormality a normal adult curve was obtained. Thus factors other than the difference in haemoglobin structures must be responsible for the foetal/maternal blood differences. It has been suggested that the difference may be related to a lower pH within the foetal red cell, to absence of carbonic anhydrase within the foetal red cell (similar curves can be obtained from adult blood when this enzyme is destroyed), or from increasing cell thickness during foetal life.

It is known that foetal cord blood has a haemoglobin content of 16–17 g-%; this gives an oxygen capacity up to 23 ml-% compared with

15–16 ml-% provided by the haemoglobin of 11 or 12 g-% present in the mother. This would favour oxygen up-take by foetal blood. More recent work has, however, suggested that the high haemoglobin levels of cord blood are, to a large extent, an expression of a response to stresses during delivery. It is known that in the human there is a comparatively small increase in haemoglobin concentration between 22 weeks and term. In animals there is a wide scatter of results for foetal blood oxygen capacity. In the rhesus monkey, rabbits and goats there is no great difference at term between maternal and foetal oxygen capacity, while in the rat the haemoglobin content is actually lower than that of the mother. Cases of severe foetal anaemia of unknown origin have been reported in live lambs of normal weight or age, and it is known that the human foetus in cases of rhesus incompatibility can survive at least to the thirty-fourth week with a haemoglobin as low as 4 g-%. Furthermore, intraperitoneal transfusion with adult blood permits survival and further growth of the foetus even though at delivery 98% of the haemoglobin detected is of maternal origin. These points have been summarized by Dawes (1967).

If it is accepted that the pH of the foetus is 7·24 whilst the maternal is 7·42, the result would be that the relevant parts of the two dissociation curves would become superimposed, so minimizing the differences between them. This point has become less relevant since the demonstration that difference in pH across the placenta in an unstressed preparation lies between 0·02 and 0·05 of a pH unit.

To summarize. By maintaining adequate flows within the foetus it is possible to provide sufficient oxygen despite the low oxygen tension. The perfusion rate on the maternal side of the placenta is also important. The pulmonary changes of pregnancy in the mother have an insignificant effect on her arterial oxygen saturation, whilst the differences between foetal and maternal blood in oxygen content and capacity are less important than was formerly believed. Finally, the Bohr effect is of the utmost importance in maintaining adequate oxygen transfer.

CARBON DIOXIDE TRANSFER

This gas diffuses through a wet membrane 20–30 times as fast as oxygen and therefore it passes much more rapidly across the placenta. Carbon dioxide carriage in blood involves three mechanisms.

(1) A small amount, probably less than 7%, is transported as carbaminohaemoglobin; this fraction, however, provides 20% or more of the carbon dioxide exchanged. Formation of carbaminohaemoglobin requires reduced haemoglobin. At a PCO_2 over 10 mmHg this mechanism is saturated.

(2) An even smaller amount is present in simple solution.

(3) The bulk of carbon dioxide is carried as bicarbonate in plasma. Dissolved carbon dioxide is in equilibrium with a minute amount which combines with water, producing carbonic acid (H_2CO_3). When this dissociates to form HCO_3^- and H^+ the latter ion is removed by a hydrogen acceptor within the erythrocyte. The bicarbonate ion now diffuses into the plasma, whilst an equivalent amount of Cl^- ion enters the cell (Hamburger shift). This chain of reactions can continue until some 90% of the carbon dioxide is eventually transported as HCO_3^-, over two-thirds of which is accommodated in the plasma. As oxyhaemoglobin is less able to accept hydrogen than reduced haemoglobin, it follows that when blood becomes oxygenated carbon dioxide will be given off (Haldane effect). At the placenta the taking up of oxygen by foetal blood helps displace CO_2 from that blood; whilst simultaneous reduction of maternal blood facilitates the up-take of CO_2 by that blood.

Nutrient function

Detailed consideration has been given to oxygen and carbon dioxide transport since, as already indicated, if the supply of oxygen to the foetus is adequate, the provision of other substances will usually be sufficient also. A liberal supply of carbohydrate is essential for foetal energy production, since a foetus derives its energy almost completely from this source. Moreover, with the exception of sucrose and lactose all dietary carbo-

hydrates are broken down to glucose on complete hydrolysis, so a brief consideration of the transport of this material across the placenta is appropriate.

The supply of glucose is all obtained by passage across the placenta. It has already been mentioned that the process by which glucose is transferred is facilitated diffusion. Rapid transfer is evident after glucose loading of the mother (Fig. 8.7).

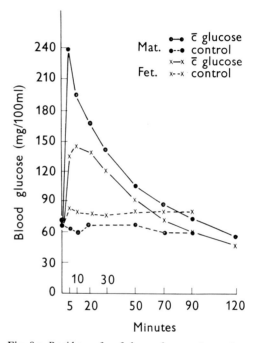

Fig. 8.7. Rapid transfer of glucose from mother to foetus following maternal glucose loading. (By courtesy of Coltart *et al.*)

Paterson *et al.* (1968a) applied the technique of foetal blood sampling to the study of glucose transfer and demonstrated very rapid passage across the placenta; this was confirmed by Coltart *et al.* (1969), at Queen Charlotte's Hospital. In this respect it appears that there is little passage of insulin from the mother to foetus and a variable response in the foetal production of insulin following the glucose loading of the mother.

Placental glycogen was at one time thought to be a source of glucose for the foetus, the amount present providing a ready store of energy for foetal activity. This is now considered unlikely (Ginsberg 1970). A very important relationship exists between the glycogen stores of the foetus and its ability to withstand hypoxia, which will be examined in Chapter 11.

Although the foetus obtains its energy almost exclusively from the metabolism of carbohydrate, lipids for growth and development must be deposited in significant quantities throughout foetal life. These lipids will be transported across the placenta, or at any rate built up from other substances so transported. The direct transport of triglycerides and fatty acids from the mother to foetus has been demonstrated in animals; from the fact that adipose tissue of the newborn contains essential fatty acids, direct transport in the human seems a probability (Bagdade et al. 1966). On the other hand, foetal tissues are able to synthesize triglycerides and fatty acids from early pregnancy onwards (Roux 1966). Which mechanism is the more important during pregnancy is uncertain; it is suggested that direct transport from mother to the foetus is probably the more common in early pregnancy, synthesis in the foetus becoming increasingly evident later in foetal life. Cholesterol is capable of direct transport across the placenta from mother to foetus in the experimental animal. However, foetal synthesis is the more important process, accounting for the majority of foetal cholesterol which can be synthesized in most tissues (Myant 1970). No direct passage of more complex lipids such as glycolipids or phospholipids has been demonstrated. These substances are quickly synthesized within the foetus.

Protein transfer is for the most part achieved by the breakdown to amino acids on the maternal side of the trophoblast, followed by active transport. Here, pinocytosis is the process chiefly involved. Direct transfer may be achieved in the case of a few proteins.

In general, it may be said that in many instances transfer of nutrient materials across the placenta is a fairly rapid process, perhaps occupying only a few minutes in substances transported by simple and facilitated diffusion; in the case of active transport, duration of 30 min to 1 hr, or less, is likely to be involved.

Hormone production

This extremely important placental function is considered in detail in Chapter 10.

The barrier function

In earlier years a good deal of attention was paid to the so-called 'barrier' function of the placenta. The placenta was thought to protect the foetus from a number of noxious substances which might be circulating in the mother if she had, say, an infectious disease or if she had been injected with a drug of some particular kind. We now believe that this barrier function is largely illusory. Many substances cross the placental barrier, by physical diffusion or by an active transport system, so much so that in practice almost any drug ingested by or injected into the mother will be found within the foetus within a fairly short time. A high molecular weight has been thought to inhibit passage across the placenta, but Apgar (1966) states that this does not interfere with transmission to the foetus, except to impose a brief timelag on the process.

That certain common infections can pass across the alleged placental barrier and affect the foetus *in utero* has been known for many years. One of the most famous of all obstetricians—Mauriceau—is said to have been born pock-marked. The occurrence of congenital syphilis has also been known for many years. It is to modern obstetrics, however, that we have to look for the most dramatic examples of the devastating effects of disease and drugs on the foetus *in utero*.

The effects on the foetus of rubella contracted by the mother in early pregnancy are now well known, and are referred to in more detail in Chapter 21. The percentage of affected children has varied considerably in reported series, suggesting that the teratogenic affect of rubella will vary from one epidemic to another, and probably between epidemic and sporadic forms of the disease. It seems probable, however, that most deformities of the foetus follow an attack of rubella during the first 12 weeks of pregnancy when organogenesis is at its height; occasionally, abnormalities may follow the disease at a slightly later period. If the mother contracts rubella during the first 12 weeks of pregnancy the chances of her giving birth to a seriously affected child may be somewhere between 15 and 50%. No other diseases have shown such devastating effects as rubella; indeed, it is by no means certain that any are teratogenic, although it has been suggested that mumps, infective hepatitis and influenza may act in a similar way (Moloshok 1966).

A number of acute infections predispose to abortion and foetal death as a result of the toxaemia and pyrexia which is usually present, but teratogenic effects are absent. Chickenpox is known to affect the foetus if contracted by the mother in late pregnancy, leading to congenital or neonatal chickenpox. As already mentioned, smallpox may be transmitted to the foetus. The relationship of smallpox to pregnancy is important so far as vaccination of the pregnant woman is concerned; this point is considered on p. 336.

The pregnant woman is apparently more liable to infection by poliomyelitis, and the disease is more dangerous if she is infected. It would appear not to be teratogenic, but the virus passing across the placenta may infect the foetus, so foetal wastage as abortion, stillbirth or neonatal death may result. Studies of Salk vaccine and orally administered, live, attenuated vaccine in pregnancy have shown no apparent foetal adverse effects, and one or other should be used if the risk of poliomyelitis is considerable.

The parasitic condition of toxoplasmosis deserves mention. This is an infestation by the parasite *Toxoplasma gondii* which may be virtually asymptomatic in the mother, but its effects may be very grave on the foetus. The parasite may pass across to the foetus during the parasitaemic phase and may give rise to serious abnormalities such as choroidoretinitis, hydrocephalus, cerebral calcification, jaundice, hepatospleno-megaly and convulsions. In some communities the disease is a significant cause of abortion, and perhaps should be more often considered in this country. Since the disease is only dangerous during its parasitaemic stage a person who has given birth to a child affected by toxoplasmosis need not concern herself in the future about a recurrence.

The appalling deformities caused by thalido-mide administered in early pregnancy should make all obstetricians acutely aware of the risks of prescribing drugs in early pregnancy and in the case of some drugs, late in pregnancy also. Whilst with no other drug has such a close relationship to foetal deformity been established as with thalidomide, several have had the finger of suspicion pointed at them. It is difficult to know whether a particular drug can be held responsible for occasional defects, and an extremely cautious approach to prescribing in early pregnancy is necessary if further calamities are to be avoided.

Some drugs, even when administered in late pregnancy, may pass to the foetus with harmful effects. Examples are a foetal goitre caused by potassium iodide or thiouracil treatment, foetal haemorrhage and death following dicoumarol treatment (heparin appears safe in this respect) and inhibition of bone growth with teeth dis-coloration following tetracycline therapy.

All things considered, the circumstances in which the placenta can really be regarded as a barrier are so few that this so-called function can be disregarded.

EARLY FOETAL DEVELOPMENT

The events of fertilization, implantation and placentation have already been examined. A little more must now be said about early develop-ment of the foetus, although no attempt will be made to deal comprehensively with embryology, for details of which standard works should be consulted.

The development of the human foetus *in utero* is usually described as falling into three stages. The first stage is from fertilization to that point at which the ovum is successfully implanted. The second stage is from then until the end of the eighth week, by which time the development of nearly all the major organs has begun; it is at this time that the embryo begins to look recognizably human. The third stage, from the eighth week until the end of pregnancy, con-stitutes largely one of organ growth.

At the end of the first week following fertilization the amniotic cavity is just making its appearance between the ectoderm and the covering of trophoblast. The embryo itself at this point is a disc composed of two layers, ectoderm and endoderm. The formation of the third embryonic layer, the mesoderm [Fig. 8.8(a)], is evident at this time; the mesoderm becomes divided into two zones, the embryonic mesoderm between

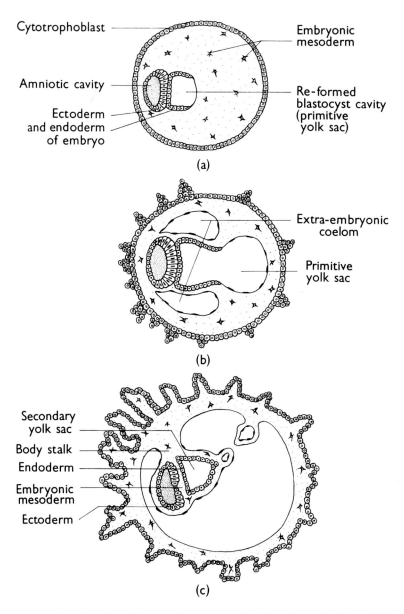

Fig. 8.8. Drawing of the formation of the mesoderm, extra-embryonic coelom and yolk sac. (Redrawn from Llewellyn-Jones, *Fundamentals of Obstetrics and Gynaecology*. London, Faber & Faber.)

the ectoderm and endoderm of the embryonic disc [Fig. 8.8(c)] and the extra-embryonic mesoderm which begins to fill the blastocyst cavity and leads to the formation of the primitive yolk sac [Fig. 8.8(b)]. A further change in the extra-embryonic mesoderm is the coalescence of numerous spaces which form the extra-embryonic coelom dividing the mesoderm into two layers: an outer layer lining the trophoblast and called the somatopleure, and an inner one lining the embryonic area and yolk sac known as the splanchnopleure.

Tremendous development now takes place in the region of the embryonic disc. Initially, the ectoderm proliferates rapidly on its posterior surface, causing the primitive streak to bulge into the amniotic cavity. The disc itself expands into a pear-shaped mass by marked development of mesoderm in the area. A groove appears throughout the length of the primitive streak, ending in the primitive pit situated anteriorly. The head process of the embryo develops from mesodermal growth anterior to the primitive pit. Further development of the head process coincides with shrinking of the primitive streak as the whole embryonic axis lengthens.

Further changes follow very quickly. In an embryo which is 3 weeks old an extension of the extra-embryonic coelom has been formed within the lateral plate, to give rise to the true coelom of the embryo. A little later, part of this is again separated off as the pericardial cavity. The heart begins pulsations. Blood vessels containing corpuscles are evident. Closure of the neural tube begins. The pronephros becomes evident and its duct begins to grow towards the cloaca. Still further development is evident in the 4 week-old embryo. Paired limb buds are evident. Abundant blood is seen in the yolk sac and circulating through the blood vessels and heart. The mesonephros and metenephros are forming. The neural tube becomes completely closed and early brain development is evident. By 5 weeks the embryo is beginning to look more recognizably human, due largely to changes in the formation of the face. Important developments take place in the eye, with the formation of the lens and choroid fissure. The genital ridges may be seen by this time, and complete formation of the mesonephros has taken place. So rapid are these changes that by the end of the first 2 months the foetus looks clearly human in form. Almost every organ has been laid down, although development is not complete. The sex of the foetus, as it is now called, cannot be determined from the external genitalia at this time, differentiation usually occurring during the period 8–12 weeks, although not until later is it easy to recognize a male from a female. It is easy to see how during this early period of rapid formation and development of primordial organs drugs such as thalidomide and diseases such as rubella can have an extremely important effect upon foetal development and can result in devastating foetal abnormalities (see p. 100).

Foetal circulation

A mass of cells, becoming so large that the inner units can no longer diffuse metabolic materials with the extracellular fluid, requires an internal transportation system. The human embryo reaches the stage by about 16 days. After this, a full vascular system is evolved to carry foetal blood to the trophoblastic surface and return it to the central body. In both foetus and adult, high blood flow is maintained to homeostatic organs while flow to other areas of the body varies with needs. The foetal and adult cardiovascular systems differ because of the alterations in homeostatic mechanisms at each phase, the placenta acting instead of the adult lung or kidney in oxygenation or catabolite excretion (Fig. 8.9).

Blood returning from the placenta is shunted along the ductus venosus directly to the inferior vena cava, so avoiding the liver. Approaching the heart, the larger portion of the blood passes from the inferior vena cava to the left atrium through the foramen ovale, without entry to the right heart (Fig. 8.10). A lesser quantity of blood from the umbilical circulation is not diverted by the crista dividens and mixes in the right atrium with the deoxygenated blood from the head of the foetus. In fact, there is very little mixing of the two streams in the right heart. Most of the blood returning from the placenta passes straight to the left atrium, for in the foetus that chamber is beneath the rest of the heart, and blood is diverted

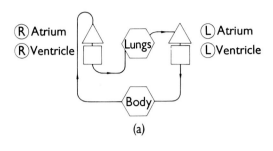

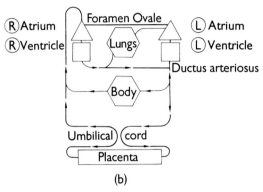

Fig. 8.9. The bypass mechanisms in the foetal circulation. (a) Shows the flow pattern of blood through the adult circulation and cardiopulmonary unit. (b) Shows the foetal situation with the added low resistance and high flow zone of the placenta and the two channels to bypass the non-functioning foetal lungs.

by the crista straight from the inferior vena cava. This simplification of ideas on foetal haemodynamics can be shown by measuring oxygen-saturation levels in superior or inferior vena cava and comparing them with the left atrial levels, and has been confirmed by injecting ^{131}I-labelled albumin into inferior or superior vena cava in turn. The first leads rapidly to a very high increase in scintillation counts in the carotid loop, the latter making no immediate change (Dawes 1968).

The blood with a higher oxygen saturation is pumped to the left ventricle and so to the aorta, from where the relatively big carotid arteries direct a larger share to the cerebral circulation. The lesser portion of oxygenated blood which actually entered the right atrium mixes with relatively deoxygenated blood from the superior vena cava and the coronary sinus, passing to the right ventricle and so to the pulmonary trunk. Pressures in the pulmonary circulation are higher than in the aorta, so most of this blood is diverted along the ductus arteriosus to join the aorta below the exit of the carotid arteries, less than 10% of the cardiac output passing through the pulmonary vessels. The blood which circulates to the foetal viscera, comes mostly from that which has circulated through the head and arms, together with a lesser quantity from the left ventricle. It passes down the aorta and about two-thirds of it is pumped along the umbilical arteries to the placenta, with a little going down the femoral arteries to the legs.

The circulation in the placenta has a low resistance, and must be sustained by high flow

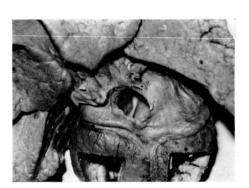

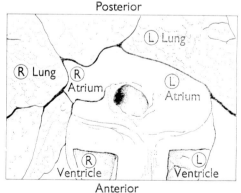

Fig. 8.10. The underside of the foetal heart with the inferior vena cava removed. The crista is clearly shown and it can be appreciated how this deflects most of the blood coming from below into the left atrium.

rates. Blood pressures drop sharply in the placenta, so that while umbilical artery pressures may be approximately 60 mmHg, those in the vein are only 10 mmHg. The effects of the flow of blood down a long vessel with numerous changing curves in the umbilical cord might be important, but most resistance to flow seems to occur in the cotyledonal vessels, while the pressure inside the villus vessels themselves is less than that of the intervillus space.

In early pregnancy more of the blood volume is outside the body (in placenta and cord) than inside but once body weight exceeds that of the placenta, at about 16 weeks, the ratio is reversed. Umbilical blood flow increases proportionally with foetal growth at a level of about 100 ml/kg/min. Alterations in flow may be due to variations in placental vascular resistance in early pregnancy, but later on are related to foetal arterial blood pressure, which by term often reaches 75/55 mmHg. Return of blood from the placenta is by *vis a tergo*, although it has been suggested that pulsations of the umbilical arteries wrapped in a spiral fashion around the vein may help to milk the blood along.

Mild hypoxia causes a rise of foetal arterial pressure, and since there is usually no alteration of the placental vascular resistance, flow rates would increase; severe hypoxia, however, can slightly increase placental vascular resistance and so might reduce blood returned to the body. Since it is probable that there is no sympathetic enervation of the umbilical vessels after they have emerged from the foetal body, this effect is probably a reflection of increased catecholamine release by the foetal adrenal glands. Under these conditions a relatively large volume of the foetal blood stays in the placental vessels, possibly exposing a greater amount of blood to the exchange of gases. It has yet to be proved that this is an advantageous response of the foetus, for the catecholamines also increase metabolic rates and so increase the usage of oxygen by the foetus, so that although there may be more blood in the region, it might be exposed to oxygen exchange for a shorter time.

Much remains to be learned about the foetal circulation and its responses. Those wishing to learn more about the interim position should consult Professor Geoffrey Dawes' volume *Foetal and Neonatal Physiology*.

IMMUNOLOGICAL CONSIDERATIONS

Theoretically, the foetus, being genetically foreign to the mother, ought to be rejected by her. That this does not happen is an extremely interesting immunological problem, the complete solution of which is yet to be obtained. The foetus appears capable of producing antigens at an early stage of development and cannot, therefore, be regarded as immunologically inert, as was at one time thought possible. The mother is equally immunologically active and capable of responding to antigenic stimuli, discounting any suggestion that an immunologically inert situation might exist in her during pregnancy which could explain the failure of the foetus to be rejected. The explanation appears to lie in the existence of some form of trophoblast/maternal barrier. Billingham (1964, 1970) suggests that in experimental animals no trophoblast antigens similar to those present in the foetus have been detected; transplantation of trophoblast can be performed between different species quite satisfactorily, whereas transplanted embryonic tissue is quickly rejected. Billingham suggests this failure of the trophoblasts to provoke an immune reaction may be concerned with a 'fibrinoid' material—sialomucin—shown to be present around the trophoblast cells. For further consideration of this problem the reader may consult Billingham (1970).

REFERENCES

ADAMSONS K. (1965) *Birth Defects*, Series 1, No. 1, p. 27.

AHERNE W. & DUNNILL M.S. (1966) *Br. med. Bull.* 22, 5.

AMOROSO E.C. (1961) *Br. med. Bull.* 17, 81.

APGAR Y. (1966) *Clin. Obstet. Gynec.* 9, 623.

BAGDADE J.D. & HIRSCH J. (1966) *Proc. Soc. exp. Biol. Med.* 122, 616.

BAKER T.G. (1963) *Proc. R. Soc. B.* 158, 417.

BARTEES H., MOLL W. & METCALF J. (1962) *Am. J. Obstet. Gynec.* 84, 1714.

BATTAGLIA F.C. (1967) *Modern Trends in Obstetrics*, 4th edn. (edited by Kellar). London, Butterworth, p. 284.

BENIRSCHKE K. & DRISCOLL S.G. (1967) *The Pathology of the Human Placenta*. New York, Springer.

BILLINGHAM W.D. (1970) *Scientific Foundations of Obstetrics and Gynaecology* (edited by Phillip, Barnes & Newton). London, Heinemann, p. 159.

BILLINGHAM W.D. (1964) *New Engl. J. Med.* **270**, 667 and 720.

CLERMONT Y. (1963) *Am. J. Anat.* **112**, 35.

CLERMONT Y. (1966) *Fert. Steril.* **17**, 705.

COLTART T.M., BEARD R.W., TURNER R.C. & OAKLEY N.W. (1969) *Br. med. J.* **4**, 17.

CRAWFORD J.M. (1962) *Am. J. Obstet. Gynec.* **84**, 1543.

DANCIS J. (1962) *Am. J. Obstet. Gynec.* **84**, 1749.

DAWES G.S. (1962) *Am. J. Obstet. Gynec.* **84**, 1634.

DAWES G.S. (1967) *Scient. Basis Med. Ann. Rev.* p. 74.

DAWES G.S. (1968) *Foetal and Neonatal Physiology*. Chicago, Year Book Medical Publishers Inc., chap. 8, p. 92.

FOX H. (1967) *J. Obstet. Gynaec. Br. Commonw.* **74**, and 881.

FREESE U.E. (1966) *Am. J. Obstet. Gynec.* **94**, 354.

FREESE U.E., RANNIGER K. & KAPLAN A. (1966) *Amer. J. Obstet. Gynec.* **94**, 361.

GINSBERG J. (1970) *Scientific Foundations of Obstetrics and Gynaecology* (edited by Phillip, Barnes & Newton) London, Heinemann, p. 343.

GROSSER O. (1927) *Fnihartwicklung, Einhantbildung und Placentation des Menschen und der Sangetier*. München, Bergnaun.

HELLMAN L.M., TRICOMIT V.M. & GUPTA O. (1957) *Am. J. Obstet. Gynec.* **74**, 1018.

LICHTY J.A., TING R.T., BRUNS P.D. & DYAR E., (1957) *Am. J. Dis. Child.* **93**, 666.

LITTLE W.A. (1960) *Obstet. Gynec., N.Y.* **15**, 109.

MARTIN C.B. (1965) *Anesthesiology* **26**, 447.

METCALF J., MESCHIA G., HELLEGERS A.E., PRYSTOWSKY H., HUCKABEE W.E. & BARRON D.H. (1962) *Quart. J. Exp. Physiol.* **47**, 74.

MOLOSHOK R.E. (1966) *Clin. Obstet. Gynec.* **9**, 608.

MYANT N.B. (1970) *Scientific Foundations of Obstetrics and Gynaecology* (edited by Phillip, Barnes & Newton). London, Heinemann, p. 354.

PATERSON P., PAGE D., TAFT P., PHILLIPS L. & WOOD C. (1968a) *J. Obstet. Gynaec. Br. Commonw.* **75**, 917.

PATERSON P., PHILLIPS L. & WOOD C. (1968b) *Am. J. Obstet. Gynec.* **98**, 958.

PAUIGEL M. (1962) *Am. J. Obstet. Gynec.* **84**, 1664.

TINDALL V.R. & SCOTT J.S. (1965) *J. Obstet. Gynaec. Br. Commonw.* **72**, 356.

VILLEE C.A. (1962) *Am. J. Obstet. Gynec.* **84**, 1684.

WILKIN P. (1965) *Patholojie du Placenta*. Paris, Masson.

CHAPTER 9

NORMAL PREGNANCY:
PHYSIOLOGY AND MANAGEMENT

From the moment of entry of the sperm, the fertilized ovum in all probability sends out messages to the fallopian tube, to the uterus, to the ovary and to the whole maternal organism. The developing ovum releases a substance, such as messenger RNA, which prepares the uterus to receive the blastocyst and ensures the continuation and development of the corpus luteum. The corpus luteum and the trophoblast and, later, the placenta, secrete hormones which circulate throughout the body and produce changes in the structure and function of the mother. There is almost no part of the maternal organism that is not adapted and prepared to accommodate and to meet the needs of the developing foetus. The mother is at the same time further prepared and adapted for the later expulsion and birth of the infant and to meet the demands of lactation and nourishment of the infant in the puerperium.

From the moment of conception the resources of the mother are mobilized, and the whole structure and function of the mother is altered and adapted so that she is maintained in good health in spite of the enormous demands imposed by the production and nourishment of a growing foetus.

This chapter describes:

(1) The changes in the mother in normal pregnancy.
(2) The duration, diagnosis and clinical changes in normal pregnancy.
(3) The management of normal pregnancy.

THE CHANGES IN THE MOTHER IN NORMAL PREGNANCY

The changes in the mother in pregnancy appear to follow three important teleological principles.

(1) *The changes in pregnancy are a temporary adaptation and produce no permanent deleterious effects in the mother.* Given adequate nutrition, the changes of pregnancy are not a strain on a woman's health. Many women feel better and happier in pregnancy and the great majority of the structural and functional changes revert to normal once pregnancy and the puerperium are complete. This is not wholly true, in that there are some minor permanent structural and functional changes which persist after pregnancy, but they do not normally produce any deleterious symptoms or effects. Pregnancy is thus physiological and not pathological and, as a fundamental part of the biological life cycle of the human female, is, in the absence of any complication, an entirely 'normal' process.

(2) *The changes in the mother prepare her to meet and anticipate any possible needs and demands of the foetus.* This preparative and positive adaptation is shown by the facts that:

(a) *The structural and physiological changes in the mother precede any possible demand by the foetus and commonly occur very early in pregnancy.* The renal blood flow, for example, has been shown to be increased by as much as 50% in some women as early as the ninth week of pregnancy (Sims & Krantz 1958).

(b) *The changes in the mother are in apparent excess of the needs of the foetus.* The cardiac output, for example, increases by between 27 and 64% in pregnancy (Kerr 1968), more than is necessary to provide for the increased blood flow to the uterus and other vital organs (Hytten & Leitch 1964). The increase is further out of proportion to the total oxygen consumption in pregnancy, which is only increased some 10% (Sinclair 1963).

(c) *The mother anticipates the future needs of the foetus and accumulates reserves.* These reserves may be accumulated to anticipate a later phase of rapid growth or increased demand by the foetus or may be to anticipate possible later periods of nutritional deprivation should the food intake of the mother become inadequate. The deposition of fat, which is characteristic of pregnancy, is thought to represent a reserve store to meet the need for energy and fat during lactation (Hytten & Leitch 1964).

(3) *The maternal internal environment is altered to create conditions favourable to the foetus.* The metabolism of the mother in pregnancy is altered to create an environment which is favourable to the foetus. These changes are most evident in the maternal arterial blood which circulates through the choriodecidual space. Maternal hyperventilation, for example, which is normal in pregnancy, lowers the PCO_2 in the maternal arterial blood. The lowered partial pressure of CO_2 in the blood on the maternal side of the placenta then facilitates the transfer of CO_2 from the foetus to the mother (Prystowsky *et al.* 1961).

At the same time the metabolic activity of the maternal tissues generally is dampened and there is a generalized relaxation of the smooth muscles of all the organs of the body (Hytten & Leitch 1964). These authors have suggested that instead of preserving the 'milieu interior, which is the most common endeavour of the body in all other situations, the physiological adaptations in the mother create a constantly changing environ-ment appropriate to the successive changes of pregnancy. The metabolism of the mother is thus adapted in pregnancy to create the conditions most favourable for the growth and development of the foetus.

The changes in the mother in pregnancy can be divided into:

(a) The changes in the genital tract to accommodate the growing foetus and to prepare for labour.
(b) The general structural changes in the mother.
(c) The physiological changes in the mother.

THE CHANGES IN THE GENITAL TRACT

Ovary

Marked positional changes of the ovary occur during pregnancy; instead of being horizontal, the long axis of each ovary becomes vertical. The ovary also becomes hyperaemic and the ovarian blood vessels enlarge to an enormous size. Further important changes occur in the corpus luteum, the stroma and the function of the ovary in pregnancy.

CORPUS LUTEUM

The ovarian changes associated with pregnancy properly begin with the alteration of the graafian follicle to form a corpus luteum. The corpus luteum begins to regress about the eighth day of its existence. By the twelfth day, however, the secretion of chorionic gonadotrophin into the blood stream by the syncytiotrophoblast is sufficient to halt the regression of the corpus luteum. Instead of shrinking, as it normally does at the end of the menstrual cycle, the corpus luteum grows and develops and becomes 'the corpus luteum of pregnancy'. At approximately the eighth week, corresponding with the increased secretion of chorionic gonadotrophin by the placenta, the corpus luteum undergoes a sudden enlargement and approximately doubles its size. After a further 2 weeks, however, once the peak of chorionic gonadotrophin is passed, the corpus luteum undergoes marked regression.

At the time of its greatest development the corpus luteum occupies at least a third of the entire ovary, but at term it is only half this size (Nelson & Greene 1953). The corpus luteum during the first half of pregnancy is composed almost entirely of granulosa lutein cells. The theca lutein cells reach their maximum development early on in pregnancy around the eighth to the tenth week, and disappear completely in the second half of pregnancy. The granulosa lutein cells contain lipoid vacuoles, colloid droplets and secretory granules. The secretory granules are present in nearly one-third of the cells up to the twenty-fourth week but disappear almost completely by term.

The corpus luteum of pregnancy is surrounded by a capsule of connective tissue containing dilated lymph vessels and blood vessels which are very prominent and engorged in early pregnancy. In the second half of pregnancy the capsule thickens, the vessels shrink and the theca lutein cells disappear (Gillman & Stein 1941).

STROMA AND FOLLICLES

Ovulation ceases during pregnancy but many follicles become temporarily active. The graafian follicles which develop at the beginning of the menstrual cycle but do not reach full maturity undergo atresia. Though the ova themselves in these follicles undergo cytolysis, the theca lutein cells of the follicles proliferate in pregnancy. These theca lutein cells, which are smaller, stain more deeply and have larger nuclei than the granulosa lutein cells, multiply to form a thick tunic around each atretic follicle. These masses of cells sometimes appear to lose their connection with the follicle, and have then been termed 'the interstitial glands of pregnancy'. Later, however, these thecal cells undergo fatty and hyaline degeneration and form irregular hyaline bodies indistinguishable from corpora albicantia.

Another change which is frequently noted on the surface of the ovary is a decidua-like reaction very similar to that seen in the endometrial stroma. The fibroblasts or mesenchymal cells underlying the germinal epithelium develop into decidual cells. This decidual reaction appears as velvety, reddish, convoluted ridges which bleed easily on touch and resemble freshly torn adhesions (Israel *et al.* 1954). Occasionally, similar decidual reactions are seen on the posterior surface of the uterus, the uterosacral ligaments, the round and broad ligaments and even on extrapelvic abdominal organs (Nelson & Greene 1953).

OVARIAN FUNCTION IN PREGNANCY

In early pregnancy up to 10 weeks the corpus luteum is probably an active and vital organ, producing oestrogen and progesterone which assists in ensuring the continuation of pregnancy and producing many of the secondary changes in pregnancy. Removal of the corpus luteum in early pregnancy in the human, however, produces abortion in only 10–20% of pregnancies (Hall 1955). The human placenta secretes, soon after implantation, enough progesterone for the maintenance of pregnancy. The corpus luteum, though necessary for implantation in the human being, is not required for pregnancy beyond the earliest stages. The continued development of the corpus luteum up to the tenth week is probably due to the secretion of chorionic gonadotrophin by the placenta. In the human, the persistence of the corpus luteum probably represents an additional safety mechanism to protect the pregnancy in the crucial period at the onset of steroid secretion by the placenta.

Fallopian tube

During pregnancy the fallopian tubes are pulled upwards out of the pelvis by the growth of the uterus. The tubes thus become stretched or suspended and come to lie almost vertically alongside the uterus, and are at the same time displaced laterally by the enlarging body of the uterus. There is, however, a disproportionate growth of the fundus of the uterus, so that in the later months of pregnancy the insertions of fallopian tubes and round ligaments are approximately half-way up the uterus.

The fallopian tubes themselves are hyperaemic and congested, though, surprisingly, there is little or no hypertrophy of the muscle of the tube in pregnancy. The epithelium is, moreover, flattened, and on microscopic examination the surface of the epithelium is irregular, due to the bulging up of the cytoplasmic processes on the non-ciliated cells (Snyder 1924). (Fig. 9.1.)

contracts rhythmically, whereas the cervix dilates to allow the passage and expulsion of the foetus and products of conception. After pregnancy, the corpus and cervix return, over a period of several weeks, to more or less their

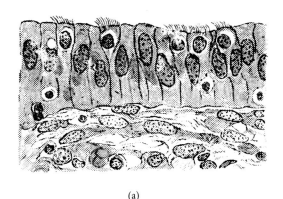

(a)

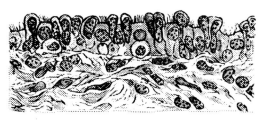

(b)

Fig. 9.1. Tubal epithelium. (a) In the mid-interval period of the menstrual cycle the tubal epithelium is tall, the ciliated cells are broad and the non-ciliated cells are narrow, closely packed and have flattened surfaces on line with surface of ciliated cells. (b) In late pregnancy the epithelium is low and irregular due to bulging of the cytoplasmic processes of the non-ciliated cells. (From Snyder (1924), by courtesy of the Editor of *Bulletin of the Johns Hopkins Hospital*.)

Uterus

The changes which occur in the uterus during pregnancy are truly remarkable. In addition to the alteration in size, shape, position and consistency which are related to the changing nature of its contents, there are also changes in its muscular arrangement, physiological behaviour and blood supply. The two parts of the uterus, the corpus and the cervix, react very differently to pregnancy and must be considered separately. The corpus, or body, of the uterus is composed essentially of muscle and undergoes growth; it is subject to distension. The cervix is composed essentially of connective tissue and, although it softens, it maintains its continuity as a relatively firm, closed, fibrous ring until the patient goes into labour. The corpus thus serves to contain the growing foetus and the products of conception, the cervix to retain them within the uterus during pregnancy. In labour the corpus

pre-pregnancy state (this period is termed the puerperium).

The corpus of the uterus

The changes in the corpus of the uterus in pregnancy may be considered under the changes in

(1) size, shape, position and consistency;
(2) muscle growth, changes in contractility and nerve supply;
(3) blood vessels, blood flow and oxygen consumption.

(1) SIZE, SHAPE, POSITION AND CONSISTENCY OF THE UTERUS

(a) *Changes in size of the uterus*

As pregnancy advances, the uterus expands rapidly to accommodate the growing products of conception. From an organ measuring approximately 7·5 × 5 × 2·5 cm and a capacity of 4 ml, it expands to an organ which at term measures 28 × 24 × 21 cm and has a capacity of 4,000 ml or thereabouts. The wall of the uterus, which is about 8 mm thick before pregnancy, grows to about 25 mm in thickness by the twelfth week. After this time, however, when the decidua capsularis fuses with the decidua vera, the wall of the uterus becomes progressively thinner as the amniotic cavity increases in size (Gillespie 1950). By the end of pregnancy the uterine wall is only 5–10 mm in thickness, though it is strong enough to develop intra-uterine pressures of 60 mmHg or so in normal labour and up to 300 mmHg in abnormal labour and the puerperium (Hendricks *et al.* 1962).

of the uterus rapidly becomes progressively more spheroid as the gestation sac enlarges, until by the twelfth week the sac completely fills the uterine cavity. Thereafter the uterus increases more rapidly in length as the foetus elongates, and its shape becomes increasingly more sac-like until term (Gillespie 1950). (Fig. 9.2).

The position of the uterus also alters as it becomes larger. Initially it is usually anteverted and anteflexed. From the twelfth week onwards it is too large to remain wholly within the pelvis, and the fundus of the uterus rises up into the abdomen. As it enlarges it progressively displaces the intestines to the sides of the abdomen and comes into contact with the anterior abdominal wall, exerting increasing pressure on the an-

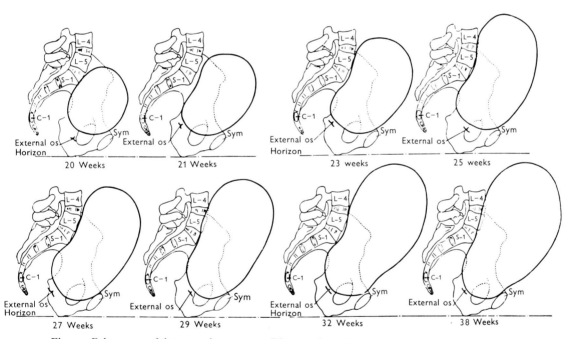

Fig. 9.2. Enlargement of the uterus in pregnancy. Diagrams drawn from lateral radiographs showing rapid elongation of uterus from twentieth to thirty-second week and increase in anteroposterior diameter thereafter. (Gillespie 1950.)

(b) *Shape and position of the uterus*

As the uterus increases in size it also changes in shape. For the first few weeks of pregnancy it retains its original 'pear' shape, but the body

terior abdominal wall and all the abdominal contents. At the same time, tension is increasingly placed on the round ligaments, which become stretched, and the broad ligaments, which 'open out'.

The mobility of the uterus depends upon the laxity of the abdominal wall, which is generally tense in nulliparae and increases in laxity in successive pregnancies in multiparae. When a woman in late pregnancy stands upright the uterus falls forwards, particularly in multi-parae [Fig. 9.3(a)]. In this position the long axis of the

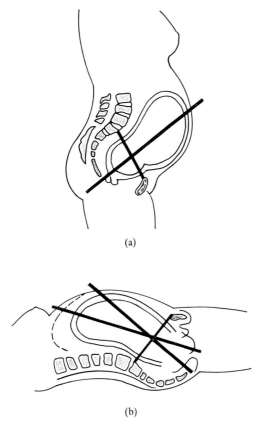

(a)

(b)

Fig. 9.3. Relation of long axis of uterus to axis of inlet in primigravida. (a) Standing; (b) lying flat.

uterus is in the same axis as the upper strait of the pelvis. When upright the fundus of the uterus rests on the anterior abdominal wall which, if it is very stretched and the rectus abdominis muscles are widely separated, may allow the fundus to bulge through, resulting in a *pendulous abdomen or herniation of the gravid uterus.*

When a woman lies supine on her back the uterus falls backwards and rests upon the vertebral column [Fig. 9.3(b)] and may compress the inferior vena cava, causing a reduction in venous return, cardiac output and blood pressure (Kerr 1968).

As the uterus grows up into the abdominal cavity it also rotates in its long axis usually to the right. This is attributed to the presence of the spinal column and sigmoid colon and rectum. This dextrorotation of the uterus is of considerable practical importance at Caesarean section.

(c) *Consistency of the uterus*

Pregnancy causes a progressive softening of the uterus starting with the isthmus or lower part of the body. This softening of the isthmus while the cervix and fundus of the uterus are still firm is most noticeable at the tenth week of pregnancy, and gives rise to Hegar's sign. After this time the cervix and fundus of the uterus become progressively softer, and the softening is said to be more marked over the site of implantation of the placenta and to be associated with the not infrequent asymmetrical growth of the uterus. After the twenty-fourth week the uterine wall is so soft that parts of the foetus may be palpated with ease.

(2) MUSCLE GROWTH, CHANGES IN CONTRACTILITY AND NERVE SUPPLY IN PREGNANCY

(a) *Muscle growth and arrangement of fibres*

In addition to alteration in size and shape, the mass of the uterus is greatly increased in pregnancy. The weight increases from 30–60 g before pregnancy to 750–1,000 g at term (Gillespie 1950). The increase in mass is due to the growth of the endometrium, hypertrophy and hyperplasia of the uterine muscle and connective tissue, and increase in size and number of blood vessels and other tissues. Most of this enormous growth is due to proliferation of the myometrium. In the first trimester there is actual hyperplasia of the muscle cells, and mitotic figures are common. Most of the increase is, however, due to hypertrophy of the muscle which occurs in the second and, to a lesser extent, the third, trimester. The individual muscle cells increase in length from 50 to 200–600 μm and grow in volume by 17 to 40 times their non-pregnant size (Stieve 1932) Fig. 9.4.

The arrangement of the muscle fibres in the uterus, both in the non-pregnant and pregnant uterus, has been studied for over 100 years or more (Helie 1864). The two chief systems of muscular fasiculi in the non-pregnant uterus result from the fusion of the two Mullerian ducts. The uterus consists of an interlacing

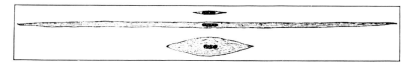

Fig. 9.4. Muscle fibres from normal non-pregnant, pregnant and puerperal uterus (Stieve 1926).

The stimulus for this growth is chiefly oestrogen and, perhaps, progesterone. Later in pregnancy the distension of the uterus and stretching of the muscle play an important role (Wood 1964). Distension is, however, by no means an essential stimulus in early pregnancy, as evidenced by the considerable enlargement of the uterus which occurs in extra-uterine pregnancy. It has been suggested that hyperplasia is primarily due to oestrogen and that as the progesterone levels increase this inhibits the hyperplasia but enhances the hypertrophy of the uterine muscle fibres.

complex of muscle fibres in which the fibres, in general, run spirally and have a bilateral symmetrical arrangement. The fibres tend to cross each other at right-angles in the fundus but obtusely in the lower segment. In pregnancy the fibres of the upper segment preserve their original arrangement, in contrast to the fibres of the lower segment which are drawn up so that the spirals adopt a more vertical course, like that of a spiral staircase (Goerttler 1930) Fig. 9.5.

The muscle fibres composing the uterine wall in pregnancy overlap one another, forming a large number of interlacing muscular lamellae,

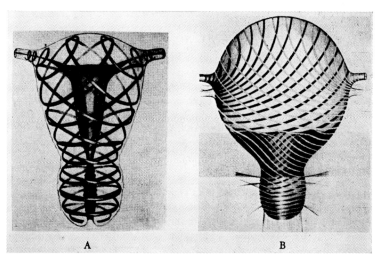

Fig. 9.5. Architecture of uterus showing arrangement of muscle fibres. (A) Non-pregnant; (B) pregnant (Goerttler 1930).

which are interconnected by short, muscular processes and are arranged in three rather indefinite strata or layers. These are:

(1) *A thin external layer* in which the muscle bundles are arranged longitudinally and arch over the fundus like a hood and extend into the round and other uterine ligaments.

(2) *A thick middle layer* of interlacing bundles, each bundle running spirally and downwards from outwards to inwards and crossing over each other at obtuse angles. These fibres form a dense network which is perforated by the spiral arterioles and other vessels. This layer provides the main muscle mass and force of the uterine contractions. It also compresses the blood vessels, forming 'living ligatures' and preventing haemorrhage when the uterus contracts and retracts after delivery.

(3) *A thin internal layer* next to the endometrium in which the fibres run obliquely upwards to the fundus and form sphincters encircling the tubal orifices and the internal os.

In addition to the changes in muscle fibres, there is a hyperplasia and hypertrophy of the connective tissue, and particularly of the elastic fibres, in pregnancy. There is a marked increase in the elastic fibres around the arteries and in the connective tissue between the muscle bundles, particularly in the external muscle layer. This increase in elastic and fibrous tissue strengthens the uterine wall, particularly in the latter part of pregnancy when the muscle elements have ceased to develop.

(b) *Changes in contractility of the uterus in pregnancy*

The intermittent contractions of the uterus which occur during the menstrual cycle and are noted especially at ovulation and during menstruation continue throughout pregnancy. The contractions are of two basic types, depending upon whether oestrogen or progesterone has a predominating effect on the uterus.

(A) *Oestrogen effect—A waves.* During the follicular phase of the menstrual cycle, when the myometrium is under the influence of oestrogen, the spontaneous activity of the uterus takes the form of contractions of low amplitude (0·2 mmHg intra-uterine pressure), and high frequency (120 per hour), and short duration (30 sec), which are known as A waves. At midcycle, corresponding with the peak of oestrogen secretion at ovulation, the frequency of the A waves increases to 240 per hour. If ovulation fails to occur and a corpus luteum is not found this pattern of spontaneous uterine activity continues throughout the cycle (Garrett 1959).

(B) *Progestogen effect—B waves.* If ovulation occurs the character of the uterine contraction changes. The contractions increase in amplitude (up to 10 times), become less frequent (30 per hour), and of longer duration (2 min), and are known as B waves (Fig. 9.6).

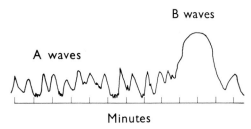

Fig. 9.6. Uterine contractions recorded by external tocography showing A and B waves (Carey 1963).

This change in behaviour and contractility of the myometrium is believed to be due to the increased secretion of progesterone, which exerts a predominating effect on the uterus in the second half of the normal ovulatory menstrual cycle. Although the secretion of progesterone drops, however, before the onset of menstruation the B wave actively continues and is maximal during menstruation and does not disappear completely until the tenth day of the next menstrual cycle.

During pregnancy from the twelfth to the fourteenth week the uterus may be felt to contract either on bimanual examination, or later, through the abdominal wall. The previously relaxed uterus becomes hard for a few minutes and the intra-uterine pressure rises to 8 cm of water or more. These contractions (known as Braxton Hicks's contractions) have been known for over

100 years or more and are characteristically sporadic, arrhythmic and infrequent until the last months of pregnancy. As pregnancy approaches term their frequency increases. They differ from the contractions of true labour only in that they are not regular and rhythmic and are not accompanied by dilatation of the cervix— and that the contractions of labour are usually accompanied by pain.

On investigation by tocodynamometry and other techniques it has been shown that during pregnancy both A and B types of uterine contractions occur (Carey 1963). For the first 30 weeks A waves occur on an average of once a minute with a rise of intra-uterine pressure of 1–2 mmHg, while the B waves (Braxton Hicks's contractions) occur on an average of once an hour with a rise of intra-uterine pressure of 10–15 mmHg. During mid-pregnancy there is a decreased uterine tone and a low level of spontaneous myometrial activity, the B waves producing rises of only 5 mmHg in intra-uterine pressure, and high doses of oxytocin are required to produce uterine contractions, which are then associated with a rise in uterine tone (Bengtson & Csapo 1962).

Over the last 10 weeks of pregnancy the B waves increase in frequency and amplitude, spread to larger areas of the uterus and have a more regular rhythm. The small, localized, uncoordinate A waves of early pregnancy tend to disappear. This period of increasing uterine activity after the thirtieth week has been designated 'Prelabour' by Caldeyro-Barcia & Poseiro (1959), and is probably one of the main factors causing the progressive 'ripening' of the cervix characteristic of late pregnancy. This period of increasing spontaneous activity is accompanied by an increasing sensitivity to oxytocin (Csapo & Sauvage 1969).

There is no clear-cut demarcation between the type of uterine activity of late pregnancy and that of early labour. There is only a gradual and progressive transition in the characteristics of the uterine contractions and in the changes in the lower uterine segment and cervix.

The initiation of labour is due to an acceleration and evolution of uterine activity, rather than some new regulatory process or stimulus (Csapo

& Wood 1968). The time of the onset of labour cannot be precisely defined. The commonly accepted clinical practice of timing the onset of labour from the beginning of regular uterine contractions may be fallacious. There is much to commend the suggestion of Caldeyro-Barcia (1965) that clinical labour should be defined as starting when the dilatation of the cervix progresses beyond 2 cm. This, admittedly, is an arbitrary point, but coincides fairly precisely with the onset of the active phase of the dilatation of the cervix, as shown in the cervical dilatation time-curves of Friedman (1956).

The increase in size and contractility of the muscle fibre as pregnancy progresses is due to the action of oestrogen and to the stretching (Csapo et al. 1965). There is an increase in actomyosin, ATP and enzyme concentration in the muscle cells, with a change in the ionic gradients and resting potential across the cell membrane. Oestrogen lowers the resting potential and makes the muscle more excitable, but progesterone tends to raise the membrane potential. The A waves are an expression of the ceaseless myogenic activity of the individual uterine muscle fibres and are primarily the effect of the increased oestrogen secretion in pregnancy. The B waves, which are present in late pregnancy, labour and the puerperium, are probably a result of the action of progesterone on the oestrogen-primed uterus. B waves differ fundamentally from A waves in that B waves involve the whole uterus and contract as one structure in peristaltic-like waves. Garrett (1959) has suggested that under the influence of progesterone the uterus behaves as one large syncytium.

The action of oxytocin and other drugs is interesting in that oxytocin has a marked action on B waves, increasing their frequency and amplitude, but has only a little effect on A waves. Ergometrine similarly increases the frequency of B waves and in large doses increases the uterine tone but has little effect on A waves. Adrenaline and noradrenaline, on the other hand, stimulate A waves and noradrenaline also stimulates B waves, whereas adrenaline actively inhibits B waves (Garrett & Moir 1958). The control of myometrial activity in pregnancy and labour, with particular reference to the factors determining onset of labour, and the effect of oxytocin and other agents on the uterus, has recently been comprehensively reviewed by Wood (1969).

(c) *The nerve supply to the uterus in pregnancy*

With the observation that paraplegic patients go into labour and that the uterus contracts normally, albeit painlessly, it has been assumed that the nervous system has little functional significance in pregnancy and labour. There is, however, a profuse nerve supply from the autonomic and central nervous system which undergoes marked hypertrophy in pregnancy, as exemplified by the increase in size of Frankenhäuser's ganglion from $2 \times 2 \cdot 5$ cm to $3 \cdot 5 \times 6$ cm.

The sensory fibres arise from the spinal cord through the sacral nerves and are distributed via Frankenhauser's ganglion. So far as is known, however, there are no sensory receptors in the uterus except the cervix, where various pacinian-type structures have been found. The only pain to arise from the body of the uterus is thought to be ischaemic in origin and to be conducted via the sympathetic nervous system.

Evidence is accumulating that motor fibres from the autonomic system may have some functional significance in the human uterus (Wood 1969). Noradrenergic nerves supplying smooth-muscle fibres in the myometrium have been demonstrated, and field stimulation and other characteristics suggest that they are of sympathetic origin (Nakanshi *et al.* 1969). Stimulation of the hypogastric nerve causes an increase in contractility in the luteal phase of the menstrual cycle and in early pregnancy (Alvarez *et al.* 1969).

In the non-pregnant uterus, noradrenergic nerves are distributed mainly to the cervix and lower part of the uterine body. Mann (1963) has shown that the isthmus of the uterus narrows during the luteal phase and opens during menstruation. The presence of the noradrenergic nerve fibres suggests that this narrowing may be due to local muscle activity resulting from nervous stimulation. Wood (1969) has suggested that this narrowing of the isthmus in the late menstrual cycle may be important in nidation and that, by closing off the lower half of the uterus,

it may help to ensure that the implantation of the fertilized ovum occurs in the fundus of the uterus. Implantation in the isthmus would result in abortion or placenta praevia.

In pregnancy, the distribution of the noradrenergic nerves alters and there is a relative denervation of the isthmus. The noradrenergic nerves supplying the smooth muscle become sparser, so that the stimulating effect of neural noradrenaline is reduced (Nakanishi *et al.* 1969). This decrease in neural noradrenaline, coupled with the increase in circulating adrenaline, results in an inhibition of uterine contractility (Wansborough *et al.* 1967). These findings suggest that the autonomic nervous system may have an important function in the control of the site of implantation and in the continuation of pregnancy.

(3) BLOOD VESSELS, BLOOD FLOW AND OXYGEN CONSUMPTION OF THE UTERUS IN PREGNANCY

(a) *Changes in uterine blood vessels in pregnancy*

The increase in the mass of the uterus, the development of the placenta and the progressive increase in blood flow through the placenta cause such an increase in the vascular system of the uterus that at term the uterus and associated blood vessels contain one-sixth or more of the total blood volume of the mother.

The uterine, ovarian and superior vesical arteries increase in diameter and length. The branches of the main vessels increase in number and size. The enlarged branches of the uterine artery are extensively convoluted and extend over the fundus and radially around the uterus, anastomosing freely in the mid-line. These branches penetrate the uterine wall obliquely inward toward the middle layer of the uterus, where they ramify in a plane parallel to the surface and are known as arcuate arteries. From these arcuate arteries radial branches, which are closely coiled and are known as *coiled arteries*, run in at right-angles toward the endometrium and branch to form the *spiral arterioles*. The spiral arterioles play an important part in the formation of the placenta and constitute the maternal arterial supply to the placenta. As pregnancy proceeds, the circulation to the placenta progressively increases, while that to the remainder of the uterus is relatively diminished (Kearns 1939).

Almost as impressive as the changes in the arteries are the changes in the veins, which follow a similar course to the arteries. The veins empty into plexuses at the side of the uterus in the medial part of the broad ligaments. The uterine and pelvic veins do not have a supportive fascial sheath such as is found in the veins of the arms and the legs. They can therefore dilate more easily and it is thought that the pampiniform plexuses of the broad ligament perform an important function and act as a reservoir when blood is forced out of the placenta, for example during a uterine contraction. It has been estimated that the capacity of the veins and the venouses increase more than 60-fold by the thirty-sixth week of pregnancy.

The spiral arterioles undergo important changes in pregnancy. In the first few weeks they grow towards the uterine lumen and become increasingly coiled. By mid-pregnancy this growth has stopped, and with the increase in size of the uterus the coils later become progressively 'paid out'. At the same time the number of arterioles communicating with the intervillous space decreases. These remaining arterioles are much straighter and have only an occasional right-angled bend (Ramsay 1949). Concomitant histological changes occur. During the early weeks the cells lining the arterioles pile up into several layers, sometimes almost occluding the lumen. This is most pronounced where the vessels enter the intervillous space. This external proliferation is followed later in pregnancy by medial and adventitial changes reminiscent of arteriosclerosis. These changes begin near the placenta and progress outwards, until by the the third trimester they may be seen in the arcuate arteries.

The spiral nature of the arterioles and the intimal fibrosis may be important factors limiting blood loss when the placenta separates at delivery. The intimal and other changes in the spiral arterioles are much more marked in pre-eclampsia and may be an important part of the pathogenesis of 'placental insufficiency'.

(b) *Uterine blood flow and oxygen consumption in pregnancy*

The growth and function of the uterus and the transport of all the essential elements for the growth and development of the foetus depend upon adequacy of the uterine blood flow and placental circulation. Our knowledge of the changes in blood flow in the uterus and placenta, however, leaves a great deal to be desired. A variety of methods have been used to measure the uterine blood flow but, owing to the technical difficulties of the various methods and the complexity of the uterine vascular system with uterine and ovarian arteries and veins on both sides and numerous anastomoses, all the results so far obtained can only be regarded as a very general indication of changes of flow. With present techniques it is also not possible to determine how much of the total uterine blood flow passes through the placental circulation and how much through the myometrium.

It has been estimated (Assali et al. 1960) that the total uterine blood flow increases from approximately 50 ml at 10 weeks to 185 ml/min at 28 weeks, and reaches a maximum of 500–700 ml/min at term. When expressed in terms of unit weight the uterine blood flow at term is of the order 100–150 ml/min/hg tissue (uterus, placenta and foetus) (Dawes 1968). It is assumed that the major increment in blood flow throughout gestation is through the intervillous space of the placenta, though there is no information regarding the distribution between myometrium and placenta at the various stages of pregnancy.

The effect of uterine contractions on uterine blood flow is of major importance for the foetus and there is good evidence that uterine contractions sufficient to cause a rise in uterine pressure of 20–30 mmHg cause a decrease of 10–50% in total uterine blood flow (Ahlquist 1950). The foetus nevertheless rarely seems to be compromised unless the uterus undergoes tetanic contraction when the blood falls over 50% (Assali et al. 1958).

Estimates of oxygen consumption are perhaps even less reliable than those of blood flow, but from the available literature Hytten & Leitch

(1964) have estimated that the average total oxygen consumption at term is as follows:

Foetus	12 ml/m
Placenta	3·7 ml/m
Uterus	3·3 ml/m
Total	19 ml/m

If it is assumed that maternal blood O_2 content is reduced on average 5 ml/100 ml blood on passage through the uterus then the total uterine blood flow necessary to supply 19 ml/m is approximately 400 ml/m, which is well within the observed total uterine blood flow at term.

Isthmus

The isthmus is, strictly, part of the body of the uterus and is defined as that portion of the uterus which joins the dense connective tissue of the cervix to the muscle fibres of the corpus. The anatomical boundaries of this zone are not well defined but its upper limit is usually considered as the constriction of the uterine cavity which marks the lower boundary of the corpus (the anatomical internal os) and its lower limit as the junction of the flattened and attenuated endometrium of the isthmus and the mucus-secreting columnar epithelium of the cervix (the histological internal os). Because the mucus-secreting epithelium of the endocervix inter-

mingles with the non-mucus-secreting glands of the isthmus, often over a relatively wide area, the lower boundary of the isthmus in particular is often ill defined (Fig. 9.7).

The isthmus of the uterus nevertheless undergoes important structural, and probably functional, changes in pregnancy. During the first trimester it hypertrophies and elongates to three times its original length. At the same time it becomes soft and extremely compressible.

This softening is so great that on bimanual examination at the tenth to twelfth week it feels as though the body of the uterus and the cervix are separate entities (Hegar's sign of pregnancy). As the gestation grows after the twelfth week the isthmus progressively opens out from above downwards and becomes shorter. This opening out continues until it is checked by the dense connective-tissue ring of the cervix. At this stage the entire isthmical canal has become incorporated in the general uterine cavity and the isthmus as such no longer exists (Danforth 1950). The walls of the isthmus thus become incorporated into, and form part of, the lower segment of the uterus. Whether it necessarily forms the whole of the lower uterine segment, however, is a matter for debate. Reynolds & Danforth (1966) have logically, and with good evidence, defined the lower uterine segment as simply that part of the body of the uterus which undergoes

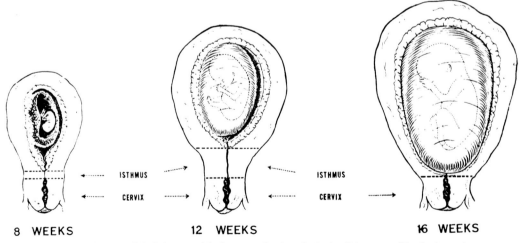

Fig. 9.7. Growth of the isthmus and its incorporation into the body of the uterus (Danforth 1950).

circumferential dilatation, whether this be in pregnancy as part of the preparation for labour, or in labour itself.

Functionally, the region of the isthmus may be of considerable importance, as the muscle fibres are arranged circularly or in a close spiral, which becomes drawn out in later pregnancy. Asplund (1952) and Youssef (1958) have presented evidence that this region functions as a true sphincter, contracting during the second half of the menstrual cycle and early pregnancy, under the influence of progesterone, and opening out at menstruation and the first half of the menstrual cycle. This sphincteric action may be of importance in helping to retain the ovum and growing foetus within the uterus and ensuring its implantation in the fundus.

Cervix

The cervix undergoes profound changes in pregnancy which assist in retaining the conceptus and maintaining a barrier between it and the vagina and at the same time enabling the cervix to dilate during labour to allow the passage of the fully developed foetus. Clinically, the cervix becomes progressively softer and blue in colour, and this constitutes one of the characteristic signs of pregnancy from the eighth week onwards.

The changes in the cervix as a result of pregnancy begin very early, even before they are clinically discernible, and affect all its components. The blood and lymph vessels increase in number and size and the connective tissue increases and alters in character. Later, the glands undergo marked proliferation so that at the end of pregnancy the mucosa is approximately one-half of the entire mass of the cervix.

(1) *Changes in stroma of cervix*

Apart from the increased vascularity and oedema, there are fundamental changes in the connective tissue of the cervix, which undergoes hyperplasia and hypertrophy. More important, however, is the loosening and dissociating of the fibrils, which cause the softening and permit the stretching and dilation of the cervix. There is a decreased amount of collagen, as evidenced by the decrease

in hydroxyproline content (Harkness *et al.* 1959) and an alteration in ground structure which binds the collagen fibres. Prior to labour, the collagen fibres are large, oedematous and loosened, but after delivery become smaller and highly branched (Danforth 1964).

(2) *Changes in epithelium and cervical glands*

The epithelium of the cervix and cervical canal, both squamous and columnar, is in a state of hyperactivity, probably as a result of the hormonal stimulation of pregnancy.

There is hyperactivity of the squamous epithelium of the portio vaginalis, which may show deviations from the normal, including:

(a) *basal-cell hyperactivity*, with irregularities in size, shape, staining and number of mitoses in the basal cells;

(b) *mid-zone hyperplasia*, with a high proportion of large, hyperchromatic, 'active' nuclei;

(c) *epithelial buds* extending into the underlying stroma with submucosal infiltration of lymphocytes and plasma cells;

(d) *occasional atypical mitotic figures*, particularly near the squamocolumnar junction.

If present in marked degree these normal pregnancy changes may resemble carcinoma *in situ*, but it is not thought that pregnancy *per se* is a cause of carcinoma *in situ* (Fluhmann 1961). It may, however, require repeated investigation after pregnancy by cervical cytology or biopsy to determine the ultimate significance of the changes.

Similar hyperactivity occurs in the columnar epithelium. The columnar cells are tall with nuclei elevated above the base and as a result of marked proliferation tend to become heaped up and form small projections. Squamous metaplasia, epidermidization, reserve-cell hyperplasia, so-called 'squamocolumnar prosoplasia' where the cells enclose clear vacuoles and produce mucus are common, particularly at the squamocolumnar junction or transitory zone, and more especially in cervical erosions, where they represent an attempt of the squamous epithelium to cover the exposed columnar

mucosa. The growth of the columnar epithelium
is so extensive in pregnancy that the endocervical
mucosa doubles in thickness from an average of
2·3 m to 4·6 m as measured in fixed histological
specimens (Fig. 9.8).

Fluhmann (1961) has claimed that the endocervix is not composed of compound racemose
glands as has been taught but instead represents
a vast accumulation of clefts running in all
directions and varying greatly in size, depth and
construction. In pregnancy, these clefts deepen
and undergo secondary changes, including the
formation of

(a) channels or tunnels which run parallel to
    the surface;
(b) secondary folds;
(c) finger-like projections or septa with spaces
    in between which are filled and distended
    with mucus.

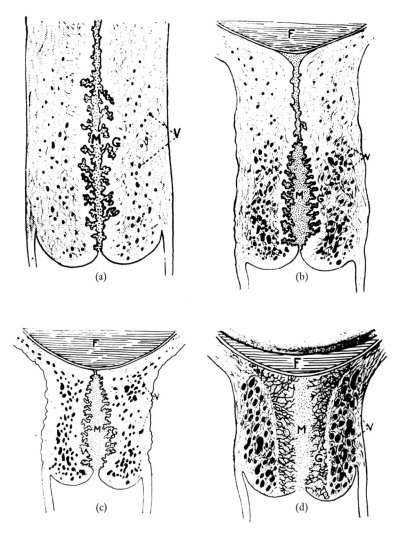

Fig. 9.8. Section through normal cervix. (a) Non-pregnant; (b) at second month; (c) at third month; (d) at term
(Stieve 1925).

These changes may be so marked in late pregnancy that the cervix macroscopically appears to be filled with a honeycomb-like structure centred around the cervical canal.

This superabundant growth of endocervical tissue may protrude from the endocervical canal, producing a physiological eversion of the cervix. At the same time, under the influence of the oestrogen stimulation of pregnancy there is extensive growth of the endocervical columnar epithelium at the squamocolumnar junction at the expense of the squamous epithelium, so that the squamocolumnar junction or transitional zone moves peripherally. This peripheral displacement of the squamocolumnar junction with the physiological eversion of the cervix and prolapse of the mucosa exposes the columnar epithelium, producing a so-called 'cervical erosion' (a misnomer) with its characteristic fiery-red 'velvety' appearance. Erosion of the cervix, which is present in more than 50% of women at term and over 80% in the puerperium, is so common in pregnancy as to be regarded as physiological and not pathological. It is probable that the majority of cervical erosions arise physiologically from the increased secretion of oestrogen either in the newborn, puberty or in pregnancy (Hellmann et al. 1950).

(3) Cervical secretions

In pregnancy the cervical mucus becomes thick, viscous and opaque and fills the honeycomb of the endocervix to form the so-called 'mucous plug of pregnancy'. At the same time there is a considerable increase in the mucous discharge from the cervix, which may be so profuse as to constitute a considerable nuisance to the patient. Cervical mucus in pregnancy characteristically has an abundance of leucocytes, cervical epithelial and vaginal cells. It is thought that the cervical secretion and the mucous plug act as an important antibacterial and mechanical barrier to the uterine cavity.

'Ferning', which normally occurs on drying of cervical mucus in patients in whom the effect of oestrogen as compared with progesterone predominates, is characteristically absent in pregnancy; in fact, if ferning is present in the first 14 weeks of pregnancy it is thought to be pathological and indicative of progesterone deficiency, as about 50% of patients abort (Ullery & Shabanah 1957).

Vagina, vulva and pelvic floor

The vagina, vulva and pelvic floor, like all other pelvic organs, undergo a profound increase in vascularity. Within a short time after the onset of pregnancy the veins become enlarged and engorged and the blood they contain is relatively deoxygenated. By the sixth to the eighth week the vagina appears cyanotic and takes on a characteristic violet, purple or deep-vein wine colour, which was previously known as Chadwick's sign of pregnancy. The vulva becomes similarly engorged and oedematous and the dilated vessels may become so large, particularly in nulliparae, as to constitute vulvar varices. These varices usually disappear completely when pregnancy is over, sometimes even before the patient leaves the delivery room.

The whole pelvic floor, including the perineum and the perineal and levator ani muscles, undergo the typical pregnancy changes, with increase in vascularity and oedema, hypertrophy of the muscles and loosening of the connective tissue. The pelvic floor thus becomes more distensible and adapted to meet the needs of pregnancy and labour.

VAGINA

The vagina increases in capacity and length by true hypertrophy and hyperplasia. The elastic fibres increase, the muscular fibres hypertrophy and the connective tissues undergo a gradual loosening similar to that which occurs in the cervix. Because of the loosening and hypertrophy, the vagina and all its supporting structures become progressively more relaxed and distensible, so that at term the vagina can readily accommodate the passage of the foetal head and trunk without rupturing. The upper part of the vagina, in particular, enlarges and is drawn up as the uterus ascends out of the pelvis as pregnancy advances. When the foetal head enters the pelvis, however, in the last month of pregnancy or in labour, the vagina may be pushed down and is sometimes thrown into horizontal circular folds. This may cause the lower part of the anterior vaginal wall to protrude to some extent through the vulval opening.

The epithelium of the vagina undergoes marked hypertrophy and hyperplasia and at term may be 500 μm or more thick. The vaginal rugae deepen and the papillae enlarge, so that the surface of the epithelium becomes rough and irregular, and presents and has a 'fine-hobnailed appearance'. The most important change in the epithelium, however, occurs in the cells of the middle layer. These cells multiply, enlarge and become filled with vacuoles, which contain glycogen. With the increased activity of the epithelium these cells quickly reach the surface and are desquamated. The cells disintegrate, releasing the glycogen, which is converted by Doederlein's bacilli (*Lactobacillus acidophilus*) into lactic acid. This results in an increasingly

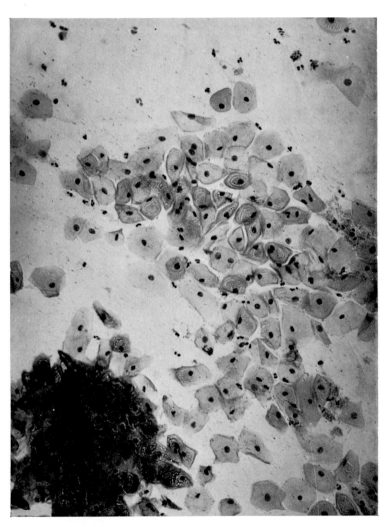

Fig. 9.9. Vaginal smear taken during pregnancy (low power).

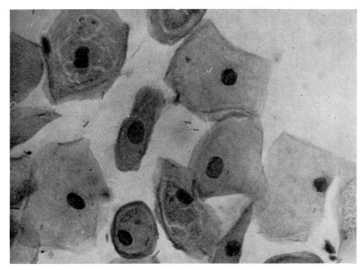

Fig. 9.10. Vaginal smear taken during pregnancy (high power).

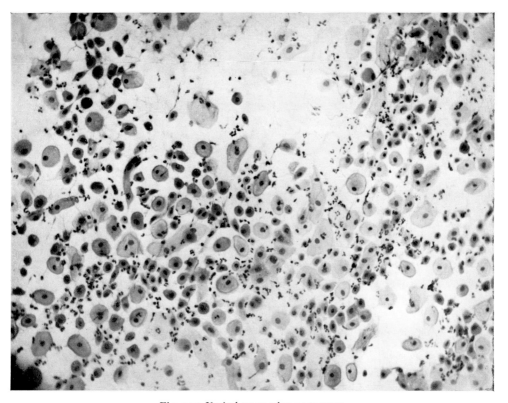

Fig. 9.11. Vaginal smear taken postpartum.

profuse, thick, white, highly acid discharge. Its pH varies from 3·5 to 6, and while Doederlein's bacilli thrive in this acid environment it probably plays an important role in keeping the vagina relatively free from pathogenic bacteria. The acid pH, on the other hand, does favour the growth of yeasts, and for this reason *Candida albicans* infection of the vagina is common in pregnancy.

The vagina shows a gradient in the number of bacteria, decreasing from the vulva inwards, the upper part of the vagina being relatively free from bacteria. This is in spite of the heavy contamination with bacteria around the rectum and the introduction of bacteria during coitus and by the fingers. The cervical mucous plug shows a similar gradient, the lower part near the external os containing a few bacteria and numbers of leucocytes and the middle part a few leucoctyes, whereas the upper part contains no leucocytes and is sterile. Thus the pregnant uterus, in the absence of interference, is kept completely free of infection.

Considerable attention has been paid to the cells desquamated from the vagina, which have been extensively studied, using the staining method of Papanicolau (1925). In early pregnancy there are increased numbers of leucocytes and basophilic cells, the latter having curled-up edges and tending to be clumped together. As pregnancy advances, the basophilic navicular cells derived from the intermediate layer, and full of glycogen, are found in increasing abundance in small, dense clusters (Wachtel 1964). These cells predominate over the superficial squamous and basal cells, and with leucocytes and Doederlein's bacilli constitute the typical smear in pregnancy. The early pregnancy changes are the same as those which occur in the second half of the normal menstrual cycle and are due to the effect of progesterones. The absence of these typical changes suggests a deficiency in progesterone secretion. Vaginal cytology has been used as a means of detecting progesterone deficiency, particularly in the case of threatened or habitual abortion (de Neef 1967). Vaginal cytology has similarly been used to determine the effect of, and to control, treatment with progesterone (de Neef 1967). It has also been used

to detect possible endocrine deficiencies at the end of pregnancy, as a guide to foetal maturity and to the prospects for labour (de Neef 1967). Postpartum, the vaginal smears typically show numerous parabasal cells. If this pattern is found in pregnancy it is thought to indicate either that labour is imminent or, if found in early or middle pregnancy, that there is a major degree of 'placental insufficiency' or intra-uterine death. A progressive increase in superficial squamous cells in pregnancy is also thought to indicate 'placental insufficiency' (Figs. 9.9, 9.10 and 9.11).

LIGAMENTS, PARAMETRIUM AND PERITONEUM LIGAMENTS

(a) *Round ligaments*

These round ligaments are continuous with the uterine muscle and hypertrophy with it and in late pregnancy may be 1–2 cm in thickness. Because of the growth of the uterus their attachment becomes relatively much nearer to the mid-line and the direction of their ligaments also becomes vertical. The round ligaments contain muscle, and it has been suggested that they contract synchronously with the uterus and thus serve to moor the uterus during labour.

(b) *Uterosacral ligaments*

These are also continuous with the uterine musculature and hypertrophy in pregnancy. It has similarly been suggested that they contract with the uterus during labour and help to keep the uterus in its proper axis.

(c) *Broad ligaments*

These are similarly strengthened by the hypertrophy of smooth-muscle cells, which thereby help to increase its usefulness as a support. The two peritoneal layers of the ligament become separated by the growth of the uterus and contain the dilated venous sinuses, arteries and other structures supplying the uterus.

PARAMETRIUM

The most striking change in the parametrium is the peculiar activity of the mesenchymal cells, which are at first particularly numerous around the blood vessels. Later they change into plasmatocytes and monocytes and acquire phagocytic properties and come to lie between the connective tissue fibres. They become more numerous towards term and are probably part of the mechanisms which protect the maternal organism against infection.

PERITONEUM

The peritoneum grows with the uterus and undergoes true hyperplasia. Over the developing lower uterine segment the peritoneum becomes loose and immediately after delivery is thrown into folds corresponding with the muscle fibres, though the folds disappear in the first few days of the puerperium. Decidual reactions, as commonly occur in the ovary in pregnancy, also occur in the pelvic peritoneum and appear as raised, velvety, red areas which may bleed to touch, particularly on the posterior surface of the uterus, the uterosacral ligaments and Douglas's pouch.

THE GENERAL STRUCTURAL CHANGES IN THE MOTHER

The structural changes in the mother vary greatly from patient to patient; in some they are trivial and not recognized clinically, in others they are severe and give rise to pathological entities.

(1) Pelvis and skeletal system

(a) *Bony pelvis*

Apart from a considerable increase in vascularity there are, surprisingly, no marked changes in the pelvic bones in pregnancy. Occasionally, there is an irregular deposit of bone under the periosteum—the puerperal osteophytes of Rokitansky.

(b) *Pelvic ligaments*

In contrast to the pelvic bones, there are marked changes in the pelvic ligaments in pregnancy. The pelvic bones are held together anteriorly by the symphysis pubis and the superior and inferior pubic ligaments, posteriorly by the sacro-iliac joints which join the sacrum to the inanimate bones on either side, and inferiorly by the sacrococcygeal joint where the coccyx is joined to the sacrum.

These joints consist chiefly of fibrocartilage with small, synovial, articular cavities. In pregnancy there is a marked softening and loosening of the fibrocartilage and there is an increase in the synovia and synovial fluid, resulting in a considerable increase in mobility in the sacrococcygeal, pubic and sacro-iliac joints, particularly in multiparae. This is readily demonstrable in the case of the pubic symphysis on vaginal examination (Budin 1897) and by X-rays (Borell 1957). The symphysis pubis increases in width during pregnancy and labour, increasing the dimensions of the pelvis, but returns to normal soon after delivery. There is also separation and movements of the sacro-iliac joints, with downward displacement of the sacrum on standing and upward displacement in the lithotomy position.

The relaxation of these ligaments in pregnancy not infrequently gives rise to pain and tenderness over the symphysis pubis and the sacro-iliac joints. In some cases the relaxation may be so great that the patient experiences incapacity, pain at the joints and finds it difficult, if not impossible, to walk, when the condition may be regarded as pathological and is known as 'pelvic arthropathy of pregnancy'. (See p. 343.)

The relaxation of the ligaments and separation of the pelvic joints may play an important part in pregnancy and labour in increasing the available pelvic diameters, but the extent to which separation normally occurs and its importance in labour has never been properly assessed.

(c) *Skeletal system*

As the pregnant uterus grows in the abdomen it protrudes anteriorly. This increasing protruber-

ance, particularly on standing, causes a progressive shift in the woman's centre of gravity
anteriorly. To prevent herself falling forwards
the pregnant woman throws her shoulders back,
straightens her back and neck, and leans backwards slightly to bring the centre of gravity
vertically over the pelvis. The cervical and
thoracic spine is thus progressively straightened
though there is, of necessity, a compensating
increase in the lumbar lordosis and, on rotation
of the pelvis, on the femurs (Fig. 9.12).

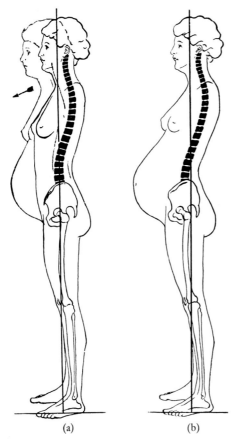

(a)   (b)

Fig. 9.12. Statics of (a) the non-pregnant woman;
(b) pregnant woman (Greenhill 1965).

The relaxation of the pelvic joints also causes
a degree of pelvic instability, so that the woman
in late pregnancy adopts a characteristic waddling

gait or strut. Because of these changes in skeleta
dynamics the pregnant woman has to make a
greater effort to maintain an erect carriage. The
unaccustomed posture may also cause backache
by placing unusual strains on particular muscles
or ligaments. These changes in skeletal dynamics
and consequent strains are much greater in
women with twins or a pendulous abdomen.

(2) Skin, face and abdominal wall

The changes in the abdominal wall are in many
ways the same as occur in the skin generally, but
the progressive distension of the abdomen gives
rise to certain features which merit separate
discussion.

SKIN

The skin generally is affected by pregnancy.
There is an increased hyperaemia and blood flow
through the skin. The sweat and sebaceous
glands increase in activity. In some women there
is an increased growth of hair and a fine lanugo
appears on the face and chest, disappearing 2 or
3 months postpartum. The subcutaneous fat
becomes thicker and in late pregnancy facial
features become coarser, partly due to increased
deposition of fat, partly to oedema.

There is very often an increased pigmentation,
particularly in specific areas—the nipples, the
vulva, the umbilicus and the abdominal skin in
the mid-line, extending from the xyphoid
cartilage to the symphysis pubis, the linea nigra.
Recent scars become heavily pigmented but old
scars do not.

FACE

The face is subject to a somewhat different form
of pigmentation in which irregular, brownish
areas of varying size appear on the cheeks, the
nose, the forehead and occasionally the neck—
so-called chloasma, or the mask of pregnancy.
Fortunately, this discoloration disappears (or at
least regresses considerably) after pregnancy,
as does most of the pigmentation. There is very
little basic knowledge of the nature of these
pigmentary changes, which are said to be due

to deposition of melanin, although melanocyte-stimulating hormone has been shown to be elevated from the eighth week of pregnancy until term. Oestrogen and progesterone, moreover, are reported to exert a melanocyte-stimulating effect (Diczfalusy & Troen 1961).

Vascular spider naevi or angiomata develop in about 60% of Caucasian and 11% of Negro women during pregnancy (Bean *et al.* 1949). They are associated with palmar erythema and are believed to be due to the effect of the high circulating blood oestrogen in pregnancy. They are identical to the spider naevi and palmar erythema seen in patients with liver disease but are thought to be of no clinical significance in pregnancy. They disappear shortly after delivery.

ABDOMINAL WALL

After the twentieth week, when the uterus has risen well out of the pelvis, the abdominal girth increases. The abdominal wall becomes stretched and thiner. The previously depressed umbilicus becomes flush with the skin around the twenty-fourth week and protrudes outwards towards the end of pregnancy. Any tendency to hernia may be aggravated, but usually the gravid uterus displaces the intestines and the omentum to one side and they are thereby kept away from the hernial openings.

Rapid and excessive stretching of the skin is accompanied by breaking of its underlying connective tissue which gives rise to characteristic, irregular, wavy, pink to purplish depressions termed striae gravidarum. These occur most frequently in the skin of the lower abdomen, over the buttocks, and along the upper parts of the thighs. They also occur on the breasts, when they are arranged radially round the nipples. Blondes are said to be more affected than brunettes, primigravidae more than multigravidae, fat women more than thin ones. Following delivery the striae become silvery-white in appearance and resemble old scar tissue. In multiparae, both the silvery-white markings of a previous pregnancy and fresh pink to purple striae of the present pregnancy are seen.

Identical striae may be seen in non-pregnant women with Cushing's syndrome and women who have rapidly accumulated subcutaneous fat. Striae of pregnancy are thus probably due to the increased secretion of adrenocortical hormones in pregnancy which cause profound changes in collagen and the ground substance of connective tissue, as well as to over-stretching.

Progressive distension of the abdomen may also affect the subcutaneous tissues and fascia, and as a result the linea alba may be greatly stretched. This effect becomes more marked with repeated pregnancies. At the same time, the rectus abdominis muscle may become stretched and separate in the mid-line, resulting in a diastasis or divarication of the recti muscles. In severe cases there is only a thin layer of skin, fascia and peritoneum covering the uterus. In rare instances there may be complete herniation of the gravid uterus.

(3) **Breasts**

Tingling, tenseness and occasional real pain in the breasts may be one of the earliest symptoms of pregnancy. These sensations are caused by increased vascularity and gland proliferation and are the same as those often noted in the week before menstruation. After the second month the breasts increase in size, partly from hypertrophy and hyperplasia of the glands and partly from increase in fat between the lobules and in the skin. As they increase in size delicate veins become visible just beneath the skin, and as they get larger appear as bluish streaks. At the same time the nipples become larger, more pigmented and erectile, and after the first few months a thick, yellowish fluid, colostrum, may be expressed. The primary areola also becomes more deeply pigmented and broader, and the base of the areola becomes puffed up and raised above the surface of the rest of the gland. Scattered through the areola are a number of small, rounded elevations which are the mouths of hypertrophied sebaceous glands and are known as Montgomery's tubercles. Later in pregnancy, around the primary areola a secondary, less pigmented, areola develops. It has been described as 'a dusky paper sprinkled with drops of water'. The clear spots without pigment occur around the opening of the sweat and sebaceous glands. The depth of pigmentation varies with the patient's complexion. In blondes the areolae and nipples become pinkish, while in brunettes they become dark brown and occasionally almost black.

The breast is made up of 15–20 distinct lobules embedded in a cushion of fat. Each lobule consists of a mass of branched glands or acini leading into tubules and eventually into one duct which opens on the nipple. There are thus 15–20 ducts opening on the nipple, each of which is dilated in the nipple to produce a sinus lactiferus. The nipple is a muscular organ surrounded by unstriped muscular fibres which unite with those of the nipple itself to produce an erectile organ.

During the first few months of pregnancy the most prominent change is the proliferation of the glandular tissue. This is followed by a marked proliferation of the ducts. About half-way through pregnancy the secretion of colostrum begins and continues slowly to term. Colostrum can normally be expressed, but the amount present is usually not sufficient to cause spontaneous leakage from the nipple. In the last month or so of pregnancy spontaneous leakage may occur, but this has no prognostic significance with regard to lactation. As the patient reaches term, breast growth is at a maximum; the ducts have hypertrophied to the point where they are ready to conduct large supplies of milk and the volume of colostrum is at a maximum. The breasts are thus fully prepared to take on the task of lactation and supplying the infant with milk once it is delivered.

OTHER PHYSIOLOGICAL CHANGES IN THE MOTHER

Widespread changes occur throughout the body during pregnancy. For the most part these are discussed in the appropriate sections dealing with different general disorders complicating pregnancy, and here they will be referred to only briefly to avoid repetition.

From the moment of conception the whole physiology of the mother is adapted and altered and all the resources are mobilized so that she is able to meet all the demands imposed by the growing foetus and is maintained in good health throughout pregnancy.

Three teleological principles govern the physiological changes in pregnancy.

(1) The physiological changes in pregnancy are a temporary adaptation and produce no permanent deleterious effects on the mother.
(2) The physiological changes in the mother prepare her to meet any demands the foetus may make. Moreover, they precede any possible need or demand of the foetus. They are in apparent excess of the needs of the foetus, and the mother accumulates certain reserves and anticipates the future needs of the foetus.
(3) The maternal internal environment is positively altered to create conditions favourable to the foetus. Instead of preserving the 'milieur interieur', which is the common endeavour of the body in all other situations, the physiological adaptation in the mother creates a constant changing environment appropriate to the successive stages of pregnancy.

The blood and its constituents

During pregnancy there is an increase in the total blood volume, the plasma volume and the red-cell mass. Increase in total blood volume is of the order of 30–40%; this peak is reached about 34 weeks of pregnancy, after which there is a gradual decrease until term. Plasma volume increase (45%) is chiefly responsible for the general increase in total blood volume, the red-cell mass increasing by some 18% only. Blood becomes more diluted as a result. These changes are further discussed on p. 291. They are summarized in Table 9.1.

There is a marked increase in leucocyte count from around 7,000 per cubic millimetre in the non-pregnant state to 10,500 per cubic millimetre in late pregnancy due to increase in neutrophil cells; lymphocytes and other cells are unchanged. Platelets increase continuously in pregnancy and the puerperium from 187,000 per cubic millimetre in the non-pregnant to 316,000 per cubic millimetre at term and 600,000

Table 9.1. Principal blood changes of pregnancy

	Non-pregnant	34 weeks	Increment
Total blood volume (ml)	4,000	5,500	1,500
Plasma volume (ml)	2,500	3,750	1,250
Red-cell volume (ml)	1,500	1,750	250
Haematocrit (whole body)	37·5%	31·5%	
Haematocrit (venous)	40%	34%	
Haemoglobin (venous)	14 g/100 ml	12 g/100 ml	
Total haemoglobin	492 g	597 g	100 g
Total iron	1,668 g	2,000 g	335 mg

per cubic millimetre in the puerperium. Haemodilution in pregnancy reduces blood viscosity (relative to water) from 4·61 in non-pregnant women to 3·84 in mid and late pregnancy. The E.S.R. (Wintrobe) rises from 9·6 mm/hr to 56 mm/hr (range 30–100 mm/hr) due to increased plasma fibrinogen and globulin.

Important plasma protein changes are seen. In general there is a fall in plasma protein concentration from the non-pregnant value to around 6 g or less per 100 ml. To some extent this is an effect of dilution, but not entirely so. There is a decrease in total plasma protein concentration and an alteration in the albumin globulin ratio from 1·5 to 1 or even less, due to a fall in the albumin fraction and a rise in the globulin fraction. These changes are summarized in Table 9.2

Table 9.2. Plasma protein changes of pregnancy

	Non-pregnant	Term
Total (g/100 ml)	7	6
Albumin (g/100 ml)	4	3
Globulin (g/100 ml)	2·5	2·5
Fibrinogen (g/100 ml)	0·25	0·4
Total protein (g)	175	215

There is a marked rise, also, in all lipids in pregnancy, with an increased ratio of β to α lipoprotein from 2:1 in the non-pregnant state to 5:1 in late pregnancy. The total lipids increase from around 600 mg/100 ml in the non-pregnant to around 900 mg/100 ml in late pregnancy. This increase is predominantly in cholesterol and triglycerides; plasma phospholipid concentration increases to a smaller extent. The cholesterol figures change from around 180 mg/100 ml in the non-pregnant state to some 270 mg/100 ml near to term.

There is a total fall of all electrolytes of the order of 10 m.equiv./l due to haemodilution.

Hyperventilation during pregnancy produces a fall in arterial blood PCO_2 from 38 to 32 mmHg. There is a partial compensatory metabolic acidosis with a fall in plasma bicarbonate. Changes in pH are of the order of 7·4 in the non-pregnant to 7·44 in the pregnant patient. Standard bicarbonate falls from some 24 m.equiv./l in the non-pregnant patient to 21 m.equiv./l in the pregnant patient. The arterial PO_2 rises from 95 mmHg in the non-pregnant to 105 mmHg during pregnancy. These changes facilitate transfer of carbon dioxide from the foetus to the mother and oxygen from the mother to the foetus.

Changes in the Cardiovascular system

Pregnancy is a hyperkinetic state, similar to hyperthyroidism. This is evidenced by increased oxygen consumption, increased cardiac output and decreased peripheral resistance.

Clinical changes which may be noted are that the pulse becomes bounding and partially collapsing; the apex beat is displaced upwards and outwards and the heart is dextrorotated; there is a prominant S-wave in lead 1 and a conspicuous Q and inverted P in lead 3; the heart is slightly enlarged in diastole; a third heart sound may be heard; haemic murmurs are common; there is a slight rise in venous pressure. Consideration of cardiac output changes is undertaken on p. 284. These changes are summarized in Table 9.3.

There is considerable discrepancy of timing of peak cardiac output in mid or late pregnancy. Many workers maintain that the fall in late

Table 9.3. Summary of cardiac changes of pregnancy

	Non-pregnant	12 weeks	36 weeks
Cardiac output (l/min)	4·5	6·0	5·5
Stroke volume (ml)	65	75	65
Pulse rate	70	80	85

pregnancy is due to the supine hypotensive syndrome. All are agreed that an increase occurs early in pregnancy and is more than sufficient to carry the increased oxygen consumption.

Further cardiac output changes occur in labour. In the first stage of labour cardiac output increases by some 30%, to 8 l/min; and in the second stage it rises by some 50%, to 9 l/min.

No significant changes occur in the blood pressure in normal pregnancy. Some workers have reported a small fall of 5–10 mmHg, particularly in diastotic pressure in the mid trimester. Venous pressure is slightly raised above the normal, except in the lower limbs where a change is greater, the pressure in the femoral veins being markedly raised up to 24 cm of water. Pulmonary artery pressures are within normal limits but show a slight rise on exercise. Peripheral vascular resistance is markedly reduced, this fall being maximal between the twenty-fifth and twenty-eighth week, due to dilatation of arteries of the uterus, kidney and skin.

Changes in the respiratory system

Mechanical changes which occur in the respiratory system are some lifting of the chest cage with upward flaring of the ribs. There is elevation of the diaphragm and increased excursion of the diaphragm, except in late pregnancy; at that time there is reduced diaphragmatic excursion, and respiratory exchange is maintained by increased thoracic movement, which may cause dyspnoea.

Physiological considerations include an unchanged vital capacity at 3,200 ml. Tidal air is increased by some 200 ml and residual volume reduced by the same amount. Increased volume of

tidal air, together with a much smaller residual volume of air in the lungs, gives a marked improvement in gaseous exchange.

Fluid balance and weight gain

In pregnancy great changes occur in fluid balance. Hytten & Leitch (1964) measured the total water increment of pregnancy at 7 l around term; of this volume it was estimated that some 5·8 l could be accounted for in the foetus, placenta, liquor amnii, enlarged uterus, breasts, plasma and the red cells, leaving 1·2 l as increase in tissue fluid.

This tissue fluid increase is closely related to the blood volume changes discussed above. The blood volume of an average-sized non-pregnant woman is approximately 4 l, 2·6 l being plasma. In pregnancy the plasma volume increases beyond this figure by some 1·3 l around 34 weeks, the increase at term being lower, of the order of 1 l. Rhodes (1970) points out that the volume of intersitial fluid must increase if the plasma volume increases, since both are part of the extracellular fluid. Escape of the fluid from the capillaries is assisted by a reduction in the osmotic pressure which accompanies the fall in plasma protein concentration during pregnancy, and, in the lower part of the body at least, from the effect of raised venous pressure.

In the face of this considerable fluid retention sodium retention is important to maintain isotonicity of body fluids. Raised aldosterone production may be responsible for this sodium-retaining effect, but this is not known for certain. Similarly, the renal function changes in respect of salt and water retention are not fully understood. The glomerular filtration rate goes up in the early part of pregnancy and this increase is maintained throughout; by contrast, renal blood flow increases to a maximum around 28 weeks, falling again towards term. In late pregnancy the ability to excrete a 'test' quantity of water is reduced, although it seems more likely that this is due to fluid collection in the tissues rather than to failure of the kidney to cope with it.

Weight gain is a crude but useful index of the changes in the mother and foetus during pregnancy. The average weight gain in a healthy patient on an adequate diet is summarized in Table 9.4.

Table 9.4. Average weight gain in healthy pregnant women on adequate diet

Weeks	Weight (kg)		
0–12	1·0		
12–16	1·0	4·0	
17–20	2·0		
			12·0
21–24	2·0		
25–28	2·0		
29–32	1·5	8·0	
33–36	1·5		
37–40	1·0		

Average net loss at delivery: 8·0 kg
Average net gain: 4·0 kg

Any weight gain in pregnancy in excess of 8·0 kg may be retained after the immediate puerperium. The distribution of the weight gain at term is shown in Table 9.5.

Table 9.5. Distribution of weight gain at 40 weeks (kg)

Foetal (approx. 5 kg)	Foetus	3·3
	Placenta	0·7
	Liquor	0·8
	Total	4·8
Mother (approx. 7·0 kg)	Uterus	0·9
	Breasts	0·4
	Blood	1·2
	E.C.F.	1·2
	Fat	4·0
	Total	12·5

The composition of this weight gain at term is shown in Table 9.6.

At delivery an infant weighing 3·3 kg contains some 400–500 g of protein, 30 g of calcium, 20 g of phosphorus, 0·5 g of iron. Two-thirds of this have been laid down in the last 3 months and one-third in the last month. Clearly, the peak demands for most nutrients therefore, is in the last months of pregnancy.

Table 9.6. Composition of weight gain at 40 weeks (g)

	Total	Water	Fat	Protein	Other
Foetus	3,300	2,335	460	435	70
Placenta	700	590	4·5	100	5·5
Liquor	800	790	0·5	5	4·5
Uterus	900	740	3·5	150	6·5
Breasts	400	300	12·0	80	8·0
Blood	1,200	1,080	19·5	130	5·5
E.C.F.	1,200	1,165	—		
Fat	3,500	—	3,500	0	0
Total	12,000	7,000	4,000	900	100

Renal changes

Marked changes occur in the renal tracts in pregnancy, these are considered in detail on p. 306. Dilation and kinking of the uterus may become pronounced, leading to stasis of urine and perhaps to urinary infection. In the kidney itself there is an increase in the renal blood and plasma flow during the first and second trimesters but a gradual fall throughout the third trimester until term, when these values have returned almost to non-pregnant levels. The glomerular filtration rate increases in a similar manner reaching a figure some 50–60% higher than that of the non-pregnant state; the fall in late pregnancy is less pronounced and the filtration rate is still significantly raised at term.

Gastro-intestinal tract

The gums of a pregnant woman become softer and bleed more easily than formerly. This gum change is usually much more pronounced and important than changes in the teeth themselves. Tooth decay may occur, but is concerned more with gum recession and increasing gingivitis than with calcium depletion from the teeth. Gingivitis of pregnancy can sometimes be a very distressing disorder which, if unchecked, may lead to the need for widespread tooth extraction.

Salivation is increased in many patients. Rarely, the increase can be so great that considerable discomfort and annoyance is experienced (ptyalism of pregnancy).

Reduction in the gastric acidity is a common finding during pregnancy, and may on occasions be pronounced. Motility of the stomach is similarly reduced; during labour this reduction of gastric emptying time may be very marked. There is a general diminution of bowel peristalsis, and troublesome constipation may be experienced in some patients. This change is no doubt concerned with smooth-muscle hypotonia associated with progesterone dominance in general, but towards the end of pregnancy a functional factor due to pressure of the very large uterus on the rectosigmoid region may also be concerned. These hormone changes may also be associated with the not uncommon symptom of heartburn which many patients suffer at some time throughout pregnancy. Entry of acid gastric contents into the lower oesophagus causes epigastric pain and discomfort which can sometimes be troublesome. In a few cases the enlarging uterus during late pregnancy appears to produce temporary hiatus hernia formation.

Biliary stasis occurs during pregnancy although it is not known how often this may be a significant change. The tendency for fertile patients to form gall stones suggest a causative effect. Increase in blood cholesterol levels may also be concerned.

Liver function is not significantly reduced during pregnancy in normal circumstances. Bromsulphthalein is a most effective way of studying liver function during pregnancy. The blood flow through the liver appears largely unchanged.

Metabolism in pregnancy

The total metabolism is increased due to the demands of the foetus, the demands of the extra work of the heart and lungs, and build-up of materials; this amount equals some 400 kcal/day, which may in part be met by economy of activity. The increase in metabolism is probably due to anterior pituitary stimulation of the thyroid. The thyroid gland hypertrophies in the majority of patients. Changes in thyroid function noted are a fall in the serum inorganic iodine from 0·2 μg/100 ml in the non-pregnant to 0·1 μg/100 ml in the pregnant patient. Thyroid uptake rises from 1·73 μg/hr in the non-pregnant to 3·0

μg/hr in the pregnant patient, and protein-bound iodine rises from 5 μg/100 ml to 10 μg/100 ml.

For the mother, pregnancy is anabolic, since she requires—and retains—extra material. Protein metabolism is notable for a markedly increased positive nitrogen balance throughout pregnancy. This nitrogen gain is greatly in excess of the needs of the foetus. During the puerperium there is a negative nitrogen balance return to the normal state, however, taking some 2–3 months before it is complete. Increase in plasma protein concentration and alterations in the albumin/globulin ratio have already been referred to.

During her pregnancy the mother deposits and stores fats and calcium, but probably not any other nutrients. Blood levels of nutrients and other substances are not increased, with the exception of those bound to β-globulins in the plasma which rise. Some nutrients are lost in the urine, namely glucose and amino acids (particularly histidine and isoleucine).

Carbohydrate metabolism is described in some detail in Chapter 20. Briefly, there is little alteration to the glucose-tolerance test or the fasting-blood sugar. Glycosuria in small amounts is common, however, due mainly to the lowering of the renal threshold for glucose to well below the normal figure of 160 mg-%. In pregnancy more glucose is utilized by the placenta, a good deal is converted into depot fat and less glycogen is probably deposited in liver and muscles.

Alterations in plasma lipids have already been referred to. Approximately 4 kg of additional fat are deposited, mostly in the abdominal wall, back and thighs during pregnancy; this deposition usually occurs before the thirtieth week. Little fat is deposited in the breasts, however. This stored fat provides energy which may be used in late pregnancy, labour and the puerperium.

There is little change in calcium levels in the blood during pregnancy, despite the increased needs of the foetus for this substance. It appears probable that a healthy mother can adequately supply her foetus with the necessary quantities of calcium required which, in late pregnancy, amounts to some 250 mg daily. Thirty to forty milligrams of calcium are deposited in the foetus during pregnancy, and this makes little alteration to the mother's calcium stores—unless she is already suffering from a malabsorption syndrome.

Folate deficiency during pregnancy can readily arise, however, and may be responsible for clinical manifestations unless precautions are taken to prevent this. Defective folate metabolism is, to some extent, responsible for this defect, especially in early pregnancy; later, the demands of the foetus aggravate the situation. The deficiency of folates is generally pronounced in patients who have had several pregnancies in quick succession, as the deficiency produced by each is not replaced between pregnancies. Multiple pregnancies provide a much greater drain on folic acid stores than single ones. Hibbard & Hibbard (1968) have written extensively on the subject. Iron metabolism is discussed on p. 291; the influence of pregnancy on the bones and the pelvic joints on pp. 125 and 343. The endocrine changes of pregnancy are dealt with in Chapter 10.

THE MANAGEMENT OF PREGNANCY

Antenatal care

The safety of our midwifery rests not only on how skilfully we manage labour, but upon the success with which we prevent the preventable diseases of pregnancy and foresee its foreseeable complications. Careful antenatal supervision will allow us to do this. Some consideration of normal antenatal practice will therefore be undertaken.

For many years it has been the practice for a patient receiving antenatal care to be seen monthly until the twenty-eighth week, every 2 weeks until the thirty-sixth week, and weekly from then until she is delivered. For a patient who develops no abnormality these intervals are satisfactory. We must, however, be prepared to change them if events make this necessary. For instance, excessive weight gain in the middle trimester of pregnancy would call for the patient to return for further examination at an earlier time, whilst the recognition of a raised blood pressure may

require her to be seen only a few days later—or, indeed, admitted to hospital forthwith.

A great deal of routine is concerned in antenatal care and it has become the practice for patients to be subjected to almost identical procedures each time they come. The blood pressure is taken, urine tested, they are weighed, abdominal palpation is carried out and the ankles are examined for oedema. Routines of this nature have both advantages and disadvantages. They prevent us from omitting some important step but if they are followed too meticulously they may be performed mechanically, and we may be distracted from some unexpected feature which should receive more attention. A point that is important here is that throughout the course of pregnancy we are not equally concerned at each visit with the same things. This is particularly true of the first visit, which is unique since it gives us an opportunity to assess a particular individual in a single pregnancy. This is a most important visit, at which most important decisions require to be taken. At the various visits from that point until late pregnancy we are more concerned with the recognition of the early signs of pre-eclampsia and of anaemia than with anything else; in late pregnancy—from, say, 32 weeks onward—the lie, presentation and position of the foetus become much more important matters.

THE FIRST VISIT

The first visit of a patient during pregnancy is an extremely vital visit. Here, we must make the diagnosis of pregnancy, we must recognize existing or pre-existing disease which might have an important influence on pregnancy or labour and we must make appropriate arrangements for confinement. More than that, however, we have the opportunity of explaining to the patient what pregnancy has in store for her, of giving her general advice, and of allowing her to question us on matters about which she may be concerned.

Diagnosis of pregnancy

Suspicion of pregnancy will arise from amenorrhoea and perhaps from some of the symptoms of early pregnancy, such as nausea, vomiting, breast tenderness and tingling and, sometimes, frequency of micturition.

The history of amenorrhoea is very important, not only in the diagnosis of pregnancy itself, but in the establishment of the duration of pregnancy at any particular time. It is necessary to determine when the patient's last menstrual period was, if it was normal, and if it was preceded by other regular periods. It is customary to calculate the expected date of confinement by adding 7 days to the first day of the last menstrual period and counting backwards 3 months. It must be emphasized, however, that elementary mistakes are often made here. Such a calculation will only be valid if the patient had regular 28-day cycles before she became pregnant. The calculation assumes ovulation 14 days after the first day of the last menstrual period, whereas it occurs 14 days before the first day of the next menstrual period. If the next menstrual period is expected after 5 or 6 or 7 weeks, and not after 4, then an alteration to the calculation will require to be made. If the patient's previous menstrual cycle is irregular it may be impossible to be certain, even within reasonable limits, of the duration of pregnancy judged from the menstrual history alone.

Other matters affect this calculation also. If the patient has recently been confined or had a miscarriage and regular cycles have not been resumed, we cannot assume that they will be precisely of the same pattern as those which preceded the pregnancy. If she has just ceased taking a contraceptive pill, we cannot assume that her next ovulation will be 14 days after the last withdrawal haemorrhage. Sometimes, instead of missing a period following conception, the patient may have a show of blood for a day or two, which she may represent as the last menstrual period; it must always be established that the period she is referring to was a normal one. These are elementary facts in history-taking, but since mistakes are made so often, emphasis is laid here.

A firm clinical diagnosis of pregnancy will rest upon the finding of an enlarged, soft uterus. The uterine fundus can seldom be palpated per abdomen for some 12 weeks in a patient's first

pregnancy, although it may be felt several weeks earlier than this if the patient has been pregnant before. In most instances it will be advisable to examine the patient vaginally at her first visit. This will enable the diagnosis of pregnancy to be confirmed, and will enable an estimate to be made of the duration of this pregnancy, an observation which may be important later if maturity is in question. A better estimate of maturity can often be made at this time than at 36 or 40 weeks. Vaginal examination will also permit the recognition of associated disorders such as the presence of a fibroid, an ovarian cyst or a cervical polyp. A cervical smear should be taken if one has not been done recently.

It will generally be unwise to make any more searching examination of the enlarged uterus to establish signs such as Hegar's sign. Softening of the cervix can easily be appreciated, so can enlargement and softening of the uterus, and these together are sufficient to permit a confident clinical diagnosis of pregnancy. Localized areas of spasm are occasionally recognized in the early pregnant uterus, which may give rise to the suggestion of a fibroid complicating pregnancy. Indeed, the uterus may be felt to contract and relax during examination, which is a certain sign that it is the uterus which is being palpated.

Occasionally, it may be wise to omit the vaginal examination at the first visit. A patient may be unusually anxious, and unless it proves possible to obtain her full confidence this examination may be withheld until the next visit. Alternatively, a patient may relate a previous miscarriage to the fact that she was examined per vaginam. This association may or may not be true, but it if is firmly fixed in her mind there may be something to be said for withholding the examination until 12 weeks have passed. In all cases, it is unwise to make any attempt to assess pelvic size at this time. This information is of limited value unless we know the size of the baby's head which will ultimately require to pass through. Moreover, the assessment of pelvic size in early pregnancy requires a vigorous examination which may be distressing, and even painful, to the patient, and we may lose her confidence.

Breast enlargement, darkening of the areola,

the presence of Montgomery's tubercles, and the expression of fluid from the nipple, are usually detectable about 12 weeks. These signs are not diagnostic of pregnancy, but are strongly suggestive of it.

The important facts of the patient's medical, surgical and obstetrical history must be recorded in detail. A general examination must be made and a blood sample should be taken for ABO and Rhesus grouping, Wasserman reaction, haemoglobin estimation, etc.

Pregnancy tests

If there is doubt about the diagnosis of pregnancy, a pregnancy test may be appropriate. Immunological pregnancy tests, such as the haemoglutination-inhibition test, have now replaced biological ones. Immunological tests are simpler and cheaper, and in general show a higher degree of sensitivity; they may be positive some 7–10 days after the first missed period, whereas a biological test will require a little

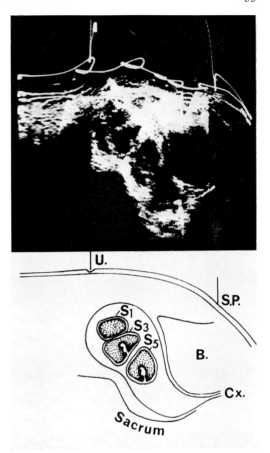

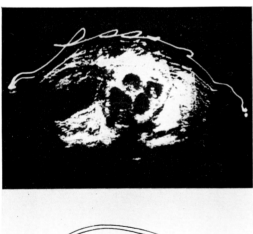

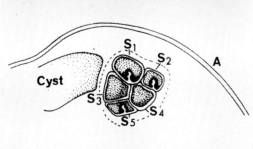

Fig. 9.13 (a)

Fig. 9.13 (a) and (b). A remarkable ultrasound picture of a quintuplet pregnancy at 9 weeks of gestation. In (a) a transverse scan of the large uterus reveals four certain gestation sacs and a probable fifth (S5). A longitudinal scan (b) establishes the presence of the fifth for certain. (By courtesy of *Lancet*.)

longer. They depend (as do biological tests) upon the presence of chorionic gonadotrophin in reasonably large quantities in the urine. These quantities may not be high enough to give a positive test within a day or two of the first missed period, nor if an early-morning specimen of urine is not provided; care should always be taken that a concentrated sample is tested if mistakes are to be avoided. Ultrasonic compound B scanning provides an alternative method of recognizing a very early pregnancy [9.13(a) and (b)]. The presence of a gestation sac may be recognizable some 6 weeks after the last menstrual period, and embryonic echoes within the sac shortly after that. These appearances continue until some 11 weeks of amenorrhoea, but between 11 and 13 weeks of amenorrhoea, the characteristic echoes disappear, probably as the result of fusion of decidua vera and decidua capsularis. The foetal head becomes recognizable, however, at about 13 weeks (Fig. 9.14). The foetal heart beat can be detected with the Doppler Foetal Heart Detector as soon as the fundus becomes palpable per abdomen.

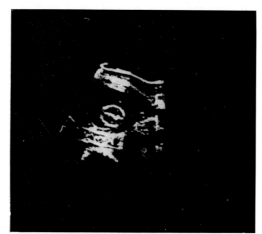

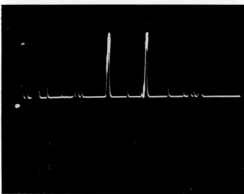

Fig. 9.14. Foetal head visualized by compound B scan (above), and measured by A scan (below), at 14 weeks' gestation.

Place of confinement

The greater safety of hospital confinement is not now disputed. If this can be arranged, even for the delivery only, it is preferable to home confinement. Home confinement, in general, does not provide the degree of safety obtainable by hospital delivery, since one cannot be certain that the appropriate attendants will be present nor that the safety measures of blood transfusion, emergency anaesthesia, infant resuscitation, etc., will be there if they are required. If the number of hospital beds does not permit every patient to be delivered in hospital, selection of those suitable for confinement outside hospital will have to be made. In general, these will be normal patients in the second, third or fourth pregnancy. The presence of any abnormality in the previous medical, surgical or obstetrical history likely to influence the confinement, or any detectable abnormality in the pregnancy itself, will indicate the need for the patient to be in hospital. Patients over 35 years of age are generally unsuitable for confinement outside hospital.

Diet in pregnancy

During pregnancy there is a need for extra energy to supply the needs of the growing foetus and to keep pace with the increased basal metabolic rate, and weight gain of the mother. The World Health Organization report entitled *Nutrition in Pregnancy and Lactation* (published in 1965) deals with these matters fully.

The pregnant woman requires a diet of some 2,500 calories daily and in this respect does not, in general, require to eat more when she is pregnant. Pregnant women in an affluent society gain weight partly as a result of fat deposition. Gopolan (1970) suggests that since this fat gain cannot be considered essential, the increased calorie requirements of pregnancy amount to only some 150 calories daily; against this, may be set the reduced physical activity common during pregnancy, so that in many cases it seems probable that little, if any, increase in calory intake is required. The WHO group recommend, however, that some 5–6 g extra protein per day should be taken during the second and third trimester. A slight increase in calcium seems desirable; a total intake of 1,000–1,200 μg daily is regarded as adequate. Iron supplements are required to the order of some 10 mg daily.

Vitamin intake is almost certainly adequate in well-balanced Western diets, although this may be by no means the case in countries where standards of nutrition are poor. Folic acid is an exception here, and deficiency is common even in reasonably well fed communities. Supplements of folic acid (300 μg/day) may conveniently be given with iron throughout the pregnancy. Fat and carbohydrate are almost always taken in adequate amounts in this country, and often in far too great amounts.

In practical terms, a patient should be told that she does not require to eat more during pregnancy, but to eat more wisely. A mixed diet, relatively high in protein (100 g) and relatively low in fat (100 g) and carbohydrate (300 g), should be her aim. In general, she should take meat, fish, fruit and vegetables, milk, cheese and eggs, and limit her intake of bread, potatoes, pastry, cakes, etc. Supplementary iron and folic acid, such as are given routinely in most antenatal clinics, will be adequate for her extra needs. It should be remembered, however, that absorption and utilization of iron and folic acid may be indifferent, and routine haemoglobin checks are essential.

General advice

Many general matters may come up for discussion when the patient starts to ask questions. It may be necessary to give advice about vomiting, heartburn, constipation, etc.; these are dealt with in appropriate chapters elsewhere in this book. Many women will be better for taking more rest during pregnancy, especially those who work as well as looking after their own home; heavy work is never in a patient's interests. If the patient does not regularly visit her dentist, then she should do so, and any treatment necessary should be carried out. Smoking has clearly been shown to be associated with limitation in foetal growth (Russell et al. 1968): although this effect will, in most patients, be an unimportant one, it may be very important in a heavy smoker with a previous history of a 'small-for-dates' baby. Intercourse can safely be continued until the last few weeks of pregnancy in normal circumstances. Patients ask such varied

questions that one can scarcely answer all of them at an early session of this kind. There is much to be said for the patient attending regular instructional talks on pregnancy and labour which most hospitals provide at the present time. These, and relaxation exercises which she undertakes later in pregnancy, will almost certainly be beneficial for her.

Visits up to 32 weeks

It will usually be satisfactory for a patient to attend monthly at the antenatal clinic until she is some 28 weeks pregnant, then every 2 weeks until the thirty-sixth week; thereafter, she should come weekly. In those cases in which no specific feature focuses our attention, we will be concerned during much of the antenatal period, with the early recognition of hypertension disorders and the prevention of anaemia. Both are important contributory causes to maternal and perinatal mortality.

Regular blood pressure recording, weighing and urine testing, and examinations for peripheral oedema, will be the methods principally used to detect the warning and early signs of pre-eclampsia, etc. These matters are discussed more fully in Chapter 16. It must be emphasized, too, that attention must be paid to the consistent growth of the foetus during these weeks. Placental insufficiency will generally be found in patients with evidence of pre-eclampsia and hypertensive disease, but in other instances there may be failure to thrive in utero without any significant maternal feature to draw attention to it. In these circumstances, only the recognition of the child that is 'small-for-dates' and growing more slowly than usual will permit diagnosis.

The patient's weight should be carefully taken each time she comes to the clinic. Excessive weight gain may be an indication of early pre-eclampsia, and advice on diet and rest may be called for (see p. 272). A patient who fails to gain weight should also be watched carefully. This patient may be deliberately attempting to limit her weight gain when, provided she is taking an adequate diet, no action need be taken. Her failure to gain weight may, however, be an indication that interference with intra-uterine growth of the foetus is taking place, and special attention should be paid to this.

Maturity is often in question late in pregnancy; is a patient overdue and therefore should she be induced, or is she still not at term? It has already been mentioned that an estimate of the size of the uterus in early pregnancy may give a more accurate estimate of the true duration of pregnancy than examination in late pregnancy. It will be advisable to note carefully, throughout pregnancy, the height of the fundus. The uterine fundus can usually be felt just above the symphysis pubis about 12 weeks in a primigravida. In a multigravida it can often be felt earlier. By 16 weeks the fundus is some 2 in above the symphysis, by 20 weeks just below the umbilicus, and by 24 weeks just above it. At 28 weeks the fundus will reach to one-third of the way between umbilicus and xiphisternum about 32 weeks to two-thirds of the way, and by 36 weeks to just below the xiphisternum. At 40 weeks, if the head becomes engaged the height of the fundus may fall a little again. If the fundus reaches to the xiphisternum, suspicion of twins or hydramnios must be entertained, since it is uncommon for the fundus to reach so high in a normal case. These levels are at the best an imprecise guide to maturity, however, and too much reliance should not be placed upon them (Beazley & Underhill 1970). Once the foetus can be palpated readily, the size of the foetus itself is a better measure of growth and maturity than fundal height.

There is much to be said for suggesting to patients that they record the date of quickening, once they are sure of it; quickening will usually be experienced between 16 and 18 weeks in a multigravid patient and between 18 and 20 weeks in a primigravid patient. In neither is the date precise, but it will be less imprecise if a record is made at the time and the patient is not asked to remember 3 months later when she first felt her baby move. The foetal heart sounds can usually be heard about 24 weeks.

Routine blood examinations to detect anaemia are called for at intervals throughout pregnancy. Most patients are given supplementary iron and perhaps folic acid as well; it must not be assumed however, that such a patient is not anaemic,

since she may not be taking the medication, may not be absorbing it, or may not be utilizing it. The problem of anaemia in pregnancy is discussed fully on p. 291.

A positive test for sugar in the urine is occasionally obtained during pregnancy, this is generally due to the lowering of the renal threshold at this time, but may be a sign of somewhat greater significance. This is discussed fully in Chapter 20.

THE LAST 2 MONTHS

During the last 2 months or so of pregnancy, attention must be focused to a greater extent upon the foetus and its relationship to the mother's pelvis. It becomes more important now to palpate the abdomen to determine the lie and presentation of the foetus, although the position of the foetus is still comparatively unimportant.

The *lie* is the relationship of the long axis of the foetus to the long axis of the uterus.

The *presentation* is that part of the foetus which occupies the lower pole of the uterus.

The *position* of the foetus is the relationship of some portion of the presenting part to the front or back, right or left of the mother; the portion of the foetus related to the mother in this way is called the denominator. For the vertex presentation the denominator is the occiput, and six positions are normally described. Left occipito-anterior (LOA); right occipito-anterior (ROA); left occipitolateral (LOL); right occupitolateral (ROL); left occipito-posterior (LOP); right occipitoposterior (ROP). When the face presents the denominator is the chin and, again, six position may be described: RMA, RMP, etc. The position is unimportant when the breech presents, although it is often described with the sacrum as denominator. The position is equally unimportant when the brow presents, since under normal circumstances this presentation is far too large for the head to pass through the pelvis.

The *attitude* of the foetus is the relationship of the different parts of the foetus to each other; normally this is one of almost complete flexion during the antenatal period, complete flexion resulting once labour pains begin.

Engagement of the head refers to the relationship of the widest diameter of the head to the pelvic brim. In the well-flexed head presentation the diameter presenting to the pelvic brim is the suboccipito bregmatic in the sagittal plane and the biparietal diameter in the coronal plane (see p. 181 *et seq.*).

Around 30–32 weeks it is not uncommon to find the foetus presenting by the breech; spontaneous version to a vertex presentation usually occurs shortly after this. In a number of instances, however, the breech presentation persists, and requires to be managed in the manner dealt with in Chapter 22.

Considerable attention must be paid at this time to the size of the abdominal swelling, the size of the foetus, and the relationship of these two things to each other. If the foetus is larger or smaller than seems appropriate for the duration of amenorrhoea, then maturity may be in question. Again, in a larger abdomen, there may be a twin pregnancy or hydramnios, or both. If the abdomen is smaller than is to be expected from the duration of amenorrhoea, we may be dealing with a foetus which is less mature than is believed, or one failing to thrive *in utero*. Very careful attention to these points is always necessary. They are all discussed much more fully in different sections of this book (see pp. 375, 378 *et seq.*).

Head–brim relationships

During the last few weeks of pregnancy, the relationship of the foetal head to the pelvic brim becomes an important matter. In patients who are pregnant for the first time, the child's head will often settle into the brim about this time, and may even be completely engaged several weeks before term. If abdominal examination reveals that the head is not already engaged in the pelvis, it can often be made to do so by downward abdominal pressure exerted on the fundus with the left hand whilst the head is palpated with the right. Some obstetricians prefer to raise the patient's head and shoulders from the bed, letting her rest back on her elbows, to bring the axis of the foetus more in line with the plane of the pelvic brim, to facilitate engagement and to exclude disproportion. Relaxation of abdominal muscles is not always complete in this position, however, and palpation may sometimes still be difficult. A bimanual pelvic examination is preferable a few weeks before term to exclude the possibility of disproportion.

The vaginal examination in late pregnancy is commonly stated to be to 'assess the pelvis'. Clinical measurement of the pelvis alone, at this point, is only partly helpful. Clearly, if an extremely small pelvis is felt, the likelihood of disproportion arises. The size of the pelvis is, nonetheless, related directly to the size of the head which has to go through it, and unless an attempt is made to fit the head into the pelvis at this bimanual examination, no satisfactory assessment of disproportion can be carried out. Assessment of the pelvis is often attempted by measuring the diagonal conjugate. In this measurement, the fingers seek to tip the sacral promontory; then the point where the upper surface of the index finger meets the lower border of the symphysis pubis is marked with the other hand, and a rough measurement be made from this point to the tip of the middle finger in contact with the promontory. An arbitrary amount, usually half an inch, is subtracted from this measurement to give some impression of the size of the true conjugate. There are a number of objections to this kind of measurement. Even if it is possible to tip the sacrum, we do not know whether we are feeling it in the region of the promontory, or some distance below this. The diagonal conjugate bears an inconsistent relationship to the size of the true conjugate. More important, however, is the fact already emphasized that measurement of the pelvis without reference to the head is of limited value.

An assessment of the size of the outlet of the pelvis is more appropriate, since the head cannot be brought into contact with this portion of the pelvis during pregnancy. Estimating the prominence of the ischial spines, assessing the size of the sacrosciatic notch, fitting the closed fist between the ischial tuberosities and palpating with two fingers beneath the symphisis pubis will give some impression of the diameter of the outlet and the size of the subpubic arch. Outlet contraction *per se* is very uncommon without some associated contraction of the upper pelvic strait, and only very rarely will the obstetrician discover really marked contraction in the outlet region.

The foetal head may remain high in a primigravid patient during the last few weeks of pregnancy for a variety of reasons. Broadly speaking, these are:

   (i) the head is too large;
   (ii) the pelvis is too small;
   (iii) something intervenes between them;
   (iv) the foetus may have far too much mobility.

The head may be absolutely large, as that of a child of 4 or 5 kg would be; it may be relatively large if deflection presents an unfavourable diameter—such as the occipito frontal diameter (11·5 cm)—to the pelvic brim; or the foetus may be hydrocephalic. The pelvis may be reduced in size in one of several ways (see p. 394). Several important structures may intervene between the head and the pelvis; placenta praevia is the most common, but ovarian cysts and fibroids are occasionally encountered. An extremely loaded pelvic colon may have a similar effect. If there is hydramnios the foetus will have unusual mobility in the uterus, and the head will probably not engage spontaneously in the last few weeks of pregnancy, although it may often be made to engage if the examination described above is carried out.

In multigravid patients the head seldom engages within the last few weeks of pregnancy, as it does in the primigravid patient. A bimanual examination should be performed nonetheless, since disproportion must be excluded in every patient in every individual pregnancy. The size of the child may differ markedly between one pregnancy and the next, and the multiparous patient may well have developed an ovarian cyst since her last confinement.

OTHER ANTENATAL CONSIDERATIONS

Several other matters can conveniently be discussed here.

Life or death of the foetus?

If a patient reports that her abdomen is not enlarging, that she has not felt quickening, or

can no longer feel movements experienced previously, suspicion of foetal death will arise. Auscultation of the foetal heart may disclose it to be beating regularly, and there may be no cause for concern. If the heart cannot be heard, this will obviously raise a strong suspicion of foetal death, but it will be unwise to conclude this too readily. The foetal heart is sometimes difficult to hear, although it may be audible if we listen shortly afterwards. If foetal death is suspected, careful auscultation with the aural stethoscope and with the Doppler Foetal Heart Detector is required. Confirmatory signs of death will not be obtainable for a week or more; a pregnancy test may not become negative for a while, and X-ray signs of foetal death do not usually develop for about a week (see below). Whenever death of the foetus cannot be confirmed, it will be wise to wait, for if the foetus is dead then there is no danger for several weeks; if it is not, interference must be avoided. Usually, the position becomes clear after a period of a week or so, and appropriate action may be taken.

Rarely, if a dead foetus is retained *in utero* for 4–6 weeks, foetal products find their way into the maternal circulation and a blood coagulation defect may result (see p. 215). This is a very uncommon complication.

Use of X-rays

X-ray examination can give helpful, and at times extremely valuable, information during pregnancy and labour. Equally, however, there are dangers inherent in radiation at this time. In practical terms the problem presented to the obstetrician is to employ X-rays when they are necessary to provide useful information which cannot be obtained in any other way, yet constantly to bear in mind the risks involved.

Radiation is at its most dangerous when directed to the pelvis during the first 2 or 3 months of pregnancy, when organogenesis is at its height and tissues are dividing rapidly. Pelvic and lower abdominal X-rays should never be utilized either during the first few months of pregnancy or when there is a possibility of pregnancy; enquiry should always be made about the date of the last menstrual period whenever such examination is contemplated. Alimentary and urinary tract series are specially dangerous in view of the exposures required. Radiological examination should not be used for the diagnosis of pregnancy. Other methods of diagnosis are available, such as immunological tests of pregnancy and ultrasound studies, both Doppler and A and B scan (Fig. 9.13), and these should be employed instead.

The dangers of irradiation are not, however, confined to early pregnancy. The possibility exists of young children developing leukaemia following X-ray of the mother during pregnancy: this risk, whilst smaller than was at first believed, cannot be disregarded, and the foetus should not be subjected to irradiation unless information of value is likely to be obtained. Another danger is the possible genetic effect on the foetal gonads of over-irradiation during pregnancy. The exposure necessary for X-ray pelvimetry makes this type of study one deserving our special consideration. The Thom's view of the pelvic brim is that delivering the highest does to foetal and maternal gonads; indeed, the dose received by foetal gonads in this view is at least three times as great as with A-P, lateral or sub-pubic arch views and the Thom's view should no longer be used.

Against these clear disadvantages are the undoubted benefits to be obtained from X-ray examinations. These are less easily measured in precise terms than radiation dosage. In cases of suspected multiple pregnancy X-ray examination is desirable to ascertain not only the number of foetuses present, but whether there is a foetal abnormality which might influence management. Even conjoined twins can be revealed in this way and it is obviously desirable for both patient and medical attendant to be as well prepared as possible for an event of this kind. Suspicion of a multiple pregnancy still remains an excellent indication for radiological examination; moreover, although the diagnosis of multiple pregnancy can be made by ultrasound scanning, the additional information about foetal normality or abnormality available by X-rays makes this method of examination desirable even when sonar has been used.

The ability of X-rays to detect a foetal ab-

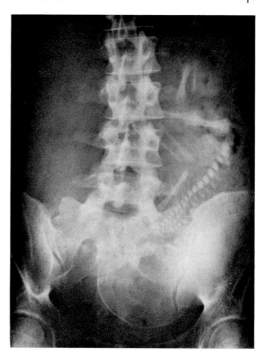

Fig. 9.15. Radiograph showing iniencephaly with a spinal abnormality.

normality remains an excellent reason for a film or films to be requested (Fig. 9.15). In the presence of hydramnios or a previous history of foetal abnormality it is most important to the correct management of the patient to know if the foetus is normal or not. The emotional situation is always highly charged when a foetal abnormality is present, but the possibility may be anticipated and appropriate action taken if we know in time what to expect. Caesarean section, which might otherwise be undertaken purely for the interests of the foetus, may be avoided and an unfortunate situation will not become aggravated.

The emotional problems present in a case of suspected intra-uterine death call for confirmation of this diagnosis as soon as it is reasonable. The foetus may be seen to occupy bizarre attitudes due to loss of muscle tone, there may be hyperflexion of the spine or overlapping of the skull bones (Spalding's sign) (Fig. 9.17). X-rays may provide the most valuable information here, and if the foetus proves to be dead there is, of course,

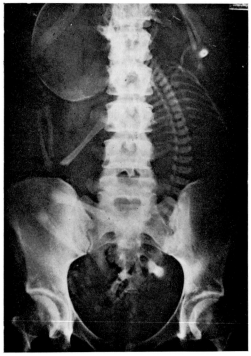

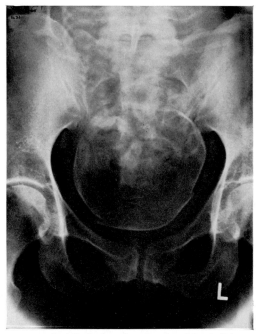

Fig. 9.17. Spalding's sign of overlapping of the skull bones in a dead foetus.

Fig. 9.16. Extension of the foetus in a footling breech presentation.

no foetal risk involved. X-rays to detect presentation will still occasionally be required for patients in whom physical signs are very difficult to elicit. If difficulty does exist clinically it is possible that some unusual foetal attitude will be present which X-rays only will detect (Fig. 9.16). A confident diagnosis of a face presentation before labour, for instance, is not easy and may be possible only on X-ray.

X-ray pelvimetry is still required in certain cases if the patient is to be managed correctly. In the case of a breech presentation, for instance, it is important to employ X-rays for pelvic measurement to permit a proper decision to be taken on treatment. Sonar is no substitute here; it may, however, be most helpfully employed as an adjunct, since the combination of X-ray pelvimetry and ultrasound cephalometry gives us the most accurate assessment yet available of the problem in a case of breech presentation. It must be stressed, too, that if X-ray pelvimetry

is to be employed it must provide all the information otherwise unobtainable. The practice of requesting standing lateral X-rays only does not do this (Rubein & Francis 1967). It should be remembered that of the various pelvic diameters and measurements, those most easily obtainable clinically are at the outlet. The A-P of the pelvic brim can, if significantly reduced, usually be detected on the clinical pelvic examination. The most difficult measurement to be obtained clinically, however, is the transverse diameter of the pelvic brim which will remain unknown if a lateral X-ray only is taken. A-P and lateral films are necessary to get the required information about the measurements of the pelvic brim; from these pictures information can also be obtained about the distance between the ischial spines and the convergence or otherwise of the pelvic walls so that a further view of the pubic arch is, in most cases, unnecessary.

It is difficult to be precise about the circumstances in which X-ray studies should be carried out in pregnancy or labour; in general terms it may be said that if there are uncertainties which cannot be solved by clinical examination and X-rays may provide helpful information the risks of omitting radiography may well be greater than those of carrying it out.

REFERENCES

AHLQUIST R.P. (1950) *J. Am. pharm. Ass. (Scient. Ed.)*, **39**, 370.

ALVAREZ H., BLANCO Y.S., PANIZZA V.G., ROSADA H. & LUCAS O. (1965) *Am. J. Obstet. Gynec.* **93**, 131.

ASPLUND J. (1952) *Acta radiol.* (Supplement) **91**, 3.

ASSALI N.S., RAUMARO L. & PELTONEXI T. (1960) *Am. J. Obst. Gynec.* **79**, 86.

ASSALI N.S., DASGUPTA K., KOLIN A. & HOLMS L. *Am. J. Physiol.* **195**, 614.

BEAN W.B., COGSWELL R.C., DEXTER M. & EMBICK J.E. (1949) *Surgery Gynec. Obstet.* 88, 739.

BENGTSSON L. & CSAPO A.J. (1962) *Am. J. Obstet. Gynec.* **83**, 1083.

BORRELL U. & FERNSTROM I. (1957) *Acta obstet. gynec. scand.* **36**, 42.

BUDIN J. (1897) *Obstetrique*, **2**, 499.

CALDEYRO-BARCIA R. & POSEIRO J.J. (1959) *Ann. N.Y. Acad. Sci.* **75**, 813.

CALDEYRO-BARCIA R.R. & POSEIRO J.J. (1965) In *Obstetrics*, 13th edn. (edited by J.P. Greenhill). Philadelphia and London, Saunders, p. 281.

CAREY H.M. (1963) In *Modern Trends in Reproductive Physiology*, 1st edn. (edited by H.M. Carey). London, Butterworths.

CSAPO A.I. & WOOD C. (1968) In *Recent Advances in Endocrinology*, 8th edn. (edited by V.H.T. James). London, Churchill, p. 207.

CSAPO A.I. & SAUVAGE J. (1969) (in press).

DANFORTH D.N. (1964) *Obstetl. gynec. Surv.* **19**, 715.

DANFORTH D.N. & CHAPMAN J.C.F. (1950) *Am. J. Obstet. Gynec.* **59**, 979.

DAWES G. (1968) *Foetal and Neonatal Physiology*. Chicago, International Year Book Publishers Inc., p. 62.

DE NEEF J.C. (1967a) In *Clinical Endocrine Cytology*. New York, Hoeber, p. 216.

DE NEEF J.C. (1967b) *Clinical Endocrine Cytology*. New York, Hoeber, p. 235.

DE NEEF J.C. (1967c) *Clinical Endocrine Cytology*. New York, Hoeber.

DICZFALUSY E. & TROEN P. (1961) *Vitams.Horm.* **19**, 229.

FRIEDMAN E.A. (1956) *Obstet Gynec., N.Y.* **8**, 691.

GARRETT W.J. (1959) *J. Obstet. Gynaec. Br. Commonw.* **66**, 602.

GARRETT W.J. & MOIR J.C. (1958) *J. Obstet. Gynaec. Br. Commonw.* **65**, 583.

GILLESPIE E.C. (1950) *Am. J. Obstet. Gynec.* **59**, 949.

GILLMAN J. & STEIN H.B. (1941) *Surgery Gynec. Obstet.* **72**, 149.

GOERTTLER K. (1930) *Gegenbaurs morph. Jb.* **65**, 45.

HALL R.E. (1955) *Bull. Sloane Hosp. Women*, **1**, 49.

HARKNESS M.L.R. & HARKNESS R.D. (1959) *J. Physiol.* **148**, 52.

HELIE M. (1864) *Recherches sur la disposition des fibres musculaires de l'uterus developpee par la grossesse.* Paris, Mellinet.

HELLEGERS A.A. & SCHTLUEFER J.J.P. (1961) *Am. J. Obstet. Gynec.* **101**, 377.

HELLMAN L.M., ROSENTHAL A.H., KISTNER R.W. & GORDON R. (1950) *Am. J. Obst. Gynec.* **67**, 899.

HENDRICKS C.H., ESKES T.K.A.B. & SAAMELI K. (1962) *Am. J. Obstet. Gynec.* **83**, 890.

HIBBARD B.M. & HIBBARD E.O. (1968) *Brit. Med. Bull.* **24**, 10.

HYTTEN F.F. & LEITCH I. (1964) *The Physiology of Human Pregnancy*, 1st edn. Oxford, Blackwell, p. 186.

HYTTEN F.F. & LEITCH I. (1964a) *The Physiology of Human Pregnancy*, 1st edn. Oxford, Blackwell, p. 206.

ISRAEL S.L., RUBENSTEON A. & MERANZE D.R. (1954) *Obstet. Gynec., N.Y.* **3**, 399.

KEARNS P.J. (1939) *Am. J. Obstet. Gynec.* **38**, 400.

KERR M.G. (1968) *Br. med. Bull.* **24**, 19.

MANN E.C. (1963) *Progress in Gynaecology*, Vol. 4. New York, Grunne & Stratton, p. 123.

NAKANISHI H., BURNSTOCK G., MCLEAN J. & WOOD C. (1969) *J. reprod. med.* **2**, 20.

NELSON W.W. & GREENE R.R. (1953) *Int. Abstr. Surg.* **97**, 1.

PAPANICOLAU G.N. (1925) *Proc. Soc. exp. Biol. Med.* **22**, 436.

PRYSTOWSKY H., HELLEGERS A. & BRUNS P. (1961) *Am. J. Obstet. Gynec.* **81**, 372.

RAMSEY E.M. (1949) *Contr. Embryol.* **33**, 113.

REYNOLDS S.R.M. & DANFORTH D.N. (1966) in Danforth D.N. *Textbook of Obstetrics and Gynaecology* (edited by D.N. Danforth). New York and London, Hoeber, p. 491.

RHODES P. (1970) In *Scientific Foundations of Obstetrics and Gynaecology* (edited by Philipp, Barnes & Newton). London, Heinemann, p. 440.

SIMS E.A.H. & KRANTZ K.E. (1958) *J. clin. Invest.* **37**, 1764.

SINCLAIR J.D. (1963) *Modern Trends in Human Reproductive Physiology*, 1st edn. p. 181.

SNYDER F.F. (1924) *Bull. Johns Hopkins Hosp.* **35**, 14.

STIEVE H. (1925) *Anat. Ang. Verhandl. anat. Gellesch.* **34**, 80.

STIEVE (1926) *Z. mikrosk.-anat. Fors.* **6**, 351.

STIEVE H. (1932) *Zentbl. Gynäk.* **56**, 1442.

TINDALL V.R. & BEAZLEY J.M. (1965) *J. Obstet. Gynaec. Br. Commonw.* **72**, 717.

ULLERY J.C. & SHABANAH E.H. (1957) *Obst. Gynec., N.Y.* **10**, 233.

WACHTEL E.G. (1964) *Exfoliative Cytology in Gynaecological Practice*. London, Butterworth, p. 77.

WANSBOROUGH H., NAKANISHI H. & WOOD C. (1967) *Obstet. Gynec., N.Y.* **30**, 779.

WOOD C. (1964) *J. Obstet. Gynaec. Br. Commonw.* **71**, 615.

WOOD C. (1969) In *Modern Trends in Obstetrics*, 4th edn. (edited by R.J. Keklar). London, Butterworths.

YOUSSEF A.F. (1958) *Am. J. Obstet. Gynec.* **75**, 1305.

CHAPTER 10

ENDOCRINE CHANGES DURING PREGNANCY

From the time of implantation, until the delivery of the placenta, there is a progressive and profound modification of a woman's hormonal environment. Much of this is immediately due to direct endocrine activity of the placenta and foetus; some of it a secondary effect of the foetoplacental hormones on the maternal endocrine glands.

Although considerable progress has been made in unravelling the hormonal interrelationships of mother–placenta–foetus, there are still large areas of ignorance. Since it is not possible to study pregnancy in the absence of the placenta, this denies to the investigator a classical method of understanding its hormonal function. Once considered endocrinologically inert, it is now clear that the human foetus is very active hormonally, and this has given rise to the concept of the 'foetoplacental unit'. The activity of this unit in turn modifies both quantitatively and qualitatively the behaviour of virtually all maternal endocrine structures.

PROTEIN HORMONES OF THE PLACENTA

During pregnancy, the placenta produces two unique hormones: human chorionic gonadotrophin and human placental lactogen. Their claim to uniqueness lies in the fact that they have never been demonstrated in the absence of trophoblastic tissue.

Human chorionic gonadotrophin (HCG)

There has been little advance in knowledge of this hormone since the subject was reviewed fully by Diczfalusy & Troen (1961). Although undoubtedly produced by the placenta, there remains lingering doubt as to just what part of the placenta produces HCG. Diczfalusy and Troen conclude that the 'cytotrophoblast is probably the major, if not the exclusive source of HCG. It appears that no definite conclusion can yet be made as to the specific cell type responsible for the elaboration of this hormone'.

HCG is a glycoprotein with a relatively high carbohydrate content. Using chemical methods, the molecular weight was found to be about 30,000, and this has been confirmed by the technique of radiation inactivation of biological activity. An international standard has been available since 1939.

Although information on the factors that may control HCG secretion during pregnancy is almost entirely lacking, the pharmacology of HCG has been fully investigated. It is free of follicle-stimulating activity. After prior exposure to FSH, HCG acts as a luteinizing hormone and is capable of inducing ovulation in FSH-primed women. Unlike human LH, it is also luteotrophic. Given early in the luteal phase of the cycle it will prolong the life span of the corpus luteum and increase luteal steroidogenesis.

It is assumed that HCG is responsible for the prominence of interstitial cells in the testes of the male foetus *in utero*; but its other physiological actions in pregnancy are unknown. 'It is indeed paradoxical that so much knowledge could accumulate on the chemistry and pharmacology of a hormone with virtually unknown physiological action' (Diczfalusy & Troen 1961).

The distribution of HCG in placenta, blood and urine throughout pregnancy has been well documented by both biological and immunological assay (Loraine & Bell 1966). Qualitatively the pattern is similar in each. Although there is still argument about the comparability of results obtained by bio-assay and immuno-assay, the latter is most widely employed now in routine laboratories. Increased plasma and urinary levels of HCG are detectable 11 days after ovulation (Marshall et al. 1968). Peak levels of urinary excretion are reached between the sixtieth and seventieth day of gestation, then decline and remain at low levels throughout the remainder of pregnancy. In the absence of retained placental tissue, HCG cannot be detected in urine, using immuno-assay, more than 4 days after delivery.

Human placental lactogen (HPL)

This polypeptide hormone, also known as chorionic growth hormone proclactin (CGP) has been the subject of review by the two groups mainly involved in its isolation and physiology (Grumbach et al. 1968; Josimovitch & Mintz 1968). It is chemically and immunologically similar to human pituitary growth hormone (HGH) and has prolactin-like and growth hormone-like activity. Although the correlation between placental weight and maternal HPL levels is slight, there is clear evidence in vitro (Gusdon & Yen 1967) and in vivo for production by the syncytiotrophoblast (Sciarra et al. 1968).

As with HCG, the factors controlling HPL secretion are obscure. Neither induced hyperglycaemia nor hypoglycaemia affects levels of

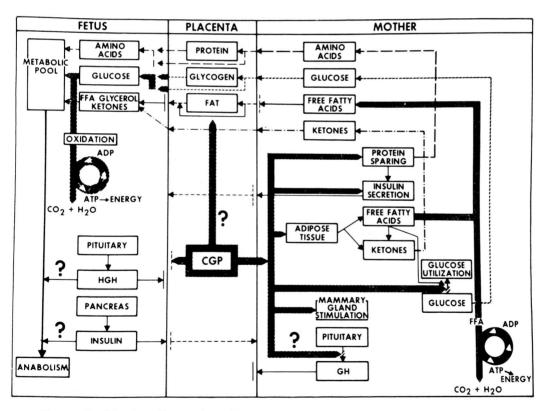

Fig. 10.1. Possible effects of human placental lactogen on foetal and maternal metabolism. (Reproduced from Grumbach et al. (1968), but courtesy of the Editor of *Annals of the New York Academy of Sciences*.)

HPL, and there is no evidence of a circadian rhythm.

Grumbach *et al.* (1968) have summarized the known metabolic effects of HPL. In acute experiments HPL causes an increase in plasma free fatty acids comparable to that produced by HGH; in chronic experiments there is nitrogen and potassium retention and increased urinary excretion of calcium and hydroxyproline. HPL causes a marked decrease in the rate of glucose disposal and an increase in plasma insulin levels; it also augments the insulin response to hyperglycaemia. To reproduce these effects in balance studies, sufficient exogenous HPL must be given to reproduce the serum levels found in the late second and early third trimesters of normal pregnancy.

Although much remains to be learnt of the metabolic effects of HPL, its actions, as postulated by Grumbach, may be summarized as follows:

(1) Rise in plasma free fatty acids and increased mobilization of fat stores.
(2) Increase in resistance to endogenous and exogenous insulin.
(3) Elevation of circulating insulin, increase in insulin response to a glucose load and islet-cell hyperplasia.
(4) Nitrogen retention.
(5) Mammary growth and initiation of lactational phase.
(6) Possible active transport of amino and certain fatty acids across the placenta.
(7) Possible maintenance of the corpus luteum of pregnancy.

Burt *et al.* (1969) have shown that HPL will cause increased hepatic incorporation of glycine into protein.

The suggested interractions of HPL on maternal and foetal metabolism are shown in Fig. 10.1.

The levels of HPL in maternal serum and urine increase progressively throughout pregnancy. Serial estimations throughout pregnancy in five women are shown in Fig. 10.2. Similar increases have been demonstrated by Saxena *et al.* (1968), and the levels during the last 10 weeks of pregnancy from a large group of women

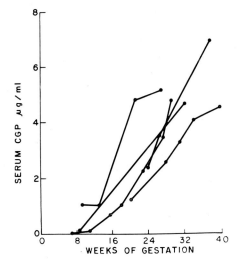

Fig. 10.2. Serial measurement of human placental lactogen (GCP in five patients). (Reproduced from Grumbach *et al.* (1968), by courtesy of the Editor of *Annals of the New York Academy of Sciences.*)

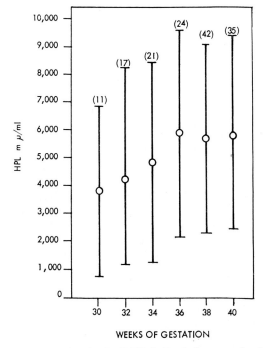

Fig. 10.3. Plasma levels of HPL during the last 10 weeks of pregnancy. (Reproduced from Gudson (1969), by courtesy of the Editor of *Obstetrics and Gynecology, New York.*)

are shown in Fig. 10.3 (Gudson 1969). Very low levels are found, on the other hand, in foetal blood, indicating that little placentofoetal transfer occurs.

STEROID HORMONES OF THE PLACENTA

Progesterone

The synthesis and metabolism of progesterone has been discussed in Chapter 3. While the maternal ovary contributes some progesterone in the very earliest stages of pregnancy, after this the placental contribution dominates, and there is no doubt that the placenta is the source of virtually all the progesterone produced during pregnancy. In addition to progesterone, two other biologically active progestogens (20α- and 20β-hydroxypregn-4-ene-3-one) are secreted, but in much lower quantities.

The placenta is able to synthesize progesterone from the same precursors as those discussed in Chapter 3 (Jaffe 1967). Unlike oestrogens, progesterone production is only very slightly affected by the foetal circulation (Cassmer 1959). These foetoplacental relationships have been fully reviewed by Solomon et al. (1967).

Although some progress has been made in determining the control of progesterone secretion in the ovary, there is very little known of the controlling mechanism(s) in pregnancy. Certainly it is independent of maternal pituitary control (Fotherby 1964), nor can any negative feed-back mechanism be demonstrated.

The metabolic effects of progesterone and its activity on the uterus have been fully reviewed by Fotherby (1964) and by Hytten & Leitch (1964). Progesterone probably antagonizes the action of aldosterone on the renal tubule, but this action is compensated for by the increased secretion of aldosterone seen in pregnancy (see p. 150). In large amounts, progesterone has a slight catabolic action and there is suggestive evidence that fat deposition may be increased.

The effects of progesterone on the uterus are complex and ill-understood. It is probable that progesterone affects the membrane potential of myometrial fibres, thereby reducing the excitability of the uterus. The effect of progesterone on the protein and collagen content of the uterus remains unresolved. It appears to increase the activity of alkaline phosphatase and succinate dehydrogenase in the uterus.

It is widely believed—but objective evidence for the belief is scanty—that the high levels of progesterone in pregnancy reduce smooth muscle tone in the ureter, colon and stomach. It is of interest that large doses of progesterone induce overbreathing with a reduction in alveolar and arterial PCO_2—changes normally observed in pregnancy.

Levels of progesterone and its metabolites in biological tissues

Unlike the evidence showing selective accumulation of oestradiol by 'target organ' (see p. 149), the only tissue which shows a very high uptake of progesterone is adipose tissue. The higher levels of progesterone in myometrial tissue directly overlying the placenta are explicable on grounds of contiguity to the major site of production in pregnancy.

Progesterone levels in blood during pregnancy have been documented by Eton & Short (1960) and Yannone et al. (1968), showing a progressive increase throughout gestation. Although the presence of urinary progesterone has been indicated in pregnancy (Ismael & Harkness 1966), there are no adequate data on excretion patterns in normal or abnormal pregnancy.

Urinary pregnanediol levels have for many years been used as a means of assessing changes in progesterone production. The limitations of such an approach need to be clearly recognized. Although there is general recognition of the poor correlation between the excretion of urinary pregnanediol and either progesterone secretion or blood progesterone levels, for both historical and technical reasons, pregnanediol assays have been wisely used in endocrinological studies for many years. Adequate data using reliable methods are well documented. Using the same method, Shearman, (1959) and Klopper & Billewicz (1963) produced very similar findings. Their results, together with those of Eton and

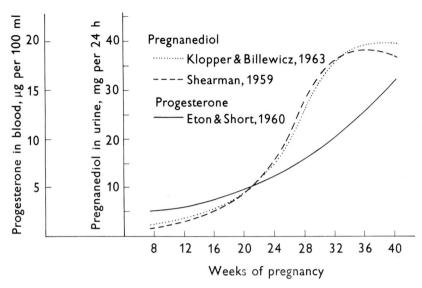

Fig. 10.4. Urinary pregnanediol excretion and blood progesterone levels during pregnancy. (Reproduced from Hytten & Leitch (1964), by courtesy of Blackwell Scientific Publications Ltd.)

Short for progesterone in blood, are shown in Fig. 10.4.

Oestrogens

In the last decade there has been a large amount of data collected on the interrelationships of the maternal, foetal and placental contributions to oestrogen synthesis in pregnancy. Much of this has been reviewed extensively during this time (Cassmer 1959; Diczfalusy *et al.* 1961; Frandsen 1963; Bolte 1967).

Although more than 25 different oestrogens have been isolated from human pregnancy urine, to simplify a complex problem only the three 'classical oestrogens'—oestrone, oestradiol and oestriol—will be discussed here.

The metabolism of oestrogens in the non-pregnant female is discussed in Chapters 3 and 7, where it will be noted that the biologically active secreted steroids—oestrone and oestradiol—are derived from androgenic precursors. Oestriol is predominantly a metabolite of these, but is secreted as such in small quantities by active steroidogenic tissue, (Barlow & Logan

1966). It is also usually accepted that a hallmark of 'secreted' as distinct from 'metabolized' oestrogen in the non-pregnant, is that they are unconjugated: conjugation under these circumstances is usually accepted as part of the biological inactivation and metabolism of the secreted parent hormone.

The picture in pregnancy is different, involving a complex of maternal and foetal precursors, the foetal contribution being very dependent on the foetal adrenal and liver, and an intact foeto-placental circulation.

In the non-pregnant individual the proportions of oestriol : oestrone : oestradiol in urine varies, but approximates 3:2:1. As indicated above most of the oestriol is derived from the metabolism of oestrone/oestradiol. In late pregnancy the urinary proportion of the three steroids is radically different—30:2:1. There is clear evidence for secretion of oestriol by the placenta during pregnancy from predominantly foetal precursors, and of oestradiol from predominantly maternal precursors (Fig. 10.5).

Studies both *in vitro* and *in vivo* indicate that there is increasing ability of the placenta to

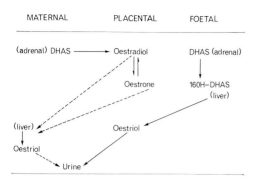

MATERNAL   PLACENTAL   FOETAL

(adrenal) DHAS ———→ Oestradiol   DHAS (adrenal)

                         Oestrone   16OH–DHAS
                                            (liver)

(liver)   Oestriol

Oestriol

Urine

Fig. 10.5. Outline of oestrogen metabolism in the foeto-placental unit.

convert maternal dehydro-epiandrosterone sulphate (DHAS) to oestradiol during pregnancy, conversion rates increasing from about 5% at 16 weeks' gestation to 40% at term (Siiteri & MacDonald 1966). Foetal DHAS also contributes to placental oestradiol production.

It is known that the placenta lacks a 16-hydroxylase, so is incapable itself of synthesizing oestriol. The particular role of the foetus in the synthesis of precursors of oestriol, suggested by the observations of Cassmer (1959) and extended by those of Frandsen & Stakemann (1963), has been amply confirmed. In essence, DHAS secreted by the foetal zone of the adrenal cortex is 16-hydroxylated in the foetal liver (16-OH–DHAS) and transported via the umbilical arteries to the placenta, where it is aromatized and hydrolized to produce free oestriol.

Apart from the clear effect that absence of the foetal adrenal zone—as may be seen in anencephaly—has on oestriol synthesis, the factors controlling oestrogen synthesis by the placenta are unknown.

Some progress has been made in clarifying the mode of action of oestrogens, and this has been reviewed by Gorski et al. (1967). The hormones of the thyroid and adrenal cortex have a catholicity of action which spreads to almost every physiological system. The oestrogens have long been remarkable for what is predominantly a selective and profound action on a few body tissues. In view of their relatively unsophisticated molecular structure, this has posed a constant problem.

Generally speaking, a hormone could have a selective action on a particular tissue for two reasons:

(i) because it is selectively concentrated in the target tissue; or
(ii) the target tissue possesses metabolic pathways or enzyme systems responsive only to that hormone, pathways not shared by less or non-responsive tissues.

Both of these factors appear to be involved in the action of oestrogens. The classical experiments of Jensen & Jacobsen (1962) show selective uptake and retention of oestradiol by target organs such as uterus, vagina and pituitary, while 'non-responsive' tissue such as liver, kidney and muscle show concentrations closely following those found in blood. A physiological receptor for oestrogens has been identified in 'target tissue' (Gorski et al. 1967).

Earlier work from Villee et al. (1960) had indicated the presence of an oestrogen-dependent pyridine nucleotide transhydrogenase, catalysing the transfer of hydrogen ions and electrons from TPNH to DPN. An essential part of this thesis is that an equilibrium must be established between oestradiol and oestrone. Utilization of oestradiol by this mechanism in vivo should allow the demonstration of the production of oestrone from oestradiol. In vivo studies have failed, so far, to confirm this. In tissues where this reversible oxidation is supposed to occur following the administration of tritiated oestradiol, no tritiated oestrone can be detected. This is true even allowing for equilibrium to lie well in the direction of reduction, i.e. in the direction of oestradiol. A specific role of oestrogens is increasing RNA synthesis by inhibiting the action of a RNA depressor has been postulated by Talwar et al. (1964).

The urinary excretion pattern of oestrogen in pregnancy is well documented, following the first accurate observations by Brown in 1956. Because of its widespread clinical use, urinary oestriol excretion has received particular attention, and there is a large amount of information dealing with levels in normal and abnormal pregnancy. The results obtained by Coyle & Brown (1963) are shown in Fig. 10.6.

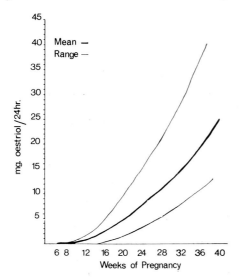

Fig. 10.6. Urinary oestriol excretion during normal pregnancy. (Reproduced from Coyle & Brown (1963), by courtesy of the Editor of *Journal of Obstetrics and Gynaecology of the British Commonwealth*.)

Other endocrine changes

THYROID

Although there is frequently enlargement of the thyroid in pregnancy and there are changes in some parameters used to assess thyroid function, normal pregnant women are euthyroid. Hytten & Leitch (1964) have shown that the increased oxygen consumption (and hence raised BMR) of pregnancy can be accounted for by the oxygen consumption of the foetus and that used by the increased cardiac output of pregnancy. There is an oestrogen dependent increase in thyroid-binding globulin (TBG) during pregnancy, causing an increase in protein-bound iodine (PBI) to between 8 and 12 $\mu g/100$ ml. Unlike the increased PBI of thyrotoxicosis, there is a concurrent fall in the resin uptake of tri-iodothyronine. Some investigators have used levels of PBI and tri-iodothyronine resin uptake to assess the 'free thyroxine index'. Uptake of [131]I—which clearly should never be administered knowingly to a pregnant woman—is normal. An excellent study of thyroid indices in pregnancy has been published by Mestman *et al*. (1969).

ADRENAL CORTEX

Aldosterone

There is a large mass of well-documented data relating to aldosterone secretion and excretion in pregnancy. The factors responsible for, and the significance of, the observed changes remain elusive.

Much of the earlier uncertainty about changes in aldosterone levels can be attributed to methodological confusion, as is so often the case. The initial observation by Venning & Dyrenfurth (1956) of an increase in pH_1-extractable aldosterone has been amply confirmed. Despite a marked increase in aldosterone secretion rate, there is no significant change in the protein binding of plasma aldosterone (Schteingart 1967). Neither the foetus nor placenta contribute significantly to the increased secretion rate.

Cortisol

Changes in cortisol secretion, transport and metabolism during pregnancy are well documented and have been briefly reviewed by Schteingart (1967). The secretion rate is doubled in late pregnancy and there is an increase in plasma cortisol. Although most of this is protein bound, there is an increase in free plasma cortisol. The plasma half-life of free cortisol is significantly prolonged in pregnancy.

PITUITARY HORMONES

Earlier confusion about changes in HGH (Greenwood *et al*. 1964) has been clarified by assays that will distinguish HGH from HPL. There is no significant increase in maternal HGH during pregnancy, but the levels in foetal blood, however, are very high (Grumbach *et al*. 1968).

There is still confusion about levels of corticotrophin during pregnancy, the consensus being that there is an increase. Although it can be extracted from placental tissue, there is no evidence that the placenta produces ACTH (Diczfalusy & Troen 1961).

Odell *et al.* (1967) have assayed thyroid-stimulating hormone by an immunological method during pregnancy, and found it to be within normal limits.

There is a significant increase in melanocyte-stimulating hormone (MSH) in pregnancy (Hytton & Leitch 1964).

INSULIN

Plasma levels of insulin, as measured by radio-immunoassay, are increased in pregnancy (Antoniades 1968; Kyle 1968). It is known that the experimental administration of HPL to non-pregnant subjects will increase plasma insulin levels and the response to hyperglycaemia (Grumbach *et al.* 1968), and it is tempting to assume that the mechanics of the observed change in plasma insulin during pregnancy are due in part to the advent of HPL.

REFERENCES

ANTONIADES H.N. (1968) In *Gynecologic Endocrinology* (edited by J.J. Gold). New York, Hoeber, p. 607.

BARLOW J.J. & LOGAN C.M. (1966) *Steroids*, 7, 309.

BOLTE E. (1967) *Clin. Obstet Gynec.* 10, 60.

BROWN J.B. (1956) *Lancet* i, 704.

BURT R.L., PEGRAM P.S. & LEAKE N.H. (1969) *Am. J. Obstet. Gynec.* 103, 44.

CASSMER O. (1959) *Acta endocr. Copenh.*, Supplement 45.

COYLE M.G. & BROWN J.B. (1963) *J. Obstet. Gynaec. Br. Commonw.* 70, 225.

DICZFALUSY E., CASSMER O., ALONSO C. & DE MIQUEL M. (1961) *Recent Prog. Horm. Res.* 17, 147.

DICZFALUSY E. & TROEN P. (1961) *Vitams Horm.* 19, 230.

ETON B. & SHORT R.V. (1960) *J. Obstet. Gynaec. Br. Commonw.* 67, 785.

FOTHERBY K. (1964) *Vitams Horm.* 22, 153.

FRANDSEN V.A. (1963) *The Excretion of Oestriol in Normal Human Pregnancy*. Copehnagen, Monksgaard.

FRANDSEN V.A. & STAKEMANN G. (1963) *Acta endocr., Copenh.* 43, 184.

GORSKI J., NOTIDES A., TOFT D. & SMITH D.E. (1967) *Clin. Obstet. Gynec.* 10, 17.

GREENWOOD F.C., HUNTER W.M. & KLOPPER A. (1964) *Br. med. J.* i, 22.

GRUMBACH M.M., KAPLAN S.L., SCIARRA J.J. & BURR I.M. (1968) *Ann. N.Y. Acad. Sci.* 148, 501.

GUDSON J.P. & YEN S.S.C. (1967) *Obstet. Gynec., N.Y.* 30, 635.

GUDSON J.P. (1969) *Obstet. Gynec., N.Y.* 33, 397.

HYTTON F.E. & LEITCH I. (1964) *The Physiology of Human Pregnancy*. Oxford, Blackwell, p. 138.

ISMAIL A.A.A. & HARKNESS R.A. (1966) *Biochem. J.* 98, 15P.

JAFFE R.B. (1967) *Clin. Obstet. Gynec.* 10, 47.

JENSEN E.V. & JACOBSON H.I. (1962) *Recent Prog. Horm. Res.* 18, 387.

JOSIMOVITCH J.B. & MINTZ D.H. (1968) *Ann. N.Y. Acad. Sci.* 148, 488.

KLOPPER A. & BILLEWICZ W. (1963) *J. Obstet. Gynaec. Br. Commonw.* 70, 1024.

KYLE G.C. (1968) In *Gynecologic Endocrinology* (edited by J.J. Gold). New York, Hoeber, p. 607.

LORAINE J.A. & BELL E.T. (1966) *Hormone Assays and their Clinical Application*. Edinburgh and London, Livingstone, p. 83.

MARSHALL J.R., HAMMOND C.B., ROSS G.T., JACOBSON A., RAYLORD P. & ODELL W.D. (1968) *Obstet. Gynec., N.Y.* 32, 760.

MESTMAN J.H., NISWONGER J.W.H., ANDERSON G.V. & MANNING P.R. (1969) *Am. J. Obstet. Gynec.* 103, 322.

ODELL W.D., WILBER J.F. & UTIGER R.D. (1967) *Recent Prog. Horm. Res.* 23, 47.

SAXENA B.N., REFETOFF S., EMERSON K. & SELENKOW H.A. (1968) *Am. J. Obstet. Gynec.* 101, 874.

SCHTEINGART D.E. (1967) *Clin. Obstet. Gynec.* 10, 88.

SCIARRA J.J., SHERWOOD L.M., VARMA A.A. & LUNDBERG W.B. (1968) *Am. J. Obstet. Gynec.* 101, 413.

SHEARMAN R.P. (1959) *J. Obstet. Gynaec. Br. Commonw.* 66, 1.

SIITERI P.K. & MACDONALD P.C. (1966) *J. clin. Endocr. Metab.* 26, 751.

SOLOMON S., BIRD C.E., LING W., IWAMIYA M. & YOUNG P.C.M. (1967) *Recent Prog. Horm. Res.* 23, 297.

TALWAR G.P., SEGAL S.J., EVANS A. & DAVIDSON D.W. (1964) *Proc. natn. Acad. Sci. U.S.A.* 52, 1059.

VENNING E.H. & DYRENFURTH I. (1956) *J. clin. Endocr. Metab.* 16, 426.

VILLEE C.A., HAGERMAN D.D. & JOEL P.B. (1960) *Recent Prog. Horm. Res.* 16, 49.

YANNONE M.E., MCCURDY J.R. & GOLDFEIN A. (1968) *Am. J. Obstet. Gynec.* 101, 1058.

ZANDER J. & MUNSTERMANN A.M. (1956) *Klin. Wschr.* 34, 944.

CHAPTER 11

THE FOETUS

From implantation to delivery, the human foetus lives for 260 days in the uterus, an encapsulated organism, shut off from the external world, dependent upon the umbilical and placental circulation. The foetus and placenta become a body compartment of the mother, the composition of foetal tissues being kept constant by the transfer function of the placenta, for while foetal homeostasis does exist, it is by and large secondary to maternal mechanisms (Fig. 11.1). Virtually all foetal intake and output occurs across the placental membrane which separates the foetal and maternal milieu interieur. Only via the maternal extracellular fluid compartment can the external environment be reached, for the foetal organs of homeostasis mostly com-

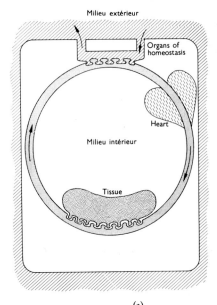

(a)

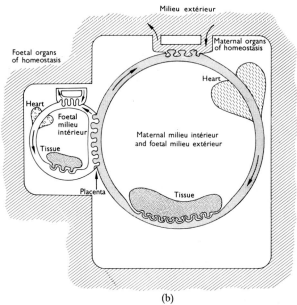

(b)

Fig. 11.1. A diagrammatic representation of the body compartments.

(a) shows the non-pregnant adult whose blood equilibrates with the tissues through the extra cellular compartment and is restored to normality at the homeostatic organs in communication with the milieu exterieur.

(b) represents the foetal situation. Although he has his own milieu exterieur in the amniotic sac, this is completely closed off and his milieu exterieur is really the maternal milieu interieur; although the foetus has his own homeostatic organs, the most effective part of this homeostatis must take place across the placenta.

municate with the amniotic cavity, which is a closed-off zone. At the placenta, the foetal and maternal circulations are close but are kept separate; it is important to remember the dual development and functional anatomy of the placenta, for any activity may be considered from the foetal or maternal side, depending on what is being measured.

Alterations in the ability of the placenta to handle the exchange of gases, fluids or nutrients leads to deprivation of the foetus, and are considered to be 'placental insufficiency'; this is a clinical concept, but many efforts are being made to measure it qualitatively. As well as its function as an exchange station, the placenta is a metabolic organ providing many hormones and enzymes. The two activities (regulation of exchange and endocrine gland) may be independent of each other, but it is the second activity of the placenta that is usually investigated when placental-function tests are performed. There may be a relationship between the efficiency of the organ in each of these functions, but if there is, it is probably a complex and altering one and there is no justification to extrapolate from one to the other. However, correlations do exist between the various placental activities and between them and the clinical state of the foetus. If these correlations can properly be assessed they are of use in foetal prognosis.

THE FOETUS IN PREGNANCY

The foetus grows in the uterus from a single fertilized cell into a complex organism, increasing his weight about six billion times. The rate of growth is the product of the rate of multiplication of cells and growth of those cells themselves. Since the former is mostly under genetic control, it is the latter which is often responsible for variations in the body size in a given species. The rate of growth of a cell depends on the availability of nutrients. In the foetus this depends upon the maternal blood in the placenta. Except in extreme conditions of starvation, the concentration of nutrients in the maternal blood is the same in most women, and so the availability of food-stuffs to the foetal cells will depend upon

the blood flow on the maternal side of the placenta and the transfer of nutrients to the foetoplacental unit.

In the first 12 weeks of pregnancy the developing embryo does not have a full placental system. For a few days it is suspended in the secretion of the Fallopian tube and the uterus. It is then implanted in the decidua as a blastocyst and all exchange of gases, food-stuffs and waste products takes place with the surrounding pool of blood and degenerating cells. Figure 11.2, showing the rate of growth of the foetus in the uterus, indicates that there is not a linear relationship between growth and maturity. By about 12 weeks, when the foetus weighs about 30 g, the placental system is evolved, and there is an acceleration of growth rate followed by a flattening in the latter weeks.

Data for charts like Fig. 11.2 are derived from two sources, weight of hysterotomy specimens in early pregnancy and birth weights in late pregnancy. The former can be accurately and reproducibly obtained but the latter are less accurate, as the time from birth to the time of weighing may be many hours, and the weight of various impedimenta may be included (such as umbilical cord clips and forceps). Further, it must be remembered that the delivery of many babies before term is for some pathological reason; induction of labour may be performed because of a hypertensive problem or the mother may go into spontaneous labour, producing a small baby because of an inefficient placenta. Hence the groups of weights in later pregnancy are less reliable when discussing normality, even when careful screening has been done to exclude all known abnormalities of pregnancy.

The variations in these groups can be defined by one of two mathematical methods. The mean curve of weight at birth is established for any gestation and curves at one and two standard deviations above and below that mean are drawn. Babies outside the second standard deviation are considered to be significantly large or small for dates. This method is used by pathologists. The other technique involves the plotting of the weights on a percentage notation when weights above the 90th or below the 10th percentile are considered to be outside normal range. Such a method of measurement is commonly used by

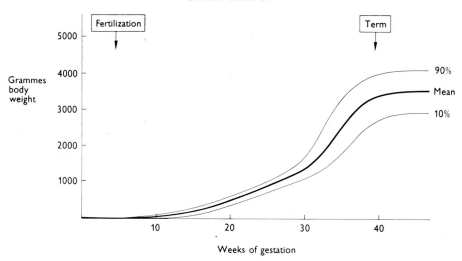

Fig. 11.2. Mean growth-gestation chart of human foetus. This is a composite chart from hysterotomy specimens in early pregnancy and from birth weights in the second half. The lighter lines indicate the 10th and 90th percentiles of the range of weights at any given gestation.

paediatricians when following babies' progress into childhood. If the distribution of babies' weights at any given maturity is random, then two standard deviations on either side of the mean contain about 96% of the population, so that both methods would give similar results. There is, however, usually a bias fractionally towards the lower weights, in which case the percentile method would be more useful in practice, but using either of these methods, two

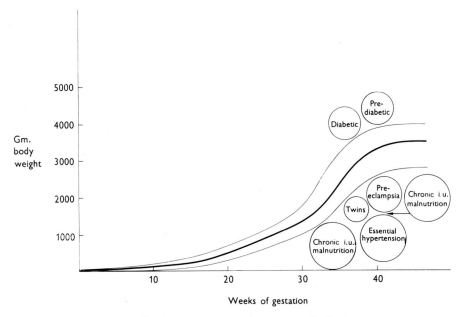

Fig. 11.3. Groups of babies recognized to be heavy—or small—for dates (see text).

groups of babies can be demonstrated (Fig. 11.3): a group that are larger, and a group that are smaller, than the expected gestation weight. Into the first group come babies born to mothers with diabetes or prediabetes. Into the latter group come the babies with congenital abnormalities (Trisomy 21 and Turner's syndrome), those with intra-uterine infections (such as the chronic rubella syndrome or toxoplasmosis), and those whose mothers are suffering from conditions known to affect placental exchange (hypertension and pre-eclampsia). Also in this group are babies born after multiple pregnancies and, sometimes, babies born to mothers who live at high altitudes. After all these recognizable groups have been identified, there is still a group of babies small-for-dates for no obvious reason.

It has long been recognized that there are variations in intra-uterine growth rate, but until recently, growth-retarded infants have been confused with premature babies. This is due partly to the weight definition of prematurity (2·5 kg or less) being used as the only criterion. The use of weight-gestation charts has differentiated these two groups—the baby born before his time, who is small but of the correct size for his gestation and the baby who may be born at any time in pregnancy but who is small for his period of gestation. The 'small-for-dates' (or growth-retarded) babies undoubtedly result from chronic malnutrition while in the uterus.

These growth-retarded babies appear long and thin with relatively large heads, as the head circumference and body length are less retarded than body weight. They show a lack of subcutaneous fat and many organs such as the liver, the lungs and the heart are smaller relative to total body weight than are those of the truly premature infant. Neurological development is mature and the brain weight is relatively greater in relation to birth weight, and so the ratio between liver and brain, which normally is 1 : 3; may be as high as 1 : 6. The reduction in organ size is due to reduction in individual cell mass rather than cell number, and is common to both the intra-uterine 'small-for-dates' foetus and the postnatal baby suffering from malnutrition.

The nutritional block to the foetus might be either in the blood supply to the placental bed,

in the placenta itself or in the foetal vessels leading from the placental mass. Experimental work in which the uterine arteries of pregnant animals were banded has shown various degrees of foetal growth retardation, the foetuses in the most hypoxic parts of the oviduct being most affected. This effect might be an exaggeration of the normal maternal constraint mechanism on foetal growth in the latter weeks of pregnancy, and taken further in certain pathological conditions when the lumen of blood vessels on the maternal side of the placenta is diminished. Thrombotic occlusion of the arteries of the placental bed in pre-eclampsia has been shown, and this is a condition well known to be associated with chronically malnourished babies. Alterations in the structure of the placental membrane are often seen in conditions associated with such babies (e.g. 'syncytial knotting'). The foetal circulation may be impaired by endothelial cushions found in the vessels on the foetal side of the placentas of growth-retarded babies, and these obstructions may affect the foetal circulation just as the thrombotic conditions can affect the maternal blood flow. Pre-eclampsia is a well-known clinical state associated with 'small-for-dates' babies, but foetal pathological conditions are only diagnosed after delivery of the placenta. Many growth-retarded babies are not so 'flagged' by any obvious clinical state of the mother, who may have a good reproductive background.

Foetal distress may now be divided into two phases: the chronic and the acute. The former is long-term malnutrition of the foetus in pregnancy, the latter the shorter reflection of this in labour, when the stress of uterine contractions is added to the chronic lack of transfer, causing the foetus to show the classical signs associated with clinical foetal distress. If exchange has been good until labour starts, the foetus can stand the extra stresses well. It is as though one wished to borrow money from the bank. To raise a debt when the account is in reasonable balance can be done without damage to the bank or the debtor. If, however, there is a chronic overdraft already, it is much harder to deal with acute debts as they arise.

Growth-retarded foetuses have a greatly increased risk of hypoxia during labour. The

National Birthday Trust Perinatal Mortality
Survey (Butler 1965), showed these babies to have
a threefold risk of asphyxia during delivery and
massive pulmonary haemorrhage in the neonatal
period. They can also be shown to have a high
risk of neonatal hypoxia. By recognizing chronic
intra-uterine malnutrition during pregnancy,
more stringent monitoring can be used in labour
to produce a less affected infant. The identification of these foetuses can be by clinical and other
estimates, and it is appropriate that a portion of
antenatal care should be devoted to the recognition of this group of babies in the uterus.

Measuring foetal activity

Management of any patient in medicine depends
on an amalgam of measurements of the current
state and knowledge of similar past situations.
Much well-documented past experience exists
in human obstetrics, but the measurement of the
foetus has been poor. Until recently, all foetal
monitoring has been by relatively coarse-scaled
clinical methods. In the last decade, techniques
have allowed more accurate measurement of the
foetoplacental unit, but most knowledge of the
intra-uterine state in the human species has been
obtained indirectly. In other animals—notably
dogs, sheep, rats and guinea-pigs—direct ex-
perimentation on, and measurement of, the
foetus has led to elucidation of many situations
in foetal physiology. Often the findings are at
variance with those in the human species, and
it may be misleading to extrapolate from one to
another. Rates of foetal development, patterns of
uterine and foetal blood flow, placental organization and membrane structure are all
different and many problems can only be resolved
by the proper study of the species that concerns
the clinical obstetrician—man.

CLINICAL ESTIMATES

The clinical assessment of any situation rests upon
data obtained from the history, the physical
examination and the results of investigations.
The first is little used when determining the
state of the foetus. Physical examination is most
useful, for it detects changes in an altering

situation, while investigations are becoming increasingly important in providing the obstetrician
with knowledge about the foetoplacental unit.

It is conventional in the Western world to
examine the patient's abdomen when she attends
for antenatal visits. This allows a rough check
to be made of the rate of growth of the uterus.
At the earlier visits the observer is measuring
hypertrophy of myometrium, and only in the
second half of pregnancy does the foetus and
his amniotic fluid become a major component
of the increase in size of the uterus. Increments
of growth are fairly easy to assess by bimanual
examination in early pregnancy until 20 weeks,
allowing an estimate of growth. Assessment of
foetal size later on is of less use, but serial
examinations, especially if done by one observer,
can indicate foetal growth retardation.

The position, presentation and number of
foetuses in the uterus can be determined, the
accuracy of any observer's examination increasing
with experience. The foetal heart can be auscultated at intervals, giving evidence of foetal
life, but the gaps between observations are
so long that this test is of little value in gauging
foetal well-being. At the very end of pregnancy,
the size and hardness of the foetal head and its
fit in the maternal pelvis can be determined. The
state of the cervix can provide a guide to the
proximity of the onset of labour, and the degree
of 'ripeness' can be gauged by a combination of
softness, dilatation and amount of reduction in
length of the cervical canal.

The briefness of this account of the clinical
assessment of the foetus should not be taken to
indicate its lack of importance. In many hospitals
it is the major method of assessing the intra-
uterine situation, but these practical matters are
best learned in the clinics and labour wards. The
subject has been very well documented, so more
emphasis is placed here on the newer and less-
well-understood investigations used to measure
foetal well-being.

RADIOLOGY

X-ray demonstration of the foetus in the uterus
was the earliest of the scientific investigations
applied in this field. Even the coarse early films

were of assistance in the diagnosis of presentation or numbers of foetuses in the uterus. The maturity of the foetus is often assessed from X-rays. Should the foetus be lying so that the sagittal diameter of his head is seen to be exactly at right-angles to the film, then a biparietal diameter can be accurately measured. This is often a chance finding. A more commonly used observation is the time of calcification in the ossification centres of various bones. The two most useful are in the lower femur appearing at 36–37 weeks, and the upper tibia at 38–40 weeks; Russell (1969) has shown a good correlation between the radiological appearance of centres of ossification and maturity prediction. Calcification of the placenta is of little use in the estimation of maturity, for while the majority of placentae show calcification when X-rayed postnatally, less than 20% present similar signs in the uterus. There is little difference between the calcification seen in pregnancies known to be at 38 weeks when compared with those of 42 weeks.

It is often desirable to know whether the foetus is grossly abnormal, for actions taken to speed labour and delivery may depend upon this. Commonly, an X-ray is requested to detect congenital malformations, but it should be stressed that usually only neuroskeletal lesions will be identified. In a recent 4-year period at Queen Charlotte's Hospital, 676 congenital abnormalities were reported in 12,900 deliveries of live and dead babies. Analysis showed that 191 (28·2%) of these malformations were capable of being radiologically identified in the later weeks of pregnancy. However, if only the major abnormalities were discussed, then 53 of 120— i.e. 52%—might have been diagnosed. These are the highest figures and show what would be theoretically possible.

The clinical diagnosis of intra-uterine death is often confirmed by X-rays; the earliest sign is the production of gas in the inferior vena cava and the venous system of the liver. This can occur within 12 hours of death, and may be accompanied by gas shadows in the umbilical cord. The classical Spalding's sign of overlapping of the cranial bones is unreliable if the head has been moulded by strong contractions of the uterus, and it may take several days to develop.

In earlier pregnancy, foetal death is often accompanied by a 'crumpling up' of the body, so that the foetus appears to be tightly packed, with acute angles of flexion seen in various parts (see also p. 140).

The risks of irradiation to the foetus have been greatly stressed, and are threefold. The first is that of teratogenesis. This could be avoided by not X-raying mothers in the first 14 weeks of pregnancy. The second risk is that of subsequent development of malignant disease in children who have been exposed to X-rays before birth. This risk has been assessed as increasing the cancer incidence of children up to the age of 10 years by about 1 in 3,000. Since some of the studies are retrospective (and even the prospective ones are looking at irradiation of past years), advances in X-ray technique may have led to a lowering of the dose of foetal radiation. The third risk of intra-uterine irradiation is to the gonads of the developing foetus, so that future generations of chromosomes may be affected. In the human species, this risk has not been fully assessed and the evidence available must come by extrapolation from other species that reproduce more quickly than the human.

ULTRASONICS

Because of the risks inherent in X-ray diagnosis, much effort has been made in other fields of physical investigation of the foetus. One of these involves the reflection of ultrasonic waves from tissue planes, and information on the general background of this science can be found in Chapter 15. The technique can be used wherever there is an interface between solid and fluid or between solids of differing acoustic density. It can be used to outline the early gestation sac, localize the placenta and diagnose hydatidiform moles, and can even detect small pieces of placenta left in a uterus after delivery. One of its more useful facets is the precise measurement of the biparietal foetal head diameter, allowing accurate assessment of foetal maturity and growth.

The sound waves are reflected back from all tissue interfaces in front of the source only if those surfaces are at right-angles to the ultrasonic beam. In order to detect all these interfaces,

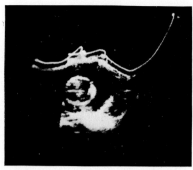

Fig. 11.4. The head of a foetus at eighteen weeks gestation. Echoes are reflected from the bony skull and from the junction between the cerebral hemispheres By retaining the image of each linear scan and by collecting a large number of these, a composite picture of the head can be built up. To measure the biparietal diameter no large number of images is required and with an A scan, the two parietal eminences and the mid line echo only are identified and the intervals measured.

the source is rocked at different angles across the abdomen. Measurement of the foetal head is accurate because the junction of the cerebral hemispheres (mid-line echo) can be detected between the parietal eminences and the same measurement can be made on each occasion (Fig. 11.4). This method has been shown to be accurate, the mean error in early and later pregnancy being less than 1 mm (Campbell 1970). Measurements taken during normal pregnancy have shown that there is a steady rate of growth of the foetal head with a narrow range of variation up to about 30 weeks (Fig. 11.5); thence the rate of growth flattens off and the range of head size widens gradually. This means that interpretations before the thirtieth week are liable to be more accurate, and work done at Queen Charlotte's Hospital has shown that it is

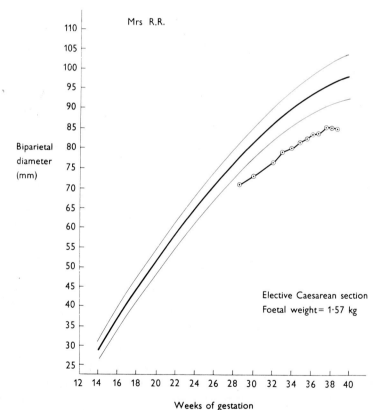

Fig. 11.5. Biparietal diameter of the foetal head throughout gestation measured by ultrasound.

The heavy line indicates the mean and the lighter lines join the limits of two standard deviations from the mean of the diameters at any given gestation. The actual readings of a growth retarded foetus are recorded on the chart.

possible to predict the expected date of confinement to ± 9 days in over 80% of cases. This accuracy compares favourably with the clinical gestation dating done on patients who are sure of their dates. Interpretation of measurements made after 30 weeks produces a less accurate prediction, but still gives a clinically useful indication of the maturity of the foetus in question.

Serial readings of biparietal diameters are of more use than a single one. The method causes the patient little inconvenience and no danger; the readings may be performed weekly to show if the foetal growth is within normal limits. At present this is the most reliable method of measuring foetal growth; it and urinary oestrogen estimation are the two main methods of antenatal foetal monitoring at Queen Charlotte's Hospital.

HORMONE ESTIMATIONS

Hormones regulate foetal growth—directly at first and later, after placental organization has occurred, through the chronic control of the uteroplacental circulation. Hormone assays therefore measure some of the basic factors in foetal well-being. The usefulness of these estimations had to await two advances in endocrinology. The former was the better understanding of hormone metabolic pathways using radio-isotopic methods; the other advance lay in the more rapid techniques of hormone measurement in biological fluids, so that the results could be obtained in time to be clinically useful in patient management. Both have stimulated a great increase in work on normal and abnormal pregnancies, and four basic hormones of the foetoplacental unit are considered briefly here in their clinical context. Full reviews of the more technical and biological aspects of this field are found in Klopper (1969).

Chorionic gonadotrophin

The hormone chorionic gonadotrophin is produced in the Langhans's cells of the placenta. Its function in early pregnancy is to prolong the existence of the corpus luteum so that ovarian steroids are produced, allowing implantation and early development of the embryo in the uterus.

Its role later in pregnancy is not certain, although it is postulated that progesterone metabolism in the placenta may be dependent upon the presence of chorionic gonadotrophin. The hormone appears in body fluids very early in pregnancy and can be detected by sensitive methods even before the first missed period, as early as the twenty-first day of the cycle (i.e. about the time of implantation). Concentrations rise rapidly to a peak by the tenth week and then fall, so that they may be low by the twentieth week. While non-pregnant levels are not found, this relative drop can give rise to the anomaly of a negative pregnancy test in the mid-trimester of a normal pregnancy. Foetal concentrations of chorionic gonadotrophin are low; ratios between maternal and foetal tissues being in the range of 20:1.

The estimation of human chorionic gonadotrophin is used in two areas of obstetrics. Firstly, the diagnosis of pregnancy through simple qualitative estimations and secondly, the detection of trophoblastic activity by quantitative assays. Since chorionic gonadotrophin is excreted in the urine, this fluid is a useful substance to assay, using the urine with the highest concentrations of hormone—the early morning specimen—although this can be unnecessary with most modern immunological techniques. While recognizable levels of chorionic gonadotrophin are present in very early pregnancy, it is usually considered of no diagnostic significance if a negative pregnancy test is obtained in the first 30 days. Since there is, however, a rough relationship between the amount of hormone produced and the volume of trophoblastic tissue present, quantitative tests done in dilution can give the clinician a rough estimate of trophoblastic bulk, for instance when there is hypertrophy of the trophoblast in hydaditiform mole and choriocarcinoma.

Most of the biological tests for chorionic gonadotrophin have been replaced by immunological ones. The former group depended on inducing ovulation in immature female rats, rabbits, mice or amphibians. They were time-consuming, expensive and demanded the maintenance of animal colonies. The modern immunological tests show positive results when

sensitized cells are exposed to chorionic gonadotrophin. They are as accurate, quicker, and
mostly more sensitive than animal tests. Radio-
immune methods do exist for assaying gonadotrophins, but with such a large amount of the
hormone present these sensitive techniques are
not commonly required.

Oestrogens

There are many hormones in this group of
steroid chemicals derived from the parent steroid
nucleus oestrane, but only three are important
in human biology. Oestradiol is the most active
naturally occurring oestrogen and is found in
conjunction with oestrone and oestriol. Although
oestriol is relatively inert, such large amounts
are produced in pregnancy it assumes an important role. Until the last decade it was considered that all oestrogens were made by the
placenta, but isotope experiments and clinical
endocrinological work (where the placenta has
survived the removal or death of the foetus),
have shown that the foetus is essential for the
production of oestriol. The majority of this
steroid's precursors are metabolized by the
foetal adrenal. They pass from this gland to the
placenta, where the first stages of oestriol
metabolism takes place.

Pregnenolone, passing to the foetus, is converted in the adrenal gland to dehydro-
epiandrosterone sulphate, which then undergoes
hydroxylation in the foetal liver. The resultant
hydroxydehydro-epiandrosterone sulphate passing back to the placenta where it is hydrolized
into the free steroid, oestriol. Although the
placenta alone cannot synthesize oestriol, it
can convert androgens such as androstenedione
to oestrone and oestrodiol. These are not used
in oestriol synthesis, for the placenta has no
hydroxylase enzymes capable of converting them
to oestriol, and less than 10% of the finally
excreted oestriol comes from these sources.
Thus in pregnancy the developing foetus is
responsible for the enormous increase in the
oestriol which shows the largest increase.
Figure 11.6 shows the concentration of the
biologically active oestrogens in pregnancy.
The function of these steroids is probably to

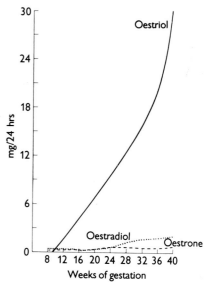

Fig. 11.6. Oestrogen excretion in pregnancy. The excretion of oestone, oestradiol and oestriol is charted showing
how this last steroid is responsible for the major part of
the increased oestrogen output in pregnancy.

stimulate uterine growth and development to
accommodate the enlarging foetus.

Although oestrogens are present in all body
fluids, they are excreted in the urine and are
present there in high concentrations. The end-
products of a whole day's oestrogen metabolism
can be measured in a 24-hour collection of the
patient's urine. Estimations are usually made of
total oestrogens (although they are often reported
as oestriol, this being the major constituent),
and the chemical methods have entirely superseded the biological ones. Hydrolosis to set the
steroid free from its conjugate is required, and
the Kober colour reaction is used. This method,
developed by Brown (1957), has been improved
by using semi-automatic techniques, whereby
one person can deal with 40 samples in a day,
producing the results within 6 hours.

As well as the experimental error in measurement, 24-hour specimens of urine used for
oestrogen estimation can be incorrectly collected,
and so give a false reading. Drugs such as
Mandelamine can affect the oestrogen levels in
the urine, while apparent increases and decreases
in oestriol excretion may be associated with high

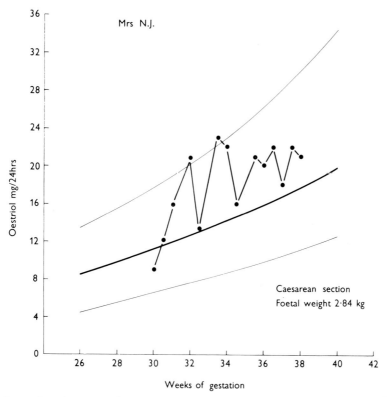

Mrs N.J.

Caesarean section
Foetal weight 2·84 kg

Weeks of gestation

Oestriol mg/24hrs

Fig. 11.7. Normal excretion of oestrogens in pregnancy. Mrs N.J., 36-year-old nullipara, had small ante partum haemorrhages at 30, 33, 35 and 38 weeks. From 34 weeks onwards she had mild pre-eclampsia despite bed rest. The oestrogen estimations (mostly twice a week) helped the obstetrician in deciding to try to maintain the pregnancy longer and caesarean section was performed when she had her last bleed at 38 weeks.

and low urinary outputs. For these reasons, and for the convenience of collection, attempts are being made to evaluate the use of single samples of either urine, blood or amniotic fluid. The problems of collection are removed by this method, but all three specimen sources must yet be shown to reflect accurately oestrogen production, while the use of blood and amniotic fluid samples increases the technical problems of assay. It does by-pass another potential source of error inherent in using urine samples— the variations produced by disease of the maternal liver and kidney in both oestrogen metabolism and secretion.

It is important for the clinician to assess the significance of any given oestrogen level before using these assays in management. There are considerable day-to-day variations in production, with a daily coefficient of variation of about 30%. This means that any given value has to be at least 60% below or above the mean of urinary values before it is outside the 5th to 95th percentile range (Klopper 1969). While single values may not be useful, a series taken twice weekly can be very helpful (Fig. 11.7). If several values are low and the trend is not increasing, this may reflect poor function of the foetoplacental unit. Conversely, a series of increasing readings is reassuring.

Any method which requires serial observations to show significant alterations is at maximum use indicating chronic abnormalities. Serial oestrogen estimations help in the management of the intra-uterine growth-retardation syndrome, pre-eclampsia and postmaturity. The first of these is a difficult syndrome to measure clinically, but

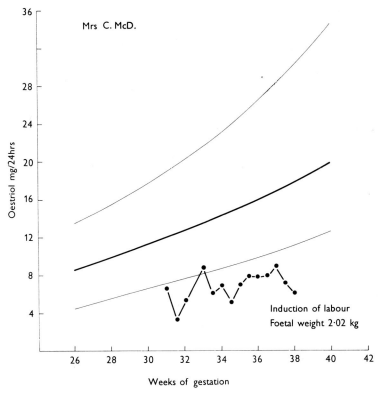

Fig. 11.8. Oestrogen excretion during a pregnancy producing a growth retarded foetus.

Mrs C.McD., a 22-year-old nullipara, was sure of her menstrual dates and examinations of growth in early pregnancy agreed with them. At 30 weeks the foetus was noted to be 'small-for-dates'; this was confirmed the following week both clinically and on foetal biparietal diameter measurements by ultrasonics. Foetal well-being was shown to be maintained by both investigations. At 37 weeks, a falling level of oestrogen was noted after a few steady readings. Cessation of foetal growth was confirmed by ultrasonic measurements and the labour was induced. She produced a growth-retarded infant after a 16 hour labour.

The value of serial observations is seen here. If the reader were to look at the position at half-way through the 31st week (cover up all but the first two readings), the situation looks hopeless, but the next few estimations were reassuring.

usually when foetal growth is retarded there is significant depression of the oestrogen output, and guidance of the optimum time for delivery can be obtained from the serial oestrogen levels. A falling series of readings indicates poor foetal adrenal function, but is not a good indication of when foetal death is likely to occur. (Fig. 11.8).

In pre-eclampsia, oestrogen excretion is usually related to the severity of the condition (Fig. 11.9), but essential hypertension often does not produce any serious alteration unless a superadded pre-eclampsia develops. Oestrogen levels may be used in these conditions to reassure the clinician of continued foetal well-being and thus

stave off induction of labour, allowing a more mature baby to be born.

The syndrome of postmaturity is generally considered to be present when a pregnancy has proceeded 14 days beyond the expected time of delivery in a patient who is sure of her menstrual dates. A decision to interfere is usually an actuarial one, based upon time intervals; to improve results some obstetricians also take into account the ripeness of the cervix. To these clinical estimates have recently been added the use of oestrogen-excretion estimations; it has been shown that so long as the excretion is normal, the babies are well. If oestrogen output

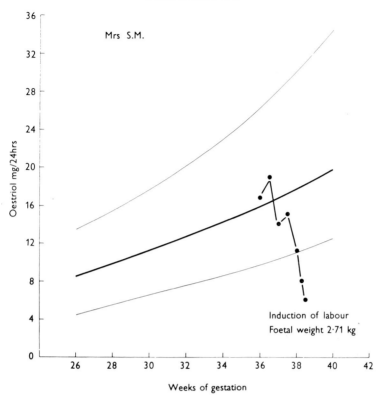

Fig. 11.9. Excretion of oestrogen in pre-eclampsia. Mrs S.M., a 27 year-old nullipara, developed pre-eclampsia at 35 weeks. This persisted mildly despite conservative therapy. Oestrogen excretion was normal for a further two weeks, but a drop indicated lower output. Induction of labour was performed.

drops there is a much higher incidence of foetal morbidity and mortality in subsequent labour. To detect these changes oestrogen estimations must be done frequently, and it is such patients who might benefit from the use of single daily urine or blood estimations.

Oestrogen assays have been of less use in the management of the diabetic pregnancy and the rhesus-affected baby. In the former, while the values may be lower than usual, they are not helpful unless the diabetic patient develops pre-eclampsia or foetal growth is poor. The rhesus-affected baby often has a hypertrophic placenta, and this may account for normal levels of oestrogen even though the foetus is standing into danger. It is possible that in the rhesus-affected pregnancy the oestrogen in amniotic fluid reflects the situation more accurately than maternal urine or blood levels. Since repeated amnio-centeses are already required in the management of the more severe of these cases, amniotic fluid oestrogen assays may prove useful in the rhesus problem.

In summary, the total oestrogen estimations by the methods currently employed are helpful in the monitoring of long-term foetoplacental problems, providing serial sampling is performed.

Progesterone

The steroid progesterone is produced early in pregnancy from the corpus luteum of the ovary and later from the cytotrophoblastic cells of the placenta, while the foetus plays little part in its metabolism. Progesterone does circulate into the foetus and can be hydroxylated in the foetal adrenal. Hydroxyprogesterone can then be transferred back into the maternal circulation, and adds to the maternal urinary levels, but most of the progesterone excreted by the mother in her urine is in the form of pregnanediol, produced on the maternal side of the placenta.

During pregnancy, levels of this hormone rise steadily until labour, when they drop sharply. In early pregnancy, progesterone helps to produce a proper implantation medium for the fertilized ovum, possibly by stimulating the production of a glycogen-rich fluid which surrounds the early blastocyst. Later, the hormone maintains the vascular bed of the endometrium. Progesterone reduces the membrane potential of cells by changing potassium levels, accounting for the well-known effect of progesterone in decreasing myometrial activity. It is possible that the onset of labour is related to a sudden drop in progesterone levels in the uterus. During labour, because of locally high levels of progesterone, the placental bed area may be spared the more vigorous myometrial efforts (and so reduction in blood flow). The hydroxyprogesterone circulating in the foetus is capable of antagonizing the potassium-losing and sodium-retaining actions of corticosteroids and might act as a foetal protective mechanism against the high concentrations of mineralocorticoids present in pregnancy.

Progesterone excretion is usually estimated by assay of its major urinary metabolite pregnanediol. This requires the collection of 24-hour specimens of urine, and suffers from the same disadvantages as mentioned previously. Plasma progesterone levels can be estimated, and may be the method of progesterone assay of the future. In addition to biochemical assay, the levels of progesterone may be estimated by its effect on tissues (biological assay). The vaginal epithelium is sensitive to hormone influences, and smears of cells of the surface layer can easily be taken and stained. When progesterone metabolism is reduced in the presence of normal oestrogen production, the pattern includes large numbers of superficial cells with pink-staining cytoplasm, and small nuclei appear, while there are fewer intermediary cells. Giving exogenous progesterone in this situation can very often convert the picture to a more normal pregnancy pattern, but this does not always improve foetal survival.

In early pregnancy the hormonal levels may be used in the management of recurrent or threatened abortions. At later gestation, serial progesterone levels are low in the presence of poor placental function and low foetal growth, thus indirectly measuring the foetus through the influence that the placenta must have on foetal well-being, but the correlations with foetal outcome are not good.

Human placental lactogen (HPL)

In the last decade a peptide hormone has been isolated in pregnancy which has both a lactogenic and a growth hormone activity. It has several names: human placental lactogen, chorionic growth hormone, prolactin, purified placental protein, human placental factor and human chorionic somatomammotrophin; the first is the time-honoured name, the last the officially accepted one. The hormone is made in the syncytotrophoblast cells of the placental villus and can be detected in the serum early in pregnancy, levels progressively rising until about 30 weeks of gestation, when they plateau until term.

HPL raises the blood glucose and insulin concentrations in humans and in animals. It has been shown to have a protective effect against insulin-induced hypoglycaemia. It increases non-esterified fatty acids and seems to be potassium and sodium sparing, whilst increasing the excretion of calcium. Some of the actions of HPL reflect some of the metabolic alterations seen during pregnancy.

Blood samples are required and the hormone is assayed by a radio-immune method. Correlations have been reported between placental weight and levels of HPL during pregnancy, but there is still no strong correlation with foetal outcome.

ENZYMES

When chronic tissue damage occurs, new enzymes can be produced and the production of others can be altered. This is the basis of the numerous investigations which attempt to find enzyme relating to placental malfunction in a quantitative way. Oxytocinases, lactic dehydro-genases, acid phosphatases and transaminases have all been examined, but none has a good correlation with alterations in placental function judged by either foetal outcome or placental pathology after delivery. Two groups of enzymes, however, deserve further consideration.

The alkaline phosphatase enzyme system consists of a group of isoenzymes, all of which will act on the same substrate and at the same pH. A fraction of this group is heat stable, and so by removing the heat-labile isoenzymes, this fraction becomes more readily identifiable; the temperature used to separate this fraction specifically from the remainder is critical. In the past 56°C has been used, but there is now some evidence that a higher temperature of 65°C may produce more specific results. Assays are performed on blood samples when the enzyme is released by hydrolysis of the serum and measured colorimetrically. As with other studies, serial readings are of more use than are individual ones. Usually in these types of test a falling value is the pointer to decreasing function, but some of the abnormal values for serum heat-stable alkaline phosphatase which are well above the normal range seem significant. It might be that in certain conditions (e.g. pre-eclampsia), there is some proliferation of the cytotrophoblast of the placenta so that the abnormal raised serum heat-stable alkaline phosphatase values indicate the increased response of the placenta to the condition which is leading to foetal danger.

A correlation can be shown between abnormal levels of heat-stable alkaline phosphatase and severe pre-eclampsia. A less significant relationship is found in pre-existing hypertension or mild pre-eclampsia. Recent reports indicate there is little correlation with the foetal outcome as judged by hypoxia in labour or Apgar score measured after delivery (Curzon 1972).

The second maternal enzyme to have been extensively investigated is diamine oxidase. This used to be called histaminase, but since it acts not only on histamines but on other diamines, the general term diamine oxidase is now in use. It is decidual in origin and its level is thought to reflect an increase in foetal production of histamine. Diamine oxidase can be measured fairly simply by a radioactive assay, using blood samples.

Steadily increasing levels of this enzyme are found in plasma as pregnancy progresses, but the increase is more constant in the earlier weeks. A declining level may indicate a decidual response to a failing foetal metabolism. It would seem that this enzyme assay is of most use in the first half of pregnancy in association with abortion. Should the levels of diamine oxidase at this time be in the normal range, it is probable that pregnancy will continue, but if the levels are falling or remain constantly low, there is a significantly increased incidence of foetal death. Again, serial estimations are of more use than individual levels.

The section on chemical assays has indicated their usefulness and limitations. They are less useful in foetal diagnosis than they are in prognosis, for, measuring as they do long-term alterations of a dynamic situation, they may be a guide to long-term treatment. Many have been considered as valid tests on inadequate grounds, alterations in hormone levels having been shown to correlate well with the severity of some disease or subsequently discovered placental pathology. The best yardstick of a test of foetal well-being must be the correlations with the foetus or baby—does the test accurately and reproducibly predict the infant's state at birth and in later life.

AMNIOTIC FLUID

Since the foetus lives surrounded by amniotic fluid, the idea has grown that examination of this milieu extérieur might give information about his metabolism, a similar philosophy to the examination of expired air or of urine in the adult extra-uterine human. It must be remembered, however, that amniotic fluid contains only a part of excretion products of the foetus, and that the vast majority of exchange takes place across the placenta. Amniotic fluid in late pregnancy, however, is largely made by the foetus and contains many products of his metabolism, but to those investigating the foetus the amniotic fluid is like the rubbish pit of an excavated site to the archaeologist. Both provide fragments of evidence about happenings, from several episodes in the past history; they are often mixed up and the time-relations require careful sifting.

The volume of amniotic fluid is used by clinicians as an estimate of the foetal state. Studies done with dye dilution techniques have shown the fluid volume to increase up to about 37 weeks' gestation in the normal patient and to diminish after this. When patients with pre-eclampsia or essential hypertension are tested, they show a similar pattern but a decline in volume may occur earlier, possibly indicating a failing placental function early in pregnancy. Clinical surveys using girth as the measure of uterine content (Elder 1970) have shown a significant correlation between liquor status and the production of a dysmature baby, particularly in the presence of essential hypertension.

Foetal urine becomes an increasingly important component of the amniotic fluid, and so content of the fluid may reflect foetal renal functions. Estimating the osmolality by the depression of freezing point is a guide to the electrolytes present in the amniotic fluid. The osmolality of liquor declines in an almost linear fashion in the second half of normal pregnancy, veering towards values in foetal urine rather than those of either maternal or foetal plasma. Deviations from this pattern are associated with an increased foetal death rate, but correlations are not yet significant and readings may be more useful in the assessment of foetal maturity; if levels of 245 mOsm/kg or below are obtained, it is probably that the foetus is beyond 38 weeks' gestation. Creatinine concentrations stay at a constant low level until the last few weeks of pregnancy when there is an abrupt increase, so that by 38 weeks the concentration is 1·5 mg–% or more. This change may indicate foetal physiological maturity, and alterations in the rate of increase of concentration might be indicative of poor renal function and thus of poor foetal metabolism.

The acid-base state of liquor has been investigated in both chronic and acute deterioration in the foetal state. As pregnancy advances, the amniotic fluid pH drops with a rising PCO_2 and a falling bicarbonate. There is a very wide variation of normal levels in pregnancy and in labour. As in blood estimations, PO_2 in amniotic fluid has a poor correlation with the foetal state; large amounts of fixed acids, high PCO_2 levels and a low pH are found in the fluid of those with hypoxic foetal distress, but the correlations have not been significant.

It is the chronic diseases and conditions which will be best diagnosed from liquor investigations. The scanning of amniotic fluid in rhesus-affected pregnancies has led to assessment of the degree of affect of the baby. This is discussed in Chapter 18. The cellular content of the amniotic fluid increasingly comes from the foetus as pregnancy proceeds. These cells are hard to obtain before 12 weeks of gestation, but once present they can be used for the investigation of chromosomal abnormalities. After cell culture, the foetal sex and certain chromosomally labelled conditions (such as Down's syndrome) can be determined. Unfortunately, very few diseases are chromosomally flagged in a manner that present methods can detect, so that the use of this technique is limited. It takes 3–6 weeks to culture cells, and pregnancy is often well advanced by the time a diagnosis is made by this method; if termination of pregnancy is to be recommended on karyometric grounds, a patient is often well into the mid-trimester before this can be done.

Cells shed by the foetus increase their lipid content rapidly in the last few weeks, and this is used as a method of assessing gestational age. Nile blue sulphate stains neutral lipids, and it has been shown that when patients are beyond the thirty-sixth week of pregnancy, 10% or more of the cells will have been stained orange, indicating their foetal origin. A large number of foetuses who are known to be at or near term do produce cells that do not take up this stain, so that while a positive result of this test is useful, a negative one may not be. The technique has been improved by the use of different staining methods and interpretation (Lind 1969) when, as well as the simple absorption of dye, the types of cells present have been analysed. These cells had been shed from the foetal skin at some unknown time previously, and their examination is limited in the prediction of gestational age. It could be important, however, as a means of assessing the level of foetal development and ability to survive, assuming the skin to be representative of other foetal body tissues.

All the methods of examining the amniotic fluid discussed so far have involved broaching the amniotic cavity. Whilst in mid or late pregnancy this is a safe procedure after the placenta has been localized, once the cervix permits, transcervical amnioscopy leaves the cavity intact. A tapered amnioscope is introduced through the vagina and manoeuvred through the cervix of the patient (Fig. 11.10). With a good light source,

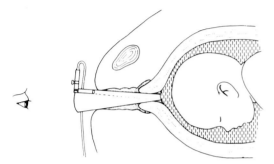

Fig. 11.10. Diagrammatic representation of amnioscopy. The sac of membranes is visualized so that its volume and contents can be examined.

a view is usually obtained through the amniotic sac of the liquor in front of the foetal presenting part. The proportion of fluid gives a very rough guide to the total quantity, and with experience oligohydramnios can be diagnosed. The colour and content of the fluid, including meconium flecks, can be seen. This method is virtually painless, and is easily done in the outpatient department with a low complication rate (in 2–3% of patients, inadvertent rupture of the membranes occurs). Its major use is for patients who have reached term by their gestational dates, and are showing no signs of labour. Those who advocate its use, perform amnioscopy every other day after term until labour occurs or until meconium is seen when action is taken. Meconium is seen in only 7% of patients, so that the surgical induction rate for postmaturity is reduced—Saling (1968) reduced his incidence of inductions from 36 to 7%, and other studies have similar figures. However, the dropping of the surgical induction rate is not the only result to be considered, for

the use of amnioscopy is associated with a significant increase in the operative delivery rate, possibly due to the association of prolonged pregnancy with abnormal uterine action. The final criterion must, of course, be the state of the foetus, and using the coarse guide of perinatal mortality, it has been shown that the use of amnioscopy alone has not caused any significant reduction in perinatal mortality rates in prolonged pregnancy (Brown & Brennan 1968).

EVOKED RESPONSES OF THE FOETOPLACENTAL UNIT

In addition to measuring the end-products of natural activity, a series of tests have evolved in which placental disposal of an exogenous substance is assayed. A variation of this tests the rate of transfer specifically to the foetus. The former group estimates placental metabolic activity, the latter examines the function of transfer to the foetus. The limitations on the use of radio-isotope-labelled substances in human pregnancy studies prevent many of the tests in the first group being used serially, or even at all. One such test used in humans measures the radioactive selenomethionine uptake in late pregnancy using this as a guide to amino-acid transfer from maternal to foetal blood. Some correlations can be shown between poor transfer and intrauterine growth retardation.

Transfer rates to the foetus must be measured by their biological effect on such foetal activities as can be monitored. The easiest of these is foetal heart rate. Atropine, a vagal blocker, produces a bradycardia followed by tachycardia, while adrenaline and isoxsuprine cause tachycardia alone. All three drugs have been given to the mother in pregnancy and the effects on the foetal heart recorded for correlation with outcome. A loose relationship has been reported (Pajutav 1968) between diminished cardiac response and decreasing placental function, especially if serial studies are done near term. However, there are many other variables effecting the concentrations of the drug presented to the placenta. Alteration of maternal size in relation to dosage and fluctuations of uterine and foetal

Table 11.1 Acid base values of 18 normal foetus and of 10 of these babies in the neonatal period (from Beard, R. W. *Ann. Clin. Biochem.* **6**, 67)

Examination of the babies in a similar series would indicate that the values of Po_2 not recorded in this study would be in the order of 73·8 (± 22·5) and 57·7 (± 22·5) at one and four hours respectively.

Timing		Mean value pH		Mean value base deficit (meq/l)		Mean value Po_2 (mmHg)		Mean value Pco_2 (mmHg)
DURING LABOUR								
Stage I		7·335		4·75		23·3		41·0
	±	0·052	±	2·55	±	5·6	±	8·2
Stage II		7·288		6·58		21·5		47·2
	±	0·058	±	2·73	±	4·2	±	10·0
AT DELIVERY								
Umbilical vein		7·301		6·65		29·5		41·8
	±	0·075	±	2·29	±	8·3	±	9·1
Umbilical artery		7·202		9·28		17·2		54·9
	±	0·075	±	3·15	±	6·0	±	9·9
AFTER DELIVERY								
1 hour		7·332		5·57		—		38·8
	±	0·044	±	2·45			±	4·0
4 hours		7·352		4·93		—		35·0
	±	0·040	±	2·34			±	4·0

blood flow rates might all effect the results more than variations in placental transfer.

Foetal response to maternal exercise is another way of examining this problem. Step tests and static bicycling have both been used as standard exercise loads and the effects on the foetus noted for later correlation. In many cases where foetal hypoxia occurred in subsequent labour there had been a bradycardia after the exercise load. Tests of this nature are crude at present but deserve evaluation, for they are assessing the transfer function of the placenta and cause no danger to mother or foetus.

THE FOETUS IN LABOUR

The foetus spends labour inside an intermittently contracting sac where pressure is uniformly transmitted as long as the membranes are intact. Once the liquor has started to drain away, uneven pressures can be applied to parts of the foetus and placenta; these vary with the uterine shape and the part of the myometrium immediately overlying each part of the foeto-placental unit. Most foetuses have a cephalic presentation, so that it is the head which first drives through the maternal pelvic tunnel. The effect of head compression can easily be shown causing vagal stimulation and alteration in the foetal heart rate.

During labour the foetus may become acidotic (Table 11.1). Since the mother is working, she often has an acidaemia, and the foetal state becomes a reflection of this. In addition, foetal acidosis can result from foetal hypoxia. The amount of carbon dioxide present rises, increasing the levels dissolved in the blood, and so producing more carbonic acid, with a further increase of carbon dioxide inside the red blood cells releasing even more hydrogen ions. This condition is foetal respiratory acidosis. If oxygen-lack continues, anaerobic respiratory mechanisms lead to the release of fixed catabolites, mostly lactic acid and pyruvic acid, and foetal metabolic acidosis follows.

If there is sufficient oxygen-lack anaerobic respiration becomes vital and foetal survival depends upon the availability of glycogen or glucose. Certain organs in the foetus (the heart and liver) contain high concentrations of glycogen which can be used in severe hypoxia, thus enabling the heart to maintain circulation. Other organs, such as the foetal brain, have very poor glycogen stores and so are almost entirely dependent upon the availability of oxygenated foetal blood. As acidosis increases, glycolysis is inhibited, so that the acidosis itself, and not the carbohydrate supply, becomes the critical factor, limiting the production of energy, and eventually restricting heart action and the circulation of blood.

With each uterine contraction the tension in the myometrium increases and the intra-uterine pressure rises. This can be sufficient to alter the haemodynamics of the placental bed during and just after the contraction. The pressure may rise above that of uterine venous pressure and so cut off venous flow; by *vis a tergo*, this will prevent flow in the placental bed and reduce the oxygen available for gas exchange at the placenta. Even higher uterine pressures may decrease flow in the afferent vessels, and so further jeopardize the placental bed circulation. It can be shown in animal experiments that foetal carotid artery blood samples taken just after the peak of the contraction consistently contain less oxygen than samples drawn during the period between. Normal uterine contractions do not last long, nor is the pressure very high, and so there is little foetal

affect, but if myometrial activity is increased, then the foetus may be in danger. It is well known that prolonged labour is associated with babies born in a poor condition, from both a clinical and a biochemical point of view. It is possible that a summation of the number and intensity of uterine contractions bears a relation to the state of the baby. It is also a fact that the foetuses born to mothers with certain high-risk situations (see Table 11.2) are also at greatly increased risk of intra-uterine hypoxia.

The uterine contraction can therefore be considered as a test of stress of the foetus, and observations of foetal behaviour in relation to this constraint may be helpful in assessing a prognosis of foetal performance in labour. Investigations at this time of maximum risk must give immediate results and be capable of rapid interpretation. Monitoring of the foetus is at its most intense during labour; both biophysical and biochemical methods will now be considered.

Foetal heart monitoring

In the early days of the stethoscope, the foetal heart was mainly auscultated to diagnose intra-uterine life, and it was not until 1843 that Bodson

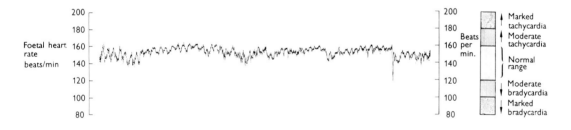

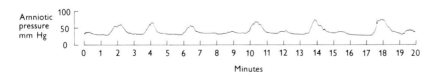

Fig. 11.11. A normal trace of foetal heart rates for twenty minutes in the first stage of labour.
The rate is fairly uniform and does not vary much with uterine contractions. Note the fine irregular variations of the trace (see text).

showed foetal bradycardia to be associated with a poor perinatal outcome. This finding was not widely used until this century, but now it is recognized that the foetal heart rate is one of the major guides to intra-uterine well-being, especially during labour. It is used by observers of differing skills and it can be reasonably accurately and reproducibly measured. The major disadvantage of clinical auscultation is that it is an intermittent measurement, so that changes can be missed in the intervals of time between measurements. Further, it is difficult to listen to the foetal heart during and just after the time of maximum stress—the myometrial contraction. Despite this, foetal heart auscultation is the commonest method used to monitor the foetus in labour. If it is assessed in conjunction with palpated uterine contractions, it gives a good guide to the state of the foetus. Continuous recording

of the foetal heart, so that no events will be missed, is better. This can be done either by recording the output of the heart (its sound or its electrical activity), or by using the Doppler principle to detect the reflected soundwave echoes produced by the heart's activity.

These methods allow a proper definition of three components of the record—baseline heart rate, heart rate irregularity, and changes in rate. The first two of these are used clinically in the recognition of foetal distress. The periodic changes in heart rate have been the subject of study over the last decade, and a considerable body of data has now been analysed showing that early foetal hypoxia can be recognized by relating the physiological stress of the uterine contraction to the foetal heart rate patterns.

Alterations of foetal heart rate can be divided into base line changes and periodic ones. The

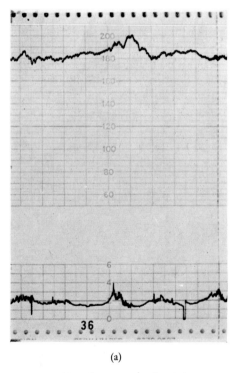
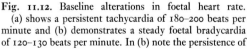

(a)

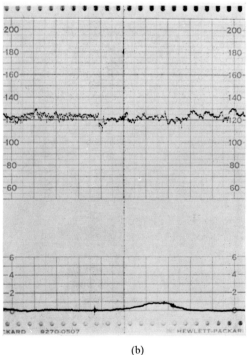

(b)

Fig. 11.12. Baseline alterations in foetal heart rate. (a) shows a persistent tachycardia of 180–200 beats per minute and (b) demonstrates a steady foetal bradycardia of 120–130 beats per minute. In (b) note the persistence of the fine beat-to-beat irregularity implying a heart still capable of responding to the minimum alteration of the controlling mechanisms. In (a) the trace is smoother, indicating a depression of this fine control mechanism.

former consists of the background rate between uterine contractions and is labelled in a similar way as are clinical foetal heart observations (Fig. 11.11). It will be noted that the trace also shows a fine baseline irregularity. (Fig. 11.12.) This is a sign of foetal health rather than the reverse, and the absence of these minor fluctuations can indicate an inability of the foetal heart to react to the varying stimuli which make up its rate control mechanism.

The periodic changes are transient ones in relation to the uterine contractions and are nearly always decelerations They may have their onset at the same time as the beginning of the uterine contraction (early deceleration), they may come

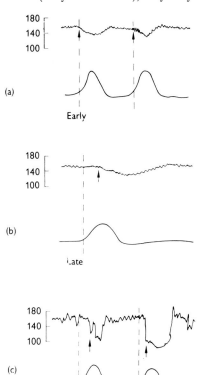

(a)

Early

(b)

Late

(c)

Variable

Fig. 11.13. Diagrammatic patterns of periodic foetal heart rate deceleration.

In each case, the foetal heart rate is drawn above and the amniotic fluid pressure below. The dotted line indicates the beginning of the uterine contraction and the arrow shows the beginning of the heart rate alteration. Compare these with Fig. 11.13a, b, c.

more than 30 sec after the beginning of the contraction (late deceleration) or the deceleration onset may bear no constant relation to the beginning of the contraction (variable deceleration). (Fig.11.13.)

The uterine contraction represents a repetitive mechanical stimulus to both the foetus and his placental circulation, and alterations in foetal heart pattern may be a response to this. The early deceleration (onset coinciding with the beginning of the contraction and a wave-form reflecting the shape of the amniotic fluid pressure curve), is probably due to pressure on the foetal head during labour. This is a normal response [Fig. 11.14(a)]. Late deceleration comes at an interval after the onset of the pressure rise inside the uterus and probably is a reflection of a decrease in the intervillous space blood flow producing an acute uteroplacental insufficiency [Fig. 11.14(b)]. Late deceleration is thought to be of more serious prognostic importance, for it may indicate early hypoxia in labour. Variable deceleration has its onset at varying times and foetal heart rate changes are not seen at all during some contractions; this is probably due to an intermittent compression of the umbilical cord during certain contractions [Fig. 11.14(c)]. Quite commonly this can be altered by change in the maternal position, and on other occasions it alters spontaneously.

Examination of a continuous trace of foetal heart rate patterns often shows that there is not a characteristic response to every uterine stimulation. Sometimes the heart rate decelerations appear unrelated to contractions, but with a little experience the obstetrician, scanning the whole trace, can pick out those decelerations which he considers to be significant and require further investigation. Since the exact mechanisms underlying these foetal heart rate changes are not known, work is currently in progress assessing them in relation to other methods of studying the foetus. Hon & Quilligan (1968) have shown a good correlation between abnormal foetal heart rate patterns and the neonatal condition, while results mentioned in the section on foetal blood sampling show that late decelerations are significantly associated with foetal hypoxic acidaemia.

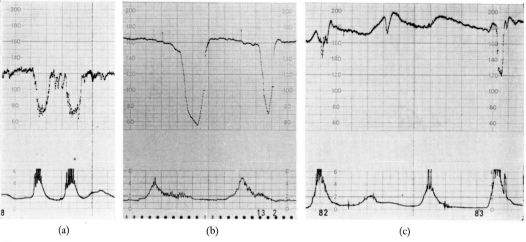

(a)   (b)   (c)

Fig. 11.14. Actual patterns of periodic foetal heart rate deceleration.

(a) shows deceleration of FHR coming on within 30 seconds of the onset of uterine contractions. Generally such heart rate patterns 'mirror' the uterine pressure traces and early decelerations are probably of no serious prognostic significance to the foetus.

(b) shows periodic bradycardia patterns coming well after the uterine pressure change. These late decelerations are of much more serious prognosis to the foetus and can be interpreted as showing an alteration in placental or placental bed blood flow.

(c) shows decelerations which bear an inconsistent time relationship with uterine contractions and which are irregular in their shape. Such variable decelerations probably reflect an alteration in blood flow in the umbilical cord and are often transient and of no serious significance.

PHONOCARDIOGRAPHY

The acoustical pick-up of the foetal heart rate allows the observer to be at a distance from the patient and permits continuous auscultation. Furthermore, the sound impulses can be converted instantly to a rate and transcribed into a permanent tracing. While phonocardiography has been used for a large amount of the basic work described above, it does suffer from several disadvantages. The microphone detecting the foetal heart sounds may also pick up borborygmi from the maternal gut, sounds from the uterine and abdominal wall musculature and even sounds from the bedclothes and the labour ward. In consequence, electronic filtering devices have been added to the circuit to improve the quality of the tracing. This can result in a loss of the foetal signal at the time of the uterine contraction so that examination of the heart rate patterns in relation to contractions can be poor, especially in late labour when the patient may be restless.

FOETAL ELECTROCARDIOGRAPHY

Cleaner traces of the foetal heart rate can be obtained by monitoring its electrical output. While this can be done through the maternal abdomen, the best results follow attachment of electrodes directly to the foetus. If the indirect method is used, a lot of interpretation is required to distinguish maternal patterns from the foetal patterns. Improved foetal records can be obtained with filtering devices to baffle the maternal output, but generally abdominal foetal electrocardiography work has been most useful in pregnancy rather than in labour.

In 1963 Hon introduced the scalp-clip electrode, since when there have been many modifications; all depend upon direct electrical continuity with foetal tissues (Fig. 11.15). With the better tracings, the patterns of alteration in foetal heart rate can be even more clearly seen, and they provide an earlier guide to foetal hypoxia. Under experimental conditions, needle

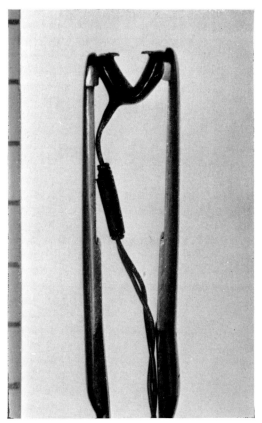

Fig. 11.15. Scalp electrode (alongside a centimetre scale).

The bipolar clip is insulated, except at its tips. When this is crimped into the foetal scalp, the bare metallic areas are inside foetal tissue and so the receiving equipment is insulated from other signals.

electrodes can be passed through the mother's abdominal wall into the foetal body, and attempts have been made to introduce fine electrodes through the cervix and membranes before labour, but these have usually been followed by leaking of the amniotic fluid. The direct method is therefore confined to the time when the cervix is dilating and the membranes have been ruptured. Once a 16 mm amnioscope can be manœuvred through the cervix, a scalp-clip can be applied.

Usually, the electrical signals are used to produce tracings of foetal heart rate and the characteristic patterns can be analysed. Analysis

of the components of the electrical signal may lead to conclusions about the metabolic activity of the muscle cells. This is well established in adult medicine, where electrocardiographic records provide diagnosis of cardiac muscle alterations, especially of tissue hypoxia. Foetal electrocardiograms have been performed for years, but clear traces had to await the attachment of electrodes directly to the foetus. There is still much interference from maternal electrical sources, and with the large number of complexes being written out it would be impossible to analyse them so that the results were useful at the time of that labour. Lee & Hon (1965) have been using a method of group averaging of a series of consecutive electrocardiogram records of each foetal heart beat to clean up the trace. Here a number of complexes are 'superimposed' upon each other by the computer, so that repetitive signals are reinforced and random activity is filtered out. Using this equipment, changes in the QRS complex of the foetus can be shown with umbilical cord manipulation. However, when the foetus is hypoxic, the foetal electrocardiograph can stay normal until just before death, with only small changes in the PR interval, and notching of the P waves. More research is proceeding into animal and human foetal heart activity, but the major bar at present to the qualitative analysis of foetal electrocardiograms is the complexity of the electronic equipment required.

ULTRASONIC DOPPLER CARDIOGRAPHY

When soundwaves are reflected from a moving object, they often travel at different frequencies from that at which they were transmitted. Ultrasonic Doppler detection of foetal heart activity has been in use for some years as small, portable units giving a signal which appears as a sound from a loudspeaker. It is possible to record these signals either as a direct record or they can be passed to a rate-meter, thus writing out foetal heart rate records and producing the patterns discussed already. The advantage of these methods of pick-up is that they are external and can be used before the membranes are ruptured. They give a good signal even in the presence of obesity and hydramnios. Their main disadvantage is that the receiving equipment must be very accurately placed on the abdominal wall to pick up the reflected sounds, so that with an active patient in labour it is sometimes difficult to maintain recording. This problem might be overcome by either modifying the angle of spread of the transmitted signal or using several receivers to pick up the reflected echo.

Doubt has been raised about the safety of soundwaves passing through human tissues, but the low-intensity of ultrasound used at diagnostic frequencies is much less than that used for cell destruction in experimental biology. Neither structural nor physiological damage to intact tissues has been demonstrated by the use of diagnostic levels of ultrasonics.

THE USE OF FOETAL HEART MONITORING

Auscultation of the foetal heart during labour is traditional and simple; it can be done by many people, the disadvantages being that the reading is an average of the beats recorded over a 15 or 30 sec interval and that the method is intermittent. Using this in conjunction with other clinical methods (meconium staining) can lead to a large number of false-positive diagnoses of foetal distress, while at the same time some babies can still be hypoxic without showing any change in these relatively coarse methods. Other methods of picking up the heart rate, detecting its beat to beat variation and recording this continuously are used at present in high-risk situations (Table 11.2). Here, either because of some pre-existing situation or something arising *de novo* in labour, the foetus is judged to be at high risk, and so continuous recording is used. Wood (1967) has shown that not all abnormalities in foetal heart rate are hypoxic, but if they are, there is nearly always a subsequent change in foetal acid base balance. It is probably wise, therefore, to monitor high-risk labour by continuous foetal heart recording, using foetal blood sampling to establish the significance of the changes in rate patterns. Neither method is perfect, the one covering the deficiences in the other.

Foetal electroencepholography

While the heart's action is a useful guide to the total body's acid base state, the brain is the ultimate organ on which hypoxia has the most serious affect. It has often been stated that the foetus shows an increased resistance to hypoxia compared with the extra-uterine baby. This is not uniform for all foetal organs. Study of foetal electroencephalographs have shown the brain to be quick to respond to hypoxia by alterations of wave frequency and diminution of electrical potential. This corresponds with the poor capacity of the brain to store glycogen. Understandable inter-uterine electroencephalograph recordings, like the electrocardiograph records, had to await a direct access to the foetus before clean traces could be obtained. Transabdominal electroencephalographs do exist, but are of complex pattern; since interpretation even of the extra-uterine electroencephalograph is difficult, the intra-uterine situation requires the cleanest trace possible to show significant changes.

Animal work with induced hypoxia shows parallel and almost synchronous alterations in foetal and maternal records (Rosen & McLaughlin 1966). Flattening of the foetal electroencephalograph traces persisted after the hypoxic insult to the mother had occurred, and been removed. The normal pattern returned more slowly in the foetal trace than it did in the mother's and long after the foetal heart rate returned to normal. During the recovering phase, the foetus often made exaggerated movements simulating respiratory activity which disappeared about the time when the brain waves became normal. These traces are similar to those found in neonatal asphyxia. Improvements in direct recording have led to foetal electroencephalographs being monitored through labour. Satisfactory traces are obtained, but at present the interpretation of the signal is easiest in relation to evoked responses, and this is not yet a method to be considered for routine use.

Foetal blood sampling

All the methods discussed so far have depended on end organ response to an altered biochemical situation, but ideally, hypoxia should be judged by its effect on the cell, especially in the acute phase. By current methods, foetal intracellular measurement is not possible, but some degree of equilibrium is maintained between the cell and the extracellular fluid and one compartment of this space is available for inspection and sampling. The capillary portion of the intravascular fluid is in close equilibrium with the rest of the extra-cellular fluid; hence if foetal capillary blood is sampled, it should give some idea of the bio-chemical status of the extracellular compartment of the foetus.

Foetal blood sampling started in the late 1950s when Saling found that at amnioscopy the membranes were occasionally accidentally rup-tured and he was given access to the underlying presenting part of the foetus, usually the scalp. From this evolved the technique of obtaining small samples of foetal blood which could be submitted to micro-analysis.

TECHNIQUE OF FOETAL BLOOD SAMPLING

The technique of obtaining a sample of blood and of measuring its acid base content is simple, once the cervix will allow the passage of a 12 mm endoscope. If the membranes are not ruptured, they can be torn and the endoscope manœuvred through the rent. Gentle pressure then allows the end of the tube to rest against the foetal presenting part, forming a coffer dam and pre-venting the seepage of amniotic fluid into the area to be examined (Fig. 11.16). This point is important, for while enough pressure has to be used to prevent leakage, not so much is applied to cut off the capillary blood supply to the area. Soon the operator learns to shift subconsciously with the small movements of the mother, and maintains a dry operating area on the foetus. A jet of ethyl chloride is sprayed on to the foetal skin for a few seconds and the reactionary hyperaemia causes arterialization of the capillary blood in the area. A film of high-tension silicone grease is spread on the operating field to allow the blood to collect as a discrete drop rather than a smear over the foetal skin. This step also allows the damp foetal hair to be smoothed to one side. A guarded, end-bearing knife blade fixed to a

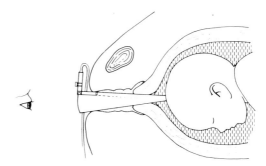

Fig. 11.16. Diagrammatic representation of foetal blood sampling.

After membrane rupture, the endoscope can be placed snugly against the foetal scalp. If pressure is correctly applied, this allows the amniotic fluid to be held back by the 'coffer dam' effect of the tube and so an uninterrupted view of the scalp is obtained.

long handle (Fig. 11.17) is used to prick the scalp. This is best done by placing the blade on the site and then with a sudden stabbing motion,

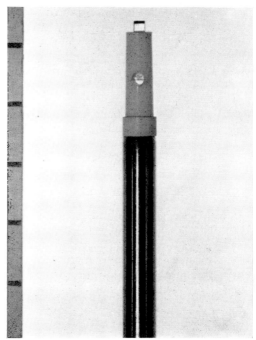

Fig. 11.17. Blade for foetal blood sampling (alongside a centimetre scale).

This is a disposable blade mounted in a plastic haft so that penetration of the foetal skin is limited to 2 millimetres and deeper structures cannot be damaged.

the skin is pierced by a wrist-flick to the handle. The plastic shoulder of the blade stops it penetrating too deeply, so that structures beneath the foetal skin are not damaged. A bead of blood collects and is drawn off in a preheparinized glass tube. The column of blood can usually be drawn into the tube by capillary action alone and negative pressure is not often required. For pH estimates about half a tube is enough (about o·1 ml of blood). If more acid-base readings are required, a full tube must be taken.

The blood is mixed with the heparin lining the tube by running a short length of steel wire up and down the lumen with a magnet from the outside. Estimates of pH should be done within a few minutes on nearby equipment, and in these circumstances no sealing of the ends of the tube is required.

The foetal scalp is compressed with a swab for a short time, allowing the stab wound to close by blood clot. The rare instance of continued foetal bleeding can be dealt with by further compression, or if necessary by securing a small metal clip to the scalp, the electrode for foetal electrocardiographic work serving well. A sample of the mother's venous blood is taken from the arm into a preheparinized syringe, for comparison of maternal and foetal acid-base studies.

The blood samples are analysed with micro-Astrup equipment. The pH is read directly on a scale and tonomotry can be easily performed using gas mixtures containing known concentrations of carbon dioxide. Two further pH readings of the foetal blood sample after exposure to known partial pressures of carbon dioxide allow calculation of base deficit, PCO_2 and standard bicarbonate by the use of a Siggaard Andersen chart. Both foetal and maternal samples can be measured in a few minutes.

The technique is easy to learn and use, but some difficulties can arise. With cephalic presentations, the head may be high and may move between the pricking and obtaining the blood sample. This can be countered by an assistant steadying the foetal head from above the pubis. Occasionally, the breech may be presenting and sampling is more difficult, not just because of the lesser vascularization, but because of the lack of bone below the skin to provide counter-pressure against the knife blade. However, samples can be obtained from the breech. Sometimes after a long labour in cephalic presentation a caput forms. If this is small, it has no effect on the foetal blood sample. Despite careful positioning, maternal blood from the cervix may enter the field and be drawn into the tube. This will give a false acid-base estimation, and the presence of maternal haemoglobin can be detected quickly in the labour ward. Several bedside tests exist, of which the metasilicate solid state test is simplest (Chamberlain & Fosker 1970).

Doctors who are not used to using electrical recorders may be a little uncertain of their abilities at first, but with a little experience the reproducibility of readings is improved, and this becomes one of the lesser sources of practical error. pH estimation should be made soon after the sample is taken, for exposure to air or keeping the blood in polythene tubing will allow diffusion of CO_2 and oxygen. The blood is best collected in a glass tube so that no diffusion takes place, and the measuring equipment is kept switched on at a steady temperature ($37°C$) in the labour ward area. Under these circumstances, the few minutes from sampling to measurement will not materially effect the pH.

VALIDITY OF ACID BASE STUDIES

Since 1958, when James showed a definite relationship between the acid base status of cord blood and the condition of the newborn, acidaemia has been recognized as a far better reflection of hypoxia than have PO_2 levels in blood or tissues. When blood became obtainable from the foetus still in the uterus, similar associations were shown. Beard (1967) demonstrated that when the pH of scalp capillary blood was above 7·20 within 30 min of delivery, the Apgar score was 7 or above in 85% of babies.

Similar comparisons can be made between foetal heart rate measurements and intra-uterine acid-base estimations. While variations of the basal rate show a poor correlation with pH alterations, late decelerations of heart rate after uterine contractions are associated with very significant drops of foetal pH, while moderate variable decelerations are also seen with a minor pH shift (Kubli 1969). Similar associations can be shown between increased foetal base deficit and late deceleration patterns of foetal heart rate (Hon & Khazin 1969).

Doubt has been raised that scalp blood is representative of the blood in the rest of the body. Capillary blood taken from the scalp during labour has values between arterial and venous samples in both animal studies when foetal rhesus monkeys were simultaneously sampled by the scalp and systemic vessels (Haworth 1968), and in human work when scalp samples were taken from cases during Caesarean section and compared these with unbilical blood taken within 60 seconds (Teramo 1969).

These and many other studies indicate that a sample of foetal blood with a pH greater than 7·20 can be reasonably assumed to come from a baby who is in good condition at that moment.

USE OF FOETAL BLOOD SAMPLING

Centres that have been sampling foetal blood for longer than an experimental period have found the method useful in clinical assessment of the foetal condition. Two groups of patients require acid-base studies and they correspond roughly to the patients mentioned in Table 11.2. The chronic group are usually identified during pregnancy, and such patients should have foetal blood sampling done every 4 hours in labour. The second group are the patients who show clinical signs of foetal distress in labour (heart rate or rhythm alterations or the passage of meconium), and they correspond with women who have the

Table 11.2. The high risk situations of pregnancy and labour
Many of the chronic group will have been identified at the beginning of antenatal care or in pregnancy. The acute group tend to arise in labour and their effects may be worsened by the pre-existing influence of one of the chronic risks.

CHRONIC RISKS	
Maternal factors	Increasing age
	Nulliparity and grand multiparity
	Low social class
	Poor obstetric history
	ABO or rhesus incompatibility
Maternal disease	Hypertensive conditions
	— chronic hypertension
	— pre-eclampsia
	Renal disease
	Diabetes
	Severe cardiac disease
	Anaemia and haemoglobinopathies
Foeto/maternal conditions	Prematurity and small-for-dates babies
	Postmaturity
	Cephalopelvic disproportion
	Malpresentations and malpositions
	Premature membrane rupture
Foetal conditions	Multiple foetuses
ACUTE RISKS	
Uterine factors	Decrease of oxygen transfer with myometrial contractions
	— prolonged labour
	— hypertonia
Umbilical cord factors	Compression and prolapse
Placental factors	Separation from placental bed
Foeto/neonatal factors	Depression of respiration
	— drugs
	— trauma

factors in the lower part of the table. In this latter group, sampling is performed when the symptoms appear. If the pH is normal, labour is allowed to progress and a check foetal blood sample taken an hour later. If the pH is depressed, the maternal sample is checked to ensure that the foetal acidaemia is not part of a generalized maternal acidosis from the work or dehydration in labour. If the pH levels are similar but low, the difference of base deficit between foetus and mother should be estimated. Should the foetus be shown to be no more acidaemic than the mother, the maternal acid-base state is corrected (intravenous 5% glucose) and the foetal blood sample re-checked after this. If, however, the acidaemia is shown to be foetal only, it may be assumed to be due to hypoxia and action must be taken to deliver the baby.

The most profitable uses of foetal blood sampling is in conjunction with continuous recording of foetal heart rate. Sampling is an intermittent measurement with all the disadvantages of discontinuous records, while the foetal heart rate records can be continuous. The use of heart rate patterns in relation to the stress of uterine contractions can show when hypoxia is suspect, so that foetal blood sampling might be employed before any coarser clinical indication of hypoxia could be detected. This is probably the most useful aspect of sampling at the moment, for it can be used to determine the significance of alterations of heart rate patterns.

The alternative use of foetal blood sampling to give warning of intra-uterine hypoxia before any other indicants in the clinically at risk group

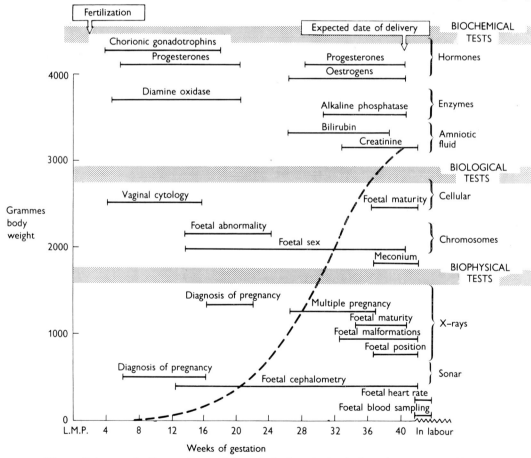

Fig. 11.18. A composite diagram of some of the methods of monitoring the foetus in pregnancy and labour.

(upper part of Table 11.2) is at present not so useful. The sample only gives information about the acid-base state at the point of time it is taken and not about what may happen in the future. It is as though one had fitted a more penetrating spotlamp to one's car; a better view is then obtained of what is on the road immediately in front, but there is still no view of what is happening round the corner.

Saling originally suggested that a foetal scalp sample pH of 7·20 or below should be considered abnormal (this corresponds approximately with two standard deviations below the mean). However, since hypoxia is a progressive event, probably the exact figure is not so important as the level in relation to the stage of labour; for example Beard (1965) has shown the merits of accepting a lower level of 7·15 in the second stage of labour.

This technique has given the first direct approach to the foetus still inside the uterus. As well as studies on the response to uterine contractions, work has been done on the foetal acid-base state in relation to over-breathing, abdominal decompression, the giving of oxygen to the mother and paracervical local anaesthetic block. The technique can also be used in other fields where micro-analytical biochemical analysis can give information on small quantities of blood. Rhesus-affected babies may have Coomb's tests and haemoglobin estimations done during the labour, thus giving longer warning of the possible affect. Carbohydrate metabolism and insulin levels have been studied simultaneously in the mother and the foetus both in diabetic and normal pregnancies.

Conclusions

Figure 11.18 shows the rough chronological spread of the methods available for examining the state of the human foetus. Some are in routine use, others are still research techniques, but the usefulness of each has to be assessed in relation to the outcome of the pregnancy. Too often an investigation is related to some biochemical or pathological criterion of the foeto-placental unit while it should be considered in relation to the condition of the extra-uterine baby.

So coarse are neonatal measuring methods, that much of what passes for normality in the new-born is only shown to be abnormal in later life; perhaps, therefore, longer-term follow-up of the children should be used in the assessment of intra-uterine investigations, for they are only screening tests to help the obstetrician detect the foetus who is at hazard in the uterus. Each must be shown to improve the purpose of obstetrics—the production of a healthy population.

REFERENCES

BEARD R.W. & CLAYTON S.J. (1967) *J. Obstet. Gynaec. Br. Commonw.* 74, 812.
BEARD R.W. & MORRIS M.D. (1965) *J. Obstet. Gynaec. Br. Commonw.* 72, 496.
BROWN J.B., BULBROOK R.D. & GREENWOOD F.C. (1957) *J. Endocr.* 16, 49.
BROWNE A.D.H. & BRENNAN R.K. (1968) *J. Obstet. Gynaec. Br. Commonw.* 75, 616.
BUTLER N.R. (1965) *Clinics in Development Medicine*, 19, 74.
CAMPBELL S. (1970) *J. Obstet. Gynaec. Br. Commonw.* 77, 603.
CHAMBERLAIN G. & FOSKER A. (1970) *J. Obstet. Gynaec. Br. Commonw.* 77, 1096.
CURZON P. & HENSEL H. (1972) *J. Obstet. Gynaec. Br. Commonw.* 79, 23.
ELDER M.G., BURTON E.R., GORDON H., HAWKINS D.F. & McCLURE BROWN J.D. (1970) *J. Obstet. Gynaec. Br. Commonw.* 77, 48.
HAWWORTH S.G., MILIC A.B. & ADAMSONS K. (1968) *Clin. Obstet. Gynec.* 11, 1183.
HON E.H. & KHAZIN A.F. (1969) *Am. J. Obstet. Gynec.* 105, 721.
HON E.H. & QUILLIGAN E.J. (1968) *Clin. Obstet. Gynec.* 11, 145.
JAMES L.S., WEISBROT I.M., PRINCE C.E., HOLADAY D.A. & APGAR V. (1958) *J. Pediat.* 52, 379.
KLOPPER A. & DICZFALUSKY E. (1969) *Fetus and Placenta.* Oxford, Blackwell Scientific Publications.
KUBLI F.W. (1968) *Clin. Obstet. Gynec.* 11, 168.
KUBLI F.W., HON E.H., KHAZIN A.F. & TAKEMURA H. (1969) *Am. J. Obstet. Gynec.* 104, 1190.
LEE S.T. & HON E.H. (1965) *Am. J. Obstet. Gynec.* 92, 1140.
LIND T., PARKIN F.M. & CHEYNE G.A. (1969) *J. Obstet. Gynaec. Br. Commonw.* 76, 673.
PAJNTAR M. & LAVRIC M. (1968) *Obstet. Gynec., N.Y.* 32, 520.
ROSEN M.G. & McLAUGHLIN A. (1966) *Expl Neurol.* 16, 181.
RUSSELL J.G.B. (1969) *J. Obstet. Gynaec. Br. Commonw.* 76, 208.
SALING E. (1962) *Arch. Gynaek.* 197, 108.
TERAMO K. (1969) *Gynaecologia, Basel,* 167, 511.
WOOD C., LUMLEY J. & RENOU P. (1967) *J. Obstet. Gynaec. Br. Commonw.* 74, 823.

CHAPTER 12

NORMAL LABOUR

Labour is the process by which the foetus *in utero* is expelled through the birth canal. Of the many factors concerned, two of the most important are the maternal pelvis and the foetal skull, and these two features and their relation to each other will be considered first.

THE PELVIS

The true pelvis is a curved, bony canal with its associated soft tissues and abdominal viscera. The posterior wall of the bony pelvis is considerably longer than the anterior one. It is customary to describe three planes of the pelvis: the plane of the brim, the plane of the cavity and the plane of the outlet (Fig. 12.1).

The pelvic brim in the normal female is slightly oval in shape with an anteroposterior measurement which is a little shorter than the widest transverse measurement; this widest transverse diameter is normally situated just behind the midpoint between the front and back of the pelvis [Fig. 12.2(a)]. In the upright position the plane of the brim forms an angle of some 60° with the vertical.

The diameters of the pelvic brim in a normal case are, approximately: anteroposterior, 11·5 cm; transverse, 13·6 cm.

The normal sacral curve ensures that the plane of the pelvic cavity, which is situated at the level of the junction of the 2nd and 3rd sacral vertebrae [Fig. 12.1(a)], is circular and capacious. The anteroposterior, transverse and oblique diameters each measure approximately 12·0 cm.

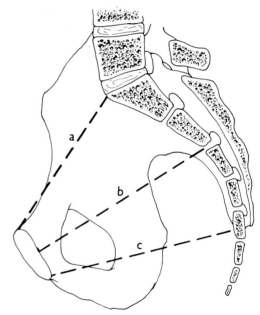

Fig. 12.1 (a). A drawing of the lateral view of the pelvis to show (a) the plane of the brim; (b) the plane of the cavity; (c) the plane of least pelvic dimensions.

The plane of the pelvic outlet is a less definitive structure than that of the brim, since it lies between a number of landmarks which are at different levels. Anteriorly is the lower border of the symphysis pubis, posteriorly the tip of the coccyx, and laterally the ischial tuberosities. Because these are at different levels, and since the coccyx is usually displaced during the delivery of the head, it is customary to describe a plane of least pelvic dimensions at the level of the ischial spines [Fig. 12.1(a)]. Here the pelvis is diamond-shaped with the anteroposterior diameter (from the lower border of the symphysis pubis to the last fixed point of the sacrum) measuring 12·5 cm; the transverse diameter, between the ischial spines, measures 10·5 cm. The shape of the pelvis changes, therefore, from above downwards, since the pelvis is wider from side to side at the level of the brim and wider anteroposteriorly at the level of the outlet.

The anterior wall of the pelvis is short, because the symphysis pubis lies immediately above the subpubic arch; this has an angle approaching

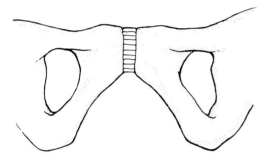

Fig. 12.1 (b). Drawing of the normal subpubic arch.

90°, although, since the walls are normally curved with the concavity inwards, an angle cannot accurately be measured [Fig. 12.1(b)].

Variations in the shape of the pelvis may be found in normal women. Four main varieties are recognized: the gynaecoid, the android, the platypelloid and the anthropoid.

The gynaecoid pelvis [Fig. 12.2(a)] has the features just described with parallel anterior and posterior pelvic walls and a wide subpubic arch. The android pelvis [Fig. 12.2(b)] has a heart-shaped brim, with the widest transverse diameter set towards the posterior part of the brim and a more acute angle of the superior pubic rami: the ischial spines are closer together and some convergence of anterior and posterior pelvic walls is evident; the subpubic arch is narrow. The platypelloid pelvis is disproportionately wide from side to side and so tends to have a kidney-shaped brim [Fig. 12.2(c)]. The anthropoid pelvis is longer anteroposteriorly than from side to side [Fig. 12.2(d)]. Mixed forms

are not uncommon. The gynaecoid and android types are much more frequent than the other two varieties.

Over the years obstetricians have been greatly concerned with attempts to measure accurately pelvic measurements. It has already been emphasized, however, that absolute measurements of pelvic diameters are of limited importance; they are only important in relation to the size of the baby's head which must pass through them. Consideration has already been given to this in Chapter 9 on the management of normal pregnancy.

THE FOETAL SKULL

The foetal skull is hard and less yielding than other parts of the body. Moreover, it must negotiate the bony pelvis without injury to the cranial contents. Important landmarks on the vault of the foetal skull are two fontanelles—the anterior, or bregma; and the posterior, or lambda. The anterior fontanelle is diamond-shaped until labour commences, when moulding will obliterate the shape; it can then be distinguished from the posterior one only by the fact that four sutures enter it—the frontal suture, the sagittal suture and two coronal sutures. The posterior fontanelle receives only three sutures, the sagittal and two lambdoid sutures. The diamond-shaped area on the vault of the skull bounded in front by the anterior fontanelle, behind by the posterior one and laterally by the parietal eminences is the vertex, and it is this area which normally forms the lowest part of the head when the foetus becomes stabilized *in utero* in late pregnancy.

The ease with which the foetal skull will pass through the pelvis will, of course, depend upon the actual size of both, but it will depend also on the relative size of the head as it presents to the pelvis; the amount of flexion or extension which is present can significantly alter the size of the head in this respect.

Normally, with the foetus in an attitude of flexion within the uterus the smallest diameters of the foetal skull present to the pelvic brim. These smallest diameters are, in the coronal

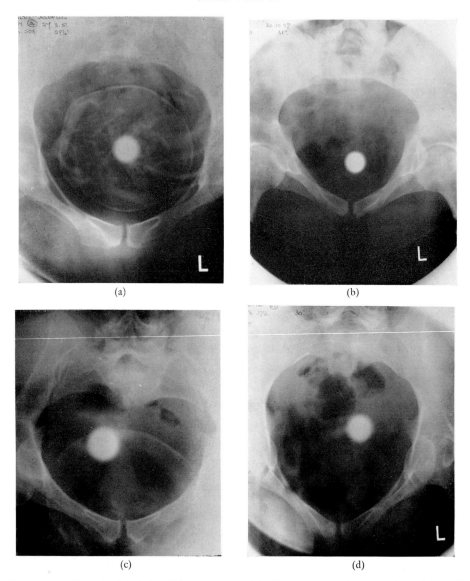

(a)   (b)

(c)   (d)

Fig. 12.2. A radiograph of the brim of (a) a gynaecoid pelvis; (b) an android pelvis; (c) a platypelloid pelvis; (d) an anthropoid pelvis.

plane the biparietal diameter, and in the sagittal plane the suboccipito bregmatic diameter; each measures some 9·5 cm, so the head presents to the pelvis as a circle of this diameter [Fig. 12.3(a)]. It is not uncommon for this attitude of flexion to become less than complete. When this happens the diameter in the coronal plane remains the same and that of the anteroposterior plane becomes the occipitofrontal, which measures some 11·5 cm. The head then presents to the pelvic brim in the shape of an oval, and may engage less readily as a result [Fig. 12.3(b)]. The vertex remains the presenting part, but now the most dependent point on the vertex will be

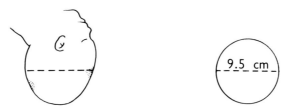

a   Sub-occipito bregmatic

Fig. 12.3 (a). A well-flexed head which presents to the brim as a circle of 9·5 cm diameter. The presenting diameter is suboccipito bregmatic.

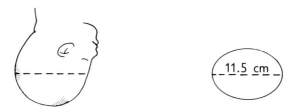

b   Occipito frontal

Fig. 12.3 (b). A deflexed head which presents as an oval with a longer occipitofrontal measurement of 11·5 cm.

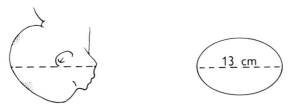

c   Mento vertical

Fig. 12.3 (c). Greater deflexion resulting in a brow presentation; the oval is still bigger, its long diameter (mentovertical) being 13 cm.

d   Submento bregmatic

Fig. 12.3 (d). A fully extended head which again presents as a circle of diameter 9·5 cm; the presenting diameter is the submento bregmatic.

immediately behind the anterior fontanelle, and not, as in the well-flexed head, just in front of the posterior fontanelle. If the head extends it presents to the pelvic brim a very large oval indeed, and it is unlikely that easy engagement, or indeed engagement at all, will take place.

Here the brow presents and the anteroposterior diameter of the presenting part is the mento-vertical, which is some 13·0 cm in size [Fig. 12.3(c)]. Complete extension results in a face presentation in which the diameters are as favourable as those of the fully flexed vertex

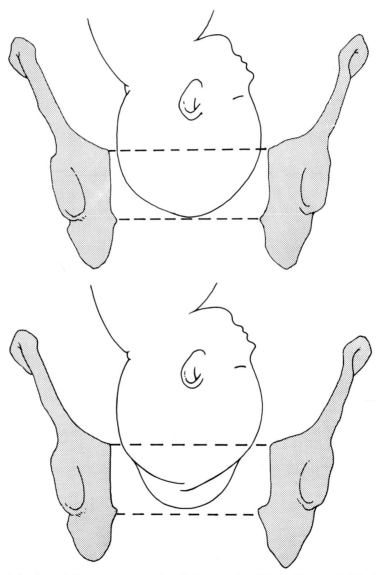

Fig. 12.4. A drawing to indicate engagement when the lowest point of the head has reached the level of the ischeal spines in most cases (above). The presence of caput and moulding may bring the lowest point to the level of the spines although the widest diameter remains above the brim (below).

[Fig. 12.3(d)]. Now the anteroposterior presenting diameter is the submento bregmatic, so that the head again presents as a circle of 9·5 cm.

The head will enter the pelvis more easily flexed than in any of the degrees of extension. Although full extension presents the same diameters as those of full flexion, the face presentation is much less favourable since, if posterior rotation of the chin occurs during labour, delivery cannot take place (see p. 359). When the largest diameters of the head have passed through the pelvis, the head is said to be engaged in the pelvis; when this has occurred a little more than half the head will probably be below the pelvis brim and on vaginal examination one will find that the lowest part of the head will be approaching the level of the ischial spines (Fig. 12.4).

THE FORCES OF LABOUR

The foetus passes through the birth canal as a result of the action of the forces of labour, which are divided into:

(i) the primary powers—these are the uterine contractions and are active throughout labour,

(ii) the secondary powers—these are the voluntary muscles of the abdominal wall and the diaphragm and are active only towards the end of the second stage of labour.

The primary powers

An account of the anatomical divisions of the uterus has already been given in the chapter on normal pregnancy, p. 112. The body of the uterus, or upper uterine segment, is the active element of labour which will force the foetus out through the combined lower uterine segment and cervix, which act together as a single functioning unit. The lower uterine segment, developed from the region of the isthmus uteri, has an extremely important function to perform. It serves as an expanding buffer between the strongly contracting uterine body and the cervix and is responsible for the slow dilatation of the cervix which takes place.

The muscle fibres of the upper and the lower uterine segments function differently during labour. The fibres of the uterine body have, in common with other muscles, the normal property of contraction; in addition, however, they have the important property of retraction. Under normal circumstances, when a muscle contracts it becomes shorter, when it relaxes it returns to its original length; uterine muscle fibres, however, have the ability to remain permanently shorter after relaxation, and this facility is called retraction. It permits the uterus to accommodate itself to a slow reduction in the size of its contents without having to remain in a permanent state of contraction; as a result of it the fibres of the upper uterine segment become shorter and thicker as labour progresses.

Fibres of the lower uterine segment function differently during labour, since they become thinned and elongated. The junction between these two segments becomes well defined and the place where the thick upper segment and the thin lower segment meet is called the physiological retraction ring. Coordinated contraction and retraction of the upper uterine segment produces, first, thinning of the lower uterine segment and then effacement and dilatation of the cervix.

The term effacement or taking up is given to the process by which the cervical canal is obliterated, the upper portions of the canal becoming incorporated into the lower uterine segment whilst the lower portion in the region of the external os remains in its previous state. Once effacement is complete, dilatation commences (see Fig. 12.5.)

Recording of uterine activity

The consideration of uterine activity undertaken in Chapter 9, indicates that no clear-cut difference exists between the type of uterine activity present in labour and that of late pregnancy. It was noted that during the last 10 weeks or so of pregnancy, B waves increased in frequency and amplitude, spread more widely throughout the uterus and occurred more regularly. These contractions may raise the resting uterine tone, normally some 5 mmHg or so, by 10–15 mmHg.

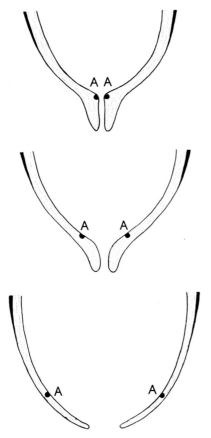

Fig. 12.5. A drawing to indicate taking up and dilatation of the cervix. The points A A indicate the position of the internal os. In the upper drawing the cervix is neither effaced nor dilated, in the middle drawing it is becoming effaced but is still undilated, in the lower drawing it is fully effaced and is becoming dilated.

Recordings of uterine activity may be made conveniently during labour by internal recording or by means of an external multichannel tocograph. Internal recordings may be obtained before membrane rupture by introducing a fluid-filled, open-ended polythene catheter between the membranes and uterine wall; this is connected via a strain gauge pressure-transducer to a moving-pen recorder. If the membranes are ruptured the catheter is inserted into the amniotic sac above the presenting part. It seems probable that comparable recordings can be obtained by either internal or external means.

The normal contractions of labour do not raise the intra-uterine tone between contractions but pressures rise with the contractions some 50–75 mmHg above the resting level (Fig. 12.6). As labour processes, increase in frequency and strength of contractions is evident. Pressures exceeding a 75 mmHg increase during contractions are seldom seen.

ONSET OF LABOUR

No one knows how labour begins. No clear-cut, abrupt changes have been demonstrated to coincide with the onset of labour. No sudden increase in oxytocic production can be shown to occur, although sensitivity to oxytocics increases as pregnancy advances. Volume changes appear to precipitate labour in some circumstances. Volume reduction has this effect since, following artificial rupture of the membranes, most patients near to term will go into labour within the next 24 hr. The opposite effect of increased uterine distension is seen in the tendency to premature labour in patients with twins and in patients with hydramnios. Similarly, an increase in the volume of the amniotic fluid by intra-amniotic injection of glucose or saline may also initiate labour. Under normal circumstances, however, significant volume changes do not occur over a short period of time.

Other possible factors involved are the effect of enzymatic changes and the role of the foetus itself. There appears to be correlation between the sensitivity of the uterine muscle to oxytocics and to 5-hydroxytryptamine. What relevance this may have to the normal onset of labour is unknown as yet. The association of prolonged gestation and anencephaly has been noted for some years. In the absence of hydramnios the anencephalic foetus may remain *in utero* well after 40 weeks if interference is withheld. The possible association with foetal pituitary/adrenal activity suggests itself, and failure in anencephaly of mechanisms normally so operating may explain delay in starting in these cases.

Recently, the possible association with prostaglandin activity has arisen. Prostaglandins E_2 and $F_{2\alpha}$ are found in liquor amnii only during or very close to labour (Karim & Devlin 1967)

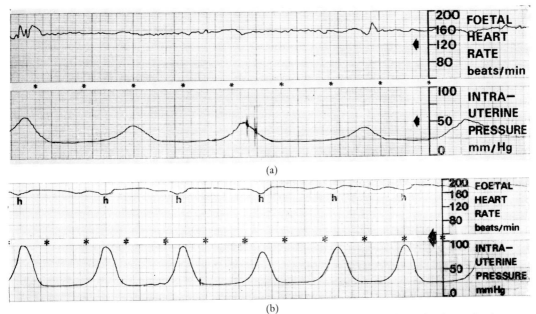

(a)

(b)

Fig. 12.6. Uterine pressure and foetal heart rate recordings in normal labour. In (a) the patient is in early labour and there is no alteration to the foetal heart rate during contraction. In (b) labour has advanced to the late 1st stage. The letter (h) indicates small dips in the heart rate during each contraction, thought to be due to head pressure (see Chapter 11). The base line between contractions is set rather high, and this reading does not indicate increased uterine tone.

whether premature or at term, and an extremely close relationship has been observed between the quantities of $F_2\alpha$ present in blood and each individual uterine contraction (Karim 1968). The significance of these findings is not known, but further work is eagerly awaited. Prostaglandins and Syntocinon appear to have a synergistic action, and this too may be concerned (Brummer 1971).

Several factors are likely to be concerned in the normal onset of labour, but until more is learnt further speculation appears unhelpful.

THE PROGRESS AND DURATION OF LABOUR

The normal duration of labour in primigravid and multigravid patients has been variously estimated by different observers. Busby (1948) reported the mean duration of primigravid labour as 13 hr and for multigravid patients 8 hr. Friedman (1955, 1956) gave figures of 14·4 and 7·8 hr, respectively. More recently, Ledger

(1969) reporting from two separate institutions gave figures of 10·9 and 9·9 hr for primigravid patients and 6·8 and 5·7 for multigravid patients.

That there is considerable variation in the length of labour is an observation which scarcely requires to be made to anyone with even a small experience of midwifery. Friedman (1955, 1956), Friedman & Sachtleban (1961, 1962, 1963, 1965) and Friedman & Kroll (1969) have made a valuable contribution to our knowledge of the progress of labour by showing graphically that labour, as judged by cervical dilatation, does not progress in a simple, straightforward fashion throughout. Friedman divided labour into a latent phase and an active phase (Fig. 12.7). During the latent phase (some 8 hr or so in primigravidae) the cervix becomes taken up and dilated to some 2 cm; this is followed by an active phase in which there is a period of some 2 hr of acceleration, a similar period of maximum dilatation and then a brief deceleration period of about 1 hr between 9 and 10 cm of dilatation. Others (Schulman & Ledger 1964; Ledger 1969)

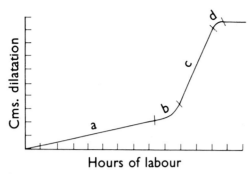

Fig. 12.7. A graph of labour modelled on Friedman, (a) indicates the latent phase (b) the phase of acceleration (c) the phase of maximum dilatation and (d) the phase of deceleration.

have confirmed these observations and have used the graphical recording for the progress of labour widely and successfully.

That labour often follows this pattern is not a new observation, and must have been familiar to generations of obstetricians. What is perhaps most valuable about the observations of Friedman and his colleagues is the fact that the practice of plotting the progress of labour in this way on an appropriate chart enables departures from the normal to be observed early in labour. Intervention, if considered appropriate, can be undertaken soon and not when labour has already lasted such a prolonged period of time that the condition of the mother is already suffering.

In present-day obstetric practice it is possible to intervene more successfully than was the case in the past and to stimulate the progress of slow labour with much greater safety. The frequency with which it may be wise to do this will remain within the judgement of individual obstetricians. All will agree, however, that the avoidance of prolonged labour with its raised foetal mortality and maternal morbidity is a desirable aim if it can be accomplished safely. O'Driscoll et al. (1969) have recently reported very successful results with active management in patients making slow progress in early labour.

CONTROL OF UTERINE ACTIVITY

Rhythmic contraction appears to be an inherent property of the uterine muscle. Thus contractions continue in isolated strips placed in physiological solutions; moreover, labour commences and continues apparently in normally paraplegic women. Nervous influences nonetheless affect labour. The anxious, emotionally unstable woman commonly suffers from less efficient, more painful uterine contractions and may have to endure a longer labour; this influence of tension on disordered uterine activity has led in the past to the aphorism 'tense mind, tense cervix'. Epidural analgesia frequently has a markedly beneficial effect in this type of case.

Another aspect of labour which may be concerned with nervous influences is the so-called polarity of the uterus. The presence of a well-flexed head fitting snugly into the cervix gives an excellent stimulus to the contractions of the upper uterine segment. By contrast, if the presenting part does not fit well into the cervix, such as when the head is extended or the breech presents, the quality of contractions tends to be poorer. This relationship is by no means an invariable one, however, since in many cases with a poorly fitting presenting part labour is nevertheless normal and rapid; in some cases in which the foetus lies transversely and no effective presenting part can be said to occupy the cervix at all, labour may progress very rapidly indeed, especially if the patient is multiparous.

The secondary powers

The secondary powers function only towards the end of the second stage and, to a much less extent, during the third stage of labour. The action of the secondary powers in expelling the child are similar to the action of defaecation. The patient fixes her diaphragm by closing her glottis and then contracts the muscles of the abdominal wall very strongly. This action may be greatly assisted if the chest and pelvis are fixed by holding some fixed object or by pushing against the foot of the bed. The greatest force of all may be obtained if the patient assumes the squatting position. This is, however, a somewhat uncontrolled situation for the obstetrician wishing to deliver the baby slowly in its final stages.

Secondary powers come into play almost involuntarily as the patient begins to feel the presenting part pressing strongly into the perineum and rectum. If this reflex is inhibited by the use of anaesthesia or heavy analgesia the patient may make no instinctive bearing-down efforts and intervention may be required to deliver the child.

THE COURSE OF LABOUR

Labour is divided into three stages, in the following manner:

First stage: The dilatation of the cervix.
Second stage: The expulsion of the foetus.
Third stage: Separation and expulsion of the placenta and membranes.

The pattern of onset of the first stage of labour will be variable. Many patients become aware of uterine contractions by experiencing pains in the lower part of the back, the pains then passing around both sides of the body to the lower abdomen. Commonly, a small 'show' of blood and mucus is noticed about this time. This is the result of separation of the mucus plus from the cervix as more and more of the cervix becomes incorporated in the lower uterine segment and dilatation begins.

The contractions, at first somewhat irregular, gradually become more regular and stronger in a normal case. In a primigravid patient some descent of the presenting part will take place even during these early stages; if the patient is multiparous, however, the presenting part may not begin to descend until well into the first stage, and perhaps even during the second stage. Progress, as judged by descent of the presenting part, is therefore a more gradual process in a primigravid patient and a much more rapid and almost terminal process in a multigravid patient.

Rupture of the membranes may occur at any time during the first stage of labour. Not infrequently, very early rupture of the membranes takes place before labour contractions can truly be said to have begun. In other cases the membranes will rupture at some point during the course of the first stage, and in still others at the beginning of the second stage, when the cervix is fully dilated. What is responsible for this variation is not precisely known. It is probable that the tensile strength of the membranes themselves is, to some extent, responsible for the time of their rupture. Another factor likely to be concerned is the application of the presenting part to the cervix; if this is a closely fitting relationship all round the circumference of the foetal head, less of the rising intra-uterine pressure with each contraction will be transmitted to the forewaters, which will have less chance of rupturing at an early stage. If the presenting part is a more irregular one, such as a transverse lie, the full force of the uterine contractions will be transmitted to the forewaters at an early stage and early rupture of the membranes is likely to take place.

Uterine contractions become much more powerful and expulsive in character during the second stage. The patient experiences this as a bearing-down sensation. The passage of the foetal head through the pelvis, which occurs predominantly during the second stage of labour, but also to some extent in the first stage, is associated with considerable displacement on the contents of the pelvis. The structures in the forepart of the pelvis are drawn upwards as the lower uterine segment stretches; the bladder becomes an abdominal organ and the urethra is elongated. In the posterior part of the pelvis the lower rectum and anal canal are thrust downwards and backwards. The muscles of the pelvic floor, the levator ani and the superficial perineal muscles are also pushed downwards and to each side to allow the baby's head to pass through. Considerable stretching of these muscles always occurs and, in many cases, tearing of portions of them as well.

When the child is born, uterine contractions cease for a short time, unless they have been provoked by an injection of an oxytocic drug towards the end of the process of delivery. If an injection of oxytocic has not been given, contractions recommence after a short resting period. One or other of these resumed contractions separates the placenta, which is then expelled from the birth canal by the combined effects of the uterine contractions and the patient's bearing-down efforts. The physiology and management of this third stage of labour is considered fully later in this chapter.

THE MECHANISM OF LABOUR AND DELIVERY

In most instances, towards the end of pregnancy the child lies in the uterus in an attitude of flexion with its head occupying the lower pole of the uterus. This is the common cephalic presentation; since the lowest portion of the head is, in most instances, the vertex, the term vertex presentation is often loosely used when it is possible to palpate the head in the lower part of the uterus.

The position of the presenting part is described by relating the occiput—known as the denominator—to the right or left side of the pelvis and to the anterior, posterior or lateral part of it. Six positions of the vertex presentation are therefore described. These are:

(1) Left occipito-anterior (LOA). Here the occiput points obliquely anteriorly towards the superior ramus of the pubis on the left side.
(2) Right occipito-anterior (ROA); occiput pointing again obliquely anteriorly, this time to the right.
(3) Right occipitoposterior (ROP); occiput pointing to the right sacro-iliac joint area.
(4) Left occipitoposterior (LOP); occiput pointing to the left sacro-iliac joint area.
(5) Right occipitolateral (ROL); occiput pointing to the right and directly laterally.
(6) Left occipitolateral (LOL); occiput pointing to the left and directly laterally.

It seems probable that direct occipito-anterior and occipitoposterior positions with the occiput pointing, respectively, directly at the symphysis pubis and the sacral promontory are very uncommon and perhaps occur only when the pelvis is of the unusual anthropoid shape (see p. 181).

Some years ago it was thought that the anterior positions were more common than posterior ones. Following the era when X-rays were more widely used to study the process of labour, it

became evident that more often the occiput is pointing directly laterally; in some cases this may be slightly in front of, and in others slightly behind, the lateral plane.

When the presenting part is not the vertex the positions and mode of delivery are as described in appropriate sections elsewhere in this book.

MOVEMENTS OF THE HEAD

During the passage of the head through the birth canal a number of changes of position, known as rotations, take place. These rotations occur for one predominant reason, namely that the pelvic floor is composed of the two levator ani muscles which present a sloping gutter directed downwards and forwards. On each side the levator ani muscles arise from a line passing posteriorly from the superior ramus of the pubis close to the symphysis, running across the white line over the surface of the obturator foramen to the ischial spine posteriorly. The muscular fibres run downwards and backwards to interdigitate with those of the opposite side in the mid-line and to surround the urethra, genital tract and rectum; posteriorly, the fibres are inserted into the coccyx. External to the levator ani sling lie the much less important superficial perineal muscles which consist of the transversus perinei passing medially from the ischial tuberosities, the bulbocavernosus surrounding the lower vagina, and the sphincter ani muscles surrounding the anal canal, all of which are inserted into the perineal body. This perineal body is the central point of the perineum, and is a small mass of fibromuscular tissue lying between the lower part of the vagina and the anal canal: it is composed predominantly of the combined insertions of the three paired muscles just described. Ischiocavernosus lying over the crus of the clitoris on each side is relatively unimportant clinically.

The important effect of the levator ani sling is that whichever part of the foetal head reaches it first will be directed forwards. When the head is well flexed, the lowest portion is in the region of the occiput. Thus, during the head's passage downwards through the pelvis, provided there is good flexion, the occiput will be directed from the transverse or oblique position towards the front. This movement is called internal rotation. Internal rotation with the head well flexed will almost always result in anterior rotation of the occiput. If the head is less well flexed, however, it is less certain which part of the head will rotate forwards. When the head presents in the occipitoposterior position a degree of deflexion is common when the sinciput may, in effect, be the lowest part and may be directed forwards, the occiput passing backwards into the hollow of the sacrum (see p. 353).

Following anterior rotation of the occiput, the head descends further and the occiput becomes free under the subpubic arch. This allows the head to move forwards and permits extension of the head from its previously fully flexed attitude. The next movement of the head, therefore, is extension.

The movement of internal rotation which the head has undergone will have had the effect of twisting the head upon the shoulders. If this has happened, the head, once free of the perineum will tend to straighten itself in relation to the shoulders by rotating backwards towards the position it occupied before internal rotation. This movement is known as restitution, and it is opposite in direction to internal rotation. Restitution, however, appears to be a movement far more often absent than present. One must conclude that the shoulders frequently follow during internal rotation of the head and any restitution mechanism is unnecessary.

Following extension and delivery of the head, there is further descent of the shoulders which meeting the sloping pelvic floor themselves. They are rotated into the anteroposterior diameter of the outlet of the pelvis also, and since the head is free, it rotates with them until the occiput points directly laterally; this is called external rotation.

Lateral flexion of the trunk occurs to allow delivery of the remaining portions of the baby.

The movements of delivery may therefore be summarized as: (1) descent; (2) internal rotation; (following the slope of the pelvic floor); (3) extension (to allow the head to become free of the subpubic arch); (4) restitution (seldom seen, but occasionally necessary to undo the twist of the head on the shoulders); (5) external rotation (as internal rotation of the shoulders occurs and the head follows); and (6) lateral flexion.

Some modification of these movements occurs during delivery if the head has been occupying a distinctly posterior position. This is discussed in detail in Chapter 22.

CHANGES IN THE FOETAL SKULL

Two very important changes occur in the foetal skull during labour; these are moulding and caput formation. The movement which is possible at fontanelles and the suture lines allows the shape of the head to be slightly altered during labour by the overlapping of these bones. This moulding process usually takes the form of the frontal and occipital bones passing beneath the parietals and one parietal passing beneath the other. When the head is flexed it is compressed around the suboccipital bregmatic diameter and becomes more elongated than normal; when it is less well flexed, compression occurs around the occipitofrontal diameter, and as a result the head becomes round.

The caput succedaneum is an area of oedema which forms in that portion of the scalp compressed by the ring of dilating cervix after the membranes have ruptured. The pressure of the cervix against the scalp by the uterine contractions delay the venous return from this area of the scalp, with resulting oedema. In practical terms, the caput is important because its presence can make the recognition of the position of the presenting part more difficult and, when marked, it appears to make the head lower than it really is (Fig. 12.4).

THE MANAGEMENT OF LABOUR

When a patient is first seen after the onset to labour, a careful history must be taken concerning the time and mode of onset of labour, the strength and frequency of uterine contractions, whether membranes have ruptured or not, if there has been a show or not, and any other relevant matter. Abdominal palpation is to be undertaken to show that there has been no alteration in the findings from the last antenatal visit. The lie, presentation, position and the relationship of the presenting part to the pelvic brim must also all be established accurately. The patient's blood pressure, pulse rate, presence or absence of oedema should all be recorded; the urine should be tested. Attention to the patient's general demeanour at this point is important. Some patients approach labour philosophically, others are naturally anxious, and still others very frightened.

Careful auscultation of the foetal heart rate is very important. Normally, the heart rate in labour is between 120 and 160 beats per minute. Occasionally, slight slowing occurs during uterine contractions, but more often than not little alteration is noted. (A further consideration of this is undertaken on p. 169.) Throughout labour, the foetal heart will require to be listened to regularly. Under normal circumstances, half-hourly intervals will probably suffice for the early part of labour, but more frequent auscultation is necessary as time goes by and during the second stage of labour, auscultation after each contraction will be desirable.

DESCENT OF THE PRESENTING PART

The progress of labour can be judged, in one respect, by the descent of the presenting part; abdominal examination alone will usually be sufficient to judge this. If the head can be felt easily on each side of the mid-line early in labour and quickly descends, so that only the sinciput is palpable, excellent progress is being made.

At intervals, however, it will be necessary to examine the patient per vaginam. Vaginal examination may be undertaken for a variety of reasons. It is often wise to make a vaginal examination when the patient is admitted in labour, to establish for certain the dilatation of the cervix, the level of the presenting part, the rupture or otherwise of the membranes and, if they are ruptured, the appearance of the liquor amnii. Whenever the membranes rupture and the head is high, vaginal examination is important to exclude prolapse of the cord.

The same examination may be undertaken to check the progress of labour at intervals, if there is uncertainty about the findings on abdominal examination, and sometimes as a guide to ap-

propriate sedation. If a vaginal examination is to be undertaken, however, it is important to obtain as much information as possible whilst doing so. We need to know:

What is the dilatation of the cervix; its consistency; its thickness; its application to the head?

What is the nature of the presenting part; its position; its degree of flexion or extension, and its station in the pelvis?

Is a caput or moulding present, or both?

Are the membranes ruptured, and what is the appearance of the liquor?

Are the vaginal and perineal tissues soft and distensible, or thick and resistant?

Is any other fault present, such as prolapse of the cord, hydrocephalus, disproportion, etc?

The station of the head will be most easily estimated by relating its lowest point to the level of the ischial spines. When this part of the head has reached the level of the spines and there is neither caput nor moulding, the widest diameter of the head will, in most cases, have passed comfortably through the pelvic brim. If the lowest part of the head is above this level then it cannot be assumed for certain that the head is yet engaged. Moreover, if there is caput or moulding, the fact that the lowest part of the head has reached the ischial spine level does not in itself, imply engagement. Whenever a vaginal examination is undertaken, abdominal palpation with the other hand must be performed at the same time, so that the amount of head above the pelvic brim can be estimated and a decision made as to whether the head is engaged or not, and how deeply. It scarcely needs emphasis that vaginal examinations during labour must be carried out with full aseptic precautions. Rectal examinations give far less information and are seldom indicated.

During the second stage of labour, the uterus itself will be quite capable of pushing the head well down into the pelvis, and the patient should not be urged to push too soon. Once we are satisfied that the head is low, then the patient may be allowed to push, if she has the desire to do so.

RELIEF OF PAIN

One very important aspect of the management of labour is to relieve the patient from the pain of her uterine contractions. It has already been suggested that antenatal education of the patient may be beneficial to her in this respect. This does not necessarily mean that a patient who has undertaken such instruction and has learnt to relax will have a painless labour, but she will probably have a less painful labour than a patient who is unduly anxious and tense throughout. In this sense education for childbirth and learning muscular control help to prevent labour from becoming a distressing process for the patient; indeed, a number of patients find it fulfilling, and even an enjoyable experience.

For most patients, however, some attention to pain relief is important throughout labour. Drugs may be given by mouth or by injection, anaesthetic gases may be inhaled, or nerve block undertaken. Each of these methods of pain relief has its advocates. Most obstetricians, however, tend to select the most appropriate means for the individual patients.

A drug which is particularly useful by injection is pethidine either alone or combined with tranquillizing preparations such as Sparine or Phenergan. Pethidine in doses of 100 mg combined with 25 or 50 mg of promazine hydrochloride (Sparine) will give excellent pain relief for a patient of average size. The dose of pethidine may be increased to 150 mg for a larger, heavier patient. This dose may safety be repeated several times during normal labour and probably has very little effect on the child unless a large amount is given shortly before delivery. It is usually wise to withhold the pethidine until the cervix is more than 2 cm dilated, to coincide with the onset of the active stage of labour. It is seldom necessary to give much sedation earlier than this, but if the patient is usually anxious a drug to relieve this anxiety—such as the alcohol derivative Oblivon—may be helpful.

A particularly distressing time for the patient in labour is the end of the first stage when contractions are strongest and the patient is not yet able to help the process by bearing down. Inhalational analgesics are often used at this time.

Formerly, Trilene and air was particularly effective; this has been largely replaced by nitrous oxide and oxygen premixed in a cylinder (Entonox). Both are effective and safe provided the patient begins to take the gas as soon as the earliest signs of pain are experienced or, indeed, when the next pain is expected.

Although these methods of relieving pain can be effective if given in sufficient doses sufficiently frequently, it has been suggested that, in practice, they do not give as much pain relief as is necessary (Beazley et al. 1967). Employing a programme of pain relief to assess its effectiveness, these workers found a satisfactory level of pain relief in only 40% of patients studied, using the conventional means described above. They concluded that there was a limit to the relief which could be obtained by techniques based upon central depression of pain by pethidine or opiates and other preparations. More effective pain relief is possible by employing a paracervical nerve block or epidural analgesia.

Cooper & Moir (1963) reported favourably on the use of paracervical nerve block in labour. The technique is an easy one to learn and will only briefly be described here. The lateral fornix is identified at vaginal examination and a special blunt-ended guarded needle is introduced and thrust against the epithelium of the fornix at 3 o'clock, then on the opposite side at 9 o'clock. The needle within the guard tube is then pushed upwards to project 7 mm beyond the blunt end into the tissues of the paracervical region. Deep penetration is therefore avoided. 10 ml of 1% lignocaine with adrenalin 1 in 200,000 was used by Cooper & Moir on each side. Good pain relief for an hour or so was obtained, when further injections were given if needed. Although good pain relief is obtained, its brief duration is a disadvantage. Use of the longer-acting analgesic Bupivicaine (Yates 1969) was undoubtedly an advance in that pain relief was prolonged for some 3 hr. A number of instances of alarming foetal bradycardia were observed, however, when 10 ml of 0·5% solution was used on each side. In an attempt to avoid this effect the strength of the anaesthetic solution was reduced to 0·25%, which appeared to allow pain relief for a comparable period without bradycardia resulting

(Gudgeon 1968). A number of obstetricians still have reservations about the complete safety of this type of analgesia, but there is no doubt that it can be most effective, and under certain circumstances would appear clearly to be indicated.

Epidural analgesia, popular in the United States since its introduction in 1943 by Hingson and Edwards, has recently become more widely used in this country. The technique of epidural analgesia will be briefly described. The patient is placed in the sitting position leaning slightly forwards. A number 16-gauge Tuohy needle is introduced between the 3rd and 4th lumbar vertebrae or between the 2nd and 3rd lumbar vertebrae. When the epidural space is entered by the needle, loss of resistance is immediately noted. After testing to ensure that the theca has not been entered, a plastic catheter with a blunt tip is passed down to the epidural space. The needle is then withdrawn and the catheter is connected with a disposable 50 ml syringe which is filled with local anaesthetic solution. The syringe may be sealed inside a transparent, sterile, plastic bag, allowing 'top-up' injections to be given without sterile precautions being required. Lignocaine 2% with adrenalin 1 in 200,000 is generally used and the dose given varies between 6 and 10 ml. 'Top-up' injections may be given as the pain returns. Moir & Willocks (1968) have reported enthusiastically on the use of this form of pain relief.

There are, however, complications to epidural analgesia, although on the whole these can be simply managed. These complications are (1) a high spinal anaesthesia; (2) high epidural anaesthesia; (3) intravascular injections; (4) cerebral irritation due to an accumulation of the drug over a long period of time; (5) hypotension; and (6) chills and shaking.

If it is known that the theca or a blood vessel has been entered the procedure should be abandoned. The hypotension noted is usually concerned with the uterus pressing on the inferior vena cava and limiting venous return to the heart (supine hypotension syndrome). It is generally easily managed by turning the patient to her right or left side.

Caudal analgesia appears to be an equally effective means of pain relief, although the technique is perhaps slightly more difficult. When epidural analgesia is employed it is necessary that an anaesthetist be present in the hospital the whole time. This seems a desirable aim in any event, but is not always achieved (Taylor 1971).

There are occasions when a patient is admitted during the night in the early latent phase of labour and whilst not yet experiencing painful contractions may require something to help her to sleep; barbiturates are particularly helpful in this situation.

The methods of pain relief discussed here seem to the author the most satisfactory. Other drugs have their advocates—morphine, heroin and, more recently pentazocine, are instances. Other methods are favoured by some. Pain control by breathing and by relaxation has its advocates; so has hypnotism (Davidson 1963). It may be that one method suits one individual obstetrician better than another and that what is required is the development by practical personal experience of a suitably effective regime with appropriate modifications for exceptional circumstances.

It must be emphasized finally that the principles of pain relief are that whatever is used should be effective, should be consistent in relieving the pain and should not interfere with uterine action or be harmful to the child, either at the time or on delivery should this occur shortly afterwards.

FLUID AND FOOD INTAKE

The problems of fluid and food intake during labour are concerned with the possible need for a general anaesthetic at a later stage. Fluids containing sugar may be dangerous if a general anaesthetic is later given and there is inhalation of gastric contents. Whereas fluid may effectively, if unpleasantly, be removed from the stomach by a gastric tube before anaesthesia, food is unlikely to be removed and may be inhaled if the patient vomits during induction of the anaesthetic. Gastric emptying time is considerably reduced in labour and it is likely that if the patient is given food in the early part of labour it will remain there for some time thereafter. In Queen Charlotte's Hospital patients in labour are allowed to quench their thirst with any beverage they wish or with water, but fluids are not forced and they are not given any containing glucose. Food is occasionally given in the early stages, but this is limited to food which will pass easily through a sieve. Patients require to take very little food at this time, and for most no food of any kind need be taken. It is possible, however, that with a regime of this kind a patient will quickly use up liver stores of glycogen and will begin to metabolize fat, with the appearance of ketone bodies in the urine. Any sign of dehydration or ketosis calls for an intravenous infusion of 10 or 20% dextrose to correct this abnormality.

OTHER OBSERVATIONS

Other observations which require to be made during labour are on the patient's pulse rate, blood pressure and, of course, foetal heart sounds, as already indicated. Attention must be paid to the urinary output. The amounts of urine passed should be measured and tested for albumin, sugar and acetone. Many patients in labour have difficulty in emptying the bladder, especially if the head fits tightly into the pelvis and the bladder is drawn up into the abdomen and the urethra elongated. Catheterization will sometimes be required, when a soft, male catheter will usually be the most satisfactory. In the early part of labour the patient need not stay in bed; when the pains begin to be more strong she will need to be nursed in bed, where she may occupy whichever position she finds most comfortable.

DELIVERY

Delivery may be accomplished in the dorsal or left lateral position, whichever the obstetrician prefers. It is not intended to discuss delivery in detail, since it is essentially one of the practical procedures which, we contend, must be learned in practice. In a primigravid patient, or one with a previous perineal tear, an episiotomy will have much to commend it. This may be quite simply performed after local infiltration of local anaesthetic along the line chosen. The episiotomy is best delayed until the head is coming up well and the perineum is thin. The blade of a pair of blunt scissors is gently inserted between the head and the posterior vaginal wall and the cut made at the beginning of a uterine contraction. If the episiotomy is made earlier than this there may be troublesome bleeding from the thick edges. The episiotomy may be median or mediolateral; in the former case the incision should be turned to the side as the anus is approached to avoid injuring that structure, and in the latter case the incision should begin in the mid-line of the perineum to avoid injury to Bartholin's duct (for other considerations see p. 422).

Most patients in this country will be delivered by their own efforts unless there is delay in the second stage of labour or maternal or foetal distress becomes evident. If epidural analgesia has been employed, however, it is less likely that the patient will succeed in delivering the baby herself. Outlet forceps delivery may then be undertaken without difficulty.

THE THIRD STAGE OF LABOUR

The third stage of labour commences with the delivery of the infant and ends with the delivery of the placenta, and is thus an event related to the process of labour. From the practical point of view, however, the efficient management of the third stage begins much earlier in labour, and some of the problems of management continue after the delivery of the placenta.

The main complication of the third stage is blood loss, and this may be excessive before the delivery of the placenta and for a period of time afterwards—this may be referred to as the fourth stage of labour. It is now agreed that the actual delivery of the placenta is of secondary importance, although its retention may lead to, or exaggerate, the haemorrhage.

Physiological mechanisms involved in delivery of the placenta

Uterine contractions have been shown to continue after the birth of the infant and, although the patient may feel little discomfort, the intra-uterine pressure continues to be rhythmically raised. Possibly during, and certainly after, delivery the uterine muscle fibres contract and retract, with a resultant reduction in the size of the upper segment. This shortening reduces the area of the uterine surface to which the relatively incompressible placenta is attached. Separation of the placenta through the spongy layer of the decidua basalis occurs as a result of this retraction, and the consequent reduction in intra-uterine volume tends to force the placenta into the relaxed lower segment, as well as assisting in the separation process. Retroplacental bleeding may play a part in this separation, but it seems that the lower edge of the placenta becomes detached first in most instances and so the concept of central separation and retroplacental bleeding is less likely (Macpherson & Wilson 1956).

When placental separation is complete and the placenta is forced into the lower segment and vagina it may be delivered spontaneously by maternal effort, the lower edge presenting first at the vulva—the Matthews Duncan method of expulsion. If traction is exerted on the umbilical cord or the uterine fundus is forcibly compressed, the foetal surface may appear first, with the membranes covering the maternal surface—the Schultze method.

The continued retraction of the uterine muscle is of paramount importance in minimizing the blood loss during and after this stage. The blood vessels supplying the placental site are compressed by the oblique fibres of the middle layer of the myometrium. This mechanism of controlling bleeding is only effective if the uterine muscle is capable of efficient contraction and retraction, and any impairment of this will predispose to haemorrhage.

Most patients can be delivered without undue blood loss, but because the consequences of severe haemorrhage are very serious—particularly in domiciliary practice—firstly, obstetric 'flying squads' were introduced, and secondly the prophylactic use of oxytocics was recommended. The *Confidential Enquiries into Maternal Deaths in England and Wales* have shown a marked decrease in the number of maternal deaths from haemorrhage after delivery, because of these and other modifications in obstetric practice.

Management of third stage

ACTION OF OXYTOCIC DRUGS

The drugs used are oxytocin and ergometrine given alone or in combination. They may be given intravenously or intramuscularly, and the injection may be administered with the 'crowning' of the head, with the delivery of the head, with the delivery of the anterior shoulder, after the delivery of the infant or after the delivery of the placenta.

Oxytocin produces rhythmical contractions of the uterus augmenting retraction, and its effect is noticeable about 3 min after intramuscular injection (Embrey 1961). An injection of 5 units of oxytocin produced effective contractions for about 15 min. Ergometrine by injection results in a more prolonged contraction with retraction, and its effect is noticeable about 7 min after intramuscular injection. When either drug is given intravenously, the uterine contraction commences in about 30–40 sec.

Obviously, the drugs will only effect the upper segment, and the uterus below the retraction ring will not respond because of the absence of muscle fibres.

USE OF OXYTOCIC DRUGS IN MANAGEMENT

The prophylactic use of oxytocic drugs is now well established, but differences in technique and in the selection of the drug used still exist. The theoretical object of prophylactic oxytocics is to ensure efficient contractions of the uterus after the delivery of the infant, thus minimizing the amount of blood loss due to failure of the compression of the blood vessels in the placental site, and to promote rapid separation and descent of the placenta. If an oxytocic drug is given before the delivery of the placenta, the routine procedure for its subsequent delivery must be strictly adhered to, otherwise the placenta may be retained and blood loss may not be prevented.

Intravenous oxytocics are given with the delivery of the anterior shoulder, and the resulting contraction should follow very soon after the one which delivers the infant. If the placenta is partially or completely sheared off the uterine wall at the time of delivery of the infant, a further contraction should complete its separation where required and encourage its descent into the lower segment or vagina. It is necessary to anticipate this process by assisting the delivery of the placenta immediately after the delivery of the infant is complete, and before the uterus clamps down preventing complete descent of the placenta as may sometimes happen. As soon as the umbilical cord has been clamped and divided, the placenta is received.

If the injection is given intramuscularly [and Syntometrine—syntocinon 5 units and ergometrine 0·5 mg (Sandoz)—is commonly used] a similar delivery of the placenta can only be achieved by administering it at the 'crowning' of the head, or after its delivery and allowing an interval of about 2 min before completing the delivery of the infant. If Syntometrine is given with the delivery of the anterior shoulder (in a vertex or face presentation) this is comparable with administering the injection after the infant is delivered. Time must then be allowed for the uterus to respond to the drug and the delivery of the placenta to be achieved.

When oxytocin is not given until after the delivery of the placenta, it is necessary to rely on the uterine contractions to separate the placenta completely from its attachment, and then to expel it into the vagina. Because the uterine contractions are sometimes inefficient and ineffective, there is a greater risk of haemorrhage in these circumstances.

Various arguments have been advanced in favour of, and against, these different methods. Hypoxia as a result of delay in delivering the infant, the possibility of difficulty in delivering the shoulders and trunk of the infant, and the problem of knowing when 'crowning' has actually occurred have been advanced as arguments against the intramuscular use of the drugs at 'crowning' of the head. If the injection is given with the delivery of the anterior shoulder, there is a latent period of around 2–3 min during which uterine relaxation may result in haemorrhage and impatience may lead to only partial separation, or, rarely, inversion, of the uterus. As objections to both these methods, advocates of the use of oxytocics only after the delivery of the placenta draw attention to the risks to an undiagnosed second twin, although the danger is less when the injection is given intramuscularly.

DELIVERY OF THE PLACENTA

Separation of the placenta may be accompanied by a little vaginal bleeding. Descent of the placenta into the vagina is followed by a narrowing of the uterine body palpable in the abdomen, increased mobility of the uterus and lengthening of the umbilical cord. However, if oxytocic drugs are given prophylactically it is not necessary to wait for these signs before effecting delivery of the placenta. When the uterus is felt to contract, the patient can be encouraged to bear down and expel the placenta by increased intra-abdominal pressure. In many patients this is not sufficient, and the hand of the attendant is required on the abdomen to counteract the divarication of the rectus muscles. Usually, this is successful in delivering the placenta.

A more active policy is often considered advisable. When the uterus is felt to contract after the delivery of the infant, it can be pushed towards the umbilicus by a hand on the lower abdomen while the cord is held taut at the vulva as described by Brandt (1933) and Andrews (1940). Alternatively, the cord may be gently and gradually pulled downwards and posteriorly with one hand while the uterus is pushed upwards (Fig. 12.8), as practised by Fliegner & Hibbard (1966). A further modification of this cord-traction technique is to initiate descent of the placenta by applying pressure to the fundus at the same time as cord traction is commenced, provided the uterus is contracting. Once the placenta is felt to be descending, the abdominal hand 'peels' the uterus off the placenta as previously described. It is essential that the uterus is contracted whenever cord traction is practised. Energetic traction of the cord with the descent of the placenta impeded may result in its avulsion from its placental attachment. This does no harm but the method of delivery of the placenta must be altered.

The necessity of clamping the maternal end of the divided cord has been questioned, as has

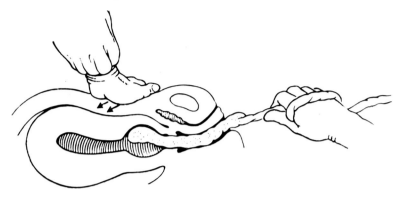

Fig. 12.8. Illustration of controlled cord traction.

the timing of clamping and dividing the cord in order to separate the infant. Botha (1968) has reported a reduction in the incidence of retained placenta and postpartum blood loss in Bantu women who squat in order to deliver their infants and later deliver the placenta without first separating the child from it. This results in an increase in the blood volume of the infant, and others have commented on the beneficial effects of this procedure. The exsanguinated placenta is thought to separate more readily and to be more easily delivered. If the infant is separated from the placenta soon after delivery, the blood in the placenta may be allowed to flow into a receptacle while a uterine contraction and the delivery of the placenta are awaited.

It has been suggested that the transfusion of placental blood to the infant is related to the development of the respiratory distress syndrome, but opinion is divided on whether early or late clamping of the cord is the more desirable. In diabetic patients, it is preferable to reduce the volume of the placental transfusion as far as possible because of the risk of vascular thrombosis in the infant. Early clamping is advocated for infants suspected of having haemolytic disease of the newborn, and in unaffected infants late clamping results in the serum bilirubin levels being higher. A higher haematocrit is to be expected in infants whose cords were clamped late.

In many centres blood from the umbilical cord—i.e. foetal blood—is collected for a variety of reasons. These include the blood grouping of the infant of an Rh-negative patient who may require an anti-Rh immunoglobulin injection, routine blood grouping of all infants and the grouping of infants in multiple pregnancies to help determine their zygosity. Blood can also be obtained from the cord and placental vessels after the delivery is completed.

EXAMINATION OF THE PLACENTA

The placenta should be examined after it has been delivered to ensure that the cotyledons are all present and that the placenta is complete. A succenturiate lobe may have been missed and retained in the uterus, and vessels ending abruptly on the foetal surface of the placenta may suggest this. Immediate exploration of the uterus is required if it is certain that placental tissue is missing, or if the nature of the delivery of the placenta makes it likely that a cotyledon is retained. The completeness of the membranes is less easy to assess, and a fragment may be detected on vaginal examination and removed with a long artery forceps or a similar instrument.

The vessels of the umbilical cord should be examined and counted, and any anomaly, including absence of an umbilical artery, should be reported to the paediatrician. If an artery is absent, the incidence of congenital abnormalities in the child is about 30% (Benirschke 1965), especially involving the renal and cardiovascular systems.

BLOOD LOSS AFTER DELIVERY OF THE
PLACENTA

Estimation of the blood lost in the third and
fourth stages is grossly inaccurate when this is
done by inspection alone. Although it is possible
to collect some of the blood lost before and during
the delivery of the patient, and allowances can
be made for contamination by amniotic fluid
and the soiling of bed linen, bleeding from
the uterus occurring during the 24 hr after
delivery is not usually measured accurately
unless the loss is considerable and replacement is required. An appreciable fall in the
haemoglobin level may occur without any
single episode of haemorrhage. An exact measurement is usually not necessary provided the
patient's blood pressure and pulse rate are
unchanged, but if there is excessive bleeding and
the patient shows evidence of shock, the amount
of blood to replace is important.

Brant (1967) described a method for calculating
the loss at delivery using a 'washing machine'
method for bed linen and drapes, and confirmed
the impression that when the actual loss was over
300 ml the attendants underestimated the volume
of the loss. A more accurate method of determining the effects of blood loss and the amount to
be replaced involves the measurement of the
central venous pressure.

Labour in special circumstances

PREMATURE LABOUR

For reasons which we are generally unable to
determine, some patients go into labour well
before the expected date of their confinement. If
labour commences more than 4 weeks before the
expected date of confinement or the infant is
expected to be less than 2·5 kg in weight special
management may be required. If pains are mild
and the membranes have not ruptured it may be
possible to stop the contractions, and the pregnancy may continue for several weeks longer.
In the past large doses of morphine were used for
this purpose, and in some instances appeared to
be effective. The disadvantage of this method of
treatment is that if labour is not prevented, and
instead proceeds rapidly, the infant is likely to

be born heavily depressed by the morphine.
More recently, other preparations have been
introduced in an attempt to inhibit premature
labour.

The drug isoxsuprine hydrochloride has been
so employed. This preparation is a stimulator of
β receptors in the uterus and has the effect of
inhibiting uterine contractions. The drug certainly appears capable of reducing uterine activity,
but whether it reduces it sufficiently to halt labour
in any particular case is uncertain. Initially the
drug is given by intravenous infusion, 40 mg
being dissolved in 200 ml of normal saline and
given at a rate of 10–15 drops per minute. An
increase to 60 drops per minute is possible
provided no hypotension is recorded. When the
threat of premature labour is under control the
drug may be given by intramuscular injection in
doses of 10 mg 3-hourly for 24 hr. On the third day
10 mg may be given 4-hourly by mouth. It is the
impression of many obstetricians that this treatment is helpful in halting the progress of premature
labours, although it is difficult to prove that the
number who do not go on into established labour
is significantly different from the number who
would have done so without this specific treatment. Better results have recently been claimed for
alcohol, an intravenous infusion of 9·5% alcohol in
5% dextrose being used (Fuchs 1967). This treatment, not unnaturally, can have a marked effect
upon the patient, who may become distinctly
inebriated or even comatose. Whether it will prove
superior to isosuprine is yet to be determined.

If we do not succeed in halting the progress of
premature labour some modification of its
management seems desirable. The premature
foetus is unusually sensitive to respiratory
depression, so if drugs are given to relieve pain
we must be quite certain that they are not used
near to the time of delivery. If such drugs are to
be employed, pethidine and Sparine in smaller
doses than usual appear the best. Nalorphine
hydrobromide in doses in 10 mg should be given
intravenously to the mother if it is clear that
delivery is imminent and there is a chance of
respiratory depression from the drugs given. A
caudal or epidural anaesthesic is preferable in
premature labour. For the actual delivery an
episiotomy should always be used to relieve

pressure on the fragile foetal skull. Delay of any kind is almost certainly better treated by a wide episiotomy and a prophylactic gentle forceps extraction which affords some protection to the foetal head.

LABOUR IN THE VERY YOUNG

There are a number of reports in the literature of pregnancy and delivery in extremely young patients. The youngest mother in the world was delivered in Peru at the age of $5\frac{1}{2}$ years. Delivery was by Caesarean section, the baby weighing 2,700 g. Other very young patients were a German girl aged $6\frac{1}{2}$ years who delivered a 3,000 g child per vaginam; a patient in Brazil delivered twins at the age of $7\frac{1}{2}$; a Mohammedan girl aged 7 was delivered by Caesarean section, the child weighing 4 lb 3 oz; the youngest mother in Britain was apparently 9 years old. These and other precocious confinements are discussed by Dewhurst (1963). In girls of 12–16 years the progress of pregnancy and labour is surprisingly normal. Pre-eclamptic toxaemia is more common at these ages and this does not appear to be due entirely to the fact that many do not come for antenatal supervision sufficiently soon. Prematurity appears slightly more common. The length of labour in very young primigravidae differs little from that of primigravidae in general. The method of delivery, too, is similar and the incidence of really difficult delivery remarkably low.

OLDER PRIMIGRAVIDAE

Whilst many older primigravidae labour extremely well, there is a distinct tendency for labour to be more prolonged. To some extent this may be concerned with anxiety which a number of such patients undoubtedly feel, since they can scarcely help being unusually concerned about the outcome. The incidence of hypertensive disorders is raised in elderly primigravidae, which may have a significant influence upon the decision to induce labour or deliver by Caesarean section before term. In those patients in whom there is no such fault and the obstetrical situation near to term is very favourable, labour may be allowed to commence, and if it proceeds rapidly,

well and good. It is unwise, however, to allow such a labour to be prolonged, and earlier resort to Caesarean section will generally be appropriate.

PRECIPITATE LABOUR

A very small percentage of women appear to have their first babies extremely rapidly. When this happens on the first occasion there is little which can be done to prevent it, and it may be a matter of chance where the baby is born. If it is known to have happened before, however, especially if labour has been extremely quick and associated with any injury to the child, it will be wise to admit the patient to hospital some time before term in order that she can be under supervision when labour commences. Induction of labour will be appropriate in some cases.

REFERENCES

Andrews C.J. (1940) Sth. Med. Surg. 102, 605.
Beazley J.M., Leaver E.P., Morewood J.H.M. & Bircumshaw J. (1967) Lancet, i, 1033.
Benirschke K. (1965) Birth Defects. (Original article series). The National Foundation, March of Dimes, p. 53.
Botha M.C. (1968) S. Afr. Jnl Obstet. & Gynaec. 6, 30.
Brandt M.L. (1933) Am. J. Obstet. Gynec. 25, 662.
Brandt H.A. (1967) Br. med. J. i, 398.
Brummer H. (1971) J. Obstet. Gynaec. Br. Commonw. (In the Press).
Busby T. (1948) Am. J. Obstet. Gynec. 55, 846.
Cooper K. & Moir J.C. (1963) Br. med. J. i, 1372.
Davidson J.A. (1962) Br. med. J. ii, 951.
Dewhurst C.J. (1963) Gynaecological Disorders of Infants and Children. London, Cassell.
Embrey M.P. (1961) Br. med. J. i, 1737.
Fliegner J.R. & Hibbard B.M. (1966) Br. med. J. ii, 622.
Friedman E.A. (1955) Obstet. Gynec., N.Y. 6, 567.
Friedman E.A. (1956) Obstet. Gynec., N.Y. 8, 691.
Friedman E.A. & Sachtleben M.R. (1961) Obstet. Gynec., N.Y. 17, 135 and 566.
Friedman E.A. & Sachtleben M.R. (1962) Obstet. Gynec., N.Y. 19, 576.
Friedman E.A. & Sachtleben M.R. (1963) Obstet. Gynec., N.Y. 22, 478.
Friedman E.A. & Sachtleben M.R. (1965) Obstet. Gynec., N.Y. 25, 844.
Friedman E.A. & Kroll B.H. (1969) J. Obstet. Gynaec. Br. Commonw. 76, 1075.
Fuchs F. (1967) Am. J. Obstet. Gynec. 99, 627.
Gudgeon D.H. (1968) Br. med. J. ii, 403.

HINGSON R.A. & EDWARDS W.B. (1943) *J. Am. med. Ass.* **121,** 225.

KARIM S.M.M. (1968) *Br. med. J.* **iv,** 618.

KARIM S.M.M. & DEVLIN J. (1967) *J. Obstet. Gynaec. Br. Commonw.* **74,** 230.

LEDGER W.J. (1969) *Obstet. Gynec., N.Y.* **34,** 174.

MACPHERSON J. & WILSON J.K. (1956) *J. Obstet. Gynaec. Br. Commonw.* **63,** 321.

MOIR D.D. & WILLOCKS J. (1968) *Br. J. Anaesth.* **40,** 129.

O'DRISCOLL K., JACKSON R.J.A. & GALLAGHER J.T. (1969) *Br. med. J.* **ii,** 477.

RUBEN E.L. & FRANCIS H.H. (1967) *J. clin. Radiol.* **18,** 213.

SCHULMAN H. & LEDGER W.J. (1964) *Obstet. Gynec., N.Y.* **23,** 442.

TAYLOR G. (1971) *Br. med. J.* **i,** 101.

YATES M.J. (1969) *Proc. R. Soc. Med.* **62,** 183.

CHAPTER 13

THE NORMAL PUERPERIUM

The puerperium is the period of time during which the body tissues, especially the pelvic organs, are returning to their previous state. It is probable that some 6–8 weeks, and perhaps even more, elapse before this return to normal is complete, or as complete as it will ever become; during the first 2 weeks of this time the changes are rapid, and become slower thereafter.

THE PELVIC ORGANS

The principal change is in the uterus, which decreases in size rapidly. After delivery the uterine fundus is usually palpable in the region of the umbilicus. Ten to fourteen days later the fundus will disappear behind the symphysis pubis, and although the uterus has not yet returned to its normal size it will no longer be palpable per abdomen. This shrinkage is achieved by the general process of involution. The mechanism by which an organ weighing at the time of delivery near 1 kg shrinks down to one some 50–60 g in weight in a few weeks is that of autolysis. The excess protein of the uterine muscle and other cells is broken down and excreted in the urine or, to some extent, utilized by the body. The body is in negative nitrogen balance during this time, for more nitrogen is being excreted than is being taken in (see p. 132).

The cervix is very flaccid and curtain-like after delivery. Within a few days, however, it is beginning to return to its original form and consistency. The external os remains sufficiently dilated to permit a finger to be introduced into it for weeks or months—and in some cases permanently—but the internal os becomes closed to a finger during the second week of the puerperium.

The vagina almost always shows some evidence of parity. In the first few days of the puerperium the vaginal walls are smooth and soft, and slightly oedematous. The distention, which has resulted from labour, remains for a few days but the return to normal capacity is quite quick thereafter. Episiotomies or tears of the vagina and perineum heal well as a rule, provided adequate suturing has been undertaken. If infection arises, or haematoma formation, healing will be interfered with and some, or all, of the wound may break down. Even if this happens healing by granulation is usually so satisfactory that it is seldom possible a few weeks later to tell that any difficulty in healing occurred at all.

Within the endometrial cavity layers of decidua begin to be cast off. As a result of ischaemia, necrosis occurs in the decidual glands and stroma, sloughing takes place and the greater part of the decidua is lost in this way as lochial flow. The lochia consist of blood, leucocytes, shreds of disintegrating decidua and organisms. The uterine cavity, at least in its upper parts, probably remains sterile for a matter of hours after delivery, but gradually organisms spread upwards from the cervix to inhabit the superficial necrotic parts of the endometrium. In the great majority of cases this produces no symptoms whatever.

The lochial flow is initially dusky red in colour, although this colour fades after the first week or so; it is not uncommon, however, for the lochia to be a reddish colour or to be tinged red from time to time for 4–6 weeks after delivery.

The new endometrium grows from the basal areas of the decidua, which retain a blood supply and do not, therefore, become necrotic, as do the superficial parts. Most of the uterine cavity is covered by new endometrium within 3 weeks; in the area of the placental attachment, however, epithelialization takes longer, and may not be complete for 6–8 weeks. There is growth of new endometrium from the sides of the placental site beneath the layer of organized fibrin on the surface of the placental site. This layer is gradually lifted off its attachments and extruded as the new endometrium replaces it beneath.

The timing of the first menstrual period following delivery is very variable and probably depends on, more than anything, lactation. If the patient breast-feeds her baby it will probably be several months before menstruation becomes re-established; in general, menstruation will remain in abeyance whilst the baby is being suckled. The period may arrive before the cessation of breast-feeding, however; moreover, since ovulation will precede this first period in the majority of instances, it is possible for the patient to become pregnant before she menstruates following her last confinement.

THE BREASTS

The changes which occur in the breasts during pregnancy have been discussed in Chapter 9. Colostrum is secreted by the breasts during the latter part of pregnancy. This is a thin, slightly yellow, turbid fluid rich in protein and in fat. Examined under a microscope it is seen to contain colostrum corpuscles in a watery, fluid medium. These corpuscles contain many fat globules.

Lactation is initiated by the secretion of lactogenic hormone (or, as it is now called, somatomammotrophin), by the pituitary. This secretion is controlled via the hypothalmus, as is gonadal stimulation. There is one difference, however. Whereas the gonadotrophic hormones of the pituitary are released by hypothalamic stimulation, hypothalamic stimulation inhibits lactogenic hormone production. The hypothalamic control of lactation is probably modified in some way by the falling levels of progesterone and oestrogen after delivery, although the precise mechanism is not known.

Milk comes quickly into the breasts about the third to the fourth day to replace the colostrum; the composition of each is seen in Table 13.1.

Table 13.1. Percentage composition of colostrum and breast milk

	Protein	Fat	Carbo-hydrate	Water
Colostrum	8·6	2·3	3·2	85·6
Milk	1·25	3·5	7·5	87·0

About this time the breasts become engorged and appear tense and distended; they feel warm and may be tender when pressed to expel milk from the nipple.

Once the hormone changes referred to have initiated lactation its continuation is dependent mainly on continued and effective suckling. This effect is brought about by the initiation of nervous impulses from the nipple which 'trigger off' the release of oxytocin from the anterior pituitary; the oxytocin stimulation of the myo-epithelial fibres surrounding the small and large ducts in the breast eject the milk from the nipple. This mechanism is often called the milk 'let-down' or 'draught'. It was formerly thought that this mechanism indicated a period of intense milk secretion in the alveoli as a result of suckling. It is now clear that milk secretion is a continuous process unless halted by congestion associated with lack of suckling or emotional disturbances, etc.; the 'draught' is concerned with milk ejection from the alveoli into the duct system and from there out through the nipple. These mechanisms have been reviewed by Cowie & Folley (1961) and Benson & Fitzpatrick (1966).

OTHER SYSTEMS

During the first few days the bladder and urethra may show evidence of minor trauma which they sustained at delivery. There may be oedema and petechial haemorrhages, or even small ecchymoses. These changes are due to displacement or bruising of the bladder base and urethra, and do not usually remain in evidence for very long. The changes which have occurred in the urinary tract itself disappear in similar manner to other involutional changes. Within 2–3 weeks the hydro-ureter and calyceal dilatation of pregnancy is much less evident, although it is probable that complete return to normal does not occur for 6–8 weeks in all. If urinary tract radiographic studies are proposed it is usually wise to wait for this period of time before carrying them out to allow possible pregnancy changes completely to subside.

There is usually a distinct diuresis during the first day or so of the puerperium. The excess tissue fluid of pregnancy is quickly eliminated in this way.

In normal cases the temperature is little, if any, raised as a result of delivery. An occasional rise in temperature during the early puerperium is not uncommon and if this is concerned with infection, as is sometimes stated to be the case, this infection is difficult to detect. A sustained or a high single rise in temperature, however, should suggest infection and call for investigation.

There is a fall in the plasma volume during the puerperium. If blood loss has been normal it is probable that no significant anaemia will be evident during this time. The disappearance of the hydraemia of pregnancy will in itself tend to increase the haemoglobin reading.

MANAGEMENT

The medical and nursing care of the puerperium seeks to return the patient as quickly as possible to normal. Since most delivered patients are well, all that is generally required is to assist their full recovery by preventing complications.

Immediately following delivery the patient must remain in the delivery room for close observation until it is clear that all is well. The uterine fundus must be checked at frequent intervals to establish that it remains contracted; its height in the abdomen is important, too, since if this is seen to be rising this indicates that the uterus is filling with blood or is being displaced upwards by a pelvic swelling—a full bladder or a haematoma. Inspection of the vulval pads is necessary to establish the amount of external bleeding. The pulse rate, blood pressure and respiration are checked; the pulse especially being checked several times during the hour after the confinement. The patient should be washed and made comfortable. She may be given a drink of almost anything she fancies. If it is thought that the bladder is full she may be allowed to try to pass urine. If she is unable to do so she may try again a little later, but if again she is unsuccessful and a considerable volume of urine is thought to be in the bladder catheterization will be wise.

During the remainder of the patient's stay in hospital attention must be paid to the prevention of infection; the care of the breasts and the establishment and maintenance of lactation; the obtaining of a suitable amount of rest, exercise and sleep; the emotional state of the patient; involution of the pelvic organs and healing of incisions and many other matters.

Infection will be prevented by gentle and careful cleansing of the vulval tissue twice-daily at first, once-daily later and whenever the bowel has moved. During the first 24 hr the vulva should be gently cleansed by the midwife with chlorhexidene solution. Thereafter the patient may be allowed up for increasing amounts and may sit in a bath or take a shower on her second day. She may then undertake vulval cleansing herself once she has been suitably instructed in its principles. Pads must be changed frequently and these should be inspected to form an opinion as to the amount and nature of the lochial flow.

If there is a perineal wound, great gentleness will be necessary or cleansing will be painful or the suture line may be injured and healing delayed. Tender episiotomies and tears may be relieved by a heat lamp used several times daily for 10–20 min at a time.

Early rising has now, quite properly, become the rule, and its value in the prevention of thrombosis and embolism—together with its positive feeling of good health and return to normal in the mother—has been amply demonstrated. Many patients may be allowed out of bed 12–24 hr after the confinement, and certainly the day after it. There are exceptions, of course, but for normal patients this should be the general rule. As the days go by she should spend more time moving gently around the ward, increasing her ambulation time each day. It is sometimes, forgotten, however, that with frequent feeding, exercising, visiting and having her own meals a recently delivered patient may have a busy time and she requires some period of time each day when she can rest quietly alone on her bed. It is helpful if some of this rest is taken in the prone position, to promote anteversion of the uterus.

Adequate sleep at night is most important to a patient's full recovery. During the first few days after delivery sedatives may be required to ensure this. Sleeplessness is a most disturbing feature, indicating the possibility of a puerperal mental disorder.

Care of the breasts is important during this time, whether the patient is breast-feeding her baby or not. The breast must be kept well supported and both breast and nipple carefully cleansed. Gentle handling at all times is imperative, since injuries will predispose to breast infections.

Daily examinations of the abdomen are necessary to ensure, in general terms, the normal progress of involution. Precise measurement of the fundal height is not required, since this is often influenced by other factors like the amount of urine in the bladder or the quantity of faecal matter in the colon. By regular abdominal examination, however, the progress of involution can be assessed and other abdominal abnormalities, such as a grossly over-distended bladder, or a previously unsuspected ovarian cyst, may be detected.

Exercises form an important part of the patient's return to normal health during the puerperium. The instruction given by a physiotherapist in exercises for the abdominal muscles, perineal muscles and limbs can be most valuable in making more complete the return of these muscular tissues to normal and in the prevention of venous thrombosis.

Before discharge from hospital careful examination must be made to ensure that there is no abnormality present. Inspection of perineal injuries should be undertaken, careful abdominal examination carried out and, of course, routine pulse and blood pressure recordings made. It is often the custom for a vaginal examination to be performed before the patient is allowed home. It is doubtful if any but a very obvious fault can be felt at this time and the value of this examination is questioned. So often it leads to a diagnosis of 'bulky uterus' and ergometrine is prescribed, the need for and the value of which are very doubtful. Moreover, vaginal examination about 6 or 7 days after delivery can be painful to the patient, and if it is to be undertaken great gentleness must be exercised.

THE POSTNATAL VISIT

Some 6 weeks or so after delivery it is advisable to see the patient again to confirm that a return to good health has been made and to give her the opportunity to ask any questions which may arise. As practised, this visit often becomes more a matter of examination of the patient's pelvic organs than of the patient as a whole, which indicates that the emphasis is being misplaced.

The patient must be questioned about her recovery and any symptoms she may have. She must be asked about the progress of her baby. She may be given the opportunity to ask questions about anything which may be troubling her, about any problems which may have arisen with intercourse, about the advisability of further child-bearing and other matters of this kind.

General examination can be briefly undertaken and must include blood pressure, pulse and temperature recording and an examination of the urine. The pelvic organs can now be examined for satisfactory healing of any perineal laceration, the appearance of the cervix, the size and position of the uterus and any other abnormality there may be. This is a convenient time to take a cervical smear for exfoliative cytological study.

Two matters have received at this time more attention than they have probably deserved, to the detriment of others. These are a 'cervical erosion' and a retroverted uterus. The subject of 'erosion' is dealt with on pp. 582–3, but it may be said here that the complete return of the cervix to the prepregnant state is often incomplete by 6 weeks postpartum. Provided that the patient makes no complaint referable to it, such as vaginal discharge, it is to be expected that thorough examination of the cervix some weeks later will show that involution has continued and the cervix returned to normal. If the patient is seen 3 months later no fault may be evident. Even if a discharge is experienced it is probably too early to undertake cautery and it will probably be wise to give the patient general advice about vulval hygiene and to see her again a few weeks afterwards. At this time, if there is no improvement, treatment may be arranged along the lines laid down on p. 584.

Retroversion discovered at the 6 weeks' postnatal examination is seldom significant. The uterus occupies the retroverted position in many patients without causing any symptoms whatever. Again it becomes a matter of what symptoms, if any, are being experienced which might be attributable to this finding; if it seems possible that these symptoms are due to the position of the uterus further attention to it may be paid. This will be the exception, and not the rule.

Many patients will ask about contraceptive advice at this visit if they have not already been given it before discharge from hospital.

REFERENCES

Benson G.K. & Fitzpatrick R.J. (1966) In *Pituitary Gland*, Vol. 3 (edited by G.W. Harris & B.T. Donovan). London, Butterworths, p. 414.

Cowie A.T. & Folley S.J. (1961) In *Sex and Internal Secretions*, 3rd edn., Vol. 1 (edited by W.C. Young). Baltimore, Williams & Wilkins, p. 590.

CHAPTER 14

ABORTION, ECTOPIC PREGNANCY AND TROPHOBLASTIC GROWTHS

ABORTION

It can justifiably be claimed that abortion (termination of pregnancy before 28 weeks' gestation) is the greatest problem in gynaecology. One in every five to ten pregnancies (no one knows the precise figure) terminates in this way and abortion now represents the most common factor implicated in maternal mortality in the United Kingdom.

Abortions may be classified in a number of different ways, but the major one is *progressive*, according to the stage:

Threatened abortion
Inevitable abortion
Incomplete abortion
Complete abortion
Missed abortion

The last category is defined as a situation in which the foetus dies *in utero* before 28 weeks but is not expelled.

Abortion may also be classed as *septic* or *non-septic* and *spontaneous* or *induced*, the last category being either legal or criminal. Finally, abortion may be graded as *isolated* or *habitual (recurrent)*.

Causes of spontaneous abortion

It is helpful to think of the causes of abortion as being conceptual, maternal and undetermined or mutual factors.

Conceptual factors include the gross malformations, chromosomal abnormalities, abnormal implantation, hydatidiform degeneration, etc. *Maternal factors* include corpus luteum insufficiency, anomalies of Muellerian fusion, cervical incompetence, metabolic diseases and infections. *Mutual factors* include immunological causes.

Abnormal conceptuses

It has long been known that in addition to the occurrence of hydatidiform mole a high proportion of aborted foetuses were grossly abnormal (Mall 1917; Rock & Hertig 1942). The latter workers reported 47% abnormal foetuses in aborted pregnancies. More recent work has indicated that a high proportion of abortions are associated with fundamental abnormality of the chromosome constitution of the conceptus (Carr 1965; Geneva Conference 1966; Schlegel *et al.* 1966; Kerr & Rashad 1966; Smith *et al.* 1969). Not all chromosome aberrations of a particular type are lethal. For example, a few individuals with a 45/XO constitution survive, though the majority are aborted. The reason for this difference is not at present known.

Wide variations in the incidence of chromosome abnormalities have been reported by different workers. In a relatively large collected series of more than 450 *induced abortions* a 2% incidence of chromosome abnormality was detected, while in 19% of 788 *spontaneous abortions* such an anomaly was demonstrated (Geneva Conference 1966). These figures are almost certainly underestimates, as in many cases cultures of the conceptus fail to yield satisfactory cells for chromosome analysis; this appears to be due to difficulties in maintaining cellular growth from trophoblastic tissues (Smith et al. 1969). The chromosomal studies have yielded interesting information about the balance of the sexes in early pregnancy. There is a slight excess of XX over XY sex chromosome complement in abortuses of normal karyotype, spontaneous and induced; there is a more marked increase of XX over XY in trisomic abortuses and an overwhelming excess of XX complements in hydatidiform moles (Geneva Conference 1966).

One factor possibly relevant to the sex ratio male preponderance at birth is related to the fact that XXY sex chromosome complement (a form of sex chromosome trisomy) is apparently usually compatible with survival while its complementary opposite XO (sex chromosome monosomy) which would be expected to be present in an equal number of conceptuses is, as mentioned above, only rarely associated with survival to maturity. A new aspect of sex-related abortion is highlighted by the recent work of Taylor (1969). In a study of 54 pregnant schizophrenics he found that all 13 who had an attack of schizophrenia within a month of conception produced female children. When the attack occurred in the second or third month the males tended to be abnormal or stillborn. Taylor postulates that some chemical factor released into the blood at the time of the acute schizophrenic attack is toxic to male foetuses.

Chromosomal abnormalities are commoner in earlier pregnancy abortions, and particularly when there is an empty sac ('blighted ovum') or a grossly malformed embryo. The almost 10-fold higher incidence of chromosome abnormalities in pregnancies which abort spontaneously than in those which are deliberately terminated supports the view that most chromosomally abnormal embryos abort.

It seems probable on the available evidence that the commonest abnormality is the presence of an extra chromosome (47), probably representing trisomy,* usually involving Group D, E and G. This was observed in 41% of the collected series referred to. Next most frequent is a monosomy for Group C, probably representing XO, found in 21%. This means that

*Trisomy—the presence of an autosome in addition to the normal homologous pair in a diploid organism.

approximately 4% of abortuses probably have the XO constitution characteristic of Turner's syndrome. A little less common (17%) is triploidy.† Carr's (1965) study shows a significant increase in mean maternal age of the mothers of trisomic abortuses as compared to those with chromosomally normal abortuses. Studies with the sex-linked Xgᵃ blood group as a marker have shown that errors in the sex chromosome constitution of the conceptus may be due to factors arising in the paternal testis, maternal ovary or the early embryo (Race & Sanger 1969). Further data is needed to complete the picture but it can be said with certainty that chromosome abnormality is a major factor in abortion.

Abnormalities of implantation may cause abortion. In many cases the precise nature of the mal-implantation is not clear. Occasionally, with low implantation, abortion occurs in late second trimester to the accompaniment of haemorrhage and it becomes clear that the situation is one of placenta praevia. Placenta praevia usually presents in the third trimester, of course; in cases in which this diagnosis is ultimately made it is found that there has been a raised incidence of threatened abortion.

Endocrine deficiencies have been suggested as a cause of abortion (see recurrent abortion, p. 219). *Luteal phase deficiency* has been postulated as a particular type of hormone deficiency in which the preparation of the endometrium (or decidua) is inadequate for the receipt of the conceptus (see Jones 1968 for review). Success has been claimed for progestational therapy but the diagnosis between pregnancy and a delayed period is often open to doubt and the consequences of ill-timed progestational therapy may be an impaired chance of conception.

Uterine abnormalities may cause abortion but, mostly in the second trimester (see middle trimester abortions, p. 216). *Retroversion of the uterus* is a rare cause of abortion. This may come about in two ways. Firstly, the retroverted uterus in early pregnancy is more liable to be traumatized at intercourse, and this may very occasionally precipitate abortion. Secondly, at the end of the

†Triploidy—the presence of three haploid sets of chromosomes, usually 69 in man.

first or beginning of the second trimester the uterus may have difficulty in rising from the pelvis, particularly if adhesions are present. In these circumstances abortion may occur. It must be appreciated, however, that *abortion is very much the exception when pregnancy occurs in a retroverted gravid uterus.* Manipulations to attempt to correct the retroversion are more likely to cause abortion than if matters are left to nature. The only action I take on discovering a retroversion in early pregnancy is to advise abstention from intercourse until the uterus has risen into the abdomen.

Maternal diseases of all sorts have been blamed for abortion in the past but while a woman 'in extremis' from any condition may abort, in these circumstances the major concern is for the mother's survival. The number of diseases which specifically predispose to abortion without the mother herself being seriously ill is, in fact, very small. Renal and hypertensive disease are rare causes of abortion.

Any infective illness accompanied by high pyrexia may be held responsible for the occurrence of abortion. Apparently, the overwhelming toxaemia and high temperature lead to uterine contractibility being stimulated. This is unlikely to happen unless the infective process is overwhelming, however, and the temperature elevation of a very high order.

There are other infective conditions in which the relationship is more specific, however, when the infective agent actually affects the conceptus. *Syphilis* is the classic example of a maternal infection which may spread across the placenta to the foetus and cause intra-uterine death and abortion. It is, however, a very rare cause today in Europe. *Brucella abortus* is the cause of abortion in animals. There is no doubt that *Brucella abortus* infection also occurs in humans. Whether it causes abortion in humans has been debated, but de Freitas (1969) concludes from a personal study and review of the published evidence that it may do so *if there is an overwhelming infection in early pregnancy.* It is, however, certainly not a common cause.

Rubella, vaccinia, acute anterior poliomyelitis, toxoplasmosis, cytomegalic inclusion body disease all possibly cause occasional abortions. *Tubercu-*

losis is also a factor for, of the few intra-uterine pregnancies which occur after treatment of endometrial tuberculosis, a very high proportion end in abortion. *South American trypanosomiasis* (Chagas' disease) and *malaria* are other uncommon causes which may operate in parts of the world where these diseases are endemic. Infection with *Listeria monocytogenes* is also probably an aetiological factor. Rappaport *et al.* (1960) found the organism in the vagina of 25 out of 35 women in Israel with a history of repeated abortion. Macnaughton (1962) reported a negative study on 78 women with threatened or incomplete abortion (not recurrent cases) in Aberdeen. Barber & Okubadejo (1965) reviewed the evidence and concluded that it may be a significant cause of recurrent abortion. They consider it likely that the diagnosis is often missed, the organism being discounted as a contaminant 'diphtheroid' or thought to be a streptococcus, or even mistaken for a Gram-negative bacillus, as it is easily discoloured. It may be harboured for long periods in the genital tract of otherwise healthy women. The diagnosis is of more than academic importance, as benzyl penicillin and demethylchlortetracycline are active against it.

Poisons may sometimes be responsible for abortion, but the dosages of such reputed abortifacients as *lead* and *quinine* which will cause abortion approximate perilously to the lethal dose. *Cytotoxic drugs,* in particular the folic-acid antagonist methotrexate will, of course, cause abortion. *Endocrine and metabolic diseases,* especially *diabetes* and *disorders* of the *thyroid gland,* have been said to predispose to abortion, but as with so many other of the alleged causes, consistent statistical conclusions are not available.

Dietetic factors have long been listed as causes of abortion, but the evidence is generally inconclusive as to which substances are specifically involved. Dietary vitamin supplements of many types have been suggested. Hibbard (1964) drew attention specifically to *folic-acid deficiency* in women who aborted, and the evidence suggesting that this vitamin is important is stronger than for any other.

Possible *immunological causes of abortion* have received attention recently as a consequence of work on the mechanisms whereby the immuno-logic rejection process towards tissue of a different antigenic constitution from the host is overcome in normal pregnancy (see Kerr 1968 for review). The best known and most clearly defined example of pathological maternofoetal immunologic antagonism is, of course, rhesus iso-immunization. As Medawar (1960) put it, this represents the 'immunological repudiation by the mother of her unborn child'. The haemolytic process involved in rhesus disease rarely causes serious foetal damage till the last trimester but when the antibody titre is very high from the start of pregnancy the baby may die *in utero* or become hydropic and be expelled from the uterus during the second trimester. In these circumstances, of course, it constitutes an abortion, but numerically this represents only a very small proportion of all abortions. ABO incompatibility plays some part in abortion (Wren & Vos 1961) and some of the minor blood group systems are probably also involved (Levine & Koch 1954). There is also evidence of increased early pregnancy wastage in the presence of maternal leucocyte antibodies (Jensen 1960; Pachi & Angeloni 1963).

Jackson *et al.* (1969) have recently put forward an interesting postulate which involves an immunological explanation for the secondary sex ratio in man which leads to the preferential birth of males. Their evidence is related to the sex-linked Xg^a blood group. They conclude that where Xg^a incompatibility exists between the mother and female foetuses there is a par-ticularly high predominance of male births. This is especially evident after the birth of the first, presumably sensitizing, daughter. They suggest that the difference in ratios may be brought about by an early rejection of Xg^a-incompatible female embryos.

These examples all concern humoral immune factors. *May cellular factors be involved?* There is no clear answer to this, but studies by Bardawil and his colleagues (Bardawil *et al.* 1962; Mitchell & Bardawil 1966) suggest that there may be an increased tendency to abortion in women who tend vigorously to reject skin grafts from their husbands. Studies with mixed lymphocyte culture techniques may also give information

on this problem (Kerr 1968). There is in normal pregnancy a specific lack of responsiveness in the maternal lymphocytes with respect to the paternal cells (Lewis *et al.* 1966c). It is possible that in certain circumstances maternal im-munologically competent cells (lymphocytes) may invade the foetal system, colonize it and cause graft-versus-host reaction and foetal death. Such invasion may be postulated if in a phenotypic male foetus XX lymphocytes are cultured in addition to the expected XY cells. Taylor & Polani (1965) record such a case, but it appears that it is a rare happening. The fact that XX, presumed maternal cells, have been found in an XY male foetus which was athymic (Kadowaki *et al.* 1965) raises the possibility that the presence of a foetal thymus may be important in preserving foetal integrity while growing in the foreign, maternal (XX) environment.

Induced abortion

Induced abortion may be legal or illegal. The precise legal situation is at present widely variable throughout the world and changing continuously. Some countries such as the United Kingdom have changed to a wider legality, while others such as Rumania, having found problems with such a policy, have moved in the opposite direction. Illegal abortion may some-times carry the capital penalty even in states where legal indications for abortion are relatively lax, as in Colorado (Droegemueller *et al.* 1969).

In the United Kingdom a revised Abortion Law was introduced in 1968 which placed on the statute what was already accepted as case-law, namely that abortion could be performed pro-vided that two doctors were, in 'good faith', persuaded that it was necessary because of risk to the life or health of the mother. In addition, it was specified that abortion could legally be performed if there was reason to suspect an abnormally high risk that the child be malformed. This situation, though unsupported by any case-law, had also been widely accepted by many in the profession as ethical prior to the Act. It was also stated that abortion could be done for the sake of the health of existing children and that social factors could be taken into account in assessing risk to health. These sections are open to wide variability in interpretation and a direct consequence was a great discrepancy in the frequency with which abortion was induced, allegedly under the Act, by different groups of doctors in different parts of the country.

The problems of legal and illegal induced abortions are similar. In large series, it should be the case that the safety of legal as opposed to illegal abortion is much greater. This is almost certainly so if the results of legal abortions carried out by trained gynaecologists in major hospitals are compared with illegal abortions performed by non-medical persons.

The abortion performed by the ill-qualified in ill-equipped premises is dangerous in two particular ways: (a) traumatic and (b) infective, in addition to the risk of haemorrhage.

(a) Traumatic

Uterine damage may lead to haemorrhage, shock and even death. Cervical tears or corporeal rupture may occur. Bladder, ureters and bowel may all be damaged and without prompt surgical intervention death may follow. Renal damage may ensue in cases not immediately fatal, especially if there is also an infective element (see abortion kidney, p. 224).

(b) Infective

Postabortal sepsis is always a risk no matter the circumstances in which abortion is performed. The further removed the circumstances are from perfect, the greater the risk. In this situation endotoxic bacteraemic shock is particularly liable to develop, constituting a grave, and often fatal, risk (see septic abortion, p. 222).

These are the immediate dangers. The long-term complications are incalculable, but relate to the same two basic factors. Damage done to the uterus—knowingly or unknowingly—at the time of induction of abortion may lead to cervical incompetence or uterine rupture in subsequent pregnancies. If there has been infection, the tubes may be blocked or adhesions around the fimbrial end interfere with the normal mechanisms

of ovum transportation, leading to infertility or tubal pregnancy when a baby is subsequently desired.

The specific *medical indications* for termination of pregnancy are now very few. In the period 1953–64 Rovinsky & Gusberg (1967) found a stable incidence of 12 per 10,000 deliveries on medical grounds and 18 per 10,000 for 'genetic' reasons (almost all the latter were for maternal rubella). The common medical indications were malignancy, cardiac disease, renal disease, and pulmonary and gastrointestinal disease, in that order of frequency. Psychiatric indications, however, rose from 24 to 56 per 10,000 deliveries in the same period of time.

TECHNIQUES OF ABORTION

The non-medical criminal abortionists have many weird methods. In the latest *Report on Confidential Enquiries into Maternal Deaths in England and Wales* (1969) in addition to instrumental techniques reference is made to the use of slippery elm, soapy water, antiseptic agents, quinine, penny royal, apiol, 'female capsules' and even the injection of parsley. These relate only to women who have died; the total range is almost certainly greater. The following remarks refer only to techniques used by the medical profession.

The most widely used medical methods are *vaginal evacuation by curette suction and sponge or ovum forceps* and *abdominal hysterotomy*. Vaginal evacuation can be an extremely hazardous procedure beyond the first 10 weeks of pregnancy. The further advanced pregnancy is, the greater the risk of making the cervix incompetent or perforating the fundus. Oxytocic preparations are, of course, administered in association with such operations. General anaesthesia is commonly employed and blood should always be available for transfusion. It may prove difficult to be certain that uterine evacuation has been complete. In these circumstances it is rash to persevere with more vigorous use of the curette. The wise course is to desist and bring the patient back to theatre for repeat curettage in a few days' time when a degree of involution has taken place.

In recent years a minor variation which has emanated from Communist countries, has been the use of the suction curette or vacuum aspirator (see Vladov *et al.* 1965; Penetz *et al.* 1967). This is little more than the old-fashioned flushing-type of curette with the machinery in reverse. It may, however, reduce the risk of foetal red blood cells entering the maternal circulation and causing iso-immunization. Matthews & Matthews (1969) showed that in procured as opposed to spontaneous abortions the incidence of transplacental haemorrhage was 25% compared with 6%. Barron (1969) reported that with a suction evacuation technique the risk of such haemorrhage is no greater than with spontaneous abortion.

If the uterus is too large for safe vaginal evacuation, *abdominal hysterotomy* is the safer procedure. If there is the slightest doubt in the operator's mind as to which method he should use, the abdominal approach should be chosen. A vertical upper segment or transverse lower segment incision may be used. If tubal ligation is indicated, as it usually will be if there are sound medical indications, the abdominal route is the one of choice, regardless of maturity. In these circumstances there is much to be said for considering the alternative of hysterectomy to the combined procedure of hysterotomy and tubal ligation. Recent claims that the mortality of combined abortion and sterilisation is greater than that for abortion alone, ignore the fact that two objectives are achieved. The alternative would be two separate operations almost certainly carrying a greater combined risk.

Patients who have had tubal ligation performed seem to have a particular tendency to menstrual symptomatology and, of course, malignancy may develop (Williams 1969). Intelligent patients will accept the explanation that no loss of hormonal activity or sexual responsiveness is involved when hysterectomy is done with conservation of the ovaries. It should also be explained that because of the elimination of the uterine cancer risk and the cessation of the menstrual blood loss, the outlook for future physical health is much better.

Another technique which has been advocated in some centres for securing interruption of pregnancy involves the *introduction of hypertonic solutions to the amniotic cavity* by the transabdominal route (see Schiffer 1969 for review). This was a by-product of the abortion laws of Scandinavia and Japan which presented gynaecologists with a large number of terminations to perform. Saline (20–33%) and glucose (50%) have been the solutions most widely employed. The mechanism of action is unknown. The idea that the solution interfered with the 'progesterone block' inactivation of the gravid myometrium has not been substantiated by critical investigation (Short *et al.* 1965). A considerable number of serious complications sometimes leading to maternal death have been described with the method. These have been grouped as due to (a) technical failures—infection or intravascular injection of the hypertonic solution; (b) aggravation of a general condition already present; (c) postpartum haemorrhage or uterine trauma; and (d) unexplained vascular collapse. This last is the most worrying group, and it may be that some of these cases are related to category (a) with unrecognized intravascular injection. This is a risk which is greater in early pregnancy, and for this reason it is advocated that the method should be avoided before 15 weeks. Confident aspiration of amniotic fluid is necessary before injection may safely be commenced. The infection risk is particularly related to the use of dextrose in the presence of a dead foetus. The combination leads to an ideal situation for pathogenic bacteria to multiply.

Wagatsuma (1965) reported Japanese experience in an American journal. He felt that due to the language barrier the English-speaking medical world was going through a phase unaware that the Japanese had had the same experience a couple of decades earlier. Japanese experience culminated in the abandonment of the method. He referred to complications in 3,148 of 6,611 pregnancies terminated by this technique. Twelve maternal deaths were reported in 1950. These horrifying figures must be considered in the light of the appalling social chaos of post-war Japan. None the less, reports such as this have ensured that the technique has not been generally adopted in this country (see also prostaglandins, p. 430).

Clinical types of abortion

THREATENED ABORTION

Threatened abortion is said to occur when a woman with an intra-uterine pregnancy experiences bleeding from the uterus prior to 28 weeks' gestation but the cervix is not dilated. This definition excludes bleeding from the lower genital tract, but it is important, as with antepartum haemorrhage, not to fall into the trap of accepting an obvious minor extra-uterine lesion as the cause of haemorrhage which has really emanated from the placental site. Prior to 12 weeks, when the decidua capsularis fuses with the decidua vera, the bleeding may occur from the decidual space. Placental bleeding is interpreted as a manifestation of some disruption of the placental attachment. The bleeding is not usually severe; if it is enough to warrant transfusion the pregnancy rarely proceeds. Severe haemorrhage may occur in relation to a low-lying placenta towards the end of the second trimester. The blood is at first bright red but later, when the placental bleeding has ceased, it comes from the vagina a brown colour. Pain is not a feature, though there may be some backache. If regular painful uterine contractions occur it must be suspected that the process is proceeding to the next stage—inevitable abortion—characterized by cervical dilatation.

Threatened abortion may proceed also to a *missed abortion*, when the foetus dies and uterine enlargement fails to progress. Confirmation may be obtained by a fall in the value of chorionic gonadotrophin excretion to non-pregnant levels or, beyond 12 or 14 weeks, failure to detect the foetal heart by means of a simple type of ultrasonoscope utilizing the Doppler effect. This can be defined as the 'apparent change of frequency of sound waves depending on the relative velocity of the source to that of the observer' (Brown & Robertson 1968). With suitable transducers the effect of pulsation in a vessel—foetal or maternal—is reproduced as a sound coinciding with the pulsation. It is not the actual sounds of the pulsation.

Management of threatened abortion is extremely difficult. In few situations in modern obstetrics is the doctor in such a state of therapeutic impotence. There is little else but rest to be offered. In a patient who is bleeding considerably per vaginam, to rest is, of course, merely common sense, and the patient would apply this unguided. If bleeding is persistent and severe in early pregnancy hydatidiform mole must be suspected, and all steps taken to exclude the possibility. The cervix should be inspected when the losses are recurrent, as a cervical lesion may be the explanation. The question of whether or not a vaginal examination should be done as a routine in threatened abortion is a matter of debate. Strictly, the diagnosis cannot be substantiated without a vaginal examination, and a gentle examination by a skilled individual should carry no significant risk of precipitating abortion. There are, however, circumstances when a very nervous patient may be acutely anxious lest vaginal examination should lead to abortion, and in these circumstances it may be prudent to defer examination until bleeding has ceased. This is designed more to protect the doctor's standing with his patient, however, than to preserve the pregnancy.

Mild sedatives, usually barbiturates, may be prescribed; they serve to make the resting more acceptable to a naturally active individual. Arrangement for grouping and cross-matching of blood should, of course, be made as appropriate. If there is only slight 'spotting', however, it is debatable whether rest has any merit. Avoidance of intercourse should be insisted upon because, quite apart from the question of a traumatic influence on the cervix, coitus stimulates uterine contractibility.

Hormone assessments on blood and urine by biological, biochemical and immunological techniques, together with assessment of hormonal status by interpretation of biological parameters such as cervical mucus and vaginal cytology, have been widely used in relation to abortion, and particularly threatened abortion. However, there is little evidence that this approach does more than reveal changes which are a consequence of the disturbance of the pregnancy, and with a few exceptions they contribute little towards rational management except when they point to the occurrence of foetal death.

When potent oral progestogen preparations became widely available, there was much enthusiasm for the use in cases of threatened abortion. This, however, was unsupported by careful, controlled trials. Such trials are particularly difficult to design for threatened abortion, which is not strictly a diagnosis but merely a term for a group of cases in which vaginal bleeding has occurred at a particular stage of pregnancy, with a particular state of the cervix. The present tendency, following upon Shearman & Garrett's (1963) controlled trial which failed to show any benefit from progestogens in recurrent abortion, is to be extremely sceptical about their value in threatened abortion. There is also a certain amount of separate evidence that threatened abortions are unresponsive to progestational agents. Overstreet (1964) records a basic 25–30% chance of threatened abortion proceeding to abortion. He observed that progestogen therapy was followed by up to 17–70% abortions in different series, and concluded that there was no evidence that it improved the chances for the pregnancy. His assessment was that, on the evidence available, it might be the case that progestogen therapy actually made the prospects worse. One added difficulty is that if the diagnosis is incorrect and the situation is actually one of missed abortion, the pregnancy may be needlessly prolonged (Cox *et al.* 1964).

Women who have threatened abortions often worry lest the pregnancy should continue and result in delivery of an abnormal child at term. They should be reassured that if the foetus is seriously abnormal pregnancy will be unlikely to continue.

INEVITABLE ABORTION

The borderline between threatened and inevitable abortion is regarded as having been crossed when cervical dilatation has developed. Pain is usually a feature. It follows that inevitable abortion presents with vaginal bleeding and pain, and on examination, in addition to the usual signs of pregnancy, it is found that the cervix is open (or opening) with products of conception possibly beginning to protrude. If the conceptus is held for any length of time in a dilated cervix,

a degree of shock out of proportion to the blood loss may develop.

Apart from necessary general measures to deal with haemorrhage and shock, the aim of treatment is to secure evacuation of the uterus as rapidly as possible. Very occasionally, especially in the second trimester, this proceeds spontaneously as a miniature labour and no action is indicated. Usually it is wise, if not absolutely necessary, to accelerate the process and the method of doing this will depend on the duration of the pregnancy. In the first trimester an injection of ergometrine malleate 0·5 mg and oxytocin 5 units intramuscularly together with 150 mg of pethidine or 15 mg of morphia is nearly always followed by control of the blood loss, and frequently by the passing of the bulk of the conceptus. As the conceptus is rarely aborted complete at this stage curettage should be performed. This can usually be delayed until the patient's general condition has been restored by transfusion, etc., further oxytocin being given as necessary. An old-fashioned type of flushing curette (used without the flushing attachment) suffices for the purpose.

If when first seen the patient is shocked and products of conception are in the cervical canal, a dramatic improvement can often be obtained by immediately removing them either by digital enucleation or under direct vision with the aid of ovum or sponge forceps. In the second trimester it is not appropriate to give ergometrine, as it may cause the cervix to clamp down on the sizeable foetus, with possible uterine damage. Rather, an oxytocin infusion is to be preferred, combined of course with morphia or pethidine as necessary. At this stage of pregnancy manual removal of the placenta may be needed but if it is expelled spontaneously and appears complete there should be no need for uterine exploration subsequently.

If blood loss and shock are severe it is occasionally necessary to utilize the service of what in the United Kingdom is known as the 'Obstetric Flying Squad', which is a resuscitation team based on a hospital and equipped to deal with acute emergencies occurring in the home when it is felt that the ambulance journey to hospital might have a seriously deleterious effect upon the patient's general condition.

INCOMPLETE ABORTION

It is often the case, particularly in the first trimester, that part of the conceptus is expelled from the uterus but that some chorionic tissue is retained. Initially, chorionic villous tissue encircles the conceptus and only after 3 months is there a discrete placenta. It is therefore not surprising that the normal placental separation mechanisms do not function effectively. The retained material is liable to cause bleeding and may prove a focus for infection. Occasionally, a placental polyp may form.

The history may or may not be a clear one of abortion. If there is such a history, in the incomplete case it is usually recorded that after passage of products of conception there is continued bleeding or blood-stained discharge, and possibly some colicky hypogastric pain. On examination the cervix is usually dilated and portions of tissue may be felt through the os. If only small fragments of material are retained the cervix may feel closed or only patulous (i.e. it tends to open on digital pressure). In cases where there has been no firm diagnosis of abortion the story is usually one of some disturbance of the menstrual cycle followed by a heavy and prolonged loss associated with some pain.

Once the diagnosis has been made surgical evacuation with curette and sponge or ovum forceps should be arranged. Bleeding should be controlled with oxytocics (see inevitable abortion, p. 214) and blood loss made good. If there is sepsis it is usually wise to delay any surgical interference until antibiotic cover has become effective (see septic abortion, p. 222).

MISSED ABORTION

Occasionally, when the foetus dies before the twenty-eighth week the uterus fails to expel it. This constitutes a missed abortion. When the dead conceptus is surrounded *in utero* by layers of blood-clot covering the chorion, the term *carneous* (or *fleshy*) *mole* is sometimes used. The death may have been preceded by vaginal bleeding (threatened abortion). The symptoms and signs of pregnancy regress and uterine enlargement ceases. Ultimately with resorption of liquor the uterine size diminishes. A brown vaginal discharge may occur. Foetal movements, if they have been felt, cease and the foetal heart, if it has been audible, is no longer to be heard. Chorionic gonadotrophin excretion levels revert to non-pregnant levels. Radiological examination, if the pregnancy has proceeded to over 16 weeks before foetal death, may reveal a collapsed foetal skeleton with all the other radiological signs of intra-uterine death.

The problems associated with the condition are complex. Not least is the psychological one. The mother eventually comes to realize that she has a dead child in her womb; she may develop a sense of revulsion and demand that it be removed. However, the great physical problem is that of sepsis. A mass of dead tissue is being incubated at body temperature; any introduction of pathogenic bacteria may lead to disastrous infection. This, however, is only likely to occur if interference is carried out with a view to encouraging uterine evacuation. The third complication which may occur is disturbance of the blood coagulation mechanism. This is rarely observed if the foetal retention is for less than a month, and usually the dead foetus is expelled after about 21 days. Even if the foetus is retained over a month from death, only one in three or four women develop the coagulation disorder (Hardisty & Ingram 1965) and many of these will have no clinical manifestations of it. The mechanism is not certain, but it has been presumed that in common with the coagulation failure found in association with abruptio placentae, it is related to entry of thromboplastins into the circulation. These may come from the degenerating placenta or the resorbed amniotic fluid (Hodgkinson *et al.* 1964).

It is impossible to lay down rules for the management of this sad situation, a complex mixture of psychological and physical problems. Provided the psychological situation does not demand immediate action it is probably wise to pursue a policy of non-intervention initially, and nature will usually solve the problem. If delivery has not occurred 4 weeks after the estimated time of foetal death then it is wise to commence checks on the coagulation mechanism. A common policy is to initiate procedures to encourage the uterus to empty itself about this time, and it is widely agreed that the most appropriate method is by intravenous oxytocin infusion, increasing the concentration until a response is obtained if necessary to as much as 200 units/l (Loudon 1959). Theoretically, this may carry some risk of increasing the tendency to coagulation disturbance if such exists; the uterine contractions induced by the oxytocin may tend to cause more thromboplastins from the dead conceptus to be forced into the maternal circulation.

Even if coagulation failure is demonstrated there is no cause for undue alarm; even with total absence of fibrinogen, haemorrhage may not be a feature. A good case can be made for continuing a policy of non-intervention indefinitely. These comments refer to missed abortion when the uterus is more than 10 weeks' size. If the uterus is smaller than this, simple vaginal evacuation can be carried out with safety as soon as the diagnosis is established.

MIDDLE TRIMESTER ABORTIONS

Most abortions occur in early pregnancy; often so early that the diagnosis is uncertain. Assessment and determination of aetiological factors is difficult. With the smaller number of abortions which occur in the second trimester, the situation is very different. The diagnosis is virtually always certain; the process is much more like a miniature labour and can be analysed to give a good idea of the mechanism involved. Factors of accommodation become particularly important at this time. The uterus in the first trimester enlarges under hormonal influence at a rate greater than the growth of the conceptus. Then the decidual space is occluded and after this the important mechanism is uterine stretching in response to conceptual growth.

The commonest accommodation problems relate to abnormalities of the uterus—*incompetence of the cervix* and *anomalies of Muellerian fusion*. Some also regard uterine hypoplasia as a factor, but the evidence on this is not convincing.

Cervical incompetence has come to be generally accepted as a factor in abortion only in the last 15 years, although many individual gynaecologists were aware of its occurrence previously (e.g. Palmer & Lacomme 1948). General appreciation of its occurrence and the prospect of surgical connection is due to the writings of Lash & Lash (1950), Shirodkar (1953) and McDonald (1957). Since then many gynaecologists have described experience with slightly different techniques. Results are hard to evaluate, as in some series the diagnosis of cervical incompetence has clearly been accepted somewhat uncritically. It is, however, beyond doubt a clinical and pathological entity for which effective treatment can be given.

The conceptus is normally retained in the uterus by a combination of hormonal and mechanical factors. One of these which operates from about the third month onwards is the constrictive influence of the circumferential fibromuscular tissue at the level of the internal os. Some authorities believe that it is not strictly the cervix which is involved and refer to 'incompetent isthmus' or 'incompetent lower segment'. If competence is lacking, the membranes are liable to herniate through the cervix. The first intimation is usually unexpected rupture of the membranes. This is soon followed by a relatively painless abortion or premature labour.

The condition may be congenital, but is usually acquired. Its production is frequently iatrogenic—by excessive gynaecological dilatation of the cervix. The circumstance in which this is done with greatest zeal is when it has the object of relieving spasmodic dysmenorrhoea. Fortunately, oestrogen–progestogen preparations now provide effective relief from dysmenorrhoea. Whatever the concern may be about their side-effects and adverse reactions when used as contraceptives, they are certainly far safer than surgery in the treatment of this condition. It can be hoped that troublesome cervical incompetence will become much less frequent as cervical dilatation for dysmenorrhoea passes from active practice. Other cervical procedures such as amputation and cone biopsy may also have the same consequence. Lacerations produced at the time of operative obstetric deliveries performed when dilatation has been incomplete may also lead to incompetence.

The classical presentation in the middle trimester of pregnancy with sudden membrane rupture and relatively painless abortion has been described. Often the presentation is atypical and it is impossible to be certain that the abortion was due to cervical incompetence. A variety of procedures can be adopted in the non-pregnant to try to confirm or refute the suspicion. Simple bimanual examination may reveal a cervix that is gaping up to internal os level and obviously incompetent. Rubovitz *et al.* (1953) described assessing the internal os competence by attempts to pass Hegar's dilators from large size downwards. If a dilator of 6–8 mm diameter goes easily through then the cervix is almost certainly incompetent. An alternative method is to fill the balloon of a Foley-type catheter placed in the uterus and assess the traction required to pull it out. Probably most helpful is to do a premenstrual hysterogram with a Leech-Wilkinson type are of cannula [Figs. 14(a) and (b)]. The films

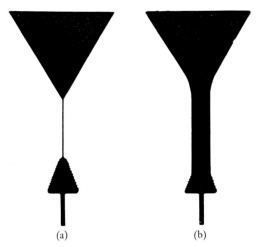

(a)   (b)

Fig. 14.1. Diagrammatic representation of the shadow obtained on hysterography in the premenstrual phase using a Leech-Wilkinson cannula (a) with a normally competent cervix, and (b) with an incompetent cervix showing the classic funnelling.

should be taken in the anteroposterior projection with the cervix pulled downwards so that the uterine body is brought into the axial position. In these circumstances the uterine cavity filled with medium shows as a triangle usually separated from the tip of the cannula by a 2–4 cm gap in which no medium is visible, or merely a tiny

threadlike shadow representing the track of the canal. If the cervix is incompetent a wider track of medium is seen running right down to the cannula from the body shadow, giving a classical 'funnel' outline. It must be remembered that *this finding is only of significance in the premenstrual phase*. Under the influence of progesterone in the second half of the menstrual cycle the internal os becomes tight; earlier in the cycle a normal cervix may give this type of appearance.

Different methods of operative treatment have been advocated but all have the aim of reinforcing the constrictive action of the cervix. Lash & Lash (1950) advocated operation between pregnancies. Shirodkar (1953), on the other hand, operated mainly during pregnancy, burying a strip of unabsorbable material in the substance of the cervix. Many different materials and variations in technique have been used. It is usually considered advisable to dissect the bladder upwards and place the stitch (or Dacron tape or other material) as close to the level of the internal os as possible. Some have claimed success, however, from a simple purse-string type of suture merely at external os level (e.g. Marshall & Evans 1967). The optimum time for operation is usually regarded as the beginning of the second trimester. Just occasionally, however, the incompetence mechanism operates earlier, and my current practice is to operate at 8–10 weeks. Where there is doubt about the diagnosis some obstetricians defer operation and inspect the cervix frequently throughout pregnancy. If the cervix shows signs of dilating or the membranes begin to bulge, operation is performed immediately. If the membranes herniate beyond the cervix into the vagina, hope of reduction and successful suturing is minimal.

The overall success rate in carrying pregnancy to maturity after this type of procedure is of the order of 50–80%, but it is unwise to read too much into the figures. When the diagnosis rate is high it is possible that unnecessary operations are being done. When the diagnosis rate is low the percentile results of treatment are usually worse, but very probably only cases really needing treatment are included. Where the cervix is seriously incompetent it is not to be expected that surgery would give 100% functional result. Some authorities discount a high incidence as *necessarily* a manifestation of over-diagnosis, and an acceptable figure of one case in 3,000 deliveries has been quoted (Greenhill 1966). This attitude fails to allow for the fact that it is the type of situation where the sins of the father are visited upon the succeeding generation. I know a gynaecologist who treated spasmodic dysmenorrhoea by *incision* of the internal cervical os. I have no doubt that his local successors in obstetric practice have a very high in-

uterine contractions occur, immediate action should be taken, otherwise severe injuries to the uterus may develop.

Anomalies of Muellerian fusion present a much more difficult problem. Failure of junction of the lower parts of the Muellerian ducts or of disappearance of the septum after fusion, may be of any degree (Fig. 14.2). There may be a completely double uterus (uterus didelphys) or there may merely be a trivial degree of persistence of a septum at the uterine fundus (uterus subseptus). Elaborate classifications with classical

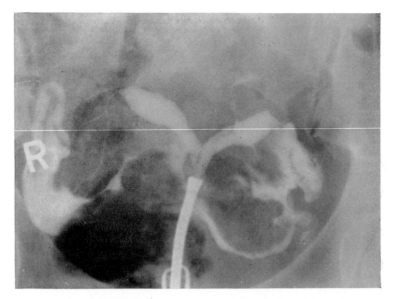

Fig. 14.2. Hysterogram in a case of imperfect fusion [compare with Fig. 1.9(b) and (c), p. 8].

cidence of true cervical incompetence to contend with!

If the suture is successful the question arises as to the course to follow to effect delivery. Many remove the suture at about 38 weeks and await the onset of labour. A good test of whether or not the suture has been functional is provided by whether labour ensues rapidly. There is often much to be said for the alternative of performing elective Caesarean section, leaving the suture *in situ* (Tacchi & Snaith 1962). It is very important to appreciate that *if at any time after insertion of the suture rupture of the membranes or expulsive*

terminologies have been invented but serve to confuse rather than clarify. A simple description in basic English or a diagram of each abnormality is preferable. If the very minor degrees are excluded the overall incidence of this type of abnormality is probably of the order of 3 or 4%.

The abortions which occur due to Muellerian fusion anomalies have no *specific* diagnostic features. They tend to occur beyond the first trimester; successive pregnancies tend to be carried longer; if a pregnancy is carried to the last trimester abnormal lie or presentation is common and there may be third stage complications. The abnormality may be discovered at the time of evacuation of an incomplete abortion or a retained placenta. It is, however, extremely difficult to be certain when removing a placenta with cornual attachment, which naturally causes a degree of sacculation, whether the cavity is truly abnormal. In cases of doubt postpartum hysterography will resolve the problem. It is important to appreciate that the gross degrees of duplication may be overlooked clinically. Most experienced gynaecologists have encountered patients with duplication of uterus, cervix and vagina in whom the anomaly had been missed despite full examination and even operation.

There are no simple rules for management of this type of lesion. The tendency is for successive pregnancies to be carried further and, if perseverance is adequate, a live child is eventually achieved. Little can be done to assist this other than prescribing rest. The whole process can prove a severe psychological strain even to women with the most resilient of personalities. Nevertheless a policy of conservative expectancy should not lightly be abandoned for there are major difficulties associated with the alternative of active surgical intervention. If, however, a patient has had three or more pregnancies without achieving a live child utriculoplasty (metroplasty or 'Strassman' operation, described by Paul Strassman 1907) is worth considering. This involves an incision into the uterus with reconstitution in such a way that the two cavities are unified. Unfortunately, it is not always possible to end up with a single 'good as new' cavity; the result of the operation may be anatomically worse than the original situation. Related to this problem is the paradox that the grossest degrees of Muellerian fusion anomalies seem less prone to be associated with clinical trouble, while with very minor degrees the surgeon cannot hope to improve on nature. The difficult clinical problem is to decide which cases would be likely to be improved by surgery. It must also be taken into consideration that the seriously scarred uterus after surgery carries with it a significant risk of rupture in a subsequent pregnancy. Elective Caesarean section late in a subsequent pregnancy is appropriate. Erwin Strassman (1966), a

descendant of the originator, reviewed 263 women who had the operation performed; 177 became pregnant subsequently and 86·4% of those pregnancies on which data were available resulted in the birth of viable children.

Uterine over-distension may also lead to late abortion in cases of *multiple pregnancy* and/or *hydramnios*. Multiple pregnancy of a high order seems likely to be an increasingly common hazard until improved methods of controlling gonadotrophin therapy for ovulation failure are achieved. *Fibroids* may also be regarded as a cause of abortion in this category.

RECURRENT OR HABITUAL ABORTION

Recurrent (or habitual) abortion is usually defined as a sequence of three or more consecutive abortions, but some writers take two or more as a standard. It usually presents in patients greatly desiring children. The challenge to the doctor is to discover the cause and correct it. This is rarely a simple matter, except in the case of middle trimester abortions referred to above.

In attempts to assess the results of management in these cases it is essential to have some idea of the chance of a subsequent pregnancy being carried to term without therapy. Unfortunately, a state of great confusion developed in the literature, as theoretical calculations were made based on unreliable data and involving false assumptions. The figures produced gave a much more pessimistic prognosis than was true. A consequence was that trials of many procedures, now accepted as valueless, were published claiming excellent results. The doubts which developed in many critical minds were epitomized by editorial comment in the *British Medical Journal* (1962). 'If a large number of golfers can beat par, then either their technique and ability is well above average or par has been set too high, or both.' The conclusion generally accepted is that 'par' was too high. The errors of these earlier calculations were palpably exposed (Warburton & Fraser 1961; James 1962) and while no precise figures are available recent estimates of the frequency of abortion after three previous abortions range from 11 to 26% (Warburton & Fraser 1961). These figures are, of course, to be considered in relation to an overall abortion risk of 10–20%. It follows that no therapy can be accepted as efficacious unless strictly controlled trials are performed. Since this realization, claims for treatment of habitual abortion have greatly diminished. Macnaughton (1961) showed that over 50% of patients aborting do so before the twelfth week. It therefore follows that any study on a group of patients of whom a considerable proportion are, at the outset, over 10 weeks pregnant is heavily biased towards success.

A careful history must be taken of the time in pregnancy the previous abortions occurred and how they commenced. Did the foetus die *in utero* before the abortion? Were there any episodes of illness about the same time? Pelvic examination may reveal a uterine abnormality. General examination and urine analysis should be done, but rarely provide any clues. Blood tests for syphilis and iso-antibodies should be done, together with a glucose-tolerance test and tests of thyroid function. Hysterography is needed, at least if the abortions have been in the middle trimester.

Many cases are seen only when a fresh pregnancy has commenced, and the investigative programme then requires to be modified. In this situation gentle assessment of uterine position and the state of the cervix, together with endocrine assessment, becomes important.

Hormonal aspects of recurrent abortion

It has long been accepted that hormones, particularly the steroid hormones produced initially by the maternal ovary and later by the placenta, play a major part in permitting the conceptus to grow within the uterus. Naturally, it was assumed that inadequate hormone production could lead to expulsion of the conceptus by the myometrium, and this suggestion was advanced particularly in relation to recurrent abortion. Many papers appeared suggesting that a wide variety of endocrine preparations were helpful—yielding salvage rates of 65–80% (see Shearman 1968). In many series, however, the dosage used was homeopathic, controlled series were conspicuous by their absence and equally good results were obtained with such disparate therapies as thyroid extract, oestrogens, chorionic gonadotrophin in addition to progestogens and oestrogen–progestogen mixtures.

The progestogen preparations have been most widely used. The reason is, of course, that progesterone has for long been regarded as the most important 'pregnancy maintaining' hormone. Investigational work to support this has been concerned with the estimation of urinary pregnanediol and plasma progesterone. There are great problems in regard to interpretation of both. Pregnanediol is merely an excretory product to which metabolized progesterone contributes, while plasma progesterone has such a short half-life that interpreting an isolated reading 'is rather like trying to assess 24-hr rainfall by glancing out of the window for a second' (Shearman 1968). Most of the information available concerns pregnanediol excretion, and as much as can be said with confidence is that with low pregnanediol levels abortion in the first trimester is more likely to occur but is by no means inevitable.

Many workers have applied therapy when the pregnanediol level was low or when other parameters such as cervical mucus crystallization (Macdonald 1963) or abnormal vaginal cytology patterns (Cox *et al.* 1964), pointed to likely progesterone deficiency. Excellent results were claimed; rises in the pregnanediol excretion were demonstrated and correction of the abnormal biological parameters reported. Shearman & Garrett (1963) however in a controlled trial which, involving treating such patients with 17-hydroxyprogesterone caproate or a placebo, showed that *significant rises in pregnanediol occurred after injection of the inert placebo* (Fig. 14.3). In a series of 50 habitual abortion patients Shearman and Garrett found as good results in the placebo group. This paper proved a turning point. Further studies (e.g. Goldzieher 1964; Klopper & Macnaughton 1965) produced similar findings. Ever since critical gynaecologists have been hesitant to accept that hormone treatment is specifically important in prevention of abortion. The current attitude is to regard biochemical or biological manifestations of endocrine deficiency as merely a sign that tropho-

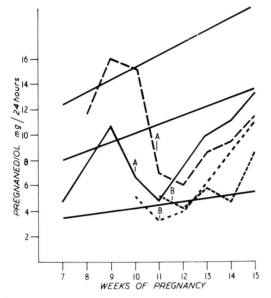

Fig. 14.3. Elevation of pregnanediol excretion levels in patients with a history of recurrent abortion and low or falling pregnanediol levels after treatment with 17-hydroxyprogesterone acetate or a placebo. One of these was labelled 'A' and the other 'B'; the letters on the chart indicate the time of first injection and the solution used. The pattern observed was similar irrespective of the solution used. (From Shearman & Garrett (1963), acknowledgements to the authors and the Editor of *British Medical Journal*.)

blastic function is inadequate. It is not believed that replacement therapy will influence correction of the trophoblastic dysfunction which may or may not occur spontaneously (Shearman 1968). The idea of giving progesterone for recurrent or threatened abortion may soon be regarded as being as illogical as the giving of hydrochloric acid to correct the underlying disorder of pernicious anaemia.

Doubtless some such therapy will continue to be administered for a time. These patients crave help from doctors and the evidence is that the psychological support of being included in any therapeutic trial—no matter what it may be and whether they receive an active or an inactive preparation—is beneficial in terms of their chances of achieving a successful outcome to their pregnancy. It is only fair to acknowledge that this was precisely the conclusion reached

by Bevis as long ago as 1951. He studied pregnanediol excretion and other hormonal aspects, but rightly deduced they were of little import. His conclusion, however, was too prosaic to have immediate popular appeal!

Accepting this situation (that the psychological support is the important aspect of treatment), it is much more intellectually honest to use a true placebo—a preparation which is completely inert. Furthermore, there is the important practical point that progestogen preparations are not devoid of ill-effects. If the mother is carrying a female foetus, large doses of certain progestogens in early pregnancy may cause a degree of virilization (Wilkins 1960). This is, of course, not progressive after birth, but can be a source of mistaken sex assignation and may cause great distress to parents and child. Norethisterone (marketed as Primolut N) appears to be the preparation most likely to be associated with virilization. The writer has recently had the unhappy experience of seeing two sisters showing virilization from this cause. The mother's first three pregnancies resulted in normal girls. She then had two first-trimester miscarriages. In her sixth pregnancy norethisterone was given from 6 to 32 weeks. In the next pregnancy another doctor refused to prescribe progestogens and abortion occurred at 5 months. In the eighth pregnancy norethisterone was again given from the sixth to thirty-second week. In both the sixth and eighth pregnancies girls were delivered at term and both showed signs of virilization. Plastic surgery will be required. Any doctor who wishes to avoid the risk of adverse legal action would be well advised to avoid such preparations in early pregnancy.

'PSEUDO-ABORTION'

Sometimes, owing to various hormone imbalances (usually an excessive or abnormally prolonged production of oestrogen or progesterone by the ovary), an expected menstrual period fails to occur and the patient imagines she is pregnant. A week or two later there is a heavy vaginal blood loss, following which menstruation returns to normal. The episode is readily labelled as an abortion by patient and doctor. It should never be assumed that a patient had had an abortion—no matter how convinced she herself may be—unless the foetus has been identified by a trained person or chorionic villi have been demonstrated microscopically. It follows, of course, that all material passed by a woman should be preserved, if possible in fixative, for subsequent pathological analysis. Failure to appreciate this condition may result in women wanting children being investigated for recurrent abortion when the real trouble is infertility associated with ovulation failure.

SEPTIC ABORTION

Any abortion is liable to be associated with sepsis, just as any term delivery may be. In certain types of abortion the risk of sepsis is very great and constitutes a major hazard to life. The spontaneous, complete abortion in the second trimester carries minimal risk of sepsis, while the criminally induced, incomplete abortion of the first trimester carries an extremely high risk. Missed abortion also carries a particular risk. The factors involved in the predisposition are several. Portions of chorionic tissue are very liable to be retained in the uterus, especially with early abortions, and form an ideal focus for infection. The same applies to the total conception in missed abortion. If the abortion is induced operatively, instruments are passed up the genital tract with the possibility of carrying bacteria into the uterine cavity. Furthermore, if the procedure is done illegally the instruments are unlikely to have been adequately sterilized. It is, however, wrong to equate septic abortion with criminal abortion; even in ideal circumstances sepsis sometimes develops.

Another factor is related to the propensity of the retained products to cause haemorrhage. For this reason the gynaecologist usually intervenes to remove them. If sepsis has developed, his intervention may lead to spread of the infection, causing septicaemia or bacteraemia. This is liable to precipitate what in the present day is the most dreaded complication of abortion —*bacteraemic endotoxic shock*. The organisms most frequently involved in abortion sepsis are *Escherichia coli*, streptococci—haemolytic, non-haemolytic and anaerobic—*Staphylococcus aureus*, *Clostridium welchii* and the tetanus bacillus.

In the majority of cases the infection is limited to the uterine cavity but it may spread to the tubes, ovaries, pelvic cellular tissue or peritoneum in addition to the disastrous spread to the general circulation. The usual signs and symptoms of infection are present together with a foul-smelling, purulent or salmon-pink vaginal discharge and tenderness over the lower abdomen and in the pelvis.

The problem of management immediately becomes a major and acute emergency when systemic shock develops in association with septic abortion. Prior to this the aim is to limit the infection. Spread to the fallopian tubes or pelvic peritoneum may be followed by secondary infertility or sterility. It is widely accepted that prompt completion of all abortions once they become inevitable is a great factor in reducing the incidence of sepsis. A policy which involves curetting a large number of uteri which turn out to be empty is one which, in the long run, will pay dividends. The problem is more difficult when the picture suggests that infection has already developed within the uterus. It is now doubly important to get rid of any retained tissue, but disturbance of the infected area may result in systemic spread. In pre-antibiotic days non-intervention was the practice. Now antibiotic agents are invariably given, and the debate concerns how long they should be given to act. Some evacuate immediately, giving the antibiotics intravenously, while others advocate a 24-hr delay. There is probably little to choose between the two schools of thought, though Ramirez-Soto *et al.* (1969) record a lower mortality with early curettage—within 8 hr of initiation of treatment. Frequently, whether to intervene immediately or delay for up to 24 hr will be dictated by other circumstances. It is particularly important when evacuating the uterus in such a case with frank infection to bear in mind that the uterus may have suffered prior damage from the manipulations of an untrained operator.

A combination of penicillin and streptomycin is usually appropriate therapy pending the availability of a sensitivity report. Large doses should be given. In serious cases this represents one of the few circumstances in which chloramphenicol is an appropriate drug to use.

Endotoxic shock

It is a well-known phenomenon that cardiovascular collapse may occur in association with bacteraemia. One particularly common predisposing factor to this is postabortal infection usually with Gram-negative organisms such as *Esch.coli*. The collapse is apparently due to reduction in the return of blood to the heart as a consequence of the endotoxin's peripheral effects. One of the great problems is that the endotoxin continues to exert its influence from dead bacteria, so that even if bacteria are killed by appropriate therapy, the toxic influence may continue. The endotoxin is said to be a lipoprotein–carbohydrate complex contained in the O-somatic antigen present in the cell wall of the Gram-negative bacteria. The endotoxin not only affects peripheral vascular tone but can also cause tissue destruction, the kidney and other viscera being particularly susceptible (Vaughn *et al.* 1967).

Also frequently implicated in the systemic disturbance of the endotoxic shock syndrome with abortion is a fundamental disorder of the coagulation system. Phillips *et al.* (1967) conclude that the initial effect is an intravascular coagulation due either to the endotoxin acting directly or secondarily following severe haemolysis. Fibrinolysis may develop subsequently. In some cases the picture is similar to the experimental generalized Schwartzmann reaction (Schwartzmann 1937)* and typical lesions are found at autopsy (Reid 1967).

The clinical picture varies. Rigors may herald the onset but the first development may be profound hypotension which will be missed if monitoring is not in operation. Pyrexia is usual, but a fall in temperature may occur. There is tachycardia. Peripheral vasodilatation is often

*In animals, if a *provocative* dose of endotoxin enters the system after a *preparing* dose, profound shock ensues associated with disseminated intravascular coagulation, especially in the glomerular capillaries. In humans pregnancy apparently acts as the *preparing* dose.

an early feature and the flushed facies may mislead as to the seriousness of the patient's general condition. Later, a cyanotic tinge develops. Oliguria is usual and jaundice may ensue. The venous return to the heart falls to an extent that cardiac output can no longer be maintained at the level necessary for the vital organs.

The management of the condition is a matter of great urgency for the mortality rate is high. Even in modern times figures of 30–90% are quoted. This range probably reflects differences in the standards for diagnosis rather than differing efficacy of various therapies. It is difficult in such a situation to secure adequately controlled trials of any therapy. There is, however, a broad measure of agreement on the general principles of management.

Firstly it is essential to *control infection*. Massive doses of intravenous penicillin (up to 100 million units per 24 hr), chloramphenicol (up to 2 g/l of infused fluid) together with intramuscular streptomycin (up to 4 g/24 hr) are used. Carbenicillin ('Pyopen', Beecham), though an expensive preparation, may possibly turn out to be of value in this situation in view of its particular activity against Gram-negative organisms. *Removal of the focus of infection* must be considered after the antibiotic cover is established. Vaginal evacuation may be hazardous and there is a place for removal of the whole uterus, carefully ligating the venous drainage before manipulation. The decision to do this, and the timing, are matters requiring great clinical judgement. Supplementary intravenous hydrocortisone is widely accepted as valuable but very large doses are required—1 g in the first hour and up to 3–4 g in 24 hr. Such therapy restores the regional blood flow and reverses the metabolic acidosis seen in the dog during the relapsing phase of endotoxic shock (Morris 1967). Much more controversial is the use of hypertensive agents which act by producing peripheral vasospasm. It is argued that such preparations may reduce still further the supply of oxygen to the vital organs and thereby, though producing a better-looking blood-pressure chart, diminish the patient's chances of survival. Possibly more logical, but requiring great courage on the part of the clinician, is the use of vasodilator agents, such as phenoxybenzamine (Martinez *et al.* 1966; Reid 1967). These, though dropping the blood pressure still further, may improve the perfusion of vital organs.

The fluid and electrolyte balance is, of course, carefully controlled. Metabolic acidosis may be reflected in the base deficit and should be corrected. Oxygen is given as necessary. Central venous pressure monitoring is essential. Frequently, blood transfusion is administered at the outset in response to the hypotension, but unless significant blood loss is occurring over-loading must be carefully guarded against. If the patient survives the acute incident of collapse and signs of renal failure develop then dialysis, etc., becomes appropriate.

Abortion haemorrhage

There is always a certain amount of blood loss in association with the delivery of any conceptus, be it abortus or mature foetus. The risk of excessive haemorrhage is, however, greater with abortion. The general principles for blood volume replacement with blood, plasma or synthetic plasma substitutes apply as with other forms of haemorrhage. The first step is to obtain blood for grouping and cross-matching. Any replacement will depend on the rate of blood loss and the patient's condition. Much more important, however, is the prevention or arrest of haemorrhage. There are a number of important measures which can be applied independently of the type of the abortion. The important points to aim for are rapid complete evacuation of the uterus and good uterine contraction and retraction. Attainment of the latter will do much to achieve the former. The administration of oxytocics is almost always appropriate if bleeding is severe; they are best given by the intravenous route. In early pregnancy instrumental evacuation of the products is appropriate; later on, manual removal of the placenta, if retained, should be done as for a third stage problem with a mature delivery.

Coagulation disorder may be a problem, particularly if it is a missed abortion or sepsis with endotoxic shock has occurred. The question may arise of specific coagulation therapy with fibrino-

gen, concentrated plasma, fibrinolysis inhibitors such as ε-aminocaproic acid, Trasylol (F.B.A. Pharmaceuticals Ltd.) or, alternatively, fibrinolytic agents such as streptokinase. These therapies are all potentially deleterious, however, and it is often impossible to say which is indicated (Scott 1968). Coagulation failure determined by laboratory methods is frequently unassociated with excessive haemorrhage. For these reasons it may be wise to withhold specific coagulation therapy.

Abortion kidney

A possible sequel of abortion haemorrhage or the combined effect of that and sepsis is *abortion kidney* (renal cortical necrosis or tubular nephrosis). Every abortion patient should be closely observed for oliguria and appropriate action taken promptly if it develops. In Smith *et al.*'s (1968) series 52 of 86 cases of renal failure due to obstetric causes followed abortion. Thirteen (25%) of these patients died, but none as a direct consequence of renal damage. The majority followed criminal interference. Hypovolaemia secondary to blood loss, together with the effects of sepsis with endotoxic shock, lead to poor renal perfusion and acute renal 'shut-down'. In addition it is possible that the bacterial toxins may cause direct damage; this has been demonstrated in animals (De Navasquez 1938). Large amounts of free haemoglobin in the circulation secondary to haemolysis may also play a part (Allen 1962). An additional factor which may be of significance is the direct nephrotoxic effect of abortifacient chemicals (Russell *et al.* 1955).

In fatal cases the histology is usually of tubular necrosis without evidence of glomerular change. Occasionally there may be patchy cortical necrosis, but this has a different distribution from the cortical necrosis of late pregnancy (Sheehan & Moore 1952).

Careful management of the fluid, protein and electrolyte balance with dialysis as necessary should ensure recovery unless there are other complications. Sometimes, mannitol 25% is given intravenously to promote diuresis, but if renal damage has occurred it would be ineffective; if the anuria is due to other causes of a prerenal nature then these should be dealt with appropriately. In particular, efforts should be made to restore the central venous pressure to normal.

Psychological aspects of abortion

A major aspect of every abortion—induced or spontaneous, isolated or recurrent—is the psychological impact on the mother. If the baby was greatly wanted there is obviously a sense of deep disappointment and this is, of course, greatest with recurrent abortions. If the pregnancy was a fortuitous one and a family of reasonable size already exists, the disappointment is less overt, but women in this situation still frequently experience a considerable degree of disturbance, presumably related to a feeling that there has been a failure of their prime feminine role. When the abortion has been induced, of course, guilt responses are common. These become exaggerated if subsequently there is difficulty in achieving or carrying a wanted pregnancy. The particular problems involved when in missed abortion a dead foetus is retained for some time *in utero* have been referred to.

No rules can be laid down for managing these aspects. Every good gynaecologist, however, will have the psychological aspect in the forefront of his mind when dealing with every case of abortion. The tendency is for this side of things to be ignored when patients who are aborting are admitted to abortion units where large numbers of abortions are dealt with on a physically efficient, rapid turnover basis. The administrative arguments for such units are strong. In terms of efficient prevention of the debilitating effects of haemorrhage and sepsis they are highly effective. Unless, however, very personal and continuous control is exercised by an experienced gynaecologist the deep personal and psychological problems of the individual patients may be ignored.

Maternal mortality and abortion

The *Report on Confidential Enquiries into Maternal Deaths in England and Wales* (1966,

1969) highlight the fact that abortion is now the commonest cause of death in relation to pregnancy. Almost three-quarters of the fatalities are associated with illegal interference. The highest proportion of deaths in the 1966 report followed injection per vaginam, usually of soapy fluid. Air embolism was most frequently the ultimate cause of death in these cases and shock, haemorrhage, *Cl.welchii* infection, etc., also contributed. The other large group of deaths was associated with instrumental interference leading to shock and haemorrhage. Other procedures responsible included the vaginal insertion of potassium permanganate crystals and slippery elm, together with the injection of quinine. The non-avoidable deaths were attributed to sepsis (25), embolism (10), concealed haemorrhage and shock (10), placenta praevia (3) and anuria (4). These figures serve to illustrate that some of the complications regarded as typical of the third trimester can still operate and carry fatal risks at earlier stages of gestation.

ECTOPIC PREGNANCY

Ectopic pregnancy is potentially the gynaecologist's most critical emergency. The site is the tube in over 95% of cases. It may, however, be the uterus (intramural, angular, cervical or in a rudimentary horn), the ovary, or the broad ligament or elsewhere in the peritoneal cavity. These latter sites are usually secondary attachments, after extrusion from the tube. Unless stated, subsequent comments can be taken to refer to *tubal* pregnancy.

The incidence in the United Kingdom is of the order of 1 per 300 mature intra-uterine pregnancies. In other communities there may be a 10-fold increase in this proportion, e.g. 1 per 28 in the West Indies (Douglas 1963). It is important to appreciate that occurrence of an ectopic pregnancy is not merely an isolated episode in a woman's life. It has very profound implications with regard to her reproductive performance. She will only have a 1 in 3 chance of ever producing a live child but a 1 in 20 chance of having another ectopic pregnancy (Grant 1962).

Aetiology

It is self-evident that the condition is due to implantation of the fertilized ovum in an abnormal site. It is a matter for debate whether this is due to the tube offering a particular enticement to the ovum or whether the ovum's passage has been delayed till it is at the stage for implantation and it merely chooses the nearest site. The weight of evidence favours the second mechanism being the common one. The precise way in which it is brought about varies in different races and communities at different times.

In some populations gonococcal salpingitis is the commonest background factor, while in others tuberculous salpingitis plays, or has played, a major role. Both these conditions are decreasing in frequency and are amenable to specific treatment, so it may be that the incidence of ectopic pregnancy will dwindle. On the other hand, the ability to treat the inflammation may mean that pregnancy can subsequently occur in tubes which would otherwise have been totally blocked. Halbrecht (1957) drew attention to the fact that of the few pregnancies which occurred after medical treatment for tuberculous endometritis about two-thirds were ectopic. Kleiner & Roberts (1967) came to the conclusion that chronic endosalpingitis was the most significant aetiologic factor. The fact that this is commonly a bilateral condition fits well with the propensity of women who have had ectopic pregnancies to have a recurrence in the opposite tube. The tissue damage from the inflammation, whatever its nature, removes the ciliated epithelium, so important in ovum transport. The peristaltic tubal action is also interfered with, and it is not difficult to appreciate how the normal progress may be impeded.

Modes of contraception also affect the incidence of ectopic pregnancy. Methods which block sperm access (sheath or diaphragm) or suppress ovulation, will obviously lower the incidence. Where a device is placed in the uterine cavity—loop, coil or whatever be in vogue—the situation is different. Sperm have access to the uterus and ova are being produced and have access to the tube. By whatever means

such devices work, they are not as effective in preventing tubal as intra-uterine pregnancies. Tietze (1966) reported that 26 ectopics were recorded in relation to 588 intra-uterine gestations occurring with intra-uterine devices *in situ* in 25,000 women-years of utilization; a 1 to 23 proportion. This figure at first suggests an alarming increase in ectopics. However, if the devices had no influence on tubal gestation 200 or 300 would have been expected in that period of exposure. Wei (1968) in a study in China found no evidence of an increase in the incidence of ectopic gestation in a population in which the intra-uterine device had come to be used extensively. It seems that there is no *true* increase in tubal pregnancies in these circumstances but, in fact, possibly a decrease. There is, however, a greatly increased ratio of ectopic to intra-uterine gestations when pregnancy occurs despite the presence of an intra-uterine device.

There is a close correlation between factors leading to infertility and those leading to ectopic pregnancy. The ectopic incidence is increased eight fold in women who have been investigated for infertility (Wyper 1962). Where tubal surgery has been performed in an attempt to correct old tubal damage, the chances of ectopic gestation are particularly high (Greenhill 1956). Any pelvic surgery, however, including tubal ligation and hysterectomy, and most types of gross pelvic pathology can be associated with ectopic gestation (Douglas 1963).

The chance of a second ectopic is relatively very high—approximately 5–10% (Grant 1962). Interestingly, ectopic pregnancy is significantly more frequent on the right side (Sandmire & Randall 1959; Grant 1962; Douglas 1963). This possibly reflects the local influence of appendicular inflammation. Ectopic pregnancy is apparently commoner in association with advancing age and gravidity order (Kleiner & Roberts 1967), but the significance of this is not clear.

Other theories include Iffy's (1963) proposition that late fertilization is important. He suggests fertilization may be too late for implantation to occur before menstruation and the ovum then passes upwards into the tube and embeds there ('reflux theory'). Transperitoneal migration of the ovum has also been claimed to be an important factor (Berlind 1960). Like Iffy's theory this is difficult to prove. Schiffer (1963) found that in 21 out of 91 salpingo-oöphorectomies performed in his series there was no corpus luteum evident in that ovary. Presumably, in these cases the ovum came from the opposite ovary.

Progress of ectopic pregnancy

The tube may rupture; tubal abortion may occur (extrusion of the gestation sac through the abdominal ostium into the peritoneal cavity); a tubal mole may form (separation of the conceptus from the tubal wall by layers of blood clot); partial rupture may occur with the conceptus surviving and the trophoblast gaining an attachment to some other structure, such as broad ligament or omentum—*secondary abdominal pregnancy*.

Presentation and diagnosis

The problem of ectopic pregnancy is essentially a diagnostic one. The first feature is usually pain; there is commonly some delay in the onset of an expected period, followed by abnormal vaginal bleeding. Syncope may also occur. The pattern may vary greatly and the categories considered in detail below represent the commoner types.

The presentation of ectopic gestation may be acute, silent or subacute. The *acute presentation* is recognizable to even the rawest novitiate. It is associated with tubal rupture and massive intraperitoneal haemorrhage leading to acute abdominal pain and cariovascular collapse. There may or may not have been some premonitory menstrual disturbance or syncope and local pain as described below under 'subacute'. Shoulder-tip or interscapular pain may be present. On examination, hypotension and tachycardia are the rule, although bradycardia is occasionally found. Generalized abdominal rigidity and rebound tenderness are present. Vaginal examination at this stage is scarcely necessary and may be unrewarding. There will usually be generalized pelvic tenderness, but the side in which the gestation has been situated may be more tender.

How do 'silent' ectopics present? Occasionally, they are detected when the patient attends the antenatal clinic for booking. Localized tenderness is elicited in one fornix, possibly with a swelling, and although there have been no symptoms, this finding is enough to raise a high level of suspicion. The question is often debated as to whether or not a bimanual examination should be performed in the early antenatal phase. In my view it should; the fact that I have recently diagnosed ectopic gestation in two women referred for routine hospital booking has confirmed me in this view. It is, however, important in this connection to differentiate between hospital examination, where all facilities for laparotomy are available should an ectopic be ruptured, and examination at home or in the consulting room where this is not the case. Ectopic pregnancy may also be discovered at laparotomy done for some quite distinct condition or at autopsy done for unexplained sudden death.

It is in the *subacute group that the great diagnostic problems arise*. There will usually have been some vaginal bleeding, but this is generally a late and secondary feature; there is no constant pattern to the loss. Syncopal attacks may occur. The precise mechanism of these in the pre-haemorrhagic state is not clear. Some degree of pain is usually the first symptom, but its degree and nature can be very variable. If free blood is in the peritoneum referred shoulder pain may be experienced. In dubious cases a worthwhile test is to lay the patient in bed with the foot raised 6 in; shoulder pain may develop over 15–30 min. Beware, of course, the leading question! Less well-documented but frequently helpful is referred discomfort from blood in the pouch of Douglas. This may cause pain on defaecation ('bathroom sign') or perineal discomfort—manifest as inability to sit square on a hard seat.

Lower abdominal tenderness and guarding may be present. *On bimanual examination localized tenderness is the most significant feature.* This may be in lateral or posterior fornix. A mass may or may not be palpable. At an initial out-patient examination the patient's general apprehension and tension may interfere with localization of the tenderness.

It is important to bear in mind that ectopic gestation can be simultaneously bilateral and coincide with an intra-uterine gestation.

The great clinical problem is what to do when the suspicion of ectopic pregnancy has been raised by some feature of history or examination yet the diagnosis cannot be made with confidence. The doctor cannot relax until he has clarified the situation with reasonable certainty one way or another. Laboratory and ancillary aids give little help. The maxim 'if in doubt look and see' is only operable if interpreted with a modicum of reasonableness. There is no disgrace in a negative peritoneal exploration for possible ectopic, but large numbers of these are a burden on hospital organization and an imposition on patients.

What can be done short of operation? Frequently, the patient has been seen amidst the tensions of a busy out-patient clinic or casualty department. Such a patient may, with benefit, be admitted to hospital and settled down for a few hours with appropriate frequent checks of pulse and blood pressure lest rupture should occur. On re-examination at leisure it is often possible to get a much better assessment. Tenderness of a general nature may have changed to specific local tenderness in a fornix. As mentioned, raising the foot of the bed may be followed by shoulder tip pain. Such measures are of much greater value than laboratory tests. The duration of such observation-assessment should, however, be carefully limited—rarely more than 24 hr. It should not be anywhere except in a hospital with staff capable of strict observation and facilities for immediate operation. Nocturnal sedation should be avoided, for it may depress the patient's response should a haemorrhage occur.

As Webster *et al.* (1965) say, 'The only laboratory test of constant value is the blood type and Rh determination which is necessary for blood transfusion'. Various types of pregnancy tests are often done, but are of little value; they are frequently negative when there is an ectopic pregnancy and positive when there is not. White cell counts may occasionally divert sus-

picion to an inflammatory lesion. Haematocrit and haemoglobin determinations may be in order but, as with blood grouping, are in no sense diagnostic.

Special clinical procedures are sometimes used. The most frequently employed, and perhaps the most controversial, is needling of the pouch of Douglas. While Webster *et al.* (1965) reported on 699 ectopics, of which 657 (94%) were subjected to needling (or 'culdocentesis') in 96·7% non-clotting blood was obtained. *The absence of clotting is important.* Other workers have been much less impressed with the method, but properly carried out and interpreted it has a place. If continuing intra-uterine pregnancy can be excluded curettage may be done but the endometrium may be of any pattern. Schiffer (1963) reported finding 28 secretory patterns, 22 proliferative, 23 decidual type and 6 atypical, including the Arias-Stella phenomenon (Arias-Stella 1954). This is characterized by atypical focal adenomatous change, the glands being in a mixed, proliferative and secretory, atypical pattern (Fig. 14.4). Intraluminal budding is evident together with atypical cell changes, nuclear hypertrophy, hyperchromatism, cellular reduplication, mitoses and nucleated syncytial masses. This pattern without chorionic villi is typical of the presence of pregnancy elsewhere in the body, but the inconstancy of it as a finding, as in the series quoted, is unfortunately the rule. To the inexperienced it may even be mistaken for carcinoma, and in one of the six cases quoted the uterus was removed on this erroneous diagnosis.

Nature, of course, may favour the conservative observer by presenting him with a decidual cast. Donald (1968) has claimed that ectopic gestation may be diagnosed as early as 6 weeks by the use of ultrasonics. Few have sufficient experience to be confident, however.

One 'aid' which tends to be the resort of the destitute in problem cases is 'E.U.A.' (examination under anaesthesia). This, in ectopic pregnancies, merely ablates the most useful physical sign—localized tenderness—and exposes the patient to the risk that the ectopic gestation with its flimsy coverings will be ruptured when examined with the protective pain response

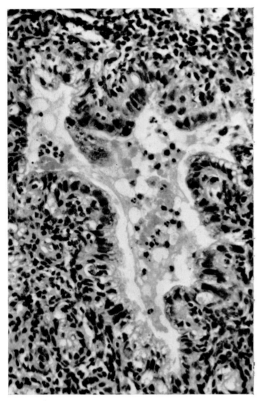

Fig. 14.4. Photo-micrograph of endometrium showing the characteristic atypical maturation pattern known as the Arias-Stella phenomenon said to be diagnostic of a pregnancy outside the uterus when found on curettage in the absence of chorionic villi. (By courtesy of Dr. P.N. Cowen.)

absent. Anyone who has seen a patient nearly die from acute intra-peritoneal haemorrhage after being passed as free from any suspicion of ectopic at E.U.A. is unlikely to resort to the manoeuvre.

Endoscopy—culdoscopy or laparoscopy—may have a small place in difficult cases when an early lesion is suspected. The help it gives is more exclusive in cases in which the suspicion of ectopic has been raised, little has been found to support it and the gynaecologist merely wishes final support in dismissing the diagnosis and discharging the patient. Out of over 500 personal culdoscopies only 4% were for possible ectopic pregnancies and all were negative, with one exception.

After full and careful consideration, taking advantage of every ancillary aid which may seem indicated in the particular case, it may still not be possible to exclude ectopic gestation with reasonable confidence. In this situation exploratory laparotomy is, without doubt, appropriate.

Treatment

As soon as the diagnosis is made immediate operative treatment is essential. Difficulties arise in relation to the patients presenting with acute collapse due to massive intraperitoneal bleeding. These patients are often so ill that the anaesthetist is unhappy about administering an anaesthetic, yet no matter how rapidly blood is transfused it does not exceed the rate of intra-peritoneal loss. In this situation conservatism holds no hope and the gynaecologist must persuade his anaesthetist colleague that *the only prospect for the patient's survival lies in getting her to theatre as quickly as possible, opening the abdomen and arresting the source of the bleeding.*

The appropriate action is to set up an intra-venous infusion capable of taking a rapid flow of blood. If the arm veins are collapsed, as may be the case, a major vein elsewhere—such as the saphenous in the upper thigh—must be used without hesitation. In the most critical cases little or no anaesthetic may be necessary. Probably the best technique in the circumstances is cyclopropane and oxygen induction followed by intubation in association with administration of suxamethonium chloride and maintenance on nitrous oxide and oxygen. Diathermy may be used within 3 min of stopping the cyclopropane. Should cyclopropane be unavailable or the anaesthetist unfamiliar with its use induction may be with nitrous oxide after pre-oxygenation.

With maximum speed the surgeon should make a vertical, mid-line subumbilical incision. Then, in the words of Lawson Tait of Birmingham, who performed the first successful operation for ectopic gestation in the 1880s, 'make at once for the source of the haemorrhage, the broad ligament, tie it at its base and then remove the ovum and debris at leisure'. Blood, uncross matched if necessary, should be given as rapidly as possible and the patient's condition should improve immediately. Usually it does. If, however, the circulatory collapse is so severe that intravenous fluid is not bringing response, intra-arterial transfusion should be resorted to. In the circumstance the internal iliac artery is probably the most appropriate to utilize. Only a small volume of blood under pressure, with precautions against air embolism, should be sufficient to restore adequate coronary circulation, and thereafter intravenous transfusion should be effective. Where adequate supplies of donor blood are not available, autotransfusion of blood collected from the peritoneal cavity may be life-saving (Douglas 1963).

TYPE OF OPERATIVE PROCEDURE

Of very much less importance than immediate arrest of haemorrhage and resuscitation is the matter of precisely what should be done surgically There is, however, wide divergence of opinion in this regard. In the early days of ectopic surgery, removal of tube and ovary was standard. Then with the Bonney era of ovarian conservation it came to be accepted that, if possible, it was right to conserve the ovary and merely perform salpingectomy. Some pressed this further and advocated that as far as possible the tube affected should be conserved—'partial salpingectomy'.

Jeffcoate (1955), however, pronounced a fundamentally different approach. It is arguable that this represents the most important modification to the traditional treatment of ectopic pregnancy which has come to the fore in the last two decades. He suggested that if the opposite appendage was normal the ovary related to the affected tube should be removed. Jeffcoate's reasoning was that (a) ova released from the contralateral ovary will only rarely undergo transperitoneal migration and reach the opposite tube; (b) approximately half the ova are released from each ovary, and in a woman with a single tube the chances of conception would be as much as doubled if it could be arranged that each ovulation occurred from the ipselateral ovary; and (c) removing the ovary with the fallopian tube

secures this effect, as the monthly pituitary stimulus for ovulation will subsequently always affect the remaining ovary which has a tube in direct relationship (see Fig. 14.5).

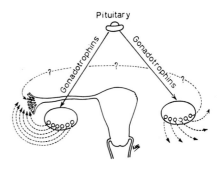

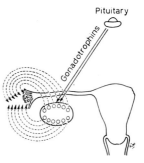

Fig. 14.5. Diagrammatic representation of the benefits of salpingo-oöphorectomy as compared with salpingectomy. With salpingectomy approximately 50% subsequent ovulations will take place from the tubeless ovary. The only chance of fertilization rests upon transperitoneal migration, accepted as a rare occurrence. If that ovary is removed, all subsequent ovulations occur from the ovary with an associated tube. (From Jeffcoate (1967), acknowledgements to the author and publishers.)

The logic of this argument has about it a Newtonian fundamentality which makes it difficult for those with preconceived ideas to accept. Many gynaecologists brought up in the gospel of 'ovarian conservation if at all possible' have what amounts to an emotional block towards this apparent contravention of their fundamental attitudes. Grant (1962), for example, dismisses the procedure with the comment that removal of one ovary usually results in a protest, places the surgeon in a defensive position and could result in a successful legal action against him: no very good reasons for any doctor to carry out the wrong treatment! Statistical proof is very difficult. Bender (1956) in a retrospective study did find a higher conception rate after salpingo-oöphorectomy than salpingectomy, but the difference was not statistically significant. He concluded, probably correctly, that the cases in which salpingo-oöphorectomy was performed were probably those with the greater pelvic pathology, and consequently the poorer fertility prospects.

The circumstances of emergency operations for ectopics, the varied background of the cases, the low overall conception rate after ectopic pregnancy and widely divergent desires with regard to subsequent child-bearing all militate against a prospective study of the problem. It is a principle, therefore, upon which every clinician must make up his mind on the basis of logical reasoning rather than statistical data. The principle has applications in other aspects of gynaecological surgery. In infertility problems it may be best to perform salpingo-oöphorectomy when there is unilateral tubal damage. The writer's personal experience in this matter is that this paradoxical operation is the most fruitful in infertility surgery! It is, of course, obvious that if at operation the contralateral tube or ovary is damaged or absent, then ovarian conservation, if at all possible, should be the rule, and if it is known that further pregnancies are particularly desired an attempt should be made to conserve the affected tube.

Where the gestation is cornual or angular, hysterectomy will frequently be necessary or, at the least, cornual resection.

Abdominal pregnancy

A difficult obstetric problem, one to which there is no completely effective answer, is the extra-uterine pregnancy which presents at an advanced stage. Though very rare in Europe, Dixon & Stewart (1960) reported ten cases occurring in relation to less than 10,000 deliveries in the West Indies. Even in modern times mortality rates are from 2 to 10% (Drury 1960 & Hreshchyshyn et al. 1961). The condition is usually suspected by persistent abnormal foetal

lie and easy palpation of foetal parts. The non-gravid uterus may be felt separate from the foetus. There may be a history of pain early in pregnancy, representing the time of transfer of the attachment from tube to peritoneum. Abdominal discomfort may persist and slight bleeding may occur.

Radiological examination may reveal shadows of maternal intestinal gas superimposed on the foetus [Figs. 14.6(a) and 14.6(b)]. A Syntocinon infusion may be employed to stimulate uterine contraction. This will, of course, only be helpful in that if the uterus is felt to contract around the foetus, ectopic can be excluded. Thermography, arteriography and hysterography may all give help, but the latter can only be justified when the diagnosis is virtually certain.

As soon as the diagnosis is made operation is usually advisable. Rarely it may be justified to continue the pregnancy for a short time to enable the foetus to have a more reasonable chance of survival.

The great problem at operation is whether or not to remove the placenta. Interference with it may lead to uncontrollable haemorrhage. If it is left *in situ* the morbidity from abscess formation is high. It must be a matter for the judgement of the individual operator whether or not removal can safely be undertaken in any given case depending upon the accessibility for ligation of the maternal vessels supplying the area. Methotrexate has been used in an attempt to inactivate the trophoblast rapidly when the placenta has been left in position (Hreshchyshyn *et al.* 1965; Lathrop & Bowles 1968) and it has been suggested it be used before operation if the baby is known to be dead.

The baby delivered from an extra-uterine sac often shows pressure malformation related to the lack of protection provided by the uterus and the fact that oligohydramnios seems to be the rule in these cases.

Maternal mortality from ectopic pregnancy

Ectopic pregnancy is a major factor in mortality due to pregnancy and childbirth. This is emphasized in the *Report on Confidential Enquiries into Maternal Deaths in England and Wales*

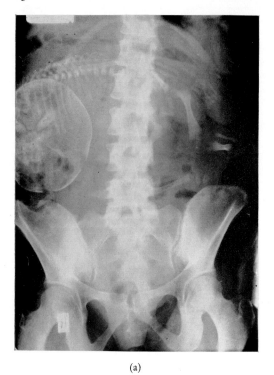

(a)

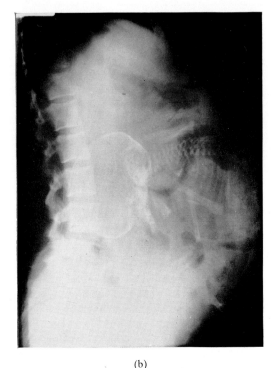

(b)

Fig. 14.6(a) and (b). X-rays of an advanced extra-uterine gestation. Note the absence of uterine contour, distorted foetal position, maternal bowel gas shadows over the foetus and, in the lateral projection, foetal skull superimposed upon the maternal spine. (Photograph by courtesy of Mr. G.A. Craig and Dr. P.P. Franklyn.)

1964–1966 (1969). Out of 579 deaths due to pregnancy or childbirth for which information was available, 42 (7%) were due to ectopic gestation. This compares with 9·2% of 920 maternal deaths in New York City. Perhaps significant in relation to the higher relative mortality incidence in New York is the fact that in the English series *at least* 30% were known to be 'coloured'; the relevant information was not available in some cases. In 29 of the 42, diagnosis was not made before autopsy. Four patients died at home and had not been seen by a doctor. Six had severe diarrhoea and vomiting, five diarrhoea alone. Cases had been wrongly diagnosed as acute appendicitis, pyelitis, cholecystitis, perforated ulcer, pulmonary embolism (twice) and cardiac failure. In seven cases (17%) avoidable factors were present. In five of these the fault was *attempting to resuscitate prior to operation.*

TROPHOBLASTIC GROWTHS

Introduction

One of the great mysteries of placentate reproduction is the mechanism whereby the trophoblastic invasion of the maternal host is halted. In the occasions when this fails the consequence may be a hydatidiform (synonym: vesicular) mole or chorionic carcinoma (synonyms: choriocarcinoma, chorionepithelioma), the latter frequently developing as a sequel to the former. While, in considering trophoblastic conditions, the usual yard-sticks of tissue malignancy are hard to apply, it is apposite to regard hydatidiform mole as the benign form of trophoblastic tumour, but at the same time the premalignant state which makes it much more probable that frank cancer—chorionic carcinoma—will develop.

Recently there has been greatly increased interest in trophoblastic malignancy, mainly because of the development of efficient chemical means of therapy; overnight a condition almost uniformly fatal came to carry a reasonable prognosis. It also became clear that there is a great variation in the frequency of these diseases in different parts of the world. Immunologic interest in cancer and the mechanism of placentate reproduction has also led to detailed study of this unique type of neoplasia. The setting up of registries—where collected pathological specimens of chorionic tumours and their clinical histories could be studied—provided profitable centres for the greater curiosity in the conditions. It is in the light of such new developments that it is proposed to consider chorionic neoplasia.

The world literature on this subject is in the words of Emil Novak (1957) 'more confusing than that pertaining to almost any other in the field of gynaecology and obstetrics'. The reasons for the difficulties and confusion are several.

(1) Trophoblastic neoplasms, especially the more malignant grades, are rare conditions in Europe and the United States, thus few Western pathologists or clinicians have substantial experience of their considerable problems and vagaries.

(2) The conditions are not strict entities as classifications suggest, but represent a spectrum of trophoblastic activity varying from benign to malignant, without precise lines of demarcation.

(3) Trophoblastic tissue is normally invasive, constituting a sort of 'physiological cancer'. There is no basement membrane, violation of which can be taken as evidence of invading neoplasm, and all the pathologists' usual criteria of tissue malignancy are inapplicable. Classification of degree of malignancy tends to be based on the *least* malignant-looking tissue seen, not the most, as in other tumour pathology.

(4) Trophoblastic tissue's normal habitat is *within* the maternal systemic vascular bed. This being so, it is not surprising that trophoblastic embolization to the pulmonary circulation is common. Attwood & Park (1961) recorded the finding of trophoblast in the lungs in 43·6% of 220 autopsies on pregnant and puerperal women.

(5) Trophoblastic tumours are heterochthonous, i.e. they are strictly homografts on the mother and they have a different genetic—and therefore antigenic—composition from their host. Immunological phenomena related to those involved in the homograft reaction may be responsible for some of the bizarre clinicopathological observations.

(6) Regression, and even disappearance, of metastases in trophoblastic neoplasia *may* occur, though it seems probable, in the view of Bardawil & Toy (1959), that the most important factor in metastatic regression in cases diagnosed as chorionic carcinoma has been misdiagnosis. These authors advise the critical investigator to regard a meticulously studied and documented example as the rarest of events. One of the factors involved in these metastatic regressions is that in cases of trophoblastic embolization haemorrhage characteristically occurs at the site. When the blood clot eventually absorbs, what has appeared an obvious metastases disappears and there may be no viable trophoblast.

(7) While trophoblastic tumours are rare they are not extremely so. This meant in the past that only those with bizarre features tended to be reported; those which behaved in accordance with expectation were deemed to be unworthy of individual recording yet few clinicians had series worthy of publication. As a result the impression got abroad that trophoblastic tumours frequently, or even usually, behaved in a bizarre fashion. This difficulty has been corrected in recent years by the trophoblastic tumour registries, which tend to collect relatively unremarkable cases of trophoblastic tumour. Analysis of their material has shown that in the great majority of the cases the tumours had behaved in an ordinary, predictable way.

It is, incidentally, proper to differentiate between 'gestational' and 'non-gestational' trophoblastic neoplasia. Non-gestational trophoblastic disease occurs rarely in relation to tumours of embryonal type. Similar as the histology and endocrine activity seems to be, it is unfortunately the case that neoplasms of this type do not share the sensitivity to chemotherapy. All subsequent remarks refer to the gestational type.

Classification and pathological characteristics

Much has been written and spoken about the pathology and classification of trophoblastic neoplasia, all to very little purpose, except that from this confusion of description and terminology there has emerged appreciation of the impossibility of applying a complex, multistage classification of trophoblastic neoplasia. This has been accelerated by the study of the pathological material collected at the trophoblastic tumour registries. Park (1959), for example, found that out of 89 cases of probable chorionepithelioma the registry panel of four or five expert pathologists only agreed that the diagnosis was chorionic carcinoma in 27 (30%). This trend away from attempts to over-classify trophoblastic tumours has also been encouraged by the advent of chemotherapy and the realization that the decisions on how to treat these lesions should not be based solely on their histology but on their behaviour as reflected clinically and by assay of their gonadotrophin production. The complete reversion from complex classification is found in the writing of Hertz and his colleagues (1963) who refer only to *metastatic* and *non-metastatic trophoblastic disease* which is the ultimate in simplicity. Most clinicians think, however, in terms of three general grades of trophoblastic disease:

(a) Simple hydropic degeneration

Dropsical villi but no evidence of trophoblastic overgrowth (synonym: hydatidiform degeneration); when the villous dropsy is evident even to the naked eye the term 'transitional mole' (Hertig & Edmonds 1940) is sometimes used.

(b) Hydatidiform mole

Dropsical villi with a very wide range of trophoblastic proliferation which may extend to invasive mole or chorionadenoma destruens, in which there is not only extreme trophoblastic overgrowth but also evidence of invasion beyond the usual limits of trophoblastic penetration and occasionally distant metastases are present; in some areas at least, however, villous structure is preserved. Tow (1966) regards this condition as merely an early form of chorionic carcinoma and uses the term *villous* chorionic carcinoma as opposed to the more advanced *avillous* grade.

(c) Chorionic carcinoma

Large masses of anaplastic trophoblast invading muscle and blood vessels and causing haemorrhagic necrosis of uterine wall; distant metastases are common, especially in the lung and around the vaginal introitus and nearly always the tumour tissue has destroyed all normal chorionic villous pattern. While it is not true to say that the presence of formed villi rules out a diagnosis of chorionic carcinoma, it must be regarded as a feature which makes the diagnosis less likely and invasive mole or chorioadenoma destruens more probable.

Brewer & Gerbie (1966) reported two cases of localized chorionic carcinoma found in otherwise normal placentae. They recorded spontaneous degeneration of the abnormal trophoblast and of formed villi. They conclude that this influence accounts for the absence of villi in the more commonly encountered advanced forms of chorionic carcinoma. They comment on the striking absence of any evidence of the malignant trophoblast invading the foetal vascular system despite its proclivity for entering maternal vessels.

It is now widely accepted that the light-microscopy appearances of trophoblastic tumour tissue do not always give a clear guide as to its malignant potential (e.g. Brewer *et al.* 1967). Several workers have therefore turned to electron-microscopy in the hope that this might give more help. The difficulties of obtaining suitably fixed material are considerable. Some of the studies have been performed on human trophoblastic tumours transplanted to the cheek pouch of the hamster which overcomes some of the technical problems. Up to the present the evidence suggests that the fine structure of neoplastic trophoblast is very similar to that of normal trophoblast (Wynn & Davies 1964a, b; Wynn & Harris 1967). Wynn (1967) postulates on this basis that the vital clue may lie in the decidua which appears less well differentiated in invasive mole.

Although Knoth *et al.* (1967) also doubt whether electron-microscopy will help with prognostication, they suggest that it may be the case that the degree of mitochondrial deformity parallels the degree of malignancy. An extensive study would, however, be needed to prove this.

The clinician faced with a situation, usually after a patient has been delivered of a mole, when he is almost certain that there is neoplastic trophoblastic activity persisting does not await histological confirmation but initiates treatment. Tow calls this *clinical choriocarcinoma*, and Park (1967) *clinical choriomatosis*.

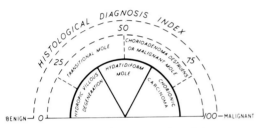

Fig. 14.7. Diagrammatic representation of the spectrum of trophoblastic neoplasia. The 'histological diagnosis index' represents the percentile proportion which might be recorded as malignant by a panel of histologists.

Figure 14.7 shows diagrammatically in simplified form the spectrum of trophoblastic neoplasia and indicates the regions in which difficulties and confusion are most likely to arise. These are the two boundaries of the hydatidiform mole segment of the spectrum, which on the benign side is straddled by 'transitional mole' and on the malignant by 'invasive mole' or 'chorioadenoma destruens'.

In the matter of histological diagnostic error it is important to appreciate that most of the mistakes are 'false-positives'—the mistaking of benign trophoblastic tissue for chorionepithelioma. 'False-negatives' are relatively rare, for the pathologist experienced in the field of general pathology will always tend to be suspicious of unusual trophoblastic elements and, if in doubt, seek a specialist opinion. The usual consequence of histological errors in the past was unnecessary removal of the uterus; very few women died because of these errors. If in the future, as at present seems likely, surgical treatment ceases to be the routine for trophoblastic malignancy, such mishaps should no longer occur.

Aetiology and geographic distribution

The aetiology of trophoblastic neoplasia is unknown. In hydatidiform mole it is widely believed that very early death or failure of development of the embryo is of importance. The chorionic villous tissue apparently survives as its source of nutrition is maternal and the cells secrete into the villi, but owing to the absence of a foetal circulation this fluid collects, distending the villi to form the classic vesicles (Edmonds 1959a). By some unexplained means the trophoblast then proliferates excessively—and this leads to the raised gonadotrophin production and the invasive tendency. Views in this area are changing as the result of cytogenetic studies.

Makino *et al.* (1964) reported a triploid (69, XXY) chromosome compliment in cells cultured from three cases of hydatidiform degeneration. Carr (1969) reported triploidy (69, XXX, XXY or XYY) in 9 of 13 cases of hydatidiform degeneration, while a tenth case was tetraploid (92, XXXX). Beischer *et al.* (1967) reported a hydatidiform mole and a coexistent foetus, both of which had a triploid chromosome constitution. It thus seems that with hydatidiform degeneration the incidence of polyploidy (more than two sets of chromosomes) is high—of the order of 70%. In frank hydatidiform mole, however, though polyploidy occurs it is relatively much less frequent—probably less than 15%.

Carr refers to the suggestion that women who have recently ceased taking oral contraceptives have an increased propensity to produce polyploid conceptuses which subsequently abort. It has been postulated that this tendency to polyploidy might be due to elevated levels of luteinizing hormone. This does have effects on the zona pellucida in certain primates, and he suggests that it might interfere with the shedding of the second polar body, predispose to polyspermy and/or affect early cleavage of the zygote.

Studies have also been done of the nuclear chromatin pattern of hydatidiform moles and these show a high proportion of chromatin-positive cells (Tominaga & Page 1966; Baggish *et al.* 1968). The question immediately arises as to whether this finding represents a predominance of female conceptuses or is merely a manifestation of polyploidy. Baggish *et al.* claim that it is not explicable by polyploidy and suggest that two cell lines develop.

Accepting the pathological concept of trophoblastic overgrowth lesions forming a spectrum with no clearly defined divisions, the question arises as to whether abnormal tissue at the most malignant extreme of the spectrum is the end result of sequential change through the progressive patterns of trophoblastic overactivity to frank cancer or whether the lesion is carcinomatous from the outset. Indirect evidence only can be offered on this point but, while the fact that the commonest precursor of chorionic carcinoma is hydatidiform mole suggests that such a progression is common, in other cases this phase may be absent or so rapid that it is of no clinical significance (Grady 1959). The report of Brewer and Gerbie previously referred to, also supports the idea that normal trophoblast may sometimes be changed directly into chorionic carcinoma.

This, and other evidence, suggests that there may be multiple methods of development of these trophoblastic abnormalities, sometimes the prime factor being foetal, sometimes maternal and, considering the complex interrelationship of trophoblastic invasion and decidual resistance which goes into the formation of the normal placenta, this is not surprising.

A unique conceptus-maternal immunological relationship is involved in placentation and the possibility exists that trophoblastic proliferative lesions may result from a disturbance of the immunological defence mechanism that normally exists because of the genetic differences between the foetal and the maternal tissues. The concept is best regarded as the reverse of rhesus haemolytic disease which is 'an immunological repudiation by the mother of her unborn child'. In chorionic carcinoma, on the other hand, it is possible that the embryonic trophoblast, through failure of immunologic response, continues to invade and brings about the death of the mother. Were there

any truth in this hypothesis chorionic carcinoma might, unlike rhesus haemolytic disease, tend to predominate in first conceptions. Scott (1962) produced evidence of such a tendency in cases of chorionic carcinoma. This data also suggested that chorionic carcinoma occurred more frequently in pregnancies resulting from fresh matings in multiparous women and that, from the limited information available, there was a higher than expected incidence of materno-conceptual blood group compatibility. Llewellyn-Jones (1967) has also reported this with a shift from O towards AB in maternal blood groups. Robinson *et al.* (1963) took this idea a stage further and demonstrated in two cases of chorionic carcinoma unusual tolerance of the paternal antigens, as represented by prolonged survival of husband-to-patient grafts as compared with foreign grafts. In both cases leuco-agglutination examinations of the serum from the patients against their husbands' leucocytes were negative. These findings are compatible with the possibility of an unusually high degree of genetic similarity between the paternal and maternal tissues in these cases. Mogensen & Kissmeyer-Nielsen (1968) studied the families of six patients with chorionic carcinoma from the point of view of tissue typing. All the husbands had one or more major tissue incompatibility with their wives but five of the matings were shown from the study of children to be capable of producing zygotes with tissue-type compatibility with the mother. They conclude that their results are compatible with the postulate that abnormal trophoblast persistence in the maternal host presupposes a high degree of histocompatibility between mother and conceptus as regards transplantation antigens. Halbrecht & Komlos (1968), on the other hand, performing mixed lymphocyte transformation studies on husband and wife, specimens found a definite increase in blast-like cell changes in cases of abortion and hydatidiform mole.

If the paterno-maternal genetic similarity is a factor of importance it would be expected that chorionic carcinoma would be commoner in association with marriages of blood relations and commonest after incestual conceptions. Data on these points, especially the latter, are very hard to obtain, though Mossanen (1963) reported that in 6 out of 40 cases of trophoblastic tumours in Tehran, the patient and her husband were blood relations. The study of Iliya *et al.* (1967) also tends to support this idea. Of their 30 cases, most came from areas where consanguinity and endogamy are common. It may be that such factors have a bearing on the high incidence of chorionic carcinoma in the Eastern and Oriental countries.

Scott's (1962) data on the relative frequency of chorionic carcinoma in first pregnancies (see later) is in contrast to Chun *et al.*'s (1964a) on hydatidiform mole which is apparently less frequent with first pregnancies. Both these studies, however, show a disproportionate occurrence of the conditions in pregnancies of high parity/gravidity order and in elderly parturients (over 39 years). The exact significance of these observations remains uncertain but suggests the operation of multiple factors. Slocumb & Lund (1969) record that in their community the incidence of trophoblastic disease appears to be highest in primigravidae and the gravida 6+ group; it was also highest in teenage pregnancies and in those in women over 35 years of age. They raise the question as to whether the disease may be transmitted by sexual contact. Similar factors are suggested by the case recorded by Scott (1962) in which chorionic carcinoma in a woman coincided with the development of embryonal carcinoma in her husband; it was suggested that the malignant taint might have been transferred to the conceptus by the spermatozoon. Brewer (1967) knows of two successive wives to one man who in turn developed chorionic carcinoma, while Iliya *et al.* (1967) report an Eastern potentate two of whose wives developed the disease virtually simultaneously.

Considerations such as these, together with the immunological factors previously referred to, serve to emphasize our ignorance of the paternal situation in most cases of chorionic carcinoma. Yet the tumour owes half its components to the father, and it is only by a cruel biological chance that the mother has to bear its ravages. It is probable that the father's constitution holds the key to many of the problems of the

disease, and there is a great need for collection of information on the paternal situation in every case of chorionepithelioma.

Suggestions as to more specific causal factors have been advanced. It was at one time claimed that a virus presumed to be the cause of hydatidiform mole had been isolated and propagated, but Bouwdizk-Bastiaanse (1957) when he tried to confirm this work came to the conclusion that the lesions produced experimentally in chicken eggs and attributed to the virus might be due rather to chorionic hormones. Bleier (1953) reported positive serologic tests for toxoplasmosis in a patient who had suffered four consecutive hydatidiform moles. Beischer & Fortune (1968), however, in recording 29 moles with coexistent foetuses report nine twin pregnancies (three monozygotic and six dizygotic). This occurrence seems against an infective factor being important.

The possibility of a significant geographic variation in the occurrence of trophoblastic tumours came to attention through the writings of Acosta-Sison *et al.* (1951, 1955, 1964) from the Philippines. Subsequent reports suggested a similar high incidence in many Eastern and Oriental as opposed to North American and European populations. The comprehensive study organized by Iverson (1959) in Asia showed that this represented a real increase and was not due to different diagnostic criteria. Edmonds (1959b) suggested that this geographic variation might be related to the distribution of a non-selective gene, but another possibility is that it may be related to malnutrition or some other environmental factor operative in the East. McCorriston (1968) writing from Honolulu found that despite good nutrition amongst Orientals, hydatidiform mole was commoner in their racial group than among Caucasians. Hawaiians, however, though having a lower socio-economic, and presumably dietary, standard, had a lower incidence of trophoblastic disease.

Hydatidiform mole

(i) PRESENTATION

Hydatidiform mole occurs with a frequency of the order of 1:2,000 or 3,000 pregnancies in

Western countries and 1:200 or 300 in Asia (Buxton 1959; Chun *et al.* 1964a). It occurs particularly in elderly gravidae of high parity and poor social and nutritional status (Chun *et al.* 1964a). The most frequent history is of amenorrhoea of some weeks' duration, associated with the usual symptoms of pregnancy and followed by vaginal bleeding; the bleeding consists of irregular, variable losses interspersed usually with a brown discharge. Vomiting seems to be more common than in normal pregnancies and uterine cramps are frequent also. Uterine enlargement which is excessive for the calculated duration of pregnancy is the commonest physical sign, but in a small proportion of cases the uterus may be the size expected from the gestation period or smaller. Toxaemia of pregnancy occurs with a frequency which is remarkable for the early stage of pregnancy. In Chun *et al.*'s 1964a Hong Kong series 135 out of 269 cases (50%) had toxaemia. Chun *et al.* noted that toxaemia was related to the size of the uterus and implied that this was similar to the distension effect which might occur in hydramnios. From the data of Scott (1958), however, it is very much more likely that this is due to the activity of the mass of trophoblastic tissue which is present rather than the uterine distension. The detection of large luteal cysts on the ovaries could help in the diagnosis, but in practice these are rarely identifiable until after the mole has been expelled. Coppleson (1958) found them in 27% of his series. These cysts are, of course, merely a manifestation of excessive HCG stimulation on the ovaries and they may be found in association with all forms of trophoblastic neoplasia. They are to be considered in the same category as the cysts sometimes found when excessive exogenous gonadotrophin is administered in the treatment of anovulation. Like these cysts they can produce an excess of pregnanetriol excretion (Stitch *et al.* 1966) and can sometimes lead to ascites (Hooper *et al.* 1966).

Absolute confirmation of the diagnosis is obtained by the observation of a typical vesicle in the vaginal discharge. If the pregnancy has passed 18 weeks, failure to demonstrate a foetal skeleton radiologically is suggestive of mole; positive demonstration of foetal parts is said to be valuable contrary evidence, but because of the occasional occurrence of mole in association with a fully formed foetus this should not be relied upon. Assay of chorionic gonadotrophin is the most commonly employed diagnostic aid and, provided the result is interpreted with appropriate caution, can be an extremely valuable one. Delfs (1959) records a maximum level of serum chorionic gonadotrophin for normal pregnancy of the order of 500,000 international units at about 65 days, but observes that in twin pregnancies, which constitute the main diagnostic problem, the peak is higher and may be delayed; but nevertheless a drop in level does eventually occur as the second trimester of pregnancy progresses. Hobson (1955) considered a urine test positive in a dilution of 1:200 or more after 14 weeks' gestation as indicative of mole, but he mentions three moles with negative biological tests, and Coppleson (1958) records a similar case. In a later publication Hobson (1958) recorded that only 6 out of 45 cases of hydatidiform mole gave tests positive in this range, while one twin pregnancy came into the same category. It follows from these observations that gonadotrophin studies must be interpreted with the greatest caution; a series of tests giving a continued high level over a period of time is much more helpful than a single test.

Acosta-Sison (quoted by Buxton 1959) claims that she can differentiate mole from normal pregnancy in doubtful cases by passing a uterine sound gently through the cervix. If the resistance of membranes is encountered then mole may be confidently excluded. This manoeuvre clearly requires a gentleness of touch which perhaps not all gynaecologists possess! Angiography of the uterine vessels performed by means of retrograde aortic catheterization is another aid to the diagnosis of hydatidiform mole and other trophoblastic tumours (e.g. Borell & Fernstrom 1961; Begg & Stichbury 1962; Bagshawe & Wilde 1964; Hirsch & Ben-Aderet 1967). The appearances found differ from normal pregnancy and it is claimed that various grades of trophoblastic neoplasia can be differentiated (Borell *et al.* 1967). Senties *et al.* (1969) describe the use of hysterography by injection of contrast medium by the transabdominal route.

Ultrasonic echo soundings (Donald 1963; Gottesfeld *et al.* 1967) are diagnostic. Two-dimensional ultrasonograms are obtained by photographing with a polaroid camera to record the display of the echoes from a transmitting and receiving probe containing a sensitive crystal. Hydatidiform mole gives a typical 'snow-storm' appearance as compared with a normal pregnancy which gives a strong echo over the foetus (Fig. 14.8).

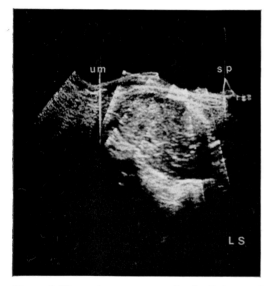

Fig. 14.8. Ultrasonic appearances at longitudinal scan of the abdomen in a case of hydatidiform mole. The umbilicus (um.) and symphysis pubis (sp.) are marked. Beneath the abdominal and uterine wall echoes is seen the multiple stippling or 'snow-storm' effect as the sound is reflected from the numerous vesicles present.

A differential diagnosis which may cause great difficulty in uniovular twin pregnancy associated with hydramnios and threatened miscarriage. In these circumstances not only may the clinical picture be classical of hydatidiform mole, but the chorionic gonadotrophin titre is greatly elevated. A pregnancy associated with fibroids which is threatening to abort may also cause confusion and the condition may simulate placenta praevia. Ultrasonic recording will readily distinguish these conditions from a mole.

Whenever trophoblastic tumour is suspected an X-ray examination of the chest should be performed, and whether this is positive or negative it should be repeated at frequent intervals for pulmonary shadows can appear and disappear with remarkable rapidity. In Coppleson's (1958) series 'benign' pulmonary metastases which resolved without therapy occurred in 2 out of 59 cases which were assessed as simple hydatidiform mole. This serves to illustrate the complexity of the clinical problem.

(ii) PROGNOSIS

The risks of hydatidiform mole are in three categories: (a) immediate from haemorrhage, sepsis or toxaemia; (b) from the occurrence of molar metastases; and (c) from subsequent development of chorionic carcinoma.

(a) Haemorrhage, sepsis and toxaemia

Treatment of all these conditions has vastly improved recently so too much reliance should not be placed on retrospective data. Chun *et al.* (1964a) recorded massive haemorrhage in 19 cases (7%) and one patient died. Sepsis is now not often a serious problem, with the range of antibiotic and chemotherapeutic agents available, while toxaemia is rarely of such severity as to cause convulsions though it may occasionally prove fatal (Acosta-Sison 1955).

(b) Molar metastases

Twenty-three out of Chun *et al'*.s (1964a) Hong Kong series of 265 clinical moles were found to be 'infiltrative' at the time of initial treatment, while 11 out of 235 cases graded as 'benign' mole later developed metastases which were not regarded as chorionepithelioma, and this incidence of approximately 5% is in accord with other figures (Park & Lees 1950; Coppleson 1958). Such metastatic lesions seem commoner in women beyond the age of 38 years who are under-nourished (Acosta-Sison 1964). It is possible that better initial management of molar pregnancies may reduce the incidence of such 'benign' metastatic lesions. Even if they do occur the prognosis with methotrexate therapy is relatively good.

(c) Chorionepithelioma

Chorionepithelioma follows a mole in from 2 to 17% cases (Hertig & Sheldon 1947; Acosta-Sison *et al.* 1951) and is the principal mortality risk. Careful follow-up to detect any trend to chorionic carcinoma at the earliest offers most to improve the prospects if followed by intensive chemotherapy (see p. 243).

(iii) MANAGEMENT

The aim of treatment is to ensure complete elimination of all the abnormal trophoblastic tissue from the maternal system. In cases where the mole is aborted spontaneously all that may be required is curettage of the uterus. Evacuation, whether spontaneous or surgical is, of course, liable to be accompanied by severe haemorrhage and possibly sepsis, and appropriate measures to control these risks in the shape of blood transfusion, oxytocic and antibiotic drugs must be prescribed as necessary. If the mole is evacuated per vaginum it is desirable to carry out a repeat curettage 7–10 days after the initial evacuation to make certain that all tissue has been removed, as at the initial evacuation the exploration may have been less than thorough for fear of rupturing the soft uterus. No treatment, of course, is required for the ovarian cysts, if present; they will regress as soon as the gonadotrophin stimulation from the trophoblast is withdrawn following evacuation of the mole.

If the condition is diagnosed yet there is no sign of spontaneous evacuation, then there are four main lines of treatment:

(a) Oxytocin stimulation
(b) Suction evacuation
(c) Abdominal hysterotomy
(d) Hysterectomy

(a) Oxytocin stimulation

This today is probably the method most widely used to secure expulsion of the mole. While oxytocin may be given by buccal, nasal or intra-muscular routes, intravenous infusion has been the most favoured in recent years. The efficacy is related to the concentration of infusion used. Loudon (1959) demonstrated that labour can be induced safely in cases where there is not a live foetus, using high concentrations, e.g. 200 units of oxytocin per litre—and as much as 350 units *in toto*. This sort of regime is effective in most cases of hydatidiform mole. In Chun *et al.*'s series oxytocin failed in only one case out of 57, and this was prior to adoption of high-concentration infusions.

Once the oxytocin has stimulated the uterus to commence the expulsion of the mole and has dilated the cervix sufficiently to permit digital or manual evacuation, then it is appropriate to complete the evacuation by this means, and finally, when the uterus is firmly contracted, gently curette the cavity with a large curette. Braga & Chun (1969), however, have recently expressed disillusionment with intravenous oxytocin induction. They suspect that it may precipitate trophoblastic embolization and thereby unfavourably affect the long-term prognosis. They, in common with Acosta-Sison (1964), Llewellyn-Jones (1967) and Tow (1966), tend to favour hysterectomy with the mole *in situ* as treatment of mole, at least in patients with a high statistical risk of subsequent trophoblastic malignancy. These include women over 40 and women with three or more children.

(b) Suction evacuation

Brandes *et al.* (1966) emptied a uterus of an undiagnosed hydatidiform mole as an abortion using a suction tube. Impressed with the meagre blood loss and other features they proceeded to use the method electively in five cases of known mole with similar good results. In view of the strong tendency for trophoblastic embolization to occur during evacuation of a mole there seems good logic behind the use of a negative-pressure method and it seems likely to be employed increasingly in the future.

(c) Abdominal hysterotomy

Prior to the use of the suction technique, surgical evacuation of the mole per vaginam was hazardous unless in the occasional case in which a mole was diagnosed while the uterus was still very small. Accordingly, abdominal hysterotomy was widely adopted. It was claimed that the uterus could be examined at the time of operation for evidence of malignancy. The attachment area, however, is always so rough and irregular that infiltration cannot be excluded by naked eye inspection. On the other hand, the uterus is left with a vulnerable scar in the event of a further pregnancy. It was also claimed that subsequent chorionic carcinoma was less likely after this method of evacuation, but this has not been substantiated and this method is now used much less frequently. There may, however, be exceptional circumstances in which it would be the method of choice.

(d) Hysterectomy

But for the single disadvantage of depriving the woman of her child-bearing function, abdominal hysterectomy with the mole in situ would constitute the ideal treatment for hydatidiform mole. Unless metastasization has already occurred, all the trophoblast is removed, and by clamping the veins from the uterus early in the procedure the operator can minimize the risk of dissemination during the operation.

The loss of reproductive function can usually be accepted in two circumstances: (i) women aged 35–40 and over (irrespective of parity), and (ii) women with three or more living children (irrespective of age). Some workers (e.g. Chun et al. 1964a, b) would extend these indications to include the cases showing infiltrative mole on the curetted specimens and those with local or pulmonary metastases attributed to infiliative mole. Scott (1964), however, found no evidence that hysterectomy was influential in the regression of metastases and, now that methotrexate is available, the removal of a uterus in the belief that this may contribute to the regression of metastases is hard to justify.

CHEMOTHERAPY

Chemotherapy has now come to be accepted as standard treatment for chorionepithelioma. More

recently it has been suggested that it has a place in other forms of trophoblastic neoplasm, including hydatidiform mole. Prophylactic chemotherapy or all hydatidiform moles was advocated (Acosta-Sison 1964; Kaku 1966) to prevent subsequent chorionic carcinoma. This, however, involves a dangerous treatment, being employed for what is only a relatively remote possibility. Fatalities from such prophylactic therapy have been reported (Braga & Chun 1969) and the method is not now favoured. Rather, it seems wise to give such therapy to particular cases that show signs of likely progression to chorionic carcinoma as described under follow-up, below.

Treatment of invasive mole, metastasizing mole or chorioadenoma destruens

The present consensus of world opinion is towards the general use of chemotherapy, as described later under chorionic carcinoma, with conservation of the uterus except in special circumstances.

FOLLOW-UP

An essential part of the management of hydatidiform mole is the follow-up for evidence of persistence of active trophoblast. A careful history particularly with regard to vaginal bleeding must be taken at each visit (Coppleson 1958) and in addition to clinical examination, it is essential that chorionic gonadotrophin (HCG) tests should be performed. At the outset it is quite in order to use the type of crude test used in the diagnosis of pregnancy provided these are positive. They measure quantities in excess of 200–500 I.U./l (Hammond et al. 1967). Once these become negative, however, or if they are negative at the outset, it is essential to use more sensitive techniques such as bio-assay on urine concentrates (Hammond et al. 1967), the mouse uterine weight method (Hertz 1967) or radio-immunoassay (Bagshawe et al. 1966; Wilde et al. 1967) which measures down to 0·001 I.U./ml. Over 30% patients with trophoblastic malignancy after hydatidiform mole will have persistently negative pregnancy tests. In interpreting these more sensitive tests it is important to remember that because of the cross-reaction between luteinizing hormone and HCG, the end-point to be aimed at is not zero but < 20 I.U./l in women with functional ovaries and < 200 I.U./l in women who have had oöphorectomy performed.

Tests should be done weekly until normal and then monthly for at least a year, for which time the patient should be advised to avoid pregnancy (Coppleson 1958; Hammond *et al.* 1967). If no further pregnancies are desired, the safe plan is to continue follow-up on a 3-monthly basis for reactivation of trophoblast may occur even after 5 years (Chun *et al.* 1964b). Such an occurrence is very rare, however, and if more children are desired it seems unreasonable to defer pregnancy for more than 1 year.

There is now general agreement that if HCG excretion levels have not reverted to normal within 6–8 weeks of evacuation of a mole that full-scale chemotherapy should be instituted (Hammond *et al.* 1967; Brewer *et al.* 1968). These are, of course, the cases of 'clinical choriocarcinoma' of Tow (1966) and 'clinical choriomatosis' of Park (1967). This type of policy seems to be preferable to prophylactic treatment with chemotherapy of all cases of hydatidiform mole. If a regime of this sort is strictly carried out Bagshawe (1967a) believes that death from postmolar chorionic malignancy could probably be eliminated—'The technology exists the clinical organization only is lacking'.

Chorionic carcinoma

(i) PRESENTATION

Marchan's (1895) original small series suggested that 50% chorionic carcinomas were preceded by hydatidiform mole, 25% by normal pregnancy and the remaining 25% by abortion or ectopic pregnancy. Subsequent studies of much larger series have confirmed this sort of distribution (e.g. Hertig 1950; Kinnunen 1952; Chan 1962a). Acosta-Sison (1962) has computed the difference in incidence between Western and Oriental communities at 1 in 30,850 pregnancies, as opposed to 1 in 1,382. It is not perhaps widely appreciated that chorionic carcinoma may present *during* rather than *after* a pregnancy; 21 (12%)

out of 175 cases recorded in the Albert Mathieu Registry presented thus. The tendency for the condition to develop with disproportionate frequency following first pregnancies has been referred to; the age may be any in the reproductive period or early postreproductive, but there is a greater incidence in relation to pregnancies in the older age group. It follows that the woman most at risk is the elderly primigravida, who has a chance of getting chorionic carcinoma 18 times higher than average (Scott 1964).

Vaginal haemorrhage is by far the commonest symptom, followed by complaint of swelling— abdominal or vaginal; amenorrhoea and chest symptoms, including dyspnoea and haemoptysis, also occur. Amenorrhoea may seem unexpected but the reason is simple. It occurs if a focus of chorionic, hormone-producing tumour is present in some site other than the uterine cavity. The hormones suppress the normal, pituitary-ovarian-uterine cycle. Akingba & Ayodesi (1966) recorded two deaths from chorionic carcinoma presenting with amenorrhoea, and 14% of Tow & Cheng's (1967) series of 80 cases had scanty or suppressed menstruation. The chest symptoms may suggest pulmonary tuberculosis, and this impression may be supported by an X-ray of the lungs simulating tuberculosis infiltration of the perivascular lymphatics (Scott 1964); in this series 13 were patients suspected of having pulmonary tuberculosis and at least three were treated on this basis. Three cases had a 'cor pulmonale' type of presentation with pulmonary hypertension (see Bagshawe & Brookes 1959). The others had frank pulmonary metastases. The frequency of intra-abdominal haemorrhage with collapse as in ruptured ectopic gestation is notable; most of the haemorrhages result from uterine perforation by the tumour tissue.

Confirmation of the diagnosis may be obtained by curettage, though this is a procedure not without risk in these cases, gonadotrophin assays, histological demonstration of the nature of metastases or by histological examination of the extirpated uterus. It is important to appreciate that the information which can be obtained by curettage is strictly limited. The most malignant tissue is likely to be in the uterine wall —this very penetration is one of the most important histological criteria and can only be assessed on hysterectomy specimens. Curettage carries with it not only the possibility of rupturing the uterus but also the considerable risk of disseminating the tumour in the blood stream. Angiography, as previously mentioned, has been used in the diagnosis of trophoblastic tumours and their extent. It seems likely to have an important place in management in the future.

(ii) PROGNOSIS

Until quite recently it was contended that chorionic carcinoma was a uniformly fatal condition, and that if a patient said to have the condition survived the diagnosis was in error (Ewing 1941), but Brewer et al. (1961) found 21 out of 147 cases in the Albert Mathieu Registry in which the diagnosis was beyond doubt yet the patients had survived for over 5 years.

The advent of chemotherapeutic agents active against trophoblast and, in particular, the folic-acid antagonist methotrexate, has revolutionized the situation. Hertz et al. (1961) reported that of 63 patients all with advanced metastatic disease and many extremely ill, 30 (48%) were free from disease as judged by clinical, radiological and hormonal assessment 6 months to 5 years after treatment. Subsequent reports have suggested that sustained remission can be achieved in 80% or more cases with vigorous and well-controlled chemotherapy (Bagshawe 1967b).

There is widespread agreement that the factor most important in prognosis, assuming the availability of full, modern, chemotherapy facilities, is the time lapse between the preceding pregnancy and diagnosis of trophoblastic malignancy. Bagshawe (1967b) considers that if this interval is less than 4 months the condition is probably always curable. It has been calculated that chorionic carcinoma metastases may have a volume doubling time of only 2–4 days, so short periods of delay in initiating treatment can make a vast difference to the bulk of tumour which has to be eradicated. Hammond et al. (1967) put it that the frequency with which sustained remission can be achieved is related to the duration of the disease and the level of gonadotrophin secretion at the outset.

CHEMOTHERAPY

It is generally accepted that chemotherapy should be the mainstay of treatment of chorionic carcinoma with surgery as a possible adjunct. While in most cancers chemotherapy is merely palliative, in chorionic carcinoma it can be curative.

The drug most used is the folic acid (pteroylglutamic acid) antagonist methotrexate (amethopterin, 4 - amino - 10 - N - methyl - pteroyl - glutamic acid). Folic acid is normally converted *in vivo* to folinic acid, the active co-enzyme, catalyzed by folinic-acid reductose. This is prevented by methotrexate. The effect of methotrexate can, in turn, be overridden by the administration of folinic acid (citrovorum factor, ^5N - hydroxyl - methyl - pteroylglutamic acid), thus short-circuiting the metabolic step involved. This folic acid–folinic acid conversion is a vital step in tissue metabolism—particularly in trophoblastic and haemopoietic tissues; in its absence there is an inability to synthesize nucleic acid and metaphase arrest of dividing cells occurs.

It is not certain whether a differential exists in the folic acid requirement of adult haemopoietic tissue and foetal trophoblast, but any such differential is small. It follows from this that the dose of folic acid antagonist which will kill all trophoblast is close to the dose which will kill the mother by complete marrow suppression. *It is fundamental to appreciate this fact, for unless the dosage is pushed near to lethal levels there can be no hope of curing established chorionic carcinoma.*

Methotrexate has been used in combination with other drugs to try to prevent drug resistance, after the fashion of combined drug therapy against bacteria. Mercaptopurine, a purine and vitamin-B_{12} antagonist, has been used as a second drug, but it is not certain whether combinations of drugs are more effective than individual drugs.

The usual type of regime advocated is oral methotrexate 5 mg three to five times daily for 5 days with, if desired, mercaptopurine 200 mg two to three times daily. Side-effects will usually have appeared before the end of the 5 days, and these usually continue to progress to a maximal level several days after completion of the course (Bagshawe 1963b). Skin rashes and gastro-intestinal tract ulceration, manifest particularly as stomatitis and proctitis, constitute the main troubles. Leucocyte depression is invariable and there is risk of complete agranulocytosis. This in turn means that infection is a serious hazard, and on these grounds it is usual to give antibiotic cover during the phase of leucocyte depression. In addition, the patients should be barrier nursed in an atmosphere of controlled asepsis. This is difficult to achieve in most general hospitals and it is with this end in view that special units have been established for the care of such cases under-going cytoxic drug therapy. Wherever possible it is desirable that patients should be transferred to such a unit for therapy. Erythropoiesis is also depressed and transfusion should be given as necessary. If facilities are available, specimens of the patient's bone marrow obtained prior to therapy may be stored under appropriate refrigerated conditions (Pegg & Trotman 1959) and then, if complete or near complete marrow suppression is caused, the autologous stored marrow can be returned to the patient.

Alopecia is another frequent and distressing side-effect; the patients can be assured that subsequent hair growth will certainly occur and be provided with a wig as a temporary measure. Jaundice associated with hepatocellular damage may occur, and liver-function tests should be performed before commencing treatment. Skin pigmentation on exposed areas occurs and the enhanced photosensitivity can readily lead to sunlight burns.

In addition to autologous marrow re-injection, a simpler corrective to over dosage with metho-trexate is the administration of folinic acid (citrovorum factor) in divided dosage of 20–40 mg per day. This, of course, not only allows renewed mitotic activity in the maternal haemopoietic tissues but also in the malignant foetal tropho-blast.

As soon as the toxic effects from the first course have subsided a further course of chemotherapy is commenced and the dosage given and the duration is adjusted in the light of the patient's reaction to the initial course. Courses are re-peated as often as necessary judged by the clinical response and the level of gonadotrophin excretion. In Bagshawe's (1963a) series the total dosage of methotrexate per course ranged from 75 to 125 mg, given over 3–5 days; the interval between courses from 5–27 days (generally 10); the number of courses in successful cases four to fourteen and the duration of treatment 2–7 months. It is desirable that two or three courses of treatment should be given *after* the HCG level has been brought down to normal limits.

There are cases in which the tumour ap-parently is, or becomes, resistant to the usual drugs and in these cases other antimitotic prepara-tions such as vinkaleukoblastine, actinomycin D, chlorambucil, 6-azauridine and nitrogen mustard may prove effective (Ross *et al.* 1962; Bagshawe 1963a).

There is some doubt as to whether metho-trexate reaches the central nervous tissues in adequate concentration, and the drug may be given intrathecally. Bagshawe (1963b) suggests that it may be best to seek neurosurgical assistance once intracranial metastases have been localized.

Sometimes, the methotrexate has been given by prolonged aortic infusion via a femoral catheter (Bagshawe & Wilde 1964). This gives a high concentration of drug in the pelvic area, and at the same time folinic acid is given systemi-cally in the hope that the unwanted effects of the methotrexate on the other sites will be diminished. By this means it may be possible to achieve more rapid regression of localized tumours with minimal toxicity. It is, of course, inapplicable to cases in which the growth has metastasized beyond the pelvis.

In addition to administering the chemotherapy, which tends to have such a debilitating influence, everything possible must be done to improve and maintain the patient's general condition by means of blood transfusion and the other general and dietetic measures.

SURGERY

Formerly, most gynaecologists faced with a case of chorionic carcinoma performed total hys-terectomy in the belief that this offered the only possible hope for the patient (Smalbraak 1957). This position no longer holds, and surgery must be assessed on the basis of how it affects the results of chemotherapy. In some cases surgery will be imperative, for example when severe haemorrhage is occurring from the uterus, but other than such obvious circumstances there is no clear evidence as to whether it is best to perform hysterectomy on women who are being treated with chemotherapy or not. Bagshawe's (1963a) opinion is that those women who have not had hysterectomy respond more favourably to chemotherapy. Chan (1962b) emphasizes the dangers of surgical manipulation causing dissemination of the malignant tissue, a fact also observed by Scott (1964). Frequently the appearance of distant metastases was apparently precipitated by surgical intervention; many of these women had symptoms which had been present for long periods and which in retrospect it could be said were due to chorionic carcinoma. All were examined for metastases prior to operation, yet in many metastases became evident shortly after the operative interference. It is, of course, not at all surprising that the surgery of trophoblastic tumours should lead to dissemination in a high proportion of cases.

To operate or not is a matter on which the clinician must, at present on slender evidence, make his own decision in each individual case; in general it can be said that if metastases are not demonstrable, rational arguments can be advanced both for and against hysterectomy, but the present trend is towards surgical non-intervention unless some emergency indication arises. Lewis *et al.* (1966b) put the situation clearly by saying that the major role of surgery is to combat complications temporarily in order to allow the patient to live long enough to respond to the chemotherapy. It is possible, by analogy with the small doses of antibacterial drugs required to prevent sub-acute bacterial endocarditis when a septic lesion is being treated surgically in a patient with valvular disease of the heart, that relatively small doses of cytotoxic therapy should prevent metastases forming compared with the dose needed to eliminate metastases once they have formed. A dose of 10 mg of methotrexate per day for 3 or 4 days commenced on the morning of the operation —curettage, biopsy or hysterectomy—would probably be adequate to prevent

metastases yet not seriously interfere with postoperative recovery. Lewis *et al.* (1966a) report using 80% of a full toxicity dose in relation to surgery. They conclude that the chemotherapy did not interfere with wound healing or cause other postoperative complications.

HORMONE CONTROL

Whatever form of therapy be employed, its success should be assessed not merely by the clinical response but particularly by the alteration in gonadotrophin level. After remission has been obtained it is important that regular checks be made by gonadotrophin assay in order that any recrudescence of trophoblastic activity may be treated as soon as it occurs.

IMMUNOLOGICAL IMPLICATIONS OF THERAPEUTIC RESPONSE

There is no clear answer as to why chemotherapy is so effective in trophoblastic malignancy. One possibility is that the peculiar immunologic situation supports the antagonistic influence of the cytotoxic drugs. Lewis (1967) carried out lymphocyte transformation studies to try to get information on this but with inconclusive results. He does consider that a low percentage transformation prior to treatment in patients with metastatic disease if associated with a normal response to phytohaemagglutinin implies a relatively poor prognosis. Davis (1967) studied the behaviour of human chorionic carcinoma transplanted to Syrian hamsters, some of which had immunological suppression with antilymphocytic serum. This group had a higher tumour incidence and tumour volume and longer tumour survival. In view, however, of the depressant effect which cytotoxic therapy has on the body defence mechanism, it would be surprising if this turned out to be the reason for chemo-therapy's success.

It is of purely historic interest that just at the time when the efficacy of methotrexate became established, immunotherapy was being tried. This was based on the observations by Schopper & Pliess (1949) and Schuster (1952) of the resemblance biologically and in terms of behaviour between chorionic carcinoma and inoculation tumours. Doniach *et al.* (1958) thought that as 50% of the conception's, and therefore the trophoblast's, genes were paternal, it was probable that any maternal antibody effect would be directed against antigens contributed by the father. Accordingly, they considered that a stronger effect might be obtained if the mother's reactivity against these paternal factors could be stimulated. They attempted to do this by means of injecting paternal leucocytes, and later demonstrated such an effect by grafting paternal skin which was rejected much more rapidly than that of an unrelated donor. Sufficient success was obtained with this apparently logical form of therapy to suggest the value of an extended trial but as the new antimetabolites had a demonstrably more impressive effect, this was never done. Occasional cases of use of this therapy have, however, been recorded after chemotherapy has failed (e.g. Cinader *et al.* 1961). It is interesting to speculate how much the pursuit of this fascinating therapeutic approach, had fate allowed it, would have stimulated progress in related fields of human immunology.

CURRENT PROBLEMS AND FUTURE TRENDS

The most fundamental problem is to discover the ultimate cause of abnormal trophoblastic growths. As it becomes evident that particular categories of pregnant women in certain parts of the world have a special tendency to develop these conditions, so does it become likely that the precise cause will be discovered. Through the geographic, demographic, biochemical and immunological studies currently being undertaken it is to be hoped that the aetiological mechanism will be elucidated and that it will prove to be one against which practical remedial action can be taken.

Until then perfection of methods of treatment is required. It is hoped that drugs will be developed which will inhibit the trophoblast without at the same time jeopardizing the life of the mother. In the meantime, this risk will be minimized by measures to achieve early diagnosis and by the development of specialized isolation units to diminish the chance of exogenous infection during leucopenia. Centralization of cases in special units is an essential for the future, not only for the reasons mentioned above, but also in order that all the investigative resources available can be brought to bear on as many cases as possible, and thus ensure that our knowledge advances.

REFERENCES

ACOSTA-SISON H. (1955) *Philipp. J. Surg. Obstet. Gynec.* **10**, 61.
ACOSTA-SISON H. (1962) *Philipp. J. Cancer*, **4**, 197.
ACOSTA-SISON H. (1964) *Am. J. Obstet. Gynec.* **88**, 634.
ACOSTA-SISON H. & BAJO-PANLILIO H. (1951) *J. Philipp. med. Ass.* **27**, 652.
AKINGBA J.B. & AYODEJI E.A. (1966) *J. Obstet. Gynaec. Br. Commonw.* **73**, 153.
ALLEN A.C. (1962) *The Kidney: Medical and Surgical Diseases*, 2nd edn. New York, Grune & Stratton.
Annotation (1962) *Br. med. J.* ii, 465.
ARIAS-STELLA J. (1954) *A.M.A. Archs. Path.* **58**, 112.
ATTWOOD H.D. & PARK W.W. (1961) *J. Obstet. Gynaec. Br. Commonw.* **68**, 611.
BAGGISH M.S., WOODRUFF J.D., TOW S.H. & JONES H.W. (1968) *Am. J. Obstet. Gynec.* **102**, 362.
BAGSHAWE K.D. (1963a) *Br. med. J.* ii, 1303.
BAGSHAWE K.D. (1963b) In *Modern Trends in Gynaecology*, Vol. 3 (edited by R.J. Kellar). London, Butterworths, p. 38.
BAGSHAWE K.D. (1967a) *Proc. R. Soc. Med.* **60**, 240.
BAGSHAWE K.D. (1967b) *Br. med. J.* ii, 178.
BAGSHAWE K.D. & BROOKS W.D.W. (1959) *Lancet*, i, 653.
BAGSHAWE K.D. & WILDE C.E. (1964) *J. Obstet. Gynaec. Br. Commonw.* **71**, 565.
BAGSHAWE K.D., WILDE C.E. & ORR A.H. (1966) *Lancet*, i, 1118.
BARBER M. & OKUBADEJO O.A. (1965) *Br. med. J.* ii, 735.
BARDAWIL W.A., MITCHELL G.W., McKEOGH R.P. & MARCHANT D.J. (1962) *Am. J. Obstet. Gynec.* **84**, 1283.
BARDAWIL W.A. & TOY B.L. (1959) *Ann. N.Y. Acad. Sci.* **80**, 197.
BEGG A.C. & STICHBURY P.C. (1962) *Aust. N.Z. Jl. Obstet. Gynaec.* **2**, 65.
BEISCHER N.A. & FORTUNE D.W. (1968) *Am. J. Obstet. Gynec.* **100**, 276.
BEISCHER N.A., FORTUNE D.W. & FITZGERALD M.G. (1967) *Br. med. J.* iii, 476.
BENDER S. (1956) *J. Obstet. Gynaec. Br. Commonw.* **63**, 400.
BERLIND M. (1960) *Obstet. Gynec., N.Y.* **16**, 51.
BEVIS D.C.A. (1951) *Lancet*, ii, 207.
BLEIER W. (1953) *Geburtsh. Frauenheilk.* **13**, 57.
BORELL U. & FERNSTRÖM I. (1961) *Acta radiol.* **56**, 113.
BORELL U., FERNSTROM I., MOBERGER G. & OHLSON L. (1967) *Lancet*, i, 144.
BOUWIDIZK-BASTIAANSE J.H.H. VON (1957) Doctoral dissertation. Leyden, The Netherlands.

BRAGA C. & CHUN D. (1969) In *Modern Trends in Gynaecology*, Vol. 4 (edited by R.J. Kellar). London, Butterworths, p. 137.

BRANDES J.M., GRUNSTEIN S. & PERETZ A. (1966) *Obstet. Gynec., N.Y.* **28**, 689.

BREWER J.I. (1967) Personal communication.

BREWER J.I. & GERBIE A.B. (1966) *Am. J. Obstet. Gynec.* **94**, 692.

BREWER J.I., GERBIE A.B. & ECKMAN T.R. (1967) In *Transcript of the Fourth Rochester Trophoblast Conference* (edited by C.J. Lund & J.W. Choate). Rochester, New York, p. 6.

BREWER J.I., RINEHART J.J. & DUNBAR R.W. (1961) *Am. J. Obstet. Gynec.* **81**, 574.

BREWER J.I., TOROK, ELIZABETH E., WEBSTER A. & DOLKART R.E. (1968) *Am. J. Obstet. Gynec.* **101**, 557.

BROWN A.D.G. & ROBERTSON J.G. (1968) *J. Obstet. Gynaec. Br. Commonw.* **75**, 92.

BUXTON C.L. (1959) *Ann. N.Y. Acad. Sci.* **80**, 121.

CARR D.H. (1965) *Obstet. Gynec., N.Y.* **26**, 308.

CARR D.H. (1969) *Obstet. Gynec., N.Y.* **33**, 333.

CHAN D.P.C. (1962a) *Br. med. J.* ii, 953.

CHAN D.P.C. (1962b) *Br. med. J.* ii, 957.

CHUN D., BRAGA C., CHOW C. & LOK L. (1964a) *J. Obstet. Gynaec. Br. Commonw.* **71**, 180.

CHUN D., BRAGA C., CHOW C. & LOK L. (1964b) *J. Obstet. Gynaec. Br. Commonw.* **71**, 185.

CINADER B., RIDER W.D. & WARWICK O.H. (1961) *Can. med. Ass. J.* **84**, 306.

COPPLESON M. (1958) *J. Obstet. Gynaec. Br. Commonw.* **65**, 238.

COX L.W., COX R.I. & SKIPPER J.S. (1964) *Aust. N.Z. J. Obstet. Gynaec.* **5**, 160.

DAVIS R.C. (1967) In *Transcript of the Fourth Rochester Trophoblast Conference* (edited by C.J. Lund & J.W. Choate). Rochester, New York, p. 186.

DELFS E. (1959) *Ann. N.Y. Acad. Sci.* **80**, 125.

DE NAVASQEZ S. (1938) *J. Path. Bact.* **46**, 47.

DIXON H.G. & STEWART D.B. (1960) *Br. med. J.* ii, 1103.

DONALD I. (1963) *Br. med. J.* ii, 1154.

DONALD I. (1968) *Br. med. Bull.* **24**, 71–5.

DONIACH I., CROOKSTON J.H. & COPE T.I. (1958) *J. Obstet. Gynaec. Br. Commonw.* **65**, 553.

DOUGLAS C.P. (1963) *Br. med. J.* ii, 838.

DROEGEMUELLER W., TAYLOR E.S. & DROSE V.E. (1969) *Am. J. Obstet. Gynec.* **103**, 694.

DRURY K.A.D. (1960) *J. Obstet. Gynaec. Br. Commonw.* **67**, 455.

EDMONDS H.W. (1959a) *Ann. N.Y. Acad. Sci.* **80**, 196.

EDMONDS H.W. (1959b) *Ann. N.Y. Acad. Sci.* **80**, 86.

EWING J.R. (1941) *Neoplastic Diseases*, 4th edn. Philadelphia, Saunders.

FREITAS J. DE (1969) Personal communication.

Geneva Conference (1966) *Cytogenetics, Basel*, **5**, 361.

GOLDZIEHER J.W. (1964) *J. Am. med. Ass.* **188**, 651.

GOTTESFELD K.R., TAYLOR S., THOMPSON H.E. & HOLMES J. (1967) *Obstet. Gynec., N.Y.* **30**, 163.

GRADY H.G. (1959) *Ann. N.Y. Acad. Sci.* **80**, 99.

GRANT A. (1962) *Clin. Obstet. Gynec.* **5**, 861.

GREENHILL J.P. (1956) *Am. J. Obstet. Gynec.* **72**, 516.

GREENHILL J.P. (1966) In *Year Book of Obstetrics and Gynaecology*, 1966–67 (edited by J.P. Greenhill). Chicago, Year Book Medical Publishers, p. 52.

HALBRECHT I. (1957) *Obstet. Gynec., N.Y.* **10**, 73.

HALBRECHT I. & KOMLOS L. (1968) *Obstet. Gynec., N.Y.* **31**, 173.

HAMMOND C.B., HERTZ R., ROSS G.T., LIPSETT M.B. & ODELL W.D. (1967) *Obstet. Gynec., N.Y.* **29**, 224.

HARDISTY R.M. & INGRAM G.I.C. (1965) *Bleeding Disorders: Investigations and Management*. Oxford, Blackwell Scientific Publications.

HERTIG A.T. (1950) In *Progress in Gynecology*, Vol. II (edited by J.V. Meigs & S.H. Sturgis). New York, Grune & Stratton, p. 372.

HERTIG A.T. & EDMONDS H.W. (1940) *Archs. Path.* **30**, 260.

HERTIG A.T. & SHELDON W.H. (1947) *Am. J. Obstet. Gynec.* **53**, 1.

HERTZ R. (1967) In *Choriocarcinoma* (edited by J.F. Holland & M.M. Hreshchyshyn). U.I.C.C. Monograph Series No. 3. New York, Springer, p. 66.

HERTZ R., LEWIS J. Jr. & LIPSETT M.B. (1961) *Am. J. Obstet. Gynec.* **82**, 631.

HERTZ R., ROSS G.T. & LIPSETT M.B. (1963) *Am. J. Obstet. Gynec.* **86**, 808.

HIBBARD B.M. (1964) *J. Obstet. Gynaec. Br. Commonw.* **71**, 529.

HIRSCH M. & BEN-ADERET N. (1967) *Obstet. Gynec., N.Y.* **30**, 498.

HOBSON B.M. (1955) *J. Obstet. Gynaec. Br. Commonw.* **62**, 354.

HOBSON B.M. (1958) *J. Obstet. Gynaec. Br. Commonw.* **65**, 253.

HODGKINSON C.P., THOMPSON R.J. & HODARI A.A. (1964) *Clin. Obstet. Gynec.* **7**, 349.

HOOPER A.A., MASCARENHAS, ANITA M. & O'SULLIVAN J.V. (1966) *J. Obstet. Gynaec. Br. Commonw.* **73**, 854.

HRESHCHYSHYN M.M., BOGEN B. & LOUGHRAN C.H. (1961) *Am. J. Obstet. Gynec.* **81**, 302.

HRESHCHYSHYN M.M., NAPLES J.D. Jr. & RANDALL C.L. (1965) *Am. J. Obstet. Gynec.* **93**, 286.

IFFY L. (1963) *Proc. R. Soc. Med.* **56**, 1098.

ILIYA F.A., WILLIAMSON S. & AZAR H.A. (1967) *Cancer, N.Y.* **20**, 144.

IVERSON L. (coordinator) (1959) *Ann. N.Y. Acad. Sci.* **80**, 178.

JACKSON C.E., MANN J.D. & SCHULL W.J. (1969) *Nature, Lond.* **222**, 445.

JAMES W.H. (1962) *J. Obstet. Gynaec. Br. Commonw.* **69**, 606.

JEFFCOATE T.N.A. (1955) *J. Obstet. Gynaec. Br. Commonw.* **62**, 214.

JEFFCOATE T.N.A. (1967) *Principles of Gynaecology*, 3rd edn. London, Butterworths.

JENSEN K.G. (1960) *Dan. med. Bull.* **7**, 55.

JONES G.S. (1968) In *Progress in Infertility* (edited by S.J. Behrman & R.W. Kistner). London, Churchill, p. 299.

KADOWAKI J., THOMPSON R.I., ZUELZER W.W., WOOLEY P.V., BROUGH A.J. & GRUBER D. (1965) *Lancet*, ii, 1152.

KAKU M. (1966) *Am. J. Obstet. Gynec.* **95**, 590.

KERR M.G. (1968) *J. Reprod. Fert.* Supplement No. 3, 49.

KERR M.G. & RASHAD M.N. (1966) *Am. J. Obstet. Gynec.* **94**, 322.

KINNUNEN O. (1952) *Annls. Chir. Gynaec. Fenn.* **41** (Supplement 3), 1.

KLEINER G.J. & ROBERTS T.W. (1967) *Am. J. Obstet. Gynec.* **99**, 21.

KLOPPER A. & MacNAUGHTON M. (1965) *J. Obstet. Gynaec. Br. Commonw.* **72**, 1022.

KNOTH M., HESSELDAHL H. & LARSEN J.F. (1967) In *Transcript of the Fourth Rochester Trophoblast Conference* (edited by C.J. Lund & J.W. Choate). Rochester, New York, p. 93.

LASH A.F. & LASH S.R. (1950) *Am. J. Obstet. Gynec.* **59**, 68.

LATHROP J.C. & BOWLES G.E. (1968) *Obstet. Gynec., N.Y.* **32**, 81.

LEVINE P. & KOCH E.A. (1954) *Science, N.Y.* **120**, 239.

LEWIS J. (1967) In *Transcript of the Fourth Rochester Trophoblast Conference* (edited by C.J. Lund & J.W. Choate). Rochester, New York, p. 205.

LEWIS J., GORE H., HERTIG A.T. & GOSS D.A. (1966a) *Am. J. Obstet. Gynec.* **96**, 710.

LEWIS J., KETCHAM A.S. & HERTZ R. (1966b) *Cancer, N.Y.* **19**, 1517.

LEWIS J., WHANG J., NAGEL B., OPPENHEIM J.J. & PERRY S. (1966c) *Am. J. Obstet. Gynec.* **96**, 287.

LLEWELLYN-JONES D. (1967) *Am. J. Obstet. Gynec.* **99**, 589.

LOUDON J.D.O. (1959) *J. Obstet. Gynaec. Br. Commonw.* **66**, 277.

MACDONALD R.R. (1963) *J. Obstet. Gynaec. Br. Commonw.* **70**, 580.

MacNAUGHTON M.C. (1961) *J. Obstet. Gynaec. Br. Commonw.* **68**, 789.

MacNAUGHTON M.C. (1962) *Lancet*, ii, 484.

MAKINO S., SASAKI M.S. & FUKUSCHIMA T. (1964) *Lancet*, ii, 1273.

MALL F.P. (1917) *Am. J. Anat.* **22**, 27.

MARCHAND F. (1895) *Mschr. Geburtsh. Gynäk.* **1**, 419, 513.

MARSHALL B.R. & EVANS T.N. (1967) *Obstet. Gynec., N.Y.* **29**, 759.

MARTINEZ J.T., FERNANDEZ G. & VAZQUEZ-LEON H. (1966) *Obstet. Gynec., N.Y.* **27**, 296.

McCORRISTON C.C. (1968) *Am. J. Obstet. Gynec.* **101**, 377.

McDONALD I.A. (1957) *J. Obstet. Gynaec. Br. Commonw.* **64**, 346.

MEDAWAR P.B. (1960) *The Future of Man.* (The Reith Lectures.) London, Methuen.

MITCHELL G.W. & BARDAWIL W.A. (1966) *Vth World Congress of Fertility and Sterility.* Excerpta Medica Foundation International Congress Series, 109, 79. (Quoted by Kerr, 1968.)

MOGENSEN B. & KISSMEYER-NIELSEN F. (1968) *Lancet*, i, 721.

MORRIS J.A. (1967) In *Advances in Obstetrics and Gynaecology* (edited by S.L. Marcus & C.C. Marcus). Vol. 1. Baltimore, Williams & Wilkins, p. 150.

MOSSANEN A. (1963) Personal communication.

NOVAK E. (1957) In *Trophoblastic Growths* (edited by J. Smalbraak). Amsterdam, Elsevier, p. xi.

OVERSTREET E.W. (1964) *Pacif. Med. Surg.* **72**, 289.

PACHI A. & ANGELONI G. (1963) *Quad. Clin. ostet. ginec.* **18**, 1028.

PALMER R. & LACOMME M. (1948) *Gynéc. Obstét.* **47**, 905.

PARK W.W. (1959) *Ann. N.Y. Acad. Sci.* **80**, 152.

PARK W.W. (1967) *Proc. R. Soc. Med.* **60**, 235.

PARK W.W. & LEES J.C. (1950) *Archs. Path.* **49**, 205.

PEGG D.E. & TROTMAN R.E. (1959) *J. clin. Path.* **12**, 477.

PERETZ A., GRUNSTEIN S., BRANDES J.M. & PALDI E. (1967) *Am. J. Obstet. Gynec.* **98**, 18.

PHILLIPS L.L., SKRODELIS V. & QUIGLEY H.J. (1967) *Obstet. Gynec., N.Y.* **30**, 350.

RACE R.R. & SANGER R. (1969) *Br. med. Bull.* **25**, 99.

RAMIREZ-SOTO E., GONZALEZ-LOYA J.P., VALENZUELA-LOPEZ S., DELGADO-URDAPILLETA J. & CASTELAZO-AYALA L. (1969) *Obstet. Gynec., N.Y.* **33**, 409.

RAPPAPORT F., RABINOVITZ M., TOAFF R. & KROCHIK N. (1960) *Lancet*, i, 1273.

REID D.E. (1967) *J. Am. med. Ass.* **199**, 805.

Report on Confidential Enquiries into Maternal Deaths in England and Wales 1961–1963 (1966). London, Her Majesty's Stationery Office.

Report on Confidential Enquiries into Maternal Deaths in England and Wales, 1964–1966 (1969). London, Her Majesty's Stationery Office.

ROBINSON E., SHULMAN J., BEN-HUR N., ZUCKERMAN H. & NEUMAN Z. (1963) *Lancet*, i, 300.

ROCK J. & HERTIG A.T. (1942) *Am. J. Obstet. Gynec.* **44**, 973.

ROSS G.T., STOLBACH L.L. & HERTZ R. (1962) *Cancer Res.* **22**, 1015.

ROVINSKY J.J. & GUSBERG S.B. (1967) *Am. J. Obstet. Gynec.* **98**, 11.

RUBOVITZ F.E., COOPERMAN N.R. & LASH A.F. (1953) *Am. J. Obstet. Gynec.* **66**, 269.

RUSSELL K.P., MAHARRY J.F. & STEHLY J.W. (1955) *J. Am. med. Ass.* **157**, 15.

SANDMIRE H.F. & RANDALL J.H. (1959) *Obstet. Gynec., N.Y.* **14**, 227.

SCHIFFER M.A. (1963) *Am. J. Obstet. Gynec.* **86**, 264.

SCHIFFER M.A. (1969) *Obstet. Gynec., N.Y.* **33**, 729.

SCHLEGEL R.J., NEU R.L., LEAO J.C., FARIAS E., ASPILLAGA M.J. & GARDNER L.I. (1966) *Cytogenetics, Basel*, **5**, 430.

SCHOPPER W. & PLIESS G. (1949) *Virchows Arch. path. Anat. Physiol.* **317**, 347.

SCHUSTER A. (1952) *Arch. Gynaec.* **181**, 477.

SCHWARTZMANN G. (1937) *Phenomenon of Local Tissue Reactivity.* New York, Hoeber.

SCOTT, J.S. (1958) *J. Obstet. Gynaec. Br. Commonw.* **65**, 689.

SCOTT J.S. (1962) *Am. J. Obstet. Gynec.* **83**, 185.

SCOTT J.S. (1964) Unpublished data.

SCOTT J.S. (1968) *Br. med. Bull.* **24**, 32.

SENTIES L., PERDOMO A. & LUNA R. (1969) *Obstet. Gynec., N.Y.* **33**, 352.

SHEARMAN R.P. (1968) In *Progress in Infertility* (edited by S.J. Behrman & R.W. Kistner). London, Churchill, p. 767.

SHEARMAN R.P. & GARRETT W.J. (1963) *Br. med. J.* i, 292.

SHEEHAN H.L. & MOORE H.C. (1952) *Renal Cortical Necrosis and the Kidney of Concealed Accidental Haemorrhage.* Oxford, Blackwell Scientific Publications.

SHIRODKAR V.N. (1953) *J. Obstet. Gynaec, India,* **3**, 287.

SHORT R.V., WAGNER G., FUCHS A.R. & FUCHS F. (1965) *Am. J. Obstet. Gynec.* **91**, 132.

SLOCUMB J.C. & LUND C.J. (1969) *Am. J. Obstet. Gynec.* **104**, 421.

SMALBRAAK J. (1957) *Trophoblastic Growths.* Amsterdam, Elsevier.

SMITH K., BROWNE J.C.M., SHACKMAN R. & WRONG O.M. (1968) *Br. med. Bull.* **24**, 49.

SMITH M., MACNAB J. & FERGUSON-SMITH M.A. (1969) *Obstet. Gynec., N.Y.* **33**, 313.

STITCH S.R., LEVELL M.J., OAKEY R.E. & SCOTT J.S. (1966) *Lancet,* i, 1344.

STRASSMAN E.O. (1966) *Fert. Steril.* **17**, 165.

STRASSMAN P. (1907) *Zentbl. Gynäk.* **31**, 1322.

TACCHI D. & SNAITH L. (1962) *J. Obstet. Gynaec. Br. Commonw.* **69**, 608.

TAYLOR A.I. & POLANI P.E. (1965) *Lancet,* i, 1226.

TAYLOR M.A. (1969) *Science, N.Y.* **164**, 723.

TIETZE C. (1966) *Br. med. J.* ii, 302.

TOMINAGA T. & PAGE E.W. (1966) *Am. J. Obstet. Gynec.* **96**, 305.

TOW W.S.H. (1966) *J. Obstet. Gynaec. Br. Commonw.* **73**, 544.

TOW W.S.H. & CHENG W.C. (1967) *Br. med. J.* i, 521.

VAUGHN D.L., BERSENTES T., KIRSCHBAUM T.H. & ASSALI N.S. (1967) *Am. J. Obstet. Gynec.* **99**, 208.

VLADOV E., IVANOV I., ANGELOV A.C. & RAKIVOSKA I. (1965) *Gynaecologia, Basel,* **159**, 54.

WAGATSUMA T. (1965) *Am. J. Obstet. Gynec.* **93**, 743.

WARBURTON D. & FRASER F.C. (1961) *J. Obstet. Gynaec. Br. Commonw.* **68**, 784.

WEBSTER H.D., BARCLAY D.L. & FISCHER C.K. (1965) *Am. J. Obstet. Gynec.* **92**, 23.

WEI P.Y. (1968) *Am. J. Obstet. Gynec.* **101**, 776.

WILDE C.E., ORR A.H. & BAGSHAWE K.D. (1967) *J. Endocr.* **37**, 23.

WILKINS L. (1960) *J. Am. med. Ass.* **172**, 1028.

WILLIAMS E.A. (1969) *Lancet,* i, 1093.

WREN B.A.G. & VOS G.H. (1961) *J. Obstet. Gynaec. Br. Commonw.* **68**, 637.

WYNN R.M. (1967) In *Transcript of the Fourth Rochester Trophoblast Conference* (edited by C.J. Lund & J.W. Choate). Rochester, New York, p. 113.

WYNN R.M. & DAVIES J. (1964a) *Am. J. Obstet. Gynec.* **88**, 618.

WYNN R.M. & DAVIES J. (1964b) *Am. J. Obstet. Gynec.* **90**, 293.

WYNN R.M. & HARRIS J.A. (1967) *Am. J. Obstet. Gynec.* **99**, 1125.

WYPER J.F.B. (1962) *Br. med. J.* i, 273.

CHAPTER 15

ANTEPARTUM HAEMORRHAGE

Antepartum haemorrhage (A.P.H.) is still one of the gravest obstetric emergencies, though thanks to improved obstetric care the maternal mortality due to haemorrhage has dropped from 220 in the 3 year period 1952–4 to 68 in 1964–6. Approximately two-thirds of these were due to antepartum haemorrhage, 7% of the total deaths (*Report on Confidential Enquiries into Maternal Deaths in England and Wales*, 1969). To maintain and improve upon this advance it is essential to be continually alert to the possibility of severe A.P.H. and familiar with the appropriate action to deal with the problems that arise. Unlike postpartum haemorrhage, which is always preceded by the adequate warning mechanism of labour, A.P.H. often occurs without warning. With dramatic suddenness a pregnant patient can become exsanguinated to the point of death. The perinatal mortality is also considerable, and in the *British Perinatal Mortality Survey* (Butler & Bonham 1963) 17·6% of the perinatal deaths were associated with A.P.H.

DEFINITION AND CLASSIFICATION

A.P.H. is customarily defined as haemorrhage from the genital tract after the twenty-eighth week of pregnancy but before delivery of the baby. The 28 week limit is a completely arbitrary one related to the legal definition of viability of the child. Precisely the same pathological types of haemorrhage can occur before 28 weeks.

Severe bleeding is relatively rare then, but when it does occur the treatment is often less intensive as it is regarded lightly as a mere threatened abortion (Baker & Dewhurst 1963; Kinch *et al.* 1969).

Cases are sometimes divided according to the anatomic origin of the blood into 'true' A.P.H. when from the placental site and 'false' when from lower in the genital tract. This is a distinction which is not of practical importance initially, for it must be assumed that every vaginal blood loss before delivery is coming from the placenta and appropriate action taken. If it eventually becomes clear that the condition is not one of the classical types of placental bleeding, then consideration of other possible pathology, particularly cervical, becomes appropriate.

Edward Rigby (1775) distinguished between *inevitable* A.P.H. occurring in association with a low-lying placenta and chance or *accidental* occurrence of haemorrhage from a normally situated placenta. This was a great advance in obstetric thinking. Unfortunately, 'inevitable' haemorrhage came to be spoken of as *placenta praevia*, while 'accidental' retained its name. The term 'accidental' when not opposed to 'inevitable' suggests a relationship to trauma, which is practically never present, and this has led to confusion of thought.

The current tendency is to use the clearly descriptive term '*abruptio placentae*' introduced by Couvelaire to describe the serious form of haemorrhage which may occur from the decidual attachment of a normally implanted placenta. This type of haemorrhage is self-extending, the accumulated blood clot causing more separation, and thus more haemorrhage, until the edge of the placenta is reached. After this, blood can escape via the potential space between decidua and chorionic membrane to the cervix. Haemorrhage may also occur from the edge of a normally situated placenta 'marginal haemorrhage' (Fig. 15.1). This was formerly referred to as 'revealed

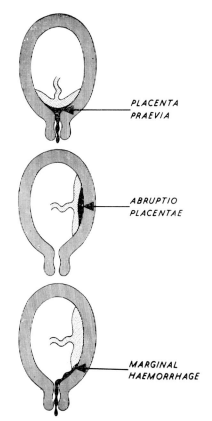

PLACENTA
PRAEVIA

ABRUPTIO
PLACENTAE

MARGINAL
HAEMORRHAGE

Fig. 15.1. A diagrammatic representation of the three anatomical types of A.P.H. (With acknowledgement to the Editor of British Medical Journal.)

accidental haemorrhage'. It does not have the same inherent process of automatic self-extension as does abruptio placentae, as it occurs from the edge of the chorionic plate. This occurs particularly frequently in association with an extrachorial (or circumvallate) type of placenta

(Scott 1960). Placenta praevia is frequently subdivided into four grades: I, lateral—when the placenta extends on to the lower segment; II, marginal—when it extends to the edge of the internal cervical os; III, complete (acentric)—when it covers the internal os but is not centrally placed; and IV, complete (centric)—covering the internal os and centrally placed. An extremely rare type of haemorrhage is that from a ruptured foetal vessel—vasa praevia bleeding. If suspected, the diagnosis can be confirmed by testing the blood for foetal haemoglobin by the Kleihauer or other technique.

The practical classification of antepartum haemorrhage as it presents to the clinician (Scott 1964) is rather different, cases falling into one of three categories:

(1) Abruptio placentae.
(2) Placenta praevia.
(3) 'Indeterminate A.P.H.'.

'Indeterminate' signifies a collective clinical category. It covers marginal haemorrhage, which has no positive features, and also other cases which cannot with confidence be diagnosed as abruptio placentae or placenta praevia. In some of these the nature and origin of the bleeding later becomes clear. It may be proved by clinical or investigative means that there is a placenta praevia, or on inspection of the placenta after delivery that there has been localized abruption. The other possibilities are that it has been a marginal haemorrhage or a 'false A.P.H.'. In this last category come local cervical and vaginal lesions and cases in which excessive 'show' has been interpreted as A.P.H.

Incidence

The frequency of A.P.H. varies with the age, parity and social status of the population, but a total incidence of about 3% is not unusual [3·1% in the Perinatal Mortality Survey total series (Butler & Bonham 1963)]. Cases are approximately equally divided between the three clinical categories: abruption, placenta praevia and indeterminate.

Clinical picture

The presentation in most cases merely accords with the definition—bleeding from the genital tract after 28 weeks. Lack of pain is typical of placenta praevia and if painless haemorrhage is associated with the physical signs of placenta praevia, such as a presenting part which is difficult to palpate or displaced, the diagnosis is fairly certain.

Abruptio placentae, however, may not be associated with revealed bleeding at the outset. The patient, usually of high parity, develops pain over the uterus and this steadily increases in severity. There is no periodicity as with the pain of labour. Faintness and collapse may occur. There are usually signs of shock; the uterus is extremely hard and tender; it does not relax; foetal parts are difficult to palpate and the heart inaudible. Unless the attendant is alert to the possibility the diagnosis may be missed until revealed bleeding eventually occurs. By this time the patient's general condition may have deteriorated seriously.

Antenatal care in relation to A.P.H.

The scope for specific prevention of antepartum haemorrhage is limited, but antenatal care has much to offer towards reducing the risks should such a complication occur. Blood-group determination is a routine procedure of obvious relevance. Other important measures include: (a) booking for hospital confinement patients judged to be particularly liable to antepartum haemorrhage; (b) prevention of anaemia; (c) suspecting the diagnosis of placenta praevia before serious antepartum haemorrhage has occurred; (d) early detection of pre-eclampsia; and (e) avoidance of trauma.

Booking for hospital confinement

If a woman booked for hospital confinement suffers an antepartum haemorrhage, either she will be admitted directly to the hospital or, if her doctor is summoned, he will be in a position to make appropriate arrangements immediately with the hospital at which she is booked. If hospital booking is not arranged the delay in ad-mission is likely to be longer, and even slight delays may prove fatal. Women who qualify for hospital booking in this connection include those who have had previous antepartum haemorrhages (most studies show a tendency to recurrence), those of parity higher than four, and those over 35 years of age. In the high-parity group the risk of antepartum haemorrhage is very great—over 10% in O'Sullivan's (1963) series. A high proportion of deaths due to abruptio placentae and placenta praevia occur in women who are having their fifth or subsequent confinement.

Prevention of anaemia

It is self-evident that the greater the degree of anaemia the lower is the ability to withstand haemorrhage. There is a strong suspicion that many maternal fatalities from antepartum haemorrhage occur in women who have been allowed to become needlessly anaemic in pregnancy. The exact policy of management of pregnancy anaemia is of less importance than the efforts which should be made to detect it at its earliest stage. Without entering into the arguments as to whether iron therapy should be given routinely in pregnancy or should always be combined with folic acid it is relevant to bear in mind the evidence suggesting a relationship between folic-acid deficiency and placental abruption (see p. 253).

Early suspicion of placenta praevia

It is now accepted that the frequency with which the presence of placenta praevia is suspected before haemorrhage has occurred is an index of the quality of antenatal care. The findings which should arouse suspicion are: (a) an abnormal or unstable foetal lie in late pregnancy—a persistent transverse lie is of the greatest significance; (b) a presenting part which has an abnormal relationship to the pelvis—for example, held high above the brim (by a central placenta praevia), deviated from the midline (by a lateral placenta praevia), pushed forward over the symphysis (by a posterior placenta praevia), or rendered difficult to define through the anterior abdominal wall (by an anterior placenta praevia). These physical signs become more significant the longer they persist, and if they have been elicited independently at two or more separate antenatal examinations in the last 6–8 weeks of pregnancy then it is usually appropriate to take steps to exclude placenta praevia by some form of placentography. If this cannot be done then hospital admission is indicated. If the physical signs are very definite it may be advisable to treat the case as one of placenta praevia on this basis alone and regard placentography as superfluous.

It is well known that with placenta praevia major bleeding is frequently preceded by small 'warning haemorrhages'. These haemorrhages or 'shows' may occur before 28 weeks and therefore be classified as threatened miscarriages. Particularly if they are repeated, they should be viewed with great suspicion and appropriate steps taken to exclude placenta praevia.

It is widely appreciated that vaginal examination is extremely hazardous in cases of possible placenta praevia, as it may provoke separation of the placenta with massive haemorrhage. Surprisingly, it is often not realized that a rectal examination is even more dangerous. Vaginally, with only the thin glove covering the examiner's finger, there is the possibility that the placenta may be felt before it is seriously disturbed. On rectal examination the gloved finger is covered by rectal wall, vaginal wall and the intervening fascia. This makes it virtually certain that the placenta will not be detected before it is separated and serious bleeding provoked.

Early detection of pre-eclampsia

Early detection of pre-eclampsia is a *sine qua non* of good antenatal care. Traditional obstetric teaching is that there is an aetiological relationship between abruptio placentae and hypertensive states and it is implied that toxaemia predisposes to abruption. If this is true, early detection of pre-eclampsia followed by appropriate management of the toxaemic process might be expected to result in a reduction in the incidence of abruption. It is remarkable, however, how infrequently abruption is seen in patients in whom a prior diagnosis of pre-eclampsia has

been made, and the existence of a significant aetiological relationship has been seriously questioned (Hibbard 1962; Hibbard & Jeffcoate 1966).

Avoidance of trauma

External version is a form of trauma in the antenatal period which occasionally cause antepartum haemorrhage. Opinion varies widely as to its place in modern obstetrics, but most obstetricians agree that, if done, it should only be attempted gently on unanaesthetized patients. If the manipulations prove difficult or cause pain, the attempt should be abandoned immediately.

Folic-acid deficiency

It has been suggested (Hibbard & Hibbard 1963; Hibbard 1964; Hibbard & Jeffcoate 1966; Streiff & Little 1967) that folic-acid deficiency is closely related to occurrence of abruptio placentae. On this basis it would seem logical to expect that administration of folic-acid supplements from an early stage in pregnancy might reduce the incidence. This does not appear to be the case (Willoughby 1967). It may be that the tendency to abruptio is due to some metabolite deficiency of which occurs *pari passu* with that of folic acid. Alternatively, it may be that folic acid exerts its fundamental ill-effect at such an early stage that commencing supplements at the time pregnancy is normally diagnosed is too late to be effective. The evidence, however, is conflicting and some workers (e.g. Pritchard *et al.* 1969) have failed to confirm a relationship between abruptio and folate deficiency.

Avoidance of sudden uterine decompression

A rare cause of abruptio placentae is the sudden release of liquor amnii in cases of severe polyhydramnios. The abrupt reduction in the area of the uterine wall to which the placenta is attached may result in placental separation in a manner similar to that which occurs in the third stage of normal labour after the baby has been expelled. Abdominal amniocentesis with a fine-bore needle and slow release of the liquor in appropriate cases may help to prevent this.

Emergency management

On first seeing a case of antepartum haemorrhage it may be possible to conclude at once that the cause is abruptio placentae or placenta praevia, but frequently the nature will be in doubt. Deliberation on causation is not a useful exercise. Whatever the mechanism the most important thing from the patient's point of view is to ensure that at the earliest possible moment she is brought within the availability of a blood transfusion service, an operating theatre, and all the other resources of a fully equipped maternity hospital. In most cases the correct procedure is to give a sedative-analgesic such as pethidine 100–200 mg by intramuscular injection and arrange immediate transfer to hospital by ambulance. It must be appreciated that the only type of hospital appropriate to receive such cases is a *major* maternity hospital with full facilities, including resident staff.

In some cases where the initial blood loss has been heavy and has produced maternal shock the question may arise whether the Obstetric Flying Squad (O.F.S.) should attend. It is hard to give categorical advice about this for, unlike the situation with postpartum haemorrhage, the amount of benefit which the patient may obtain from the O.F.S. service is strictly limited. For example, with the torrential haemorrhage which sometimes occurs with placenta praevia, Caesarean section at the earliest opportunity is life-saving; attempts at blood replacement prior to this may be futile and the delay can jeopardize life. In abruptio placentae, blood transfusion is unlikely to make a great contribution to improving the patient's condition unless combined with amniotomy and other measures designed to bring about speedy termination of the abruption process, which can only be performed satisfactorily in hospital.

For these reasons it is often preferable to get the patient into hospital immediately rather than delay until she has been attended by the O.F.S. At Leeds Maternity Hospital, out of 186 consecutive attendances by the O.F.S. only four were for antepartum haemorrhage. During the same period 137 antepartum haemorrhage cases were admitted directly to the hospital—without a fatality.

Management after admission

No matter what the type of haemorrhage, blood replacement by transfusion is always indicated if there has been more than a slight loss or if there is any degree of shock. Blood should immediately be obtained for cross-matching and confirmation of grouping. Whether to delay administration of blood until a full cross-match has been completed, to give uncross-matched group O Rhesus-negative blood or blood of the patient's group, is a matter for decision by the individual clinician in charge of a particular case. Very rarely in cases of any severity will it be justifiable to await completion of the full cross-match. Other measures depend upon the type of haemorrhage. In the cases where there is urgency about action the diagnosis is, fortunately, almost always obvious.

(a) ABRUPTIO PLACENTAE

In the case with frank clinical abruption the appropriate treatment in hospital is (1) liberal blood transfusion; (2) sedation; (3) vaginal amniotomy; and (4) oxytocin infusion.

The first and third measures are the most important. Amniotomy encourages the onset of labour and reduces the uterine tension which may contribute to two of the complications of abruption most liable to cause maternal death. These are (a) *renal cortical necrosis*, possibly mediated through the co-called uterorenal reflex, and (b) *coagulation disorder*. Blood transfusion is also instrumental in preventing ischaemic renal damage by maintaining the blood pressure and circulating red cell mass, and, of course, it ensures that the patient is in a better position to withstand any postpartum haemorrhage. In recent years blood has been given on a much more liberal scale in cases of abruption, and it is probable that this has contributed to the greatly improved maternal mortality figures. Only 22 maternal deaths occurred from this cause in England and Wales 1963–6, compared with 78 in the 1952–4 period.

The mere fact that abruption can be confidently diagnosed clinically means that there has been considerable concealed blood loss and justifies the transfusion of a minimum of 1 l of blood regardless of the patient's general condition. The blood pressure is a notoriously unreliable guide to the extent of blood loss in these cases, as a severe degree of vasospasm or capillary bed blockage is a common response to the abruption, leading to elevated readings. Attention has recently been drawn to the fact that the best answer to the problem of securing adequate blood replacement rests in the use of central venous pressure (C.V.P.) monitoring as a guide (O'Driscoll & McCarthy 1966; Muldoon 1969). The average C.V.P. in the third trimester is around 10 cm of water. This may be taken as an appropriate figure up to which patients should be transfused. Using this as a guide Muldoon (1969) found that 80% more blood was transfused, that the postnatal haemoglobin concentration was higher and that the incidence of postpartum obliguria was less. It is also possible that this policy may result in a lower incidence of coagulation disorder, for there is evidence that fibrinogen conversion is more likely to occur in the presence of hypovolaemic shock (Hardaway 1966).

With renal failure in mind, all patients with placental abruption should have careful records kept of fluid balance. Abruptio is by far the most important haemorrhagic cause of obstetric renal failure (Barry et al. 1964; Smith et al. 1968) and all the evidence suggests that hypovolaemia is the major aetiological factor. The treatment of established renal failure is a separate problem (see Chapter 19) which has to be tackled after the haemorrhage has been arrested, and other than avoiding fluid overloading is not a concern during the period of active bleeding.

Coagulation disorder should always be in the clinician's mind when managing a case of abruptio. The nature of the coagulation disturbance is discussed in Chapter 18. The precise mechanisms may seem of purely academic interest, but this is far from being the case, as rational clinical management should be related to the mechanism.

Ideally, the clinician would also like to know which changes in the coagulation situation are harmful and which represent a beneficial function of the defence system. Unfortunately, this is not possible. The clinician is also faced with the problem that the process is developing so swiftly that results obtained from even the most rapidly efficient laboratories may bear no relationship to the situation existing when they become available.

Fibrinogen replacement was at one time recommended whenever coagulation failure became manifest, then fibrinolysis inhibitors such as epsilonaminocaproic acid or Trasylol (FBA Pharmaceuticals Ltd.), a polypeptide extracted from animal parotids, were advised. More recently it has been suggested that it may be wise to avoid specific coagulation therapy (Scott 1968; Bonnar et al. 1969; Basu 1969, personal communication.)*

It is not sufficient that a particular therapeutic weapon should be capable of changing a pathological disorder such as the coagulation state found with abruptio placentae; *it must be reasonably certain that the change is likely to be beneficial.* This is not the case with regard to the therapies referred to. If fibrinogen is given during the thromboplastic or consumptive phase it will undergo conversion to fibrin, with possible capillary blockage. Giving it at this stage may be compared with 'attempting to rebuild a house on fire rather than summon the fire-brigade' (Scott 1968). Conversely, giving fibrinolytic inhibitors may interfere with the mechanism by which nature is preventing intravascular occlusion (Bonnar et al. 1969).

A wise approach in relation to the coagulation disorder of abruptio seems to be to concentrate on the haemorrhage *per se.* If the uterus is encouraged to empty itself rapidly, if blood replacement is adequate, then coagulation disorder is much less likely to occur (Basu 1969; Bonnar et al. 1969). The mere fact that the blood is in an incoagulable state should not be taken as

*It will be seen that the opinions expressed here on treatment are similar but not precisely the same as those expressed on p. 298, Chapter 18. Clearly, there is still room for differences of opinion in this field. Both points of view are printed to give the reader a more general impression.

an indication for therapy. The one situation in which it does become of specific relevance is the rare occasion when Caesarean section is contemplated (see below). In a surgical procedure the haemostasis is much more dependent upon the coagulation mechanism.

Caesarean section has possibly a small, though hotly disputed, place in the management. The baby is nearly always dead in the severe case and for the mother vaginal delivery is safer than Caesarean section. If the child is still alive it may sometimes be felt that a Caesarean section would be justified in the remote hope that it will survive. Unfortunately, most such babies if born alive die in the early neonatal period, often displaying the respiratory distress syndrome of the newborn. Hibbard & Jeffcoate (1966) calculated that in their series three baby lives *might* have been saved if 60 mothers had been exposed to the risks of Caesarean section, which are considerable in these circumstances. If Caesarean section is considered then it will usually be advisable to proceed only if the clotting is effective. If coagulation failure is present, the question of the risks of specific coagulation therapy must be weighed against the risks of not performing the operation.

In general, the best therapy—as well as the best prophylaxis in relation to coagulation failure —is liberal blood transfusion. If it can be obtained, fresh blood would be ideal (Bonnar *et al.* 1969), though the problems of achieving this, even with an efficient transfusion service, are considerable, and blood transfusion should certainly not be delayed to await the availability of *fresh* supplies.

Usually, with the measures outlined, vaginal delivery is rapidly achieved. The most dangerous stage of labour for any patient is the third, and this is particularly true if there has been significant antepartum bleeding of any type; the management described later must be rigorously applied. Frequently, the placenta has been completely separated by the abruption, and foetus and placenta are delivered spontaneously. After vaginal delivery the arrest of bleeding from the placental site is mainly dependent on myometrial retraction, and liberal doses of oxytocics should always be given.

(b) PLACENTA PRAEVIA

If the case is obviously one of placenta praevia the management depends upon the duration of the pregnancy and the extent of the haemorrhage. If the pregnancy is of less than 37–38 weeks' duration, the usual aim is to allow it to continue until the baby has grown to a size which will give a reasonable chance of survival *ex utero*. This policy, introduced by Macafee (1945, see also Macafee 1960) has done more than anything else to reduce the foetal mortality in placenta praevia, which was mainly due to prematurity. The Macafee regime requires, for safety, strict adherence to several vital principles. From the time of the initial diagnosis of placenta praevia until delivery the patient *must* remain in a fully equipped and staffed maternity unit. This means one in which *blood is immediately available* for transfusion, in which full facilities for Caesarean section exist and in which there is, continuously throughout the 24 hr, a member of staff available to perform the operation should it prove necessary. All steps necessary must be taken to correct any anaemia that may be present, in view of the likelihood of further haemorrhage.

This all sounds simple, but in practice it can tax to the limits the combined resources of obstetrician, midwives, family doctor and social service staff. The lives of such patients can be saved by the whole-hearted cooperation of all concerned towards keeping the patient contented during the period of what seems to her unreasonable detention in hospital while feeling perfectly well.

Once the pregnancy has advanced to 37–38 weeks, or if the first haemorrhage occurs then, opinion differs as to whether vaginal examination under anaesthesia should be performed followed by Caesarean section if a major degree of placenta praevia is encountered, or a decision made on the available evidence without vaginal examination to perform elective Caesarean section. In minor degrees of placenta praevia, vaginal amniotomy may be sufficient to allow the head to control any bleeding in labour by pressing on the placental edge. It must be appreciated, however, that Caesarean section is usually the ultimate method of delivery of choice whenever there is more than a very minor degree of placenta praevia and the baby is alive. Macafee *et al.* (1962) attribute the improved perinatal mortality in their hospital, at least in part, to a greater use of Caesarean section.

The Caesarean section done for placenta praevia is much more hazardous than that done for many other indications. It always tends to be haemorrhagic and a number of different dilemmas may present which demand great experience in their solution. It follows that the experience of the operator is of great importance. If severe haemorrhage is taking place it may be wise to open the abdomen with a vertical midline incision rather than the normally preferable Pfannenstiel. Seconds *may* be vital. The next decision is whether to perform the conventional lower segment operation or elect for the classical uterine incision. The inexperienced operator may be daunted by the massive vessels sometimes evident over a lower segment on which the placenta is implanted. The experienced operator, however, will rarely regard the classical incision with its consequent disadvantages as justified. If it is felt that the time-factor should influence the decision in this regard, the patient's condition must indeed be parlous.

The next problem, if the lower segment approach is adopted, is how to deal with the placenta if it is encountered deep to the incision. If the placenta is incised with a view to delivering the baby through it, loss of foetal blood may occur and, of course, even a small quantity of this may prove fatal to the baby. On the other hand, if attempts are made to deliver the baby round the placental edge difficulties may arise which can lead to foetal death from asphyxia. As long as both hazards are borne in mind it is unlikely that either will give rise to serious trouble.

After delivery of the baby, removal of the placenta from the lower segment may prove difficult. As a consequence of the relative lack of decidua, marked adherence tends to occur. Bleeding at this juncture may be profuse. The policy is to proceed expeditiously with placental removal and closing of the uterine incision. Often a remarkable degree of haemostasis is secured with one continuous, astraumatic suture. If control of bleeding proves difficult despite precise suturing, pressure with warm packs, oxytocics,

etc., then a time will come when hysterectomy has to be contemplated. This is a decision concerning which no precise rules can be formulated. The experienced operator will know when further attempts are likely to hazard the mother's life and he will opt for the drastic action of hysterectomy before she is *in extremis*. Manœuvres such as bipolar version and traction with Willett's forceps on the foetal scalp have little place in modern obstetrics where hospital facilities are available.

Hibbard (1969b), dealing with a relatively poor population in Los Angeles, reports little improvement in the perinatal mortality with the use of expectant management—24·9% compared with 24·7%. This is not general experience, and Gordon's (1969) figure of 5% perinatal mortality (corrected for foetal abnormality) gives a better idea of what this approach has to offer in modern obstetrics. Macafee *et al.* (1962) reporting the Belfast figures for 1953–60 give an uncorrected foetal loss of 11·1%.

(c) INDETERMINATE A.P.H.S

In cases in which the nature of the haemorrhage is not clear in the initial stages, the blood loss is not usually of an extent to cause serious concern. In all cases the usual assessment is made of the general condition and blood is taken for grouping, cross-matching and haemoglobin determination. Further action depends on the maturity of the pregnancy. If this is 37–38 weeks, induction of premature labour by vaginal amniotomy is usually regarded as wise as the baby will almost certainly be sufficiently developed to survive. The chances are that the placenta has been to some extent damaged by the haemorrhage and its functional reserve reduced; there is also the possibility that further, more serious, haemorrhage will occur. If there is the slightest suspicion that the bleeding may be due to placenta praevia, the amniotomy should be done in theatre under anaesthesia. A blood transfusion should be running and full preparations made for immediate Caesarean section should this be necessary.

In other cases, in which the maturity is less than 37 weeks, conservative management is indicated. The patient is kept strictly at rest in bed in the hope that bleeding will cease, which it usually does. Any anaemia is corrected and after the patient has been free from bleeding for 4 or 5 days an attempt is made to determine the source of bleeding. The possibility of a degree of placenta praevia is always the first thing to be excluded, and this can sometimes be done with moderate certainty by abdominal palpation. Usually, some form of placentography is necessary to confirm the placental position.

If placenta praevia is diagnosed or the suspicion of it cannot be excluded, then management is that outlined under placenta praevia. If, on the other hand, the placenta can be demonstrated convincingly on the upper segment of the uterus, it *may* be considered safe to allow the patient home. Before doing so a speculum may be gently passed to exclude a cervical cause for the bleeding. Be it noted that speculum examination is *not* recommended initially. Exposure of the pregnant cervix is difficult and could easily result in further bleeding if the placenta should be low-lying; also, a cervical polyp or vascular erosion may be observed and the haemorrhage attributed to this, though the real source of the trouble has been a placenta praevia.

If this policy is implemented it must be remembered that the baby is still particularly at risk. Regular tests of placental function may be helpful and it will usually be appropriate to deliver the child when reasonable maturity is reached.

The commonest source of bleeding in the cases in this category proves to be the edge of a normally implanted placenta. In the American literature this is frequently referred to as 'haemorrhage from the marginal sinus', an apparently suitable description but for the single drawback that the weight of anatomical opinion is against the existence of such a structure. This type of haemorrhage is particularly common if the placenta is circumvallate or 'extrachorial' (Fig. 15.2) (Scott 1960). In these placentae there is a fibrous ring round the edge of the chorionic plate which retracts, often causing repeated haemorrhages. This history of these repeated haemorrhages is, in fact, highly suggestive of placenta praevia, but the physical signs are

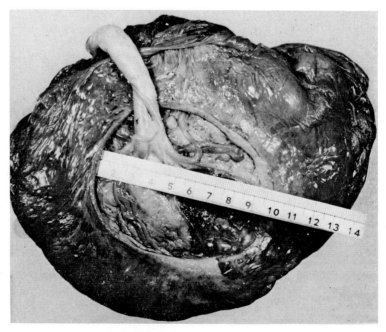

Fig. 15.2. A circumvallate (or extrachorial) placenta with which A.P.H. is particularly common. The fold at the edge of the chorionic plate, indicated by the ruler, is the site at which bleeding tends to occur.

absent. Though the condition may be suspected antepartum, the diagnosis cannot be made with certainty until the placenta has been delivered and inspected. Fortunately, haemorrhages from this condition carry little risk to mother or baby.

MANAGEMENT OF THE THIRD STAGE

'It's the A.P.H. that weakens and the P.P.H. that kills' is a true aphorism. Not only is the woman who has suffered an A.P.H. likely to be relatively anaemic when she reaches the third stage of labour, there are also several factors which make it much more likely that she will have a postpartum haemorrhage. If she has suffered a placental abruption the whole uterus, owing to intramuscular haemorrhages or a circulating inhibitor of the myometrium (Basu 1969), may not contract and retract efficiently to control the blood loss. In addition, should this happen, or should there be any lacerations, bleeding may be aggravated by failure of blood coagulation. If the A.P.H. was due to placenta praevia, the postpartum bleeding may be excessive owing to the fact that the lower segment to which the placenta has been attached contracts and retracts less efficiently than does the upper segment.

The third-stage management is therefore critical in the case of the patient who has suffered an A.P.H. By administration of an oxytocic drug such as 0·5 mg ergometrine maleate intravenously with the birth of the trunk, supplemented by oxytocin 5 units if necessary, every effort is made to obtain maximal uterine contraction. If need be, these drugs may be repeated several times. At the same time an intravenous infusion should be running and cross-matched blood available so that, if postpartum haemorrhage occurs, blood administration can be commenced immediately.

With regard to cases showing coagulation disorder, the arguments for withholding specific coagulation therapy cease to be as strong after delivery, as the consumptive phase of the disorder is presumably over. In the relatively small proportion of cases with coagulation failure which develop postpartum haemorrhage (30%, Basu 1969) fibrinolytic inhibitors and/or fibrinogen may be given.

If despite these measures haemorrhage occurs and continues, bimanual compression of the uterus may be attempted after excluding traumatic causes for the bleeding. The most important factor in the control of postpartum blood loss is uterine retraction; redoubling of the efforts to secure this usually pays the best dividends.

Very large doses of oxytocic drugs intravenously may be effective when the traditional doses have failed, and occasionally a hot intra-uterine douche has a miraculous effect. Very rarely, hysterectomy may have to be resorted to as the only means of controlling the haemorrhage, but in the presence of coagulation failure this is fraught with danger.

Placental localization

The one area in relation to placenta praevia and indeterminate A.P.H. in which there have been significant developments in recent years is that of placental localization. The profusion of methods in existence make it clear that there is as yet no ideal one available. The current situation is reviewed in detail by Gordon (1969). The techniques most used involve X-rays, radioactive isotopes, ultrasonic scanning or thermography.

X-RAY TECHNIQUES

One advantage of the several methods of localizing the placenta by X-rays is that pictures of the foetal skeleton are obtained. Knowledge of gross skeletal abnormalities may have a bearing on the ultimate management of the case.

Positional method

In this technique films are taken which may show deviation of the presenting part from its natural position in relation to the pelvis (Reid 1951). More detailed information may sometimes be obtained by injecting radio-opaque material into the bladder or amniotic cavity (cystography and amniography) and by manual pressure on the presenting part in an attempt to close any apparent gap between it and the pelvis.

This method is not reliable until the later weeks of pregnancy, when it is least needed. It does not positively localize the placenta; it merely shows that there is or is not a space between foetal and pelvic bony landmarks which *could* be occupied by a placenta praevia of normal thickness. A placenta of abnormal thinness can easily be missed. The technique reveals very little that it is not possible to elicit by means of careful abdominal palpation.

Soft tissue method

In this technique X-rays of low penetration are used to demonstrate the placental shadow (Reid 1949; Whitehead 1953; Hartley 1959). In some cases in late pregnancy this is aided by the fact that the placenta has undergone calcification. In some hands it is a reliable method of placental localization and, unlike the positional technique, gives positive localization. It is, however, dependent on first-class radiographic technique and if this is lacking, as is all too often the case, it merely involves useless exposure to radiation.

Aortography

Following retrograde injection of radio-opaque dye through a catheter into the aorta, direct demonstration of the arterial blood passing through the placenta may be obtained by X-rays taken a short interval later (Fig. 15.3). This method was at one time painful and hazardous, but retrograde aortographic catheterization is now a routine procedure in X-ray departments and with modern media injections are virtually painless. There is positive demonstration of the placenta and where *precise* localization is important or where localization is required particularly early in pregnancy (Sutton 1966; Herlinger 1968). It may be indicated if ultrasonics are not available.

ISOTOPE PLACENTAL LOCALIZATION

By the injection of a radioactive isotope into the maternal circulation, followed by counting the intensity of radiation over the uterus, the site of the placenta may be localized. Most techniques utilize albumen labelled with radioactive iodine

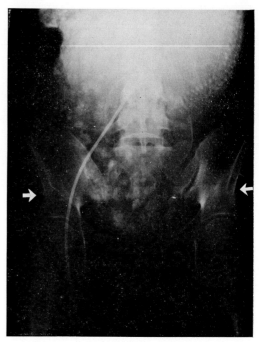

Fig. 15.3. Aortographic placentography with angled view showing a major degree of right-sided placenta praevia. The shadow of the rods indicating the uterine intersegmental junction lies between the arrows.

(^{132}I) or technetium (99^mTc). These isotopes have half-lives of $2\frac{1}{2}$ and 6 hr, respectively. The radiation involved is minimal and very much less than that with X-ray methods.

Aiers *et al.* (1969) found a high level of accuracy using ^{132}I-human serum albumen (HSA). Kohorn *et al.* (1969) report similar observations; the isotope they used was 99^mTc. Jacoby *et al.* (1969) also report favourably on the 99^mTc HSA technique. Kinch *et al.* (1969) avoided labelling HSA by using technetium-99^m in the form of pertechnetate (99^mTcO$^-_4$). This is eluted direct from the parent radiomolybdenum and is always available for emergencies. The pertechnetate is freely diffusible, but with a gamma-ray scintillation camera scans can be obtained within 8 min of intravenous injection. By this technique the placenta is readily visualized in the second trimester—a most important point as it is the early placentography which is of most help.

Hibbard (1969a) described a simple isotope technique using 99^mTc and a light-weight, hand-held scintillation counter and a portable ratemeter. It can be performed by resident obstetric staff with minimal technical knowledge and the radiation dose is low. A complete apparatus for bedside use may be bought for approximately £250; many of the other techniques involve the use of much more expensive apparatus.

ULTRASONIC TECHNIQUES

The value of ultrasound in obstetric diagnosis is now generally accepted. This technique is extremely valuable for placental localization, not only in cases of antepartum haemorrhage but to identify the placental site prior to amniocentesis in cases such as rhesus incompatibility and when there is doubt about foetal maturity.

Ultrasound methods were introduced into obstetrics and gynaecology by Donald in Glasgow in 1958. The name is given to sound-waves of a frequency greater than 16,000 Hz which is the upper audible limit. In medical practice, however, frequencies of $1\frac{1}{2}$–$2\frac{1}{2}$ million Hz are employed. Very high-frequency sound can be transmitted as a beam like a beam of light, unlike audible sound which radiates outwards from its source in a circular fashion. This beam of ultrasound can be projected in any desired direction and like a beam of light it can be reflected, refracted or absorbed. Solids and fluids, such as those present in various body tissues, allow the passage of ultrasound waves, although attenuating them to a varying extent depending upon the consistency of the tissue concerned; each tissue then has what is called its 'specific acoustic impedance'.

The ultrasound beam is reflected from interfaces between tissues of different acoustic impedance, and by suitably displaying the reflected beam information can be obtained about, for instance, the depth and nature of a swelling under review. As the ultrasound beam is greatly attenuated by air, some means of excluding air from between the probe emitting the wave and the body surface must be used; this is achieved by applying a layer of oil to the skin.

In clinical use the ultrasound beam is pulsed. Donald uses 300 pulses per second each of the very short duration of $1\frac{1}{2}$–2 μs, after which there is a 3 ms interval before the next pulse of ultrasound. Accordingly, in 1 hr of scanning there are only 2 sec of sound passage. The reflected sound is displayed in one of two ways: (1) 'A' *scan*, which is uni-dimensional, in which the reflected beam is recorded as a verticle deflection on the horizontal time base sweep of the cathode-ray tube, and (2) '*B*' *scan* in which the reflected wave is represented as a dot corresponding to the position of the echo. In 'B' scanning the probe emitting the ultrasound is moved linearly across the body surface. In 'compound B' scanning the probe is rocked through an arch so that many more tissue interfaces are crossed by the sound; finally, an 'echogram' of the relevant area is produced (Figs. 15.4 and 15.5).

Ultrasound placentography compares favourably with other methods so far as the correct recognition of placental site in cases of antepartum haemorrhage is concerned. Donald & Abdulla (1968) and Campbell & Kohorn (1968) report a 94% accuracy, and Gottesfeld *et al.* (1966) one of 98%. The method has, however, advantages over others in its simplicity, its lack of any discomfort or danger to the patient, and in the extremely clear picture it gives in most cases of the precise relationship of the lowest point of the placenta to the internal os. An important part of the technique is to carry out the ultrasonic scan with the patient's bladder full, so that this relationship between the lowest point of the placenta and the cervix can readily be appreciated (Figs. 15.4 and 15.5).

Ultrasound techniques are valuable in accurate measurement of the foetal biparietal diameter (Chapter 11), the prediction of maturity (Chapter 11), the diagnosis of hydatidiform mole (Chapter 14) and in the early recognition of multiple pregnancy (Chapter 22).

THERMOGRAPHY

Another technique which has been experimented with is thermography—the pictorial representation of body-heat patterns. Results, however, are not encouraging in some hands (Millar 1966), though others have reported reasonable success (Birnbaum & Kliot 1965).

Placenta   Head

(a)

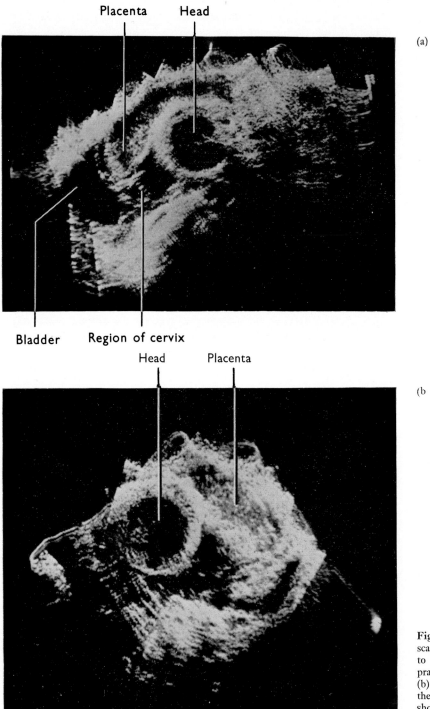

Bladder   Region of cervix

Head   Placenta

(b

Fig. 15.4.(a) Longitudinal
scan of lower abdomen
to demonstrate placenta
praevia (anterior type 2).
(b) Transverse scan above
the symphysis pubis
shows placenta displacing
head.

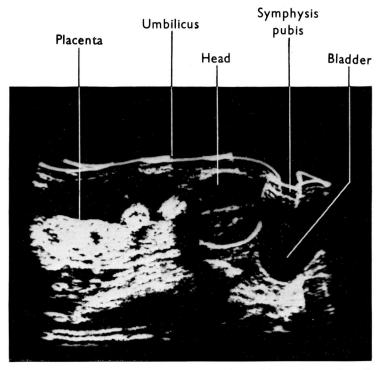

Fig. 15.5. A longitudinal scan of the abdomen to demonstrate a placenta lying on the posterior wall of the upper uterine segment above the head.

CONCLUSION

Current attitude to placentography is that it has a place in selected cases and that probably more than one technique should be available. In many cases a sufficiently accurate localization will be obtained by one of the techniques which, from the patient's point of view, is relatively simple, such as ultrasonic or radio-isotope scanning. The latter gives an indirect impression of the placental situation, the former being far more precise.

REFERENCES

BAKER J.L. & DEWHURST C.J. (1963) *J. Obstet. Gynaec. Br. Commonw.* **70**, 1063.

BARRY A.P., CARMODY M., WOODCOCK J.A., O'DWYER W.F., WALSH A. & DOYLE G. (1964) *J. Obstet. Gynaec. Br. Commonw.* **71**, 899.

BASU H.K. (1969) *J. Obstet. Gynaec. Br. Commonw.* **76**, 481.

BIRNBAUM S.J. & KLIOT D.A. (1965) *Obstet. Gynec., N.Y.* **26**, 515.

BONNAR J., McNICOL G.P. & DOUGLAS A.S. (1969) *J. Obstet. Gynaec. Br. Commonw.* **76**, 799.

BUTLER N.R. & BONHAM D.G. (1963) *Perinatal Mortality.* Edinburgh and London, E. & S. Livingstone.

CAMPBELL S. & KOHORN E.I. (1968) *J. Obstet. Gynaec. Br. Commonw.* **75**, 1007.

DONALD I. (1968) *Br. med. Bull.* **24**, 71.

DONALD I. & ABDULLA U. (1968) *J. Obstet. Gynaec. Br. Commonw.* **75**, 993.

GORDON H. (1969) *Modern Trends in Obstetrics*, Vol. 4. London, Butterworths, p. 257.

GOTTESFELD K.R., THOMPSON H.E., HOLMES J.H. & TAYLOR E.S. (1966) *Am. J. Obstet. Gynec.* **96**, 538.

HARDAWAY R.M. (1966) *Syndromes of Disseminated Intravascular Coagulation.* Illinois, Thomas.

HARTLEY J.B. (1959) *Proc. R. Soc. Med.* **52**, 559.

HERLINGER H. (1968) *Clin. Radiol.* **19**, 59.

HIBBARD B.M. (1962) *J. Obstet. Gynaec. Br. Commonw.* **69**, 282.

HIBBARD B.M. (1964) *J. Obstet. Gynaec. Br. Commonw.* **71**, 529.

HIBBARD B.M. (1969a) *Br. med. J.* iii, 85.
HIBBARD B.M. & HIBBARD E.D. (1963) *Br. med. J.* ii, 1430.
HIBBARD B.M. & JEFFCOATE T.N.A. (1966) *Obstet. Gynec.,
    N.Y.* 27, 155.
HIBBARD L.T. (1969b) *Am. J. Obstet. Gynec.* 104, 172.
JACOBY H., ARNOT R.N., JEYASINGH K., GLASS H.I. &
    BROWNE J.C.M. (1969) *Obstet. Gynec., N.Y.* 33, 358.
KINCH R.A.H., ROSENTHALL L. & COLLINS J.A. (1969)
    In *Controversy in Obstetrics and Gynaecology* (edited by
    D.E. Reid & T.C. Barton). Philadelphia, Saunders, p. 55.
KOHORN E.I., WALKER R.H.S., MORRISON J. & CAMPBELL S.
    (1969) *Am. J. Obstet. Gynec.* 103, 868.
MACAFEE C.H.G. (1945) *J. Obstet. Gynaec. Br. Commonw.*
    52, 313.
MACAFEE C.H.G. (1960) *Lancet*, i, 449.
MACAFEE C.H.G., MILLAR W.G. & HARLEY G. (1962)
    J. Obstet. Gynaec. Br. Commonw. 62, 203.
MILLAR K.G. (1966) *Br. med. J.* i, 1567.
MULDOON M.J. (1969) *J. Obstet. Gynaec. Br. Commonw.*
    76, 225.
O'DRISCOLL K. & MCCARTHY J.R. (1966) *J. Obstet.
    Gynaec. Br. Commonw.* 73, 923.

O'SULLIVAN J.F. (1963) *J. Obstet. Gynaec. Br. Commonw.*
    70, 158.
PRITCHARD J.A., WHALLEY P.J. & SCOTT D.E. (1969)
    Am. J. Obstet. Gynec. 104, 388.
REID F. (1949) *Br. J. Radiol.* 22, 81.
REID F. (1951) *Proc. R. Soc. Med.* 44, 703.
*Report on Confidential Enquiries into Maternal Deaths in
    England and Wales*, 1964–66 (1969) London. Her
    Majesty's Stationery Office.
RIGBY E. (1775) *An Essay on the Uterine Haemorrhage.*
    London, Johnson.
SCOTT J.S. (1960) *J. Obstet. Gynaec. Br. Commonw.*
    67, 904.
SCOTT J.S. (1964) *Br. med. J.* i, 1163, 1231.
SCOTT J.S. (1968) *Br. med. Bull.* 24, 32.
SMITH K., BROWNE J.C.M., SHACKMAN R. & WRONG O.M.
    (1968) *Br. med. Bull.* 24, 49.
STREIFF R.R. & LITTLE A.B. (1967) *New Engl. J. Med.*
    276, 776.
SUTTON D. (1966) *Br. J. Radiol.* 39, 47.
WHITEHEAD A.S. (1953) *Br. J. Radiol.* 26, 401.
WILLOUGHBY M.L.N. (1967) *Br. J. Haemat.* 13, 503.

CHAPTER 16

PRE-ECLAMPSIA, ECLAMPSIA, HYPERTENSION AND CHRONIC RENAL DISEASE

Pre-eclampsia, eclampsia, hypertension and chronic renal disease have been considered together for some years in obstetric writing. This is not to say that we cannot distinguish one from the other, although it is probable that pre-eclampsia, hypertension and chronic renal disease cannot always be distinguished on ordinary clinical grounds. These conditions are considered together because they share the very important clinical features of raised blood pressure and proteinuria; because they may be present in association with each other, as when pre-eclampsia becomes superimposed upon hypertension; and because their effect upon the course of pregnancy and the welfare of the mother and child is similiar.

These disorders constitute at the present time one of the major threats to the mother's life during pregnancy, labour and the puerperium; a glance at Table 29.1 on p. 448 will confirm this. Moreover, they constitute one of the chief contributors to perinatal mortality (p. 453). Eclampsia is a desperate, acute, obstetric emergency. It seldom occurs now, but when it does it is generally preceded by signs of pre-eclampsia occurring either *de novo* or in association with pre-existing hypertension; the duration of pre-eclamptic changes may be very short or of several weeks' duration.

A brief word must be said about terminology. These conditions had been referred to for years as toxaemias of pregnancy. This term is still frequently used either to refer in general terms to hypertensive disorders or to refer more specifically to pre-eclampsia. There is no certain evidence that even pre-eclampsia itself is due to the production of any toxic substance, despite numerous speculations on the matter. The word toxaemia has, however, been used for so long that when it is used in the context of pregnancy it is understood to be referring to the triad of raised blood pressure, oedema and albuminuria, and not to any 'toxaemic state'. By common usage, therefore, it may be continued. Pre-eclampsia and eclampsia are here preferred, however. Pre-eclampsia has the merit that it indicates the state preceding eclampsia, and the fact that modern treatment prevents this unhappy circumstance in no way diminishes the potential risk of untreated pre-eclampsia. Chronic hypertensive disease is often known to be present in a patient before, during and after pregnancy, and every effort to separate this condition from pre-eclampsia should be made. Chronic renal disease may also be the underlying cause of the clinical features.

The mother may lose her life from the various complications of eclampsia or, less commonly, from pre-eclampsia alone (see Table 29.2, p. 450). The foetus may die of anoxia *in utero* either in association with pre-eclampsia or its occasional complication accidental haemorrhage; alternatively, foetal loss may result from slowly increasing placental infarction—placental insufficiency; death in the neonatal period may occur from prematurity and its complications.

GENERAL CONSIDERATIONS

Despite extensive investigations over many years into almost every aspect of pre-eclampsia and its relationship to hypertension and chronic renal disease, many matters remain unsolved. Some of these will be examined in further detail later in this chapter. Meanwhile, we will consider in general terms some of what is known about these disorders and their probable relationship to each other.

Pre-eclampsia is disease of the pregnant or very recently delivered woman. It is characterized by three principal physical signs: raised blood pressure, oedema and, later, albumin in the urine. These signs seldom appear before the twenty-fourth week or so of pregnancy, and are often much later than this. Once one or other does appear the disease may run a slow course, any increase in severity being gradual over several weeks, or deterioration may be rapid over a few days. Following delivery, the signs disappear fairly quickly. Rarely, the first signs appear only during labour or after delivery, when they are usually of short duration, although they may be of marked degree.

Eclampsia is the occurrence of epileptiform convulsions in a patient previously affected by pre-eclampsia. Usually, clear evidence of pre-eclampsia is present for weeks—or, less commonly, days—before convulsions. Rarely, the eclampsia is fulminating, signs of pre-eclampsia appearing only hours before the fits commence. Eclamptic fits may be seen postpartum only, when they are usually confined to the first 48 hr; very rarely indeed, the fits may appear, or may recur, later than this, although whether they can then be regarded as eclamptic is uncertain.

Hypertensive disease may be present in a patient before she becomes pregnant. The level of blood pressure may be largely unaltered during pregnancy but, more often, increased blood pressure readings are obtained, and in some of these patients the additional signs of oedema and albuminuria indicate a state of pre-eclampsia superimposed upon the existing hypertension. Eclampsia may supervene here as in the case of uncomplicated pre-eclampsia, although it is less common. If the level of the patient's blood pressure before pregnancy is unknown a distinction between chronic hypertension and pre-eclampsia can often be made by noting blood pressure levels in early pregnancy. If these are raised before the twenty-fourth week, even though a subsequent fall occurs, it is probable that the diagnosis is hypertension and not pre-eclampsia. The return to normal, or otherwise, of the blood pressure after delivery should help in this respect to confirm or refute the diagnosis.

Chronic renal disease, such as nephritis or the nephrotic syndrome complicating pregnancy, is generally considered uncommon. Here, raised blood pressure and albuminuria are frequently present for a large part of pregnancy, and in this sense differentiation from pre-eclampsia or pre-eclampsia superimposed upon hypertension may be difficult unless the existence of the previous renal lesion is known.

In a subsequent pregnancy a patient, previously pre-eclamptic, may remain entirely normal—indeed, she is more likely to do so than otherwise. The chances of such a patient developing similar features again in the next pregnancy are, however, greater than those of the patient who has never suffered from pre-eclampsia at all. This may then be called 'recurrent toxaemia', although whether this is truly so, or whether the case should not more correctly be regarded as one of chronic hypertension aggravated by a succeeding pregnancy, cannot be stated with certainty, since often the blood pressure levels between pregnancies are unknown. It seems likely that the latter is the case and that most patients with apparent recurrent pre-eclampsia are in reality patients with chronic hypertension aggravated by pregnancy. As already mentioned, the levels of blood pressure in early pregnancy may be a good guide to diagnosis.

For many years the possibility of pre-eclampsia causing subsequent hypertension or renal damage was hotly debated. It is clear that a number of patients with pre-eclampsia will subsequently develop chronic hypertensive disease, but so will others who have never had pre-eclampsia or, indeed, ever been pregnant at all. It seems unlikely that pre-eclampsia causes hypertension, but it may expedite the appearance of hypertension sooner than would otherwise have been the case. This tendency to aggravation of hypertension by pre-eclampsia may mean that some cases of apparent recurrent pre-eclampsia in patients with normal blood pressure levels between pregnancies may still be manifestations of a hypertensive tendency appearing only under the stress of pregnancy. Browne & Dodds (1939), Platt (1958) and especially Chesley and his colleagues (1962, 1964), have reported important work in this field.

It seems very unlikely that pre-eclampsia alone causes chronic renal damage.

It will be clear that these conditions are very closely related to each other. Attempts at precise diagnosis should always be made, however, in order that progress in their understanding will continue to be made.

A classification of these disorders suggested by the American Committee on Maternal Welfare is in keeping with the views expressed above. It was advocated that four categories be employed: acute toxaemia of pregnancy; chronic hypertensive vascular disease; recurrent toxaemia and unclassified toxaemia.

The term pre-eclampsia (or acute toxaemia of pregnancy) would then be applied to a patient more than 24 weeks' pregnant who developed hypertension, proteinuria or pathological oedema.

Eclampsia is the occurrence, in a pre-eclamptic patient, of convulsions and coma—rarely coma alone.

Chronic hypertensive vascular disease requires the presence of a raised blood pressure before 24 weeks and evidence of hypertension persisting thereafter.

Chronic hypertensive vascular disease with superimposed toxaemia requires an increase in the blood pressure of 30 mmHg systolic or 15 mmHg diastolic, or poteinuria.

Recurrent toxaemia can be diagnosed if, in a pregnancy, following one complicated by pre-eclampsia, there is a recurrence of the same physical signs, the blood pressure having been normal between pregnancies and remaining normal thereafter.

Unclassified toxaemia refers to conditions which cannot be classified by the above criteria. This term does not, however, refer to chronic renal disease, which, it was felt, could be recognized by clinical investigation.

These views, although similar in substance to those just expressed in this section, differ slightly from them. Specifically, the view is preferred here that recurrent toxaemia, even if known to be associated with normal blood pressure levels between pregnancies, is more likely to be a manifestation of chronic hypertensive disease which is not yet overt except during the stress of pregnancy.

Having surveyed the field in this general manner a more detailed examination of each condition will now be undertaken.

PRE-ECLAMPSIA

Clinical features

The principal features of pre-eclampsia have already been stated; they are a raised blood pressure, oedema (or excessive weight gain) and albuminuria. It will be noted that these are physical signs. There are no symptoms of mild or moderate pre-eclampsia. With severe degrees of pre-eclampsia, symptoms of headache, spots before the eyes, diplopia, dizziness, epigastric discomfort and vomiting may make their appearance. These symptoms are commonest in rapidly progressing or fulminating pre-eclampsia, when the first sign of the disease may have been noted only a day or two earlier. They are an indication of imminent eclampsia unless urgently treated. A further rise in the level of blood pressure, more generalized oedema, and a larger quantity of albumin in the urine, generally accompany these symptoms, which are often called the pre-eclamptic state.

RAISED BLOOD PRESSURE

The level of blood pressure commonly required before a diagnosis of pre-eclampsia can be entertained is not universally agreed. A level of 140/90 mmHg in a patient with previously normal levels of blood pressure in early pregnancy is regarded as abnormal by all. A few authorities, however, accept a lower figure of 135/85 mmHg. There are, occasionally, circumstances in which a lower figure must be considered abnormal, as when the blood pressure in early pregnancy has been very low—such as 100/60 mmHg. In general, however, the level of 140/90 mmHg seems a realistic one, justifying a diagnosis of pre-eclampsia. At levels lower than this advice may well be given to the patient in an attempt to halt the blood pressure rise and to prevent the onset of pre-eclampsia, which cannot yet be said to exist.

OEDEMA

Oedema is a physical sign which should always suggest the diagnosis of pre-eclampsia, although not all patients with oedema will be proved to be pre-eclamptic. Oedema of the legs is a not uncommon sign in late pregnancy. In some patients ankle oedema is doubtless a pressure effect and may be evident when the abdominal swelling is very large, when varicose veins are present, in hot weather, or if the patient has been on her feet a great deal; some patients have a tendency to ankle oedema when they are not pregnant. Whilst some cases of ankle oedema in pregnancy may therefore be accepted as not 'toxaemic', care must be taken to establish for certain that other signs of pre-eclampsia are absent before accepting this as so.

Hytten & Billewicz (1967) have recently reviewed oedema in pregnancy and its significance. They stress that greater significance should be attached to generalized oedema than to oedema of the lower limbs, which may be, in some cases, physiological. Oedema itself is not an ominous sign, but must be considered carefully before deciding that significance need not be attached to it.

Weight gain in pregnancy is closely related to oedema. Hytten & Billewicz demonstrated that women who were overweight for their height and gained more rapidly during the second half of pregnancy developed oedema more readily than others. Weight gain during pregnancy is, in part, due to fluid storage and partly due to the increased weight of the uterus and its contents; a patient who eats a great deal will, of course, gain weight from over-eating and fat deposition. Whatever the precise relationship between weight gain, oedema and pre-eclampsia, efforts to control weight gain by dietary advice can only be beneficial. Any patient gaining more than 1 lb per week between the twelfth and fortieth weeks of pregnancy must be considered to be gaining abnormally. Even this degree of weight gain can, with benefit, be far less.

ALBUMINURIA

Albuminuria is, in almost all instances, the third physical sign to appear. Before the disease process is fully established and whilst it still remains, to some extent at least, a reversible condition, albumin is absent from the urine, or is present only occasionally and in small amounts. Once albumin is regularly present the disease can seldom be reversed, although it may be held in check for a few weeks. As in the case of oedema, the mere presence of albuminuria is not in itself an indication of pre-eclampsia. Clearly, albuminuria may be present if there is chronic renal disease such as nephritis or the nephrotic syndrome; or in certain cases of pylonephritis. In a number of normal people albuminuria may be present without detectable renal disease. Orthostatic albuminuria is sometimes seen. It has been suggested that the occurrence of a recent placental infarct, via the mechanism of the so-called uterorenal reflex, may precipitate a transient episode of albuminuria; the evidence in favour of this is slender, if indeed any exists.

The appearance of albuminuria is generally a sign of increase in the severity of the disease. It must not be assumed, however, that this is the case until a urinary infection has been eliminated. Microscopic examination of a mid-stream sample of urine should be undertaken. If features of the case suggest doubt about the diagnosis of pre-eclampsia renal function tests may also be employed. In pre-eclampsia itself there is seldom any significant deterioration in renal function apart from the acute episodes of renal failure complicating fulminating pre-eclampsia and eclampsia.

COURSE OF THE DISEASE

The progress of events in patients with pre-eclampsia is extremely variable. In most cases occurring in this country, where a high standard of antenatal care is almost universally practised, recognition of the early signs of pre-eclampsia results in treatment which tends to delay further deterioration. Even many untreated cases run a slow course over some weeks, or longer. Less commonly, despite treatment the blood pressure continues to rise, and albuminuria to increase, over a few days. Occasionally, the whole process occurs so rapidly that oedema may appear almost visibly, the blood pressure climbs steeply and the symptoms of the pre-eclamptic state are complained of perhaps even before a specimen of urine containing albumin is actually passed. These symptoms—headache, visual disturbances, etc.—may appear in any advanced case, although the opportunity to recognize deterioration in the more chronic type of case allows more time for action to be taken before these symptoms arise.

In advanced cases, especially in those progressing rapidly, oliguria may be a notable feature.

Incidence

It is difficult to be precise about the incidence of pre-eclampsia, but it seems probably that it complicates some 5% or so of all pregnancies. This incidence is increased in some circumstances however.

Pre-eclampsia is predominantly a disease of primigravid patients, especially young primigravidae. When pre-eclampsia affects multiparous patients it is usually superimposed upon hypertension or, less often, is associated with one of the features described below.

Twin pregnancies are especially prone to be complicated by pre-eclampsia, the incidence being increased by two or three times, or even more.

Diabetes carries a similar increased risk, which is greater if the disease is not well controlled (Peel 1962).

Perhaps the greatest increase in incidence occurs in cases of hydatidiform mole, when up to 50% of pregnancies may show evidence of pre-eclampsia. Also, in the presence of this disease the pre-eclampsia may appear unusually early, providing perhaps the only exception to the general rule that pre-eclampsia commences after the twenty-fourth week of pregnancy.

Pre-eclampsia is more common in certain patients with hydramnios. Hibbard (1962) pointed out, however, that not all cases of hydramnios were associated with this increased incidence; hydramnios occurring in association with twins, diabetes or hydrops foetalis was associated with a raised incidence of pre-eclampsia, whereas hydramnios due to a foetal abnormality such as spina bifida, anencephaly or oesophageal atresia was not. The association with hydramnios appears, therefore, to be more with the cause of the hydramnios than with the uterine distention from the increased volume of fluid.

Some authors (Jeffcoate & Scott 1959) stress the frequent association of hydrops foetalis and pre-eclampsia, suggesting that as many as 50% of cases of hydrops foetalis may be so complicated. It is not in the author's experience that the frequency of pre-eclampsia in hydrops foetalis is anything approaching this. Like pre-eclampsia, however, hydrops foetalis is not always a very precise diagnosis. Many seriously affected foetuses demonstrate hydropic features which may not be accepted by all as constituting hydrops foetalis *per se*; in many of these pre-eclampsia is not a specially pronounced feature. Furthermore, an acute maternal syndrome of oedema, albuminuria and hypertension rarely appears very suddenly in association with serious rhesus disease (Beazley 1965). Whether this condition is the same as, or different from, pre-eclampsia is uncertain at the present time.

Aetiology

It is doubtful if even now, after very many years of study, speculation and theorizing, a really helpful account of the aetiology of pre-eclampsia and eclampsia can be written. Any attempt to cover the subject in detail would inevitably involve very prolonged discussion indeed. This complex has been called 'the disease of theories', since so many have been advanced in an attempt to explain it. So far none has done so satisfactorily. Objections may be raised to all in one respect or another, usually because well-recognized facts in the clinical associations of pre-eclampsia and eclampsia cannot be explained by the theory in question. Since so many objections may be raised to all theories and since, happily, we have none to offer in their place, the interested reader is referred to detailed accounts of the aetiology of these conditions by Platt (1958), Browne (1958), Lewis (1964) and Jeffcoate (1966).

Pathological features

Reduced to the simplest terms, the essential pathological features of pre-eclampsia are vascular spasm associated with salt and water retention. It is only in fairly recent times that more information has become available concerning the pathological changes in non-fatal cases of pre-eclampsia. Previously, a great deal of work had been done but, with few exceptions, on fatal cases in which the essential features might have been obscured by terminal events or post-mortem changes. Sheehan (1950) reviewed this earlier work. More knowledge has become available following the greater use of kidney biopsy (Altchek 1961, 1964; Pirani *et al.* 1963; Pike *et al.* 1966; Altchek *et al.* 1968). The renal lesions proper will be discussed presently, but it can be mentioned here that in their studies of renal biopsy material by both light- and electron-microscopy, Altchek *et al.* noted marked spasm of glomerular arterioles with, in some cases, a lumen so narrowed that only one red cell could pass through at a time. Even larger arterioles showed similar vasospasm with an increased ratio of wall thickness to lumen diameter. Assuming these lesions to be representative of vascular activity elsewhere, a picture of vascular spasm with increased peripheral resistance emerges. Blood pressure elevation therefore occurs to compensate for this spasm and to maintain the blood flow through the tissues.

Blood flow through the placenta, however, is generally considered to be reduced in most cases of pre-eclampsia, the amount of reduction depending upon the severity of the case. This reduction through the placenta is mediated by vascular spastic changes in the spiral decidual arterioles. The blood flow to the myometrium is reduced also.

Cerebral blood flow is probably little, if any, affected, except for the terminal stages of severe cases.

The kidney is affected by marked reduction of plasma flow resulting in reduction of the glomerular filtration rate. The blood flow through the arm tends to be increased in pre-eclampsia, and liver blood flow may be increased also.

The renal changes are probably of the greatest significance, since they account directly for the proteinuria, and in all probability for the salt and water retention also. Altchek *et al.* (1968) have studied renal changes in considerable detail. Reporting on renal biopsy studies in 76 patients with pre-eclampsia they described lesions recognizable by light-microscopy in all. These lesions comprised (1) glomerular lesions, (2) juxtaglomerular cellular hyperplasia, (3) lesions of Henle's loop, and (4) afferent arterular spasm.

The glomeruli were slightly enlarged and cellular; all glomeruli appeared affected, but the distribution within a single glomerulus was patchy. There was an increase in the number of cells between capillaries (Mesangial cells). An appearance of splitting of the basement membrane of the glomerular capillary walls, seen by light-microscopy, was found at electron-microscopy to be due to an increase in the Mesangial matrix. Capillary endarterial cells were swollen and many lumina appeared empty or absent. A deposition of fibrillary protein strands was found within Bowman's capsule. This material was found connecting capillary loops to capsular epithelium, within the capsular space, and in the lumina of the proximal convoluted tubules. There was an increase in the number and size of juxtaglomerular cells with cytoplasmic swelling and vacuolation.

The epithelium of Henle's loop was severely desquamated, with fragments of nuclei and cells evident. Swelling of the cytoplasm and vacuolation were pronounced. In other areas regeneration was evident.

Afferent glomerular arterioles showed marked vasospasm as already indicated.

After delivery these changes largely disappeared, only occasional traces remaining of increased mesangial matrix. Altchek *et al.*'s article should be consulted for further details.

Salt and water changes, whilst not completely understood, doubtless result from the renal changes described; they may be the result of changes in the glomerular filtration/tubular re-absorption ratio. In normal pregnancy tubular reabsorption is increased to counteract the increase in glomerular filtration which usually occurs. Reduction in the glomerular filtration rate which occurs as a result of the arteriolar changes above referred to, will result in reduced filtration of sodium through the swollen glomeruli, the net result being increased sodium retention and, consequently, water retention also.

The part played by the adrenal cortex in this retention is uncertain. An increase in aldosterone production which normally occurs in late pregnancy is probably a compensatory mechanism for the raised progesterone levels present, since progesterone inhibits the salt-retaining effects of aldosterone. It is not yet known if this mechanism is directly concerned with the salt and water changes of pre-eclampsia. The general endocrine effects of pregnancy are discussed in detail in Chapter 10, p. 144. It is still uncertain if alterations in the activity of the maternal endocrine glands, as distinct from the activity of the placenta and foetus, is in any way concerned with pre-eclampsia. Oestrogen excretion in many toxaemic patients is normal, reflecting, in a general way, the well-being of the foetus; maintenance of normal levels of pregnanediol excretion has similar implications. These matters are discussed in greater detail in Chapter 11, p. 152.

Renal function in pre-eclampsia appears somewhat reduced as judged by the clearances of uric acid and inulin. Plasma uric acid is thought by some to be as reliable a guide as any to deterioration in the pre-eclamptic process. Uric acid appears normally to be filtered completely by the glomeruli, reabsorbed completely by the proximal tubules, and then secreted into the distal convoluted tubules. It seems likely that the glomerular changes described may lead to less filtration and reabsorption of uric acid, and thus to an increase in the plasma levels.

Plasma volume changes result in progressive haemoconcentration, as there is a flow of fluid into the tissue space. There is increased viscosity of blood as a result. Venous pressure does not, however, rise until cardiac failure supervenes in serious cases.

The pathological features of various organs in fatal cases are similar to those seen in fatal cases of eclampsia, and are considered in that section on p. 276.

Effects on the foetus

No one knows how often the foetus is significantly affected in cases of pre-eclampsia, or indeed in hypertensive disease in general. The fact that placental changes indicative of pre-eclampsia are noted does not in itself indicate that the total effect of these changes is sufficient to reduce oxygenation and nutrition below adequate levels. Under normal circumstances, the placental reserve is probably large and when pre-eclampsia arises it may be some time before this reserve is absorbed by the process.

It is a matter of common observation, however, that, in many cases of pre-eclampsia of several weeks' duration, foetal growth is interfered with; the foetus may die in utero from hypoxia, may develop foetal distress as the contractions of labour further reduce oxygenation, or may be born severely asphyxiated. A child born alive under these circumstances is small, with little subcutaneous fat because of interference with nutrition and growth in utero. Not all foetuses are so affected especially in mild cases, or even in acute severe cases, if induction is not delayed, since no chronic interference with foetal development may have yet taken place. Further consideration of the foetus in these circumstances will be found in Chapter 11, p. 152.

The placental changes giving rise to this interference with foetal growth and oxygenation are generally referred to as infarcts. There is increasing fibrosis replacing the highly vascular villi or interfering with the free transport of materials from the choriodecidual space into the foetal blood. Paine (Russell et al. 1957) has described in detail the pathological processes taking place in pre-eclampsia and hypertensive disease. The main features indicating ageing of a normal placenta are slow, but progressive, thinning of syncitium with a gradual thickening of blood vessels in the villus stalks and villi (Figs. 16.1–16.4); there is also progressive conversion of foetal-type mesoderm to fibrous tissue. These ageing changes are accelerated in toxaemia and hypertension. In pre-eclampsia it is the syncitial atrophy which is the most marked feature and the vascular and stromal changes which are most evident in essential hypertension. Paine's paper should be consulted for further details.

The perinatal mortality associated with pre-eclampsia is raised partly as a result of these processes and partly as a result of prematurity and its complications if delivery is necessary to halt the pre-eclamptic process (see Chapter 29, p. 451).

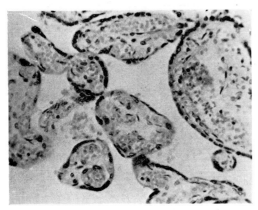

Fig. 16.1. Normal term placenta showing sinusoid formation beneath the trophoblast at the periphery of the villi. (By courtesy of C.G. Paine and the Editor of *Journal of Obstetrics and Gynaecology of the British Commonwealth*.)

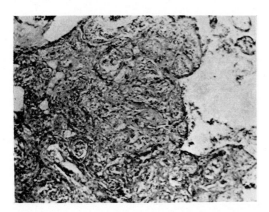

Fig. 16.2. Placenta in a case of pre-eclampsia. Intervillous fibrin deposition has occurred following trophoblastic atrophy. (By courtesy of C.G. Paine and the Editor of *Journal of Obstetrics and Gynaecology of the British Commonwealth*.)

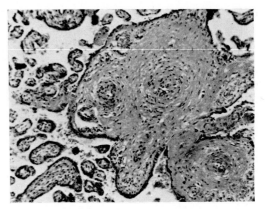

Fig. 16.3. Villus stalk in a case of hypertension complicating pregnancy. There is vascular thickening, obliterative change and stromal fibrosis. (By courtesy of C.G. Paine and the Editor of *Journal of Obstetrics and Gynaecology of the British Commonwealth*.)

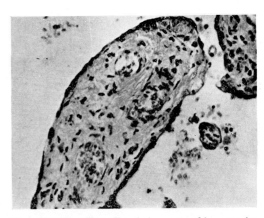

Fig. 16.4. Intravillous fibrosis in a case of hypertension complicating pregnancy. Sinusoid formation has been interfered with, and such as have formed are towards the centre of the villus. Compare with Fig. 16.1. (By courtesy of C.G. Paine and the Editor of *Journal of Obstetrics and Gynaecology of the British Commonwealth*.)

Clinical management

PROPHYLAXIS

Pre-eclampsia is to some extent a preventable disease—but only to some extent. The more carefully we carry out antenatal supervision the sooner the warnings of the disease and its early physical signs will be noticed. The more often prophylactic advice is given, and taken, the more successful we will be in reducing the amount and severity of pre-eclampsia. Initially, therefore, it is the antenatal care that is of the utmost importance.

A blood pressure reading of 140/90 mmHg or more at the first visit must be an indication to give advice then and there about the patient's own activities during the remainder of her pregnancy, since such a patient is at risk from superimposed pre-eclampsia.

Rest and diet

These are, predominantly, the two facets of ante-natal care which require most emphasis. The patient must be informed of the need for increased rest, starting at once. A person does not need to go to bed to rest; given the willingness to rest she may then be able to organize her everyday life to do less physical work, to sit down and to lie down more than previously. Not every one will be able to do this, of course, but the advice must be given, which they should take to the best of their ability.

Diet and weight limitation are subjects which have many advocates in the medical profession. It is by no means certain that reducing weight gain by dietary measures will, *per se*, reduce the incidence of pre-eclampsia. Hamlin (1952) and his colleagues, however, achieved spectacular results in preventing severe degrees of pre-eclampsia by limiting weight gain. It is the author's view that pregnancy presents a golden opportunity to educate a person in the importance of a correct diet. A diet high in protein and low in fats and carbohydrate should be the patient's aim. She should be urged to eat meat, fish, fruit, vegetables, milk, cheese and eggs and to limit her intake of fats, bread, cakes, potatoes, pastry, etc. This type of regime can only be beneficial in pregnancy. What purpose is served in the regular weighing of patients in ante-natal clinics if no effort is made to reduce weight gain?

This kind of advice on diet is appropriate also to patients who are already grossly overweight. It is believed by many that the patient who is overweight at the beginning of pregnancy is prone to pre-eclampsia. Some individuals appear to have a raised blood pressure more frequently than others. It is possible that increase in blood pressure recordings is due, in part, to taking the pressure with a relatively narrow cuff attached to a fat arm. This effect was described by Ragam & Bordley (1941). Pickering *et al.* (1954) described a correction factor which might be made in the case of very fat patients, but they gave their opinion that such corrections, although worth-while for large numbers of patients, were not indicated in individual cases, since arm circumference accounted for only one-quarter of the difference between direct and indirect blood pressure readings. Dietary advice for the overweight is clearly indicated in any event. Such patients can often remain the same weight throughout pregnancy, or limit the gain to a few pounds.

TREATMENT OF MILD TO MODERATE CASES

An increase in the level of the blood pressure recorded in early pregnancy or excessive weight gain or ankle oedema, call for advice to be given as described above, even though pre-eclampsia cannot yet be said to be present. Nevertheless, by emphasizing in particular the need for more rest, some patients can be prevented from becoming overtly pre-eclamptic.

Rest

Rest remains still the cornerstone of treatment in pre-eclampsia. This can be taken at home in the earliest cases with blood pressure levels of the order of 140/90 mmHg, but increases beyond this figure call for rest under supervision; unless the patient can be visited regularly at home this means rest in hospital. The effect of rest on the blood pressure is usually evident quite soon, and this simple treatment may be all that is required to keep it under control. Sedation with phenobarbitone, sodium amytal, etc. is of very doubtful value indeed in most early cases of pre-eclampsia. Many patients without symptoms at all may feel worse from the effects of sedation than they did before. If a patient is unusually anxious, of course, sedation or a tranquilizing drug may well be helpful.

The effect of rest on oedema is also evident if the patient is weighed regularly whilst in hospital.

Disappearance of oedema from the ankles is not in itself sufficient evidence of improvement, since the sacral area may become oedematous instead, the excess fluid merely having been redistributed. By regular weighing, however, a definite reduction in weight can be demonstrated in the first few days of treatment.

Diuretic therapy

It is questionable if the use of diuretics is of direct therapeutic value. Undoubtedly they will result in the loss of much fluid whilst they are being used, but some of this fluid will reaccumulate, perhaps quite quickly, after they have been stopped. More important than this, however, are doubts about their effect on the underlying toxaemic process. Some consider that harm may be done by the patient, who is less oedematous, appearing to be improved, whereas she is, in effect, no better, and may be worse. It is difficult to accept that diuretic therapy has more of a small place in the management of pre-eclampsia. A survey by Kraus et al. (1966) failed to demonstrate any beneficial effect in a large series of patients. In a patient with symptoms due to pronounced leg oedema, short-term therapy with diuretics may, however, be effective in relieving discomfort.

Salt and fluid restriction

It is equally questionable if restriction of salt or fluid has any beneficial effect on the course of pre-eclampsia. In practice it is difficult to reduce salt in a diet without very special precautions being taken. A personal survey carried out a few years ago failed to demonstrate any sign of deterioration in a group of pre-eclamptic patients treated with extra salt; it has even been suggested by some that extra salt is beneficial. Salt restriction can be irksome to many patients, and lack of any clear beneficial effect accruing suggests it to be unnecessary. Fluid restriction is even more distressing, and since again no clear benefits are demonstrable little can be said in its support. An intake and output chart should always be kept during the treatment of a patient with pre-eclampsia.

Abdominal decompression

Blecher & Heynes (1967) have reported favourably on the use of abdominal decompression in preventing pre-eclampsia and treating early cases. One would like to see these results confirmed on larger numbers and in other units to be convinced of the value of this treatment.

Induction of labour

The conservative management of mild to moderate cases of pre-eclampsia may be continued for many weeks in so far as the mother is concerned. Unless there is a marked increase in physical signs the risk of eclampsia is very small and the risk of permanent hypertension or renal damage need not be considered. The effect of chronic pre-eclampsia on the foetus, however, is another matter. Even in relatively mild pre-eclampsia placental infarction may be progressive. Induction of labour may be indicated in the interests of the foetus under these circumstances.

It is difficult to give precise advice about the timing of induction of labour in this condition. In general terms the severity of the pre-eclampsia must be balanced against the risks of prematurity. Since the condition of the mother is giving little cause for concern, the assessment of the condition of the foetus in utero is all important. Induction too early will hazard the foetus from prematurity; delayed induction in the presence of placental insufficiency may lead to foetal death in utero.

Various methods of assessment of the condition of the foetus in utero have been employed. Clinical methods alone are unreliable. The level of the blood pressure, oedema and albuminuria do not necessarily reflect the degree of foetal affection; an increase in physical signs usually indicates a raised foetal risk, but the foetal environment may be deteriorating despite the mother's condition remaining unchanged.

Hormone assay, enzyme measurement, ultrasonic study of the foetal biparietal diameter, amnioscopy and perhaps continuous foetal heart auscultation may be employed in assessing foetal well-being (see Chapter 11, p. 144).

In those cases in which there is no deterioration in the condition of the foetus in utero, induction of labour probably need not be considered until term or close to term. There seems little to be gained, however, by allowing the pregnancy to continue beyond the expected date of confinement, and induction of labour is then indicated. Induction of labour before 35 weeks is associated with considerable foetal risk and should only be contemplated in the type of case under discussion if there is clear evidence of imminent danger to the foetus. Most patients with mild to moderate pre-eclampsia will be managed by induction of labour between these times. Provided the foetus remains in good condition the nearer to term the pregnancy can be continued the better, but if the various methods of assessment indicate a deteriorating situation induction must be performed quickly.

SEVERE AND FULMINATING
PRE-ECLAMPSIA

Rapid deterioration in an established case of pre-eclampsia, or fulminating pre-eclampsia appearing over a very short time, calls for urgent and effective management. Here the threat of eclampsia is prominent and action must be taken at once in the mother's interests. Initially, control of the pre-eclamptic condition in order to reduce the likelihood of eclampsia is essential. Once this threat has been diminished and the progress of the pre-eclampsia is halted, delivery of the patient must be achieved quickly by the most appropriate means.

Heavy sedation with tribromethol, magnesium sulphate, Valium, etc. is indicated as if the patient were already eclamptic (see p. 277). If a satisfactory state of sedation is achieved and blood pressure levels come down, induction of labour, or Caesarean section, is required regardless of the duration of pregnancy or the condition of the foetus. The mode of delivery in these circumstances will depend upon various factors— the parity of the patient, the mode of delivery of previous children, the duration of the pregnancy, the state of the cervix, and other matters of this kind. Delivery soon is necessary, and the circumstances of individual cases will vary so much that rules cannot easily be laid down for how this is to be achieved. Caesarean section will

in many cases be the most satisfactory method of treatment; provided vaginal delivery can be anticipated quickly, however, this will sometimes be a suitable alternative.

Complications

Accidental haemorrhage has, for many years, been regarded as a special threat in pre-eclampsia and eclampsia. Even now, despite suggestions to the contrary, some obstetricians, the author included, are reluctant completely to relinquish this association as one of clinical significance. More recently, Hibbard & Hibbard (1963) have incriminated folic-acid deficiency as the causative factor and have sought to show pre-eclampsia and eclampsia *per se* not to be predisposing features Coyle & Geoghegan (1962) report the frequent finding of megaloblastic erythropoesis in accidental haemorrhage, which lends support to this view. Raised blood pressure and albuminuria found in association with the accidental haemorrhage may be an effect, and not the cause, of the condition.

URINARY SUPPRESSION

Oliguria is sometimes a marked feature of pre-eclampsia and eclampsia. For the most part a diuresis occurs shortly after delivery and this coincides with excellent recovery of the patient. In a minority of cases the oliguria becomes a definite pathological feature and a cause for real concern.

Tubular necrosis or more widespread acute cortical necrosis may be present in the kidney. In clinical terms a distinction cannot be made between them, and the management called for is the same in either event. This complication is not confined solely to pre-eclampsia and eclampsia, but occurs with accidental haemorrhage, septic abortion and poisoning with abortifacients such as mercuric chloride as well.

Management is similar to that advocated in Chapter 14, p. 224. Mannitol, 500 ml of a 20% solution, may be used once after delivery if the oliguria shows no sign of being corrected spontaneously. If this does not produce a prompt response fluid intake should be restricted to

500 ml per day plus the volume of urine passed, if any.

Carbohydrate only should be given by mouth, but to aim at a high-calorie intake in an attempt to reduce endogenous protein metabolism seems unnecessary. Early transfer to a renal dialysis unit will be the best mode of management.

ECLAMPSIA

Happily, eclampsia is an uncommon condition in Britain at the present time, although in those parts of the world without an effective system of antenatal care this is, unfortunately, not the case. Eclamptic convulsions may be antepartum, intrapartum or postpartum. In former times postpartum eclampsia was comparatively uncommon, accounting for some 10–20% of cases. Nowadays, with effective antenatal care and prompt treatment of severe and fulminating pre-eclampsia, antenatal eclampsia is relatively less common, and postpartum eclampsia relatively more so. Presumably the stress of labour occasionally aggravates a moderate situation which then progresses to eclampsia. In Queen Charlotte's Hospital during 1967, 1968 and 1969 there were twenty-eight eclamptics, the first fit occurring before labour in one, during labour in eight and after delivery in nineteen.

Eclamptic convulsions are epileptiform in type. There is a tonic phase of generalized muscular contraction during which the patient loses consciousness and becomes cyanosed, with a suffused face and frothing mouth. She may assume an attitude of opisthotonous, so marked may be contractions of her dorsal muscles. This phase lasts perhaps half a minute and is followed by the clonic phase of convulsive, jerky, muscular contraction which may last a minute or longer, after which the patient passes into a brief period of coma. Immediately preceding the tonic phase the patient may become confused, the eyes turn upwards and fibrillary twitching of muscles may be evident. During the convulsions the patient may inhale vomit, bite her tongue, fall from the bed or injure herself in some other way. A fit may be followed rapidly by a second or a third, but more often with effective treatment the

disease is quickly controlled before more than one or two fits have occurred. The blood pressure usually reaches very high peaks indeed immediately before and during a convulsion. Oedema, if not marked before, quickly becomes generalized and albumin heavier in the urine.

DIAGNOSIS

A convulsion of the variety just described is easily recognizable to a trained medical person; such a feature developing in a pre-eclamptic patient provides no difficulty in diagnosis. The fit is not always witnessed by a medical or nursing individual, however, and the preceding state of the patient may be unknown. One may be confronted by a comatose patient breathing stertorously, and various other diagnoses should at least be considered.

Epilepsy, a cerebral accident, uraemia and diabetic coma are possibilities which may require to be eliminated. A history of epilepsy may be obtained; without it, diagnosis will not be easy. A helpful sign is that an epileptic patient is usually incontinent and an eclamptic seldom so; this distinction has, surprisingly, been little emphasized. The recognition of a raised blood pressure, oedema and, as soon as a specimen of urine can be obtained, albuminuria, will go a long way to confirm eclampsia; without all these features it will be wise to keep an open mind about diagnosis. The blood pressure shortly after the end of the fit may be lower—even within normal limits; the oedema, although developing rapidly, may not yet be marked; albumin can, rarely, be absent or present only in traces in the urine sample present in the bladder at the time, although a subsequent specimen may be heavily loaded with it. These are exceptions, however, and one can expect all the physical signs in the majority of patients with eclampsia. Prolonged coma will raise the possibility of a cerebral accident, as will the presence of localizing signs when recovery begins.

Pathological features

The pathological changes found in fatal cases of eclampsia are, for the most part, the result of the vascular spastic effects mentioned already. The renal lesions have been described in some detail on p. 270. More extensive renal damage of similar nature is evident in fatal eclamptic cases. The liver shows subscapular haemorrhages and haemorrhagic infarcts throughout its substance. Periportal haemorrhages and necrosis are a prominent feature. The brain demonstrates similar vascular changes. Oedema is often marked. Tiny haemorrhages are frequently observed; sometimes, much larger ones are present and are the likely immediate cause of death. The heart and adrenals show similar haemorrhagic areas. The lungs often demonstrate congestion, infection or aspiration of vomit.

Management

For many years the principles of management in eclampsia have been (1) control of fits and (2) induction of labour. These principles are still valid now, especially if we substitute 'early delivery of the patient' for 'induction of labour'. In the early years of this century, before Strogonoff introduced his conservative regime for the management of eclampsia, early intervention to achieve delivery was widely practised. This scheme of management sprang from the reasoning—sound, it appears, in principle—that since the condition occurred only in pregnancy, ending the pregnancy would allow recovery to occur. The mortality was, however, very high. Strogonoff's regime of heavy sedation with morphia by injection and chlorol and bromide per rectum gave infinitely better results. In addition to drugs the patient was nursed in a darkened room and stimulation was reduced to an absolute minimum. Once the convulsive tendency was fully controlled the membranes were ruptured. Mortality figures improved markedly.

The essential aspects of Strogonoff's management have since been practised, with little alteration, until very recent times. Changes have been made in the drugs employed. Tribromethol and magnesium sulphate have become extremely popular. The 'lytic cocktail' of Phenergan, Largactil and pethidine has also been widely used with success. More recently, Valium and

Librium have been acclaimed as particularly effective. All authorities, however, seek to control the hyperexcitable state and prevent convulsions. Nursing under quiet, dim surroundings is the rule in most hospitals.

Control of fits is still essential to effective management of the eclamptic patient. Whatever drugs are employed they must be given in large doses and repeated at intervals as judged by the blood pressure levels and the excitability of the patient. Tribromethol, preferred by the author, is given per rectum in doses of 0·09 ml/kg. In practice, since the weight of the patient is seldom known, an estimate must be formed of it, and the dosage becomes less precise than is suggested by this formula. Between 4·5 and 6 ml of tribromethol solution are diluted to 220 ml. This is quickly tested with Congo red to ensure that no deterioration of the tribromethol has occurred with formation of toxic products; the solution is then heated to almost 40°C and instilled into the rectum. An excellent sedative effect is quickly obtained. Blood pressure levels fall. The patient may remain well controlled for several hours, when a further rectal injection is likely to be required. After a while, intervals between injections become longer.

Magnesium sulphate, which was later introduced into his regime by Strogonoff, is also popular. It may be given intravenously in doses of 20 ml of a 50% solution which can be repeated approximately 4-hourly. Magnesium sulphate is particularly effective in reducing central nervous system irritability and cerebral oedema.

The 'lytic cocktail' is one of several variations also popular. Mitra et al. (1958) employed an immediate injection of 12·5 mg of chlorpromazine and promezathine; this was given intravenously in 50 ml of 5% glucose solution. After the immediate effect of this had been observed a drip infusion of 50 mg of each in 540 ml of 5% glucose was given to maintain the sedative effect and control blood pressure. Pethidine 100–200 mg was given intramuscularly if difficulty was experienced in controlling fits. Menon (1961) and others have also used this technique, or its variations, with considerable effect.

Drugs to lower the blood pressure have been employed more extensively by some workers than others. Apresoline may be used, 20 or 30 mg being given slowly intravenously or 50–100 mg in 1 litre of 5% dextrose given in drip form. Reserpine has been employed similarly. This form of therapy may be more necessary when magnesium sulphate is used, which is less likely to reduce the blood pressure than tribromethol. With tribromethol specific hypotensive therapy is generally unnecessary.

Lean *et al.* (1968) have reported excellent results with large doses of Librium or Valium. With Librium, an initial intravenous injection of 200 mg is followed by a continuous infusion of 200 mg in 500 ml of 5% dextrose given at 30 drops per minute. Valium is used in initial doses of 40 mg intravenously, a further 40 mg in 500 ml of dextrose being given at 30 drops per minute. In addition, whenever there is difficulty in controlling blood pressure a hypotensive agent is used.

NURSING CARE

The nursing care of an eclamptic patient remains a very important feature of treatment. A quiet room is desirable with a medical or nursing attendant always present. Pulse rate, respiration, blood pressure, colour, restlessness, etc. must be all constantly observed. Oxygen must be available. A mouth gag and airway must be handy. The patient must be turned at hourly intervals from one side to the other, and always nursed on her side to prevent the inhalation of vomit. A catheter may be left in the bladder to give an accurate assessment of the amount of urine secreted and to prevent restlessness from this cause.

OBSTETRIC MANAGEMENT

Once convulsions are definitely under control attention must be directed to delivering the patient. It will nearly always be advisable to allow 2 or 3 hr of observation to ensure that satisfactory control of fits has, in fact, been achieved before any further stimulation of the patient is undertaken by way of vaginal examination or artificial rupture of the membranes.

In the past, Caesarean section has been strenuously avoided, but in more recent years there has been a greater tendency to use this technique more freely; sometimes this has been used very soon after the patient has been sedated. Whilst agreeing that Caesarean section may now, with benefit, be more freely used, there seems little to be gained by very early resort to it in most cases. Some patients will be found already to be in labour; others will start quickly once the membranes are ruptured. Labour should not present a problem if further sedation with pethidine is employed to relieve restlessness from pain. Efforts should be made to achieve delivery within 24 hr of the first fit, and in all cases in which progress is not being made Caesarean section must be seriously considered.

If delivery within this period of time can be achieved, little further therapy will be needed. Attention need not be paid to the electrolyte position nor to the patient's nutritional requirements. The volume of fluid given intravenously should not be large, bearing in mind the oliguria which is often a pronounced feature of this disease. Urine output must be scrupulously measured and any suggestion of pathological oliguria immediately treated (see below).

POSTPARTUM CARE

Once a patient is safely delivered the above sedative regime should be maintained over the first 24 hr and gradually withdrawn. Diuresis is an excellent sign of recovery and if large volumes of urine are passed there will probably be little further cause for concern. Failure to achieve a diuresis is a serious sign, to which considerable attention must be paid. In recovering patients, lighter levels of sedation may be continued for a few days.

Prognosis

Eclampsia occurs with such different degrees of severity and conditions of obstetric care are so variable that comparisons of results of treatment are only helpful in a very general way. A few reported series from very recent times will, however, give an impression of the seriousness of the disease and the effectiveness of treatment.

Dewar & Morris (1947), employing tribromethol, had a 4·5% maternal mortality in a largely rural and extensive area of Scotland.

Mitra *et al.* (1958), using the 'lytic cocktail', reported no maternal deaths in 125 cases of eclampsia.

Menon (1961) described a 2·2% mortality in 402 cases using a similar regime.

Kyank *et al.* (1964), reporting on the results of a questionnaire sent to a large number of clinics in Germany, gave a 5·3% mortality in 1,013 cases.

Lopez Llera (1967), reporting from Mexico, had a 10·3% mortality in 107 patients; two women were, however, moribund on arrival in hospital. Magnesium sulphate was employed as the chief sedative, and fairly early Caesarean section resorted to.

Pritchard & Stone (1967), in the United States of America, reported no deaths in 69 patients over a 12-year period; magnesium sulphate was chiefly used.

Harbert *et al.* (1968) had a 4·7% mortality in 168 eclamptics over a 25-year period also employing magnesium sulphate.

Lean *et al.* (1968) had a 3·3% maternal mortality in 90 cases with treatment with Valium and Librium.

It must be emphasized again, however, that many of the circumstances surrounding these eclamptic patients varied so much that differences in success cannot directly be attributable to one drug or to one method of management or another. It will be evident, however, that eclampsia remains a most serious disorder with too high a mortality. Prevention is, once again, far better than cure.

Perinatal mortality has similarly varied from 11·1% in the series reported recently by Lean *et al.* (1968) to 32·1% described by Mitra in 1961. It is tempting to consider the improvement in the foetal results to be concerned to a large extent with the wider and earlier use of Caesarean section in Lean's unit, but this is merely one of the factors concerned and it will be prudent to reserve judgement on it. Crichton *et al.* (1968) are also in favour of the fairly free use of Caesarean section, and they employed it in 240 of 358 eclamptics. Their maternal mortality rate of 4·2% in those treated by Caesarean section and 4·8% in those delivered vaginally does not demonstrate special superiority; moreover, the perinatal mortality rates of 35·4% in the section group and 47% in the vaginal delivery group are so high that, taking into account the many other factors present, this cannot be regarded as strong evidence in favour of early Ceasarean section.

REMOTE PROGNOSIS

A patient having once had eclampsia is more likely to have a raised blood pressure and oedema and albuminuria in a subsequent pregnancy than one who has never suffered from pre-eclampsia at all. However, it is more likely than not that she will remain normal next time she becomes pregnant. If the blood pressure remains raised between pregnancies, of course, the chances of it going still higher and of pre-eclampsia becoming superimposed are much increased.

HYPERTENSION COMPLICATING PREGNANCY

Some of the associations between chronic hypertensive disease and pre-eclampsia have already been examined in the earlier part of this chapter. If it is known that a patient had a raised blood pressure before her pregnancy, or that the blood pressure is raised early in the pregnancy, the diagnosis of hypertension complicating pregnancy is clear-cut. A further rise in the level later, plus oedema and albuminuria, indicates the superimposition of pre-eclampsia.

If the patient is not seen until 20 weeks or so of pregnancy and is then found to have about a normal blood pressure level which subsequently goes up and is accompanied by oedema and albuminuria, we cannot say for certain whether we are dealing with pre-eclampsia alone or pre-eclampsia superimposed upon existing hypertension. It is common for the blood pressure of a patient with mild or moderate chronic hypertension to fall to normal levels during the second trimester of pregnancy only to rise again later; if a patient is seen for the first time only during this second trimester, a confident diagnosis cannot be made until blood pressure levels during the year or so after delivery are studied.

In practice, so far as the management of an individual patient is concerned it matters little which is the correct diagnosis, since the patient can be regarded as having pre-eclampsia or as being so likely to develop it that her management is the same.

Consequently, the recognition of a raised blood pressure in early pregnancy calls for the prophylactic advice about increased rest and weight restriction already outlined on p. 273. In more severe degrees of raised blood pressure, of the order of 160/100 mmHg or above, a more positive line will need to be taken.

The effect of a previously raised blood pressure on the foetus is variable, but the danger is that progressive fibrosis will first eat away the placental reserve and then begin to encroach upon essential respiratory and nutrient functions. The foetus is, in essence, affected as in some cases of preeclampsia discussed on p. 271. This is not always the case, however, and in some patients with a raised blood pressure levels throughout pregnancy the foetus does not appear to suffer much, and occasionally not at all. What influences whether the foetus is affected or not is unknown.

The placental pathology shows an acceleration in ageing processes. In particular, the blood vessels of the villus stalks and the villi themselves thicken, and foetal-type mesoderm becomes replaced by adult-type fibrous tissue (Fig. 16.3). The blood sinusoids in the villi, normally closely adjacent to the trophoblast and thus to the maternal blood in the choriodecidual space, become fixed in the substance of the villus (Fig. 16.4), with consequent interference with the exchange of gases and nutrient materials (Russell *et al.* 1957). The superimposition of pre-eclampsia will produce syncitial atrophy also (see p. 270).

The risk of accidental haemorrhage was once thought to be high in essential hypertension. Hibbard & Hibbard (1963) suggest this association to have been exaggerated; they believe the main predisposing feature to be folic acid deficiency. Barnes (1970) found accidental haemorrhage in only 3 of his 145 cases of essential hypertension complicating pregnancy.

DIAGNOSIS

The distinction between hypertension and preeclampsia has already been referred to several times (for example, pp. 266 and 267) and need not be repeated again. The possibility of hypertension being concerned with an underlying renal artery stenosis should be entertained, and auscultation over the renal artery area should be carried out to detect a systolic bruit. A midstream sample of urine must be examined for any suggestion of renal disease and, if appropriate, renal function tests performed. Inspection of the retinae is appropriate. Palpation of the femoral arteries to confirm a pulse of good volume is required to eliminate the possibility of coarctation of the aorta, although this is nowadays almost always recognized during childhood. The heart must be carefully examined for evidence of cardiac enlargement.

A pheochromocytoma of the adrenal is a possible diagnosis accounting for a raised blood pressure; whilst it need not frequently be considered seriously, it must be borne in mind on occasions. Gemmell's paper in 1955 surveyed pheochromocytoma and child-bearing by analysing 55 cases. The hypertension here is usually intermittent, by not always so. Recognition of increased catacholamine excretion in the urine should provide the diagnosis; a raised excretion of vanillyl mandelic acid in the urine may also be detected (Thiery 1967).

Management

In comparatively minor degrees of hypertension the general advice on rest and diet given for the prevention of pre-eclampsia and for the treatment of early pre-eclampsia will be applicable. Provided the patient is warned in early pregnancy of the need to organize her everyday life on quieter lines, this should be possible. A rise in the blood pressure level—the systolic over 150 mmHg the diastolic to 95 mmHg—will be an indication to admit the patient for rest in hospital. This will usually result in a slight fall in blood pressure and, if the fall is maintained over several days of simple ambulation in the ward, this response can be assumed if the patient goes home. It may be necessary for her to spend short periods of time in hospital and other short periods at home to maintain supervision and to ensure rest.

The foetus requires to be monitored carefully by the various means discussed in Chapter 11. Hormone assay, ultrasound measurement, etc. will recognize the threatening situation for the foetus and allow the appropriate time for delivery to be selected.

In more severe cases of hypertension the outlook for a successful pregnancy is less satisfactory. If the diastolic blood pressure level is 100 mmHg or more in early pregnancy this is a poor sign, suggesting that considerable rest will require to be taken and careful observation carried out.

In such a case admission to hospital to determine the effect of rest alone and to allow further investigation of renal function, re-examination of the optic fundi, etc. should be carried out. The response to rest alone is often excellent, even in more severe cases of this kind. With the expected mid-trimester fall in blood pressure to come, this simple management may be all that is required.

The place of hypotensive drugs in the treatment of the more severe forms of hypertension complicating pregnancy is not an easy one to decide. Barnes (1970) in Queen Charlotte's Hospital reserves them for patients who do not have the mid-trimester fall in blood pressure. Reserpine in doses of 0·25 mg b.i.d. is suggested by Barnes; he emphasizes the depletion of adrenalin which may occur here and stresses that there may be alarming falls in blood pressure during anaesthesia. The drug should be stopped 7–10 days before delivery if possible. Methyl dopa 250 mg three times a day is a suitable alternative. Similar considerations also apply here to anaesthesia. Ganglion-blocking agents appear to be much less satisfactory. Kincaid-Smith *et al.* (1966) and Leather *et al.* (1968) report favourably on the use of methyl dopa in severe hypertension complicating pregnancy. Propanalol has recently been advocated as an alternative to methyl dopa by Pritchard *et al.* (1969). Whichever hypotensive agent is employed, care and attention to detail are required and rest in hospital for some weeks is still likely to be necessary.

It is doubtful if diuretic therapy is much more help here than in pre-eclamptic patients.

There will occasionally be an indication to interrupt the course of pregnancy early in the mother's interests if the levels of blood pressure remain high despite rest and intensive treatment. Usually, however, the maternal condition can be controlled, and delivery is sought in the interests of the foetus.

The timing of delivery will be governed by those considerations already referred to in relation to pre-eclampsia (p. 274). Here, since we are dealing with a more chronic situation, the opportunities to monitor foetal progress for some weeks will almost always be available. Whilst foetal well-being *in utero* is assured, delivery is to be withheld until term approaches; if evidence is obtained of failure to thrive *in utero* the time for interference must be chosen carefully. In cases of severe interference with foetal growth and oxygenation early delivery, even before 35 weeks, may be preferable to waiting longer.

The mode of delivery will be influenced, as always, by the age, parity, previous obstetric history, maturity, state of the cervix, etc. Caesarean section in the interests of the very fragile, premature baby seems to have much to commend it (see p. 439).

COARCTATION OF THE AORTA

Coarctation of the aorta complicating pregnancy will call for careful assessment of the situation in consultation with a physician and a thoracic surgeon. Many patients have gone through successful pregnancies apparently unscathed, yet it cannot be denied that serious risks exist. Rosenthal (1955) reviewed 91 cases and added five more; he recorded eleven patients whose death was directly due to pregnancy the cause being rupture of the aorta in six. Goodwin (1958) reviewed an even larger series—136 in all. The maternal mortality concerned with pregnancy was 13 (9·5%).

All the circumstances of a case will require very careful consideration before it is decided what must be done. If an operation seems indicated for the coarctation, the pregnancy need not be considered a barrier. Mode of delivery constitutes a problem which will be approached, as always, by consideration of age, parity, maturity and other factors of this kind; but if the blood pressure reaches very high levels serious consideration of Caesarean section is recommended.

Prognosis

The relationship of pre-eclampsia and eclampsia to the subsequent development of hypertension has been dealt with on p. 266. Once chronic hypertensive disease is present it is likely to be a problem in every pregnancy. It is not always the case that a subsequent pregnancy is more severely complicated, but generally speaking a pattern, once established, is repeated. Future child-bearing should be carefully considered with this point in mind.

CHRONIC RENAL DISEASE

In the past it has been thought that chronic renal disease seldom complicated pregnancy. There can be no doubt that it is uncommon to see pregnant patients with a clear-cut history of previous nephritis or the nephrotic syndrome and with evidence of impaired renal function. It is possible, however, that chronic renal disease is more common than this but is not recognizable as such without renal biopsy. McCartney (1966) records that a clinical diagnosis of chronic renal disease was reached in only 1·1% of a large series of patients with hypertensive disorders at the Chicago Lying-in Hospital. Following renal biopsy, interpreted by both light- and electron-microscopy, the frequency of unrecognized chronic renal disease was found to be about 20%. It may be that greater experience with, and wider use of, renal biopsy and electron-microscopy will elucidate this problem further.

In the presence of a known history of renal disease it becomes a matter of considerable importance not only to assess the patient's renal function carefully, but to evaluate every aspect of the case. Concentration and dilution tests, creatinine clearance, microscopy for casts, red blood cells and white blood cells will all give valuable information. The retinal vessels should be examined on several occasions. The blood pressure must be carefully monitored twice daily over a week or so to establish the pattern present. If albuminuria is present the daily protein loss should be estimated. Full-blood examination is very important.

On the basis of the results of these tests an estimate can be made of the chances of the patient carrying her baby towards term and of delivering a live child. With little hypertension, and renal damage reduced to a minimum, the outcome will probably be good—perhaps there will be foetal salvage in the order of 80–90%. Definitive hypertension appears to increase the risk of abortion or foetal death at an early stage of pregnancy. Barnes (1970) quotes a foetal loss of almost 40% in patients with chronic renal disease whose blood pressure was 150/100 mmHg in early pregnancy. Undoubtedly, if a patient has evidence of chronic renal damage with protein loss and a grossly raised blood pressure the chances of a successful foetal outcome are very slender and the risk to the patient correspondingly increased. In these cases termination of pregnancy will seem appropriate if the risk to the patient's life is to be reduced. If an attempt is to be made to carry the baby through towards term, rest, observation in hospital and foetal monitoring as in the case of pre-eclampsia and hypertension will all be essential.

THE NEPHROTIC SYNDROME

Again, this condition is uncommonly seen in the pregnant patient. When it is present oedema is often a marked feature and the loss of albumin in the urine may be great. The approach to treatment will be similar to that in the other cases discussed in this chapter. The foetal results may be better than other forms of chronic renal disease, however. Studd & Blainey (1969) reported only one neonatal death in 31 pregnancies complicated by the nephrotic syndrome. Diuretics may be more effective here than in the other disorders. Efforts to replace some of the heavy protein loss may be helpful. Cortisone therapy does not appear to give improved results.

REFERENCES

ALTCHEK A., ALBRIGHT N.L. & SOMMERS S. (1968) *Obstet. Gynec., N.Y.* **31**, 594.

ALTCHEK A. (1961) *J. Am. med. Ass.* **175**, 791.

ALTCHEK A. (1964) *Circulation*, **30** (Supplement 2), 43.

BARNES C.G. (1970) *Medical Disorders in Obstetric Practice*, 3rd edn. Oxford, Blackwell Scientific Publications.

BEAZLEY J.M. (1965) *Br. med. J.* **ii**, 919.

BENNETT M. & MATHER G. (1959) *Lancet*, **i**, 811.

BLAIR R.G. (1963) *J. Obstet. Gynaec. Br. Commonw.* **70**, 110.

BLECHER J.A. & HEYNS O.S. (1967) *Lancet*, **ii**, 621.

BROWNE F.J. (1958) *Lancet*, **i**, 115.

BROWNE F.J. & DODDS G.H. (1939) *J. Obstet. Gynaec. Br. Commonw.* **46**, 443.

CHESLEY L.C., ANNITTO J.E. & COSGROVE R.A. (1964) *Obstet. Gynec., N.Y.* **23**, 874.

CHESLEY L.C., COSGROVE R.A. & ANNITTO J.E. (1962) *Am. J. Obstet. Gynec.* **83**, 1360.

COYLE C. & GEOGHEGAN F. (1962) *Proc. R. Soc. Med.* **55**, 746.

CRICHTON D., NOTELOVITZ M. & HILLER I. (1968) *J. Obstet. Gynaec. Br. Commonw.* **75**, 1019.

DEWAR J.B. & MORRIS W.I.C. (1947) *J. Obstet. Gynaec. Br. Commonw.* **54**, 417.

GEMMELL A.A. (1955) *J. Obstet. Gynaec. Br. Commonw.* **62**, 195.

GOODWIN J.F. (1958) *Lancet*, **i**, 16.

HAMLIN R.H.J. (1952) *Lancet* **i**, 64.

HARBERT G.M., CLAIRBORNE H.A., McGAUGHEY H.S., WILSON L.A. & THORNTON W.N. (1968) *Am. J. Obstet. Gynec.* **100**, 366.

HIBBARD B.M. (1962) *Clin. Obstet. Gynec.* **5**, 1044.

HIBBARD B.M. & HIBBARD E.D. (1963) *Br. med. J.* **62**, 1430.

HYTTEN F.E. & BILLEWICZ W.Z. (1967) *J. Obstet. Gynaec. Br. Commonw.* **74**, 1.

JEFFCOATE T.N.A. (1966) *Proc. R. Soc. Med.* **59**, 397.

JEFFCOATE T.N.A. & SCOTT J.S. (1959) *Am. J. Obstet. Gynec.* **77**, 475.

KINCAID-SMITH P., BULLEN M. & MILLS J. (1966) *Br. med. J.* **i**, 274.

KRAUS G.W., MARCHESE J.C. & YEN S.C. (1966) *J. Am. med. Ass.* **198**, 1150.

KYANK H., SCHUBERT E. & GYONGYOSSY A. (1964) *Germ. med. Mon.* **9**, 108.

LEAN T.H., RATNAM S.S. & SHIVASAMBOO R.R. (1968) *J. Obstet. Gynaec. Br. Commonw.* **75**, 856.

LEATHER H.M., HUMPHREYS D.M., BAKER P. & CHADD M.A. (1968) *Lancet*, **ii**, 488.

LEWIS T.L.T. (1964) *Progress in Clinical Obstetrics and Gynaecology*, 2nd edn. London, Churchill, p. 137.

LOPEZ-LLERA M. (1967) *J. Obstet. Gynaec. Br. Commonw.* **74**, 379.

MENON M.K.K. (1961) *J. Obstet. Gynaec. Br. Commonw.* **68**, 417.

McCARTNEY C.P. (1966) *C in. Obstet. Gynec.* **9**, 864.

MITRA S., BHOSE L. & DE K. (1958) *J. Obstet. Gynaec. Br. Commonw.* **65**, 988.

PEEL J. (1962) *Am. J. Obstet. Gynec.* **83**, 847.

PICKERING G.W., ROBERTS J.A.F. & SOWRY G.S.C. (1954) *Clin. Sci.* **13**, 267.

PIKE R.L., MILES J.E. & WARDLAW J.M. (1966) *Am. J. Obstet. Gynec.* **95**, 604.

PIRANI C.L., POLLAK V.E., LANNIGAN R. & POLLI G. (1963) *Am. J. Obstet. Gynec.* **87**, 1067.

PLATT R. (1958) *J. Obstet. Gynaec. Br. Commonw.* **65**, 385.

PLATT R., STEWART A.E. & EMERY E.W. (1968) *Lancet*, **i**, 552.

PRITCHARD J.A. & STONE S.R. (1967) *Am. J. Obstet. Gynec.* **99**, 754.

PRITCHARD B.N.C. & GILLAM P.M.S. (1969) *Br. med. J.* **i**, 7.

RAGAN C. & BORDLEY J. (1941) *Bull. Johns Hopkins Hosp.* **69**, 504.

ROSENTHAL L. (1955) *Br. med. J.* **i**, 16.

RUSSELL C.S., PAINE C.G., COYLE M.G. & DEWHURST C.J. (1958) *J. Obstet. Gynaec. Br. Commonw.* **64**, 649.

SHEEHAN H.L. (1950) In *Toxemia of Pregnancy: Human and Veterinary*. A Ciba Symposium (edited by J. Hammond, F.J. Browne & G.E.W. Wolstenholme). Philadelphia, Blakiston, p. 16.

SIMS E.A.H. (1965) *Am. Rev. Med.* **16**, 221.

STUDD J.W.W. & BLAINEY J.D. (1969) *Br. med. J.* **i**, 276.

THIERY M. (1967) *Am. J. Obstet. Gynec.* **97**, 21.

CHAPTER 17

HEART DISEASE IN PREGNANCY

Before discussing the problems of heart disease and pregnancy, it is necessary to consider the haemodynamic changes which occur during pregnancy in the healthy patient.

HAEMODYNAMIC CHANGES IN PREGNANCY

It is difficult to obtain accurate and consistent information about the haemodynamic changes which occur during the course of normal pregnancy, because the methods used in measuring these changes are complex and rather limited in value. Serial estimations throughout pregnancy on a few patients are probably of more value than a large number of isolated tests at different weeks of gestation in many patients, particularly if there is a common trend in the results.

It has been known for some time that there is an increase in blood volume during pregnancy. The blood volume falls to below the non-pregnant level at about 8 weeks' gestation due to a fall in red cell mass, but thereafter there is a steady increase until between the twenty-eighth and thirty-fifth week, when it is about 35% greater than the non-pregnant volume. Both the plasma volume and the red cell mass are altered, but the plasma volume is increased by about 40% while the increase in red cell mass is only about 18%. The total blood volume falls by 15–20% from its highest figure by term, because of a reduction in the plasma volume. The actual circulating volume may be reduced, but it is possible that the fall may be related to the posture of the patient during the estimation.

The increase in the blood volume is just one factor which is likely to alter the haemodynamics in pregnancy. The presence of an abdominal swelling of increasing size with elevation and 'splinting' of the diaphragm and compression of the inferior vena cava when the patient is in the supine position also causes circulatory and respiratory changes, and the marked increase in circulating steroid hormones, particularly oestrogens, may have an effect. As the changes are occurring throughout pregnancy, some adaptation is possible, provided the functional ability and reserve capacity of the heart are satisfactory.

CARDIAC OUTPUT

For many years it was believed that the cardiac output rose progressively during pregnancy until the thirty-second week and thereafter decreased until term. Work by Walters *et al.* (1966) suggested that there was a marked rise in output by the twelfth week of pregnancy, after which the level was maintained until there was a further rise at 28–30 weeks. The output then fell until term.

Scott & Kerr (1963) showed that compression of the inferior vena cava by the gravid uterus with the patient in the supine position may cause complete occlusion in late pregnancy, and that a collateral circulation by means of the paravertebral veins may be opened up. Most studies of cardiac output were carried out with the patient in the supine position and this explained the apparent fall in cardiac output after the thirty-

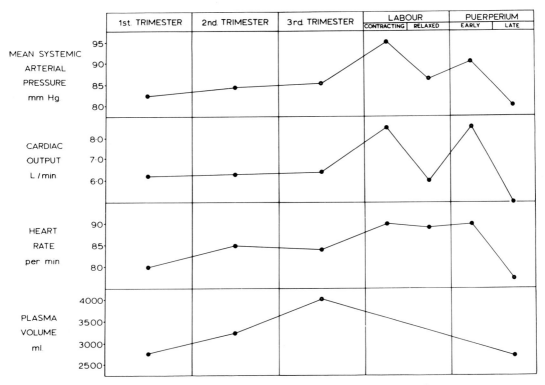

Fig. 17.1 Blood pressure, cardiac output, heart rate and plasma volume during pregnancy, labour and the puerperium.

second week. Before the third trimester, the uterine pressure on the inferior vena cava was of less consequence, but during the last 8 weeks the venous return by the inferior vena cava was reduced or completely obstructed. If the collateral circulation proved to be inefficient, these patients felt faint when lying on their backs and were said to have exhibited 'the supine hypotension' syndrome.

Lees *et al.* (1967) using an indicator-dilution method and indocyanine green as indicator studied a number of patients serially during pregnancy and showed that the maximum cardiac output was attained at the end of the first trimester, with only slight and variable changes thereafter. The maximum output was an increase of between 30 and 40% over non-pregnant levels. In late pregnancy a fall in the output occurred when the patient was in the supine position, but no change

in output was demonstrated when the tests were carried out with the patient lying on her side (Fig. 17.1). The authors have suggested that the early dramatic increase in cardiac output might be due to the increased production of ovarian and placental sex steroids.

During labour the cardiac output rises due to an increase in the stroke volume. The rise is about 40% above the late pregnancy level by the end of the second stage of labour (Kerr 1968), although the output falls when the uterus is not contracting. A further rise in the cardiac output occurs after delivery, associated with an increase in the stroke volume, a consistent bradycardia being observed. Posture, blood loss and the administration of ergometrine may complicate the haemodynamic changes after delivery, but the relief of venal caval compression is an important factor.

OTHER CHANGES

The heart rate as measured by the electro-cardiograph seems to alter very little during pregnancy, and recent studies have shown that there is little change in the arterial blood pressure under normal circumstances. The stroke volume must therefore be increased during pregnancy as well as after delivery.

The oxygen consumption is increased during pregnancy but respiratory excursion is impaired in the later weeks of pregnancy. The respiratory rate increases and dyspnoea, even on mild exertion, is a normal finding in late pregnancy.

The average changes are shown during the three trimesters of pregnancy (with the patients on their sides during the third trimester for cardiac output estimations), during labour with the uterus contracting and relaxed, and in the early and late puerperium in Fig. 17.1. The mean systemic arterial pressure, the cardiac output, the heart rate and the plasma volume changes are recorded. Healthy pregnant women are usually able to tolerate these various changes and can determine readily their own exercise tolerance. They also avoid lying on their backs because of feeling faint, and learn to sleep with extra pillows under their shoulders because of wakefulness and dyspnoea. Heart murmurs are frequently detected, the intensity of the first sound may be increased and a third heart sound may be heard. Cardiac enlargement may be detected on an X-ray and the electrocardiograph pattern may be altered, because of elevation of the diaphragm.

HEART DISEASE AND PREGNANCY

Rheumatic fever is still the most common aetiological factor in pregnant women with heart disease. However, in recent years the incidence of rheumatic heart disease has fallen, in general, because of the use of antibiotics and perhaps the presence of less virulent strains of streptococci. The number of women with congenital heart disease who reach child-bearing age has increased because of better methods of early diagnosis and management and the advent of cardiac surgery

for some of the congenital conditions. The overall incidence of heart disease in pregnancy has fallen while the ratio of rheumatic to congenital heart disease has altered from 9 : 1 to 3 : 1 or 4 : 1 at the present time in Great Britain.

Examination of the patient in early pregnancy may uncover unsuspected heart disease, sometimes without any suggestive history. Conversely, patients labelled as having heart disease may be found to have normal hearts. Close cooperation between the obstetrician and the cardiologist is therefore essential and most centres now have 'combined' clinics.

It is not the purpose of this chapter to discuss the diagnosis and treatment of all the cardiac disorders which may be found in the pregnant woman, but merely to consider the obstetrical management of these patients and to indicate some of the advances in cardiological management in recent years.

RHEUMATIC HEART DISEASE

The maternal mortality rate from rheumatic carditis has fallen dramatically during the last 30 years, as shown by the *Ministry of Health Reports on Confidential Enquiries into Maternal Deaths in England and Wales, 1932–1966*. This fall is due to the early diagnosis of the condition and close supervision during pregnancy, prolonged medical treatment in hospital or cardiac surgery before or during pregnancy and the prevention and management of the complications of heart disease.

Mitral stenosis, alone or along with other valvular disease, is the most important feature of this condition and will be considered in some detail.

MITRAL STENOSIS

The increase in work done by the left atrium in mitral stenosis is directly proportional to the degree of stenosis. As the cardiac output depends on the stroke volume and the heart rate, a reduction in the volume of blood entering the left ventricle has to be compensated for by tachycardia. The heart rate can be raised by a limited extent only. As the maintenance of arterial blood pressure depends on the cardiac output and peripheral resistance, a reduction in cardiac output will result in an increase in peripheral resistance, or hypotension.

As the work of the left atrium may increase enormously in this condition, it is not surprising that complications should occur if it is unable to carry out its function satisfactorily. The right ventricular output may be increased to compensate for left atrial inefficiency, with resultant pulmonary arterial or venous hypertension, and pulmonary oedema. Failure of the right ventricle will result in congestive cardiac failure.

In pregnancy the increased circulating blood volume and raised cardiac output puts an additional strain on the heart with mitral stenosis. If the heart is able to compensate for this, it is obvious that any additional strain or stress will readily precipitate failure of heart action. These factors include anaemia, tachycardia as a result of pyrexia or emotional upsets, exertion especially in labour, upper respiratory tract infections and any increase in circulating blood volume, particularly after the delivery of the infant and placenta.

Antenatal management

Antenatal care is concerned with the assessment of possible complications and their management. The previous medical and obstetrical history are considered, along with changes in the heart size and shape, auscultatory evidence of valve damage, the rate and rhythm of the heart, and the blood pressure as well as the condition of the lungs, anaemia, and the response to exercise and intercurrent diseases. Radiological examination of the heart and lungs—including cineradiology, electrocardiography and, sometimes, cardiac catheterization—may be required in evaluating the condition of the patient.

The severity of heart disease is commonly graded according to the classification of the New York Heart Association (1964). This is considered useful as a guide to the severity of the symptoms but need not bear any relationship to the extent of the heart lesions present.

Grade I is applied to patients with cardiac disease but no limitation of physical activity.

Grade II includes patients with heart disease and slight limitation of physical activity. Fatigue, palpitations, dyspnoea and pain may all occur with ordinary activity and result in inclusion of the patient in this grade.

Grade III refers to patients with marked limitation of activity, symptoms arising with minimal exertion.

Grade IV is present when the patient is unable to carry out any physical activity without discomfort, and has orthopnoea.

This classification is not accepted as reliable by all cardiologists, and Turner (1968) considers it potentially dangerous, as the majority of maternal deaths occur in patients who have been placed in Grades I or II in early pregnancy on account of absent or minimal symptoms. Certainly careful supervision of *all* cardiac patients during pregnancy is required to detect any deterioration in the symptoms and grading of the patient.

TERMINATION OF PREGNANCY

This may be necessary because of the danger of deterioration in the heart condition in early pregnancy. Other factors, including the patient's age and parity as well as her domestic situation, should also be taken into account in reaching a decision. Early vaginal evacuation of the uterus is preferable to termination after 12 weeks' gestation, and sterilization by tubal diathermy and the laparoscope can be performed later.

With improved methods of medical and surgical management of rheumatic heart conditions, the indications for termination of pregnancy on purely cardiological grounds are becoming fewer.

MITRAL VALVOTOMY

This operation is sometimes indicated during pregnancy, but is better performed prior to pregnancy. It has been emphasized by many writers that assessment for operation must be made for each patient and that generalizations can only be made as to the indications. The main indication is the presence of severe or 'tight' mitral stenosis which would have necessitated operation in the non-pregnant patient. If there is undue dyspnoea prior to pregnancy, or if there is evidence of pulmonary venous hypertension or right ventricular hypertrophy, operation is considered advisable. The optimum time for operation is as soon after the twelfth week of pregnancy as possible, but operations later have been successfully carried out. While most authorities agree that operation during pregnancy is sometimes indicated, they also agree that surgery should be avoided if there is any doubt about the anatomical severity of the lesion, and medical treatment is to be preferred. Ueland (1965) reported a mortality rate of 1·7% in 515 operations for mitral stenosis during pregnancy.

MEDICAL TREATMENT

This includes the prevention and prompt treatment of anaemia, antibiotic therapy for any infection, especially respiratory infection, and adequate rest and sleep. Disorders of cardiac rhythm may require digoxin therapy, fluid retention is treated with oral diuretics, measures being taken to compensate for potassium loss, and immediate admission is necessary if pulmonary congestion or oedema is suspected.

Pulmonary oedema may occur without warning and be very serious. The venous return to the heart is effectively reduced by the application of inflatable cuffs to the upper and lower limbs. Morphine derivatives are excellent in moderate dosage to relieve anxiety and the resultant increased respiratory rate. Tachycardia or fibrillation may necessitate immediate digitalization, and the administration of diuretics reduces the circulating volume after the cuffs have been removed. Oxygen therapy is beneficial and, when the patient's condition warrants it, surgical relief of the stenosis may be undertaken.

Admission to hospital for rest and treatment is imperative if there is any deterioration in the patient's condition, and for a few days at least before term. The dangers of venous thrombosis and pulmonary embolism must be guarded against, and while anticoagulants are not routinely recommended, they should be given if embolism occurs and possibly prophylactically during the puerperium, particularly if prolonged confinement to bed is required.

MANAGEMENT OF LABOUR

During labour, the patient should be propped up with pillows in order to assist respiration. Oxygen must be available and may be given intermittently, or continuously if there is dyspnoea or cyanosis. Effective sedation and analgesia with morphine derivatives is of great benefit. Continuous epidural anaesthesia has been used to good effect in these patients. There is no evidence that patients with cardiac disease have easy labours, but this impression may have resulted from the increased attention and sedation which these patients receive, along with a more active approach to their management. There is no merit in inducing labour because of the presence of cardiac disease, but sometimes a patient who has responded to treatment for cardiac failure might have her labour induced by artificial rupture of the membranes around term before a further circulatory crisis developed. Caesarean section is usually avoided but is not contra-indicated for obstetrical complications. If labour is likely to be prolonged, early Caesarean section is preferable to a vaginal delivery in a dehydrated and potentially infected woman. The use of the vacuum extractor has been advocated in order to hasten the first stage of labour, but this seems unnecessary provided satisfactory progress is being made or unless there is some other sound obstetrical indication for using the instrument.

In the second stage of labour, bearing-down with breath-holding is to be avoided, as the increase in cardiac output which has been recorded during expulsive efforts should not be permitted for any longer than is strictly necessary. The early application of obstetrical forceps is therefore to be recommended.

The use of ergometrine is contra-indicated, especially when given intravenously and after elective Caesarean section, because of the tonic uterine contraction produced, with the return of about a litre of blood to the effective circulation. If the uterus relaxes and profuse bleeding occurs, oxytocin by intravenous infusion or by intramuscular injection is probably safer and should be tried in the first instance. After completion of the third stage, careful observation for congestive failure or pulmonary oedema is of the greatest importance, as this is probably the most critical time of the pregnancy.

PUERPERIUM

Active movement in bed, early rising and early ambulation are to be encouraged, depending on the cardiac state of the patient. Alternatively, anticoagulant therapy should be instituted because of the dangers of venous thrombosis and pulmonary embolism. Antibiotics are required if there is any evidence of infection, or prophylactically if the labour has been long or the delivery complicated, because of the danger of subacute bacterial endocarditis developing.

The question of sterilization should be considered in the puerperium, laparoscopic tubal diathermy being a particularly suitable method of achieving this 6–8 weeks after delivery. If a further pregnancy is inadvisable for some time, perhaps to allow cardiac surgery to be performed, effective contraceptive advice should be offered.

Congenital heart disease

There are a number of different forms of congenital heart disease, some of the conditions being of relatively minor importance. Major forms in which there is a reversal of blood flow or in which oxygenation of the blood is inadequate, may result in abortion or the birth of small infants as a result of foetal hypoxia.

Among the conditions found are *pulmonary stenosis* with right ventricular hypertension and eventually failure of the right side of the heart. Stenosis may occur at the pulmonary valve or at the conus of the right ventricle. A harsh systolic murmur and thrill is found in the second left intercostal space, and the pulmonary second sound may be accentuated. Cyanosis is not present, but the features of cardiac failure may develop. Surgery may be indicated but is better performed before pregnancy.

A *patent ductus arteriosus* leads to the presence of a permanent arteriovenous shunt with an increase in the work of the left ventricle and pulmonary hypertension. In moderately severe cases dyspnoea on exertion will be present and gradually cardiac failure will develop. A 'machinery' murmur is heard maximally in the second left intercostal space, near the sternum, both systolic and diastolic accentuation being present. The diastolic blood pressure is low and the pulse pressure is increased with exercise. In pregnancy, the cardiac output is increased and the likelihood of failure is therefore greater. Treatment by ligation of the patent ductus can be performed in pregnancy if not diagnosed previously, but is better carried out at an earlier age, or before pregnancy.

Coarctation of the aorta is found in the region where the ductus arteriosus joins the aorta. There may be no symptoms, or headaches and dizziness associated with hypertension. The blood pressure is higher in the arms than in the legs, and the femoral pulses are weaker and more difficult to obtain. A collateral circulation may be seen, with a systolic murmur heard over the collateral vessels or at the base of the heart. Caesarean section is the preferred method of delivery because of the increased strain on the heart during labour, and surgical correction by resection of the narrowed area may be required during pregnancy.

An *atrial septal defect* may be of importance, giving rise to a shunt from the left to the right side of the heart with gradual enlargement of the right side of the heart and pulmonary artery. If the pressure is increased on the right side the shunt may be reversed. The diagnosis is then made because of breathlessness and cyanosis and later, cardiac failure. The pulmonary second sound may be accentuated, with a murmur to the left of the sternum. In Lutembacher's syndrome mitral stenosis is associated with an atrial septal defect. Treatment is medical during pregnancy, with closure of the defect at a suitable time after delivery.

When a *ventricular septal defect* is present, there is a shunt from the left to the right side and a harsh systolic murmur is heard in the fourth left intercostal space. If cardiac enlargement and reversal of the shunt occurs, congestive cardiac failure will result. Operative treatment should be avoided during pregnancy.

In *Eisenmenger's complex*, there is an inter-ventricular septal defect, with right ventricular hypertrophy and dextrorotation of the aorta, overlying the septal defect. Cyanosis is a late feature when blood passes from the right ven-tricle through the left ventricle into the aorta. Pregnancy should be avoided in this condition because of the danger of severe cardiac failure, and prepregnancy sterilization may be con-sidered after the problems have been discussed with the patient, her husband and the cardiolo-gist.

In the *tetralogy of Fallot*, the features of Eisenmenger's complex are present, along with stenosis of the pulmonary artery. Dyspnoea and fatigue are the principal symptoms, made worse by pregnancy; cyanosis, polycythaemia and finger-clubbing are found. A loud systolic murmur is maximal to the left of the sternum, with a weak pulmonary second sound and en-largement of the heart. While surgical correction of this condition is possible, the operative risks are considerable. Pregnancy is again best avoided, but can be undertaken with particular attention to the avoidance of excess weight gain, prompt treatment in hospital of even minimal evidence of failure, oxygen therapy during labour and antibiotic therapy if infection occurs.

In all patients with congenital heart disease the risk of subacute bacterial endocarditis is present, and steps must be taken to treat in-fection with antibiotics. The other general provisions recommended for the antenatal care and the management of labour and of the puerperium are applicable. In general, surgical correction of the congenital defects is to be avoided during pregnancy and continuous medical support is preferable. In the severe conditions the question of prepregnancy or even premarital sterilization should be considered.

Cardiomyopathy

Cardiomyopathy or myocarditis has been des-cribed, particularly in the puerperium. This condition presents with cardiac enlargement, tachycardia, disproportionate increase in dia-stolic pressure and oedema. Pulmonary em-bolism may result in the death of the patient.

The condition may not be a definite entity, but has been found in patients with an inadequate dietary intake. Virus infection and fibrinogen disturbances have also been implicated.

REFERENCES

KERR M.G. (1968) *Br. med. Bull.* **24**, 19.
LEES M.M., TAYLOR S.H., SCOTT D.B. & KERR M.G. (1967) *J. Obstet. Gynaec. Br. Commonw.* **74**, 319.
Ministry of Health Report on Confidential Enquiries into Maternal Deaths in England and Wales, 1932–1966. London, H.M.S.O.
SCOTT D.B. & KERR M.G. (1963) *J. Obstet. Gynaec. Br. Commonw.* **70**, 1044.
TURNER R.V.D. (1968) *Br. Med. J.* ii, 383.
UELAND K. (1965) *Am. J. Obstet. Gynec.* **92**, 148.
WALTERS W.A.W., MACGREGOR W.G. & HILLS M. (1966) *Clin. Sci.* **30**, 1.

CHAPTER 18

BLOOD DISORDERS IN PREGNANCY

The most commonly encountered haematological disorder in pregnancy is anaemia. Recently, attention has been drawn to coagulation disorders and, in the last decade, advances in the prevention and management of Rh immunization have been made. These three conditions will therefore be considered in this chapter.

ANAEMIA IN PREGNANCY

Changes in the blood in pregnancy

It is clearly established that the total blood volume, the plasma volume and the red cell mass increase in pregnancy. The total blood volume is maximal at about 34 weeks, the increase being of the order of 35% over the non-pregnant level. A decrease in volume is then thought to occur until term. Most of the increased total blood volume is due to an increase in the plasma volume of 45% at 34 weeks, while the red cell mass has only increased by less than 15% at this time and by 18% at term (Hytten & Leitch 1964). The mean corpuscular haemoglobin content is not affected in normal circumstances and so there is a definite increase in red cell production, especially in late pregnancy.

The differing ratios of total blood and plasma volumes and red cell mass result in a progressive lowering of the haemoglobin concentration and the haematocrit in the peripheral venous blood. The haemoglobin level may fall to 11 or 12 g/100 ml until the plasma volume is maximal, and then it increases slightly with the reduction in plasma volume to term. This gives rise to the 'anaemia' detected in many patients in pregnancy, and is often described as being 'physiological'.

In view of the recent work on cardiac output in late pregnancy (Chapter 17) it is interesting to speculate on the effect of the supine position on estimations of the plasma volume. Possibly, occlusion of the inferior vena cava interferes with the mixing and transportation of the marker 'dyes' used to determine plasma volume, and the fall may not be a real one.

If iron tablets are taken during pregnancy, many workers have shown that the mean haemoglobin concentration rises to almost nonpregnant levels. The packed cell volume and the red blood cell count are also modified by iron therapy, and it seems clear that iron can provide a temporary stimulus to erythropoiesis. Iron also stimulates the synthesis of protein acceptor, apoferritin, in storage cells with the formation of ferritin and later haemosiderin. The serum iron level falls in pregnancy, but is raised by the administration of iron. The iron-binding capacity, which depends on the amount of β-globulin transferrin, is raised in pregnancy but the reason for this is not clear. As Hytten & Leitch pointed out, the 'normal' situation in pregnancy cannot be readily related to the non-pregnant state. The 'normal' dilution anaemia of pregnancy reduces the viscosity of the blood and compensates for the increased cardiac output by allowing the blood pressure to remain within reasonable limits. On the other hand, it is desirable that the red cells and plasma are in the optimum condition for the transport of oxygen to the maternal and foetal tissues. Whether artificially raising the haemoglobin level above 'normal' reduces the likelihood of postpartum haemorrhage or increases the ability of the patient to withstand the complications of antepartum or postpartum haemorrhage, has not been established. Excessive lowering of the haemoglobin level, however, must be prevented.

Other changes noted in the blood in pregnancy include a leucocytosis, with a rise in polymorphonuclear leucocytes and a slight rise in lymphocytes. The erythrocyte sedimentation rate is raised and is unreliable in pregnancy as a guide to inflammatory changes. The rise is possibly related to the increase in plasma fibrinogen, while the albumin in plasma protein falls markedly.

Iron-deficiency anaemia

Most of the 4–5 g of iron in the body is in the haemoglobin, while about one-fifth is stored in the liver, spleen and marrow. Between 3 and 15 mg of elemental iron are required each day to ensure a positive iron balance as pregnancy progresses, but only about 10% of the 10–20 mg taken in a normal diet is absorbed. If there is an iron-deficiency anaemia more may be absorbed and utilized, but unless the patient's stores of iron are satisfactory, additional iron is required. The plasma transferrin level is raised and iron probably crosses the placenta to the foetus by means of transferrin and ferritin, the ferrous form being utilized. The foetus obtains the iron it requires, in spite of maternal anaemia.

Iron-deficiency anaemia in pregnancy is associated with multiparity, pregnancies in quick succession, prepregnancy menorrhagia and inadequate dietary intake. In early pregnancy, anorexia, nausea and vomiting result in a reduction in the dietary iron intake. If the patient is urged to take oral iron in these circumstances, it is unlikely either to improve her appetite or to increase the amount of iron ingested during the remainder of her pregnancy.

CLINICAL FEATURES

The most reliable method of detecting anaemia is to obtain frequent haemoglobin-concentration estimations, these being performed accurately in a laboratory. Many of the symptoms experienced by an anaemic patient may occur during pregnancy without anaemia being present—tiredness, lassitude, dyspnoea, and pallor, etc. If the patient has chronic anaemia and the changes associated with this prior to pregnancy, she will of course continue to exhibit these features.

The level of haemoglobin concentration at which the patient is considered to be anaemic is subject to variation depending on a number of factors. Certainly, a level of 10 g/100 ml or less indicates anaemia. Examination of a blood film in iron-deficiency anaemia may show varying degrees of hypochromia, microcytosis, anisocytosis and poikilocytosis. The serum iron level is low—below 50 μg/100 ml—and the bone marrow shows normal blood precursor cells but little evidence of iron. Iron deficiency in pregnancy may accompany other forms of anaemia, especially megaloblastic anaemia.

PREVENTION AND TREATMENT

The provision of oral iron tablets is widely practised as a routine measure in antenatal clinics, and in moderation is probably beneficial. If the haemoglobin level is over 12 g/100 ml and the red cells appear normochromic and normocytic, it is doubtful if the patient derives much benefit (unless her stores of iron are low), and she may be subjected to unnecessary, unpleasant side-effects such as nausea, vomiting, constipation or diarrhoea. Iron tablets should not be taken during the first trimester, because of the prevalence of gastrointestinal symptoms. If severe anaemia is present, parenteral iron is indicated at this time. The gradual introduction of iron tablets to supplement the diet, with the patient being encouraged to take the tablets during or after a meal, may be beneficial.

Ferrous sulphate 200 mg, ferrous fumerate 200 mg, ferrous gluconate 300 mg or ferrous succinate 300 mg may be used in prophylaxis, while in the treatment of iron-deficiency anaemia three tablets are given each day. When intolerance is observed, it may be necessary to give enteric-coated tablets or to use other forms of treatment. A rise in haemoglobin concentration of 1 g/100 ml is anticipated after 25–30 mg of elemental iron have been absorbed. Parenteral iron may be used if the patient is unable to tolerate iron tablets, if absorption is interfered with because of gastrointestinal disorders or infections, or if a rapid response is required. A serum iron estimation should be performed in these patients, and the iron-binding capacity should be estimated also, particularly if there is a possibility of the sickle-cell trait being present. The presence of even small amounts of ionized iron may overwhelm a binding mechanism and lead to haemosiderosis. For this reason, oral iron should be discontinued for 2 or 3 days prior to the administration of parenteral iron. Iron–dextran complex may be given intramuscularly in doses of 2 or 5 ml (1 ml contains 50 mg iron) but it is now more frequently given intravenously in saline as a total-dose infusion. Saline is a safer medium than dextrose because there is less likelihood of ionized iron being formed. Although there are risks in the administration of intravenous iron, attention to the above points will reduce them considerably. Anaphylactic shock is very uncommon, and the severity of allergic reactions such as skin rashes, pruritus and vomiting may be reduced by adding antihistamine to the infusion. An iron–sorbital citric acid complex with dextran is sometimes used intramuscularly or intravenously, 1 ml of solution containing 50 mg iron. Saccharated oxide of iron may be injected intravenously daily, an 0·5 ml ampoule containing 100 mg of iron and producing a haemoglobin rise of about 0·6 g/100 ml.

Blood transfusion is very rarely necessary and in chronic anaemia, when the volume of blood required to raise the haemoglobin to a satisfactory level is considerable, it may be dangerous. Packed red cells given slowly are recommended, and diuretics such as frusemide may help to prevent overloading of the circulation and myocardial failure. The other risks of blood transfusion, such as hepatitis and incompatibility, should also be considered.

After delivery, oral iron therapy should be continued until the haemoglobin level is shown to have returned to normal. If possible, the iron stores should be replenished by a diet containing meat and green vegetables, and excessive menstrual loss should be treated before a further pregnancy.

Megaloblastic anaemia

Megaloblastic anaemia in pregnancy is frequently due to a deficiency of folic acid, but sometimes of vitamin B_{12}. There are usually adequate stores of both in the liver, but during pregnancy the demands of the foetus and uterus may deplete the stores and the dietary intake is insufficient to replenish them. This form of anaemia is therefore the result of excessive demand, defective absorption and utilization and, most important, of inadequate dietary intake. Because of anorexia and nausea in early pregnancy it is unlikely that adequate amounts of liver, kidney and green vegetables can be taken in the diet. Defective absorption of folic acid may be associated with atrophy of the jejunal mucosal villi (Whitfield & Love 1968). The foetus will usually obtain sufficient folic acid to meet its requirements, if necessary at the expense of the mother, and the serum folate level is found to be higher in umbilical cord blood than in the maternal blood at delivery.

Folic acid is essential for the formation of nucleic acid, and so the demand for it in pregnancy is considerable, especially in multiple pregnancy, because of the larger amount of new and growing tissue present. A deficiency of folic acid in pregnancy will eventually give rise to megaloblastic anaemia, but Hibbard *et al.* (1965) have suggested that abruptio placentae, abortion, premature delivery and foetal malformations may also result.

CLINICAL FEATURES

As in the diagnosis of any anaemia, routine examination of the blood is frequently required. A low haemoglobin level associated with megaloblasts in the 'buffy coat' of peripheral blood is diagnostic. Coincidental iron deficiency may mask the megaloblastic element, but a leucopenia with an increase in the multilobar polymorphonuclear leucocytes is very suggestive. The serum vitamin B_{12} level may be lowered during pregnancy but, as with the haemoglobin level. this may not be due to a deficiency. Estimation of the level of folate in the serum is the most useful diagnostic aid, but the detection of formimino-glutamic acid in the urine after histidine loading is very suggestive.

Although some writers have suggested a relationship between the low serum levels of iron and folic acid and infants of low birth weight and pregnancies of less than normal duration (Whiteside *et al.* 1968), Chanarin *et al.* (1968) were unable to find a correlation between the folate status and birth weight, antepartum haemorrhage, abortion or urinary tract infection.

PREVENTION AND TREATMENT

As megaloblastic anaemia of pregnancy is also a deficiency disease, the addition of small quantities of folic acid to supplement the diet is now considered acceptable. The dose recommended by Willoughby & Jewell (1968) is 300 μg per day, and they have shown that, while a smaller dose may seem to be satisfactory during pregnancy, megaloblastic anaemia may not become apparent until 6 weeks after delivery unless this larger dose is given. A tablet containing 100–150 mg of a ferrous iron preparation and 150 μg of folic acid is therefore satisfactory for prophylaxis if taken twice daily. An initial period during which only one tablet is taken daily is advisable.

In the treatment of established megaloblastic anaemia, folic acid in doses of 15 or 20 mg per day should be given. If absorption is inadequate, intramuscular injections of folic acid 15 mg daily for 5 days is recommended.

The danger of prolonged treatment with folic acid is that it may mask the features of Addisonian pernicious anaemia. The nature of the anaemia may be differentiated by performing a maximal histamine secretion test or measuring the uptake of cobalt-labelled vitamin B_{12}. In pregnancy these are not desirable, and as folic-acid treatment may precipitate subacute combined degeneration of the cord, it is probably easier and safer to give an intramuscular injection of vitamin B_{12} (cyanocobalamin) in a dosage of 250 μg monthly during the pregnancy, along with folic acid. The

patient should be investigated after delivery for Addisonian pernicious anaemia. Because of the risk of neurological complications, large doses of folic acid must not be given as a prophylactic measure (Armstrong *et al.* 1968).

Haemolytic anaemia

This may be due to an intrinsic abnormality in the red cell or to an extracorpuscular or extrinsic mechanism which is in the plasma. In the intrinsic group are included a number of hereditary conditions such as congenital spherocytosis and the haemoglobinopathies, including sickle-cell anaemia and thalassaemia. In the extrinsic group there are a number of haemolytic conditions, including those associated with other diseases and drugs. In pregnancy, the hereditary haemoglobinopathies are of importance.

Haemoglobinopathies

In these conditions the formation of normal adult haemoglobin is impaired. In sickle-cell anaemia abnormal variants of haemoglobin are present, while in thalassaemia there is inhibition of the formation of normal adult haemoglobin and increased amounts of other normally occurring haemoglobins are found.

Haemoglobin consists of four haem chains attached to a globin molecule. The globin may vary but the different types of haemoglobin found depend on the numbers of different haem chains which are present. Adult haemoglobin (HbA) contains two α and two β chains, while foetal haemoglobin (HbF) consists of two α and two γ chains. There are a number of abnormal haemoglobins designated by letters and other means, the types being genetically determined. The genes for haemoglobin are paired, one for each type being obtained from each parent, thus accounting for heterozygous forms of haemoglobinopathies.

(1) SICKLE-CELL DISEASE

In this condition the red cells contain HbS, which is much less soluble than normal HbA, and in its reduced state causes the red cells to become deformed and sickle or crescent shaped. Haemoglobins S and C are due to alleles of a gene and are found most frequently in Negroes. In pregnancy there are variable reports on the maternal mortality rates in association with sickle-cell anaemia, but the perinatal mortality rate is increased and is reported as being between 15 and 30%.

There are two complications of this disease. Haemolytic anaemia is due to the accelerated removal of abnormal cells from the circulation. Vascular obstruction results from the impaction of the sickle-cells in capillaries and small veins where the oxygen tension is lowest. The reduced HbS results in slowing of the circulation because of the increased viscosity, and this ultimately leads to ischaemia and necrosis.

Complications in pregnancy

The abortion rate is high and Curtis (1959) reported an increase in the premature delivery rate. The incidence of infection is increased, particularly pneumonia and pyelonephritis. Aseptic necrosis of long bones may also occur because of vascular obstruction.

There is usually a severe anaemia near term and megaloblastic anaemia is common because of the increased rate of red cell destruction and the disordered haemopoiesis when folic-acid intake is deficient.

Management

Abel *et al.* (1969) treat their patients with folic acid 15 mg daily and with transfusions of packed red cells during the third trimester, or earlier if the anaemia is severe. They consider that the transfusions correct the anaemia and thus relieve the cardiopulmonary symptoms, and by diluting the abnormal cells reduce the likelihood of thrombosis also. The increase in the circulating red cell mass suppresses the abnormal haemopoiesis also. Antibiotics are required in the treatment of any intercurrent or chronic infections.

Iron therapy, particularly the parenteral administration of iron, can be dangerous if the serum iron level is normal or raised with a low iron-binding capacity present. As trace amounts of ionized iron may be injected when iron preparations are given, the iron-binding capacity must be adequate to remove this iron from the circulation, otherwise it may become deposited in the marrow or reticulo-endothelial system, with resultant haemosiderosis.

The likelihood of the complications of sickle-cell anaemia developing are increased in the presence of maternal hypoxia. It is particularly important, therefore, to avoid hypoxia during labour, and the use of caudal or epidural analgesia for pain relief has much to commend it. Alternatively, Caesarean section may sometimes be indicated.

(2) THALASSAEMIA

This hereditory disease is most common in Italy and Greece, and is often referred to as Mediterranean disease. There is a defect in erythropoiesis because the cells contain abnormal amounts of HbA_2 and HbF, with a reduction in the amount of HbA. The red cells are thinner and mis-shapen, and have a shortened life-span. The increased destruction of the abnormal cells leads to anaemia.

In the minor forms of thalassaemia, the anaemia is not necessarily severe but a failure to respond to iron therapy in the presence of hypochromic, microcytic cells in patients of Mediterranean origin requires electrophoretic identification of the haemoglobin pattern. The serum iron level is likely to be high and iron therapy is contraindicated.

Complications in pregnancy

Apart from anaemia, pregnancy does not present a problem, and the perinatal mortality rate is not increased (Freedman 1969). In thalassaemia due to Hb Bart's, foetal hydrops has been reported, and in Asian countries where this form of the disease is found, hydrops is more commonly due to this complication than to blood group immunization. An amniogram is indicated if hydrops is suspected, and if confirmed intra-uterine transfusions with normal blood are required. Exchange transfusion of the infant after delivery may also be indicated.

Management

Again, folic-acid therapy is important, and transfusions of packed cells may be required if the haematocrit is low or there is an excessive blood loss at delivery. Hypoxia should be avoided because of the haemoglobin deficiency.

DISORDERS OF THE COAGULATION AND FIBRINOLYTIC SYSTEMS IN PREGNANCY

For some years the dangers of hypofibrinogenaemia in obstetric disorders have been well known, and more recently the complications involving the fibrinolytic system have been recognized. Knowledge concerning the interrelationship between the two systems has also been increasing, and the subject is well reviewed for the obstetrician by Bonnar *et al.* (1969).

The coagulation system and the fibrinolytic system

The platelets and fibrin network are the first line of defence when damage to the vascular endothelium occurs. The fibrin network traps platelets to form a clot and to prevent further haemorrhage. When the fibrin has served its purpose, it is removed by fibrinolysis. Failure of the fibrinolytic system might permit excessive intravascular clotting, while failure of the coagulation process results in prolonged haemorrhage. If both fail, as is more usual in pathological states, haemorrhage persists despite blood transfusion, because there is good evidence that the two systems are interrelated.

The coagulation system is principally concerned with the formation of fibrin by the activation of the plasma protein, fibrinogen (factor I). This activation is accomplished by means of calcium (factor IV) and thrombin, which in turn is produced by the action of thromboplastin (factor III) and the protein, prothrombin (factor II). Thromboplastin is formed by two mechanisms, the intrinsic or blood constituents system and the extrinsic or tissue system.

Injury allowing contact to be made between the blood and wound surface stimulates a number of blood factors (XII, XI, IX, VIII and X) by the 'cascade' mechanism, where one activates another, so that these and a combination of factor V and phospholipid released by damaged platelets in contact with the wound are available to convert prothrombin to thrombin. This is the intrinsic system.

Tissue damage allows activation of factor VII from the blood and phospholipid may be released from the damaged area or from platelets, as in the intrinsic system. With factor V, these form prothrombin and constitute the extrinsic system.

The dissolution of fibrin from clots or in the plasma is performed by the proteolytic enzyme, plasmin. The basis of the fibrinolytic system is the activation of the plasma protein, plasminogen, which is widely distributed in the body. Plasmin is able to digest fibrin, fibrinogen, prothrombin, factor V and factor VIII. The activator of plasminogen is found in most body tissues, particularly in the uterus, and its level rises in response to stress.

The plasma also contains inhibitors of plasmin and plasminogen activator. Antiplasmins are present in the serum in excess of plasminogen, in order to prevent excessive plasmin activity should this be formed from its precursor.

When a clot is formed with platelets and fibrin, plasminogen is deposited in it also and as the antiplasmin level in the clot is low, lysis of fibrin will occur when sufficient activator has entered the clot also from the plasma. Any excess of plasmin would normally be removed by circulating antiplasmin or possibly by the platelets which have antiplasmin activity.

Under conditions of stress, the amount of circulating plasminogen activator released into the circulation is increased and the delicate balance between plasmin and antiplasmin is upset, free plasmin appearing in the circulation. This results in fibrinogen being destroyed by plasmin and the breakdown or degradation products interfere with normal fibrin formation. Clot formation is therefore imperfect and delayed, with prolongation of the clotting time and inadequate coagulation.

The plasma fibrinogen increases during pregnancy to a level of 500–600 mg/100 ml in the later weeks and in labour. There is also an increase in the levels of prothrombin, factors VII, VIII and IX, platelets and phospholipids to a varying degree.

Reports on the changes in the fibrinolytic system are at variance, and the differences may depend on the methods of assay used. Nilsson & Kullander (1967) found a definite decrease in fibrinolytic activity during pregnancy, with low levels being obtained in the third trimester and in labour. A rapid rise in activity was found within a few hours of delivery. Brakman & Astrup (1963) suggested that plasminogen activator is inhibited during pregnancy, but Shaper *et al.* (1968) were unable to demonstrate any reduction in plasminogen or in the antiplasmin content of the blood. Woodfield *et al.* (1968a) found that some women were unable to produce as much plasminogen activator following a moderate physiological stress, such as exercise in late pregnancy, as others, regardless of the amount of plasminogen activator present in the circulation in the resting state. This might be of importance in conditions in which there is extensive intravascular coagulation. Woodfield *et al.* (1968b) also found that there was a steady, progressive increase in the amount of fibrinogen and fibrin breakdown products throughout pregnancy, and while there are many possible explanations for this observation, it would appear that fibrinolysis is increased in pregnancy. This may perhaps be related to the vasodilatation of pregnancy and the increased area of endothelium over which fibrin may be deposited, with a resultant increase in the amount of fibrin available for breakdown and a relative increase in the amount of degradation products in the circulation.

Recently, Wardle & Menon (1969) found that urinary fibrinolytic activity is reduced more in patients with hypertension and toxaemia. They postulate that in these conditions there is a persistent low-grade intravascular coagulation and that increased fibrin deposition is related to the renal changes which are reported. The fibrin may persist because of the reduction in fibrinolysis.

The rising level of oestrogens in pregnancy is thought to be important in the changes in the two systems, especially in the inhibition of normal fibrinolytic activity. The fall in oestrogen level after delivery may explain the rapid return of the fibrinolytic system to normal (Shaper *et al.* 1968). The kidneys and uterus, as well as other tissues, may contribute to the maintenance of circulating levels of plasminogen activator.

CHANGES IN PREGNANCY DISORDERS

If the delicate balance between the coagulation and the fibrinolytic systems is upset, a haemorrhagic diathesis may develop. This can give rise to alarming and uncontrollable bleeding unless prompt action is taken. The most common conditions in obstetrics associated with defibrination are abruptio placentae and intra-uterine death, along with missed abortion, and the syndrome is also reported in association with amniotic fluid embolism, septic abortion, placenta praevia and following Caesarean section.

Abruptio placentae (see Chapter 15)

The most usual explanation for the haemorrhagic diathesis is that of intravascular coagulation, and in some instances fibrinolytic activity is increased. It has been suggested that local fibrinolysis at the placental site might also explain the sequence of events. With separation of the placenta, damage to the decidua and to the placenta itself must occur, with the release of thromboplastin into the circulation. This will trigger off widespread intravascular coagulation with the deposition of fibrin in the retroplacental clot and in the blood vessels. The fibrinolytic enzyme system is secondarily stimulated by this, otherwise fatal thrombo-embolism in the pulmonary and renal vessels would occur. Removal of the excessive fibrin causes the release of fibrin degradation products, which in turn interferes with the conversion of fibrinogen to fibrin, and also with the adhesiveness of the platelets (Coopland *et al.* 1968). Thus the haemorrhage is uncontrolled and may prove fatal. If the haemostatic defect is due to primary excessive fibrinolytic activation, as a result of premature placental separation, the management of the patient will be different.

Intravascular coagulation may be treated with heparin given intravenously in an infusion, while excessive fibrinolysis may be inhibited by epsilon aminocaproaic acid (EACA).* It has been suggested that EACA might give rise to widespread vascular occlusion, but in normal dosage this should not happen. In the management of this condition, fresh whole blood may be all that is required, and if it is not, fibrinogen depletion should be replaced with 6 g of fibrinogen intravenously in 15–30 min. Alternatively, fresh frozen plasma will also replace factors V and VIII, which may also be deficient. If the haemorrhage is still not controlled, then heparin 1,500 units per hour may be useful; also, EACA in an intravenous drip may be given in a dose of 1 g/hr after an initial dose of 4 g. Apart from determining the plasma fibrinogen level, which is time-consuming, laboratory control of the level of plasminogen and fibrin degradation products is not usually readily available.

The obstetrical management is considered in Chapter 15, but generally, early vaginal delivery offers the best prognosis.

INTRA-UTERINE DEATH AND MISSED ABORTION (SEE CHAPTER 14)

Intravascular coagulation is thought to occur as a result of thromboplastin release from the dead foetus and placenta, and this in turn will result in fibrinogen depletion. The plasma fibrinogen level begins to fall after the dead foetus has been retained for about 3 weeks, and dangerous levels may be reached 5 weeks after death or later. Spontaneous expulsion has occurred in most instances by then, but if it has not and the fibrinogen level is approaching 150 mg/100 ml, this is an additional indication for emptying the uterus. Fibrinolysis will be stimulated by the intravascular coagulation, and the release of fibrin breakdown products may result in failure to form fibrin and therefore haemorrhage. Platelet damage and depletion is also reported in some instances. If labour is induced when the

*See footnote on p. 255, Chapter 15.

plasma fibrinogen level is below 150 mg/100 ml, intravenous fibrinogen can be given. The potential coagulation defect should be corrected by this but, if not, the use of heparin may be considered.

AMNIOTIC FLUID EMBOLISM

This condition occurs during or after labour or at Caesarean section and has to be fatal for a firm diagnosis to be made—lesser degrees may be associated with 'unexplained' postpartum haemorrhage. Amniotic fluid enters the maternal circulation and causes intravascular clotting with thrombosis of the pulmonary vessels. If it is not fatal, there is a fall in the level of fibrinogen, other blood factors and platelets, and fibrinolytic activity is increased. Treatment of the coagulation upset consists of administering heparin because of the intravascular coagulation.

SEPTIC ABORTION OR UTERINE INFECTION

Infection of the uterus following criminal abortion may result in a serious coagulation disorder with thrombocytopenia, fibrinolysis and heavy bleeding. Initially, there may be profound shock with a pyrexia or a subnormal temperature and minimal bleeding. The course of the condition resembles that found in the Schwartzmann reaction in experimental animals, pregnancy replacing the primary injection of endotoxin. Intravascular coagulation occurs with micro-embolism to the renal glomerular capillaries and to other sites. Phillips et al. (1967) found that heparin given early may minimize the intravascular clotting process, but not when its administration is delayed. EACA, on the other hand, could cause renal cortical necrosis if given early, as it may prevent the removal of the thrombi by fibrinolysis. The best method of treatment, apart from antibiotic therapy and local treatment of the uterus, is fresh blood with fibrinogen and perhaps heparin.

CAESAREAN SECTION OR HYSTEROTOMY

Occasionally, the defibrination syndrome has been reported following these operations.

Thromboplastic material may be released into the maternal circulation during the operation. The writer has seen this occur in a patient undergoing hysterotomy following a missed abortion. The fibrinogen level was normal and the defibrination syndrome was attributed to the release of thromboplastin when the uterus was compressed to expel clots after the procedure. Both fibrinogen depletion and increased fibrinolytic activity were found, and treatment with blood, fibrinogen and EACA was successful.

RH IMMUNIZATION

Major advances in the management of Rh immunization in recent years include its prevention by the injection of anti-Rh immunoglobulin G, assessment of the affect of the antibodies on the foetus by examination of the amniotic fluid, intra-uterine intraperitoneal transfusion of the foetus and improved techniques of management of the infant with haemolytic disease. More is also known about the natural history of Rh immunization and Rh haemolytic disease of the foetus and newborn.

Development of Rh immunization and its prevention

When red blood cells containing the Rh_0 or D (Rh) antigen enter the circulation of a woman who does not possess this antigen on her red cells, the development of Rh immunization is possible. A transfusion or injection of blood which is incompatible in the Rh system with the recipient's blood may stimulate the production of antibodies to that factor, most usually the Rh_0 or D factor. However, antibodies to rh' (C) and hr″ (e) may also be formed and multiple immunization may occur. Immunization as a result of pregnancy is nearly always due to the Rh_0 (D) antigen, and this one will be considered here.

Rh-positive red cells enter the maternal circulation during pregnancy, and although the amount of foetomaternal haemorrhage is usually small, it is likely to increase as pregnancy progresses. Foetal cells can be demonstrated and counted in a maternal blood film by means of the

acid-elution technique. Red cells containing adult haemoglobin are unable to withstand the citric-acid buffer in which the blood film is immersed, while cells containing foetal haemoglobin are unaffected by the buffer. The haemoglobin in adult cells is eluted and when the film is counterstained, the cells appear as ghosts. Foetal haemoglobin-containing cells take up the counterstain and are clearly seen when the film is examined (Fig. 18.1). Certain obstetrical

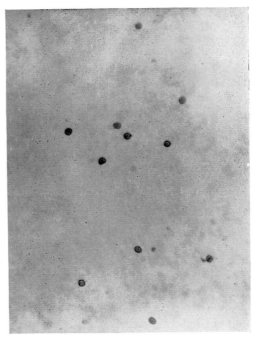

Fig. 18.1. Foetal red blood cells in maternal blood film (acid-elution technique). Foetal cells appear dark and adult cells are 'ghosts'.

complications are known to be associated with an increased risk of foetomaternal haemorrhage and thus of Rh immunization, but these may both occur during an uncomplicated pregnancy and with a normal delivery. Both spontaneous and therapeutic abortion may give rise to foetomaternal haemorrhage (Matthews & Matthews 1969), and also external cephalic version, pre-eclampsia, antepartum haemorrhage, Caesarean section and manual separation of an adherent placenta. Some of these complications are known to be associated with an increased incidence of Rh immunization.

A woman who is Rh negative and whose foetus is ABO incompatible with her, is usually protected from immunization because the anti-A or anti-B antibody circulating in her blood will remove rapidly the A- or B-positive cells entering from the foetus. The Rh antigen is probably not brought into contact with immunologically competent cells and the chance of Rh immunization is very small. The development of Rh immunization appears to depend on the volume of foetal cells present in the maternal circulation, and the Combined Study from Centres in England and Baltimore (1966) found that a foetal cell count below a critical number resulted in one patient in twenty becoming immunized, while a count above this number increased the rate to one in five.

It is generally agreed that cells enter the maternal circulation throughout pregnancy, but as immunization is rarely found during a first pregnancy, either the volume of foetomaternal haemorrhage is insufficient to stimulate an antibody response, or the mother is unresponsive to the stimulus, or immunization occurs but is not detectable during the pregnancy. The foetal cells continue to circulate in the maternal circulation, if there is no ABO incompatibility, until they age and are removed by the reticulo-endothelial system, and this process may take weeks or months. The largest number of cells are found in the maternal circulation at the end of pregnancy, after delivery and in the first few days of the puerperium. The count may continue to increase during the puerperium, especially after Caesarean section, presumably because of spillage into, and subsequent absorption from, the peritoneal cavity.

Immunization nearly always develops after the immunizing pregnancy. As patients are rarely examined for the presence of antibodies in their blood until a subsequent pregnancy, the true incidence of immunization has not been revealed until controlled studies were undertaken in order to prevent its development. It has now been shown that 6 months after delivery, about 10–12% of those at risk develop antibodies, and an additional 10% exhibit antibodies during a

subsequent pregnancy as a probable consequence of the immunizing one. The ability to detect small quantities of antibody is very important in attempting to obtain the true incidence. After a further Rh-positive pregnancy, the Rh-negative woman appears to be at the same risk of immunization.

The antibodies formed are of two types. Immunoglobulin M (IgM) or 19S antibody is of large molecular size and weight and does not cross the placenta. It therefore has no effect on the foetus but will remove foetal Rh-positive red cells entering the maternal circulation. Immunoglobulin G (IgG) or 7S antibody is smaller and can be actively transported across the placenta, and so is the antibody which causes haemolytic disease.

PREVENTION

The theoretical concepts involved in the development of the method of prevention of Rh immunization by using anti-Rh IgG have been described by Clarke (1967) and by Pollack et al. (1969). Clinical trials in Europe, North America and Australasia have been published to show that the method is successful in preventing immunization on nearly all occasions. The procedure is that blood is obtained from the umbilical cord and from the mother at delivery. The infant's blood is grouped—ABO and Rh—and the mother's blood is again grouped and screened for the presence of Rh antibodies. If the foetus is Rh positive and the mother is Rh negative but not immunized, an intramuscular injection of anti-Rh immunoglobulin is given within 48–72 hr of delivery. This injected antibody causes the removal of any foetal red cells in the maternal circulation and possibly competes with the antibody-forming cells for Rh antigen released from the destroyed cells. The injected antibody will eventually be destroyed in the normal process of protein breakdown in the body, but the stimulus to immunize will have been removed until the patient has another Rh-positive pregnancy.

Variations in the above procedure depend on the availability of anti-Rh IgG, the volume of foetomaternal haemorrhage and the dosage of material considered necessary. In Canada,

Zipursky & Israels (1967) gave injections of IgG during the third trimester without ill-effects being noted in the infants. This was done to prevent immunization developing late in pregnancy before the postdelivery injection was given. In certain European centres, intravenous IgG has been given to hasten the removal of the foetal cells with a smaller dose of IgG. The usual dose recommended at the present time is between 200 and 300 μg protein per millilitre, but further dosage studies related to the volume of foeto-maternal haemorrhage are required.

Anti-Rh IgG is obtained from naturally immunized women, with or without 'boosting' their antibody titre by the injection of Rh-positive cells, and by deliberately immunizing Rh-negative volunteers by the same process. Plasmapheresis is performed on the donors, whole blood being withdrawn, the red cells being retransfused, and the plasma being processed into anti-Rh IgG. Frequent donations are possible without detriment to the donor's health by this method.

When sufficient material is available, all Rh-negative women can be protected after every pregnancy in which the infant is Rh positive, but at present, because of economic considerations, some countries have to select patients on the basis of parity, foetal-cell counts and ABO grouping. Failures have been reported in protection programmes, and the reasons for these are not yet certain. Most usually, antibodies are already present when the patient receives her injection after delivery, either because the testing has been inadequate or the antibodies are incapable of detection. Whether an injection of IgG in these circumstances enhances the immune response has not yet been established. The possibility of IgG, given to protect against the effects of rubella, containing anti-Rh IgG has been considered in two known failures, but the association with enhancement has not been proven.

While this method of prevention should reduce considerably the incidence of Rh immunization, it is accepted that there will be some failures, and some patients will be immunized during their first pregnancies. Also, a number of women already immunized will have pregnancies for the next 10 or 20 years, so the management of the immunized patient is still very important.

CONSEQUENCES AND MANAGEMENT OF RH IMMUNIZATION

Usually, a patient who 'develops' antibodies during her pregnancy was immunized by a previous pregnancy, and the titre was so low that the initial antibody screen failed to detect its presence. As the concentration increases during pregnancy, the antibodies are more likely to be discovered. For this reason, blood should be tested from all pregnant women and an antibody 'screen' carried out. If the patient is Rh negative and a primigravida, repeat tests at 32 and 38 weeks are advisable, and certainly blood should be tested at delivery prior to the injection of anti-Rh IgG. In a multiparous Rh-negative patient, screening for antibodies should be repeated at 20, 28, 32–34 and 36–38 weeks as a minimum, and again at delivery.

If antibodies are discovered, more frequent tests are indicated if it is considered that the height of the antibody titre or changes in the titre are of significance. There are limitations in the use of antibody titres in the management of patients, particularly if premature induction of labour and intra-uterine transfusion are being considered. Many writers, however, have recommended that amniocentesis should be performed only after a critical titre has been reached, this titre being determined by the outcome at similar titres in pregnancies investigated by the particular laboratory. Tovey (1969) has recently reviewed their place in management.

If the antibody is IgG and crosses the placenta, the Rh status of the foetus is important. If the foetus is Rh negative (the father being Rh negative or heterozygous Rh positive), the antibodies will have no effect. If the foetus is Rh positive, the IgG molecules become attached to the antigen sites on the cell surface. Only a small percentage of these sites need to be occupied for the cell to be rapidly removed from the circulation by the reticulo-endothelial system. The foetal cells coated with antibodies give a positive direct antiglobulin or Coombs's test. The removal of varying numbers of foetal red cells—the number depending on the amount of antibody in the foetal circulation and the ability of the foetal tissues to remove 'coated' cells—results in two separate, but related, processes.

The removal of red cells from the circulation results in anaemia and a compensatory haemopoiesis occurs. A number of immature red cells or erythroblasts enter the circulation and the haemopoietic centres are stimulated. If the anaemia can be adequately compensated for, the haemoglobin level remains satisfactory and the infant at birth may be slightly anaemic or develops anaemia during the first few weeks of life. A single transfusion is sufficient to deal with this.

Excessive removal of circulating red cells leads to definite anaemia with hypoxia affecting the brain, the heart and other tissues including the placenta. Placental hyperplasia occurs to increase the transfer of oxygen, but as the anaemia tends to be progressive, the immature cells being Rh positive also, the number of oxygen-carrying cells continues to fall. At some stage as a consequence of hypoxia, cardiac and circulatory failure develops with oedema of the tissues and ascites, as well as oedema of the placenta, and of perhaps equal importance, metabolic failure with acidosis occurs. The foetus then has hydrops foetalis and is unlikely to recover despite intra-uterine or extra-uterine treatment. The definition of hydrops foetalis is very difficult in the 'border-line' case, as recovery has been reported after the treatment of ascitic and oedematous foetuses and infants. However, if severe metabolic failure has occurred, recovery is unlikely. A follow-up study on the neurological state of severely hydropic but surviving infants is necessary to evaluate the benefits of treating this group. Treatment before the development of irreversible hydrops or acidosis is well worth while.

Excessive red cell destruction results in the level of unconjugated bilirubin rising, but luckily this can be excreted into the maternal circulation by an efficiently functioning placenta. A small percentage of this bilirubin enters the amniotic fluid, perhaps from the foetal lung or through its skin, as well as from the cord and placenta. After the delivery of the infant and clamping of the umbilical cord, the bilirubin circulates in the infant and jaundice develops. This is icterus gravis neonatorum. The bilirubin level rises because of the inability of the liver to conjugate the excessive amount in the circulation. If the level rises too high—perhaps above 15–20 mg/100 ml—bilirubin crosses the blood-brain barrier and the basal ganglia of the brain are damaged. This is kernicterus, and it is prevented by maintaining the bilirubin concentration below the danger level by means of exchange blood transfusion.

MANAGEMENT

Once a diagnosis of Rh immunization has been made, the aim of management is to deliver the patient of a living infant without hydrops foetalis and hypoxia, and with a reasonable chance of survival. Thus, delivery should be as near term as possible. It is obvious that the longer the foetus is exposed to antibodies, the greater the amount of red cell destruction. Therefore, the earlier it is removed from this hostile environment the better. A compromise depending on the predicted severity of the haemolytic disease is necessary. The most useful method of evaluating the condition of the foetus is by examination of the amniotic fluid, this being obtained by transabdominal amniocentesis. Various sites have been used for obtaining the fluid, the most popular being the site opposite the foetal back between the foetal limbs. It is also possible to obtain fluid by pushing the small foetus towards the fundus and inserting the needle suprapubically. Local anaesthetic is injected into the skin at the site of puncture and a 22-gauge-$3\frac{1}{2}$-in spinal needle is inserted. As little as 5 ml of fluid is sufficient for testing, but up to 30 ml can be removed without complications. The reader is referred to two excellent reviews on this subject by Queenan (1967) and Liley (1968).

Because of its close proximity to the foetus, the amniotic fluid contains many products of foetal metabolism. If excessive breakdown of red cells is occurring in the foetus with a rise in the circulating bilirubin level, the bilirubin content of the amniotic fluid would be expected to bear some relationship to the haemoglobin level remaining in the foetus. This need not be a close relationship, and foetuses react differently to the same haemoglobin level. However, the foetal haemoglobin level is rarely available at the time of amniocentesis, the volume of amniotic fluid is not constant for a particular gestation and contamination with meconium and blood may cause inaccuracy. The amount of bilirubin is small and the standard biochemical methods of estimation are inaccurate at low concentrations. However, a number of methods have been described for biochemical estimation, and Black et al. (1969) reported good results.

The most usual method of estimating bilirubin involves spectrophotometry. A number of methods of determining the bilirubin content have been described and are reviewed by Robertson (1969a). Having obtained a value for the bilirubin content of the amniotic fluid, this is then used to predict the severity of the haemolytic disease (Liley 1961), to report on the state of the foetus (Freda 1965) or to indicate the appropriate management (Robertson 1969b). Results tend to correlate poorly when very accurate predictions in terms of haemoglobin levels, bilirubin changes or numbers of exchange transfusions required are made. Basically it is necessary to know if and when the test should be repeated, when the foetus should be delivered—at term, between 38 and 40 weeks, between 35 and 38 weeks or before 35 weeks—and when intra-uterine transfusion is required.

Other methods of assessing severity include amniography and radiology (Queenan et al. 1968), oestriol estimation in the amniotic fluid (Schindler et al. 1967) and urine, but these tend to indicate only the very severely affected foetuses.

The management of patients with Rh antibodies by removing or neutralizing the antibodies has not proved very successful. Rh hapten, D-glucosamine and corticosteroids have all had variable success.

The induction of labour as indicated by the tests employed is probably the most useful method of management and instead of the very early inductions sometimes performed, the use of intra-uterine, intraperitoneal transfusion is preferred.

This involves the injection of Rh-negative red cells into the peritoneal cavity of the foetus prior to delivery. Radio-opaque material may be injected into the amniotic fluid some hours prior to the transfusion and subsequent radiographs will show the outline of the foetus and placenta more readily; also, swallowing of the material allows a 'target' of bowel (Fig. 18.2) to be seen

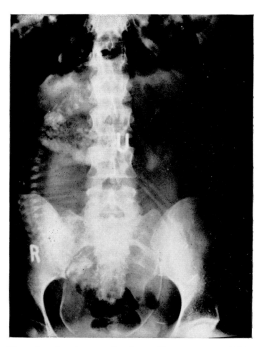

Fig. 18.2. Amniogram showing radio-opaque material in foetal gut.

more easily on fluoroscopic screening. If the radio-opaque material is swallowed, gross hydropic change can be excluded.

With the patient sedated and under the image intensifier, a long needle is inserted through the skin into the uterus and then into the peritoneal cavity of the foetus (Fig. 18.3). If the foetal back is anterior, external version may be carried out to make the insertion easier by turning the back posteriorly. A little radio-opaque solution is injected through the needle, and a characteristic 'pattern' is seen (Fig. 18.4). Blood may then be injected slowly through the needle or through a catheter inserted before the removal of the needle. The blood should be freshly drawn with some plasma removed so that its haematocrit is about 70. The volume injected depends on the

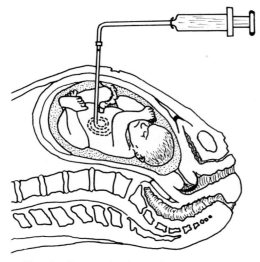

Fig. 18.3. Intra-uterine, intraperitoneal transfusion.

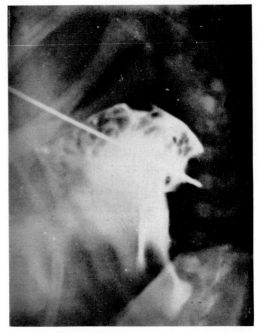

Fig. 18.4. X-ray of foetal abdomen after injection of radio-opaque material. Material seen outside foetal gut, and thus in peritoneal cavity.

maturity of the foetus, and it is preferable to inject too little rather than too much blood. At 20 weeks, 20 ml is recommended by Queenan (1967), and at 33 weeks he suggests no more than 75 ml. Certainly no more than 100 ml should ever be given. Transfusions must be repeated every 2 or 3 weeks, depending on the condition of the foetus and the gestation. Delivery at 36 weeks is desirable, but not always possible.

Among the complications to the foetus are trauma, the liver, pericardium and bowel all having been penetrated. Maternal complications include infection, trauma to maternal tissues and premature onset of labour. Hepatitis of the foetus and mother has been reported and there is the possibility of 'graft-versus-host' disease.

The technique and complications have been described by Liley (1968), who also considered the other forms of intra-uterine transfusion which have been attempted. In skilled hands, a 50–60% survival rate has been achieved, but the selection of patients is of great importance. The results are best when the foetus shows no evidence of ascites or hydrops and the first transfusion is performed after 28 weeks' gestation. They are worst when the foetus is hydropic and the first transfusion is given before 28 weeks. In the latter, more transfusions are required, less blood must be given during the early transfusions and the condition

of the foetus is poor, if not hopeless, at the commencement of treatment. Digoxin, diuretics and electrolytes have been tried in hydropic infants and peritoneal dialysis was reported to have had some success.

After delivery, prompt paediatric assessment and treatment may be required in the seriously affected infant. This may include the rapid removal of blood, the injection of bicarbonate and packed red cells, albumin infusions and small, frequent transfusions. Recent work with ultra-violet light has been successful in treating infants with icterus gravis neonatorum, and this may reduce the number of exchange transfusions required.

REFERENCES

ABEL H.R., BRADLEY T.B. & RANNEY H.M. (1969) *Clin. Obstet. Gynec.* **12**, 39.
ARMSTRONG B.K., DAVIS R.E., MARTIN J.D. & WOODLIFF H.J. (1968) *Br. med. J.* iv, 158.
BLACK J.A., PENNINGTON G.W. & WARRELL D.W. (1969) *J. Obstet. Gynaec. Br. Commonw.* **76**, 112.

BONNAR J., McNICOL G.P. & DOUGLAS A.S. (1969) In *Modern Trends in Obstetrics*, Vol. IV (edited by R.J. Kellar) London, Butterworths, p. 162.

BRAKMAN P. & ASTRUP T. (1963) *Scand J. clin. Lab. Invest.* **15**, 603.

CHANARIN I., ROTHMAN D., WARD A. & PERRY J. (1968) *Br. med. J.* **ii**, 390.

CLARKE C.A. (1967) *Br. med. J.* **iv**, 7.

Combined Study from Centres in England and Baltimore (1966) *Br. med. J.* **ii**, 907.

COOPLAND A.T., ISRAELS E.D., ZIPURSKY A. & ISRAELS L.G. (1968) *Am. J. Obstet. Gynec.* **100**, 311.

CURTIS E.M. (1959) *Am. J. Obstet. Gynec.* **77**, 1312.

FREDA V.J. (1965) *Am. J. Obstet. Gynec.* **92**, 341.

FREEDMAN W.L. (1969) *Clin. Obstet. Gynec.* **12**, 115.

HIBBARD B.M., HIBBARD E.D. & JEFFCOATE T.N.A. (1965) *Acta obstet. gynec. scand.* **44**, 375.

HYTTEN F.E. & LEITCH I. (1964) *The Physiology of Human Pregnancy*. Oxford, Blackwell Scientific Publications.

LILEY A.W. (1961) *Am. J. Obstet. Gynec.* **82**, 1359.

LILEY A.W. (1968) *Advances in Pediatrics*, Vol. XV (edited by S.Z. Levine). Chicago, Year Book Medical Publishers, p. 29.

MATTHEWS C.D. & MATTHEWS A.E.B. (1969) *Lancet*, **i**, 694.

NILSSON I.M. & KULLANDER S. (1967) *Acta obstet. gynec. scand.* **46**, 273.

PHILLIPS L.L., SKRODELIS V. & QUIGLEY H.J. (1967) *Obstet. Gynec., N.Y.* **30**, 350.

POLLACK W., GORMAN J.G. & FREDA Y.J. (1969) In *Progress in Haematology*, Vol. VI (edited by E.B. Brown & C.V. Moore). New York, Grune B Stratton.

POLLACK et al. (1968) *Progress in Hematology*. New York, Grune & Stratton.

QUEENAN J.T. (1967) *Modern Management of the Rh Problem*. New York, Evanston and London, Hoeber Medical Division, Harper & Row, p. 56.

QUEENAN J.T., GAL H.V. VON., KUBARYCH S.F. (1968) *Am. J. Obstet. Gynec.* **102**, 264.

ROBERTSON J.G. (1969a) In *Modern Trends in Obstetrics*, Vol. IV (edited by R.J. Kellar). London, Butterworths, p. 202.

ROBERTSON J.G. (1969b) *Am. J. Obstet. Gynec.* **103**, 713.

SCHINDLER A.E., RATANASOPA V., LEE T.Y. & HERRMANN W.L. (1967) *Obstet. Gynec., N.Y.* **29**, 625.

SHAPER A.G., KEAR J., MACINTOSH D.M., KYOBE J. & NJAMA D. (1968) *J. Obstet. Gynaec. Br. Commonw.* **75**, 433.

TOVEY L.A.D. (1969) *J. Obstet. Gynaec. Br. Commonw.* **76**, 117.

WARDLE E.N. & MENON I.S. (1969) *Br. med. J.* **ii**, 625.

WHITESIDE M.G., UNGAR B. & COWLING D.C. (1968) *Med. J. Aust.* **i**, 338.

WHITFIELD C.R. & LOVE A.H.G. (1968) *J. Obstet. Gynaec. Br. Commonw.* **75**, 844.

WILLOUGHBY M.L.N. & JEWELL F.G. (1968) *Br. med. J.* **iv**, 356.

WOODFIELD D.G., COLE S.K., ALLAN A.G.E. & CASH J.D. (1968a) *Br. med. J.* **iv**, 665.

WOODFIELD D.G., COLE S.K. & CASH J.D. (1968b) *Am. J. Obstet. Gynec.* **102**, 440.

ZIPURSKY A. & ISRAELS L.G. (1967) *Can. med. Ass. J.* **97**, 1245.

CHAPTER 19

URINARY TRACT DISORDERS
IN PREGNANCY

In recent years, disorders of the urinary tract in pregnancy have aroused considerable attention, particularly urinary infection and renal failure. Studies have also been undertaken to examine the physiological changes produced by pregnancy and to relate these to the conditions which are encountered by the pregnant woman.

PHYSIOLOGICAL CHANGES IN THE URINARY TRACT DURING PREGNANCY

Pregnancy is a severe test of a patient's renal function, and appropriate investigations during and soon after pregnancy may reveal defects in functional ability.

In early pregnancy the enlarging uterus presses upon the bladder, and in certain circumstances, such as retroversion and incarceration of the uterus, may displace the bladder into the abdomen, with consequent pressure upon the urethra. As pregnancy progresses the production of progesterone increases, and this hormone in particular has a relaxing effect on the uretero-vesical sphincter. As the pressure of fluid in the bladder exceeds that in the ureter in pregnancy, there is a reflux of urine from the bladder into the ureter and renal pelvis.

As the uterus increases in size and rises out of the pelvis, it will eventually press against the ureters at the pelvic brim. This pressure is more likely on the right side than on the left because of dextrorotation of the uterus and the sharp angulation of the ureter as it passes over the right common iliac vessels, while the left ureter crosses the left common iliac vessels obliquely. The pelvic colon and its mesentery protect the left ureter whereas the right is exposed more directly to uterine pressure.

The ureter in the pelvis is muscular, and therefore less distensible, even under the influence of hormones. The abdominal portion of the ureter, however, has more connective tissue in its wall and therefore is more liable to dilate. As the ureter is only loosely bound down to the underlying muscle, it can be displaced and is liable to undergo 'kinking'.

The renal pelvis becomes dilated in pregnancy and the pressure in it rises so that the renal parenchyma has to secrete urine against increased pressure. The capacity of the ureter also increases but, because of dilatation and kinking or tortuosity, it takes longer for urine to reach the bladder, and a state of stasis of urine occurs. Peristalsis is diminished because of the progesterone effect, while towards the end of pregnancy, oestrogen appears to improve the tone of the ureter by producing hyperplasia of its smooth-muscle fibres.

Urinary stasis is maximal at about 24 weeks' gestation and then lessens until a few weeks after delivery. As pregnancy proceeds and the presenting part enters the pelvis, the bladder is compressed against the symphysis pubis. This may give rise to frequency and incontinence of urine. During labour, the bladder is forcibly compressed between the foetal head and the symphysis pubis. Part of the bladder rises out of the pelvis but the pelvic portion is emptied of urine and subject to pressure and trauma.

TESTS OF RENAL FUNCTION

The renal plasma flow and renal blood flow have been shown to increase during pregnancy until about 1 month from term, when they fall almost to the non-pregnant level (Hytten & Leitch 1964). This fall, as term approaches, may be related to the pressure of the uterus on the renal blood vessels when the patient is studied in the supine position. The glomerular filtration rate is raised during pregnancy by about 60% using the method of inulin clearance. Creatinine clearance was considered to be a measure of the glomerular filtration rate, but has been found to be unreliable in pregnancy although it shows an increase in rate over the non-pregnant state. The clearance of urea is increased in pregnancy and while this results in a lowered blood urea nitrogen, compared with the non-pregnant level, it can also be used as a test of the glomerular filtration rate.

During pregnancy it seems that the ability to excrete a 'test' quantity of water is increased until late in pregnancy when the amount excreted is reduced. With the increase in glomerular filtration rate, the amount of sodium filtered will also be raised. Sodium, however, is reabsorbed by the tubules to a very large extent and the amount in the urine is not generally greater than in the non-pregnant state. Glycosuria is common in pregnancy and may again be the result of an increased filtration of glucose with a failure of complete reabsorption. The excretion of amino acids and folic acid is also increased, probably as a result of the increased glomerular filtration rate.

URINARY TRACT INFECTION

Acute pyelonephritis is a common disease in association with pregnancy. However, from the pioneer work of Baird (1935) and the later work of Kass (1956) it is apparent that the disease should not be considered merely as an episode in pregnancy which can be corrected by a course of antibiotics.

Aetiology and pathogenesis

This can be considered in two ways: (i) the causation of acute pyelonephritis in pregnancy, and (ii) the development of overt urinary tract infection during a pregnancy. During pregnancy, *Escherichia coli* is the most common infecting organism of the urinary tract, and is responsible for over 90% of infections. Other organisms causing a urinary tract infection include enterococci, *Staphylococcus aureus*, *Pseudomonas pyocyanea* and *Bacillus proteus*.

The organisms may gain access to the kidneys and the urinary tract by haematogenous and lymphatic spread, particularly if there is obstruction to the urinary flow—as may occur if the ureters are kinked. As a general rule, however, the presence of coliform organisms in the blood will produce a systemic upset prior to the onset of the renal infection. Lymphatic spread from the large bowel has not been convincingly shown to be an important cause. The most likely route of infection is by the reflux of infected urine from the bladder to the renal pelvis and parenchyma. The female urethra has been shown to contain bacteria, including *Esch.coli* (Cox 1966), and it seems possible that these organisms may enter the bladder by pressure on the urethra as in coitus and by instrumentation, particularly catheterization. The presence of organisms in the bladder need not result in cystitis unless there is an obstruction, with delay in the emptying of the bladder. However, if infected urine in the bladder is forced into the ureters because of laxity at the vesico-ureteric sphincter, organisms will reach the renal pelvis and medulla, and the infection can spread to the cortex from there. That reflux is demonstrable in some women is beyond doubt, and the hormonal and anatomical changes in pregnancy would certainly suggest this route of infection to be likely.

It is possible, and indeed probable, that many women have chronic pyelonephritis or renal abnormalities which predispose to infection without these necessarily having been diagnosed prior to pregnancy. As about 6% of women attending antenatal clinics in different centres in Britain, Australia and North America have asymptomatic but significant bacteriuria (i.e.

10^5 organisms per millilitre of urine, or more, without definite symptoms of urinary tract infection), renal infection must have been present before they became pregnant. The incidence of significant bacteriuria in school-girls is reported as around 1%, and this incidence rises with increasing age. In a small series of nulliparous women attending an infertility clinic, an incidence of 8% was found. Thus pregnancy may be an aggravating factor in the natural history of chronic pyelonephritis, but it is responsible for the disease being diagnosed and treated.

DETECTION OF BACTERIURIA

As the use of the catheter to obtain urine for bacteriological examination is deprecated, it is necessary to ensure that the technique for obtaining mid-stream or clean specimens of urine is satisfactory. Much has been written about the necessity of, and the methods for, preparing the patient to give the specimen. Certainly obvious contamination by vaginal discharge should be avoided. Beard and his colleagues (1965) described a technique for obtaining uncontaminated urine by puncturing the bladder transabdominally. As there is no possibility of contamination by this method, a significant count can be obtained from one specimen if it is present. The urine should be sent to the laboratory within 3 hr so that it can be placed on the appropriate culture medium without delay, or alternatively the urine should be refrigerated until laboratory examination can be performed. The multiplication of contaminant organisms makes the count inaccurate and must be prevented.

The methods available for detecting 'significant' numbers (i.e. 10^5) of bacteria in a millilitre of urine have been well outlined by Constable (1967). Obviously, bacteriological culture methods are the most reliable, but are time-consuming and expensive. Patients in hospital undergoing investigations for urinary tract infection should always have the benefit of the most accurate method. For screening purposes, semi-quantitative methods such as the one described by Brumfitt & Percival (1964) are of practical value, even although bacteriological facilities are necessary. In this test, a piece

of blotting-paper of known dimensions is immersed in the urine to be tested and then applied to the surface of a special MacConkey agar plate. After incubation the number of colonies, and therefore organisms, is counted. A standard curve is used to determine how many organisms per millilitre are represented by the colony count. Chemical tests—the Griess nitrite test as modified by Sleigh (1965) and the triphenyl tetrazolium chloride test—are less accurate but possibly easier to perform in a busy clinic, although incubation in a water-bath is required for 4 hr.

The 'Uricult' (Orion Labs.) technique permits both qualitative and quantitative examination of the urine. A slide is covered on one side with nutrient agar and on the other with MacConkey's medium. This is dipped into the freshly voided specimen of urine to be tested, the excess of urine is shaken off and the slide is replaced in the container provided. Culture takes place if the slide is maintained at 37°C or even at room temperature (Arneil et al. 1970). A chart is supplied for comparison with the test slide and an estimate of the bacterial count per ml. is obtained. The nature of the colony and the characteristics of the organisms as seen in a suitably stained film should identify the cause of the infection.

The leucocyte count is considered by some to be of value but this may only be confirmatory, as a high bacterial count is of greater importance. A 'stress' situation can be reproduced by the injection of prednisolone with a resultant increase in the leucocyte count. Significant urinary tract infection is not always accompanied by an increased excretion of white cells, and there are other causes of a raised white cell count in the urine that are not directly related to renal infection.

The detection of a rising or significantly high titre of agglutinating antibodies to *Esch.coli* strongly suggests a diagnosis of renal tissue infection. According to Percival et al. (1964), it permits a distinction to be made between lower urinary tract infection and renal infection. They also found a raised titre in 32% of women with asymptomatic bacteriuria in early pregnancy, confirming the presence of renal tissue damage.

Acute pyelonephritis

CLINICAL FEATURES

It is uncommon to find a patient who presents with the classical features of acute pyelonephritis during pregnancy, namely marked pyrexia, loin pain, rigors and severe dysuria. More frequently, the patient has a slightly elevated temperature with dysuria, frequency and nocturia, nausea with vomiting, backache and some loin tenderness on palpation. She may merely feel unwell and be anaemic without localizing features being apparent, and it is only by routinely examining the urine of patients with vague symptoms during pregnancy that significant bacteriuria may be detected.

TREATMENT

Various factors must be considered in the treatment of acute pyelonephritis, the most important being the causal organism and its degree of sensitivity to the available therapeutic agents. In general, it is advisable to use bactericidal rather than bacteriostatic drugs, and to avoid those known to have unpleasant side-effects. It is essential that a full course of treatment is given, this being a minimum of 10 days, and preferably 14 days (Whalley 1967). The urine should be examined bacteriologically at the completion of the course of treatment and should be free from organisms. The patient should be kept under surveillance during the remainder of her pregnancy and examined again some weeks after delivery.

Prophylactic drug therapy may be successful in preventing reinfection or in suppressing acute episodes in a patient with chronic pyelonephritis. This does not always happen, but it is probably worth-while in order to control the symptoms of the infection and to prevent readmission to hospital during the pregnancy. The drugs used must not be harmful to the foetus.

Drugs used in treatment include ampicillin 500 mg 6-hourly, sulphadimidine 2 g followed by 1 g 6-hourly, nitrofurantoin 100 mg 6-hourly, nalidixic acid 1 g 6-hourly, cycloserine 250 mg twice daily and kanamycin 250 mg 6-hourly by intramuscular injection. In prophylactic therapy, ampicillin 250 mg twice daily, cycloserine 250 mg daily and sulphadimidine 250 mg twice daily may be given.

General treatment with analgesics and oral or intravenous fluids is given, an adequate intake and output being of importance.

Asymptomatic bacteriuria

By routinely examining the urine of women attending antenatal clinics, significant bacteriuria has been found in the absence of symptoms in from 2 to 10%. The variation is related to the socio-economic status of the women being examined (Whalley 1967). The importance of detecting this bacteriuria is threefold. It has been shown by many workers that about 50% of these patients will develop acute pyelonephritis during their pregnancies, and this can be prevented in many cases by early treatment. Secondly, some of the patients who do not have acute symptoms may have lesions in their renal tracts which are detrimental to their health. These lesions may be diagnosed after pregnancy by further investigation of the patient (Robertson *et al.* 1968). Thirdly, Kass (1960) and others have found an increased incidence of prematurity and perinatal mortality in women with bacteriuria. Other studies have not supported this view, but an association with anaemia and hypertension in pregnancy has been made in some series. The whole subject has been well reviewed by Whalley (1967).

Treatment of the infection should follow a regime similar to that described for acute pyelonephritis, and prophylactic therapy is also necessary.

Obviously, every patient with bacteriuria will not have chronic pyelonephritis or congenital renal abnormalities. However, many do, and drug treatment of urinary infection during pregnancy is unlikely to have a curative effect, and at best can only suppress the infection. It is not possible to diagnose the extent of the disease with certainty during pregnancy, but full investigation of the patient is indicated soon after delivery.

The renal tract should have returned to its prepregnancy state by 3 months after delivery. While the abnormal radiological changes associated with pregnancy may still be found at that time, it is more likely that they are the result of some pathological lesion and further investigation by a urologist is indicated.

Screening of the patient should include a further urine examination for the presence of bacteriuria and this should be repeated if there is any doubt about the significance of the result. In asymptomatic bacteriuria, and when there has been a recurrence of pyelonephritis during the pregnancy, an intravenous pyelogram is essential and if any abnormality is found, full urological investigation is indicated. This may include renal-function tests, renogram studies, ureteric catheterization and retrograde pyelography, and when necessary, renal biopsy.

The number of patients found to have renal disease or anomalies varies with the method of selection for investigation, but some studies have reported quite appreciable numbers. The writer found each of two women to have a non-functioning kidney due to chronic pyelonephritis in a group of ten patients followed-up because of asymptomatic bacteriuria during pregnancy. It can be concluded that this type of follow up is fully justified.

OTHER DISORDERS OF THE URINARY TRACT DURING PREGNANCY

Urinary calculus

This is not common in pregnancy, but if it occurs it can give rise to serious complications. Acute pyelonephritis is very likely as a result of obstruction to the urinary flow with a resultant increase in the amount of damage to the kidney tissue. Attacks of pain may occur but because of the dilated state of the ureters, a stone may pass more easily or its arrest may cause few symptoms. However, repeated attacks of acute pyelonephritis may draw attention to the obstruction.

Diagnosis in pregnancy may be difficult because of the problem of detecting the calculus on radiographs and the reluctance to perform intravenous pyelography during pregnancy. Haematuria is not always present. A stone may be passed in the urine or recurrent infections may be suggestive.

In early pregnancy it is possible to remove the calculus, although radiological investigation may perhaps be harmful to the foetus. In later pregnancy, antibiotic therapy for the infections may be sufficient until after delivery, when extraperitoneal ureterolithotomy should be carried out. It is preferable to remove any stones present before or between pregnancies.

Haematuria

Blood in the urine during pregnancy is most usually caused by contamination and a 'clean' specimen of urine should be obtained. Urinary tract infection and urinary calculus are the most important causes, but on very rare occasions a renal neoplasm may be present, and renal tuberculosis must not be forgotten. The lesion may be in the bladder in which case cystoscopy should reveal the cause, but if it is in the kidney or ureter, further investigation is required during pregnancy or after delivery. It has been suggested that spontaneous bleeding may occur from renal veins as a result of the increased level of oestrogens, and the bleeding stops after delivery. Bleeding because of vitamin C deficiency and hypoprothrombinaemia is possible, and may also be caused by drugs such as sulphonamides. In late pregnancy, in the presence of a lower-segment Caesarean section scar, haematuria may be due to rupture of the scar with involvement of the bladder. Haematuria may also be encountered when a large volume of retained urine in the bladder is released by a catheter; this complication may follow bladder drainage of urinary retention in a case of retroverted incarcerated gravid uterus.

The treatment is that of the cause and is otherwise expectant, with sedatives and an adequate fluid intake to ensure a satisfactory urinary output and to prevent clotting in the urinary tract, if possible. It may be necessary to wash out the bladder by catheter if the bleeding is severe.

Renal failure and pregnancy

Acute renal failure is a serious complication of pregnancy. In early pregnancy it is usually a complication of abortion, frequently criminally induced, and is related to acute blood loss with consequent hypotension, and to infection, *Clostridium welchii* and *Esch.coli* being the organisms most commonly incriminated. In later pregnancy, hypertension is frequently present in patients who develop renal failure. Pre-eclampsia and eclampsia, and abruptio placentae, are the most common causes. Renal cortical necrosis may develop with the prognosis grave, but more usually the condition is one of tubular necrosis.

In the phase of oliguria the patient may appear to be quite well and to be recovering from the precipitating cause of the renal damage. Her output is low, and this can only be detected by routinely recording the fluid intake and urinary output in patients who have aborted, especially if criminal abortion is suspected, and in those who have moderate or severe pre-eclampsia, eclampsia, or accidental haemorrhage, especially of the concealed type.

In management, early diagnosis is of the utmost importance and early referral to a renal unit is advisable. Fluid restriction and careful control of the plasma electrolytes is mandatory, as death can be hastened by overloading the circulation with fluid which cannot be excreted, and by hyperkalaemia and uraemia. Peritoneal dialysis is advocated by Smith *et al.* (1965), but if this is unsuccessful, haemodialysis may be performed. Chronic renal failure may require repeated dialysis or renal transplantation.

Prevention of renal failure involves the careful replacement of blood loss and the vigorous treatment of infection in patients with abortion, and the restoration of the circulatory blood volume in patients with abruptio placentae even if the blood pressure is raised, together with prompt emptying of the uterus and attention to coagulation disorders.

Robson *et al.* (1968) reported four patients who had puerperal renal failure with possible cardio-myopathies and described distinctive light- and electron-microscopic changes found in the kidneys. They suggested that an adverse reaction may have developed to ergometrine or oxytocin given at delivery.

Pregnancy and renal disease

The opinion of the obstetrician is sometimes sought as to the advisability of a patient with renal disease having a pregnancy or continuing with a pregnancy. No general ruling can be given, as each patient must be considered individually. However, certain principles can be laid down.

While it is accepted that pregnancy may cause or aggravate renal disorders, there is a considerable physiological reserve as regards renal function. The risk, therefore, will depend on the existing ability of the kidneys to perform their normal tasks as well as their ability to respond to the stresses caused by pregnancy. A patient with one healthy kidney may well be in a better position to have a pregnancy than a patient with two diseased kidneys. The long-term prognosis must also be considered because of the risk to the patient's life and health and her ability to care for her child or children.

In chronic pyelonephritis controlled by continuous antibiotic therapy, with or without previous surgery, the number of pregnancies should be kept to a minimum, and if advice is sought, pregnancy should be discouraged. However, the enthusiasm with which this is done depends on the parity of the patient and the extent of detectable renal damage, assessed by renal-function tests, bacteriological examination of the urine, intravenous pyelogram and renogram studies and, possibly, by retrograde pyelography. On the other hand, a patient with congenital absence of a kidney or anomalies of one which have resulted in its removal may have a normally functioning remaining kidney, and one or two pregnancies are a reasonable risk.

If a patient has had renal failure because of a previous obstetric accident, or for other reasons, pregnancy should be avoided if there is a possibility of recurrence of the precipitating cause, and because there may be a degree of bilateral renal damage. Although pregnancy has been reported after successful renal transplantation, the circumstances for permitting this are likely to be exceptional and dependent on the reasons for the renal failure.

REFERENCES

ARNEIL G.C., McALLISTER T.A. & KAY P. (1970) *Lancet* i, 119.

BAIRD D. (1936) *J. Obstet. Gynaec. Br. Commonw.* **42**, 774.

BEARD R.W., McCoy D.R., NEWTON J.R. & CLAYTON S.J. (1965) *Lancet*, ii, 610.

BRUMFITT W. & PERCIVAL A. (1964) *J. clin. Path.* **17**, 482.

CONSTABLE P.J. (1967) *J. Coll. gen. Practurs Res. Newsl.* **13**, 290.

COX C.E. (1966) *Sth. med. J., Nashville,* **59**, 621.

HYTTEN F.E. & LEITCH I. (1964) *The Physiology of Human Pregnancy.* Oxford, Blackwell Scientific Publications, p. 114.

KASS E.H. (1956) *Trans. Ass. Am. Physns,* **69**, 56.

KASS E.H. (1960) *Archs. intern. Med.* **105**, 194.

PERCIVAL A., BRUMFITT W. & DE LOUVOIS J. (1964) *Lancet*, ii, 1027.

ROBERTSON J.G., LIVINGSTONE J.R.B. & ISDALE M.H. (1968) *J. Obstet. Gynaec. Br. Commonw.* **75**, 59.

ROBSON J.S., MARTIN A.M., RUCKLEY V.A. & MACDONALD M.K. (1968) *Q. Jl Med.* **37**, 423.

SLEIGH J.D. (1965) *Br. med. J.* i, 76.

SMITH K., McCLURE BROWNE J.C., SHACKMAN R. & WRONG O.M. (1965) *Lancet*, ii, 351.

WHALLEY P. (1967) *Am. J. Obstet. Gynec.* **97**, 723.

CHAPTER 20

DIABETES, THYROID DISEASES AND ADRENAL DISEASES COMPLICATING PREGNANCY

DIABETES IN PREGNANCY

There is no clear definition of diabetes today, because it has become increasingly apparent that there is a slow gradation from normal carbohydrate metabolism to clinical diabetes with its recognizable features of glycosuria, hyperglycaemia and a tendency to keto-acidosis due to a deficiency, or diminished effect, of insulin. When causing symptoms, this combination is termed, clinical diabetes; when not causing symptoms, it is termed chemical or asymptomatic diabetes. In terms of the most commonly employed diagnostic procedure—the oral glucose-tolerance test (G.T.T.)—diabetics will exceed the normal upper limits for true glucose in capillary blood after a 50-g glucose load, i.e. fasting 100 mg/100 ml, 1 hr 160 mg/100 ml and 2 hr 120 mg/100 ml. Broadly speaking, there are two clinical types of diabetes. The younger ketosis-prone diabetics, who have little or no circulating insulin, and the older, milder, obese diabetics who may have normal fasting levels of insulin which, however, respond more slowly than normal to a glucose load, so that hyperglycaemia, but not ketosis, results. Dietary restriction alone will often improve the insulin response to glucose in these obese patients. A number of population surveys have been carried out to determine the incidence of diabetes in a general population, but these have shown variable results depending on the criteria used to diagnose the condition.

GLYCOSURIA

This is found in 3–5% of the general population when random samples of urine are examined. A higher incidence of glycosuria is found when urine is examined after a glucose load. Thus, in the Bedford diabetes survey (Butterfield 1964) the incidence of glycosuria in women of different age groups after a 50-g glucose load varied between 6·3% in the 18–24 age group and 10·9% in the 35–44 age group. Older women showed a higher incidence still. Apart from glycosuria produced by hyperglycaemia, glycosuria may occur as a result of a low renal threshold. Normal people excrete 0–15 mg glucose per 100 ml urine; in renal glycosuria much larger amounts are passed, as much as 50 g or more being passed in 24 hr. Renal glycosuria does not give rise to the symptoms of diabetes, and is not thought to be a precursor of this condition. The renal threshold rises with age, so that whereas 90% of the glycosuria found in women in the 20–29 age group is due to a low threshold, in women over 70 glycosuria is almost always due to hyperglycaemia. Pregnancy lowers the renal threshold for glucose, a factor of considerable practical importance (see below).

GLUCOSE TOLERANCE

Glucose tolerance as measured by the standard oral G.T.T. is found to be abnormal in a surprisingly high proportion of a random population, even amongst those not showing glycosuria;

17% of one study group (Butterfield 1964) had a 2-hr capillary blood glucose level exceeding 120 mg/100 ml, age being the most important single factor in determining the abnormality.

INSULIN RESPONSE TO GLUCOSE

The characteristic response of normal people to the oral administration of glucose is a rise in the level of blood insulin. The fasting level of less than 25 micro-units per millilitre rises to a peak of about 50 micro-units per millilitre 30 min after the ingestion of glucose, falling progressively thereafter, to return to fasting levels after 2 hr. The ketotic type of diabetic lacks circulating insulin and shows no response. The milder obese diabetic, on the other hand, shows a delayed response, but the insulin then rises to abnormally high levels, indicating a slower but excessive response of the islet cells.

Pregnancy and carbohydrate metabolism

Pregnancy imposes a strain on the mechanism for the control of carbohydrate metabolism, which is of importance both in relation to each individual pregnancy and in relation to the effect of pregnancy on the later development of diabetes in the parous woman.

GLYCOSURIA IN PREGNANCY

Glycosuria is a common occurrence in normal pregnancy, especially in the second and third trimesters. In random samples the amount of glucose passed by individual patients is not great, and it may occur on one occasion only. Glycosuria was present in 9% of normal pregnant women (Peel & Oakley 1968). It was rarely present before the twentieth week and reached a peak incidence at 30–34 weeks. The mechanism of glycosuria in these cases is uncertain; the lowered renal threshold found in pregnancy may be due to defective tubular absorption of glucose or to increased glomerular filtration. The renal threshold returns quickly to normal after delivery. Lactosuria may occur during late pregnancy or lactation. The distinction between glycosuria and lactosuria can be made by using the specific urinary glucose test 'Clinistix'. In an attempt to elucidate the significance of glycosuria, Campbell (1969) gave fasting normal pregnant women a 50-g oral load of glucose and studied the incidence of glycosuria and the level of blood glucose and serum insulin 2 hr later. Of 314 women tested before the twentieth week, 29 (9·3%) had glycosuria. The mean 2-hr blood glucose level in this group was higher than in the normal group, as was the serum insulin. These findings were repeated in a group of 208 patients studied after the thirty-second week of pregnancy, although the differences between the glycosuria group and the normals was less marked. Detailed examination of these findings revealed that women who have glycosuria are much more likely to have a 2-hr glucose level over 90 mg/100 ml than women without glycosuria. High 2-hr levels of glucose are associated with a high 2-hr level of insulin. Glycosuria was more frequently seen in women over the age of 30, and Campbell suggests that the stress of pregnancy may produce a situation which reflects what the subject's carbohydrate metabolism may be in later life, and to this extent may have a limited prognostic value.

GLYCOSURIA IN PREGNANCY AND FOETAL PROGNOSIS

Although patients exhibiting glycosuria in pregnancy may develop defective carbohydrate metabolism in later life, the obstetrician is primarily concerned with its possible effect on the foetal outcome. By itself, glycosuria does not seem to have any special significance, but it is often an indication to investigate a particular patient further. Glycosuria occurring on one occasion before the sixteenth week, or on more than one occasion thereafter, should be followed by a standard 50-g oral G.T.T. Glycosuria occurring at any time in pregnancy in a patient who has a positive family history of diabetes or a past obstetric history of a baby weighing 4·5 kg (10 lb) or more should be similarly investigated. If the 2-hr blood glucose level is 90 mg or more, the patient has a definite tendency to have a baby larger than average. She also runs a slightly increased risk of being delivered by Caesarean section and also of having a stillborn baby. The difficulty in assessing the significance of the last two correlations lies in the fact that impaired glucose tolerance is more likely to occur in the older age groups. These are the patients who in any case are more prone to operative delivery and perinatal mortality. In some patients the 2-hr figure will be even higher or the curve be frankly diabetic (gestational diabetes), with all that this implies in therapeutic and prognostic terms.

GLUCOSE TOLERANCE IN PREGNANCY

In pregnancy, although the fasting glucose level is decreased the oral G.T.T. curve is shifted in a diabetic direction, especially in the last trimester. Wilkinson & O'Sullivan (1963) found abnormal G.T.T.s in 6·2% of 752 unselected pregnancies. There was a definite rise in the postglucose values in the 215 women tested in successive trimesters, and abnormal glucose tolerance was related to age and parity. An important practical point in this connection is that a normal G.T.T. in early pregnancy may be converted to an abnormal G.T.T. in later pregnancy as glucose tolerance becomes impaired. An abnormal G.T.T. in pregnancy is associated with a higher incidence of diabetes in later life; the greater the abnormality the greater the chance of developing diabetes. If any of the following levels of glucose (in milligrammes per 100 ml) are exceeded—fasting 90, 1 hr 165, 2 hr 145, 3 hr 125—there is a 21·6% chance of the patient developing diabetes after 7 years (O'Sullivan & Mahon, 1964). A similar figure was found for a group of patients followed-up for 7 years after an abnormal cortisone glucose-tolerance test (C.G.T.T.) by Conn & Fajars (1961). The C.G.T.T. has been extensively used in the study of glucose tolerance, but has no great advantage over the ordinary G.T.T. The intravenous G.T.T. involves the injection of 25 g of glucose as a 50% solution into an ante-cubital vein over a period of 4 min, after first obtaining a sample of blood for a fasting glucose level. Blood samples are then taken every 10 min for the next hour. The result of the test depends upon the slope of the decline in blood glucose. In diabetes the glucose is removed from the blood more slowly than in normal subjects. This test has been applied to the pregnant patient and is more sensitive than the oral G.T.T., giving a higher incidence of abnormal results. It has also confirmed the shift of glucose tolerance towards diabetes that occurs in normal pregnancy, especially where there are other features suggestive of diabetes. Thus, of 197 pregnant women with a family history of diabetes, 31% showed impaired intravenous glucose tolerance (Silverstone et al. 1961). The disadvantages of the intravenous G.T.T.—the need for frequent sampling and accuracy in timing the sampling, together with the occasional occurrence of venous thrombosis—have made it less popular in the detection of abnormal glucose tolerance than the standard oral G.T.T., which remains the most usual way of detecting this condition in both the pregnant and non-pregnant subjects.

INSULIN SENSITIVITY IN PREGNANCY

Hand in hand with impaired glucose tolerance in pregnancy, there is a decreased sensitivity to insulin which develops particularly in the later months of pregnancy. This is reflected in an increased insulin response to glucose in the normal woman and the almost invariable increase in insulin requirement in the diabetic woman. There is as yet no satisfactory explanation for the changes in either glucose tolerance or insulin sensitivity, but it is possible that they may both result from the production by the placenta of a diabetogenic hormone, human chorionic somatomammotrophin (HCS), otherwise known a placental lactogen.

BLOOD GLUCOSE AND INSULIN RELATIONSHIPS IN MOTHER AND FOETUS

Maternal–foetal glucose and insulin relationships have been investigated by Coltart et al. (1969) and Beard et al. (1970) by means of foetal-scalp blood-sampling after rupture of the membranes, but before the onset of labour. Maternal and foetal serum levels of glucose and insulin were measured before and after the administration of an intravenous glucose load to the mother.

In non-diabetic pregnancies there is a close relationship between the concentrations of glucose in mother and foetus, and an immediate rise in foetal insulin occurred after glucose loading. In diabetic pregnancy there is a greater difference between foetal and maternal glucose levels, so that in spite of maternal hypergly-caemia the foetal glucose levels are relatively normal. The insulin response in the diabetic foetus was delayed, although neither the fasting concentration nor the overall increase of insulin after glucose loading was significantly different in either group. The mechanism by which the diabetic foetus maintains a relatively normal blood glucose in the face of recurring maternal hyperglycaemia is not known, but it may be that placental regulation of glucose transfer is an important factor (Beard *et al.* 1970). It is usually held that maternal hyperglycaemia is responsible for the commonly found foetal islet β-cell hypertrophy, which may cause foetal and neonatal hypoglycaemia. The control of maternal blood sugar during pregnancy reduces this risk.

HUMAN CHORIONIC SOMATOMAMMOTROPHIN. PLACENTAL LACTOGEN

This is a protein hormone produced by the syncytiotrophoblast (Higashi 1967; Josimovich & MacLaren 1962). It has a structure similar to that of growth hormone and a molecular weight of approximately 19,000. Detectable levels of HCS appear in the maternal plasma by the sixth week, and thereafter the level rises steadily to a plateau during the last trimester. The physio-logical role of HCS is not yet clearly understood, but its actions resemble those of growth hormone in many respects. It is growth-promoting, lactogenic and luteotrophic, and in addition exerts a diabetogenic action on carbohydrate metabolism. Both haemagglutination and radio-immunoassay methods have been used to measure HCS levels, the latter being more time-consuming but more accurate. There is a wide variation in HCS levels in normal pregnancy and conflicting reports on the levels in diabetic pregnancy, one group of workers (Sarcena *et al.* 1969) reported a higher level than normal, and others

(Samaan *et al.* 1969; Teoh 1970) found no change. If it is ultimately found that changes in the levels of HCS in diabetics are reflected by changes in insulin requirement, support will be given for the hypothesis that it is responsible for the exacerbation of diabetes that occurs in pregnancy.

DIABETOGENIC EFFECT OF PREGNANCY

The majority of women survive repeated preg-nancies without becoming diabetic, but a small proportion do not do so. As a result, the incidence of diabetes in later life in parous women is greater than in nulliparous women (Pyke 1956). When a family history of diabetes, the bearing of large babies or a past history of unexplained perinatal death is added to parity, the incidence of diabetes in later life is increased still further, especially in obese women of parity 4 and over. The influence of parity seems to be limited in the absence of maternal obesity, and in a modern society with low average parity the importance of pregnancy as a factor leading to the develop-ment of clinical diabetes will be relatively small. It is possible that the declining importance of this potentially diabetogenic factor could be associated with a genuine fall in the incidence of diabetes in women, and that this is the cause of the apparent change in the sex ratio for newly diagnosed cases of clinical diabetes in Britain (Malins *et al.* 1965).

Potential and latent diabetes

(1) POTENTIAL DIABETES

A potential diabetic is a person with a normal glucose tolerance who has, nevertheless, a greater risk of developing diabetes than normal. The two major features in a woman which place her in this category are a positive family history and a past history of overweight babies.

Family history of diabetes

The evidence that diabetes is, at least in part, inherited is very strong, but the exact mode of inheritance is not clear. It is no longer held that a single autosomal recessive gene is responsible.

A claim has been made (Vallence Owen 1965) that an insulin antagonist is inherited as a dominant factor and that this results in the individual developing diabetes if other adverse factors affecting carbohydrate metabolism operate. The significance of this observation is, as yet, not clear. Approximately 7% of all offspring of a diabetic may be expected to develop the disease themselves (Pyke 1968)—an incidence of between five and ten times that of a child of non-diabetic parents. When both parents are diabetic the incidence of diabetes in the offspring rises, depending upon the age at which the parents became diabetic (Cooke et al. 1966). The greatest risk of diabetic offspring occurs where one or both parents develop the disease before the age of 40. Even so, not more than 25% of their children will become diabetic, and the figure is lower in children of parents with diabetes of late onset. The extent to which a positive family history makes an individual a potential diabetic, will therefore vary with circumstances.

Previous heavy baby

The incidence of babies weighing 4·5 kg or more is about 1·5% of all births. Among the children of women who later develop diabetes the figure is much higher, varying in different reports from 4 to 31% (Pyke 1962). The tendency to bear heavy babies is present for 40 years or more before clinical diabetes appears. There is no clear-cut evidence to support the idea that the proportion of heavy babies increases as the time of diagnosis draws near, suggesting that genetic factors are more important than environmental (such as maternal hyperglycaemia). That maternal environmental factors can influence birth weight is shown by the fact that the mean birth weight of women whose diabetes is very carefully controlled is less than similar women who are less well controlled (Pyke 1968). Furthermore, women who develop an abnormal glucose tolerance in pregnancy can normally be expected to produce a baby heavier than average, but if treated with diet and insulin they do not (O'Sullivan et al. 1966). Apart from the genetic and environmental influences exerted by the mother, the father might, theoretically, exert a genetic influence on the birth weight of his offspring. There is no convincing evidence that men who subsequently become diabetic father heavier babies than normal in their prediabetic phases or indeed once they become actual diabetics.

Follow-up of mothers of heavy babies

A number of studies have been carried out to discover the fate of women who bear babies weighing much more than normal. It is clear that such women have an increased risk of becoming diabetic but it is not easy to assess the extent of the risk for the individual woman. In the Birmingham study (Fitzgerald et al. 1961) one-third of the women who had given birth to a baby of 4·7 kg or over 13 years earlier were clinical or chemical diabetics. In another study of women 20 years after the birth of a 4·5 kg baby, 44% were clinical or chemical diabetics. In both studies it is likely, since the women were only in their forties and fifties, that the incidence of diabetes will ultimately be higher. This means that a woman who has a 4·5 kg baby has a 50% chance of developing diabetes sometime in later life.

(2) LATENT DIABETES

The latent diabetic is an individual who has a normal carbohydrate tolerance in normal conditions, but in conditions of stress develops chemical or clinical diabetes. The cortisone-stressed G.T.T. has been widely used to detect this type of individual, many of whom, but not all, will become full-scale diabetics in later years. Pregnancy is another stress, and reveals a group of latent diabetics (gestational diabetics) who are of particular interest to the obstetrician. In practical terms these patients are treated according to the degree of their abnormal glucose tolerance by diet with or without insulin during the pregnancy, with a similar outcome to that in established diabetics. Most latent diabetics revert to normal once the pregnancy is over. They may, or may not, follow a similar pattern in a subsequent pregnancy. A considerable proportion of women with gestational diabetes will later develop diabetes, although in some cases impaired glucose tolerance remains unchanged or even improves, so that gestational diabetes cannot be regarded as an inevitable precursor of diabetes.

The interaction of pregnancy and diabetes

The effects produced by the two conditions on each other vary considerably, according to the exact status of the maternal carbohydrate metabolism and the duration of the pregnancy. As indicated above, the effect of pregnancy on carbohydrate metabolism is considerable, especially in relation to the lowering of the renal threshold and diminishing sensitivity to insulin as the pregnancy advances.

Renal threshold

A high proportion of diabetics have a lowered renal threshold to glucose in pregnancy, and this makes control of maternal diabetes more difficult.

Insulin response

Little or no change in insulin requirement is seen in early pregnancy, but in the majority of cases the dose of insulin required to maintain normal blood glucose levels rises from about 16 weeks onwards. Not all diabetics show this need for more insulin, but the majority do so, and in many cases the insulin dose at the end of pregnancy is several times that seen in the non-pregnant state.

Diabetic complications

The commonly occurring medical complications of diabetes—retinopathy, diabetic nephropathy and vascular disease—may be seen in association with pregnancy. In the majority of cases, pregnancy does not have a deleterious effect on these conditions, which individually do not usually constitute a contra-indication to a diabetic woman becoming pregnant (or when pregnant, an indication for termination).

Pregnancy complications in diabetes

SPONTANEOUS ABORTION

In the well-controlled diabetic the incidence of spontaneous abortion does not seem to differ from the non-diabetic woman. Badly controlled diabetes may bring about foetal death at any stage of pregnancy, and so may be responsible for abortion.

PREGNANCY VOMITING

Diabetic women are not more likely to have this complication, but because of the effect it may have on diabetic control it is potentially more serious. Nausea, which reduces carbohydrate intake, and vomiting, which disturbs the maternal acid-base balance, may prove disastrous to the foetus. Such a serious situation is, fortunately, rare, but the possibility should always be borne in mind.

URINARY TRACT INFECTION

This complication is more prone to occur in pregnant diabetics than in non-diabetics (Pedersen & Pedersen 1965). Screening for asymptomatic bacteriuria, and its treatment with urinary antiseptics, should be part of routine antenatal management. The differentiation between urinary infection and diabetic nephropathy may present difficulties in the patient seen in pregnancy for the first time.

MONILIAL VAGINITIS AND VULVITIS

The presence of glycosuria seems to make the pregnant diabetic more prone to infection with *Monilia albicans* than the non-diabetic, and early recognition and treatment with nystatin pessaries and ointment will save the patient much discomfort.

HYPERTENSION, PROTEINURIA AND OEDEMA

A blood pressure of 140 mmHg systolic and 90 mmHg diastolic on two separate occasions occurs in about a quarter of diabetic patients in early pregnancy, a higher incidence of hypertension than seen in non-diabetics. *Proteinuria* may be a manifestation of diabetic nephropathy or a urinary tract infection. *Oedema* is commonly present in diabetic patients in the later stages of pregnancy and is, partly at least, a pressure effect, being most noticeable in patients with large babies or hydramnios. The occurrence of hypertension and either proteinuria or oedema will, nevertheless, most often be due to pre-eclamptic toxaemia, although care must be taken to exclude the above alternatives before making a firm diagnosis. The reported incidence of toxaemia in diabetes varies, but is it considerably higher than in non-diabetic women, especially bearing in mind the fact that most diabetic women are delivered before the thirty-eighth week. Oakley (1965) reported an incidence of 8% in 226 cases. Different criteria for diagnosis, and different methods of management, account for the variation in incidence in different series, as does the proportion of long-standing diabetics in the series. Long-standing diabetics—especially those with renal lesions and hypertension—are very prone to get an increase in blood pressure and proteinuria. This 'superimposed pre-eclampsia' is not, strictly speaking, the same as pre-eclampsia arising in a previously normotensive, protein-free woman, but in practice the distinction is somewhat academic, since hypertension, proteinuria and oedema, from whatever origin, are associated with an increased perinatal mortality (Peel 1963), making mandatory the non-specific treatment of rest and sedation.

ECLAMPSIA

Whilst pre-eclampsia toxaemia is common in diabetics, eclampsia is only very rarely seen in modern obstetric practice. Pedersen (1967) reported an incidence of 2 per 1,000 diabetic pregnancies in a collected series, but this is too high for cases treated by intensive antenatal supervision and early delivery.

HYDRAMNIOS

The clinical diagnosis of excessive liquor amnii is not very precise, but definite clinical hydramnios

can be diagnosed in a high proportion of diabetic patients examined at about 30 weeks of pregnancy. Thereafter, in properly managed patients, the degree of hydramnios diminishes in individual patients, so that by 37 weeks the incidence of hydramnios is much reduced. Diabetics behave differently from non-diabetics in this respect, in that in non-diabetic pregnancy the maximum liquor volume is found before 36 weeks, diminishing thereafter. In a series of 26 cases investigated by the Coomassie Blue technique (Elliott & Inman 1961) only three had a liquor volume in excess of 1200 ml just before delivery. There is no satisfactory explanation for the high incidence of hydramnios in diabetic pregnancy, beyond the fact that it is usually associated with a large baby and a large placenta. The quality of the liquor amnii in diabetics does not seem to differ from that of the non-diabetic, except that it has a higher glucose content related to the maternal hyperglycaemia. There is no direct relationship between the concentration of glucose in the liquor and its amount, so that a raised glucose concentration is not the explanation for the hydramnios.

MATERNAL MORTALITY

Allowing for the high incidence of operative delivery, the risk of maternal mortality in diabetic women is probably very little greater than in non-diabetic women.

PERINATAL DEATH

The most striking effect that diabetes has upon pregnancy is the increased incidence of perinatal foetal death. Starting at a level in excess of 50% in the pre-insulin days, the perinatal mortality in most large, modern series is about 10%, a dramatic reduction, but still four to five times the perinatal loss in the non-diabetic. To the 'recognized' perinatal mortality should be added an uncertain additional number of perinatal deaths which occur in women who develop diabetes for the first time in pregnancy and, the condition not being recognized, produce an unexpected stillbirth or early neonatal death. The only pointers to diabetes as the cause of such foetal losses after delivery may be the large size of the foetus or the demonstration of abnormal maternal glucose tolerance. In some cases the development years later of diabetes in the mother gives the only clue to the cause of a previously unexplained perinatal loss.

STILLBIRTH

Intra-uterine death of the foetus is most likely to occur in the last 4 weeks of pregnancy. It may result directly from an acute episode of diabetic keto-acidosis or, more commonly, without such an episode. In the latter case it is probable that the diabetic control, whilst being adequate to keep the mother from serious biochemical disturbance, is, nonetheless, sufficiently abnormal to bring about foetal death. The exact mechanism is not understood, but there is a clear correlation between high perinatal mortality and poor diabetic control (which in turn is likely to be related to the severity and instability of the maternal diabetes). Foetal anoxia due to placental insufficiency, birth trauma and congenital abnormality may all cause stillbirth in a diabetic woman, but not to a significantly greater extent than in non-diabetics; the greatest known danger the foetus faces *in utero* is that of maternal biochemical imbalance.

EARLY NEONATAL DEATH

Once it was realized that there was an increased risk of intra-uterine death in the last 4 weeks of a diabetic pregnancy, delivery at or about the thirty-sixth week was widely adopted. This resulted in a fall in the number of stillbirths but an increase in the early neonatal deaths, so that the total perinatal loss was not at first much reduced.

RESPIRATORY DISTRESS SYNDROME

The commonest cause of early neonatal death in babies born to diabetic mothers is the respiratory distress syndrome, which occurs in up to one-quarter of such babies (Grellis & Hsia 1959; Farquhar 1959). There is no clear reason why this increased incidence occurs. Prematurity plays a part but is not by itself a sufficient explanation, since the incidence in 'diabetic' babies resembles that in a much earlier gestational age group of 'non-diabetic' babies. The improved results of treatment of the respiratory distress syndrome have contributed considerably to the improvement in perinatal mortality (see below).

NEONATAL HYPOGLYCAEMIA

Glucose levels in the cord blood of babies at birth vary widely, but in general are slightly lower than the maternal level. For this reason the initial glucose levels in babies born to diabetic mothers may be higher than in those born to non-diabetic mothers (McCann *et al.* 1966). Thereafter, however, the glucose levels in the diabetic drop more quickly, and to a lower level, than in the non-diabetic. This together with the faster rate of disappearance of injected glucose in babies born to diabetic mothers (Baird & Farquhar 1962) and their higher levels of insulin-like activity support the idea that islet β-cell hyperactivity is a feature of these babies. Although the physiological findings support the pathological findings of an increased number, size and granularity of β-cells in the islets of babies examined *post mortem*, the hypothesis requires more direct observations on foetal insulin levels before it can be accepted without reservation. Unfortunately, when insulin concentration is measured as immunologically detectable insulin the presence of insulin antibodies may lead to the findings of excessive insulin values. The significance of neonatal hypoglycaemia in relation to survival and future well-being is uncertain, but cerebral damage from hypoglycaemia may occur in babies born to non-diabetic mothers. It seems unlikely that the baby born to a diabetic mother is uniquely protected against prolonged, severe hypoglycaemia, so for this reason steps are usually recommended to correct the low level (see below).

THE BABY

The baby born to a diabetic mother presents characteristic features. It is heavy for its period of gestation, due to the presence of an excessive amount of fat, which also gives it a rounded, cherubic face with buried eyes. The skin is often red and the hair abundant. The body length is increased but only in proportion to the excessive weight. The classic description of the diabetic baby by Farquhar (1959) bears reproducing in full: 'The infants are remarkable, not only because, like foetal versions of Shadrach, Meshach and Abednego, they emerge at least alive from within the fiery furnace of diabetes mellitus, but because they resemble one another so closely that they might be related. They are plump, sleek, liberally coated with vernix caseosa, full faced and plethoric. The umbilical cord and the placenta share in the gigantism. During their first 24 or more hours of extra-uterine life they lie on their backs, bloated and flushed, their legs flexed and abducted, their lightly closed hands on each side of the head, the abdomen prominent and the respiration sighing. They convey a distinct impression of having had such a surfeit of both food and fluid pressed upon them by an insistent hostess that they desire only peace so that they may recover from the excesses. And on the second day their resentment of the slightest noise improves the analogy while their trembling anxiety seems to speak of intra-uterine indiscretions of which we know nothing.' The extent to which a particular baby shows these characteristics seems to depend, to some degree, on the efficiency of the treatment of the maternal diabetes (Peel & Oakley 1968). More effective control of the maternal diabetes in the latter part of pregnancy seems to lead to lower average birth and placental weights. Nevertheless, some apparently well-controlled diabetics produce very large babies with all the characteristics described above. Among the babies coming to post mortem examination, the most constant feature is the hypertrophy of the pancreatic islet-cell tissue (Cardell 1953). The degree of hypertrophy is related to the birth weight and is made up by an increase in the number, size and granularity of the insulin-producing β cells. Other organs are increased in size correspondingly to the increased weight, but the weight of the brain is constantly less than that of 'non-diabetic' controls of similar birth weight and gestational age, respectively. The bone structure is normal but the ossification centres in the legs correspond to gestational age or less, rather than to the birth weight (Pedersen & Osler 1958), although Russell & Rangcroft (1969) have reported on accelerated radiological maturation. (This conflict of view suggests a wide normal variation, and accounts for the lack of accuracy in most radiological estimates of foetal maturity in maternal diabetes.)

CONGENITAL MALFORMATION

There is an increase in congenital abnormality in babies born to diabetic mothers compared with babies born to non-diabetics (Pedersen 1964). This applies to major abnormalities (5·2 : 1·2%) fatal abnormalities (2·1 : 0·3%) and multiple abnormalities (1·6 : 0·2%). The worse the diabetes, the greater the likelihood of congenital malformation. There is no characteristic malformation in these babies, but ventricular septal defect and malformation of the femora and lower spine are more common than in babies born to non-diabetic mothers. There is no convincing explanation for the cause of the increased congenital malformations.

THE PLACENTA

The diabetic placenta is large, like the baby it supplies. It works efficiently in the majority of cases and placental insufficiency is not caused by diabetes *per se*. Uterine muscle blood flow, oestriol excretion levels in urine, serum HCS levels, foetal blood oxygen levels and pH studies in labour have not revealed any difference from the non-diabetic placenta, except where the maternal diabetes has been complicated by hypertension or vascular disease. Placental insufficiency may then arise, as it does in the non-diabetic woman. A great deal of effort has been directed toward the investigation of the hormone production of the diabetic as compared to the non-diabetic placenta. The original observation by Smith & Smith (1937) that there was an increased excretion of chorionic gonadotrophin and a decreased excretion of oestriol, led to a widespread use of oestrogen in the treatment of pregnant diabetic women (White 1949). There is now general agreement that such treatment does not improve the clinical results. The production of progesterone and its excretion in the urine as pregnandiol were also claimed to be of value in monitoring the foetus *in utero* (White 1965). However, most observers have felt that the fall in pregnandiol excretion is not sufficiently constant to provide a reliable guide as to when to deliver a particular foetus. It will be seen, therefore, that placental-function tests have not, so far, proved more valuable in diabetic then in non-diabetic pregnancy.

The management of pregnancy complicated by diabetes.

CLINICAL DIABETES

There are three major problems in the management of the pregnant diabetic: (i) the careful control of the patient's diabetes, (ii) the choice of time and method of delivery of the baby, and (iii) the expert care of the baby in the first few days after birth. Essentially, therefore, a team composed of diabetic physician, obstetrician and paediatrician is called for, and good results can only be expected if each member of the team plays his part in cooperation with the other members. During the antenatal period it is helpful if the patient can be seen jointly at her visits to the antenatal clinic by both diabetic physician and obstetrician, so that any problems that arise can be discussed by both clinicians together. Frequent antenatal visits, and early recourse to hospital admission if diabetic stability is threatened, ensure careful control of the patient's diabetes and the early detection of obstetric abnormalities. The routine admission to hospital of all patients from the thirty-second week onwards remains the policy at King's College Hospital, and certainly brings a precision to diabetic control and the detection of obstetric complications which cannot easily be achieved on an outpatient basis. Most diabetic women know that pregnancy complicated by diabetes entails a greater risk of perinatal loss and accept any extra restrictions willingly for the sake of the baby. An explanation of the likely course of events early on in the pregnancy will ensure cooperation later.

Diet

The patient's usual diet will be sufficient in early pregnancy. Later in pregnancy the carbohydrate intake may need to be increased. The normal range of carbohydrate intake for a pregnant diabetic will be between 150 and 250 g. No restriction is placed on fat or protein intake, unless the patient seems to be putting on weight excessively.

Insulin

Changes in insulin requirement do not usually occur in the first trimester, but thereafter there is usually a steady rise. The need for extra insulin is best judged on the results of blood-sugar estimations and urine testing for ketosis, since glycosuria is not a reliable guide in the second and third trimesters. The aim of treatment is to prevent significant hyperglycaemia, (i.e. blood sugar not higher than 160 mg/100 ml) and ketosis. A regime of morning and evening doses of soluble insulin is preferable to a single mixed dose of soluble and a longer-acting insulin. Hyperglycaemia and ketosis are most likely to occur in the early morning and the late afternoon. This tendency is best corrected by the addition of a small dose of zinc protamine insulin, 4–16 units to the evening injection, which is then given before tea time. As an alternative, a dose of isophane insulin (NPH insulin) may be combined with both morning and evening injections, which are then given before breakfast and the evening meal. Where the renal threshold for glucose is very low, ketosis may occur in spite of well-controlled blood-sugar levels. This may be overcome by the addition of up to 15 g of sugar (1 tablespoon) at each of the main meals. Good control of the blood sugar and avoidance of ketosis is the overriding consideration, and the method by which this is achieved is less important. For this reason, oral hypoglycaemic agents (e.g. sulphonylureas may) be used in mild cases. Suggestions that such substances may be teratogenic have not so far been substantiated, but because they cross the placenta their use in the 48 hr before delivery is contra-indicated, so as to avoid hypoglycaemia in the newborn baby.

Admission to hospital

As noted above, pregnant diabetic patients are admitted to King's College Hospital at the start of the thirty-second week of pregnancy. This policy ensures close control of the diabetes and allows for the early detection of obstetric complications, particularly hypertension, oedema and proteinuria. Arguments have been put forward that equally close diabetic control can be achieved on an outpatient basis, and in some patients this may be so. Nevertheless, as a general policy admission to hospital is still preferred at thirty-two weeks, and at other any time during the pregnancy when other complications arise which may interfere with diabetic control. Urinary tract infections and gastrointestinal upsets causing vomiting quite commonly occur, and are best treated on an inpatient basis. Whilst in hospital awaiting delivery the patient spends a good deal of her time resting, but in uncomplicated cases is allowed to be up and about for meals, washing and toilet purposes and reasonable recreational activities. Urine is collected for testing on a 4-hourly basis during the day and blood-sugar estimations are performed as required. A routine estimation of blood sugar before breakfast, lunch and supper and at bedtime is carried out at least once a week. These findings, together with twice-daily blood pressure recordings and twice-weekly estimations of oestriol output in the urine, are entered on to a special chart which gives a composite picture of the patient's progress (Fig. 20.1). A plain X-ray film of the abdomen is taken at about 36 weeks in all cases to detect any bony foetal abnormality and as a check on maturity. Ultrasound measurement of the foetal biparietal diameter is probably a more valuable method of measuring maturity and has been added to the routine investigation of these patients.

Timing of delivery

The premature delivery of the diabetic pregnant woman is designed to avoid the unexplained incidence of intra-uterine foetal death in the last 2 or 3 weeks of the pregnancy. Although the risk of intra-uterine death is reduced by careful diabetic control, it is by no means eliminated, and may occur even in uncomplicated, well-controlled patients. The exact timing of delivery needs to be decided for each individual patient according to circumstances, but would generally be during the thirty-seventh week, i.e. between 14 and 21 days before the calculated expected date of delivery. When all is going well the end of the thirty-seventh week is preferable to the beginning. Earlier delivery than the thirty-seventh week may be indicated where the pregnancy is complicated by hypertension or pre-eclampsia, by severe hydramnios which is increasing, or by evidence of placental insufficiency as judged by the clinical findings of a small-for-dates foetus and falling oestriol excretion levels. A sudden drop in insulin requirements has been thought to be an indication of impending intra-uterine foetal death, but by itself it is unreliable. Foetal death may occur without a change in insulin requirement and, on the other hand, a falling requirement be associated with the later delivery of a normal infant. Minor falls can be safely ignored if all else is proceeding satisfactorily. A persistent slow fall or a sudden major fall calls for careful reappraisal of the situation, and possible early delivery. The risks of prematurity and respiratory distress have to be weighed against the risks of intra-uterine death and, since in some measure both risks are unknown, a final decision may have to be made on the rather insecure basis of clinical evaluation and experience.

Method of delivery

Vaginal delivery is to be aimed at in diabetic patients as in non-diabetics, but a high incidence of Caesarean section is common in most series because of the practical difficulties involved in the successful induction of labour and subsequent successful vaginal delivery. The uterine response to rupture of the membranes at 37 weeks is less reliable than that at full term, and the same applies to stimulation with oxytocin. Nevertheless, labour can usually be initiated by a combination of amniotomy and oxytocin. The subsequent success of the induction depends on the ability of the uterus to deliver what is often a large baby without causing foetal distress and

DIABETIC ANTENATAL INPATIENT CHART

ADMITTED: NO:

NAME: WARD:

DATE	GEST	BP	OED	WT	FH	TIME	URINE			BLOOD	INSULIN		URINE
							ALB	SUG	KET	SUGAR			OESTRIOL

Fig. 20.1.

in a reasonably short time, so that the maternal diabetes does not become unstable. Vaginal delivery should be abandoned in favour of Caesarean section if reasonable progress toward full dilatation has not been made 12 hr after induction. Careful monitoring of the foetal heart rate throughout labour is essential, and a foetal scalp blood-sample should be examined for pH level if variation from the normal range occurs. Maternal keto-acidosis will be reflected by similar changes in the foetus, so that diabetic control of the mother must be as careful as possible. On the morning of the induction a reduced dose of insulin, commonly half the normal dose, is

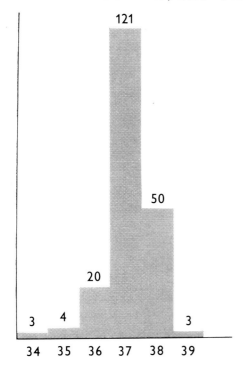

121

50

20

3   4   3

34   35   36   37   38   39

Diabetic pregnancies K.C.H. 1964-69
Duration of pregnancy at C/S or induction
(201 cases)

Fig. 20.2. The timing of delivery in pregnant diabetic patients delivered at King's College Hospital in the years 1964–9. It will be seen that the majority (60%) of the patients were delivered during the thirty-seventh week.

given and the carbohydrate intake is in the form of an intravenous glucose drip. Thereafter, glucose intake and insulin dosage are decided on a 4-hourly basis, depending upon the results of urinary tests for glucose and ketones and blood glucose estimations. By this flexible approach ketosis and hyperglycaemia can usually be avoided. If they do occur delivery should be expedited. The decisions to abandon attempts at vaginal delivery in favour of Caesarean section should be made early by 'non-diabetic' standards, and certainly before the patient's general and bio-chemical condition shows any appreciable deterioration.

Table 20·1 shows that 42·9% of a series of 226 cases were induced, but that the induction

Table 20.1. Diabetic pregnancies at King's College Hospital, 1964–9 (266 cases)

Induction	97 (42·9%)
Vaginal delivery after induction	56*
Caesarean section after induction	41

* This means that induction was unsuccessful in 41·2

succeeded in only 58·8% of the 97 women induced. Elective Caesarean section is indicated in all patients who have had a previous Caesarean or a difficult vaginal delivery (especially if the foetus did not survive). Obstetric complications—severe pre-eclampsia, malpresentation or disproportion—call for elective operation, and this method of delivery is recommended in primigravida over the age of 30. When a patient's diabetes is difficult to control it may be better to do a set operation than risk the additional control problems posed by labour. The high elective Caesarean section rate, together with the Caesareans following failed induction, result in a total operative delivery rate of about 60%.

Table 20.2. Diabetic pregnancies at King's College Hospital, 1964–9 (226 cases)

Elective Caesarean section	104 (46·0%)
Caesarean section after induction	41
Total Caesarean section	145 (64·1%)

The management of the patient's diabetes on the day of operation is similar to that employed when the patient is being induced. It is best to perform the operation early in the day, and in this case the patient receives her normal morning carbohydrate intake in the form of intravenous glucose, together with half the usual morning insulin dose. These are usually given 1 hr before operation, together with the premedication. Postoperatively, the patient is managed on an emergency diabetic regime based on 4-hourly urine testing with blood sugar estimations as required until such times as she is able to take carbohydrate by mouth. The immediate post-partum insulin requirement is likely to be about half of the predelivery dose. All procedures carried out on the pregnant diabetic which need a general anaesthetic call for the services of a skilled anaesthetist, bearing in mind particularly the possibility and dangers of vomiting at this time.

MANAGEMENT OF DIABETICS TREATED BY DIET ONLY

The dangers to the foetus are not related to the severity of the maternal diabetes, but only to the efficiency of diabetic control. For this reason the treatment of the 'mild' diabetic in pregnancy should not differ from that given above. The same arguments apply to gestational diabetics, and good overall foetal results can only be achieved if the rules of management are applied strictly to all pregnant women with a definite disturbance of carbohydrate metabolism.

MANAGEMENT OF GLYCOSURIA IN PREGNANCY

Glycosuria on a single occasion before the sixteenth week of pregnancy, glycosuria on a single occasion associated with ketonuria, or glycosuria on two occasions after the sixteenth week, call for further investigation. A family history or suggestive past obstetric history in association with a solitary episode of glycosuria should similarly be investigated. The most valuable urine specimen for testing for glucose is the second specimen passed after rising but before the patient has had breakfast. The first specimen passed on rising may be 'contaminated' by urine secreted after the previous evening's meal and so not be a true fasting sample. The second specimen passed before taking in any food is a true fasting specimen. Glycosuria in this sample is of infinitely greater significance than postprandial glycosuria, which is much more likely to be the result of a low renal threshold. When further investigation is indicated it should take the form of a full oral glucose-tolerance curve. If the investigations are negative in early pregnancy the patient should be carefully observed as the pregnancy progresses, bearing in mind that the strain on carbohydrate metabolism increases up to approximately the thirty-fourth week. If the investigations show an impaired carbohydrate tolerance the patient should be seen in

consultation with a diabetic physician and the significance of the findings assessed. Once the diagnosis is established immediate steps should be taken to control hyperglycaemia and any tendency to keto-acidosis. These patients require a period of inpatient supervision until they are stabilized.

MANAGEMENT OF THE NEWBORN INFANT

If the care of the foetus during labour has been satisfactory, the newborn infant should not require special resuscitative measures at birth. Nevertheless, it is as well to have the paediatrician who is to take over the care of the baby present at the delivery so that he may supervise the baby from the start. If he is not skilled at resuscitation the services of the obstetrician or anaesthetist should be immediately available, especially if endotracheal intubation is necessary. The most important step after delivery is the rapid and efficient clearing of the air-passages by means of a sucker. If hydramnios has been present and the baby delivered by Caesarean section, considerable quantities of liquor may be removed. Once respiration is established the baby should be transferred in an incubator to the special-care baby unit, where it should invariably spend the first 24–28 hr of life under constant observation. The importance of early, expert paediatric care cannot be over-emphasized, and in this environment careful watch is kept for signs of respiratory difficulty or hypoglycaemia. A sample of blood is taken soon after birth and examined for oxygen content, pH and glucose levels to give a base-line for comparison with repeat samples if these are felt necessary later. Acidosis is treated by an intravenous drip of sodium bicarbonate solution (8·4%) given through the umbilical vein or a scalp vein. Oxygenation of a hypoxic baby can be improved by increasing the oxygen content of the air in the incubator, but if respiratory distress seems to be developing early consideration should be given to assisting the baby's respiration through an endotracheal tube connected to a respirator. A critical situation may quickly develop, therefore the oxygen and pH levels in the baby's blood should be carefully monitored and oxygen and bicarbonate therapy adjusted accordingly. Hypoglycaemia is common in the diabetic neonate but does not require treatment unless symptoms and signs develop or the blood sugar remains at 20 mg or less 2 hr after birth. Glucose is administered by the intravenous route in a 10% solution. If the baby's general condition is satisfactory early oral feeding is a satisfactory alternative and avoids any danger of overloading the circulation. Hyperbilirubinaemia, like hypoglycaemia, is prone to occur in infants born to diabetic mothers for reasons that are not always clear, although cephalhaematoma and bruising following a difficult vaginal delivery seem sometimes to have been responsible. Early oral feeding has much reduced the incidence of hyperbilirubinaemia and exchange transfusion is not now usually necessary.

Once the early hazards of respiratory distress, hypoglycaemia and hyperbilirubinaemia have been overcome the baby's progress in uneventful and it can be treated normally. There is no contra-indication to breast feeding, although lactation seems to be slightly less good in diabetic mothers—perhaps as a result of operative delivery and the need to keep the baby in a special care unit for the first few days of life. With regard to the ultimate fate of babies born to diabetic mothers, there is no evidence that they fare less well in later life than their 'non-diabetic' fellows, although there may be a slightly greater mortality in infancy due to congenital malformations. Whether they have an increased liability to develop diabetes themselves is a question which has not so far been satisfactorily answered. Theoretically, hypertrophied islet β-cells may be damaged, and more easily undergo later degeneration. If this were so, the badly controlled pregnant diabetic would be more likely to have an offspring which would itself develop diabetes in later life, and even more force be thus given to the need to control maternal hyperglycaemia in pregnancy. No direct evidence on this point exists at the present time.

RESULT OF TREATMENT

Although the perinatal mortality in infants born to diabetic women remains much higher than

normal, the loss can be reduced to 10% or less by careful attention to the detailed management outlined above. The results obtained at King's College Hospital in the 6 years 1964–9 are shown in Table 20.3. There was a considerable variation

Table 20.3. Diabetic pregnancies at King's College Hospital, 1964–9 (299 cases)

Maternal mortality	0	
Stillbirths	5	(2·2%)
Neonatal deaths	11	(4·8%)
Perinatal mortality	16	(7·0%)

in the perinatal loss from year to year, as is inevitable with small numbers, but the overall figure represents an improvement on the previous results and a considerable improvement when compared with the results obtained before patients were admitted to hospital for rest and stabilization from the thirty-second week onwards. An analysis of stillbirths (see Table 20.4) reveals

Table 20.4. Diabetic pregnancies at King's College Hospital, 1964–9 (229 cases)

Stillbirths: 5 (2·2%)

Causes of stillbirths

Macerated	3
Intrapartum asphyxia	1
Subdural haematoma	1

that two might have been avoided by more vigilant obstetric care in labour and one macerated stillbirth apparently resulted from a temporary loss of diabetic control and a consequent episode of keto-acidosis at 35 weeks. In the remaining two macerated stillbirths the diabetic control was good and no explanation can be given for the intra-uterine death. There were eleven first-week deaths in 229 babies, of which three were due to severe congenital abnormality (see Table 20.5), a surprisingly low figure and comparable with the incidence in non-diabetic babies.

Prematurity (two cases, 29 and 31 weeks) and placental insufficiency (two cases) were complications associated with respiratory distress, but there were eight 'uncomplicated' cases of this

Table 20.5. Diabetic pregnancies
at King's College Hospital, 1964-9
(299 cases)

First-week deaths: 11 (4·8%)	
Causes of first-week death	
Respiratory distress	8
Congenital abnormality	3

condition, indicating the importance it still has in diabetic perinatal mortality. Among the eight 'uncomplicated' cases four were delivered vaginally and four by Caesarean section, so that the mode of delivery did not seem to be an important factor.

CONCLUSIONS

Recent studies have clarified some of the changes that take place in carbohydrate metabolism in pregnancy both in the diabetic and non-diabetic woman. There is a need for the recognition of potential diabetes and the early detection of gestational diabetes in the antenatal clinics. Once diagnosed, all grades of diabetes in pregnancy require careful control, since the foetus shares any abnormality in the maternal biochemical status. In the absence of more precise knowledge of the cause of the raised perinatal mortality in pregnancy complicated by diabetes, good foetal results can only be obtained by close co-operation between diabetic physician, obstetrician and paediatrician. The importance of the latter is emphasized by the fact that respiratory distress is now the most important single cause of perinatal loss.

THYROID DISORDERS IN PREGNANCY

The control of thyroid activity

The thyroid gland synthesizes and releases tetraiodothyronine (thyroxine) and tri-iodothyronine which exert a powerful effect on metabolic processes and growth. The formation of these two hormones by the thyroid is normally under the control of the pituitary thyroid-stimulating hormone (TSH). This in turn is secreted under the influence of a tripeptide-releasing factor (TRF) formed in the hypothalamus and transported to the anterior pituitary via the portal vessels. The action of TRF on the pituitary and the release of TSH by that gland are inhibited by tri-iodothyronine and thyroxine, so that a feed-back controlling mechanism operates which keeps the secretion of TSH constant under normal conditions. Radio-immunoassay of plasma TSH has shown raised levels in patients with primary hypothyroidism and undetectable levels in patients with hypothyroidism secondary to pituitary disease. In thyrotoxicosis, plasma TSH is almost always undetectable, confirming the importance of abnormal stimulators or autonomous hyperfunction as the main factors in this disorder. A long-acting thyroid stimulator (LATS) has been detected in patients with thyrotoxicosis (Adams 1958) and the fact that this substance is a γ-globulin suggests that it may be an auto-antibody to a thyroid antigen (Mackenzie 1968). The ability of LATS to cross the placenta is the probable explanation of neonatal thyrotoxicosis in infants of thyrotoxic mothers.

Thyroid function in pregnancy

The total amount of circulating thyroid hormone is 6–8 μg/100 ml. Of this, only about 0·3 μg is in the form of tri-iodothyronine, the remainder being thyroxine. Circulating thyroxine is strongly associated with plasma-binding proteins, and free plasma hormone only makes up a small fraction of the total circulating level. The major binding protein is thyroxine-binding globulin, whose production by the liver is increased when the blood oestrogen level rises. When this happens in pregnancy (or on oestrogen therapy, e.g. the contraceptive pill) the proportion of protein-bound thyroxine rises and that of free thyroxine falls. The feed-back mechanism now comes into play, with an increase in TRF activity and TSH production by the anterior pituitary. This in turn leads to thyroid hyperplasia and a consequent return of the free thyroxine level to normal, although the protein-bound thyroxine level remains above the normal level.

Thus the free thyroxine available to the tissues is unaltered by pregnancy, in spite of the hyperplasia of the gland and the raised protein-bound thyroxine. Clinically, enlargement and increased vascularity of the thyroid is noted in over 50% of normal pregnancies. The basal metabolic rate rises after 12 weeks to up to +20% of normal by the last trimester. This rise is nowadays attributed to oxygen consumption by the foetus rather than an increase in maternal metabolism.

MEASURING THYROID FUNCTION IN PREGNANCY

A common problem facing the clinician is to detect minor degrees of hyperthyroidism. This may be difficult, because the pregnancy itself may lead to thyroid enlargement, tachycardia, emotional lability and warm extremities. Nevertheless, a careful clinical assessment, including the sleeping pulse rate counted by the husband (Barnes 1970), will often be of great value. Measurement of the basal metabolic rate is unreliable, as noted above, and similarly the protein-bound iodine (PBI) level, usually taken as a measure of the protein-bound thyroxine, is increased because of the oestrogen-induced rise in protein-binding globulin. The normal non-pregnant level of PBI is $4\cdot5-8\cdot5$ μg-%, whilst the range in the pregnant patient after the first 8 weeks is $6\cdot5-11\cdot5$ μg-%. The uptake of radioactive [132]I, which is commonly used in the non-pregnant patient, is not suitable for use in pregnancy because of the possible dangers of irradiating the foetal thyroid. Total serum-thyroxine can be measured by displacement binding assay in a system including thyroid-binding globulin and labelled thyroxine (Murphy 1969), but the most useful laboratory test of thyroid function in pregnancy at the present time is an *in vitro* uptake test in which the uptake of labelled tri-iodothyronine to resin is used to provide a reflection of the free thyroxine in the plasma. A raised level of free thyroxine is indicative of thyrotoxicosis, but low levels are less reliable in the diagnosis of hypothyroidism. In all cases the results of laboratory investigations need to be interpreted carefully in the light of the clinical findings.

Non-toxic thyroid enlargement

SIMPLE GOITRE

A simple colloid goitre such as occurs in districts where iodine deficiency is endemic usually enlarges considerably during pregnancy and may cause pressure symptoms if there is a retrosternal extension of the gland. The cause of the enlargement is thought to be the fall in plasma-inorganic iodine which results from the increased renal clearance of iodine during pregnancy (Crooks *et al.* 1964). In order to take up its normal amount of iodine in the face of this relative deficiency the thyroid has to clear much more blood than usual, and the increased size is a measure of the increased vascularity. These patients should use iodized salt in place of ordinary salt with food and in cooking. As mild degrees of hypothyroidism may occur in association with this form of thyroid enlargement a small dose of L-thyroxine should also be given (0·2 mg daily). This will not harm the foetus and will protect against the ill-effects to the pregnancy of hypothyroidism. If surgical treatment is needed to relieve pressure symptoms it can be safely carried out in pregnancy but extra thyroxine should then be given, since hypothyroidism may well develop for a time postoperatively.

HASHIMOTO'S DISEASE

Auto-immune thyroid disease can be differentiated from simple goitre by the finding of an antibody to thyroglobulin in the patient's serum. Although this antibody can cross the placenta it does not seem to affect the foetal thyroid. The importance of making the diagnosis in the pregnant woman is that the characteristic firm enlargement of the gland can be reduced without the need for surgery by the administration of adequate amounts of L-thyroxine.

Hyperthyroidism

Mild hyperthyroidism is compatible with conception, and pregnancy complicated by this condition is not uncommon, an incidence of about 0·04% being commonly quoted (Hawe &

Francis 1962). Severe hyperthyroidism is associated with infertility. Pregnancy does not cause hyperthyroidism, although the condition may be first manifested in pregnancy. In the majority of cases seen in pregnancy the hyperthyroidism is due to overactivity of the whole gland, and not the result of a toxic adenoma. The effect of the condition on the pregnancy is unremarkable in the mild case but if it becomes more severe, abortion or premature labour may occur. A rare complication is neonatal hyperthyroidism, which occurs as a result of the transplacental passage of LATS from mother to baby (see above). The baby returns to normal thyroid function within 2 or 3 weeks of birth.

Diagnosis

The difficulty in detecting mild degrees of hyperthyroidism has been indicated. Careful clinical assessment, together with measurement of the PBI and a tri-iodothyronine resin uptake test, will usually enable a firm diagnosis to be made.

Treatment

Very mild cases may respond to simple sedation alone, but the majority will require specific treatment. Since the use of radioactive iodine is not advisable in pregnancy, the choice of treatment lies between antithyroid drugs and thyroidectomy. Treatment with iodine alone causes a rapid but transient improvement by blocking the release of thyroid hormone, and is used during preparation for surgery. Medical treatment is generally favoured at the present time (Herbst & Selenkow 1963), although good results have been obtained by means of thyroidectomy (Hawe & Francis 1962).

Antithyroid drugs

In treating the pregnant hyperthyroid patient with these substances care must be taken not to render the baby hypothyroid. Carbimazole, thiouracil and potassium perchlorate, the three drugs in common use, all pass the placenta, whilst thyroxine only does so slowly. Maternal hypothyroidism may lead to impairment of foetal brain development which cannot be corrected postnatally by the administration of thyroxine. Providing the mother is kept euthyroid, however, no foetal damage will occur, although slight enlargement of the foetal thyroid may be noted at birth and for 2 or 3 weeks thereafter. Carbimazole given in a dose of 15 mg t.d.s., reducing to 5 mg b.d. when the patient is euthyroid, is a satisfactory regime. The drug acts by blocking thyroid-hormone synthesis. Propylthiouracil, which acts in a similar way, may be used as an alternative in a dose of 100 mg t.d.s. reducing to 50 mg daily. Potassium perchlorate, which interferes with the uptake of iodine by the thyroid, is given in a dose of 250 mg t.d.s. reducing to 300 mg daily once the patient is euthyroid. All the antithyroid drugs are excreted in the milk, so breast feeding is contraindicated. Toxic reactions occasionally occur and, rarely, agranulocytosis. Unexplained fever, or a skin rash, is an indication to discontinue the drug being used and carry out a full blood count.

Thyroidectomy

Partial removal of the thyroid is a rapid and effective way of controlling thyrotoxicosis, but is followed in a significant number of cases by hypothyroidism. Providing the operation is done by an expert in the field, excellent results can be obtained, and where for any reason antithyroid drugs are unsuitable operation can be safely carried out at any time between 14 and 36 weeks. Pre-operatively, the patient is prepared with a course of iodine, whilst postoperatively L-thyroxine 0·2 mg daily should be given to avoid possible maternal hypothyroidism.

Hypothyroidism

Severe degrees of hypothyroidism are usually associated with infertility, and in the few recorded cases of myxoedema and pregnancy, abortion has usually occurred unless the patient was given replacement therapy. Patients who become pregnant when being successfully treated for hypothyroidism will require an increased dose of thyroxine to meet the increased requirements of pregnancy. The increase in dose in these patients should not be less than 0·1 mg daily. The extent to which subclinical hypothyroidism is associated with infertility and abortion, especially recurrent abortion, has been much debated and in some patients there is little doubt that deficient thyroid secretion is a factor in both these conditions. With modern laboratory methods of investigation, however, thyroxine should be only administered to those cases where a definite deficiency can be demonstrated.

DISORDERS OF THE ADRENAL GLAND IN PREGNANCY

The secretion of steroid hormones by the adrenal cortex involves biosynthetic pathways leading from cholesterol through progesterone and 17-α-OH progesterone to the two major adrenal steroids—cortisol (hydrocortisone) and aldosterone. In addition, the adrenal produces small amounts of progesterone, testosterone, androstenedione and dihydroepiandrosterone. During pregnancy the adrenals enlarge and increase their output of hormones. The rise in cortisol production is doubled by the last month of pregnancy (Cope & Black 1959). As with thyroxine, much of the cortisol is bound to a globulin (cortisone-binding globulin, CBG) which is inactive. The production of CBG is increased when the level of plasma oestrogen rises, so that the increase in plasma cortisol is partly due to the increased production by the adrenal and partly to the rise in CBG. Disorders of adrenal secretion include adrenal failure (Addison's disease) and excessive adrenal secretion (Cushing's syndrome). Both these conditions may rarely occur in association with pregnancy.

Addison's disease

In the majority of the hundred or more cases of Addison's disease complicating pregnancy which have been described, the patient has become pregnant as a known sufferer under replacement therapy. In a small number of cases the disease has developed during pregnancy. Most cases of the condition nowadays are due to atrophy of the gland and not to tuberculosis as in the past. Pregnancy constitutes a special strain for the patient with Addison's disease, especially during the stress of labour or at other times when vomiting or a diuresis cause sodium loss, a fall in blood volume and hypotension. Without adequate replacement therapy with cortical hormones there is a high mortality (Davis & Plotz 1953).

Management

The average stabilizing dose of hydrocortisone of 30 mg daily, together with fludrocortisone 0·1 mg for its salt-retaining properties, is continued in pregnancy but may be increased up to double these amounts if abnormal loss of sodium occurs. Intramuscular or intravenous administration may be necessary when the patient is vomiting. The high production of oestrogen and progesterone by the placenta in late pregnancy may improve the patients salt-retaining capability and allow a reduction in fludrocortisone. To cover the stress of labour, 200 mg of hydrocortisone is given intramuscularly at the onset, followed by 100 mg every 6 hr until labour is completed, when the administration of hydrocortisone should be tailed off. Labour should be kept as short as possible, forceps being used to expedite the second stage. Morphine and other opiates are badly tolerated, and so should be used cautiously at a reduced dosage. The baby is not adversely affected and there is no indication to deliver it by Caesarean section unless obstetrical complications arise.

Cushing's syndrome

Excessive secretion of adrenal steroids may result from adenoma or carcinoma of the adrenal cortex, or bilateral adrenal hyperplasia due to excessive stimulation of the adrenals by ACTH secreted by the pituitary. Pregnancy very rarely occurs in these patients because they usually develop anovulatory amenorrhoea early on in the disease. In the few cases described the hypertension characteristic of the condition has provided the main danger to mother and baby. Placental insufficiency, intra-uterine death and premature onset of labour are the main complications noted.

The management of case is essentially that of the condition itself, the pregnancy being ignored in this respect. Bilateral adrenalectomy is often needed and these patients then require replacement therapy post operatively, as for Addison's disease.

The administration of corticosteroids in pregnancy

Patients who are receiving corticosteroids for medical conditions can safely continue to do so when they become pregnant. With the increased output of their own corticosteroids as pregnancy advances the dose of administered hormone can often be decreased. It should not be drastically reduced or withdrawn, however, because the patients' adrenals may then fail to respond adequately when faced with stress, for example in labour. The slow recovery of normal adrenal function after a course of administered corticosteroids means that patients who have received such a course of treatment in the preceding 12 months should be given hydrocortisone cover in labour. If more than a year has elapsed such treatment is unnecessary, but careful watch should be kept on any patient who has had previous corticosteroid therapy in times of stress. Unexplained failure to respond to such stress calls for the immediate administration of hydrocortisone.

Teratogenic effect

A few cases of cleft palate and hare-lip have been reported in women receiving corticosteroids in early pregnancy [like the experimental rats similarly treated (Davis & Plotz 1956)]. Although the incidence of this deformity may be higher in such women, modern experience suggests that the normal doses of corticosteroids (50–100 mg hydrocortisone or 5–20 mg prednisolone) employed in the long-term medical treatment of such conditions as asthma, rheumatoid arthritis and the collagen diseases can be safely continued through early pregnancy with minimal risk.

ACUTE ADRENAL FAILURE

Apparent acute adrenal failure may occur rarely in association with obstetric complications themselves producing shock. Septicaemia, haemorrhage and amniotic fluid embolism may be associated with a failure to respond by the patient and, post mortem, widespread haemorrhage and thrombosis in the adrenal glands. The significance of these findings is not clear, but hydrocortisone should be freely administered in large doses when pregnant patients do not quickly respond to normal resuscitative measures in these conditions.

REFERENCES

ADAMS D.D. (1958) *J. clin. Endocr. Metab.* 18, 699.

BAIRD J.D. & FARQUHAR J.W. (1962) *Lancet*, i, 71.

BEARD R.W., TURNER R.C. & OAKLEY N.W. (1970) In *Proceedings of the Symposium on Foetal Biochemistry, Detroit, U.S.A.*, April 1970 (edited by A. Hodari). Springfield, Thomas.

BUTTERFIELD W.H. (1964) *Proc. R. Soc. Med.* 57, 196.

CAMPBELL N. (1969)

CARDELL B.S. (1953) *J. Path. Bact.* 66, 335.

CONN J.W. & FARJARS S.S. (1961) *Am. J. Med.* 31, 834.

COOKE A.M., FITZGERALD M.G., MALIUS J. & PYKE D.A. (1966) *Br. med. J.* ii, 674.

COPE C.L. & BLACK E. (1959) *J. Obstet. Gynaec. Br. Commonw.* 66, 404.

CROOKS J., ABOUL-KHAIR S.A., TURNBULL A.C. & HYTTEN F.C. (1964) *Lancet*, ii, 334.

DAVIES M.E. & PLOTZ E.J. (1956) *Obst. Gynec. Surveys.* 2, 1.

ELLIOTT P.M. & INMAN W.H.W. (1961) *Lancet*, ii, 835.

FARQUHAR J.W. (1959) *Archs. Dis. Childh.* 34, 76.

FITZGERALD M.G., MALINS J.M. & O'SULLIVAN D.J. (1961) *Lancet*, i, 1250.

GELLIS S.S. & HSIA D.Y.Y. (1959) *Am. J. Dis. Child.* 97, 1.

HAWE P. & FRANCIS H.H. (1962) *Br. med. J.* ii, 817.

HERBST A.L. & SELENKOW H.A. (1963) *Obstet. Gynec.* 21, 550.

HIGASHI (1961) *Endocr. jap.* 8, 228.

JOSIMOVITCH J.B. & MACLAREN J.A. (1962) *Endocrinology*, 71, 209.

McCANN M.L., CHEN C.H., KATIGBAK E.B., KOTCHEN J.M., LIKLY B.A. & SCHWARTZ R.F. (1966) *New Engl. J. Med.* 275, 1.

MACKENZIE J.M. (1968) *Physiol. Rev.* 48, 252.

MURPHY B.E.P. (1969) *Rec. Prog. Horm. Res.* p. 563.

O'SULLIVAN J.B. & MAHON C.M. (1964) *Diabetes*, 13, 278.

PEDERSEN J. (1954) *Acta endocr., Copenh.* 15, 333.

PEDERSEN J. (1967) *The Pregnant Diabetic and her Newborn.* Copenhagen, Munksgaard.

PEDERSEN J. & PEDERSEN L.M. (1965) *Acta endocr., Copenh.* **50**, 70.

PEEL J.H. (1963) *Proc. R. Soc. Med.* **56**, 1009.

PEEL J.H. & OAKLEY W.L. (1968) In *Clinical Diabetes* (edited by J.H. Peel, W.L. Oakley & K.W. Taylor). Oxford, Blackwell Scientific Publications, p. 653.

PYKE D.A. (1956) *Lancet*, **i**, 818.

PYKE D.A. (1963) *Disorders of Carbohydrate metabolism.* London, Pitman Medical Publishing Company.

PYKE D.A. (1968) In *Clinical Diabetes* (edited by W.G. Oakley, D.A. Pyke & K.W. Taylor). Oxford, Blackwell Scientific Publications, Chapter 9.

RUSSELL J.G.B. & RANGECROFT R.G. (1969) *J. Obstet. Gynaec. Br. Commonw.* **76**, 497.

SAMAAN N.A., BREDBURY J.T. & GOPLERAD C.P. (1969) *Am. J. Obstet. Gynec.* **104**, 781.

SAMAAN N., YEN S.C.C., GONZALEZ D. & PEARSON O.H. (1968) *J. clin. Endocr. Metab.* **28**, 485.

SAXENA B.N., EMERSON K. & SELENKOW H.A. (1969) *New. Engl. J. Med.* **281**, 225.

SELTZER H.S. & SMITH W.L. (1959) *Diabetes* **8**, 417.

SILVERSTONE F.A., SOLOMONS E. & RUBRICIUS J. (1961) *J. clin. Invest.* **40**, 2180.

SMITH O.W. & SMITH G.V. (1937) *Am. J. Obstet. Gynec.* **33**, 365.

TEOH E.S. (1970) *Blair Bell Lecture.* London, Royal College of Obstetricians and Gynaecologists.

VALLANCE-OWEN J. (1965) In *On the Nature and Treatment of Diabetes* (edited by B.S. Leibel & G.A. Wrenshall). Excerpta Medica Foundation.

WHITE P. (1949) *Am. J. Med.* **7**, 609.

WILKINSON H.L.C. & O'SULLIVAN J.B. (1963) *Diabetes*, **12**, 313.

CHAPTER 21

MISCELLANEOUS DISORDERS
COMPLICATING PREGNANCY

INFECTIOUS DISEASES

Reference has been made already to the significance of various infectious diseases complicating pregnancy in Chapter 8, p. 100. A number of further points must be discussed, particularly with reference to rubella.

Rubella in pregnancy

Effects on the foetus of rubella contracted during pregnancy are now well known, so that only a brief account of them is necessary. Since the earliest report by Gregg (1941) from Australia drawing attention to the fact that congenital cataract and congenital heart disease were associated with maternal rubella during pregnancy, this association has been confirmed many times. We now know that serious affections are confined almost exclusively to cases in which the maternal infection has occurred during the first 12 weeks of pregnancy. The teratogenic effects of rubella probably vary between epidemic and sporadic forms and between one epidemic and another, but a mother having rubella during the first 12 weeks of pregnancy runs a 15–50% chance of having a severely affected child.

After the twelfth week of pregnancy the chances of malformation in the foetus are far smaller, although the risk may remain increased until about the sixteenth week. Recently, it has been reported that even later infection of the mother may be associated with abnormalities in the offspring (Hardy *et al.* 1969); gross lesions are absent but hearing defects and retardation in physical and mental growth were detectable some years later. These observations were made following the United States epidemic of 1964, which may have been unusually virulent in its foetal effects.

The clinical features of rubella are not always pronounced, and consideration must be given to the possibility of an affected child in a mother showing few, if any, signs of the disease. Viral isolation and neutralizing antibody studies indicate that there are some subclinical cases of rubella without a rash, but in general it seems unlikely that a mother who has not demonstrated a fairly typical rash of the disease has any serious risk of giving rise to an affected child.

The abnormalities produced in the foetus are congenital cataract, other ocular abnormalities such as microphthalmus and glaucoma, congenital heart disease, deafness, microcephaly, mental deficiency, cleft palate and hare-lip, and various minor dental anomalies. In the United States epidemic of 1964 more widespread lesions were evident, which have been referred to as the 'expanded rubella syndrome'. The additional features here were hepatosplenomegaly, thrombocytopenic purpura and defective calcification of bone. It is also established, and this was a matter of some importance, that the affected infant continued to shed the virus from the pharynx for many months after birth. In addition to producing serious foetal malformations it seems probable that the virus of rubella has other effects too, producing a small increase in the abortion and stillbirth rate.

The virus of rubella is present in the throat perhaps as early as 7 days before a rash and for 21 days after it. Viraemia occurs as early as a week before, and always 2–3 days before, the attack. It disappears quickly once the rash comes out. It is during the viraemic stage that the foetus will be affected.

An important problem clearly presents, therefore, when a patient who is in the first trimester of pregnancy reports being a rubella contact. Fortunately, the measures available to investigate this situation are more satisfactory now than they were a few years ago. It is realized that nearly all cases of congenital rubella are the result of the disease attacking the pregnant nonimmune woman, and although re-infection is a possibility it is so remote as scarcely to be worth consideration. We know, too, that so far as the mother is concerned the injection of gamma globulin following exposure to possible infection is of little or no value in preventing her from contacting the disease (Report of Public Health Laboratory Service Working Party 1967, 1968). This is not to say, however, that there might not be modifications of the manifestation of the disease in the patient and, more important still, that the severity of any effect on the child might not be reduced; any reduction of the foetal effect might make a profound difference to the ultimate disability of the child.

Examination of a specimen of blood from a pregnant woman exposed to possible disease may indicate that she is already immune to rubella, and therefore neither she nor her foetus is at risk. To be certain of this, however, rubella antibodies require to be detected in the patient's blood within some 10 days of the exposure. After that time it might not be possible to say that the antibodies detected were not the result of a recent infection; indeed, if the titre were found to be rising this would seem likely. It is of the utmost importance, therefore, to arrange for an examination of the patient's blood for antibodies at the earliest possible moment following the exposure; in this way we can at least know if the patient is immune or not and if there is cause for concern or not.

If the infection is confirmed in the mother who is less than 12 weeks pregnant the chances of an affected child are high and therapeutic termination of pregnancy is legally permissible.

In the future it will be possible to vaccinate susceptible members of the population before the child-bearing age (Dudgeon et al. 1969). For those within the child-bearing age who are still susceptible vaccination can also be employed—although, since vaccination is with live attenuated vaccine (the effects of which in pregnancy are not yet known), vaccination during pregnancy should be avoided. In Queen Charlotte's Hospital vaccination of susceptible patients has been practised effectively after delivery (Hurley et al. 1970).

Other infections

It must first of all be asked: Do any other infections have similar teratological effects to rubella? It is not yet certain what is the correct answer to this question. Certainly if any other diseases have teratological effects they cannot be compared in frequency and severity to those of rubella. It is possible, however—and not at this stage more than possible—that mumps, infective hepatitis and influenza act in a similar but less profound manner. Hyatt (1961) surveying 90 published cases of mumps in pregnancy quoted a 16% incidence of foetal abnormality; again, the first 3 months of pregnancy appeared to be the dangerous time. It is suggested that virus A of infective hepatitis does not cross the placenta but virus B—the virus of homologous serum jaundice—may do so. If congenital malformations can be attributed to viral hepatitis it is likely that they will vary from one epidemic to another. Moloshok (1966) quotes two series of viral infections occurring in the first trimester of pregnancy; in one, five abnormal foetuses and three abortions occurred in 21 pregnancies, but in the second there were several premature deliveries but no foetal abnormality in 29 pregnancies. So far as influenza is concerned, the evidence is less certain still, although Coffey & Jessop (1959) have reported that a group of patients afflicted with Asian influenza had a rate of congenital malformation 2·4 times that of a control group. It will be wise to adopt a cautious view of all these findings, however, until further evidence is available.

Teratogenic effects apart, it must be pointed out that abortion and late foetal death may be the result of maternal pyrexia and general toxic state. Measles does not appear to be teratogenic, but may cause foetal deaths or abortion in this way. Moloshok suggests that if a pregnant woman who has not had measles is exposed to the disease, gamma globulin in a dose of 0·1 ml/lb body weight should be given at once.

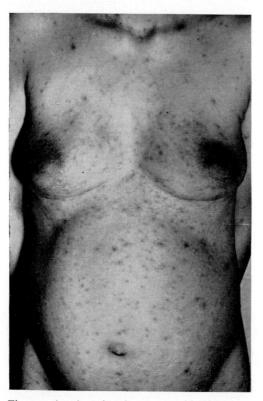

Fig. 21.1. A patient 36 weeks pregnant with chickenpox.

Similarly, chickenpox (Fig. 21.1) is not teratogenic, but several reports concerning mothers who have developed the disease late in pregnancy refer to congenital or neonatal chickenpox. The infant is probably infected during the mother's viraemic stage; most infants survive but the disease may be fatal in a premature child.

Smallpox may be transmitted to the foetus. Moloshok (1966) quotes a mortality among infected foetuses of some 50% as abortion or stillbirth. Infants may be born pox-marked or with active lesions present. The relationship of smallpox to pregnancy is important so far as vaccination of the pregnant woman is concerned. More and more people are now travelling abroad to countries which require a valid vaccination certificate, and the problem arises much more frequently as to whether a pregnant woman can safely be vaccinated or not. The situation was reviewed by Green et al. (1966). They make it clear that foetal death from generalized vaccinia is a rare but serious complication of vaccination. It is clear that primary vaccination of the mother is mainly responsible for foetal vaccinia; 11 of 15 reported cases of foetal vaccinia in Green et al.'s paper followed primary vaccination; two were revaccinations whilst in the remainder the type of vaccination was unknown. The authors suggest that all women of child-bearing age presenting themselves for vaccination should be asked specifically about the time of their last menstrual period. They further suggest that when vaccination cannot be avoided during pregnancy specific protection to ensure against foetal vaccinia is desirable. Hyperimmune gamma globulin can be given at the same time as vaccination or revaccination or, alternatively, a suitable inactivated vaccine may be given before vaccination, although the time required for this to be effective may contra-indicate its use.

The effect of poliomyelitis has been considered (see p. 101).

Cytomegalic inclusion disease is a condition which is now attracting more attention. The foetus may be affected directly from the mother if she becomes infected herself during her pregnancy. Microcephaly, thrombocytopenic-purpura, mental retardation and other lesions may result. The cytomegalovirus is very widespread and most adults have antibodies present, indicating former infection. It is likely that there are no specific clinical features permitting diagnosis when the disease affects an adult, so no indication of its presence in a pregnant woman will arise. The first suggestion may be the condition of the newborn or young child. It now seems likely that foetal infection may result from intra-uterine transfusion or exchange transfusion after delivery in cases of rhesus incompatibility. Whether such infections are always serious, however, is another matter. In all probability some children will recover from them and continue to develop normally, although some will be retarded. Further work on this subject is awaited with great interest.

Bacterial infections appear free from risk of teratogenicity. Maternal toxaemia and pyrexia may cause abortion, stillbirth or premature labour in a similar manner to acute infectious fevers. Malaria may act similarly. Intra-uterine infection of the child may occur when the mother is affected by malaria, although this is exceptional.

RESPIRATORY DISORDERS

Nearly every kind of respiratory disorder can occur in association with pregnancy. For the most part the course and management of the disorder are little affected by the pregnant state. The pregnancy may, however, be affected by certain chest diseases, especially the more acute infections with high fever. Since much of what is appropriate to respiratory disorders in the non-pregnant is appropriate to the pregnant woman also, little is to be gained by considering these general aspects—with which most obstetricians are familiar and which can readily be referred to in standard works of medicine. The special features pregnancy introduces will be discussed in more detail.

Acute infections such as pneumonia may cause abortion, foetal death or premature labour if the infection is severe and there is a marked febrile reaction. Considerable respiratory embarrassment may cause significant foetal hypoxia, which may also lead to foetal death. Intensive antibiotic therapy is required, although the tetracyclines are best avoided in view of the risk of foetal bone and teeth lesions. Oxygen therapy may be indicated if breathing is severely embarrassed and it is thought the foetus might suffer. Similar considerations will apply to less severe respiratory infections, but to a much less extent.

Bronchitis, bronchiectasis, emphysema, etc. may be somewhat aggravated in later pregnancy,

dyspnoea becoming marked especially at night. More rest is desirable and the patient should sleep propped up on several pillows for greater ease.

Pulmonary tuberculosis should be managed in a similar way to that in which it would be managed in the non-pregnant patient. The one modification which might be introduced is the withdrawal of streptomycin therapy if this can be achieved without significantly affecting the correct management of the mother. There *may* be a small risk of foetal nerve deafness if this drug is given for prolonged periods of time, although this association is far from proved. Treatment of the mother must be the first consideration, and if streptomycin would otherwise be indicated it should be used. BCG vaccination must be given to the baby and segregation from the mother for some 6–9 weeks is important in open lesions. If the lesion is not open, segregation may be dispensed with. Breast feeding is better avoided however. A word must be said about the special position of 'routine' chest X-rays during pregnancy. It is probable that the pick-up rate of significant abnormality—tuberculous or otherwise—on X-ray screening of a complete obstetrical population will be small; moreover, the number of other organizations offering mass X-rays to employees, etc. is so large that some patients would be X-rayed too frequently if chest films were demanded of all pregnant patients. The report of the Joint Tuberculosis Committee on the Control of Tuberculosis in Special Groups, Hospitals, Schools, Infants and Expectant Mothers, however, took the view that it was still necessary to X-ray a number of pregnant women if mistakes were to be avoided. Among the recommendations of the report was the general policy that a full-sized chest film of all expectant mothers should be taken unless reliable evidence of normal recent chest X-rays or a successful B.C.G. vaccination could be provided. The film should be taken between the twelfth and twenty-fourth week of pregnancy and a lead apron should be placed around the mother. Miniature radiography was to be avoided. Attention was drawn to several important groups of patient for whom chest X-ray during pregnancy was specially desirable. These were immigrants, diabetics, patients living in bad home conditions and patients with one of the following indications: a recent family history of tuberculosis, a past history of tuberculosis, recent contact with tuberculosis, persistent respiratory symptoms, or unexplained ill-health and recent tuberculin conversion or a large reaction. It may be mentioned, too, that a number of non-tuberculous lesions are sometimes found, and the committee considered there was good reason for continuing to advise X-ray during pregnancy in many individuals. Stanton (1968) has reviewed the practice at Queen Charlotte's Hospital.

Asthma is variably influenced by pregnancy, but as a rule little increase in symptoms is observed. Again, the treatment normally given may be continued. Cortisone therapy if employed will call for careful observation, however, during and immediately after labour. An increase in the dose normally taken should be considered or hydrocortisone should be given intravenously when the stress of labour begins. This increased dosage may be tailed-off over 2–3 days postpartum.

NERVOUS DISORDERS

Chorea gravidarum

This disorder has always been an uncommon complication of pregnancy. Nowadays in Britain it is very rare indeed. In Queen Charlotte's Hospital there has been no case in the last 20,000 admissions. Lewis (1966) and Clinch (1967) review the condition in some detail.

The precise cause of chorea gravidarum is unknown. It is probable, however, that the disease is closely related to Sydenham's chorea. Indeed, a previous history of chorea or rheumatic fever was obtainable in more than 50% of cases by Beresford & Graham (1950) and was probably present even more frequently.

The disease varies in severity from mild cases with such minor manifestations that close scrutiny of the patient is necessary to detect abnormal muscular activity, to very severe ones with violent, constant, uncontrollable movement. In simple cases slight athetoid hand movements and minor facial grimaces may be all there is to be found;

both tend to increase when the patient is examined or agitated. Evidence of a cardiac lesion may complicate any case, increasing the seriousness of the prognosis.

Treatment is by sedation with appropriate drugs such as barbiturates or tranquillizing agents, and the establishment of complete rest in quiet, peaceful surroundings. Salicylates may be employed also, although their value is open to question.

In extremely severe cases if the violent movements cannot be controlled by therapy and there is deterioration of the patient's condition consideration may be given to termination of the pregnancy. This is rarely the case now.

The disorder is now so uncommon that it is difficult to form a correct impression of the risk involved. In 1950, Beresford & Graham reported two maternal deaths in 144 patients, with a foetal loss of 3·3%. Nearly 20 years earlier, Willson (1932) reported a maternal mortality rate of 33% in severe cases treated by therapeutic termination of pregnancy, and 13% in those allowed to continue with pregnancy and deliver per vaginam. It seems likely that similar further improvement of mortality has occurred in recent times. Clinch (1967) reviewed 24 recent cases. There was no maternal mortality; 19 babies were delivered normally, two by forceps extraction and one by the vacuum extractor. Intra-uterine death occurred in one patient with pre-eclampsia and one patient miscarried.

Epilepsy

The effect of pregnancy on epilepsy is uncertain; indeed, the disease is a good example of the aphorism concerning the effects of pregnancy on a particular general disorder that 'some get better, some get worse, some stay the same'. Advice should be sought from a physician when an epileptic patient becomes pregnant. Careful observation is desirable to detect any change in the epileptic pattern, in order that alteration to treatment may be made. In general, the drugs employed to control epilepsy in the non-pregnant patient are used during pregnancy also. Barbiturates and Epanutin provide the mainstay of treatment. It is worthy of mention that

Epanutin is an anti-folic acid agent, and megaloblastic anaemia is more likely when this treatment is being given.

If attacks are at all common it will be wise to ensure that the patient is carefully supervised during the feeding of her baby and during the changing, bathing, etc. Breast feeding is not contra-indicated *per se*.

Poliomyelitis

Reference has already been made (p. 101) to the raised incidence of poliomyelitis in pregnancy. Despite this apparent increased susceptibility of pregnant women to the disease, prognosis for the mother is similar to that in the non-pregnant individual. There is, however, a significant foetal mortality, largely on account of hypoxia. The risk from hypoxia may be reduced by adequate ventilation of the mother on a respirator. Little is to be gained by early termination of pregnancy, and since labour is likely to be normal—the uterus not being affected by the disease—Caesarean section will only occasionally be indicated for some unusual circumstance. Forceps delivery is likely to be required, however, and local analgesia should be chosen if possible. The possibility of foetal affection by poliomyelitis is remote, although some cases have been reported (Shelokov & Weinstein 1951). Horne (1958) has reviewed many aspects of the management of poliomyelitis in pregnancy.

Myasthenia gravis

As is the case with epilepsy, the effect of pregnancy on myasthenia gravis is uncertain; patients have exacerbations or remissions or remain unaffected with more or less equal frequency. Generally, however, pregnancy can be managed easily and safely, although alterations to the dosage of neostigmine may be required. Early consultation with a physician is desirable and careful observation will be required to establish what changes in therapy are to be made and to confirm that these adjustments have been satisfactory. Once a suitable regime is established the patient is likely to remain well throughout her pregnancy. Only in exceptional cases will it be necessary to consider termination of pregnancy. Labour, too, is likely to be normal, since the uterine action is unaffected by the weakness involving the voluntary muscles. Delivery may need to be assisted, however, by the vacuum extractor or by forceps. Local analgesia should then be employed whenever possible.

The disorder tends to be aggravated by infection, which should be treated at once, and thoroughly. Moreover, patients with myasthenia are often unduly sensitive to narcotics, tranquillizers or sedatives, which should be used cautiously.

The main problems are likely to be encountered during the puerperium. Postpartum relapse is common and may be severe. Very careful observation indeed is imperative.

Myasthenia gravis may affect the newborn child of an afflicted mother, so very careful nursing is required to detect early manifestations of the disease. Chambers *et al.* (1967) have recently reviewed the subject.

Disseminated sclerosis

Disseminated (multiple) sclerosis is a progressive, demyelinating disorder. Progression, however, is often slow and is characterized by spontaneous remissions and exacerbations. This uneven course of the disease sometimes seems to suggest a cause-and-effect relationship which does not exist; a remission coinciding with a particular treatment may be thought, incorrectly, to be due to that treatment, or a relapse may be similarly—and wrongly—attributed to other changes in treatment or to some circumstance such as pregnancy. There is little, if any, evidence to suggest that pregnancy has an immediate or a permanently deleterious effect upon the disease. For this reason, termination of pregnancy need seldom be considered. Termination is not uncommonly employed, however, the decision being influenced by the difficulty the patient may already have in looking after her existing family, let alone another child.

Labour and delivery are likely to be normal in most cases. If there is significant weakness, however, or contractures, problems may arise. The foetus is not affected.

Parasthesia of the hand

Feelings of numbness and tingling in one or both hands in pregnancy are not uncommon symptoms. In most cases they are brief and mild and cause the patient little disturbance. Occasionally these symptoms are more troublesome and pain is experienced which may be quite distressing to the patient during the day and interfere with sleep at night. The fingers feel stiff and swollen and their movements are difficult and clumsy. These symptoms mostly make their appearance during the third trimester. Impaired sensation may or may not be present. Oedema of the hand and fingers is common.

The condition appears to fall into two categories: one in which symptoms are confined to the distribution of the median nerve (the thumb, index and middle fingers), and one in which all the hand (and perhaps the forearm, too) are involved. Wood (1961) reviewing the condition in outpatients at Queen Charlotte's Hospital found 23 patients in 2 years with troublesome symptoms confined to the hand; of these, 12 had symptoms corresponding to the median nerve distribution, 10 complained of involvement of all the fingers and thumb, and one patient had symptoms confined to the inside of the forearm and the little finger. If the numbness and tingling are restricted to the distribution of the median nerve the condition is usually referred to as the carpal-tunnel syndrome. It is regarded as being due to compression of the median nerve beneath the flexor retinaculum at the wrist. The explanation of more generalized paresthesia is less certain. In Wood's cases, X-ray examination for a cervical rib or a cervical spine abnormality was negative. Oedema of the fingers was present in most patients, however, suggesting that fluid retention may be involved in the etiology of either variety.

The most satisfactory form of treatment is diuresis. Hydrochlorthiazide 50 mg daily or twice daily for a week was effective in all but two of Wood's patients. Soferman et al. (1964) suggest that splinting of the hand in a neutral position may sometimes be helpful, especially at night. In severe cases when relief is not obtained by these measures hydrocortisone in-

jections into the flexor sheath may be considered in those patients who have a clear-cut carpal-tunnel syndrome. Surgical division of the flexor retinaculum is seldom, if ever, required during pregnancy.

Mental disorders

A patient with an existing mental disorder may, of course, become pregnant. When this occurs it is likely that she will already be under the care of a psychiatrist, who will consider the situation at once. If it is thought that the condition will be affected adversely by pregnancy or if it is already a very serious disorder in itself, termination of pregnancy may be advised.

Mental symptoms can appear for the first time during pregnancy. In a proportion of these patients a previous episode may be disclosed when the history is taken more fully. In others there may be a positive family history; sometimes, no previous history of any kind can be discovered.

Every patient's personality will influence her mental approach to pregnancy. In general, however, during early pregnancy her reactions are labile and she may be prone to quick mood changes. Some anxiety is not uncommon. Baker (1967) stresses this lability, pointing out that some patients may show obvious ambivalence to their pregnancies, being clearly delighted at one time and depressed shortly afterwards. This rapid fluctuation of mood is not uncommonly seen in patients referred for consultation in connection with termination of pregnancy; one minute they are wishing it to be done and the next they have changed their minds completely. Assessment can be very difficult under these circumstances.

After the first 3 months of pregnancy patients usually become more stable emotionally, even those who had been excitable and anxious before they became pregnant. This situation often prevails until delivery. Some patients, however, tend to become depressed as pregnancy continues and they complain that it seems never-ending; others may worry about the possibility of something going wrong or their child being abnormal. These are, of course, natural reactions; whether they should be regarded with concern or not is dependent on their degree.

Puerperal mental disease is briefly discussed on p. 418. The varieties of mental illness which may occur then are similar in their clinical features to those which can occur, although less frequently, during pregnancy. Psychiatric advice at an early stage will always be wise.

VENEREAL DISEASE

Syphilis

Syphilis is an important disorder at any time; during pregnancy there are no adverse maternal effects, but it is particularly serious for the foetus. The manifestations of syphilis in the patient herself are similar whether she is pregnant or not. In most cases the foetus will become affected by the disease, and this affect will vary with the stage of the infection in the mother. In a recently acquired infection it is almost certain that the foetus will be so markedly involved that foetal death *in utero* will occur. The infection does not appear to reach the foetus until the second trimester or later, so that syphilis need rarely be considered as a cause of early abortion. If the maternal disease has been present for a while, foetal death may occur later in pregnancy. In maternal disease of still longer duration the foetus may be born alive either with obvious lesions of syphilis on the skin or without apparent abnormality. In this latter event the child will demonstrate a positive serological test for syphilis and, untreated, will develop clinical features weeks, months, or even years, later.

The diagnosis of syphilis in the mother will be made in the same way as in the non-pregnant patient. Spirochetes may be detected in cutaneous lesions or a positive serological test may be obobtained. The Wassermann reaction, although almost always an indication of the disease, can rarely be positive in other circumstances. The reaction may remain positive in patients formerly affected, although it seldom does so at a high titre; it may also be positive in patients who have previously suffered from other disorders such as yaws; rarely, it seems that it is positive in a patient who does not have syphilis and never has had. A single positive Wassermann reaction should not,

therefore, be taken as certain evidence of syphilis. Such a patient must of course be thoroughly investigated by other serological means, such as the treponemal immobilization test.

Treatment must be started as soon as the diagnosis is certain. Even if it is begun in late pregnancy protection of the baby is still a possibility. Penicillin should be given to a total of 10 million units, a daily injection of 1 million units being satisfactory. Alternatively, a long-acting penicillin can be used; procain penicillin G in oil with 2% aluminium monostearate is given initially in a dose of 2·4 mega-units, and 1·2 mega-units are repeated every 3 or 4 days to a total of 10 million units in all. Follow-up studies on the mother and child are essential and other members of the family should be investigated also.

Gonorrhoea

Gonorrhoea in the mother presents in the same way as if she were not pregnant. Diagnosis is approached similarly, by the examination of urethral or cervical smears and serological tests. In suspicious cases it will be advisable to carry out several tests to be assured that no infection exists. The gonococcal complement-fixation test is not a completely reliable indicator of gonorrhoea, although it may be useful in some cases. The child may develop ophthalmia neonatorum due to ocular infection during passage through the birth canal.

Treatment should be given by injections of penicillin, 600,000 units of crystalline penicillin being given twice daily for 3 days or, procain penicillin, 1·2 mega-units being given daily for 3 days. The possibility that there may have been a coincident infection with syphilis must always be remembered, and adequate tests taken to ensure that syphilis is not present before the above treatment—which could mask the manifestations of syphilis—is started.

JAUNDICE IN PREGNANCY

Jaundice is not common during pregnancy. Sheehan (1961) suggested a frequency of 1 in 2,000–3,000 pregnancies. Haemmerli (1966) gives a slightly higher figure of 1 in 1,500. Various causes, of which a viral hepatitis is the most common, are found to explain the symptom. Other conditions include haemolytic jaundice, recurrent cholestatic jaundice of pregnancy, jaundice occurring in association with treatment with drugs such as chlorpromazine and, rarely, jaundice in severe cases of excessive vomiting or eclampsia.

Viral hepatitis does not appear to occur more frequently in pregnancy than at other times, nor is it significantly different in its course or management so far as the mother is concerned. The disorder may occur at any stage of pregnancy. Adams & Combes (1965) suggest the disease runs a fairly benign course, and they do not confirm the increased mortality during pregnancy which has sometimes been described. It seems probably that in well-nourished individuals the resistance of the pregnant woman will be similar to that of others who are not pregnant; in areas of poor nutrition, however, an increased mortality has been reported (Naidu & Viswanathan 1957).

Management of the patient is not influenced by pregnancy, and similar treatment should be given then as in the non-pregnant.

The outcome for the foetus may be a little less favourable. Prematurity and stillbirth are more common if the disease occurs later in pregnancy; if jaundice occurs earlier, however, it appears to be less harmful.

Jaundice due to gallstones obstructing the common bile duct is perhaps less frequent than would seem likely, since fat, fertile females are prone to this disorder. If jaundice does occur from this cause, however, and an operation for removal of a stone would otherwise be indicated, it should be carried out and the pregnancy disregarded.

A variety of jaundice which is now more widely recognized than formerly is recurrent jaundice, which may be seen towards the end of several pregnancies. Moore reported that 3 out of 33 patients with jaundice during pregnancy seen at the Rotunda Hospital had recurrent jaundice in subsequent pregnancies. The jaundice is accompanied by considerable itching, and occasionally this pruritus may be the only feature. If the condition has been present in the previous pregnancy its recurrent nature, combined with pruritus, will be sufficient to permit the diagnosis on purely clinical grounds. The most consistent abnormality on liver-function testing is a slightly raised serum bilirubin and a definitely raised alkaline phosphatase. The jaundice is clearly obstructive in origin and the prevailing view now is that it is due to intrahepatic cholestasis. It is generally stated that this type of jaundice is benign for both mother and child, but Dewhurst (1968) questions that it is always innocent as far as the child is concerned; he reports foetal loss possibly due to this cause. After delivery the pruritus disappears quickly and the jaundice more slowly.

Acute hepatic failure in pregnancy

Rarely, in late pregnancy, a patient will develop vomiting, upper abdominal pain and jaundice; these features are quickly followed by headaches, mental confusion, coma and death. The whole duration of the disease may be merely a few days. The urine is bile-stained and the stools are pale, indicating the jaundice to be obstructive in type. Obstetric acute yellow atrophy and the acute fatty liver of pregnancy are names which have been applied to this condition. Whether pregnancy can, in any way, be considered an essential feature of the disease is open to question however. Acute liver failure of this type arises at other times following (although not by any means immediately following) drugs or various poisons; tetracyclins have been incriminated (Kunelis et al. 1965). In other cases, however, a cause may not be discovered.

The most prominent histological feature is fatty degeneration in the centre of the liver lobule; necrosis of liver cells is not a marked feature and the picture is not the same as that of acute hepatic necrosis of viral origin.

The progress of the condition is so rapid that effective treatment may be almost impossible. Early delivery is indicated at the first appearance of jaundice.

It would be wise to apply names such as acute fatty liver of pregnancy only to those cases in which this fatty infiltration is pronounced, in order that this diagnosis may not be widely used for different types of case.

THE PELVIC JOINTS IN
PREGNANCY AND LABOUR

The effect of pregnancy on the pelvic joints has been investigated with considerable thoroughness in the past. The radiographic studies of Heyman & Lundqvist (1932) and Abramson et al. (1934) demonstrated than an increase in the width and mobility of the symphysis pubis takes place in every pregnancy, a similar decrease occurring postpartum. Whether the decrease is always equal to the increase is in question, but if there is a permanent increase in the size of the symphysis pubis with repeated pregnancies it must be very slight. Widening and increased mobility

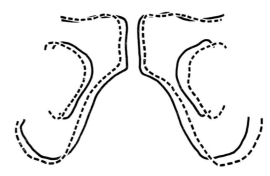

Fig. 21.2. A tracing of an X-ray of the pubic arch at 36 weeks of pregnancy (dotted line), and 6 weeks after delivery (continuous line), to show increase in size resulting from relaxation of pelvic joints.

(a)

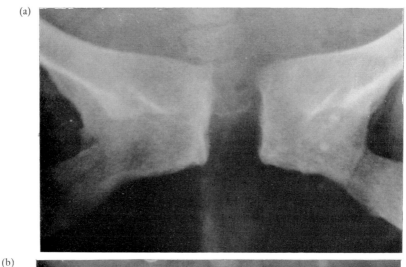

(b)

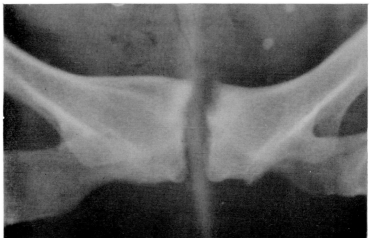

Fig. 21.3. An example of relaxation of the symphysis pubis with considerable increase in the size of the joint: (a) at 36 weeks, (b) 6 weeks postpartum.

of the sacro-iliac joints occur also, but to a smaller degree; moreover, it is more difficult to demonstrate clearly even on careful radiographic studies. It must be stressed that these changes occur during pregnancy and probably begin in the early months, the maximum increase being reached sometime before term. During labour no further increase in size occurs, although the greater mobility of the joints may have obvious beneficial effects (Fig. 21.2) (Russell, 1969).

The increase in the width and mobility of the symphysis pubis can sometimes be marked (Fig. 21.3). Greater mobility may give rise to a certain measure of instability which can sometimes become pronounced, when it is referred to as pelvic arthropathy. In mild cases there will be backache, which may be referred to one or both sacro-iliac joints, and discomfort and tenderness in the symphysis pubis. More severe cases will complain of considerable pain, especially in the pubis. It may be very difficult for the patient to move about, and walking, if it is possible, will be with a 'waddling' type of gait. In the most marked cases the patient may have little freedom from pain even whilst at rest in bed; turning over in bed alone may be agonizing, and is sometimes

described by the patient as feeling as if one half of the body is left behind. Cases occurring during pregnancy are seldom so severe as this, the most marked cases usually appearing during the puerperium. Moreover, the onset of symptoms in pregnancy is gradual, whereas in the puerperium it is likely to be sudden and excruciating. On examination there will be tenderness in the symphysis pubis and perhaps over the sacro-iliac region, and if there is a large symphysial gap (which need not always be the case) this may be palpable clinically.

Treatment is by rest and pelvic support. In one marked case (Fig. 21.4) it was necessary to sling the patient from a beam to achieve pain-relief. Young (1940), who wrote at length on this subject, recommended this kind of treatment for severe cases. Usually, however, it is unnecessary to go to these lengths, and simple rest will be sufficient. A tight roller-towel wrapped around the pelvic region may give excellent relief until symptoms subside. Usually, the condition settles well within a few weeks. It may recur in subsequent pregnancies.

Traumatic rupture of the symphysis pubis during normal or instrumental delivery is also described, with similar symptoms and signs.

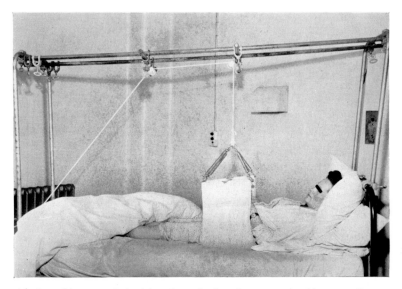

Fig. 21.4. A patient with very marked pelvic arthropathy slung from an overhead beam to relieve severe pelvic pain.

Whilst this undoubtedly appears at times, it is probable that many cases so reported are examples of pelvic relaxation, minor injury during delivery precipitating the clinical features. Indeed, it is possible that features of pelvic arthropathy are caused by minor trauma, to which such relaxed joints will certainly be more liable.

GENITAL TRACT LESIONS

Various lesions of the genital tract occurring in association with pregnancy are discussed elsewhere in this book. Fibroids complicating pregnancy and labour are dealt with on p. 610, ovarian tumours on p. 654, carcinoma of the cervix on p. 619, fusion deformities on p. 346 and cervical incompetence on p. 216. The few remaining genital tract lesions will now be discussed.

Vulval lesions

Condylomata accuminata of the vulva are found during pregnancy at least as often as in the non-pregnant state, and their management is similar. Podophylin may be applied or the lesions removed surgically.

Varicose veins of the vulva, perhaps in considerable number and reaching a large size, may occasionally be encountered. Alarming though their presence is, the prospect of serious bleeding is hardly ever borne out. For the most part they can be ignored, but if bleeding does arise, due to injury during delivery or at some other time, pressure alone may be sufficient to control it; failing that, simple surgical ligation may be carried out.

Bartholin cysts or abscesses may be observed during pregnancy. They can be managed by marsupialization as effectively then as at other times.

Vaginal lesions

The general problem of vaginal discharge is considered on p. 579. During pregnancy, greater pelvic vascularity and raised oestrogen production cause an increase in the amount of vaginal discharge. Not infrequently, patients mention their awareness of this discharge but they are seldom worried once they know the reason for it. *Candida albicans* infection is more common in pregnancy than at other times, presumably due to the tendency for the pregnant woman to pass sugar in the urine from time to time. Nystatin pessaries or similar treatment will deal with the infection swiftly and effectively.

An infestation with *Trichomonas vaginalis* may occur during pregnancy, but probably does not do so with any increased frequency. Physical signs and investigation are the same as in the non-pregnant patient. Treatment, too, can effectively and safely be carried out with metranidazole after the twelfth week of pregnancy. It is probable that this treatment can safely be given before this time, but this is not conclusively established and alternative treatment with an arsenical pessary is preferable.

Uterine lesions

Retroversion of the gravid uterus is nowadays thought to present fewer problems than was at one time believed to be the case. As a cause of infertility it is unlikely that retroversion has a significant effect in any but one specific area—this is when the uterus is very markedly retroverted and the cervix is displaced forwards and upwards to occupy a position just behind the symphysis pubis it may be so removed from the discharge of seminal fluid at coitus that the chances of fertilization are greatly reduced.

Once the pregnancy occurs, however, the likelihood of abortion, once thought to be high, is now believed to be little, if any, increased. Even granted a slight increase in the chance of abortion from this cause it is probable that attempts to antevert the uterus manually or by the use of a pessary will make abortion more, and not less, likely. The clinical diagnosis of pregnancy may be more difficult, since the retroverted uterus cannot so easily be felt bimanually; a vigorous vaginal examination should not then be made, but a pregnancy test should be preferred for confirmation.

INCARCERATION OF THE RETROVERTED GRAVID UTERUS

Most retroverted uteri will correct themselves without any difficulty as pregnancy advances. As the uterus enlarges it grows upwards out of the pelvis between the twelfth and the sixteenth week. Rarely, incarceration of the retroverted gravid uterus may arise. When this happens the first symptoms are urinary. Between the twelfth and the sixteenth week of pregnancy the patient may become aware of difficulty in passing urine, leading eventually to an episode of acute retention. During this fourth month the uterus becomes large enough to fill the pelvis, and the urethra may become mechanically obstructed or may be unduly elongated upwards with the displaced cervix.

The physical signs will be the presence of a lower abdominal cystic swelling, the over-distended bladder and there will be a swelling palpable vaginally in the posterior fornix, the retroverted fundus. The cervix may be so high that it is elevated beyond reach.

The management of this state of affairs is to pass a catheter to empty the bladder. Complete and immediate emptying of the bladder can be employed quite safely without fear of complications. The catheter must then be left *in situ* and the patient nursed in a prone position. It is extremely uncommon for this simple treatment not to be successful. If the bladder is kept empty by continuous drainage the enlarging uterus will raise itself out of the pelvis and become palpable abdominally within 24–48 hr in nearly all cases. If it is ever necessary to employ other measures this contingency must be very unlikely. Digital pressure with the patient occupying the knee/chest position has been described, but how frequently this is really necessary is open to conjecture. It has never been necessary in the author's experience to carry out measures other than the simple treatment by continuous bladder drainage as described above.

Abortion may complicate incarceration of the retroverted gravid uterus, but is likely to be more common if vigorous digital attempts at replacement have been performed; employing continuous bladder-drainage only, abortion is rare.

FUSION DEFORMITIES

Fusion deformities of the uterus have been referred to in several sections already. In particular, their possible association with recurrent abortion has been considered on p. 218, and their association with transverse lie on pp. 7 and 369. The management of fusion deformities giving rise to transverse and oblique lie is the same as that arising from, say, multiparity. Since, in general, the obstetrician is unaware of the uterine fault the problem must be approached along general lines, mainly correction of the transverse lie or, failing that, Caesarean section. Even if it has been previously established that the uterus is bicornate, similar management is indicated. The obstetric problems arising from the presence of a vaginal septum are considered on p. 12.

UTERINE PROLAPSE

Minor degrees of prolapse frequently exist in association with pregnancy. Rarely do they give rise to a difficulty at any stage. If stress incontinence is marked this may cause soreness and discomfort from which some relief should be sought. If a urinary infection is present treatment for this may be helpful. Otherwise a simple mechanical aid offering some relief is the introduction of a Hodge pessary upside down. A fairly large pessary is likely to be required; this sits with its prominent bar firmly against the region of the bladder base, and some patients achieve considerable relief as a result.

Major degrees of prolapse are seldom seen complicating pregnancy. When they are they may present a problem during the first 16 weeks or so, when a large part of the uterus and the cervix are outside the body. There may be discharge and bleeding as the exposed areas rub against underclothes, bed-clothes, etc. Some relief may be obtained by inserting a plastic ring pessary. After 16 weeks or so the enlarging uterus gradually lifts the exposed cervix back into the vagina and fewer symptoms are experienced.

If a patient has previously undergone successful repair for a prolapse or stress incontinence of urine the question arises as to the most satisfactory form of delivery in any other pregnancy. Following a Manchester-type of repair un-complicated vaginal delivery is not uncommon. However, in a significant proportion of cases there may be delay in cervical dilatation, or tearing of the cervix and the vault of the vagina may occur. Whether simple or complicated vaginal delivery results, the risk of recurrence exists. It seems likely that the best interests of many patients will be served by performing elective Caesarean sec-tion; this may be particularly the case of cervical scarring and rigidity are evident when the patient is examined towards the end of her pregnancy.

Similarly stress incontinence cured by a previous operation may recur if vaginal delivery is undertaken. It may of course recur if Caesarean section is carried out although the chances of this seem reduced. Here, too, Caesarean section is preferred in most instances.

Massive breast enlargement

Rarely, the normal breast enlargement of preg-nancy proceeds so rapidly and excessively that enormous hypertrophy results (Fig. 21.5). This may give rise to considerable physical and mental distress. The breasts become so heavy that they can scarcely be supported by any brassiere, how-ever large. The patient may have difficulty in finding any comfortable position and her sleep may become disturbed. Her embarrassment at possessing such gigantic disfigurement may be pronounced. The reduction in size of the breasts after delivery may be incomplete and the patient may be left with very large breasts indeed, for which plastic surgical treatment should be con-sidered.

SKIN DISORDERS

Changes in pigmentation of the skin are an almost universal finding in pregnancy. There is darkening of the primary areolar and the appearance of the secondary areolar in the breast, the linea nigra in the lower abdomen and the chloasma on the forehead and cheeks. These changes are almost certainly due to an increase in melanaphore-stimulating hormone, in common with increases

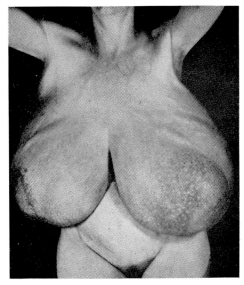

Fig. 21.5. An example of enormous breast hypertrophy complicating pregnancy.

in other trophic hormones in pregnancy. They are physiological manifestations which cause no symptoms nor call for treatment. Skin disorders do occur, however, which can cause extremely troublesome symptoms on occasions.

HERPES GESTATIONIS

This is one of the most distressing skin diseases directly associated with pregnancy. It is, fortu-nately, an infrequent one, Russell (1962) quoting an incidence of 1 in 4,500 pregnancies. It may appear at any time from mid-pregnancy onwards. Itching is one of the earliest manifestations, to be followed shortly by patches of erythema, papules and bullous eruptions (Fig. 21.6). These various lesions appear in groups at intervals throughout pregnancy and may cause much distress by their itching, by the soreness of lesions which become infected, and by the lack of sleep caused. In severe cases considerable constitutional upset may occur.

General treatment for herpes gestations is important whatever specific therapy may be employed. An adequate diet must be ensured, although it may be necessary to tempt the patient

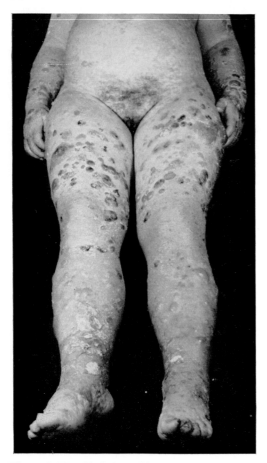

Fig. 21.6. The skin lesions of herpes gestationis in late pregnancy. (By courtesy of Professor C.S. Russell.)

with tasty portions if she is disinclined to eat. Rest, too, is important; drugs to ensure relief from discomfort and to promote sleep at night will be necessary in many instances. Local lesions may be bathed in potassium permanganate 1 in 10,000 or in saline, or treated with simple dusting powder when they are dry. Antibiotic therapy may be required if secondary infection is widespread; again, tetracyclines should be avoided. For the treatment of severe cases corticosteroid therapy is indicated. Whatever preparation is employed increase in the dosage or the use of hydrocortisone intravenously is desirable during labour. Herpes gestationis has a tendency to recur in subsequent pregnancies,

so the desirability of further child-bearing may require to be discussed with the patient.

PAPULAR DERMATITIS OF PREGNANCY

Spangler *et al.* (1962) described a generalized papular eruption occurring widely over the legs, arms and even, in some instances, scalp and face. Itching is intense as in the case of herpes gestationis, but the papules in Spangler's cases were covered with a hemorrhagic crust and bullous lesions did not form. The foetal mortality in their series was raised in those cases which were not treated by corticosteroids. They employed prednisolone in doses as high as 100 mg daily.

PREGNANCY PRURIGO

Various names have been given to a condition in which a patient in late pregnancy develops an irritating rash in the form of tiny papules. The toxic eruption or toxaemic rash of pregnancy have been names used; more recently, the phrase prurigo of pregnancy has been introduced. Bourne (1962) and Nurse (1968) have both described series of cases. The abdomen, hands and feet are the most common parts affected. Itching is pronounced and the patient may loose a great deal of sleep. Many cases occurring late in pregnancy may be controlled by giving sedatives to the patient at night and applying a local oily calamine lotion to the lesions. Systemic corticosteroid therapy is seldom required and is best avoided unless symptoms are very severe and occur earlier in pregnancy.

IMPETIGO HERPETIFORMIS

This is a much more serious disorder, in which widespread pustular eruption is present in association with marked constitutional disturbance. It is difficult to obtain reliable information on the occurrence or management of this condition. Corticosteroids, gonadotrophins and antibiotics are mentioned by various authors (Main 1969; Jenner 1970).

Skin disorders not specifically associated with pregnancy may, of course, occur at that time. Similar management is, in general, indicated as in the non-pregnant patient.

THROMBOSIS AND EMBOLISM

The problem of thrombosis and embolism complicates the puerperium more frequently than pregnancy. It is considered, therefore, in the chapter on puerperal disorders on p. 410. Thrombotic and embolic lesions do, however, occasionally occur during pregnancy, when they give rise to special problems. These accidents occurring during pregnancy appear to be more dangerous than those in the puerperium, if we are to judge by maternal mortality statistics. Despite the comparative infrequency of antenatal deep venous thrombosis, one-quarter of all fatal cases of pulmonary embolus considered in the *Confidential Enquiry into Maternal Deaths in England and Wales, 1964-1966* occurred before delivery. This may be because embolism is a more likely sequel to thrombosis at that time, although it seems more probable that the greater mortality rate is related to the failure to diagnose antenatal deep venous thrombosis soon enough, and perhaps to treat it adequately.

The clinical features are similar to those described on p. 410. Treatment is more difficult, however. Heparin has a large molecule and probably does not pass the placenta. Coumarin derivatives do, however, and the foetus may suffer from bleeding complications and may die. Heparin, therefore, is the drug of choice and should be employed whenever possible, despite its difficulties of prolonged administration intravenously. If these difficulties are too great over a long period of time it may be a difficult decision to know whether to run the risks involved with coumarin drugs or not. Anticoagulants should be stopped during labour and resumed at once after delivery. Coumarin derivatives may then be used.

ALIMENTARY TRACT DISORDERS

Pregnancy is accompanied by a general diminution is smooth-muscle tone which affects the alimentary tract. It is responsible for the incompetence of the gastro-oesophageal sphincter and for the delay in gastric emptying, especially in labour. Constipation of greater or lesser degree is similarly the product of diminished bowel activity; it is also often due to the effect of administered iron. As pregnancy advances the enlarging uterus may make constipation worse by pressing on the colon as it crosses the pelvic brim, and may also increase the occurrence of acid reflux from the stomach into the oesophagus, causing 'heartburn', a very common symptom in pregnancy. Vomiting in early pregnancy, the other very common gastrointestinal upset, seems less troublesome nowadays than it apparently was. The progression from the simple nausea and vomiting of early pregnancy to the hyperemesis gravidarum syndrome of intractable vomiting and biochemical disturbance is comparatively uncommon. Nevertheless, the occasional patient may not respond to simple antinausea drugs such as meclozine hydrochloride (ancolan), and require admission to hospital for correction of dehydration and ketosis by the administration of intravenous fluids.

Hiatus hernia

When acid reflux into the stomach occurs frequently and heartburn is severe, it is probable that the patient has developed a sliding hernia of the stomach through the oesophageal hiatus. The existence of such a hernia can only be diagnosed with certainty by radiological examination, a barium swallow carried out with the patient tilted into the head-low position. Two-thirds of a series of patients with reflux had some degree of hiatus hernia (Gorbach & Reid 1956). Radiological examination should be avoided in most cases, however, the diagnosis being assumed from the severity of the patient's symptoms. Exacerbation of the heartburn on bending or lying flat is a useful confirmatory symptom. Vomiting and eructations are common, and occasionally small haematemeses may occur as a result of superficial ulceration of the lower oesophagus. The symptoms disappear very quickly after delivery.

MANAGEMENT

The patient should avoid adopting any position which brings on the symptoms, and in particular should avoid bending over, and should prop herself up with several pillows under the head and shoulders when in bed. Small, frequent meals and the use of antacid agents will help to relieve what is often considerable discomfort. Magnesium trisilicate mixture in a dose of 15–30 ml usually provides rapid relief. The use of magnesium trisilicate powder is recommended in intractable cases, a level teaspoonful provides a coating for the lower oesophagus which protects it for some hours. Another preparation which often acts for several hours is aluminium glycinate, which is prepared in tablet form (Proxedin), one tablet is dissolved under the tongue as required.

Peptic ulcer

The association of peptic ulcer and pregnancy is not uncommon, but the symptoms rarely develop for the first time during pregnancy. Most patients with established peptic ulcers who do become pregnant experience relief of their symptoms during the pregnancy and a relapse within 6 months of delivery. Fortunately, haematemesis and perforation do not often occur during pregnancy, but if they do so are most likely to happen during labour or the early puerperium. Very occasionally, maternal death from the complications of peptic ulcer may occur; two such cases were recorded in the *Confidential Enquiry into Maternal Mortality in England and Wales, 1964-1966*. The management of the condition should be along normal medical or surgical (in the case of perforation or haematemesis) lines. Lactation is accompanied by an increase in acid secretion by the gastric mucosa, so breast feeding should be avoided in patients with a long past history of ulceration or of perforation or haematemesis. The probability of an exacerbation of symptoms in the 6 months following delivery should be borne in mind.

Small-bowel lesions

Intestinal obstruction due to the incarceration of small bowel in hernial sacs or around intraperitoneal bands may occur during pregnancy as at other times. Care must be taken to exclude obstruction in pregnant patients who present with abdominal pain and vomiting. Although rare in pregnancy, intestinal obstruction is the commonest disorder of the alimentary tract to cause death in pregnancy. Regional ileitis—Crohn's disease—tends to pass from a quiescent to an active phase during pregnancy, and if the disease is already active it gets worse at this time. When the disease develops first during pregnancy it tends to take an acute form. The management of this condition, as of other small-bowel lesions, should follow the treatment for the non-pregnant patient although, clearly, the presence of the pregnant uterus may make some surgical procedures more difficult.

Acute appendicitis

Although acute appendicitis is only a very rare cause of maternal mortality in this country at the present, it may nevertheless be a source of worry to the clinician from both diagnostic and therapeutic viewpoints. The combination of central abdominal pain, fever, vomiting and constipation may occur in a number of conditions, especially pyelonephritis or, rarely, cholecystitis. Early in pregnancy, incomplete abortion and ectopic pregnancy may cause diagnostic difficulty, whilst later on torsion of an ovarian cyst and complications arising in fibroids may be confusing. In patients with sickle-cell disease mesenteric infarction must be added to the list. Once the possibility of acute appendicitis is admitted, however, the difficulties in making the diagnosis are not too great, especially when the pain moves from the centre to the right iliac fossa. The tendency of the enlarging uterus to displace the caecum and appendix upward and laterally has perhaps been over-emphasized in the past, and in most cases—except in late pregnancy—the site of maximal pain and tenderness is little different from that in the non-pregnant patient. This has an important practical bearing, for when operation is decided upon the incision should be placed over the site of maximum tenderness, and not a hypothetical position indicated by a textbook diagram of where the appendix ought to be for the particular stage of gestation concerned.

The presence of an enlarged uterus does seem to make localization of appendicular inflammation by the omentum less efficient, so that peritonitis is a more common complication than appendix abscess. Appendicitis is prone to cause abortion, especially if the diagnosis is delayed and peritonitis occurs. The risk of abortion or premature labour in the uncomplicated case is of the order of 5%, whilst if peritonitis develops 50% or more of patients abort (Barnes 1970). An early decision to operate should be taken in all cases where there is a reasonable suspicion that the patient may have acute appendicitis in pregnancy. The removal of a mildly inflamed (or normal) appendix through a McBurney incision, adjusted if necessary to the point of the patient's maximal tenderness, carries little risk to the patient or the foetus. Delay, however, may result in a rapid deterioration of the patient's condition as peritonitis develops. The free use of antibiotics and intravenous fluids help in all but the mild cases, and the patient should be kept well sedated to reduce the chance of abortion or premature labour. If either ensue shortly after appendicectomy extra analgesia will be necessary for the patient because of the additional discomfort of the abdominal incision.

Ulcerative colitis

Ulcerative colitis in pregnancy is not uncommon. Dombal et al. (1965) described 107 pregnancies in 72 patients with the disease. Most of the patients were in a quiescent phase when they became pregnant, and for this group the chance of a relapse developing (48%) was no higher than in non-pregnant controls. When relapse did occur it was most likely to do so during early pregnancy or in the puerperium. Rising levels of plasma cortisol may protect patients to some extent during the second and third trimesters. The sudden fall in cortisol levels following delivery might, equally, be the precipitatory factor in the relapses occurring during the puerperium. When the disease is active at the start of a pregnancy 50% of the patients will deteriorate further. The reason for this is obscure, for a proportion of the acute cases seem actually to improve during the pregnancy. As the out-

come cannot be predicted in an individual case, patients should be encouraged not to become pregnant during the active phase, but need not be discouraged when the disease is quiescent. When a patient first develops ulcerative colitis during pregnancy or the puerperium it is likely to be severe, and patients who do badly in one pregnancy are likely to repeat the performance in subsequent pregnancies. The disease has little effect on the outcome of pregnancy and most patients proceed uneventfully to produce healthy offspring. The abortion rate is no higher than normal, even in those patients who relapse. Termination of pregnancy is not indicated unless there are other medical or social factors.

MANAGEMENT

Radical surgery is, fortunately, very rarely needed during pregnancy. The patient's symptoms can usually be controlled with codeine phosphate 30 mg two or three times daily and sulphasalazine 1 g four times daily. In the more severe cases oral ACTH or adrenal steroids can be used and prednisone retention enemas given. A nourishing, low-residue diet is essential, and systemic iron or blood transfusions used to combat anaemia. Labour is usually uncomplicated even in women who have had a previous proctocolectomy. There is no special indication for Caesarean section in this latter group of patients, but perineal scarring may call for a generous episiotomy and forceps delivery. Although patients with this condition seem to do well, they should be advised to have small families, and attention to contraception or sterilization postpartum is an important part of the management.

Acute pancreatitis

This is an uncommon complication of pregnancy but its occurrence in a younger age group than is normal for the disease makes it likely that the association is not coincidental. There is no constant aetiological factor, but about half of the patients have gallstones. Rarely, alcoholism or the administration of thiazide diuretics may play a part in causing pancreatitis, and it is possible that the raised level of blood lipids in pregnancy

may be a factor. Primigravidae between 20 and
30 years of age make up the bulk of the cases, and
the disease may occur at any time during the
pregnancy or puerperium. The presenting symptom is of severe upper abdominal pain radiating
to the back and made worse by food. Nausea
and vomiting may be severe and the patient
become dehydrated and ketosed as a result.
Mild obstructive jaundice is sometimes seen. The
diagnosis may be difficult on clinical grounds,
but elevation of the serum amylase level points
strongly to pancreatitis. The normal level of
180 Somogyi units per 100 ml may be exceeded
many times in severe cases. The management of
the condition is conservative in the first instance
with adequate analgesia (pethidine is preferred
to morphia, which may cause spasm of the sphincter of Oddi) and intravenous fluids. Gastric
suction is indicated if the patient is vomiting
badly, and a broad-spectrum antibiotic should
be given systemically. Once the acute phase
has passed and the pregnancy has been concluded
any necessary biliary tract investigations and
surgery should be carried out. Abortion or
premature labour may occur in the severely ill
patient, but in the majority of cases the pregnancy
continues undisturbed.

REFERENCES

ABRAMSON D., ROBERTS S.M. & WILSON P.D. (1934)
    Surgery Gynec. Obstet. **58**, 595.
ADAMS R.H. & COMBES B. (1965) *J. Am. med. Ass.* **192**, 195.
BAKER A.A. (1967) *Psychiatric Disorders in Obstetrics.*
    Oxford, Blackwell Scientific Publications.
BARNES C.G. (editor) (1970) *Medical Disorders in Obstetric
    Practice*, 3rd edn. Oxford, Blackwell, p. 140.
BERESFORD O.D. & GRAHAM A.M. (1950) *J. Obstet. Gynaec.
    Br. Commonw.* **57**, 616.
BOURNE G. (1962) *Proc. R. Soc. Med.* **55**, 462.
CHAMBERS D.C., HALL J.E. & BOYCE J. (1967) *Obstet.
    Gynec., N.Y.*, **29**, 597.
CLINCH J. (1967) *Hosp. Med.* **2**, 317.
COFFEY V.P. & JESSOP W.J.E. (1959) *Lancet*, **ii**, 935.

DEWHURST C.J. (1968) *Br. med. J.* **i**, 253.
DIMSDALE H. (1959) *Br. med. J.* **ii**, 1147.
DOMBAL F.T. DE, GOLIGHER J.C., WATTS J.M. & WATKIN-
    SON G. (1965) *Lancet*, **ii**, 595.
DUDGEON J.A., MARSHALL W.C., PECKHAM C.S. &
    HAWKINS G.T. (1969) *Br. med. J.* **ii**, 271.
GORBACH A.C. & REID DE (1956) *New Engl. J. Med.*
    255, 1131.
GREEN D.M., REID S.M. & RHANEY K. (1966) *Lancet*,
    i, 1296.
GREGG N.M. (1941) *Trans. ophthal. Soc. Aust.* **3**, 35.
HAEMMERLI U.R. (1966) *Acta med. scand.* **197** (Supplement)
    444.
HARDY J.B., McCRACKEN G.H., GILKESON M.R. &
    SEVER J.L. (1969) *J. Am. med. Ass.* **207**, 2414.
HEYMAN J. & LUNDQVIST A. (1932) *Acta obstet. gynec.
    scand.* **12**, 191.
HORN P. (1958) *Clin. Obstet. Gynec.* **1**, 127.
HYATT H.W. (1961) *Am. Practnr. Dig. Treat.* **12**, 359.
JENNER F.J. (1970) In *Medical Disorders in Obstetric
    Practice* (edited by C.G. Barnes). Oxford, Blackwell
    Scientific Publications, p. 241.
KUNELIS C.T., PETERS J.L. & EDMONDSON H.A. (1965)
    Am. J. med. **38**, 359.
Leading Article (1965) *Lancet*, **ii**, 118.
LEWIS B.V. & PARSONS M. (1966) *Lancet*, **i**, 284.
MAIN R.T. (1969) *Br. J. clin. Pract.* **23**, 47.
MILLAR J.H.D. (1961) *Proc. R. Soc. Med.* **54**, 4.
MOLOSHOK R.E. (1966) *Clin. Obstet. Gynec.* **9**, 608.
MOORE H.C. (1963) *Lancet*, **ii**, 57.
NAIDU S.S. & VISWANATHAN R. (1957) *Indian J. med. Res.*
    45, (Supplement), 71.
NURSE D.S. (1968) *Aust. J. Derm.* **9**, 258.
Report of Public Health Laboratory Service Working
    Party (1967) *Br. med. J.* **iii**, 638.
Report of Public Health Laboratory Service Working
    Party (1968) *Br. med. J.* **iii**, 203.
RUSSELL B. (1962) *Proc. R. Soc. Med.* **55**, 464.
RUSSELL J.G.B. (1969) *J. Obstet. Gynaec. Br. Commonw.*
    76, 817.
SHEEHAN H.L. (1961) *Am. J. Obstet. Gynec.* **81**, 427.
SHELOKOV A. & WEINSTEIN L. (1951) *J. Pediat.* **38**, 80.
SOFERMAN N., WEISSMAN S.L. & HAIMOV M. (1964)
    Am. J. Obstet. Gynec. **89**, 528.
SPANGLER A.S., REDDY W., BARDAWIL W.A., ROBY C.C.
    & EMERSON K.J. (1962) *J. Am. med. Ass.* **181**, 577.
STANTON S.L. (1968) *J. Obstet. Gynaec. Br. Commonw.*
    75, 1161.
WILLSON P. & PREECE A.A. (1932) *Int. med.* **49**, 471.
WOOD C. (1961) *Br. med. J.* **ii**, 680.

CHAPTER 22

MALPOSITIONS OF THE OCCIPUT, MALPRESENTATIONS, MULTIPLE PREGNANCY, HYDRAMNIOS, OLIGOHYDRAMNIOS AND POSTMATURITY

INTRODUCTION

Perinatal mortality is increased both by malposition and by malpresentation. So, too, is perinatal morbidity. In the minority of cases the malposition actually results from intra-uterine foetal death or congenital malformation. In other instances associated prematurity or multiple pregnancy may cause an increase in foetal loss. Furthermore, any malpresentation will predispose to prolapse of the cord, abnormal uterine action and prolonged or obstructed labour, all of which can cause foetal hypoxia. Intra-uterine infection and meconium aspiration can follow prolonged rupture of membranes. Finally, manipulative vaginal delivery, maternal hypoxia during anaesthesia, and maternal ketosis and dehydration may further compromise the foetus.

Equally important are the increased risks to the mother. Early diagnosis, skilled assessment, careful supervision of labour and planned delivery by experienced staff working in proper surroundings are necessary to achieve the best results. Any of these patients may require a general anaesthetic at short notice, and this should be remembered throughout labour. Suitably experienced anaesthetists should be available for this most difficult group of cases. Finally, the dangers of infection must be appreciated in prolonged rupture of membranes, and the risks to the mother of Caesarean section in labour and of difficult vaginal delivery. These points are emphasized by the figures in the *Report on Confidential Enquiries into Maternal Deaths in England and Wales, 1964–1966*. Forty-seven

mothers died after Caesarean section for malpresentation, disproportion, foetal distress and prolapsed cord. Most of the 20 deaths from sepsis following Caesarean section in labour involved cases with prolonged labour, where membranes had been ruptured for a considerable time. Twelve deaths from traumatic uterine rupture occurred in cases of brow, shoulder and compound presentation, difficult forceps, internal podalic version, and the unwise use of oxytocin in older maultiparous patients who had often been attended by less experienced obstetricians.

These considerations provide a background against which one must consider the descriptions of individual malpresentations which follow.

OCCIPITO POSTERIOR POSITIONS AND DEEP TRANSVERSE ARREST

The occiput is usually found to be lateral during engagement of the head, but in labour it will rotate anteriorly in four cases out of five. Very rarely, the head will be born in the occipito-transverse position, and occasionally it will rotate to an occipitoposterior position.

In about one-fifth of cases in early labour the occiput is posterior and the sagittal suture in one or other oblique diameter, usually the right. Left occipitoposterior position is rare, because the colon occupies the left posterior pelvic quadrant and dextrorotation of the uterus is usual. With increasing flexion the occiput may become the leading part and anterior rotation ensues. Should deflexion be maintained, or should it increase, the bregma will be the part which first reaches the pelvic floor, and it will rotate forwards so that the occiput will rotate backwards.

In cases where the foetus is very small and the pelvis capacious the head may enter the brim with the occiput directly posterior. This also occurs in the anthropoid pelvis, with a long, oval inlet and capacious measurements, especially in the hind pelvis. In these circumstances the head descends without rotation and is born, with ease, face to pubis. In such cases the perinatal mortality and morbidity and the duration of labour are no greater than with occipito-anterior positions, nor does the incidence of operative delivery rise (Calkins 1953).

Aetiology

An anteriorly situated placenta or a pelvic brim which is longer anteroposteriorly than transversely will predispose to an occipitoposterior position. If the back of the foetus comes to lie along the front of the maternal spine its normal flexion will be decreased, and the resulting deflexion of the head tends to maintain the occipitoposterior position. This effect will be less evident in a multipara with lax abdominal musculature.

Two main pelvis types have an inlet whose anteroposterior diameter equals or exceeds the transverse: the anthropoid and the android.

The anthropoid pelvis has a long, oval inlet, large measurements (especially the posterior sagittal diameters), wide greater sciatic notches and an adequate subpubic arch. Even if there is associated high assimilation a direct occipito-posterior position must be regarded as normal and delivery face to pubis confidently expected. The same will apply with any capacious pelvis and a small baby. In 266 consecutive face-to-pubis deliveries at Queen Charlotte's Hospital between 1961 and 1969, there were four deaths of normal infants ($1 \cdot 5\%$), of which three weighed less than 2,000 g.

The android pelvis, however, favours an oblique occipitoposterior position. The relatively flat sacrum, reduced posterior sagittal diameters, small sacrosciatic notches and prominent ischial spines make anterior rotation less likely, and cessation of progress with the occiput posterior or transverse will occur much more frequently.

Diagnosis

There may be visible flattening of the abdomen below the umbilicus, and in direct occipito-posterior positions a dip may be palpable. Limbs are felt anteriorly, the anterior shoulder being palpated at some distance from the mid-line. The back is often difficult to define but can usually be identified well round in the flank. Here also, the foetal heart is best heard. Deflexion is revealed when the prominences of sinciput and occiput can both be felt at the same level above the symphysis pubis (Fig. 22.1). If the occiput is directly posterior the head will feel relatively small from side to side. Extreme deflexion may result in the foetal heart tones being best heard anteriorly, albeit faintly.

Vaginal examination in early labour reveals a high deflexed head, the anterior fontanelle being felt in the centre of the pelvis whilst the posterior lies at an higher level and is more difficult to reach. The sagittal suture may occupy an oblique diameter or may run anteroposteriorly.

Anterior rotation is preceded by increased flexion so that the posterior fontanelle comes to lie more centrally in the pelvis, the anterior fontanelle coming to lie at a higher level. Continued deflexion, with the anterior fontanelle central and evident, is associated with posterior rotation.

In late labour, landmarks may be difficult to identify because of moulding and caput. It must then be remembered that the occipital bone is the only one which is overriden by both its neighbours. If one finger is placed on each side of the sagittal suture and they are then drawn along the length of that suture the fingers must either cross the lambdoid suture and come to rest on the occipital bone or, alternatively, cross the coronal suture and reach the frontal bone. Unlike the occipital, the latter is composed of two halves separated by the frontal suture, and the two halves can be made to move on one another. If doubt still exists an ear should be sought, both tragus and pinna being identified.

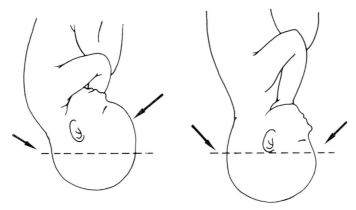

Fig. 22.1. The hands palpating a well-flexed head (left) are at different levels; those palpating a deflexed head (right) are at the same level.

A final opportunity to correct a misdiagnosis is presented when forceps are applied. With an uncorrected occipitoposterior position the forceps will lock with difficulty, or not at all. With traction, which will need to be greater than anticipated, the perineum will stretch and the anus gape while the presenting part is still high, and the forceps will not sweep forwards as the head descends.

Features of labour

Labour has often been stated to be slow, with incomplete cervical dilatation. Backache and incoordinate uterine action are not infrequent, but Friedman (1967), using his graphostatistical method, has emphasized that these abnormalities are more often indicative of associated disproportion. Premature rupture of membranes is not rare, with its associated problems of prolapsed cord and possible infection. Forty years ago, Miller (1930) emphasized that membranes ruptured prematurely in only 27% of cases, but that in this group spontaneous delivery occurred in only one-quarter. Deep perineal laceration may occur unless the child is small and the patient multiparous. Early distension of perineum and dilatation of anus with the head comparatively high will suggest that face-to-pubis delivery is likely.

Treatment

Antenatal correction by pads and binders has been abandoned as inefficient and unnecessary.

During labour, interference may be called for because of foetal distress, cessation of progress or incidental complications. The most important of these are prolapse of the cord and cephalopelvic disproportion. Cessation of progress is usually associated with failure of internal rotation. In many of these cases continued deflexion of the head has resulted in posterior rotation of the occiput, and this is most likely if the back of the child lies posteriorly. In others, the head may have become impacted with the occiput posterior in a constricted hind pelvis before reaching the pelvic floor. In cases with occipitotransverse arrest this may have resulted from failure of rotation of a head which has entered the pelvis with the occiput laterally or because prominent ischial spines and a restricted bispinous diameter have prevented forward rotation from an occipitoposterior position.

All patients must have careful assessment of progress, adequate intravenous fluid replacement with prevention of ketosis, and foetal monitoring by the best available method. In cases where backache or incoordinate uterine action are evident, disproportion having been excluded, epidural analgesia or paracervical block may be especially helpful.

OPERATIVE DELIVERY

This may take several forms.

(1) *Caesarean section*

This may be necessary for foetal distress, cord prolapse or disproportion, and will always be the method of choice if the cervix is less than half dilated. In the discussion on difficult vaginal delivery at the Glasgow British Congress 1965, an incidence of 7·3% of cerebral damage was associated with difficult forceps delivery, so that in developed countries the tendency is towards fewer such deliveries and more Caesarean sections.

(2) *Ventouse delivery*

In a series presented by Chalmers (1968) instrumental delivery was necessary in 11·1% of occipitotransverse or occipitoposterior positions. The ventouse takes up none of the space necessary for rotation and does not demand general anaesthesia. By encouraging flexion it produces better cervical stimulation with improved uterine contractions, and allows the occiput to rotate in the direction most suitable for delivery through a particular pelvis. Thus 5% of occipitotransverse and one-third of occipitoposterior positions rotate to direct occipitoposterior, and are delivered as such. The ventouse alone was successful in 85·8% of occipitoposterior and 89·6% of occipitotransverse position. The ventouse was not employed if the head was high, disproportion present, or the cervix less than half dilated. A reduced perinatal mortality has been claimed for the ventouse as compared to the obstetric forceps [1·19%, as compared to 5·2% (Bergman & Malmstrom 1962)].

(3) *Forceps rotation and extraction*

Kielland's forceps have been deservedly popular with those obstetricians trained to use them properly. They can be used with local anaesthesia, but epidural, spinal or general anaesthesia are preferable. Correct cephalic application is followed by disimpaction and rotation at the level of optimal diameters and extraction without re-application. For the android pelvis it is a disadvantage to rotate until the presenting part is

very low (D'Esopo 1941). Contrary to general teaching, it is not necessary to perform episiotomy before application, or even before rotation. Indeed, it is an advantage to defer episiotomy until rotation has been performed, the danger of spiral vaginal tears being lessened.

Recently, Parry-Jones (1968) has reviewed the use of Barton's forceps for the occipitotransverse position.

These instruments must be used only by properly trained operators, but so used are safe. In Queen Charlotte's Hospital between 1960 and 1967, in 607 deliveries using Kielland's forceps the corrected perinatal mortality was 0·99%.

Other types of forceps demand more than one application in a Scanzoni manœuvre. They include Shute's forceps, which are little used in Britain.

(4) *Manual rotation and forceps delivery*

This method, favoured by some because they feel it is more gentle than rotation with forceps, suffers from the disadvantage that deep general anaesthesia is necessary and the hand must take up more than a little of the available space. Displacement of the head can only be upwards and it can never be drawn down to a more favourable level for rotation. Excessively high displacement of the head can favour cord prolapse or may have to be followed by a high forceps delivery. These disadvantages have meant that in Queen Charlotte's Hospital it has been used in only 112 cases, compared with 607 cases of Kielland's forceps between 1961 and 1967. Rotation of the head may be possible or the anterior shoulder can be grasped and rotated by the internal hand.

Manual rotation and forceps delivery of a right occipitoposterior position will be facilitated by putting the patient in the exaggerated left lateral position, if the operator is familiar with the technique.

FACE PRESENTATION

Face presentation was found once in 556 deliveries among 392,035 cases reviewed by Kenwick (1953), while Friedman (1967) calculated an incidence of 1 in 496 when reviewing 19 reports in the literature totalling 1,645 face presentations.

In Queen Charlotte's Maternity Hospital from 1958 to 1965 inclusive, the incidence of 1 in 335 births corresponded closely to the 1 in 380 and 1 in 305 described by Posner et al. (1963) and Mostar et al. (1966), respectively.

AETIOLOGY

In early labour, deflexion attitudes are common, especially with occipitoposterior positions and multiparity (Fig. 22.2). In such cases uterine contractions often cause increased flexion, but occasionally the extension will increase and the presentation will pass through brow presentation to the fully extended face. Thus, most face presentations are secondary, becoming evident only in established labour.

Anencephaly, stated by earlier authors to be one of the commonest causes, has since been reported in not more than 10% of cases (Kenwick 1953; Martyn 1956). Should a face be felt during vaginal examination the possibility of anencephaly must be considered, but when discussing the management and outcome of face presentation it is usual to exclude anencephalics.

In some series no cause could be found in almost half the cases.

Prematurity is a definite association, occurring in 12·4% of Kenwick's (1953) series and 34% of the cases of Posner et al. (1963). Friedman (1967) quoted a 25% incidence of prematurity in his patients with face presentation, against an expected incidence of 9·8%.

A large baby (8 lb or over) was noted in 10·9% of Kenwick's cases and in 28·4% of those reported by Morris (1953). Among 97 cases personally reviewed in Cardiff hospitals, however, the proportion of large babies was no greater than in the hospital as a whole.

Contracted pelvis was diagnosed in 15% of Kenwick's cases and 39·4% of those described by Hellman et al. (1950). Chen & Wei (1960) also found this association.

Multiple pregnancy is frequently seen (Posner et al. 1963). This may act by causing hyper-extension, although other factors are clearly concerned.

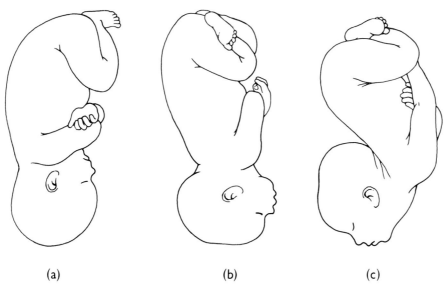

(a)   (b)   (c)

Fig. 22.2. Deflection attitudes. In (a) the child is in the military attitude of early deflection often associated with the occipitoposterior position; in (b) there is more deflection amounting almost to brow presentation; in (c) extension is complete and the face presents

Other causes suggested include the presence of several loops of cord coiled round the neck, tumours such as goitre or branchocoele, and an unduly large thorax. Hydramnios, pelvic tumours, bicornate uterus or uterine obliquity and placenta praevia may each account for an occasional case. Primary extensor tone is well documented, but the proportion of cases thought to be caused by it varies widely.

The importance of multiparity in producing face presentation is difficult to assess. Rudolph (1947) described equal numbers of multiparae and primiparae among his cases, but in Queen Charlotte's Hospital (1958–65) 63% were multiparae compared with 54% of the hospital population. Kenwick (1953) quoted similar figures and Posner *et al.* (1963) found that over 70% of their patients were multiparae. Increasing numbers of face presentation have been reported as maternal age rises.

Dolicocephaly is probably a result of face delivery and not its cause. Recovery of normal skull shape after birth is rapid.

POSITIONS

In 1953 Kenwick found that mento-anterior positions were diagnosed three times as often as mentoposterior ones, whilst in only 1 case in 10 was the denominator lateral. In the series of Posner *et al.* (1963) 77% were mentoanterior, and the figure of 81% quoted by Morris (1953) for Queen Charlotte's Hospital has not altered for 8 years up to 1965. The results of X-ray examination suggest that more mentotransverse positions would be present if diagnosis were made earlier (Borell & Fernström 1960).

DIAGNOSIS

The majority of face presentations are secondary and arise in labour from other deflexion attitudes. Primary face presentations will occasionally be diagnosed on antenatal radiographs because of a high head or bizarre abdominal findings (Fig. 22.3).

In half the cases the diagnosis is not made until delivery is imminent (Dede & Friedman 1963; Posner *et al.* 1963).

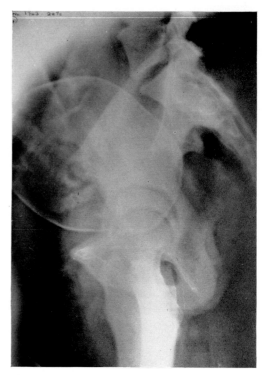

Fig. 22.3. A lateral X-ray showing a foetus presenting by the face. Note the narrower bifrontal diameter at the lowest level and the wider biparietal diameter above the pelvic brim.

Abdominal findings

The well-rounded breech is prominent in the fundus. The foetal back can be felt easily near the breech but recedes from the examining hand and is difficult to define in the lower half of the uterus. Limbs are felt anteriorly, usually to one side of the mid-line. In vertex presentations one can distinguish a triangular pool of liquor bounded by the foetal arms, legs and back, but in face and brow presentation this triangle is absent. Between the anterior shoulder and the head prominence there is a characteristic deep depression in which no foetal part can be felt. A large amount of head is palpable on the same side as the back, but no cephalic prominence can be felt on the same side of the pelvic inlet as the foetal limbs. Foetal heart sounds are transmitted through the foetal thorax and are heard most clearly on the same side as the limbs, which is also the side opposite that of the maximum cephalic prominence. Palpation of the lower pole of the foetus may be rendered difficult by overdistension, spasm or tenderness of the lower segment.

Vaginal findings

During this examination one should avoid damaging the eyes by trauma or antiseptics. In early labour the presenting part will be high. Landmarks to be distinguished are the mouth, jaws, nose, malar and orbital ridges. The presence of jaws distinguishes the mouth from the anus. It also helps to remember that mouth and maxillae form the corners of a triangle, whilst the anus is on a straight line between the ischial tuberosities. This is especially valuable when much oedema is present. Vaginal examination must conclude with a search for cord presentation or prolapse.

Labour in face presentation

The face is incompressible and of irregular outline and therefore would be expected to exert little stimulus on the lower segment and to predispose to inertia. However, Friedman (1967) suggests that abnormal uterine action usually results from associated bony dystocia and not the presentation itself. The poor line of thrust between body and head of the foetus usually results in prolongation of the second stage of labour. Early rupture of membranes may occur.

Descent occurs followed by internal rotation, the chin passing anteriorly. It must be remembered that the biparietal diameter is 7 cm behind the advancing face, so that even when the face is distending the vulva the biparietal diameter has only just entered the pelvis. Descent is thus always less advanced than vaginal examination would suggest, even when one allows for the gross oedema which is usually present. The value of abdominal examination in such cases cannot be overstressed. Anterior rotation having occurred, the neck comes to lie behind the symphysis and the head is born by flexion, causing considerable perineal distension in the process. The shoulders and body are then born in the usual way.

In cases of persisting mentoposterior position the neck is too short to span the 12 cm of the anterior aspect of the sacrum. Delivery is impossible unless, as can happen with a very small foetus or one which is macerated, the shoulders can enter the pelvis at the same time as the head. With satisfactory uterine action and a mento-anterior position, spontaneous or easy 'lift out' assisted delivery ensues in 80% or more (Dede & Friedman 1963; Hellman *et al.* 1950). Even with mentoposterior positions, anterior rotation will occur in from 45 to 65%, so that persistent mentoposterior position or mentotransverse arrest are encountered in only 10% of face presentations.

Management

Foetal abnormality and contracted pelvis must first be excluded. This done, one considers: the patient's age and parity; the previous obstetric history; whether a Caesarean section or myomectomy has been performed previously; whether complications such as pre-eclampsia are present and, finally, whether the child is thought to be larger than 3·5 kg. It may now become evident that elective Caesarean section is necessary. Antenatal conversion is unreliable even if the diagnosis has been made sufficiently early for it to be considered.

In cases where elective Caesarean section is not necessary, labour is carefully supervised, progress being assessed by careful examination of the abdomen as well as per vaginam.

With mento-anterior positions no interference is necessary whilst satisfactory progress continues and there is no foetal distress or cord prolapse. Generous episiotomy is always necessary. Attempts at conversion to a vertex presentation by Thorn's manœuvre fail in half the cases, and if only partly successful result in brow presentation. They are seldom employed.

In a mentoposterior position conversion would be even more difficult. Assistance is required only if the mentoposterior position persists or if foetal distress occurs. The choice then lies between forceps rotation and extraction or Caesarean section. The Caesarean section rate in this type of case is from 25 to 30%, and a vertical lower segment incision may be found useful.

In the neglected case with an impacted dead foetus, the choice between craniotomy and Caesarean section is influenced by local conditions.

Internal version and breech extraction are dangerous both to mother and child. They have no place in treating face presentation.

After birth, the oedema and bruising of the child's face can persist for some days and may make feeding difficult.

Increasing use of Caesarean section and the avoidance of complicated vaginal manœuvres have reduced the perinatal mortality to a figure similar to that for the occipitoposterior positions of the vertex. The mother is liable to all the puerperal complications which can follow prolonged labour, instrumental delivery and deep perineal laceration and bruising.

BROW PRESENTATION

This is an extension attitude between deflexed vertex and face presentation. Incidences of 1 in 1,039, 1 in 1,796 and 1 in 2,314 deliveries are quoted by Mostar *et al.* (1966), Posner *et al.* (1963) and Kenwick (1953), respectively, whilst Berger *et al.* (1967) reviewing the literature of the last 30 years calculated an incidence of 0·08%. Many brow presentations are transient, proceeding to full deflexion or, alternatively, undergoing spontaneous flexion and correction to vertex.

AETIOLOGY

The causes are those of face presentation, and will not be repeated. Prematurity, noted in 64% of cases by Posner *et al.* (1963), has been less frequent in other series (12–14%), though this is still twice the expected incidence. (Berger *et al.* 1967; Meltzer *et al.* 1967). Contracted pelvis occurred in over half the cases described by Hellman *et al.* (1950) and Mostar *et al.* (1966), though others have found it in only 10·9% (Meltzer *et al.* 1967). Even this was four times the expected incidence in their practice.

DIAGNOSIS

Abdominal findings resemble those of face presentation. The foetal back is very difficult to feel except near the breech, the foetal heart is best heard on the same side as the limbs, whilst the maximum head prominence is on the side opposite to the limbs. Unlike face presentation, however, a head prominence is palpable on the same side as the limbs and the groove between anterior shoulder and head, though distinct, is less marked. The head feels large from side to side, so that hydrocephaly may be suspected. Many cases are diagnosed by X-ray for 'high head' at term or in early labour (Fig. 22.4).

On vaginal examination a hard, high, rounded part presents, the bregma occupying the centre of the dilating cervix. Frontal suture, anterior fontanelle, orbital ridges and nasion can be identified, but nose, mouth, and chin cannot be felt. In labour a large caput succedaneum may

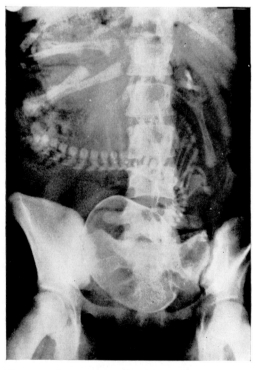

Fig. 22.4. An anteroposterior X-ray showing marked deflexion of the foetus and a brow presentation.

make diagnosis almost impossible. The nasion is more often found anteriorly than posteriorly.

Course of labour

Prolonged and complicated labour has often been described (Madden 1956; Morris 1953; Posner et al. 1957). More recent studies suggest that prolongation of the second stage and of the phase of deceleration in the first stage are the only consistent features and that other abnormalities in the first stage such as incoordinate action or arrest of dilatation are indicative of disproportion (Posner et al. 1963; Friedman 1967). There is a slightly increased incidence of premature rupture of membranes.

In persisting brow presentation the mento-vertical diameter has to engage. Engagement may be possible with a capacious pelvis and a small foetus, which becomes markedly moulded. In patients with contracted pelvis or, when a large or average size foetus is present, with a normal pelvis, engagement may prove impossible. The case then becomes one of obstructed labour. Following engagement, anterior rotation will occur and the forehead, orbital ridges, and nasion will appear at the vulva. The maxilla then becomes fixed against the lower part of the symphysis pubis, and by flexion of the head, brow, anterior fontanelle, vertex and occiput successively appear. Finally, the face and chin slip out from behind the symphysis. Occasionally, following engagement spontaneous correction to a vertex will occur in the pelvis.

PROGNOSIS

Should the brow presentation be transient, the first stage of labour of average length, and moulding not excessive, the prognosis for the infant is that of the face or vertex presentation which ensues. In persistent brow presentation the outlook is best where the foetus is small and the pelvis large. With a term foetus of average size the factor of disproportion is all-important and foetal mortality will rise because of gross moulding, early rupture of membranes, long labour, and the need for operative delivery. These will also contribute to maternal morbidity.

Management

Foetal abnormality and pelvic contraction must first be excluded. This done, no treatment is necessary if labour progresses normally, especially if the infant is small. In all 11 such cases described by Posner et al. (1963) vaginal delivery proved possible. In assessing progress, however, it must be remembered that increasing caput succedaneum can produce a false impression of descent of the presenting part.

Pelvic contraction, associated disease, or a term infant persisting as a brow presentation are best treated by Caesarean section. Should delay in labour or foetal distress become evident then, again, Caesarean section is probably the best treatment.

OTHER POSSIBLE COURSES OF ACTION

(1) Conversion manœuvres

Thorn's manœuvre attempts a radical conversion to vertex presentation. It is performed under general anaesthesia and demands not only an adequate amount of liquor so that membranes should be intact or only recently have ruptured, but also a sufficiently dilated cervix to allow a hand to be introduced into the uterus. The occasions on which it can safely be attempted are therefore extremely rare. Conversion to a face presentation is feasible even less often. Both manœuvres have largely been abandoned.

(2) Forceps or ventouse extraction

By rotation with Kielland's forceps, with which is associated an increasing flexion of the head, or through the increased flexion produced by the ventouse, delivery of the deeply engaged brow presentation is often possible. In Queen Charlotte's Hospital between 1958 and 1965 there were 41% brow presentations so delivered (16 of 39), but this method should be used only when full dilatation has been achieved and there is no disproportion present.

(3) Craniotomy

This is used in cases of foetal abnormality. It is otherwise reserved for cases which have passed unrecognized, resulting in obstructed labour with a dead foetus under circumstances where Caesarean section is to be avoided if at all possible. Such conditions should not occur in properly supervised cases (Lawson & Stewart 1967). In developed countries Caesarean section is usually safer than craniotomy even when the foetus is dead.

Internal podalic version has no place in the management of brow presentation.

BREECH PRESENTATION AND LABOUR

Among cases in the Perinatal Mortality Survey of 1958 the infant presented as a breech at delivery in 2·13%. A similar incidence (2·23%) was found for singleton pregnancy in the North West Metropolitan Region (Law 1967). In the United States, Hall *et al.* (1965) quoted 3·17% in 190,661 deliveries between 1955 and 1959, while Morgan & Kane (1964) in 404,847 patients found 16,327 breech births (4·04%); their series, however, including a high percentage of twin pregnancies.

Aetiology

One foetus in four will present by the breech at some stage of pregnancy, but at the thirty-fourth week most have undergone spontaneous version to a head presentation. Subsequent reversion to breech is rare, occurring in 4% (Vartan 1945). It is therefore hardly surprising that premature infants comprise up to a quarter of babies born as breech presentations. In patients who reach term with breech presentation the cause must be sought among conditions which have prevented spontaneous version. These include multiple pregnancy, oligohydramnios and abnormalities of uterine shape whether congenital or the result of attachment of the placenta in the cornual region or the lower uterine segment (Hay 1959; Hall *et al.* 1965). The latter point out that in a multipara with a breech presentation there is a 14% incidence of previous breech delivery. The proportion of frank breech increases markedly towards term, suggesting that

extended legs also hinder spontaneous version. The frequency of extended legs in primiparae may account also for the disproportionate number of breeches often noted in these patients (Law 1967; Friedman 1967; Hall 1965).

Other conditions which favour breech presentation include hydrocephaly, polyhydramnios, intra-uterine foetal death and, very occasionally, pelvic tumours. Opinion is divided over the extent to which breech presentation can be caused by contracted pelvis. Vartan (1945) stated that this was of slight importance in aetiology, though of vital interest when deciding the mode of delivery. In 1966, Beischer could demonstrate contracted pelvis clinically in only 3% of his series, though this figure rose sharply in the small group in whom X-ray pelvimetry was performed. Friedman (1967) found disproportion of twice the expected frequency, but commented that with breech presentation this was more carefully sought and evaluated than with head presentations.

Diagnosis

There is no characteristic finding on abdominal inspection. Palpation reveals the hard, round, ballottable head occupying the fundus uteri, with the back on one side and limbs on the other. The rather narrow and softer breech may be mobile above the pelvic brim or may dip through it. When the head is strictly in the mid-line it is probable that the legs are extended, and a frank breech is also suspected if the presenting part is deeply engaged. The foetal heart will be heard best above the umbilicus. On vaginal examination prior to labour the presenting part is usually high, of softer consistency than the head, and may be irregular in outline. Confirmation of the diagnosis can be obtained by sonar, which will also exclude placenta praevia and multiple pregnancy, or by radiography, which will also exclude multiple pregnancy and reveal major skeletal abnormality. Both methods will show up hydrocephalus, and X-ray examination will reveal the degree of flexion or extension of the head.

In labour, the presenting part will be high initially, but rapid descent is to be expected and at full dilatation the station should be comparable with that of a vertex presentation. Even when the presenting part is high a deliberate effort must be made to exclude cord presentation. Later, with a frank breech the tuber ischii, sacrum, and anus are palpable and the external genitalia may be identified. During prolonged labour or with slow cervical dilatation the marked oedema which results may make the distinction difficult between breech and face presentation. Here, abdominal examination is helpful. Whilst the diagnostic features of face presentation are the maxillae and jaws meconium may soil a finger inserted into the foetal anus.

In complete breech presentation the feet may be felt alongside the buttocks, and in foot and knee presentations the appropriate parts are evident. Though the hard projection of the heel identifies the foot, the examiner should follow the limb in continuity to the buttock before diagnosing a footling breech presentation, as it is possible for a foot to present alongside the head in one form of compound presentation.

Early diagnosis of breech presentation allows time for adequate assessment and delivery under optimal conditions.

TYPES OF BREECH PRESENTATION

(1) *Frank breech*

The lower extremities are fully flexed at the hip and fully extended at the knee (see Fig. 22.5). The feet are thus high in the uterus, leaving a smooth, well-fitting presenting part which tends to engage early, so making external cephalic version less easy. The snug fit results in a low incidence of cord prolapse with a foetus of average size. The frank breech occurs in 60–70% of cases, being more frequent in primiparae and as term approaches. Difficulty in delivering the aftercoming head would be expected less often than in footling breech, because with a foetus of average size the passage of the combined mass of both thighs and the foetal abdomen is only possible through a fully dilated cervix. It was an unexpected finding in Law's (1967) series that, except in primiparae, in premature labour the perinatal mortality was uninfluenced by the position of the legs, and that both first and

second stages of labour were actually longer than in cases with flexed legs.

(2) *Complete or flexed breech*

Here the hips and knees of the foetus are flexed, the feet being closely applied to the dorsal aspect of the thighs (see Fig. 22.5). The presenting part is more irregular and less pointed, so that early engagement is less likely and prolapse of the cord is four times as common as in frank breech (Law 1967), occurring in 4–6·3% of flexed mature breech births; Hay (1959) found prolapse of the cord in 20% of flexed breech and in no cases of frank breech.

(3) *Incomplete breech—knee or footling presentation*

These are self explanatory, presentation of one or both feet being more common than knee presentation (Fig. 22.5). Not only is there a high risk of presentation or prolapse of the cord, but delivery of the infant up to the level of the thorax may occur through an incompletely dilated cervix. This is especially liable to occur if the obstetrician is foolishly tempted to deliver the baby vaginally prior to full dilatation because one or both lower limbs have appeared at the vulva or because of clinical foetal distress or cord prolapse.

The dangers of breech delivery

Risks to the mother include sepsis, tears of the vagina or cervix and uterine rupture due usually to unskilled attempts at vaginal delivery with inadequate facilities. Though Hay (1959) described an increased incidence of postpartum haemorrhage and of 'subinvolution' (35%), the former is not as obvious when active management of the third stage is employed.

The main dangers are to the child. Perinatal mortality figures provide a crude measurement of the efficiency of obstetric management. In considering breech delivery it is usual to correct the figure by excluding antepartum deaths, congenital malformations incompatible with life, cases of haemolytic disease and first-week deaths unconnected with the mode of delivery. When this was done for the North West Regional Board (Law 1967) the figures for multiparae

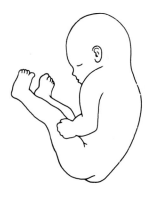 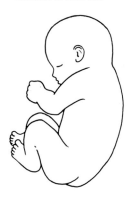 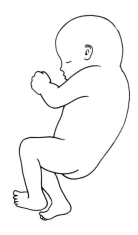

Frank breech   Flexed breech   Footling presentation

Fig. 22.5. Types of breech presentation.

and primiparae were 10·5% and 6·6%, respectively. The increased perinatal loss in multiparous patients agrees with the findings of Methuen (1958), who produced figures of 6·4% and 2·8%, respectively. Potter *et al.* (1960) and Wulff *et al.* (1960) found the reverse. If one corrects for prematurity (22·9% of cases in Law's series) the corrected perinatal mortality for mature infants is still greater in multiparae (4·7%) than primiparae (2·2%). Law suggested that increasing maternal age alone is directly related to an increase in foetal loss.

Stillbirth may result from asphyxia if delivery is too slow or from traumatic intracranial haemorrhage if delivery of the aftercoming head is rapid and uncontrolled. Prolapse of the cord is a risk inherent in the malpresentation, and medullary coning through the foramen magnum has occurred in cases where efforts have been made to deliver the head with traction and forceful abdominal pressure. Other injuries caused by unskilled efforts at delivery include fractures of the femur, humerus and clavicle or the more serious epiphyseal separation of these bones. A sterno-cleido-mastoid haematoma and brachial plexus injury can occur. Injury to abdominal viscera can result from rough handling, and fractured skull and fracture dislocation of the spine have also been reported. To these must be added risks inherent in premature rupture of the

membranes. Hall & Kohn (1956) maintained that this trebled the perinatal mortality. More recently, Law (1967) was unable to show any increased risk to the foetus in cases where membranes ruptured prematurely.

Consideration of the above hazards, and a natural reluctance to perform Caesarean section in the days when it was a less safe operation, led obstetricians to employ external cephalic version in an attempt to reduce the number of cases of breech delivery.

External cephalic version

The breech is turned to a head presentation by manipulation through the mother's abdominal wall. The presenting part must be disengaged and the uterus neither tense nor irritable. There must be sufficient liquor and the abdominal wall must be thin and relaxed. The last requirement may be facilitated by general anaesthesia, which is itself not without risk. Advocates of external version do not attempt it in the presence of moderate or severe hypertension, in patients who have experienced antepartum haemorrhage, or in those who have placenta praevia, uterine scars and ruptured membranes. It is contra-indicated in twin pregnancy, when delivery by Caesarean section is planned, and when major foetal deformity has been demonstrated.

A failure rate of only 3% in 706 cases was claimed by Friedlander (1966), though he found it necessary to use general anaesthesia in 13% after the thirty-third week. The average number of versions per patient after this stage of pregnancy was 2·6, with a rate of reversion to breech of 11·2%. Others have quoted lower success rates even when using general anaesthesia—72% (Neely 1961) to 87% (Peel & Clayton 1948) with a perinatal mortality due to the version itself of 1 and 1·7%, respectively. Spontaneous cephalic version can occur just prior to term in cases which have previously defied all attempts at external cephalic version, whilst Vartan (1945) showed that following external version 22% of cases reverted to breech. It has been suggested, therefore, that successful external cephalic version merely anticipates the spontaneous cephalic version which would have occurred naturally. The incidence of breech delivery is similar in clinics where version is avoided and in those where it is routine (Hay 1959).

The complications of general anaesthesia, accidental haemorrhage, premature labour with prolapsed cord, and ruptured uterus have all followed attempts at external version, whilst the significance of the bradycardia which often follows the procedure is unknown.

Considerations such as these led White in 1956 to calculate that if one assumed success rates of 70 and 88% in primigravidae and multiparae respectively, with a foetal loss due to version itself of not less than 1%, then the procedure could only be justified in places where the perinatal mortality of breech delivery exceeded that of cephalic presentation by more than 2·5%. In units such as those of Cox (1955) and Hay (1959), with skilled obstetric teams and ready recourse to abdominal delivery, corrected perinatal losses of 2·4 and 1·2%, respectively, mean that external version is no longer justified. Indeed, Husslein (1965) in a survey of Continental units showed that the perinatal mortality was greater in those units where external version was most practised.

It was well argued by Neely (1961) that external cephalic version, including that under general anaesthesia, might still have a place in areas where facilities are less good, and he claimed

to have produced a decrease in the incidence of breech delivery to 1·2% in his small series. The same argument may be applicable also in those countries where Caesarean section is to be avoided because of the risks of a scarred uterus in subsequent pregnancy. Here the suggestion by White (1956) may be relevant, that external cephalic version could be used selectively in cases where minor pelvic contraction was suspected, as the subsequent cephalic presentation would allow of trial labour.

Antenatal assessment of cases

The case of breech presentation which persists and in which associated diseases do not demand abdominal delivery, must be assessed carefully and the route of delivery planned accordingly. It is important that this should be done in the multipara with the same care as in the nullipara, because it is possible that the higher perinatal mortality of breech births in multiparae may be contributed to by failure in this respect (Law 1967; Hay 1959; Daly & Michael 1953).

Pelvic shape and capacity must be judged by past obstetric history where applicable and thorough clinical assessment, with especial reference to outlet shape and anteroposterior diameter. The value of X-ray pelvimetry has been questioned by Law (1967), though Beischer (1966) revealed unexpected mid-plane contraction in nearly one-quarter of the 11·3% of his small series who were subjected to the procedure. Most obstetricians employ clinical assessment in conjunction with a single upright X-ray lateral pelvimetry (see comments on p. 142).

It has been shown by Cox (1950) and others that a large infant is at increased risk. Estimating foetal size is difficult, but if the baby is clinically large, then elective Caesarean section should be considered. X-ray cephalometry is of limited help in this regard, but ultrasonic cephalometry is far more precise and is indicated if facilities are available. X-rays may give other useful information, however (Fig. 22.6).

Zatuchni & Andros (1965) awarded prognostic scores based on parity, gestational age, estimated foetal weight, previous breech presentation, cervical dilatation and station. Scores range from

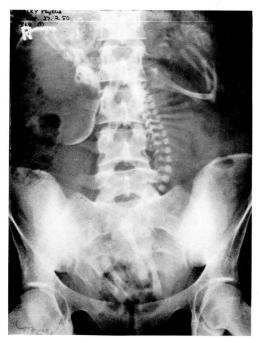

Fig. 22.6. Gross extension of the foetus in a case of breech presentation.

0 to 11. Patients with a score of 3 or less should be delivered abdominally. This prognostic index has proved of value in the hands of its authors (Zatuchni & Andros 1967). Friedman (1967) has stressed the especial prognostic value of cervical dilatation and of station in late pregnancy or early labour.

Elective Caesarean section in breech presentation

Abdominal delivery may be chosen because of associated conditions such as diabetes mellitus, moderate or severe hypertension, fulminating pre-eclampsia and in selected cases of rhesus immunization. It may be indicated following accidental antepartum haemorrhage or in the presence of placenta praevia. Abdominal delivery must also be considered in the small-for-dates syndrome. When disproportion is present, as with a contracted pelvis at any level or when the infant is assessed as 3,750 g or more, elective section should be employed. It should also be

considered in multiparae with a poor obstetric history, in patients who have experienced difficulty in conceiving, and in the primigravida over 35 years of age. In patients with a previous Caesarean section a vaginal breech delivery should be considered only when the malpresentation is the sole abnormality present, the uterine scar is considered sound, the section was performed for a non-recurring indication, and when with a small or average size foetus there are no unfavourable features of pelvic shape and size. A Caesarean section rate from 15 to 20% in breech presentation is reported in recent series, of which 85% have been elective. Vaginal delivery will be decided upon in primigravida under 35 years of age and multiparae with a good obstetric history with no indication for elective Caesarean section.

Mechanism of labour

Contrary to older teaching, the first stage of labour is not usually prolonged. In only 10% of cases reported by Hay (1959) did it exceed 20 hr, and was found to be less than 12 hr in 53% of primiparae and 77·2% of multiparae with mature singleton breech delivery reviewed by Law (1967). When labour was premature the percentages were even higher. Friedman (1967) showed that at term there was no difference between flexed and extended breech presentations and vertex delivery in the duration of the first stage, a shortening of the latent phase in nulliparae being explained by the increased incidence of premature rupture of membranes in this group. There was prolongation of all phases with increasing infant weight. In multiparae all phases of labour were slightly longer. Perinatal mortality rises when the first stage exceeds 24 hr.

The presenting part will usually engage with the bitrochanteric diameter occupying an oblique or the transverse diameter with the sacrum anterior. The anterior hip leads and on meeting the pelvic floor is rotated anteriorly beneath the pubic arch. Should the posterior hip reach the pelvic floor first, it usually undergoes long anterior rotation. The hip is now held up at the pubic arch, lateral flexion allowing the posterior hip to be born. The child then straightens as the anterior hip is born, the legs and feet following. As the shoulders enter the brim in the oblique or transverse diameter, the trunk undergoes external rotation. The shoulders then undergo their own internal rotation to bring them into the anteroposterior diameter of the outlet, the trunk following. The third and final part to enter the pelvis is the head, which rotates until the posterior part of the neck becomes fixed under the subpubic arch and the head is born by flexion, the chin, mouth, nose, forehead, vertex and occiput appearing progressively. It is obvious that every attempt must be made to keep the back of the foetus anterior and to maintain flexion of the foetus by avoiding premature or unwise traction, so allowing heads of smaller diameter to engage.

THE SECOND STAGE OF LABOUR

The length of this is determined largely by the degree of intervention by the obstetrician so that Hay (1959) quoted averages of 39 min for primigravidae and 20 for multipara, whilst Law (1967) found that the stage exceeded 60 min in 45·9% of primigravidae with mature infants, though in only 7·1% of multiparae with mature infants. It is probably unwise to allow the second stage to exceed 1 hr in primiparae or 30 min in multiparae.

THE THIRD STAGE OF LABOUR

This is usually managed actively following administration of an oxytoxic drug, but there is still a tendency to excessive blood loss in cases of premature labour and in multiparae (Law 1967).

Conduct of vaginal breech delivery

All cases should be delivered in a unit equipped for Caesarean section and should be attended by an experienced obstetrician and an anaesthetist who is skilled at obstetric anaesthesia. Both must be present at delivery.

FIRST STAGE

These patients may require general anaesthesia urgently and should receive adequate fluid and dextrose or fructose intravenously to avoid ketosis. For the same reason, oral intake should be of water only, with administration of antacid 2-hourly to maintain a high pH of the gastric contents. Particular care should be taken to observe signs of clinical foetal distress, optimally by continuous foetal heart monitoring, and in every case at least one vaginal examination should be performed by an experienced attendant prior to rupture of the membranes to seek a cord presentation. Should incoordinate uterine action or inertia be noted the case must be reviewed, lest previously unsuspected mechanical difficulty is present. Administration of oxytocin should be avoided if possible.

SECOND STAGE

Delivery may occur in one of three ways:

(A) Spontaneously.
(B) Assisted breech delivery.
(C) Breech extraction.

(A) Spontaneous breech delivery

This is rare, except in multiparous patients in premature labour. Such cases carry a high perinatal mortality and occur when skilled help is not available.

(B) Assisted breech delivery

The patient should be in the lithotomy position with her bladder empty. Full dilatation of the cervix must be confirmed by vaginal examination, at which one must exclude cord prolapse and also ascertain that the child is not astride the cord. In the latter situation the cord should be displaced over the thigh or if this is not possible with a tense cord a general anaesthetic should be given, the cord cut between ligatures and full breech extraction performed without delay.

In most cases the infant's sacrum will be anterior or lateral, but in the few cases where the back is posterior it will usually rotate spontaneously to an anterior position. Especially with a frank breech, the perineum becomes progressively more distended by maternal effort during contractions. Cox (1955) emphasized that delivery should not begin until the foetal anus becomes visible. Latterly, the tendency has been to commence delivery somewhat earlier, but only when the perineum is distended and thinned by a breech which is 'climbing' the perineum. At this time a generous episiotomy is essential. This may be performed after infiltration of the perineum with local anaesthetic but may be usefully combined with transvaginal pudendal block anaesthesia. No further anaesthesia is necessary in the majority of cases. Epidural and spinal anaesthesia are less satisfactory, being associated with high uterine tone. In the Liverpool technique (Cox 1950; Hay 1959) general anaesthesia is induced when the infant has been born as far as the umbilicus, extended legs being delivered by the Pinard manœuvre before the shoulders and head are extracted. Pudendal block and perineal infiltration are being used increasingly with fewer general anaesthetics (Law 1967). This trend is encouraging in view of the increasing proportion of maternal deaths ascribed to anaesthesia in the *Confidential Report into Maternity Mortality, 1964-1966*.

Unexpected difficulty in delivery in a well-chosen case should arouse suspicion of foetal ascites or of tumours of kidneys or other organs. The arms will usually be found flexed on the anterior chest wall and will be delivered with the thorax without difficulty. No attempt should be made to deliver an arm until the scapula and one axilla are visible. Extended arms and the rare nuchal displacement usually result from unwise traction by the obstetrician and his failure to keep the foetal back anterior during all manœuvres. If the baby is unexpectedly large it may be wise to deliver an arm before the shoulders become wedged in the pelvis. For this operation general anaesthesia is necessary. In most instances, however, the Lovset manœuvre is employed, and only rarely is it necessary to insert a hand into the uterus. If the back has remained anterior and the case is well selected, the head will enter the pelvis and descend without difficulty under the influence of gravity, the attendant merely allowing the body to hang for as long as is necessary to rinse the hands. The process can be facilitated if an assistant places the palms of his hands above the symphysis pubis and draws

up the uterus as in the Brandt-Andrews method for delivery of the placenta.

When the nuchal region is seen, delivery of the head may be conducted by the Burns-Marshall manœuvre or, more usually, with obstetric forceps. Any straight forceps can be used, though the Piper forceps was especially designed for this purpose. Forceps provide better control than the Mauriceau-Smellie-Veit method. When the head is unexpectedly delayed in the pelvic cavity, adequate vaginal retraction may permit the infant to breathe before the nose and mouth are visible. Once the face appears the airway is cleared and extraction of the head proceeds smoothly, without haste. The third stage will be actively managed following administration of an oxytocic, delivery being completed by inspection of vagina and cervix and episiotomy suture. If by carelessness or accident the head enters the pelvic cavity with the occiput posterior, delivery may be effected by using the Prague grip in reverse, the direction of shoulder traction being downwards and backwards.

One other technique of breech delivery should be mentioned. This, the Bracht manœuvre, is popular on the Continent and has been described at length by Plentl & Stone (1953).

(C) Breech extraction

The obstetrician delivers the whole infant without assistance from the mother. The method is used to expedite delivery in cases of foetal distress or prolapsed cord, and occasionally when progress ceases in the second stage or for delivering the second twin. Before starting one must know that the cervix is fully dilated and that there is enough liquor to allow intra-uterine manipulation. The uterus must be fully relaxed by suitable general anaesthesia. The operator must be confident that there are no mechanical obstacles to delivery, and in particular that progress has not been arrested by unsuspected disproportion. A footling presentation is easier to extract than a breech with extended legs, in which the foot must first be delivered by inserting a hand into the uterus and using Pinard's manœuvre. This should not be attempted before full dilatation. Breech extraction may prove necessary with a premature infant if the perineum fails to distend, but should be avoided with a large infant and should never be performed if a uterine scar is present. Breech extraction is especially dangerous in the multipara because of the high risk of uterine rupture. Those who electively adopt breech extraction for full-term infants obtain a corrected foetal mortality of 0·9%, but for the majority of obstetricians it is less safe than assisted breech delivery.

Caesarean section may become necessary in labour for cord prolapse or foetal distress prior to full dilatation, and should be seriously considered in cases of incoordinate uterine action or prolongation of the first stage of labour.

TRANSVERSE AND OBLIQUE LIE —SHOULDER PRESENTATION

This occurred once in every 322 deliveries at the Mayo Clinic (Johnson 1964), and Yates (1964) quoted an incidence of 0·5%. In the decade ending December 1967 the abnormality was noted during labour in 92 cases at Queen Charlotte's Hospital among 30,941 babies born, an incidence of 1 in 336 births.

Aetiology

Most of the patients are multiparae with lax, pendulous abdomens (74% of the cases at Queen Charlotte's Hospital). Transverse and oblique lie can occur when engagement of the head is prevented by contracted pelvis, pelvic tumour or placenta praevia. The latter was diagnosed in 11% of cases by Hall & O'Brien (1961). In others hydrocephalus or foetal hyperextension prevents engagement. Prematurity, hydramnios and intra-uterine foetal death are other possible causes.

Twin pregnancy is commonly associated and usually involves the second twin, though the very rare double transverse lie should suggest conjoined twins. Of the 92 cases at Queen Charlotte's Hospital, the foetus was one of twins in 37.

Abnormal lie can result from abnormal uterine shape, either congenital as in arcuate or subseptate uterus, or caused in the current pregnancy by insertion of the placenta either in the fundus or in the lower segment. The placenta was so situated in 92·3% of cases reported by Stevenson (1949).

In transverse and oblique lie the back is usually anterior, so maintaining foetal flexion. The head is most often on the left side. Dorso-posterior positions are less common; extension is inevitable and, consequently, prolapse of an arm is more likely, with associated twisting of the foetal spine. Rarely, the back can be inferior or superior.

Diagnosis

In pregnancy the uterine outline is broad and often asymmetrical, the fundus being less high than expected. The long axis of the foetal ovoid may be transverse but is more often oblique, the head being felt in the iliac fossa or flank. The firm, smooth surface of the back, or the more irregular prominences of limbs, can be felt in the central abdomen in dorso-anterior and dorso-posterior positions respectively. There is no foetal pole occupying the fundus. The pelvic inlet may appear empty or one will feel there the prominence of shoulder and arm.

Vaginal examination reveals an empty pelvis or, occasionally, a limb presentation. Pelvic contraction or pelvic tumour might be evident. This examination is best avoided until placenta praevia has been excluded.

In early labour abdominal findings are unchanged. An elongated bag of forewaters can be felt and may contain a limb or a loop of cord. The presenting part is high, irregular and difficult to define. Membranes rupture early. Later in labour the shoulder descends, and in cases first seen at this stage the landmarks to be identified are the ribs on the medial wall of the axilla, the clavicle and the acromion. They may be obscured by oedema. Where the foetus is very small or macerated, the lowest part palpable may be the thorax or back. In other cases a hand, or hand and foot together, may present, and in all cases prolapse of the cord is likely.

In very late labour abdominal signs are those of obstructed labour, whilst the considerable oedema which ensues may make it hard to differentiate shoulder presentation from breech, face and brow.

Features of labour and the possible outcome

Inertia or incoordinate uterine action are seen as a response to the obstruction which is inevitable in cases of transverse lie unless the foetus is very small or macerated. Membranes rupture early, much liquor is lost and infection becomes a hazard. There may follow a period in which contractions cease and uterine tone is normal. Still later (or, more often, with no preliminary respite) uterine tone increases, contractions become violent, the lower segment is thinned and the pathological retraction ring is detected as it ascends in the abdomen (Fig. 22.7). Meanwhile, the bladder becomes thick and easily felt. Ketosis, dehydration and infection are now evident and the foetus dies of asphyxia. Such an outcome

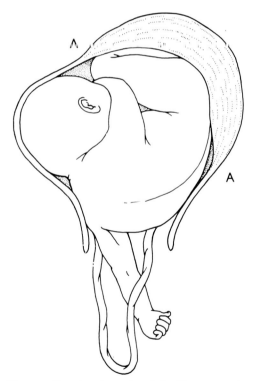

Fig. 22.7. Drawing of a neglected shoulder presentation. The line AA represents the line of the pathological retraction ring.

represents *obstruction and neglected shoulder presentation*. It will lead almost inevitably to uterine rupture though, very rarely, secondary inertia is seen once intra-uterine infection with gas-forming organisms occurs. Other possibilities must be recorded but their occurrence should never the relied upon:

(a) Spontaneous reversion to a longitudinal lie can occur only when membranes are intact or very recently ruptured. It is unlikely to occur in established labour.

(b) Spontaneous expulsion is seen when the foetus is so small or macerated that it can be doubled up by strong uterine action. The first part born is the back, the head and abdomen being expelled together and the feet last.

(c) Spontaneous evolution usually involves very small infants (though one of 3,300 g has been reported) and violent uterine action. It usually follows prolapse of an arm in dorso-anterior positions. The neck elongates and the presenting shoulder is fixed at the outlet. Continuing contractions result in extreme lateral flexion of the spine. If this occurs with its concavity to the same side as the leading shoulder then the breech will next be born, having been thrust down behind the shoulder. The abdomen, thorax, second shoulder and head follow in order. When the lateral flexion has its convexity to the side of the leading shoulder then birth of the shoulder is followed by that of thorax abdomen, breech and legs in sequence, the second shoulder and head appearing last.

It must be emphasized that these are matters of interest only, having no part in a properly managed case.

Management

ANTENATAL

After 34 weeks' gestation in a multipara gentle external cephalic version in the clinic may be followed by engagement of the head. When the abnormal lie recurs in a multipara, and whenever it is diagnosed in a nullipara, the first steps are to exclude twin pregnancy, foetal abnormality, placenta praevia and contracted pelvis. Radiography, sonar and radio-isotope placental localization may be essential. Such abnormalities having been excluded, the patient must be told to come to hospital at once should contractions start or should she lose liquor. Recurrent 'unstable' lie justifies hospital admission at 37 weeks to await the onset of labour. If the lie is still unstable at the forty-first week in a multipara it is occasionally reasonable to induce contractions with dilute Syntocinon infusion, after performing external version and then rupturing the forewaters. In primigravidae or in any case where complications are present—such as pelvic tumour, placenta praevia, contracted pelvis or associated disease—then elective Caesarean section is the best treatment.

IN LABOUR

Treatment will depend principally on the cause and on the time in labour that the diagnosis is made. With this will be associated the problems of uterine thinning or rupture, intra-uterine infection and foetal death. Prolapse of cord may demand Caesarean section. It occurred in 14 out of 92 cases in the series at Queen Charlotte's Hospital.

(1) *External version*

This is applicable to cases in very early labour having weak contractions and with intact membranes in whom there is no indication for rapid delivery and in whom pelvic contraction, placenta praevia and pelvic tumour have been excluded. Such cases are rare. External version, rupture of membranes and ventouse delivery is, however, useful for delivery of the second twin.

(2) *Caesarean section*

This should be the most frequently employed method of delivery. It includes all cases having another indication for abdominal delivery, any primigravidae in early labour and all cases of pelvic contraction. The value of longitudinal lower segment incision is emphasized, as this can be extended upwards if necessary.

In cases of established labour where uterine thinning is suspected or the woman has borne four children, Caesarean section is the preferred method of delivery if the child is alive, and may be the safest even when the child is dead. With severe infection a Caesarean hysterectomy may be considered.

(3) *Decapitation*

Using the Blond-Heidler saw, this is performed for neglected transverse lie with a dead foetus when practising among developing peoples, where every effort must be made to avoid section. In Western practice it is rarely used.

(4) *Other methods*

Internal version has little place in the treatment of transverse and oblique lie in labour. It is the commonest cause of ruptured uterus and carries a perinatal mortality of between 40 and 50% (Yates 1964; Wood & Forster 1959, Harris & Epperson 1950; Chapman 1967). The sole indication for this operation in modern obstetrics is probably for delivering the second twin. If it is so used it must be effected immediately the membranes of the second sac have been ruptured. Even so, in the cases of transverse lie at Queen Charlotte's Hospital, which included many twins, the perinatal mortality with internal version and breech extraction was 30%.

Results

Maternal mortality and morbidity rise because of the age and multiparity of the patients, their liability to associated conditions such as hypertension, the risks of early membrane rupture and obstructed labour, and finally the frequent need for operative interference.

Foetal mortality and morbidity will rise with early rupture of membranes, from trauma due to unwise manipulative delivery, and hypoxia due to obstructed labour or prolapse of the cord. It is disappointing that in Queen Charlotte's Hospital the perinatal mortality corrected for antepartum death, congenital anomalies incompatible with life and death from haemolytic disease was still 19%, and this illustrates the folly of continuing to use internal version and breech extraction, with which were associated 16 of 17 deaths and which were used in 52 out of 92 babies. Hall & O'Brien (1961) quoted a foetal mortality of 28% with vaginal and 7·2% for abdominal delivery.

COMPOUND PRESENTATION

This term describes cases of head presentation when one or more limbs lie alongside and present with the head, and includes also breech presentation where one or both arms present with the breech.

The causes are similar to those of prolapsed cord, which can complicate the compound presentation in some 17% of cases (Chan 1961).

Compound presentation can occur if engagement of the head is prevented by contracted pelvis,

hydramnios and pelvic tumours. Deflexion attitudes of the head, or a dead and macerated foetus, may also predispose to the condition. The most common associations are with prematurity, which was found in 45% of cases reviewed by Sweeney & Knapp (1961), and twin pregnancy, which formed 39·7% of their cases.

The incidence of compound presentation is variously given as 1 in 652 (Goplerud & Eastman 1953) 1 in 743 (Fields & Nelson 1959) 1 in 1,293 (Sweeney & Knapp 1961), and 1 in 1,321 (Chan 1961).

Presentation of an arm with the vertex (Fig. 22.8) accounts for about three-quarters of such cases. Next in frequency, a foot presents with the head, or the breech with an arm (11% each), and least common is presentation of arm, foot and vertex (Sweeney & Knapp 1961).

Diagnosis is usually not difficult once the membranes have ruptured. Only 2 of 74 of Sweeney & Knapp's cases were diagnosed when membranes were intact, and in 62 of the remainder the cervix was over 6 cm dilated, full dilatation having been achieved in 50 patients.

TREATMENT

This will depend upon the type of presentation, the stage of labour and state of the membranes. It will depend upon the condition and size of the infant and whether singleton or twin pregnancy is involved. Efforts are made to diagnose congenital abnormality, cephalopelvic disproportion and contracted pelvis. Finally, the presence of prolapsed cord will take precedence over the presentation if the foetus is alive.

In general, expectant treatment is preferable to more aggressive management, as in the majority of cases the extremity will recede as the presenting part descends, labour ending with a low instrumental or a normal delivery. Replacement of an arm is rarely necessary, and is quite superfluous if head and limb engage together. When the arm appears to rise into the uterus with a contraction this is a favourable sign and encourages further expectancy. Both maternal and foetal deaths rise threefold when active interference is routinely practised. More active treatment is, of course, necessary in cases of cord

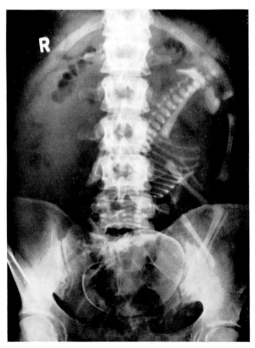

Fig. 22.8. A compound presentation. A hand and a foot, respectively, lie below and alongside the head.

prolapse with a live foetus or pelvic contraction, when Caesarean section is the procedure of choice. Intranatal radiography is valuable in the assessment of these cases. The most dangerous manoeuvre which has been employed is that of internal version and breech extraction. This is hazardous both to mother and foetus. Even in the case of the second twin, compound, presentation is to be treated expectantly unless prolapse of the cord occurs, when the rule invoked is that of immediate delivery by the least traumatic method.

The perinatal mortality in term infants where there was no prolapse of cord or traumatic operative delivery has been between 3 and 4% (Goplerud & Eastman 1953; Sweeney & Knapp 1961). With more general adoption of expectant treatment this can be expected to fall further.

PROLAPSE AND PRESENTATION OF THE UMBILICAL CORD

This occurs once in every 200–300 deliveries, the lower frequency being derived from American papers (Goldthorp 1967; Pathak 1968). Whilst the membranes remain intact the condition is that of presentation of the cord, which becomes cord prolapse when the sac ruptures. The foetal mortality will be slightly lower with cord presentation but the problems of presentation and prolapse are very similar and they must be considered together.

Aetiology

More than one factor may contribute.

(1) *The presenting part does not fill the lower segment and is poorly applied to it*

Such cases include: transverse lie, breech presentation, especially with flexed legs (Hay 1959), and face or brow presentation (though Clark *et al.* 1968 disagree). Occipitoposterior positions, cephalopelvic disproportion and, rarely, pelvic tumours, predispose to cord prolapse as will be excessive foetal mobility in polyhydramnios. In over 53% of cases reported by Clark *et al.* (1968) a malpresentation was present.

(2) *Prematurity*

This relationship is, again, highly significant because of the small foetus, relatively copious liquor and high incidence of associated malpresentation. Similar considerations apply in multiple pregnancy.

(3) *Multiparity*

Four-fifths of cases occur in multiparous patients. In them the head remains free until labour has begun, though the cervix may be somewhat dilated before that time. In one series only was it suggested that primiparae were at increased risk, because they need a greater number of operative procedures (Mengert & Longwell 1940).

(4) *Operative manoeuvres*

Forewater amniotomy or manual rotation prior to forceps extraction have been responsible for up to 20% in various series.

(5) *Abnormality of the cord*

A long cord, or low placental insertion, have been contributory in some series.

(6) *Foetal hypotension*

It has been suggested that the normally turgid cord will not prolapse and that the occurrence is more likely in cases such as abruptio placentae, in which foetal hypotension ensues (Seligman 1961).

Diagnosis and Anticipation

All patients must be told to come to hospital at once if they notice a leak of liquor, even if they feel no contractions. This must be emphasized particularly to women who have malpositions and malpresentations and when minor cephalopelvic disproportion exists. Cases of unstable or oblique lie may with advantage be admitted electively at 37–38 weeks.

Before performing a surgical induction the level of the presenting part must be assessed and if it is not engaged one may, with advantage, initiate contractions by oxytocin infusion prior to amniotomy. Every patient for amniotomy is a potential candidate for Caesarean section, and must be prepared accordingly. The cord should be felt for diligently both before and after amniotomy, especially if foetal heart rate variations follow the procedure.

In any labour, vaginal examination and careful auscultation should be carried out when the membranes rupture. This is equally important in multiple pregnancy. Whenever foetal distress becomes evident in labour, cord prolapse should be suspected; in the condition of occult prolapse (Niswander *et al.* 1966) one may feel coils of cord within the forewaters, when the distinction from toes may not be easy unless pulsation is evident. The cord may be visible through an endoscope or may appear within an elongated sac of membranes. In such *presentation of cord* it is important to keep the membranes intact whilst preparing for early delivery. Cord compression is possible if liquor is scanty and the head presents. Once the membranes have ruptured the case is one of *cord prolapse*. The strength and frequency of pulsation and its response to uterine contractions must be noted. Further information necessary before selecting treatment includes the stage of cervical dilatation, the nature and station of the presenting part, coexistent pelvic abnormalities, any associated diseases, and knowledge of the facilities available. The foetus should not be thought to possess a major congenital abnormality.

Treatment

Postural treatment involves keeping the fingers in the vagina and placing the patient in Sims's position or Trendelenburg's position, which are easier to maintain than the knee-elbow position. These measures aim to keep pressure from the cord. It is of equal importance that the cord should be replaced within the warm, moist vagina, so preventing the vasospasm which results from cold and local irritation (Rhodes 1956).

DEFINITIVE

If the foetus is dead, cord prolapse can be ignored, the problem being the mechanical one of the associated malpresentation. With a living foetus the aim is immediate controlled delivery by the appropriate route. (Cox 1951; Fenton & D'Esopo 1951). For example, if the cervix is fully dilated then forceps or ventouse delivery or breech extraction may be wise. In 110 cases reported by Suraiya & Fernandez (1966), the cervix was fully dilated in 36% at the time of diagnosis.

When the cervix is less than 7 cm dilated, Caesarean section is safest, and a section rate of 30–35% is usual in recent series. A possible exception would be a case of cord presentation with a longitudinal lie in a multipara where labour is progressing rapidly and the foetus is not distressed. In these circumstances, it may be reasonable to keep membranes intact until vaginal delivery becomes possible. Alternatives such as manual reposition and the use of Voorhees's bag no longer have a place in the well-equipped unit.

The most difficult cases are those in which the cervix is approaching full dilatation, the foetus is alive and the lie is longitudinal. This group produced the highest mortality in Goldthorp's series (1967), and the choice between Caesarean section on the one hand and manual dilatation of cervix with breech extraction or forceps ventouse delivery on the other may tax the judgement and skill of the most experienced operator. Internal version and breech extraction produces a damaged or dead baby in up to 40% of cases (Daly & Gibbs 1968), in addition to the risks to the mother. It should be abandoned.

Foetal mortality

Recent series have shown a corrected mortality of from 10·7% (Goldthorp 1967) to 16·8% (Clark *et al.* 1968). Prompt diagnosis at amniotomy induction results in a low mortality, as does a short diagnosis/delivery interval. Among cases reported by Clark *et al.* 1968 the mortality was only 5·5% if delivery was effected within 10 min. Prematurity quadrupled the perinatal mortality in the group described by Daly &

Gibbs (1968). Even when the cervix is approaching, but has not attained, full dilatation, the perinatal mortality is lower in cases delivered abdominally than in vaginal delivery.

MULTIPLE PREGNANCY

Twins occur about once in 80 European pregnancies. In negroid races the incidence is once in 25 pregnancies due to a higher incidence of spontaneous superovulation. Triplets occur once in 6,000 pregnancies. The recent use of gonadotrophins to stimulate ovulation is attended by a 25% risk of multiple pregnancy, and the incidence of superovulation and multiple births is on the increase.

There appears to be a familial tendency to multiple births, and the paternal and maternal influence on twinning is about equal. The frequency of twins increases with maternal age.

Binovular twins develop from two ova, and thus each foetus has its own placenta, chorion and amnion.

Uniovular twins develop from a single ovum, and thus there is only one placenta. There may be one or two chorionic membranes, but the amniotic sacs are always separated—at any rate initially (Fig. 22.9). Incomplete division of the germinal area will result in conjoint twins (Fig. 22.10). There is a communication between the placental circulations in uniovular twins, and this may cause unequal development of the foetuses, or even death of one foetus. The retained dead foetus becomes macerated and compressed, when it is known as foetus compressus or foetus papyraceous. Genotyping can accurately determine the zygosity of twins in 45% of cases (Cameron 1968).

Diagnosis

The first suspicion of twin pregnancy is usually the finding of a uterus which is too large for the period of gestation. Many of the symptoms and signs of pregnancy, including nausea and vomiting, are more pronounced. The increased requirement of iron and folic acid may lead to anaemia unless these are given as a supplement to a normal mixed diet. The increased abdominal distension may be further exaggerated by the complication of hydramnios associated with uniovular twins.

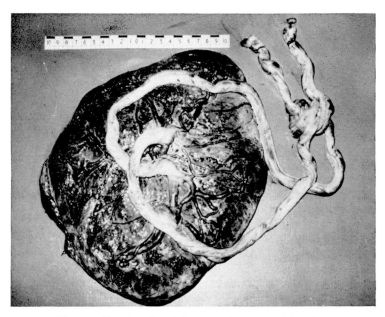

Fig. 22.9. Knotting of cords in a case of mono-amniotic twins.

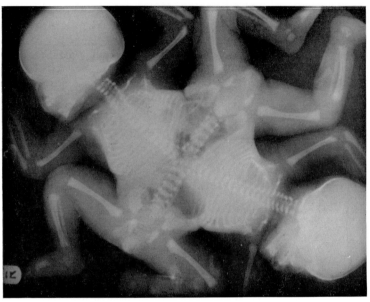

Fig. 22.10. Conjoined twins.

Oedema of the legs, varicose veins and haemorrhoids are common. Pre-eclampsia occurs in 25% of cases, and may be severe and of early onset. Both accidental antepartum haemorrhage and placenta praevia are more common.

A certain diagnosis will be made when two foetal heads can be easily palpated, but this should be verified by ultrasound (Fig. 22.11). Later in pregnancy radiological examination will confirm the diagnosis, and may also reveal evidence of bony malformation.

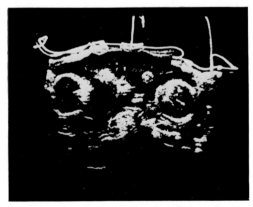

Fig. 22.11. An ultrasonic picture of a twin pregnancy.

Labour in twin pregnancy

In 70% of cases the first foetus will present as a vertex; in 40% both will be vertex. Nevertheless, malpresentations are very common, but serious difficulties are seldom encountered as the foetuses are small (Fig. 22.12).

Prematurity constitutes the greatest foetal hazard and prolonged rest from 30 to 36 weeks should be encouraged, or even enforced, in an effort to prolong pregnancy. Towards term the added complication of pre-eclampsia may necessitate premature induction of labour. The first stage of labour is not usually prolonged, as the infants are small and there is seldom any disproportion. Delivery should be conducted in a well-equipped hospital with an anaesthetist present. Infiltration of the perineum with lignocaine hydrochloride or a full pudendal block is all that is usually required, but general anaesthesia may be necessary for internal version, manual removal or other internal manipulations. The cord of the first foetus is divided and the clamp on the placental end replaced by a ligature to facilitate delivery of the second foetus and to eliminate risk of foetal haemorrhage from a common placenta. Malpresentation of the second

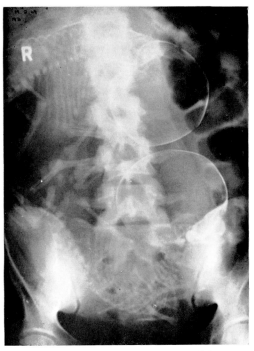

Fig. 22.12. A twin pregnancy, both foetuses lying transversely.

foetus is, if necessary, corrected by external version, which is easily performed through the lax abdominal wall. If the mother is conscious she can easily push the presenting part through the pelvic brim as soon as the membranes have been ruptured. It matters little whether the second foetus is delivered as a vertex or as a breech; the birth canal has been already stretched and in either event there is no opportunity for the head to undergo moulding. If, on the other hand, the mother has been anaesthetized for the birth of the first foetus, then the uterus will remain atonic until delivery is completed and the presenting part will remain above the pelvic brim. Under these circumstances it is better to perform an external podalic version, then to rupture the membranes and pull down a leg. This breech extraction proves easier and safer than attempts at high forceps with the head above the brim. On rare occasions even when the mother has not been anaesthetized the uterus becomes completely inert after the birth of the first

infant. This is usually overcome by rupturing the membranes, but a continuous intravenous oxytocin drip may prove useful.

Twins predispose to postpartum haemorrhage, and this risk should always be minimized by giving ergometrine 0·5 mg intravenously with the birth of the second twin or with a continuous intravenous oxytocin drip.

Occasionally, the diagnosis of twins is missed until the birth of the first infant. Under these circumstances the situation may be complicated by the giving of ergometrine, to prevent postpartum haemorrhage. The vigorous uterine contraction which follows may expel the second twin, may cause tonic uterine spasm and death of the foetus from anoxia, or may even cause rupture of the uterus. If the foetus is retained general anaesthesia is rapidly induced, amyl nitrite 2 ml is given as an inhalation in an effort to effect some uterine relaxation. The membranes are then ruptured and the foetus delivered by forceps or breech extraction. Under no circumstances should internal version be attempted, as this may easily effect uterine rupture.

When there are three or more foetuses present, (Fig. 22.13) the pregnancy is frequently complicated by severe pre-eclampsia and placental insufficiency. It is very important to avoid foetal anoxia and rapid delivery by Caesarean section is sometimes preferred.

The second of twins appears to be at greater risk than the first. This can in part be accounted for by the higher incidence of malpresentation (Law 1967), internal manipulations (Behrman 1965), placental insufficiency (Hubbard *et al.* 1964), and congenital abnormality (Hendricks 1966).

Difficult cases of twins

Interlocking of twins is rare and is most likely to occur when the first foetus is delivered as a breech and the head of the second twin descends into the pelvis alongside the neck of the first. It may be possible to push the head of the second twin upwards and out of the pelvis, and this will permit delivery of the first twin. If this fails the first twin will have died from cord compression, and decapitation is necessary. The second,

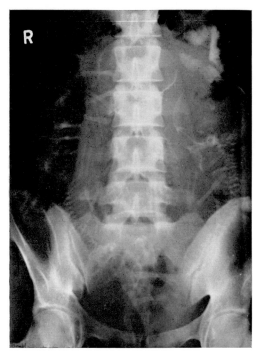

Fig. 22.13. A triplet pregnancy. Note the legs of the middle foetus below the head of the leading one. Locking may result.

surviving twin is then delivered, followed by the free head of the first twin.

Occasionally, two heads both presenting may become locked at the level of the pelvic brim, but this can usually be overcome under anaesthesia by pushing up the higher head until it is free of the brim.

Conjoint twins should be suspected if the X-ray of the mother reveals two heads lying at the same level within the uterus. Oblique films will usually clarify the diagnosis. Since it is now possible surgically to separate many of these twins, the mother should be delivered at or near to term by Caesarean section.

Twin transfusion syndrome

An interesting abnormality which occasionally calls for urgent treatment of one or both twins shortly after birth is the twin transfusion syndrome. One twin appears to 'bleed' into the other, so that one plethoric and one anaemic baby are born. Monochorial twins only are affected.

The plethoric twin is usually a larger, red, deceptively healthy looking infant, compared to the smaller, pale, anaemic one. Both, however, are at risk, for the plethoric child may quickly develop signs of cardiac decompensation, due to hypervolaemia, whilst the anaemic twin may be at risk for the opposite reason. Hydramnios generally affects the sac of the plethoric baby and oligohydramnios that of the anaemic one.

Rausen (1965) reported on 19 cases (14·6%) out of 130 monochorial twin pregnancies studied; the diagnosis was arrived at following haematological, morbid anatomical and clinical studies, and it is unlikely that this frequency reflects the clinical frequency of cases severe enough to call for treatment. Rausen suggests that a haemaglobin difference of 34% (5 g/100 ml) is necessary to establish the diagnosis, since differences of haemaglobin up to this figure have been found in dizygotic twins.

If treatment is required as a matter of urgency, the plethoric twin may be bled through the umbilical vein in amounts of 5 ml/30 min until the venous pressure is reduced to normal levels (Conway 1964). Whole blood or packed cells in amounts consistent with the body weight may be given to the anaemic twin.

The precise placental features leading to this unusual state of affairs are still not fully explained, although it seems clear that a placental vascular shunt of some kind is involved. Strong & Corney (1967) and Aherne *et al.* (1968) review this aspect of the subject well.

LIQUOR AMNII AND ITS ABNORMALITIES

Comparatively little is known about the mode of production and disposal of liquor amnii. Various suggestions as to its source have been made, without its origin being unequivocally established. Foetal urine has been shown to contribute (Jeffcote 1932), and in the sheep, fluid is produced from the nasopharynx (Reynolds 1953). Macafee (1950), in fact, suggested the respiratory system as a possible source in man, although this seems unlikely, since the newborn produces only small quantities of fluid from the nasopharynx.

It seems probable that the production and disposal of a large quantity of fluid is involved, since Vosburgh *et al.* (1948) claimed that the water content of the fluid was changed every 3 hr. The validity of this work has been questioned, but further studies by Hutchinson *et al.* (1959) appear to substantiate it. Bevis (1967) believes that the evidence supports the production of liquor amnii on the membranes covering the foetal surface of the placenta, perhaps from exposed vessels at this site. Bourne's observations (1962), suggest that large quantities of fluid, including substances in solution, may be passed through the foetal membranes. Hibbard (1962), favours the likelihood of the majority of this fluid transfer occurring at the region of greatest vascularity; that is, the placental surface. He points out that histochemical studies have demonstrated that the amniotic epithelium in this area shows marked secretory activity.

Disposal in late pregnancy is, to some extent, the result of foetal swallowing. It seems unlikely that this mechanism could dispose of much liquor, however, and in early pregnancy may not operate at all. A to-and-fro passage of fluid through the membranes into the circulation seems likely. Imbalance between production and disposal may quickly give rise to abnormalities of the quantity of liquor present.

VOLUME OF LIQUOR AMNII

The volume of liquor amnii increases as pregnancy advances towards term, when there is some decline. Rhodes (1966) found liquor volumes of around 30 ml at 10 weeks; this had risen to around 100 ml by 13–14 weeks, and to 150 ml by 15 weeks. Gadd (1966) reported similar values. Liquor volumes continue to rise until late pregnancy; they reach a peak between 34 and 37 weeks and then decline until delivery. Gadd found volumes in normal pregnancy which varied from 500 to 1100 ml between 30 and 37 weeks, and between 600 ml and zero by 43 weeks. In mild to moderate cases of pre-eclampsia Gadd found normal liquor volumes, and in severe cases

considerably reduced volumes. Amounts varying between 1,500 ml and more than 6,000 ml were recorded in association with foetal abnormalities.

COMPOSITION OF LIQUOR AMNII

The liquor amnii composition is some 97% water, with small quantities of minerals and organic materials. The chief minerals are chlorides and sodium, the chief inorganic constituent is protein. A further consideration of the substances present in liquor amnii and their application to foetal maturity is given on p. 165.

Hydramnios

Hydramnios is a recognizable excess of amniotic fluid. Usually, the hydramnios is chronic, the excess fluid accumulating slowly during the last trimester of pregnancy; occasionally, the condition is subacute, the increase taking place over 2 or 3 weeks; rarely, in acute hydramnios the accumulation of fluid is extremely fast, a week (or perhaps only a few days) being sufficient for great distress to be experienced by the patient. This variety of acute hydramnios is usually associated with a uni ovular twin or triplet pregnancy.

Hydramnios is important clinically because of the conditions which may be associated with it, the discomfort it may produce, the increased difficulty it causes in abdominal examination, and the effect it may have on the course of labour.

ASSOCIATED CONDITIONS

We do not know the precise reason for hydramnios, but we may find it in association with either maternal or foetal abnormalities. The chief maternal lesion is diabetes, which is not infrequently complicated by hydramnios, especially if the diabetes is not well controlled. A common foetal association is multiple pregnancy, when the accumulation of fluid may be of the usual chronic variety, or in uni ovular multiple pregnancy it may be acute. Such acute examples are rare, but are very serious, not only because of the distress they cause the patient, but also because they occur unusually early—26–30 weeks—and are likely to be followed by premature labour with foetal loss. Foetal abnormalities associated with hydramnios are either those affecting the central nervous system—anencephaly or spina bifida— or obstructions to the upper part of the gastro-intestinal tract—eosophageal or duodenal atresia. Hydramnios is sometimes seen in association with rhesus incompatibility, especially the more serious examples of the condition. Very rarely, a chorio-angioma of the placenta may be associated with hydramnios.

ABDOMINAL DISCOMFORT

The size of the abdomen may be a source of some distress to the patient, who may find it difficult to rest in a comfortable position for any period of time. Dyspnoea may be troublesome, as may oedema of the ankles.

ABDOMINAL EXAMINATION

The quantity of fluid present usually makes abdominal examination more difficult. The foetus is unusually ballottable and frequent changes of lie and position occur. It may be difficult to ascertain on clinical grounds if a single foetus or a multiple pregnancy is present.

The diagnosis of hydramnios is not made merely by finding a large abdomen. This may have several explanations, which will be enumerated below. If there is a real excess of liquor, a fluid thrill should be recognizable, which, together with the increased ballottement of the foetus, permits a confident diagnosis. In marked examples, this thrill is very easily elicited, the abdomen is very tense, and the skin stretched and shiny.

Other causes of a larger abdomen than is in accord with the period of amenorrhoea are:

(i) A mistake in dates, the pregnancy being more advanced than appears to be the case.
(ii) Multiple pregnancy, which may, of course, be associated with hydramnios.
(iii) Fibroids or an ovarian cyst complicating pregnancy.
(iv) An unusually large baby.

COMPLICATIONS OF LABOUR

A greater mobility of the foetus in the uterus increases the likelihood of abnormal lie or presentation at the time of the onset of labour. Labour, is, not infrequently, so complicated, and the problems which arise may be still further aggravated by early rupture of the membranes and prolapse of an arm or the cord. Premature labour is more frequent, especially with severe degrees of hydramnios. Labour is often said to be prolonged, but if so, it is less frequently the case than was previously believed.

OBSTETRIC MANAGEMENT

The association of hydramnios with multiple pregnancy and foetal abnormalities is an indication for X-ray examination whenever the condition is recognized. In the absence of any important associated condition, the discomfort experienced by the patient will be our chief concern, at first. Increased rest in a semi-reclining attitude will be helpful; sedatives at night may be required if there is difficulty in sleeping.

In more severe degrees of hydramnios with abdominal discomfort, relief can sometimes be obtained by giving a diuretic; occasionally, this appears to keep the condition in check, even if it does not markedly reduce the amount of fluid present. More severe degrees, still, should be considered for amniocentesis to remove sufficient fluid to relieve discomfort. It will first be wise to localize the placenta, so that this can be avoided. Then a needle of the type used for lumbar puncture may be inserted into the amniotic sac at any convenient point, and liquor removed. The fluid does not emerge rapidly, and a system of suction may be helpful to take off sufficient fluid to produce relief. One to two litres of fluid may be all that can be removed, however, even after several hours, and although this may bring temporary relief there is likely to be re-accumulation during the next few days. Paracentesis uteri is seldom a really helpful measure, but must be tried on occasions.

Towards the end of pregnancy the mobility of the foetus is a matter of some concern, and the patient must be kept in hospital, so that if the lie is abnormal when pains begin, it may be corrected instantly. Alternatively, an attempt may be made to induce labour by artificial rupture of the membranes. There are, however, two disadvantages to this; the lie may still revert to an abnormal one, even after much liquor has been removed, and separation of the placenta may occur as the volume of the uterine contents is greatly reduced by the removal of the fluid. If the membranes must be ruptured, it will be advisable to take off fluid as slowly as possible; a Drew-Smythe catheter has advantages here. Moreover, oxytocic stimulation to establish uterine contractions quickly will help to prevent recurrence of the abnormal lie.

Hydramnios associated with anencephaly (Fig. 22.14) is best managed by artificial rupture of the membranes, when labour usually begins shortly afterwards. In the unusual circumstance of anencephaly being recognized at a very early stage of pregnancy—say 28–30 weeks—this surgical intervention may be less certain to be followed by early labour. Induction with prostaglandins should prove effective here.

Postpartum haemorrhage must be prevented. Hydramnios is one of the conditions which has been held to be frequently associated with this complication. It is likely that the association is less common than has been suggested in the past, but it is an important associated condition nonetheless.

A baby born of a mother with hydramnios should be suspected of having atresia of the upper gastrointestinal tract, if no other visible abnormality exists. This will be particularly likely if the infant produces increased amounts of fluid from his mouth and nose; here, a tracheo-oesophageal fistula is a distinct possibility. A gastric tube should be passed to establish that there is no oesophageal obstruction and feeding witheld until this fact is proved with reasonable certainty.

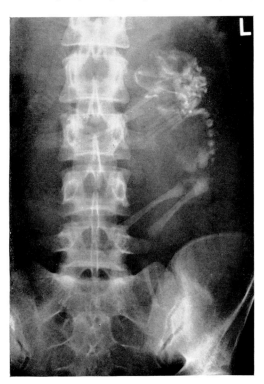

Fig. 22.14. An anencephalic foetus in association with hydramnios.

Oligohydramnios

This condition, although less frequent than hydramnios, is not so uncommon as was thought in the past. The increasing awareness of the association of low volumes of amniotic fluid and the foetus failing to thrive *in utero*, has led to the more frequent recognition of oligohydramnios. Low liquor volumes do not have the same maternal significance as high ones, but they are associated with considerable foetal risks.

Oligohydramnios is evident clinically in two particular circumstances: in association with a small-for-dates baby, and with severe renal anomalies of the foetus. The baby failing to thrive *in utero*, whether or not this is associated with obvious hypertensive disease, is likely to be surrounded by a small volume of liquor amnii. This fact may be evident on abdominal examination or may become apparent for the first time when an attempt is made to induce labour by artificial rupture of the membranes. Indeed, failure to release a quantity of fluid on attempted forewater rupture should be regarded as a suspicious sign, and the case should be reviewed

with foetal dysmaturity in mind. The oligohydramnios itself will not influence management

beyond drawing attention to the foetus in
danger.

The association between oligohydramnios and
renal agenesis was emphasized by Jeffcoate &
Scott (1959) and Bain & Scott (1960). In this
condition the infant fails to grow during late
pregnancy. The presentation is often breech,
and premature labour is common. An X-ray
examination of the foetus may indicate that it
is closely confined within the uterus (Fig. 22.15),
and an ultrasonic scan may confirm the very
small volume of liquor that is present. When born,
the child has the characteristic facies described by
Potter—low-set ears, epicanthic folds, flattening
of the nose and micrognathous; this appearance
is not diagnostic of renal agenesis, and may be
seen in other cases of oligohydramnios where
there is no renal anomaly. Pressure effects may be
concerned in some of these facial changes.

Another condition associated with oligohydramnios is amnion nodosum (Fig. 22.16).
The amnion shows areas containing small
nodules, a millimetre or two in size, and yellowish
in colour. They are formed by aggregations of
squames in an amorphous matrix, and are often
seen in cases of oligohydramnios whatever the
cause.

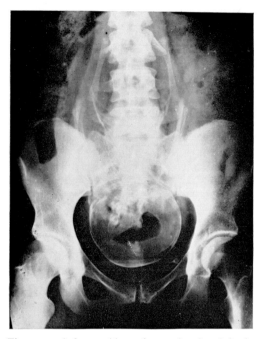

Fig. 22.15. A foetus with renal agenesis gripped firmly
within the uterus in a case of oligohydramnios.

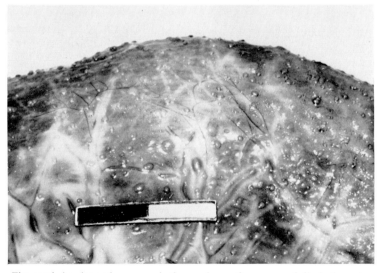

Fig. 22.16. Amnion nodosum seen in the membranes from a case of oligohydramnios.

POSTMATURITY

Postmaturity is a difficult subject to assess, since our yard-sticks of maturity are so imprecise. Various aspects of maturity and its assessment by clinical and other means have been undertaken in Chapter 11. In this section, the management of a patient who passes the expected date of confinement without going into labour will be considered.

Many patients, of course, fall within this category and relatively few of them require intervention. Postmaturity and 'postdate pregnancy' are not synonymous. The estimation of the expected date of confinement which we normally employ assumes that fertilization occurs 14 days after the last menstrual period, which will not always be the case. It further assumes that all pregnancies last the same length of time, which is unlikely to be so. It is only reasonable, therefore, to regard a short interval following the expected date of confinement as within the limits of normal, and unless there is some other abnormality present, to take no action.

Postmaturity can, in general, be said to be present when the pregnancy has continued so long beyond term that an extra risk to the foetus exists. This risk will usually arise from the ageing of the placenta and its consequent inability to nurture the foetus; less commonly, danger may be associated with an increase in foetal size and increasing ossification of the foetal skull bones, and thus with greater difficulty during passage of the head through the pelvis.

The problem clinically is to determine the appropriate time to intervene if labour has not begun. Since foetal mortality associated with prolongation of pregnancy beyond 42 weeks is almost double that between 37 and 41 weeks (Walker 1965; Beischer *et al.* 1969), most obstetricians are reluctant to allow pregnancy to continue beyond this date. In some cases, however, there may be danger earlier, and even to wait so long may result in loss of the child's life.

A helpful clinical approach to postmaturity is to seek first to establish the accuracy or otherwise of the calculation of the expected date of confinement. This presupposes a known date for the first day of the last normal menstrual period; and it presupposes previous regular periods at about 28-day intervals. If the date given was not associated with a normal period, the calculation may not be valid. If previous periods were not every 28 days, but at longer intervals, the calculation will have be to revised. If the cycle was not regular at all, no valid calculation can be made.

Having considered these facts, other landmarks of maturity may be sought. Is the history known? Was quickening felt at approximately the correct time and was this in accordance with the uterine size? Quickening is a variable feast, but can give a general guide to maturity, especially if a note is made shortly after the patient is first aware of it. Uterine size and growth can be helpful, and can give an approximate, but only approximate, guide to maturity.

So often, however, these facts are unknown, and the patient is seen for the first time apparently beyond term, when a decision must be made. In this situation, X-ray examination and liquor amnii studies may be helpful if there is reason to doubt dates or maturity. Ultrasonic assessment is less helpful after 30 weeks, although an absolute reading for the biparietal diameter may be useful if this is very large or very small.

Having assessed all the facts obtainable, it remains to decide if any other feature should influence a decision to induce labour. The importance of a raised blood pressure or of pre-eclampsia in accelerating placental ageing, and causing foetal loss from placental insufficiency, has already been stressed. The association of these factors, even in a mild form, will almost certainly call for induction of labour about term or shortly afterwards, rather than at 41–42 weeks. A history of loss of a previous child in similar postmature circumstances will call for early induction also. The age of the patient may be regarded as a reason for induction sooner rather than later. Patients over 35 years of age are thought by many to be more at risk than younger patients; moreover, if increasing age is associated with a degree of subfertility, or if the patient has no living child, foetal loss, should it occur is more tragic. Induction at or soon after term has obvious advantages.

If, however, there is doubt about maturity—let alone postmaturity—if the foetus appears small but is surrounded by a normal quantity of liquor and is apparently growing, a little time may be taken to assess the situation more fully by the investigations outlined in Chapter 11 before intervening. If there are no special features calling for early induction, nor reasons seriously to doubt maturity, induction 10–14 days after the expected date of confinement will usually be indicated. A casual decision should never be made, however, since if induction is to be performed a good indication must exist. Browne (1963) has stressed the problems of postmaturity and of interference, and has emphasized the degree of clinical skill which must be used.

REFERENCES

AHERNE W., STRONG S.J. & CORNEY G. (1968) *Biologia Neonat.* **12**, 121.

BAIN A.D. & SCOTT J.S. (1960) *Br. med. J.* **i**, 841.

BEHRMAN S.J. (1965) *Postgrad. med.* **38**, 72.

BEISCHER N.A. (1966) *J. Obstet. Gynaec. Br. Commonw.* **73**, 421.

BEISCHER N.A., BROWN J.B. & TOWNSEND L. (1969) *Am. J. Obstet. Gynec.* **103**, 483.

BEISCHER N.A., BROWN J.B., SMITH M.A. & TOWNSEND L. (1969) *Am. J. Obstet. Gynec.* **103**, 483.

BERGER M., HEIMANN H. & WICK A. (1967) *Bibl. Gynaec.* **45**, 1.

BERGMAN P. & MALMSTROM T. (1962) *Gynaecologia*, **154**, 65.

BEVIS D.C.A. (1967) *Trans. N. Engl. obstet. gynaec. Soc.* p. 56.

BORELL U. & FERNSTROM I. (1960) *Acta obstet. gynec. scand.* **39**, 626.

BROWNE J.C. McC. (1963) *J. Am. med. Ass.* **186**, 1047.

BUTLER N.R. & BONHAM D.G. (1964) *Perinatal Mortality.* Edinburgh, Livingstone.

CALKINS L.A. (1953) *Obstet. Gynec., N.Y.* **1**, 466.

CAMERON A.H. (1968) *Proc. R. Soc. Med.* **61**, 13.

CHALMERS J.A. (1968) *J. Obstet. Gynaec. Br. Commonw.* **75**, 889.

CHAPMAN K. (1967) *J. Obstet. Gynaec., India*, **17**, 368.

CHEN H.Y. & WEI P.Y. (1960) *J. int. Coll. Surg.* **34**, 756.

CLARK D.O., COPELAND W. & ULLERY J.C. (1968) *Am. J. Obstet. Gynec.* **101**, 84.

CONWAY C.F. (1964) *Obstet. Gynec., N.Y.* **23**, 745.

COX L.W. (1950) *J. Obstet. Gynaec. Br. Commonw.* **57**, 197.

COX L.W. (1955) *J. Obstet. Gynaec. Br. Commonw.* **62**, 395.

COX L.W. (1951) *Lancet*, **i**, 561.

DALY D. & MICHAEL A.M. (1953) *J. Obstet. Gynaec. Br. Commonw.* **60**, 492.

DALY J.W. & GIBBS C.E. (1968) *Am. J. Obstet. Gynec.* **100**, 264.

DEDE J.A. & FRIEDMAN E.A. (1963) *Am. J. Obstet. Gynec.* **87**, 515.

D'ESOPO D.A. (1941) *Am. J. Obstet. Gynec.* **42**, 937.

FENTON A.N. & D'ESOPO D.A. (1951) *Am. J. Obstet. Gynec.* **62**, 52.

FIELDS H. & NELSON P.K. (1959) *Am. J. Obstet. Gynec.* **78**, 539.

FRIEDLANDER D. (1966) *Am. J. Obstet. Gynec.* **95**, 906.

FRIEDMAN E.A. (1967) *Labor. Clinical Evaluation and Management.* New York, Appleton-Century-Crofts.

GADD R.L. (1966) *J. Obstet. Gynaec. Br. Commonw.* **73**, 11.

GHAN D.P.C. (1961) *Br. med. J.* **ii**, 560.

Glasgow Congress (1965) *J. Obstet. Gynaec. Br. Commonw.* **72**, 866.

GOLDTHORP W.O. (1967) *Br. J. clin. Pract.* **21**, 21.

GOPLERUD J. & EASTMAN N.J. (1953) *Obstet. Gynec., N.Y.* **1**, 59.

HALL J.E., KOHL S.G., O'BRIEN F. & GINSBERG S. (1965) *Am. J. Obstet. Gynec.* **91**, 665.

HALL J.E., COUNSELMAN R. & BROOKS J. (1956) *Obstet. Gynec., N.Y.* **7**, 277.

HALL J.E. & KOHL S.G. (1956) *Am. J. Obstet. Gynec.* **72**, 977.

HALL S.C. & O'BRIEN F.B. (1961) *Am. J. Obstet. Gynec.* **82**, 1180.

HARRIS B.A. & EPPERSON J.W.W. (1950) *Am. J. Obstet. Gynec.* **59**, 1105.

HAY D. (1959) *J. Obstet. Gynaec. Br. Commonw.* **66**, 529.

HELLMAN L.M., EPPERSON J.W.W. & CONNALLY F. (1950) *Am. J. Obstet. Gynec.* **59**, 831.

HENDRICKS C.H. (1966) *Obstet. Gynec., N.Y.* **27**, 47.

HIBBARD B.M. (1962) *Clin. Obstet. Gynec.* **5**, 1044.

HUBBARD W.F., LEIB L. & KANTOR H.I. (1964) *Sth. med. J., Nashville*, **57**, 69.

HUSSLEIN H. (1965) *Zentralb. Gynak.* **87**, 682.

HUTCHINSON D.L., GRAY M.J., PLENTL A.A., ALVAREZ H., CALDEYRO-BARCIA R., KAPLAN H. & LIND J. (1959) *J. Clin. Invest.* **38**, 971.

JEFFCOATE T.N.A. (1932) *J. Obstet. Gynaec. Br. Commonw.* **38**, 814.

JEFFCOATE T.N.A. & SCOTT J.S. (1959) *Can. med. Ass. J.* **80**, 77.

JOHNSON C.E. (1964) *J. Am. med. Ass.* **187**, 642.

KENWICK A.N. (1953) *Am. J. Obstet. Gynec.* **66**, 67.

LAW R.G. (1967) *Standards of Obstetric Card.* Edinburgh, Livingstone.

LAWSON J.B. & STEWART D.B. (1967) *Obstetrics and Gynaecology in the Tropics.* London, Arnold.

MACAFEE C.H.G. (1950) *J. Obstet. Gynaec. Br. Commonw.* **57**, 171.

MADDEN L.H.Jr. (1956) *Am. J. Obstet. Gynec.* **72**, 31.

MELTZER R.M., SACHTLEBEN M.R. & FRIEDMAN E.A. (1967) *Am. J. Obstet. Gynec.* **100**, 255.

MENGERT W.F. & LONGWELL F.H. (1940) *Am. J. Obstet. Gynec.* **40**, 79.

MILLER D. (1930) *Br. med. J.* **i**, 1036.

METHUEN D. (1958) *Proc. R. Soc. Med.* **51**, 169.

MORGAN H.S. & KANE S.H. (1964) *J. Am. med. Ass.* **187**, 262.

MORRIS N.F. (1953) *J. Obstet. Gynaec. Br. Commonw.* **60**, 44.

MOSTAR S., AKALTIN E. & BABUNCA C. (1966) *Obstet. Gynec., N.Y.* **28**, 49.

NEELY M.R. (1961) *J. Obstet. Gynaec. Br. Commonw.* **68**, 490.

NISWANDER K.R., FRIEDMAN E.A., HOOVER D.B., PIETROWSKI H. & WESTPHAL M.C. (1966) *Am. J. Obstet. Gynec.* **95**, 853, 1099.

PARRY-JONES E. (1968) *J. Obstet. Gynaec. Br. Commonw.* **75**, 892.

PATHAK U.N. (1968) *Am. J. Obstet. Gynec.* **101**, 401.

PEEL J.H. & CLAYTON S.G. (1948) *J. Obstet. Gynaec. Br. Commonw.* **55**, 614.

PLENTL A.A. & STONE R.E. (1953) *Obstet. Gynec. Surv.* **8**, 313.

POSNER A.C., FRIEDMAN S. & POSNER L.B. (1957) *Surgery Gynec. Obstet.* **104**, 485.

POSNER L.B., RUBIN E.J. & POSNER A.C. (1963) *Obstet. Gynec., N.Y.* **21**, 745.

POTTER M.G., HEATON C.E. & DOUGLAS G.W. (1960) *Obstet. Gynec., N.Y.* **15**, 158.

RAUSEN A.R., SEKI M. & STRAUSS L. (1965) *J. Pediat.* **66**, 613.

REYNOLDS S.R.M. (1953) *Nature, Lond.* **172**, 307.

RHODES P. (1956) *Proc. R. Soc. Med.* **49**, 937.

RHODES P. (1966) *J. Obstet. Gynaec. Br. Commonw.* **73**, 23.

RUDOLPH S.J. (1947) *Am. J. Obstet. Gynec.* **54**, 987.

SELIGMAN S.A. (1961) *Br. med. J.* i, 1369.

STEVENSON C.S. (1949) *Am. J. Obstet. Gynec.* **58**, 432.

STRONG S.J. & CORNEY G. (1967) *The Placenta in Twin Pregnancy.* Oxford, Pergamon Press, p. 68.

SURAIYA U. & FERNANDEZ W. (1966) *J. Obstet. Gynaec., India*, **16**, 188.

SWEENEY W.J. & KNAPP R.C. (1961) *Obstet. Gynec., N.Y.* **17**, 333.

VARTAN C.K. (1945) *J. Obstet. Gynaec. Br. Commonw.* **52**, 417.

VARTAN C.K. (1958) *Proc. R. Soc. Med.* **51**, 170

VOSBURGH G.J., FLEXNER L.B., COWIE B.B., HELLMAN L.M., PROCTOR N.K. & WILDE W.S. (1948) *Am. J. Obstet. Gynec.* **56**, 1156.

WOOD E.C. & FORSTER F.M.C. (1959) *J. Obstet. Gynaec. Br. Commonw.* **66**, 75.

WULFF G.J.L., TRUEBLOOD A.C. & HOLLAND R.C. (1960) *Obstet. Gynec., N.Y.* **16**, 288.

WHITE A.J. (1956) *J. Obstet. Gynaec. Br. Commonw.* **63**, 706.

YATES M.J. (1964) *J. Obstet. Gynaec. Br. Commonw.* **71**, 245.

ZATUCHNI G.I. & ANDROS G.J. (1965) *Am. J. Obstet. Gynec.* **93**, 237.

ZATUCHNI G.I. & ANDROS G.J. (1967) *Am. J. Obstet. Gynec.* **98**, 854.

CHAPTER 23

ABNORMAL UTERINE ACTION AND PROLONGED LABOUR

Prolonged labour is a progressively serious obstetrical problem fraught with maternal hardship, suffering and potential injury. It strongly predisposes to postpartum haemorrhage, intrauterine infection and foetal anoxia, and the timing and conduct of labour and delivery may call for the best obstetrical judgement and clinical skill.

INNERVATION OF THE UTERUS

During pregnancy the uterus increases its mass sixfold by hypertrophy of the muscle fibres and enlargement of the blood vessels. With this enlargement there is a progressive sensitization of the myometrium to oxytocin, which is probably in the main responsible for controlling the onset and progress of labour and coordinating uterine contractions. Although the uterus possesses an inherent rhythmicity and is capable or regular contractions independent of any extrinsic nerve supply, it is nevertheless influenced by nerve impulses received via the autonomic nervous system and by hormonal blood levels.

The sympathetic nerve fibres are derived from the 5th to 8th thoracic spinal segments. It is generally held that these fibres conduct impulses responsible for vasoconstriction and pain, and some observers believe they inhibit both circular and longitudinal muscle fibres. In support of this view is the relaxation by adrenalin of circular muscle fibres in a constriction ring, and the easy and rapid labour which follows resection of the presacral nerve.

It is now generally agreed that the uterus receives no parasympathetic nerve supply, but some of the efferent sympathetic fibres are adrenergic and others cholinergic. Since caudal analgesia may result in painless labour, sensory impulses must enter the spinal cord at a lower level, possibly via the sacral nerves (S.2.3.4).

Much is owed to Csapo (1960) for demonstrating that uterine plain muscle resembles, rather than differs from, striated muscle. Schematically, it is possible to regard the myometrial cell as a contractile system enclosed by an excitable membrane. The myofibrils contain the thin filaments of the complex protein actomyosin, which effects the contraction.

Between the myofibrils, spaced like beads in a row, are the mitochondria containing the high-energy phosphates. Thus the sites of energy production and expenditure are in close propinquity.

The potential of the surrounding membrane is of the order of 50 mV, and depolarization of it precedes the development of the action potential. The spread of the contraction is due to an electric current which passes from fibre to fibre at those points where the membranes of contiguous cells come into close contact, or are actually fused. Some authorities think that there may even be lacunae in the membranes at these points. Thus does the whole organ contract almost as if it were one giant cell.

UTERINE CONTRACTION

Caldeyro *et al.* (1950) and Helman *et al.* (1950) pioneered much of the fundamental measure-

386

ments of intra-amniotic pressure and uterine muscle tone during labour. They showed a gradient of diminishing activity from the fundus to the lower segment in normal uterine action, and this increases as labour advances. This so-called fundal dominance is not obvious in prolonged labour and may be lacking in false labour.

In brief, the features of good, quick labour are:

(i) Large absolute intensity of contraction with an intra-amniotic pressure of over 24 mmHg.
(ii) Strong fundal dominance.
(iii) Good synchronization between different parts of the uterus.
(iv) Regularity in rhythm, intensity and form of contractions.
(v) During uterine relaxation the intra-amniotic pressure descends to the level of normal tones (10 mmHg).
(vi) The trough of the wave resembles the troughs of adjacent waves.

The features of prolonged labour are:

(i) Absolute intensity of contraction in less than normal (15–24 mmHg.)
(ii) No frank fundal dominance.
(iii) No good synchronism.
(iv) Irregularity of rhythm, intensity and form of contraction.
(v) Lack of descent to the level of normal tone between contractions.

The features of false labour are:

(i) Absolute intensity of contraction in less than 15 mmHg.
(ii) Absence of fundal dominance.
(iii) Good synchronism.
(iv) Regularity in rhythm of contractions, but irregularity in intensity.
(v) Normal descent to the level of normal tone between contractions.

Although an individual in normal labour possesses a contraction pattern which persists throughout her labour, this contraction pattern is peculiar to herself and differs from those seen in other women in normal labour. Neither the character nor the frequency of Braxton Hisks's contractions in any part of the uterus prior to the onset of labour can foretell the characteristics which the uterus will exhibit when it is in labour.

Definition of prolonged labour

Previously, labour was defined as prolonged if it exceeded 48 hr, but abnormal uterine action can be recognized much earlier, and it is now usual to accept 36 or even 24 hr. During the 10 years from 1939 to 1948 at Queen Charlotte's Maternity Hospital, London, there were 19,745 deliveries with a maternal mortality of 1·2 per 1,000 deliveries 3·2% of labours lasted more than 48 hr, and of these mothers 4·7 per 1,000 died. Of the 19,745 deliveries, 30 infants per 1,000 deliveries were stillborn and 16·5 infants per 1,000 deliveries died in the neonatal period. In the cases of inertia, however, 98 infants per 1,000 deliveries were stillborn and 22 infants per 1,000 deliveries died in the neonatal period. Half of the foetal deaths occurred during the first stage of labour, and were attributed to placental insufficiency (MacRae 1949). In more recent years, there has been a steady trend towards the freer and earlier use of Caesarean section. In the same hospital in 1968 there were 3,425 deliveries, of which only 19 labours lasted more than 36 hr, with no maternal or foetal deaths.

Clinical causes of prolonged labour

PARITY

The majority of cases are primigravida (about 96% of hospital bookings), and the resistance of the soft tissues of the pelvic floor and cervix may contribute towards the difficulty. Lack of familiarity and fear of labour may have an inhibiting effect upon uterine contractions.

AGE

This does not appear to have much influence, although labour of more than 24 hr is seldom permitted in primigravida over 35 years.

MALPOSITION

The occipitoposterior position is a very common association and this, together with disproportion, will be discussed later in more detail.

POSTMATURITY

The average duration of pregnancy is 40·8 weeks, and this tendency towards postmaturity is commonly associated with a large foetal head, the occipitoposterior position and a mild degree of brim disproportion.

OTHER FACTORS

Pre-eclampsia, antepartum haemorrhage, surgical induction, overdistention of the uterus by twins or hydramnios, uterine fibroids, uterine malformations and cervical fibrosis have all been claimed as factors responsible for prolonged labour, but these are now largely discounted.

CLASSIFICATION

Until such time as we have a clearer understanding of uterine action and the mechanism of cervical dilatation, the classification of prolonged labour must remain arbitrary. Lack of progress sometimes appears to be due to feeble uterine contractions, and on other occasions to lack of coordination. These will be discussed further.

Hypotonic uterine inertia

The time of onset of labour is indefinite. The contractions are weak and infrequent, and are of normal distribution in the hypogastrium and flanks. The membranes may rupture early in labour, but this is unusual. The cervix is soft and pliable and if normal labour supervenes it becomes fully dilated without difficulty. The mother is not distressed but may become impatient and anxious because of lack of progress. If the condition is allowed to continue for more than 24 hr the bladder and colon may share in the general atonia and become distended. Provided the foetus is mature, it is usual to stimulate the uterus to achieve normal progressive labour. The bowel is emptied with an enema. The membranes are ruptured, and if this fails a continuous intravenous oxytocin drip is usually effective. This type of labour may be associated with an overdistended uterus, as in twins and hydramnios.

Incoordinate uterine action

This is a condition in which the uterus contracts vigorously, but the cervix dilates very slowly. The time of onset of labour is often indefinite and there is a tendency for several days of false labour pains of a colicky character, felt mainly over the sacral region and in the hypogastrium. Because the intra-amniotic pressure between contractions approximates to, or exceeds, 25 mmHg (the threshold level for pain), the patient has a constant backache, which during uterine contractions is accentuated by distressing, colicky, irregular pains felt mainly over the sacral region and radiating forwards into the hypogastrium. By palpation it is often difficult to time the onset of each uterine contraction, and the clinician is given the impression that painful sensation precedes and outlasts each contraction. Vomiting and distension of the bowel are common. The membranes frequently rupture early in labour and this leads to a progressive uterine retraction and embarrassment of placental circulation, and foetal hypoxia. The condition is seen most frequently in the primigravida.

The uterus is tender to the touch and highly irritable. Abnormal stimulation by intra-uterine manipulations, bags and recording devices, abdominal massage and oxytocic drugs may easily produce local uterine constriction and contraction rings, and although these may occur at any stage of labour they are most frequently seen during the second and third stages.

Achalasia of the cervix has been described as a separate entity (MacRae 1949), but it now appears to be just a manifestation of incoordinate uterine action. The cervix is taken up but the os fails to dilate completely. The edge of the cervix has a wire-like edge which resists attempts at mechanical dilatation. No abnormal amount of fibrous tissue has been discovered in this cervix (Dill 1950), and it is probably neurological in origin. Careful digital palpation will often detect a contraction of the internal cervical os with each uterine pain. If labour is allowed to continue the cervix may eventually become completely taken up posteriorly, but as a result of pressure between the foetal head and the symphysis pubis the anterior cervical lip becomes elongated and oedematous, and eventually spontaneous laceration of the cervix may permit delivery.

On rare occasions it would seem that the external os fails completely to dilate, and this is known as conglutination of the external os (Carter 1926). In these cases, spontaneous annular detachment of the cervix, probably at the fibro-muscular junction, may occur as a result of ischaemic necrosis from the downward thrust of the foetal head.

Incoordinate uterine action is very often associated with the occipitoposterior position, which is responsible for changing the uterine axis pressure (Arthure et al. 1961). With each contraction the foetal head is pushed downwards and forwards against the back of the pubis instead of directly downwards on to the cervix. In early labour the cervix is felt posterior to the foetal head, which attempts to sacculate the anterior wall of the lower segment. Later in labour the same pressure causes progressive oedema of the anterior lip of the cervix. If the head can be rotated and maintained in the anterior position cervical dilatation is then usually normally progressive. When the mother has her second confinement the resistance of the muscular pelvic floor is less, the foetal head undergoes spontaneous rotation to the occipitoanterior-position early in the first stage, and labour is rapidly progressive.

Cephalopelvic disproportion must always be suspected in prolonged labour, and this may or may not be associated with the occipitoposterior position. The recognition that a prolonged first stage often precedes a difficult and traumatic delivery has lead to the freer use of Caesarean section. Where maternity services are inadequate obstructed labour will occasionally be seen. The normal physiological retraction becomes exaggerated, so that a marked ring develops between the thinning lower segment and the thick upper segment. This pathological retraction ring of Bandl is pathognomonic of advanced obstructed labour. Occasionally, however, a full and oedematous bladder will create a transverse ridge in the lower abdomen which can be confused with a Bandl's ring. In obstructed labour, however, the presenting part is usually high, the cervix is oedematous, badly applied and hangs

like a curtain below the head. There is often dehydration, ketosis, intra-uterine infection and signs of foetal distress. Radiography will often confirm the disproportion. In the primigravida the uterus eventually becomes exhausted and ceases to contract (secondary inertia), but in the multigravida progressive thinning of the lower segment will result in uterine rupture.

MANAGEMENT OF PROLONGED LABOUR

Prophylaxis

Careful physiological antenatal preparation for labour of all pregnant women, especially primigravida, can play a helpful role in reducing the incidence of prolonged labour. Each antenatal interview should be conducted with an air of reassurance and pleasant anticipation. A simple explanation should be given of the physiological mechanism of labour and the associated bodily sensations, and the patient should be taught to relax and should be familiar with the various forms of available analgesia. Kartchner (1950), however, emphasizes that training education and indoctrination will be of benefit to those patients already well motivated for childbirth, but will have little effect on those with more severe emotional conflicts and upon unconscious motivating factors.

Since cephalopelvic disproportion is a strong predisposing factor, every effort should be made to exclude pelvic contraction before the onset of labour, and if an X-ray pelvimetry has not been performed it should be taken as soon as the delay is recognized. Breech presentation is corrected by external cephalic version after the thirty-second week.

Unless the indications are such that immediate termination of pregnancy is essential, surgical induction of labour is often best avoided. Where the foetus appears to be unduly large, induction after term is now often preferred, and in many centres the induction rate is between 12 and 20%

General treatment during the first stage

Because of the high incidence of instrumental delivery and morbidity, it is desirable that the entire labour should be conducted in hospital. This has, in addition, the advantage of removing the patient from a possible environment of over-anxious and fear-inducing relatives.

Routine swabs are taken from the throat and vagina. Urine is tested for acetone and albumen and after 24 hr of labour sent for culture. It is usual to give prophylactic antibiotics to patients whose membranes have been ruptured for more than 24 hr, to reduce the incidence of intra-uterine and foetal infection.

Every effort should be made to keep the fluid intake at not less than 2 l, and if this becomes difficult or acetonuria appears then a continuous intravenous 4% glucose–N/4 saline infusion is preferred.

During the early part of labour it is customary to provide pain relief with pethidine 150 mg given intramuscularly every 2–3 hr. This may be supplemented with chlorpromazine 50 mg intramuscularly. If more prolonged analgesia is required then morphine 15 mg intramuscularly is given, but after 24 hr of labour regional blocks are often used.

Special methods of treatment

OXYTOCIN

The use of posterior pituitary extract in ob-stetrics was pioneered by Hofbauer (1911) and later by Watson (1913), but the large doses used resulted in ruptured uteri, but Theobald *et al.* (1947) introduced the more physiological drip. It is now usual to give about 3 milli-units/min of oxytocin. Dosage above 5 milli-units/min is uncommon and it is very rare to use more. The rate of administration is regulated by the uterine response, and regular contractions (one every 3 min, say) with good relaxation of the uterus between contractions is ideal. Administration with a simple continuous intravenous drip is usually satisfactory, but when fluids and electro-lytes should be limited a continuous-infusion Palmer pump is helpful. Tocograph control and frequent or continuous recording of the foetal heart rate increases its safety. During the first few hours of the infusion the uterine contractions are often strong but painless. During this time

there is little cervical dilatation and the patient should not be relied upon to time the contractions. Labour tends to be shortened (O'Driscoll 1969), and this is a reflection of the more frequent con-tractions. Oxytocin is of particular value in hypotonic uterine inertia, and artificial rupture of the forewaters will increase its efficiency. In cases of incoordinate uterine action the uterus is liable to go into tonic spasm, and oxytocin is of little value and is potentially dangerous to the foetus.

Recently, O'Driscoll *et al.* (1969) have tried to eliminate prolonged labour by an active stimulation of the uterus in all cases where pro-gress appears to be slow. There were 1,000 primigravida of which 119 were stimulated—84 by low artificial rupture of membranes, 35 by membrane rupture and oxytocin drip, and 85 by oxytocin drip alone. Only one labour lasted more than 24 hr, although there were several patients admitted in a state of dehydration and ketosis which was attributed to narcosis, and who, it was claimed, were not in labour. Caesarean section was necessary in 40 cases (4%) and forceps or ventouse extraction in 189 cases (18·9%). There were three foetal intra-uterine deaths from hypoxia and one neonatal death, all of which could possibly have been due to the method. Some observers would question O'Driscoll's criterion of labour, which he defines as progressive dilatation of the cervix, but nevertheless, one must be impressed by these results. It is clear that the doctrine of masterly inactivity should be replaced by a more active therapy accompanied by careful personal supervision.

Other oxytocic substances including ergo-metrine and dihydro-ergotamine do not appear to have any advantages over synthetic oxytocin.

EPIDURAL AND CANDAL ANALGESIA

Following the pioneer work by Hingson & Edwards (1943) epidural analgesia has been used extensively in America for the relief of labour pain. In Great Britain it has never been popular, as its safe management requires the presence of a skilled anaesthetist throughout labour, and the abolition of the reflex expulsive efforts of the second stage demands a high forceps delivery rate. Nevertheless, Hellman (1965) reported 26,000 cases without maternal mortality and very low morbidity. More recently, Moir & Willocks (1967) have analysed the use of continuous epidural analgesia using 2% lignocaine with 1:200,000 adrenalin in 100 cases of incoordinate uterine action. Complications included dural puncture (2%), puncture of epidural vein (3%), and paravertebral passage of the catheter and hypotension (15%). Other series have reported retention of broken catheter, permanent paresis attributed to toxic effect of analgesic drug, and infection. It is common experience to find that when the block is maintained for more than 10 hr the repeated injections of lignocaine become progressively less effective (tachyphylaxis), and for this reason it would seem wise not to induce the epidural block too soon, but to await at least 4 cm cervical dilatation. The block appears to increase the rate of cervical dilatation one and a half times, in addition to providing complete analgesia free from narcosis. A continued slow rate of dilatation after the block suggests disproportion, and in Moir & Willocks series 26% required Caesarean section. There is no increased incidence of postpartum haemorrhage and there is some evidence that maternal placental site blood flow is increased (Johnson 1957). Candal analgesia is preferred by Johnson, but in the obese patient this may prove technically difficult and the risk of sepsis may be increased.

PARACERVICAL NERVE BLOCK

Cooper & Chassar Moir (1963) reported the use of 1% lignocaine in paracervical block, but the main disadvantage was the short duration of 1–2 hr. Gudgeon (1968) reports the use of bupivacaine 0·25% with adrenalin 1:400,000, which provides pain relief for about 3 hr in 87% of cases. Cervical dilation is not delayed and the block may be repeated. Gordon (1968), however, has shown that the foetal bradycardia which is sometimes observed is due directly to a high foetal blood level of bupivacaine, and this constitutes a foetal hazard. Murphy *et al.* (1970) have reported 118 cases with foetal bradycardia in 11% and two foetal deaths.

THE VACUUM EXTRACTOR IN THE FIRST STAGE

The concept of assisting delivery using a suction device was first used by Yonge (1706), since when there have been many developments. The metal cap devised by Malmstrom (1957) is now widely used, and in many countries has largely replaced the use of forceps. It is not without its potential dangers, including the risk of intracranial haemorrhage (Ahuja *et al.* 1969). As an instrument for delivery at full dilatation of the cervix it has its limitations. Chalmers (1964) reports a 10% failure in cases that were subsequently delivered successfully with forceps.

When labour has progressed for more than 24 hr and the cervix is more than 5 cm dilated, the application of a small Malstrom cup may prove useful. The perineum is infiltrated with local analgesic and the small cup carefully introduced through the cervix. A vacuum of 0·7 kg/cm² is established slowly over 10 min. Traction is applied intermittently for a maximum of 40 min. Each traction effort should last not longer than 5 sec and this is followed by a pause. Every 5 min the vacuum is reduced to 0·2 kg/cm² for 1 min; and then returned without delay to 0·7 kg/cm². By using this technique the risks of cephalohaematoma, scalp necrosis, retinal haemorrhage and tearing of the tentorium cerebelli are reduced to a minimum. The head is pulled down progressively on to the cervix, which should dilate rapidly with each uterine contraction. The resistance of the pelvic floor may encourage rotation of the head to the occipito-anterior position, but this tends to occur very late when the outlet has been reached, and this is a serious disadvantage. Excessive traction may cause tearing of the cervix, but detachment of the cup usually provides some measure of safety.

ROTATION IN THE FIRST STAGE

If the head is in the occipitoposterior position and the cervix has reached 7 cm dilatation, rotation to the occipito-anterior position will, in most cases, effect immediate full dilatation and permit safe vaginal delivery. This type of delivery should be conducted in an operating theatre under general anaesthesia. The rotation and extraction is performed slowly, and is most easily accomplished with Kielland's forceps. If undue difficulty is encountered there should be no hesitation in proceeding to immediate Caesarean section. Rotation at 3–4 cm dilatation of the cervix has been used successfully (Arthure *et al.* 1961) but this should only be attempted by those highly skilled in use of Kielland's forceps. Following the rotation the forceps are removed and labour will then often progress rapidly. Any signs of foetal distress or a return to the occipito-posterior position demands immediate Caesarean section.

CERVICAL INCISIONS

Duhrssen's cervical incisions are now rarely employed, but may still have a place in carefully selected cases, especially when facilities for Caesarean section are poor. The duration of the first stage should not be less than 36 hr, and this will insure that the cervix is completely taken up and the vault of the vagina is dilated sufficiently to accommodate the head. Under general anaesthesia the head is rotated with Kielland's forceps to the occipito-anterior position and pulled well down on to the cervix. The forceps are steadied by an assistant, who will also retract the lateral vaginal walls. Straight, round-ended scissors are guided through the cervix along the upper edge of the forceps blade and two incisions 1 inch in length made at 10 o'clock and 2 o'clock. This creates a small, anterior cervical flap, and slow extraction of the head is then possible. Under no circumstances should cervical incisions be employed in the presence of foetal distress or cephalopelvic disproportion. After delivery the cervix is successfully repaired with interrupted catgut sutures. The application of the vacuum extractor nowadays appears preferable.

CONSTRICTION RING DYSTOCIA

A constriction ring around the foetal neck is most likely to develop following prolonged labour, stimulation with oxytocin, and any form of intra-uterine manipulation. It should always be suspected in the multigravida who experiences delay in the first stage and who has had a previously easy labour. Diagnosis is usually made when attempts to deliver with forceps fail. The head can be pulled down by the forceps but returns immediately to its previous level when traction is released. An inhalation of amyl nitrite 2 ml placed beneath the anaesthetic mask will, in most cases, effect rapid relaxation of the constriction ring and permit easy delivery. Rarely, the amyl nitrite may have to be repeated and the anaesthesia deepened. In the event of complete failure the child is likely to be dead, in which case perforation of the head and heavy forceps traction may be necessary. Should the child still be alive delivery by Caesarean section, using a longitudinal incision to divide the contraction ring, would be permissible under antibiotic cover.

CAESAREAN SECTION

The development of general anaesthesia, the blood transfusion service, potent antibiotics, and a clearer understanding of fluid and electrolyte balance, together with a more extensive training of obstetric specialists, has effected a progressive fall in both maternal and foetal mortality and morbidity. Caesarean section is now employed more freely, and has rendered many of the more difficult vaginal manipulations almost obsolete.

The use of foetal scalp blood sampling to detect early respiratory and metabolic acidosis (Beard 1968); foetal heart monitoring (Huntingford *et al.* 1969) and amnioscopy (Henry 1969) have all proved useful in selecting patients for Caesarean section, and have helped to avoid unnecessary operations. If, however, after 24 hr of incoordinate uterine action the cervix is no more than 3 cm dilated, or after 36 hr in labour no more than 5 cm dilated, and especially if the head is still high in the pelvis, then lower-segment Caesarean section is indicated. It must be remembered that uterine action improves with each pregnancy, and when Caesarean section is performed in the first pregnancy the outcome of the second is largely dependent upon the degree of cervical dilatation reached at the time of the first operation. Where the patient is young, and will in all probability become pregnant again, a slightly more conservative policy may be adopted in an effort to obtain vaginal delivery, but this should not be permitted at the expense of undue maternal hardships of foetal morbidity.

REFERENCES

AHUJA G.L., WILLOUGHBY M.L.N., KERR M.M. & HUTCHINSON J.H. (1969) *Br. med. J.* ii, 743.

ARTHURE H. & HOLMES J.M. (1961) *J. Obstet. Gynaec. Br. Commonw.* 68, 82.

BEARD R.W. (1:68) *J. Obstet. Gynaec. Br. Commonw.* 75, 1291.

CALDEYRO R., ALVAREZ H. & REYNOLD S.R.M. (1950) *Am. J. Obstet. Gynec.* 91, 1.

CARTER P.J. (1926) *Am. J. Obstet. Gynec.* 11, 828.

CHALMERS J.A. (1964) *Br. med. J.* i, 1216.

COOPER K. & CHASSAR MOIR J. (1963) *Br. med. J.* i, 1372.

CSAPO A., WOLSTENHOLME G.E.W. & CAMERON M.P. (editors) (1961) *Progesterone and Defence Mechanism of Pregnancy.* London, Churchill.

DILL L.V. (1950) *Am. J. Obstet. Gynec.* 59, 785.

GORDON H.R. (1968) *New. Engl. J. Med.* 279, 947.

GUDGEON D.H. (1968) *Br. med. J.* ii, 403.

HELLMAN K. (1965) *Can. Anaesth. Soc. J.* 12, 398.

HELLMAN I.H., HARRIS J.S. & REYNOLDS S.R.M. (1950) *Am. J. Obstet. Gynec.* 60, 47.

HENRY G.R. (1969) *J. Obstet. Gynaec. Br. Commonw.* 76, 790.

HINGSON R.A. & EDWARDS W.B. (1943) *J. Am. med. Ass.* 121, 225.

HOFBAUER J. *Zentbl. Gynäk.* (1911) 35, 137.

HUNTINGFORD P.J. & PENDLETON H.J. (1969) *J. Obstet. Gynaec. Br. Commonw.* 76, 586.

JOHNSON G.T. (1957) *Br. med. J.* ii, 386.

KARTCHNER F.D. (1950) *Am. J. Obstet. Gynec.* 60, 19.

MacRAE D.J. (1949) *J. Obstet. Gynaec. Br. Commonw.* 56, 785.

MALMSTROM T. (1957) *Acta obstet. gynec. scand.* 36 (Supplement 3), 27.

MOIR D.D. & WILLOCKS J. (1967) *Br. med. J.* ii, 396.

MURPHY P.J., WRIGHT J.D. & FITZGERALD T.B. (1970) *Br. med. J.* i 526.

O'DRISCOLL K., JACKSON R.J.A. & GALLAGHER J.T. (1969) *Br. med. J.* ii, 477.

THEOBALD G.W., GRAHAM A., CAMPBELL J., GRAINGE P.D. & DRISCOLL W.J. (1948) *Br. med. J.* ii, 123.

WATSON B.P. (1913) *Can. med. Ass. J.* 3(NS), 739.

WILLIAMS B. (1942) *J. Obstet. Gynaec. Br. Commonw.* 49, 412.

YONGE J. (1706) *Phil Trans. R. Soc.* B25, 2387.

CHAPTER 24

CONTRACTED PELVIS, DISPROPORTION AND OBSTRUCTED LABOUR

Disproportion exists when the relative sizes of head and pelvis are such that the one cannot pass through the other. With pelvic bony disease less common than formerly, significant disproportion is encountered less frequently than it was in the past. Minor degrees are not uncommon, however, and the search for disproportion is a most important part of antenatal care during late pregnancy.

Labour may become obstructed for reasons of disproportion or for a variety of other reasons to be considered in this chapter.

There has been a gradual improvement in the standards of antenatal care and many of the underlying causes of obstructed labour can be recognized, and serious difficulties are now frequently prevented or anticipated before the onset of labour. Furthermore, the freer use of Caesarean section has rendered obsolete many of the more difficult and potentially dangerous vaginal manipulations that were often performed late in labour in the presence of a thin lower segment and an infected uterine cavity.

Common causes of obstructed labour include contraction or deformity of the bony pelvis, persistent posterior or lateral position of the foetal head, shoulder presentation, and a large foetus.

Uncommon maternal causes include tumours of the uterus, ovary, rectum, bladder and bony pelvis; pelvic kidney; stenosis of the vagina or cervix; congenital septum of the vagina; contraction ring of the uterus and sacculation of the uterus.

Uncommon foetal causes include breech, face, brow and compound presentations; locked twins; hydrocephaly; iniencephaly; hydrops foetalis, foetal tumour, etc.

CONTRACTED PELVIS

The pelvis can be classified according to the shape of the pelvic brim (Caldwell *et al.* 1940) (Fig. 24.1). Although less importance is now attached to these parent types, some knowledge of them and the differences between them may be helpful in the management of individual cases.

The gynaecoid pelvis (Fig. 24.1) is the normal female pelvis, with a slightly oval brim, the largest transverse diameter lying mid-way beween the front and the back of the pelvis. The anterior and posterior walls of the pelvis are parallel and the subpubic arch is wide. The android pelvis, or male pelvis (Fig. 24.1) has a heart-shaped brim in which the widest transverse diameter is situated towards the back of the brim; the pelvic walls tend to converge so that the outlet is somewhat narrowed, the ischial spines are prominent and the angle of the arch is more acute. The majority of female pelves tend to resemble one or other of the two above types. There are, however, two less common varieties: the platypelloid, or flat, pelvis, and the anthropoid pelvis. In the former (Fig. 24.1) the pelvic brim is narrowed from front to back, giving it a flat, kidney-shaped appearance, whilst in the latter the opposite is the case, the brim being narrower from side to side than anteroposteriously. These variations may have some influence upon the manner in which the

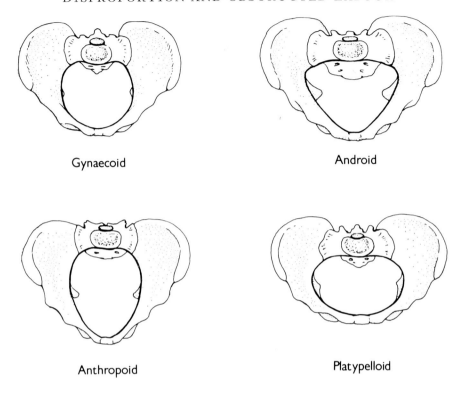

Gynaecoid

Android

Anthropoid

Platypelloid

Classification of pelvic brim shape

Fig. 24.1. Illustrations of the four parent types of female pelvis.

head passes through the pelvis. In the android pelvis, for instance, in which the widest part of the brim is at the back, the occipitoposterior position is often found, and late in labour deep transverse arrest of the head may occur at the level of the prominent ischial spines. In the anthropoid pelvis, on the other hand, the head will tend to engage with the occiput directly backwards or forwards, and will remain in this position throughout delivery.

Pelvic bony disease may significantly alter the pelvic size of shape, although such diseases are now, fortunately, rare in this country. At one time rickets was common and rachitic flattening of the pelvis caused serious obstetric problems. In this condition the sacral promontory is thrust forwards by the weight of the upper part of the body, causing contraction to the anteroposterior diameter of the pelvic brim, and the ilia are flared outwards so that the inter-spinous and intercristal external diameters are virtually the same. The transverse diameter of the brim tends to be fairly large. As the sacral promontory is carried forwards, the lower part of the sacrum is rotated backwards, so that the outlet of the pelvis may be larger than usual. Osteomalacia, again extremely rare in Britain, may give rise to a similar type of deformity.

Local disease of the hip (tuberculosis, sup-purative arthritis, Perthes's disease, etc.) may interfere with growth and mobility of one side of the pelvis, imparting an obliquity to the brim—this, however, does not usually cause significant contraction, nor interfere with the normal process

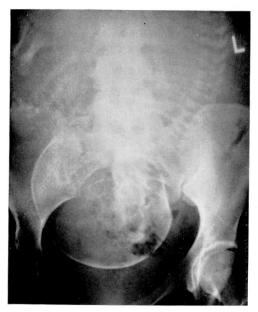

Fig. 24.2. Obliquity of the pelvic brim resulting from foetal abnormality of the right hip; note absence of the head of the femur from the right acetabulum.

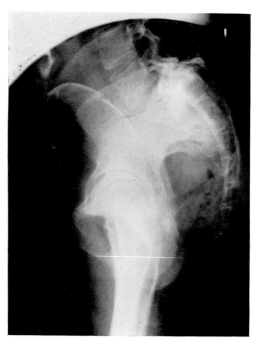

Fig. 24.3. A radiograph in a case of spondylolisthesis.

of delivery (Fig. 24.2). A significant reduction in the anteroposterior diameter of the brim may, however, be found in the somewhat uncommon condition of spondylolisthesis (Fig. 24.3), in which the lumbar vertebrae slide forwards on the sacral promontory, curtailing, perhaps markedly, the space available.

Alterations to the pelvic shape and the pelvic brim inclination may be associated with kyphoscoliosis or poliomyelitis. Kyphoscoliosis affecting the thoracic spine is likely to be compensated by a lumbar lordosis which greatly increases the angle of inclination of the brim, so as to make it almost vertical (Fig. 24.4). Lumbar kyphosis, however, may have the opposite effect of reducing the brim angle (Fig. 24.5). The problems associated with kyphoscoliosis are not all mechanical ones affecting the pelvis and head, however; cardiovascular complications may be just as important, or more so (Dewhurst 1953). Poliomyelitis affecting one leg may produce a type of oblique contraction similar to that seen with hip disease. Manning *et al.* (1967) and Chau & Lee (1970) have also reviewed this subject.

Caldwell *et al.*'s terms are still often used when describing radiological appearances, although the shape of the brim does not bear any consistent relationship to either the shape or size of the cavity, or the outlet of the pelvis. Brim appearances alone are of little assistance in the clinical management and, indeed, efforts to forecast the outcome of labour by radiological pelvimetry in borderline cases of disproportion have not been successful (Williams *et al.* 1949). Nevertheless, a full pelvimetry—including a lateral film with the patient standing, an anteroposterior of the pelvis and a film of the subpubic arch—can be of great value. Serious difficulties can be anticipated before the onset of labour, the level of rotation can be selected before attempts are made to effect instrumental delivery, and a lateral film taken late in labour will reveal much useful data (including the degree of moulding and asynclitism), as well as confirming the position of the head and the relative size of the pelvis.

A reduction in the true conjugate to below 10 cm is most often seen in the simple flat pelvis or, more rarely, in the rachitic, flat pelvis. The

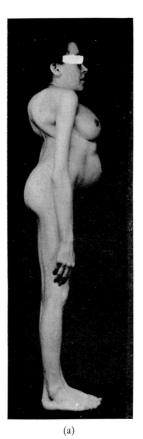

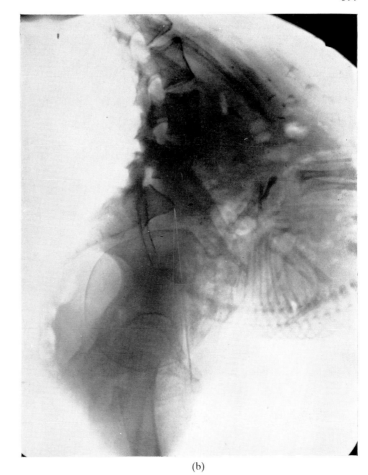

Fig. 24.4. (a) A patient 4 ft tall with thoracic kyphoscoliosis. (b) A radiograph of the patient seen in (a). Note vertical brim and engaged head.

head engages with its long axis in the transverse diameter of the brim. The head is shifted towards the side of the pelvis to which the occiput is directed, and this, together with slight extension of the head, brings the wide biparietal diameter nearer to the occipital pole and away from the forward projection of the sacral promontory. The head is tilted towards the posterior shoulder (anterior asynclitism or anterior parietal presentation). The diameter of engagement becomes the super-subparietal diameter, 8·6 cm (3½ in), and the anterior parietal bone may then be able to slip down into the pelvis, before the posterior parietal bone is forced past the sacral promontory.

The cavity and outlet of the flat pelvis is usually adequate, and once the head has negotiated the pelvic brim a rapid and normal delivery can be anticipated soon afterwards.

The funnel pelvis is commonly seen with an android brim. The fore part of the pelvis is diminished and this tends to encourage an occipitoposterior position. The head engages after the onset of labour and is often arrested at mid-cavity. The associated flat sacrum and prominent ischial spines cause deep transverse arrest at or near full dilatation. Delivery is made more difficult by the narrow, subpubic arch, which reduces the effective anteroposterior diameter

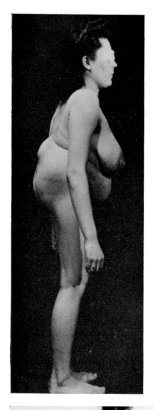

(a)

(b)

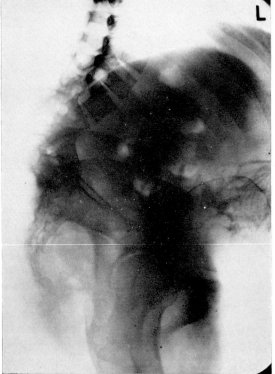

Fig. 24.5. (a) A patient 4 ft 5 in tall with lumbar
kyphoscoliosis. (b) A radiograph of the patient seen in
(a). Note flat plane of the brim.

of the pelvis and forces the head backwards against the perineum and rectum.

Women of large stature (over 5 ft 9 in) usually have a large pelvis with an anthropod-shaped brim. The 5th lumbar vertebra is often fused to the sacrum (high assimilation pelvis), and this may cause a false promontory and a brim inclination of 80°. The head engages in the occipito-posterior position and spontaneous delivery face to pubes is common.

MANAGEMENT OF SUSPECTED DISPROPORTION

If the head has failed to engage in the pelvic brim by the thirty-sixth week, contracted pelvis should be suspected. This can usually be safely excluded by clinical pelvimetry, and an internal examination made by an experienced obstetrician will often spare the patient unnecessary exposure to radiation. In cases of doubt, the size of the pelvis and foetal head will be assessed by X-ray pelvimetry and ultrasonic methods. If the true conjugate is 8 cm or less and the foetus of average size, an elective Caesarean section is indicated. Between 8 and 9·5 cm considerable difficulty can be anticipated. Over 9·5 cm a relatively easy vaginal delivery is usual, but the progress of labour depends very much upon the size and position of the foetal head. No amount of investigation can accurately forecast the strength of the uterine contractions, the elasticity of the pelvic joints, the resistance of the pelvic floor, the degree of moulding of the skull, the rate of cervical dilatation, the efficiency of the placenta in maintaining adequate foetal requirements, and the emotional and physical fortitude of the mother. It is for these reasons that cases of borderline pelvic contraction are submitted to trial of labour.

Trial of labour

Induction of labour is best avoided, and the spontaneous onset of labour is awaited until at least 10 days over term unless the baby appears to be exceptionally large. Frequent vaginal examinations are made to exclude presentation and pro-lapse of the cord. Progress is assessed by noting the descent of the head on abdominal palpation and, on vaginal examination, the characteristics of the cervix—including dilatation and taking up and position in relation to the head; a lateral X-ray of the pelvis may be of considerable value. The membranes are to be ruptured at half dilatation, the appearance of the liquor amnii noted and, if necessary, a foetal scalp blood sample taken. If after a further 6 hr of strong labour the head has failed to engage in the pelvic brim insuperable disproportion can be diagnosed, and a lower-segment Caesarean section is performed without delay. Even when the head engages, delivery with forceps will usually be required. Unfortunately, it is not always possible to exclude absolute disproportion, as threatened foetal distress may demand immediate delivery by Caesarean section. Nevertheless, every effort should be made to prove the pelvis during the first labour, as the presence of a Caesarean section scar will always weaken the uterus and render subsequent trial of labour more hazardous.

Hawksworth (1952) reported on 124 cases of trial of labour delivered at Oxford from 1948 to 1951. Only 29 (23%) had a normal delivery, 44 (36%) had a forceps delivery and 51 (41%) required a Caesarean section.

Trial of forceps

This method of management (Jeffcoate 1953) is reserved for those unusual cases of contracted outlet. The head engages in the pelvic brim, but only after the onset of labour and eventually becomes arrested high mid-cavity. Under general anaesthesia the head is brought into the anterior position and moderately heavy traction is applied intermittently with forceps. If the head fails to descend the forceps are removed and Caesarean section performed. This type of delivery should be conducted in an operating theatre, and only by the highly experienced obstetrician.

SYMPHYSIOTOMY

This operation is rarely performed in Great Britain, where repeated Caesarean section is more acceptable. In underdeveloped countries, where communications are poor and the population is widely scattered, there may be difficulty in reaching hospital. The patient will eventually arrive late in labour, which is obstructed by cephalopelvic disproportion. The birth canal is often infected and the soft tissues are friable and oedematous. Attempts at difficult forceps delivery will add trauma to the already ischaemic bladder base and may easily cause a vesicovaginal fistula. Caesarean section could disseminate intra-uterine infection, and will leave the patient with a vulnerable uterine scar for future pregnancies. Symphysiotomy skilfully performed will enlarge the pelvis at all levels, will overcome the obstruction, and will permit safe vaginal deliveries both immediately and in future pregnancies. It is contra-indicated when the true conjugate is less than 8 cm, the brim is less than 70 cm², or when the foetus is over 4·3 kg

($9\frac{1}{2}$ lb). The cervix should be at least half dilated. Previous Caesarean section for pelvic contraction, sacro-iliac instability, and locomotor disturbances are also contra-indications.

The pubic area is infiltrated with 0·5% lignocaine. A No. 20 Foley catheter is inserted into the bladder. The fibrocartilagenous disc of the symphysis is identified with a needle. Two fingers in the vagina displace the catheter and urethra away from the mid-line. While the symphysis is divided with a one-piece, handle-bladed scalpel (Fig. 24.6). If the cervix is nearly fully dilated, early delivery can be anticipated and a pudendal block and deep episiotomy will reduce stretching of the vaginal walls and the risk of bladder fistulae. If there is delay a large, Malmstrom vacuum extractor cup may be applied and intermittent traction effected for not more than 10 min (Bird *et al.* 1967). This is much safer than forceps delivery, and either manual

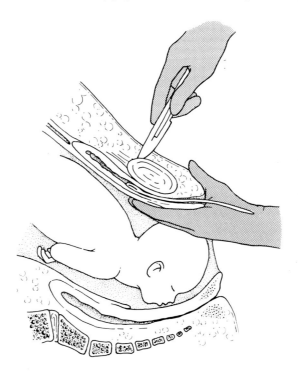

Symphysiotomy

Fig. 24.6. A drawing of the procedure of symphysiotomy.

or Kielland forceps rotation is particularly dangerous under these circumstances. Following delivery, open bladder drainage is maintained for 3 days, and the legs are kept strapped together for 24 hr (Iseedat *et al.* 1962). Haematoma, sepsis, stress incontinence, pubic pain and backache are occasional complications.

Seedat & Crichton (1962) report 505 cases of symphysiotomy performed on Bantu women with pelvic disproportion. Of the 478 cases in which the operation was undertaken for a planned trial of labour there were 23 perinatal deaths. No maternal death was attributable to the operation. Complications attributable to the operation were uncommon; in the whole series of 505 cases these consisted of ambulatory difficulty in 16 and stress incontinence in 5.

Pubiotomy is an obsolete operation attended by a high risk of osteomyelitis.

DYSTOCIA DUE TO SOFT-TISSUE OBSTRUCTION

FIBROIDS

Fibroids situated in the upper segment may undergo red degeneration during pregnancy, but do not cause obstruction during labour. Even those situated in the lower segment and below the presenting part are usually drawn up during the first stage, and permit unobstructed vaginal delivery. If the fibroid is situated in the cervix, then Caesarean section is necessary. Fibroids can become ischaemic and infected during the puerperium. If the fibroid mass is large and the family is complete an elective Caesarean/hysterectomy is sometimes indicated.

OVARIAN CYSTS

Ovarian cysts will only obstruct labour if they are situated below the pelvic brim. It is sometimes possible, in early labour or before, to push the cyst out of the pelvis by gentle digital pressure through the vagina. A steep Trendelenburg position and a short, general anaesthetic may assist this manipulation. The cyst often has a long pedicle, and torsion is particularly likely to occur in the puerperium. For this reason, removal 2 days after delivery is recommended. A cyst which is within the pelvis and which cannot be pushed above the presenting part will obstruct labour, and Caesarean section is necessary. Under no circumstances should the foetal head be pulled past the obstructing cyst.

CICATRIZATION OF THE CERVIX

Severe scarring of the cervix may follow amputation of the portio vaginalis, deep cauterization, trachelorrhaphy and other operations. Adhesions may follow lacerations of previous labour. Failure of the cervix to dilate under these circumstances is most likely to be seen where there has been a prolonged interval between pregnancies and the patient is reaching the end of her fertile life. When the scarred cervix has thinned out in response to labour it may be possible to effect safe delivery after cervical incisions, but in other cases Caesarean section will be preferred.

CARCINOMA OF THE CERVIX

Carcinoma of the cervix during pregnancy tends to be highly malignant with poor prognosis, and this demands treatment without delay. The uterus is evacuated by hysterotomy or classical Caesarean section performed under antibiotic cover, followed 10 days later by full radium therapy. Occasionally, classical Caesarean section is followed by an extended Wertheim's hysterectomy.

VAGINAL ABNORMALITIES

Cicatricial contraction may follow previous lacerations or ulceration. Severe stenosis is sometimes seen in underdeveloped communities following the insertion of rock salt into the vagina immediately after delivery. This is done in an effort to reduce the vagina to its premarital size.

Resistant perineal muscles, oedema of the vulva, haematoma from rupture of varicose veins within the vaginal wall, adhesions of the labia, and rigid hymen can be incised. In cases of haematoma formation the clot is evacuated by digital pressure, and following delivery the bleeding is arrested either by undersewing or by a vaginal pack left *in situ* for 24 hr.

A vaginal septum does not usually cause obstruction, but may have to be divided and the edges subsequently oversewn.

PENDULOUS ABDOMEN

This condition is usually seen in the multigravida of short stature and with a contracted pelvic brim. Previous vaginal deliveries may have been possible, but if the foetus is larger then complete obstruction may occur. An abdominal binder will support the abdomen and may encourage engagement if the pelvis is adequate.

RETROVERSION OF THE FULL-TERM, GRAVID UTERUS

This is a rarity which is treated by Caesarean section. Labour leads to complete obstruction, foetal death and, possibly, uterine rupture.

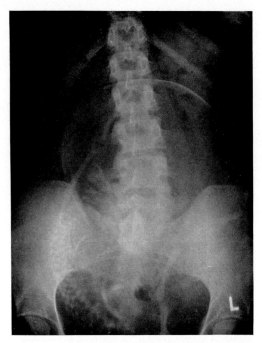

Fig. 24.7. A radiograph showing a large hydrocephalic head in a foetus presenting by the breech.

FOETAL ABNORMALITIES CAUSING OBSTRUCTION

HYDROCEPHALY

The diagnosis may be easy. The large head is felt above the pelvic brim, the widely separated cranial bones are felt through the dilating cervix, and an X-ray will confirm the wide separation and thinning of the cranial vault bones (Fig. 24.7). An ultrasonic scan will give the true size of the head (Fig. 24.8). Mild degrees of hydrocephaly may be overlooked or cause difficulty in forceps extraction. In cases of doubt, Caesarean section will always be preferred to destructive operations.

When diagnosis is certain, a cephalic presentation renders treatment easier, since the head can then be perforated at 3 cm dilation of the cervix, using a Simpson's perforator. The hole is kept open with a short length of pressure rubber tubing while the head collapses. Some obstetricians prefer a wide-bore needle, and claim

there is less risk of maternal injury. If the perforator has been used it is important to pass a sponge holder through the hole and to destroy the medulla, before delivery is completed.

If the foetus is delivered as a breech the head cannot be perforated until the trunk is delivered through the fully dilated cervix. Gross hydrocephaly may cause uterine rupture before full dilatation is reached, and in this case a needle should be inserted under local anaesthetic through the abdominal and uterine wall. Lesser degrees may be dealt with at the time of delivery. If there is an associated spina bifida, a metal cannula can be inserted into the open spinal canal. Otherwise, a small, transverse incision is made between the cervical vertebrae, and the dilated spinal canal exposed. Direct perforation of the aftercoming head is difficult, and may lead to severe maternal injury. The Catholic obstetrician is reluctant to perforate, but Caesarean section may prove difficult. A very large uterine incision is necessary, and this may cause damage to the uterine vessels, with loss of the uterus by hysterectomy.

the spine. Induction of labour at 32 weeks may permit vaginal delivery of a small foetus; otherwise, Caesarean section is necessary.

DOUBLE MONSTERS

Diagnosis is made by antenatal X-ray. If foetal survival and subsequent surgical separation seem possible, then Caesarean section at 38 weeks is the delivery of choice; otherwise, surgical induction at 30 weeks may permit vaginal delivery.

OTHER FOETAL ABNORMALITIES

Hydrothorax, ascites, full bladder and spina bifida are reduced by needle aspiration. Congenital cystic kidneys and protrusion of enlarged viscera may, rarely, require evisceration.

SHOULDER DYSTOCIA

One of the most exasperating complications of the actual delivery of a baby is that of shoulder dystocia. It usually occurs without warning, often during an otherwise uncomplicated confinement and at nearly the last moment of delivery when the baby is almost born and a successful outcome seems assured. The complication is generally associated with the presence of a much larger baby than has been suspected. This is well illustrated by a most dramatic case of shoulder dystocia recorded by Gould & Pyle (1901).

In 1871 Captain Martin Bates and Miss Anne Swan, calling themselves the tallest couple in the world, were married at the church of St. Martin-in-the-Fields in London. Miss Swan was 7 ft $5\frac{1}{2}$ in tall, Captain Bates 7 ft $2\frac{1}{2}$ in. During Mrs. Bates's second confinement great difficulty was experienced. Forceps were used for the delivery but could not be easily applied owing to the height of the head and the length of the vagina. When the head was born insurmountable shoulder dystocia was encountered. Finally, after another physician had been summoned by telegram and after 'a laborious siege', the patient was delivered of a stillborn male child weighing 23 lb 12 oz.

Few of us are likely to be faced with a problem of this degree, but the difficulties encountered in shoulder dystocia can be great nonetheless.

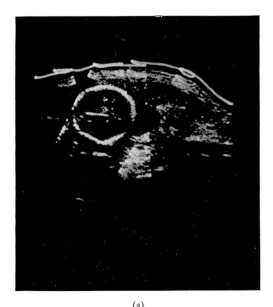

(a)

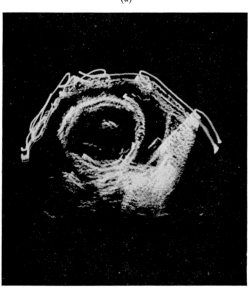

(b)

Fig. 24.8. (a) An ultrasonic picture of a normal head of about 36 weeks' gestation. (b) A greatly enlarged hydrocephalic head; same gestation as (a).

INIENCEPHALY

The soft tissues over the occipital and sacral regions are fused and there is gross extension of

It has already been emphasized, advisably, that the complication occurs when the baby's head is *almost* born, because the very first sign of shoulder impaction is failure of the head to extend fully over the perineum. Only with difficulty is the mouth exposed and the chin freed. If the attendant at the confinement fails to appreciate the significance of this sign then he will wait in vain for further advance, the baby's head all the time becoming more and more congested. Finally when it is clear that arrest has occurred some desperate measure is necessary in an attempt to deliver the child.

This physical sign of failure of the baby's head fully to extend at the last moment is a very important point. It suggests that the shoulders are a very tight fit and are even becoming impacted. One of the attendants should then exert strong downward pressure on the mother's lower abdomen to thrust the anterior shoulder down behind the symphysis pubis, if necessary, climbing on the bed to do so. At the same time another attendant takes the baby's head and draws it posteriorly to exert traction on the same shoulder (Fig. 24.9). This combination of abdominal and vaginal manœuvres will usually release the shoulder in time. But time is the one thing we do not have if this complication arises, which is why it is so important to recognize at once the significance of the physical sign described of failure of the head fully to extend at the last moment of delivery.

Some authorities suggest that to relieve the obstruction the hand be placed into the vagina and the shoulders rotated or the posterior shoulder brought down (Kinch 1962). This may be successful but it is a very difficult manœuvre indeed, because the baby's head seems so to fill the lower part of the pelvis and vagina that manipulation alongside it is well-nigh impossible. Sometimes, the pressure necessary to delivery the baby is very great, and in one recent personal case during attempts to deliver a baby $11\frac{1}{2}$ lb in weight bilateral Erb's baby was produced which, happily, recovered spontaneously. This complication arises infrequently [0·15% of all deliveries, according to Kinch (1962)], but because it occurs so unexpectedly a high foetal mortality results from it.

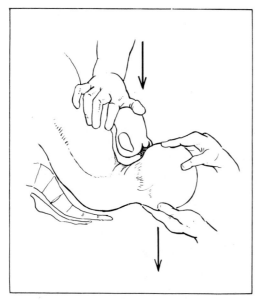

Fig. 24.9. Manœuvre for relief of shoulder dystocia.

REFERENCES

BIRD G.C. & BAL J.G. (1967) *J. Obstet. Gynaec. Br. Commonw.* **74**, 266.

CALDWELL W.E., MOLOY H.C. & D'ESOPO D.A. (1940) *Am. J. Roentg.* **40**, 558.

CHAU W. & LEE K.H. (1970) *J. Obstet. Gynaec. Br. Commonw.* **77**, 1098.

GOULD G.M. & PYLE W.L. (1901) *Anomalies and Curiosities of Medicine*. Philadelphia, Saunders.

HAWKSWORTH W. (1952) *Proc. R. Soc. Med.* **45**, 527.

JEFFCOATE T.N.A. (1953) *Br. med. J.* ii, 951.

KINCH R.A.H. (1962) *Clin. Obstet. Gynec.* **5**, 1031.

MANNING C.W., PRIME F.J. & ZORAB P.A. (1967) *Lancet*, ii, 792.

SEEDAT E.K. & CRICHTON D. (1962) *Lancet*, i, 554.

WILLIAMS E.R. & ARTHURE H.G.E. (1949) *J. Obstet. Gynaec. Br. Commonw.* **56**, 560.

CHAPTER 25

COMPLICATIONS OF THE THIRD STAGE
OF LABOUR

Some of the complications which arise after the birth of the infant can be anticipated and avoided, while others result from complications during the actual delivery.

Haemorrhage

This may be traumatic or atonic in origin.

(a) Trauma

Bleeding from a perineal laceration or episiotomy is likely to be obvious, and prompt ligation of the damaged vessel and repair of the wound is usually sufficient. Vaginal or cervical lacerations may be suspected if there has been any difficulty during the delivery or if it was precipitate. If the bleeding continues when the uterus is well contracted, particularly after an oxytocic drug has been administered, traumatic haemorrhage is confirmed. Immediate exploration is required, and this is best undertaken under general anaesthesia. Vaginal lacerations are readily seen if a good light is available and if the cervix can be grasped and pulled away from the bleeding area. Repair of the laceration with deep sutures will usually control the haemorrhage. When the cervix is being examined, a vaginal speculum is inserted and the anterior lip of the cervix is lightly grasped with sponge-holding forceps. By using two or three pairs of these forceps it is possible to examine the whole of the loose cervix and to identify the bleeding area. This should be ligated and deep cervical lacerations should be repaired with interrupted catgut sutures, al-

though there is some controversy about the subject of cervical repair in general.

Haemorrhage from a lacerated or ruptured uterus should be suspected if bleeding persists even when the uterus appears to have responded to ergometrine and when no vaginal or cervical cause can be found. Full exploration under general anaesthesia, with blood available for transfusion, is then required. If a vaginal delivery has followed a previous Caesarean section, exploration of the site of the previous incision is required, particularly if there is excessive bleeding or if the labour and delivery have been complicated. Rupture of the uterus is nearly always treated by hysterectomy, but it may be possible to control the haemorrhage and repair the rupture. Whether a subsequent pregnancy will be possible with safety depends on a number of factors, but generally, pregnancy should be avoided.

A haematoma may form in the broad ligament as a result of damage to the uterus, but this can usually be managed conservatively with blood transfusion, and antibiotics to prevent secondary infection. The diagnosis of this complication is not always easy, a progressive anaemia in association with tenderness and a swelling in one or other iliac fossa possibly being the only features. Acute symptoms may not be present because of limitation of the haemorrhage by the broad ligament.

(b) Atony

Atonic haemorrhage is associated with the inability of the uterus to contract effectively and efficiently. This may be due to a number of factors:

(i) Retained products of conception. A placental cotelydon or fragment, or even membranes, may prevent efficient contraction of the uterine muscle.

(ii) Prolonged labour with inertia of the uterus.

(iii) General anaesthesia, especially if halothane or cyclopropane have been used.

(iv) Over-distension of the uterus, as is associated with hydramnios and, possibly, multiple pregnancy.

(v) A large placental site, as is found in multiple pregnancy and hydrops foetalis; perhaps over-distension is present, and there may also have been disordered uterine action.

(vi) Multiple fibromyomata, especially of the interstitial type, because of the resulting ineffective uterine contraction and retraction.

(vii) Placenta praevia, because of the inability of the lower uterine segment to retract.

(viii) Abruptio placentae, where there is interstitial uterine haemorrhage and later hypofibrinogenaemia.

(ix) Grand multiparae, with an increase in the fibrous tissue of the uterine wall and a decrease in the muscular tissue.

The uterus increases in size because of the retained blood and feels soft and 'boggy'. However, it may be very difficult to palpate the uterus and the uterine fundus because it is completely flaccid. The patient has a rapid, thready pulse with a fall in blood pressure and she is pale and apprehensive.

PREVENTION

Patients at special risk should be singled out for particular attention during labour and delivery, with the administration of intravenous ergometrine when the anterior shoulder is delivered. Prolonged labour should be avoided or the prophylactic use of an oxytocin intravenous drip considered prior to delivery, so that rapid retraction of the uterus after delivery may be ensured. If coagulation disorders are anticipated, adequate countermeasures should be available, including fibrinogen or fresh frozen plasma, epsilon amniocaproic acid and fresh blood.

MANAGEMENT

The bleeding must be stopped as rapidly as possible, oxytocic drugs being given in the first instance. Intravenous ergometrine 0·5 mg may be followed by intramuscular injections of Syntometrine or oxytocin, whether or nor the placenta has been delivered. If the placenta is still within the uterus an attempt may be made to deliver it when the uterus contracts, but if this is not successful, it is important to control the blood loss while resuscitative measures are taken and arrangements made for general anaesthesia. When the condition of the patient permits, the placenta is manually removed, further oxytocic drugs being given as required, either by injection or intravenous infusion.

If the placenta has been delivered and atraumatic causes have been excluded, the patient is resuscitated, if necessary by blood transfusion, and uterine contractions are stimulated by oxytocin in an intravenous infusion, by ergometrine parenterally, or temporarily by uterine massage and bimanual compression. If the uterine fundus is pushed firmly downwards and posteriorly and a pad is placed at the vulva, the blood loss is restricted to the amount filling the pelvis. When the uterus is satisfactorily contracted, the vaginal clots can be allowed to escape, and resuscitation continued. Packing of the uterus and vagina requires a general anaesthetic to be effective and should not be performed.

Retained placenta

If the placenta cannot be delivered by the methods described, it is 'retained'. With an active policy for the management of the third stage, no time-limit need be exceeded before arriving at this diagnosis. If there is associated bleeding despite the administration of oxytocic drugs, partial separation has certainly occurred, and therefore prompt measures to remove the placenta are required. If there is no vaginal bleeding and the uterus is contracted, the placenta has either completely separated or no separation has taken place.

If the placenta has separated it will be pushed into the lower segment or vagina, provided it is not caught by the 'retraction ring' at the junction of the upper and lower segments. This is more likely following an ergometrine injection than when syntometrine or oxytocin has been given, and most likely with intravenous ergometrine. The placenta may be wholly or partially trapped by the retraction ring, and if the latter, the lower edge can be felt on vaginal examination. In these circumstances it is advisable to await uterine relaxation before removing the placenta, provided there is no bleeding. If there is excessive bleeding, however, the uterus must be relaxed by a general anaesthetic, and a further oxytocic injection, either intravenously or intramuscularly, will be required after the removal of the placenta.

If the placenta is adherent to the uterine wall it should be removed under general anaesthesia by digital separation through the spongy layer of the decidua basalis. The other hand should be placed on the uterine fundus to maintain its position in the abdomen and to allow counter-pressure to be exerted. After the removal of the placenta, more oxytocin will be required.

There is no place for the use of vigorous fundal compression in an attempt to expel the placenta. This is very painful and may cause complications, including inversion of the uterus, particularly if cord traction is applied at the same time.

If an active policy of management for the third stage is not practised, the indication to remove the placenta manually is vaginal bleeding or intra-uterine bleeding with relaxation of the uterus. If there is no bleeding, it is a matter of convenience as to when the placenta should be removed. An intravenous injection of ergometrine may stimulate a uterine contraction, and an attempt at placental delivery by cord traction may be made at this time. If it is unsuccessful, it is usually advisable to prepare the patient for a general anaesthetic.

Placenta accreta

When it is impossible to separate the placenta from the uterine wall, placenta accreta may be present. This arises because implantation of the ovum occurred in an area of the uterus in which the endometrium was deficient or damaged, possibly as a result of previous scarring or a congenital anomaly. The chorionic villi readily penetrate the endometrium and reach the myometrium. As there is no satisfactory plane of separation, complete or partial placenta accreta is found.

Placenta increta refers to penetration of the myometrium by the chorionic villi, and when the villi reach the serosal aspect of the uterus, this is *placenta percreta*. Some instances of placenta accreta have been found in association with placenta praevia (James & Misch 1955), but the condition is rare.

Hysterectomy is the safest method of treatment. If uterine function must be preserved, it is possible to leave the placenta *in situ* and hope that complete autolysis will occur. Further pregnancies have been reported after this form of management, but the risk of uterine infection is considerable. Antibiotic therapy would certainly be required to prevent this. No attempt at 'piecemeal' removal of the placenta should be contemplated, because of the danger of severe haemorrhage.

Inversion of the uterus

In this condition, the fundus of the uterus descends through the uterine body and cervix into the vagina, and sometimes protrudes through the vulva. It will not occur if the uterus is contracted, and is most likely when vigorous attempts are made to expel the placenta, or cord traction is used with the uterus in a relaxed state.

It is worthy of emphasis that the use of controlled cord traction to deliver the placenta is certain to result in the occasional case of acute uterine inversion despite efforts to prevent it by counter-pressure upwards on the uterine fundus as illustrated in Fig. 12.8. Fell (1966) referred to three such cases occurring in his own hospital in a period of 16 months.

In its mildest form, the uterus is 'dimpled'; the ease with which this can occur is demonstrated at Caesarean section when the placenta is removed. Incomplete inversion occurs when the uterine fundus descends through the cervix and comes to lie in the upper part of the vagina. With complete inversion the endometrial aspect of the uterus is seen outside the vulva, sometimes with the placenta still attached. The vagina may be pulled out partially or completely. The abdominal organs, particularly the small bowel, may be found in the funnel produced by the inversion.

The condition may be diagnosed in various ways. Acute complete inversion resulting from cord traction is immediately obvious. Incomplete inversion should be suspected when a state of shock develops in a patient whose blood loss is insufficient to account for it. This is particularly so if the usual means of resuscitation fail to produce improvement; inversion should always be suspected under these circumstances and a vaginal examination made. Theoretically, incomplete inversion may be recognized by the fundus of the uterus being felt at a lower level in the abdomen; the fundus is also described as feeling 'dimpled'. Neither of these two physical signs is helpful in the diagnosis. The fundus in incomplete inversion is rarely significantly lower in the abdomen than usual, perhaps because as the fundus goes down, the vault of the vagina is drawn up; characteristic 'dimpling' is frequently masked by lower abdominal guarding.

If the condition is diagnosed immediately it occurs, replacement should be carried out instantly. At this time the pelvic soft tissues will be relaxed and there will be no spasm preventing replacement (Dewhurst & Bevis 1951). Delay by only a few minutes, however, will allow shock to develop and spasm at the neck of the sac will effectively prevent manual replacement. In this type of case when the inversion occurs with the attendant present at the bedside instant replacement can be life-saving.

Once shock has developed it is better to commence resuscitative measures, but it is not likely that real improvement will occur until a uterus has been replaced. Digital replacement under general anaesthetic may be carried out, but the hydrostatic method described by O'Sullivan (1945) is probably more effective and safer. Warm, sterile fluid is gradually instilled into the vagina by means of a douche can and tubing (Fig. 25.1), as much as 4 or 5 l being required. The fluid pressure reverses the inversion and results

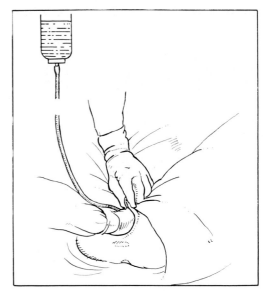

Fig. 25.1. Diagrammatic representation of hydrostatic replacement.

in the uterus being distended, so returning to its normal intra-abdominal position. The fluid is then drained off and ergometrine is given, a hand remaining in the uterus until the fluid has escaped and the uterus is contracting satisfactorily. If the placenta is still adherent, it is probably better to remove it after the uterus has been replaced and conditions are optimal for retraction of the placental site.

Sheehan's syndrome

In any variety of postpartum collapse with very low blood pressure there is an urgent need to replace blood loss and restore blood pressure to normal, not only to save the patient's life, but to prevent pituitary necrosis (Sheehan's syndrome). The pituitary, enlarged as a result of pregnancy, is most susceptible to the effects of profound and prolonged hypotension. Sheehan (1943) demonstrated pituitary necrosis, partial or complete, in association with severe cases of postpartum haemorrhage and collapse. In extreme cases the whole anterior lobe may be destroyed.

One effect of this pituitary damage is failure of menstruation due to a lack of gonadotrophin secretion. If widespread destruction occurs there may be atrophy of breasts and genital organs, weight loss, premature ageing, etc.— effects of almost total loss of pituitary function. Early and complete replacement is essential to help to prevent this catastrophe. For further consideration see Chapter 6.

REFERENCES

DEWHURST C.J. & BEVIS D.C.A. (1951) *Lancet*, i, 1394.
FELL M.R. (1966) *Br. med. J.* ii, 764.
JAMES D.W. & MISCH K.A. (1955) *J. Obstet. Gynaec. Br. Commonw.* **67**, 551.
O'SULLIVAN J.V. (1945) *Br. med. J.* ii, 282.
SHEEHAN H.L. (1943) *J. Obstet. Gynaec. Br. Commonw.* **50**, 27.

CHAPTER 26

ABNORMALITIES OF THE PUERPERIUM

The puerperium, although frequently uncomplicated, and therefore nowadays little regarded, may see the first appearance of serious, and sometimes fatal, disorders. The main cause of loss of life during this time is thrombosis and embolism, as a glance at the maternal mortality statistics in Chapter 29 will show. Sepsis, once the predominant killer, is less common and less serious when it does occur, but can still lead to maternal deaths. Breast infections urinary complications and mental disturbances can cause much ill-health for weeks, months or years to come.

THROMBOSIS AND EMBOLISM

Thrombosis in the legs and pelvic veins is not confined to the puerperium, being seen occasionally during pregnancy (see Chapter 21). It is far more common in the puerperal patient, however, when it may present in one of several forms.

Aetiology

Three important factors are concerned in puerperal thrombosis. These are infection, stasis of blood, and alterations in its constituents. Infection usually occurs at the time of delivery and spreads to the lateral pelvic wall. If the external iliac vein is involved the striking clinical features of phlegmasia alba dolens will occur.

Venous return from the foot and calf is retarded during late pregnancy and the puerperium; the rise in venous pressure in the lower limb during late pregnancy has already been indicated (p. 130). This effect will be more evident in patients who have been at rest in bed for pre-eclampsia before delivery or for pyrexia or some other complication after delivery. The importance of physical leg exercises in the prevention of thrombotic episodes in patients confined to bed has already been mentioned. The important changes in the constitution of the blood have been described already in Chapter 9. There is a considerable rise in the platelet count, occasionally reaching readings of 600,000 per millilitre. Furthermore, there is an increase in fibrinogen concentration, from some 250 mg/100 ml in the non-pregnant state to 400 mg/100 ml or more at term.

A factor of some importance here is that of oestrogen administration for the suppression of lactation. The possibility that oestrogens administered to suppress lactation might be an important aetiological factor in the onset of thrombo-embolism was first suggested by Daniel et al. (1967). They reported that the incidence of puerperal venous thrombosis was increased 10-fold in mothers aged 25 or more whose lactation was suppressed. It was concluded that oestrogen must play a part in this association. Later, Daniel et al. (1968) showed that a raised level of factor IX in the blood followed administration of high doses of oestrogen. Jeffcoate et al. (1968) reviewing consecutive cases of puerperal thrombo-embolism concluded that the administration of oestrogen to inhibit lactation was associated with a threefold increase in this complication. The effect was most marked in women over 25 years of age whose delivery was assisted by operative means; in women over 35 years of age with an assisted delivery inhibition of lactation was associated with a 10-fold increase in thrombosis. Age and operative delivery have already been shown to be factors increasing the risk of thrombosis; Jeffcoate et al. point out that it is these women who are likely also to receive oestrogen to suppress lactation. These authors stress the difficulty of interpretation of various findings in this field, and they conclude that administration of oestrogens is probably not in itself a cause of thrombosis but may constitute an additional factor sufficient to tip the scales against those patients who by reason of age, parity, operative delivery or previous history are already liable to this complication. The evidence supports a much more selective approach to the use of oestrogens to suppress lactation in the puerperium. If the drug is to be used at all it should probably be limited to those people in whom no increased risk of thrombosis already exists.

There are other factors sometimes concerned. One is trauma to leg veins during delivery. This may occur from pressure on stirrups if the legs have been inadequately padded at the point of pressure. It should be mentioned, too, that although early ambulation is, to a degree, protective against thrombosis, the patient who merely gets out of bed and sits motionless in a chair with her knees at right-angles is, if anything, more at risk than the patient who exercises her limbs correctly in bed. Mode of delivery is also concerned, patients delivered by Caesarean section or by operative means per vaginam having a higher rate of thrombosis than those delivered by natural means. Older patients are more at risk than the younger ones; the risk is increased in anaemic patients.

Clinical features

Venous thrombosis presents in several ways.

SUPERFICIAL THROMBOPHLEBITIS

This condition is somewhat misnamed. To refer to it as superficial thrombophlebitis suggests it to be predominantly infective, which it is not. It is concerned with venous stasis in varicose veins and the altered blood constituents already referred to; the presence of reddening which surrounds the affected vein is a reaction to clot and not to bacterial infection.

An area of varying size surrounding a varicose vein, usually in the lower leg, is painful, reddened and tender. Sometimes, the long saphenous vein may be affected. Apart from the discomfort experienced there is little cause for concern, since this form of superficial thrombosis is very seldom serious. It is sometimes suggested that if the long saphenous vein is affected spread to the femoral vein might occur, but if this is so it must be infrequent. Treatment consists of relief from weight-bearing with the continuation of free movement in bed until pain free, when the patient may be allowed up. Applications of glycerine and icthyol are commonly applied, but their value is in doubt.

DEEP VENOUS THROMBOSIS

This condition occurs in two forms: phlebothrombosis and iliofemoral thrombophlebitis. The former affects the veins of the foot or the calf initially, although spread to the thigh may occur later. The aetiology of this condition is concerned predominantly with venous stasis and altered coagulability of the blood. Pressure on the veins of the calf or region of the knee at delivery is a further factor.

Iliofemoral thrombosis—once called phlegmasia alba dolens—is predominantly of infective aetiology in association with pelvic sepsis, although the same factors which operate in phlebothrombosis will have an effect also.

Many cases of deep venous thrombosis during the puerperium fall fairly clearly into one or other category, although sometimes a clear distinction is not possible. Iliofemoral thrombosis may be due to spread upwards from the lower leg in some cases, and may not be directly associated with pelvic infection.

Phlebothrombosis presents with pain in the calf. Examination shows calf tenderness on deep pressure and a positive Homans's sign—pain in the calf on dorsiflexion of the foot. Swelling is variable but seldom pronounced; a little puffiness of the ankles may be evident but is more often absent. It must be emphasized that the first sign of phlebothrombosis may be a pulmonary embolus, perhaps a fatal one; although some patients apparently presenting in this way are found on closer scrutiny to have had minor symptoms earlier, it must be admitted that thrombosis in the deep veins of the calf can be present with few, if any, definitive features and can easily be overlooked.

Iliofemoral thrombosis presents with more dramatic local features. It is commonest during the second week of the puerperium. Mild pyrexia often precedes it for 4–5 days. Quite suddenly the patient complains of pain in the leg, which is seen to be swollen throughout its length (Fig. 26.1). The degree of discomfort and the physical signs in the leg are related to each other. If there is great pain it is likely that there will be the classical signs of phlegmasia alba dolens type of abnormality. The leg is swollen, painful, white and cold. The great pain is due to arterial spasm,

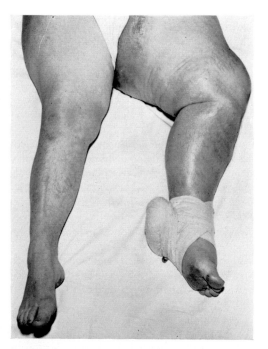

Fig. 26.1. The typical swollen leg of phlegmasia alba dolens.

which in turn is due to irritation from the nearby clotted vein. The pallor and coldness of the leg are similarly explained by this arterial spasm. In other cases the discomfort is much less and the leg is swollen, blue and warm. Pain is here mainly due to swelling and tenseness of the limb; the blueness and the warmth are due to venous thrombosis in association with unimpaired arterial supply.

Either phlebothrombosis or iliofemoral thrombophlebitis may give rise to pulmonary embolus formation. There may be a minor episode of chest pain, followed, perhaps, by a second accompanied by blood-stained sputum; more serious emboli are frequent, however, and there may be sudden collapse with dyspnoea and hypotension due to a massive embolus in the main pulmonary vessel.

Investigation

It must be admitted that the clinical diagnosis of deep venous thrombosis is imprecise. The assessment of the sign of pain in the lower leg on clinical grounds alone can be very difficult; if tenderness is minimal and discomfort slight on dorsiflexion of the foot, what are we to conclude? The physical signs in iliofemoral thrombosis are more definite, and diagnosis here is easier, at any rate once the condition is fully established. Recognition of either variety in its earliest stage, however, is well-nigh impossible clinically.

If we are to attempt to reduce mortality from thrombosis and embolism, more precise and earlier diagnosis is essential in order that spread of the thrombotic process can be halted and emboli prevented.

Three relatively new methods of investigation have been introduced which help to make more precise the diagnosis of deep venous thrombosis. These are phlebography, the use of ^{125}I-labelled fibrinogen, and ultrasound scanning.

Phlebography may be employed by injecting a radio-opaque dye into a vein on the dorsum of the foot. Using variations of the technique it is possible to visualize the calf, popliteal, superficial femoral, common femoral and iliac veins. Alternatively, an injection of dye may be given at a higher level to demonstrate the common iliac vein and inferior vena cava. The application of this technique, along with television monitoring during the injection of the dye, gives the best results, since films can be taken at the correct time. This is not an easy technique to perform and unless it is done well, poor results will be obtained. If it is used correctly, however, Browse (1969) believes that it displays 90–95% of existing venous thrombi.

[131]I-labelled fibrinogen was shown some years ago (Hobbs & Davies 1960) to be taken up preferentially in fresh thrombi in rabbit leg veins. This action has now been utilized as a useful test for the recognition of venous thrombosis (Flanc et al. 1969); 100 μc of ^{125}I fibrinogen are given intravenously and pass into existing thrombi. Radioactivity can be detected with a scintillation counter. The uptake by the thyroid must be blocked first with potassium iodide. Counts of radioactivity at fixed points in the legs are then taken. If the count in one area is significantly raised a deep venous thrombosis can be confidently diagnosed. Trauma or oedema may account for some false-positive results. [125]-labelled fibrinogen is most valuable for thrombosis in the lower leg, of doubtful value in the upper thigh, and of no value above the inguinal ligament.

Ultrasound techniques utilizing the Doppler effect have also been applied to the diagnosis of deep venous thrombosis (Evans & Crockett 1969; Evans 1970). The Doppler effect recognizes alterations in frequency of an ultrasound beam passing through a moving column of blood or against a beating surface like that of an artery or the heart. A standard Doppler instrument, such as a Sonicaid or Doptone machine, can be used to detect flow in a major vein and will indicate whether the vessel is patent or blocked. This technique is best employed when there is a suspicion of thrombosis in the upper thigh.

Browse (1969) suggests an approach to accurate diagnosis which many will find helpful. Patients are divided into two groups, those with a pulmonary embolus and those without. A patient with an embolus is investigated as an emergency with a phlebogram to obtain the maximum information about site and extent of the thrombus so that future emboli can be prevented. Patients in whom there is a suspicion of deep venous thrombosis but so far no embolus are investigated by both ultrasound and labelled fibrinogen techniques. The ultrasound technique is first utilized to confirm or refute thrombosis in large veins. If there is none, fibrinogen is given and the legs are scanned the following day to look for thrombi in smaller vessels. As soon as the diagnosis is confirmed treatment is started. If further scanning with the scintillation counter indicates progress of the thrombus a phlebogram is undertaken.

Management

Since diagnosis has been so imprecise in the past, and to a large extent still is, we have had no firm basis on which to judge the success of various treatments employed. Certain measures, however, appear to be indicated in specific cases.

ANTICOAGULANTS

Anticoagulant therapy has been employed for some years with reasonable success. The drugs used have been heparin for 24–36 hr, accompanied by a drug of the coumarin series, which takes a little while to reach its maximum effect. Heparin is administered intravenously. Doses of the order of 15,000 units are given initially, followed by 10,000 units 4- to 6-hourly for four to six injections; once blood coagulation has been depressed to the therapeutic levels the heparin may be stopped and the coumarin drug continued. Heparin's principal effect on the blood coagulation mechanism is to inhibit the action of thrombin on fibrinogen, and so to prevent fibrin formation; it also inhibits plasma thromboplastin formation. Over-dosage may cause bleeding, which will call for immediate inactivation of the heparin with protamine sulphate. Protamines combine rapidly with heparin and neutralize its anticoagulant effect.

When the first dose of heparin is injected, a drug of the coumarin series—or one of the indanediones—is given at the same time by mouth. These drugs act by depressing the synthesis in the liver of factors II (prothrombin), VII, IX and X. Warfarin or dicoumarol are commonly employed. The initial dose of the former is

30–50 mg, and of the latter 300 mg. Dicoumarol reaches its peak effect within 36–48 hr, warfarin takes slightly longer. Each has an effect which lasts for 5–6 days, so continuation of the same dosage will inevitably lead to greater anti-coagulant effect and to haemorrhage. For this reason laboratory studies on prothrombin activity must precede each daily coumarin dose, which is judged from the laboratory results obtained. Richards (1966) suggests that there is little to choose between the various laboratory methods of judging prothrombin activity. If the Quick's one-stage prothrombin time-test is employed, a level two to three times above normal must be achieved. Prothrombin concentration must be reduced to some 20% of normal, but not be allowed to go much lower. Vitamin K is the pharmacological antidote to these drugs; 20 mg should be given intravenously if there is bleeding or if it is feared. There may, however, be a latent period of 6–8 hr before the full effect is obtained, so a dangerous situation may exist for a while.

Other possible forms of anticoagulant-type treatment are with Arvin—an enzyme extracted from the venom of the Malayan pit viper (Reid & Chan 1968; Flute 1969)—or with fibrinolytic drugs. Arvin acts on plasma fibrinogen and produces micro-clots which are rapidly removed from the circulation. The margin of safety of this drug is high, and it may prove to be a useful adjunct to treatment. Streptokinase is a fibrinolytic agent which has been effectively employed. Bleeding is a somewhat greater danger with this preparation and, again, daily laboratory control is necessary. Direct injection of strepto-kinase into a thrombus has been employed with good results (Kakkar *et al.* 1969). Flute (1969) has reviewed these various methods of the treatment.

Anticoagulant therapy must be continued whilst there are signs or symptoms of thrombosis. Whilst pain and tenderness are present the patient must be kept in bed with the leg relieved from pressure by a cage. Movements in bed are continued. Once pain and tenderness subside the patient may get up and begin to move around the ward. Anticoagulant therapy is continued throughout this time and should only be stopped when it is clear that all evidence of the disease has

disappeared. Treatment for several weeks will be required.

ANTIBIOTICS

Antibiotic therapy will be required for deep venous thrombosis associated with pelvic infection. If an organism can be isolated from a high vaginal swab the antibiotic to which it is sensitive may be employed. Usually, however, we are in the dark as to the nature of the infecting organism, when antibiotic therapy must be used arbitrarily.

SYMPATHETIC BLOCK

In the variety of iliofemoral thrombosis associated with spasm of the iliac artery—phlegmasia alba dolens—pain is intense in the early stages. This pain may be greatly relieved by lumbar sympathetic block provided this is done within the first 24 hr, and the sooner the better.

SURGICAL TREATMENT

The place of surgery in the management of deep venous thrombosis is a subject about which there is little general agreement. Without effective visualization of the clotted segment by phlebography no proper assessment of the situation is possible, so precise methods of diagnosis, such as those referred to above, must be more widely used. Mavor (1969), who reviews the subject well, suggests that thrombectomy is the surgical procedure of choice, if any is indicated, and that this is better employed for clot in the iliofemoral segment than in the lower part of the limb. Caval thrombectomy may be feasible but caval ligation is seldom indicated. The majority of published accounts chiefly consider postoperative thrombosis, and the real place of these methods in puerperal thrombosis is yet to be determined.

TREATMENT OF THE PULMONARY EMBOLUS

Chest pain, dyspnoea and blood-stained sputum indicate the presence of a peripheral pulmonary embolus. An X-ray of the chest may provide confirmation of this in some cases, but does not always do so. If the diagnosis is likely it will be weil to treat the patient's deep venous thrombosis with a view to preventing further emboli. Specific therapy for a small embolus of this kind is unnecessary in most cases.

A massive pulmonary embolus lodged in the main pulmonary vessel will cause collapse, and perhaps death, so quickly that no treatment is possible. If there is time, surgical assistance should be sought urgently, since removal of the embolus from the vessel may be the patient's only hope. In this kind of circumstance all the resources of the hospital must be marshalled immediately—anaesthetists, physicians, surgeons and the staff of the intensive care unit accustomed to dealing with emergencies of this kind. Adequate anticoagulant therapy is necessary whatever other treatment is employed. Miller (1970) and Paneth (1970) have reviewed the medical and surgical management, respectively.

PUERPERAL INFECTION

A raised temperature in the puerperium may have several explanations and careful examination and investigation are required to elucidate the cause.

The patient must be examined clinically for evidence of any extragenital infection—pharyngitis, influenza, bronchitis, otitis etc. These sometimes appear coincidentally. Careful abdominal and pelvic examination, and examination of the legs, is required too. The presence of foul-smelling lochia, lower abdominal and pelvic tenderness, loin tenderness or tenderness in the calves, etc. will help to isolate a possible cause. The breasts should be examined carefully. A high vaginal swab and a mid-stream sample of urine must be taken and sent for bacteriological examination as soon as possible. We are searching for a source of infection which calls for clinical skill, care, and attention to detail.

PELVIC INFECTION

If pathogenic organisms have been introduced into the upper genital tract during labour they will find an ideal culture medium in which to become established. Acute pelvic infection may take several forms—a localized intra-uterine infection with organisms of low virulence, when the uterus will remain bulky and the lochia foul-smelling; an infection with more virulent organisms likely to spread more rapidly through the pelvis to produce greater constitutional upset but less local physical signs; more widespread infection still, with septicaemia and a positive blood culture. Puerperal infection is fully discussed on p. 467.

BREAST INFECTIONS

With effective prenatal attention to breasts, cleanliness and avoidance of trauma, breast infections are less common than formally. Engorgement of the breast may be pronounced by the third or fourth day and it is best to ensure emptying of the breasts by effective sucking, gentle expression or a pump. If engorgement is marked a single dose of 1 mg of stilboestrol will relieve it and will prevent failure of lactation from the engorgement itself. An engorged segment of breast must be emptied gently, or infection is likely to develop.

When evidence of early infection is seen—reddening of a wedge-shaped segment with tenderness and pain—immediate and large doses of chemotherapy must be given to abort it. Penicillin in doses of 1–2 million units daily will be effective if given soon enough. Breast feeding may be continued or the breast may be emptied by other means. Unless chemotherapy is employed very early, however, the infection may not be stopped but the process converted to a more chronic one without effective pus formation. It is better to withhold chemotherapy if it is thought too late to halt infection, to stop breast feeding, and to incise the abscess later once pus has formed.

Breast infections of this nature are seldom seen in the hospital patient, since they usually occur after the tenth to fourteenth day.

Infection in the urinary tract is a common cause of puerperal pyrexia; it is considered below.

Urinary complications

RETENTION OF URINE

This is a common complication following delivery and is attributable to bruising of the bladder base, discomfort from an episiotomy wound, etc. Usually, a patient will be able to pass urine eventually by being allowed to sit out of bed on a bedpan stool. If this, combined with drugs to relieve local pain, fails, however, catheterization is necessary to prevent over-distention of the bladder.

The bladder may easily become over-distended during the early puerperium. It will hold a litre or more of urine without difficulty and may become gradually still more distended, culminating in retention with overflow. This situation may remain unrecognized, since the unwary attendant may imagine the patient to be passing urine well. The quantities passed, however, will be small— 50–150 ml or so, at frequent intervals. If this is noted it should call first for an abdominal examination, when the distended bladder may be readily palpable; if the bladder cannot be felt for certain, a catheter must be passed after the patient has voided urine to determine the quantity of residual urine present. In a case of retention with overflow a litre or more of urine may be retained in this way.

Treatment is by the insertion of an indwelling catheter, which must be left draining constantly into a bag; the patient may carry this around with her whilst walking round the ward. Antibiotics should be given for 5–7 days. After the bladder has been kept completely empty for 48 hr the catheter may be removed and a check kept on the quantities of urine passed. If these are reduced and suspicion of further retention with overflow is aroused, the volume of residual urine must again be measured. If necessary, the indwelling catheter must be replaced for a further period of 2–3 days and the procedure repeated.

SUPPRESSION OF URINE

Retention and suppression of urine must be clearly distinguished from each other. If the volume of urine passed in the first 24 hr is reduced to 400 ml or less, suppression of urine must be suspected and prophylactic measures adopted This subject is discussed on pp. 224 and 311.

INCONTINENCE OF URINE

This is, fortunately, an infrequent symptom following confinement. Stress incontinence may

well follow later, but it is seldom marked in the early stages. It must first be established whether the incontinence is urethral or via a fistula. Careful examination of the patient may establish this, since the fistula or the obvious escape of urine from the urethral orifice may be seen. A three-swab test will usually detect the presence of a fistula.

Three small swabs are inserted into the vagina one at the top, one in the middle and one by the introitus. A small amount of methylene blue is then instilled into the bladder through a catheter. Staining of any of the swabs by the blue dye will indicate the presence of a fistula. The site of the fistula will be demonstrated by which swab is stained; if the upper swab is stained with urine, but is not blue, a ureteric fistula is present.

Urinary fistulae are uncommon in obstetric practice in Britain, although they are still seen in other parts of the world. Direct injury with the obstetric forceps or some other instrument may be responsible, when the leak of urine will be almost immediate. Sloughing following prolonged pressure from the head during an intractable second stage of labour may also cause fistula formation. Incontinence will not then occur for some 8–12 days, which is the time necessary for the slough to separate.

The management of the vesicovaginal or urethrovaginal fistula is a specialized subject, of which few obstetricians have but a small experience. Continuous bladder drainage should be undertaken at once, for if the fistula is very small spontaneous closure may occur. This happy result is uncommon, however, and surgical repair later will nearly always require to be performed. Immediate surgery is hardly ever successful and should seldom even be attempted unless the injury is a single, clean hole made at Caesarean section. This, of course, must be repaired at once and bladder drainage instituted.

Specialized treates, such as those by Moir (1961) and Russell (1962), should be consulted for a more detailed consideration of this subject (see also pp. 686–8).

URINARY INFECTIONS

This is one of the chief causes of puerperal pyrexia. It may be a recurrence of a pyelonephritis of pregnancy or a recently acquired lower urinary tract infection secondary to urine retention and catheterization. Cystitis following catheterization is not uncommon in the puerperium. The constitutional upset of these infections is nowadays seldom great. Mild pyrexia and tachycardia, with some pain and frequency of passing urine, will probably be the only features present. Rarely, a more pronounced temperature rise with shivering, headaches, etc. may be observed. The infection can usually be confirmed easily by examination of a mid-stream sample of urine. Treatment should begin at once, before waiting for sensitivity studies. Many of the organisms responsible still respond well to sulphonamides, which should usually be the first drug of choice.

It is most important to ensure that a patient who has suffered from a urinary tract infection during the puerperium, or during pregnancy, is fully recovered before she is discharged. A mid-stream sample of urine must be obtained following treatment and another course of a different antibiotic employed if it is clear that there is still infection present. If such a patient is allowed out of medical supervision without completely curing her infection she may have recurrent troubles for a very long time thereafter.

Secondary postpartum haemorrhage

Bright bleeding during the puerperium is abnormal, since the lochial discharge is of a dull-red colour. Secondary postpartum haemorrhage may occur at any time after the first 24 hr following confinement until the 6 weeks of the puerperium are completed. Bleeding is more common, however, between the eighth and the fourteenth day after confinement. Dewhurst (1966) reviewed 97 cases of this complication and found 18 occurring between days 1 and 7, 60 between days 8 and 14, 7 between days 15 and 21, and 12 after the twenty-second day. The amount of loss is seldom large enough to threaten the patient's life, unless the bleeding occurs in circumstances which prevent effective early treatment. The haemorrhage may, however, be of sufficient severity to cause some deterioration of the patient's general condition and to call for blood transfusion. Often, however, the loss varies from

100 to 500 ml before treatment brings it to an end.

Secondary postpartum haemorrhage is usually attributable to retention of small pieces of placental tissue. The amount of apparent placental tissue removed at surgical evacuation of the uterus seems to confirm this. However, if the removed tissue is examined histologically in the laboratory, chorionic villi will often be found to be absent. In Dewhurst's series placental fragments were confirmed histologically in only 29 of 89 patients from whom material was obtained. There appears to be no reason why separation of large pieces of decidua alone should not be associated with some bright bleeding, which would be in keeping with the lack of histological confirmation of villi in many patients.

Infection alone seems unlikely to cause bleeding. A further possible cause, however, is bleeding following the use of oestrogens to suppress lactation. If a considerable amount of this hormone has been prescribed, especially when endometrial regeneration is well under way, stopping the drug may later lead to pronounced withdrawal haemorrhage. Other possible causes which have been mentioned are retention of small pieces of membrane, but if these ever do cause trouble it must be extremely infrequent. In later cases the possibility of a chorionepithelioma must be remembered.

TREATMENT

This condition is best managed actively. If the amount of bright bleeding has been very small it may be permissible to procrastinate for a while (24 hr or so) to await events. The patient should remain in hospital, of course, during this time. This may be one of the very few situations in which ergometrine 0·5 mg given during the puerperium might have a beneficial effect; at any rate, it may be prescribed without evident disadvantage. If there is further loss, however, or the initial loss is somewhat greater, it is better to take the patient to the operating theatre and to remove any retained tissue—placental or otherwise—which may be inside the uterus.

This procedure must be approached with some caution. Blunt instruments only may be used and the more fragments which can be removed by the finger the better. Ideally, the uterine cavity should be explored with the finger, then a pair of sponge-holding forceps introduced to remove loose matter, and finally the cavity gently scraped with a blunt curette. It must be emphasized that injury to the uterus is a special risk of this operation. The uterus was perforated on three occasions in the 89 patients treated surgically in Dewhurst's series. It may be stressed, too, that injury with an instrument to a recently pregnant uterus calls for immediate operation to establish the extent of the damage and to deal with it appropriately (Fig. 25.2). It may be thought that a tiny injury

villi may have led to the bleeding in the first place and may have predisposed to injury with the instrument. It is better to open the abdomen and be certain of the extent of damage than to risk a ruptured uterus at the next confinement (see Fig. 27.4, p. 425).

Whether or not fragments of placenta are removed from the uterus, bleeding almost always stops and no further treatment is necessary.

It may be mentioned finally that chorion-epithelioma can occasionally follow fairly soon after a normal confinement. This should be remembered if there is an unusually long duration of red lochial flow which increases during weeks

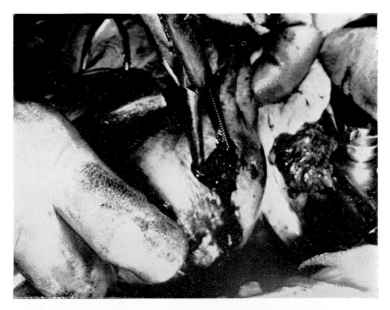

Fig. 26.2. A uterus injured by an instrument at operation for secondary postpartum haemorrhage. The blades of a pair of artery forceps are spread to show the extent of the damage.

from a single dilator will cause minimal uterine damage. There are two arguments against this, however. The uterus is hardly ever injured by a single dilator, for if there is a suspicion that a perforation has occurred a second will inevitably be passed to make sure that it is; moreover, we can never be certain of the condition of the uterine wall at the point where the perforation occurred, since unusually deep penetration of chorionic

5 and 6 rather than disappears. Radio-immuno-assay of chorionic gonadotrophin, with or without curettage, should be arranged to exclude this possibility.

Puerperal mental disorder

Puerperal mental disorder is not an easy subject to grasp in all its intricacies. In more general terms, however, most obstetricians are aware of the normal and abnormal mental reactions throughout pregnancy and labour. Reference to mental disorder during pregnancy has been made on p. 340.

Neurotic reactions are far more common than psychotic ones during the puerperium. Indeed, minor neurotic symptoms are very common, although these seldom justify concern.

The anxiety state is perhaps the commonest neurosis to be observed. This anxiety may be evident as minor symptoms of pain, nervousness, irritability or worry about the child, who is nonetheless physically well. Unreasonable fear that some serious problem has arisen is common. Depression is comparatively common in minor degrees during the early puerperal days. The onset of breast discomfort, early troubles with breast feeding and other minor matters of this kind may precipitate a feeling of depression, which is usually mild and temporary. The success story is over and the patient is in contact with reality again. Her husband may not visit her often enough or be less attentive when he does so. Other family problems may obtrude. For a while she may be depressed by these events but usually, with a little consideration and patience, this reaction will diminish. Obsessional states are sometimes observed, but not so often in the early puerperium as they are later when the patient is back in her own home.

Psychotic illnesses are, fortunately, less common. Occasionally, these will have some organic basis, such as puerperal infection. Baker (1967), who has written admirably on this subject, suggests that marked anaemia may also be a possible cause. These patients may show confusion or delirium with pains and discomforts; mood-changes may be pronounced.

Schizophrenia may become evident during the early puerperium. There will usually be earlier evidence of this in the patient herself or a family history in one of her parents. Its manifestations are extremely valuable.

Depressive psychoses are the most common of the psychosis in the recently delivered patient; mania is a less pronounced feature. Baker suggests that mania is very rare indeed in the puerperium, although it must remain a possibility. The

clinical picture presented by these various conditions will be variable. Features that should always be regarded as danger signs are confusion, delirium, extreme wakefulness at night, hallucinations and delusions. It is disconcerting if the patient dwells for very long on the discomfort she experienced during delivery and continues to complain about how unpleasant this experience was. Sometimes the patient believes that she may injure her baby, and if this is so it must be taken very seriously, since it is precisely what may happen. Brooding on some imagined abnormality of the child is common. So is the belief that patients and staff are together discussing her case and withholding important information from her. These features are generally sufficient to demand psychiatric advice at once, and if it is thought that she might attempt suicide or may try to kill her baby, to arrange for the transfer of the patient to a psychiatric institution.

Management in the early stages will involve examination of the problems the patient believes herself to have, to decide if they are real or imaginary. Sleep and relief from anxiety must be achieved. Sedatives will be helpful and tranquillizers are often employed; heavy doses must be given, however, for an effect in some patients. It will be wise to check temperature, pulse and general condition of the patient to eliminate physical cause, which may be at least contributory. The help of the husband should be sought; he may come to see the patient more often and remain longer in order to relieve her anxiety and remove her to some extent from the hospital atmosphere.

A history of any previous mental disorder should always be sought whenever the reaction of the patient is beyond the common mild anxiety or depression found briefly in the early puerperium.

In the more serious cases of mental disorder the assistance of a psychiatrist is necessary at once. Effectively treated, puerperal mental disorder responds well, but it is better that treatment be given early if possible. The advisability of future childbearing must be seriously considered, although in general a previous episode of mental disorder does not definitely rule it out.

Other puerperal abnormalities

RAISED BLOOD PRESSURE

Not uncommonly, the patient will be found to have a slightly raised blood pressure immediately after delivery. The precise explanation of this is open to dispute; sometimes it is clearly an exacerbation of a raised blood pressure in a patient already mildly pre-eclamptic, but this is not always the case. Provided the level remains within moderate limits, however, avoidance of too much excitement and a little sedative may be all that is required. If the diastolic blood pressure reaches 100 mmHg heavy sedation will be called for, and if still higher levels are recorded the patient should be managed as a potential eclamptic, as outlined in that section on p. 275.

EPISIOTOMY BREAKDOWN

Episiotomies and perineal tears do not always heal completely. There are several possible explanations for this—infection, haematoma formation, imperfect suturing, etc.—and it may not always be evident why it has occurred. If the whole suture-line breaks down early in the puerperium and the wound looks clean it may be resutured after gently freshening the edges (Stallworthy 1956). It is important in this procedure not to excise too much of the wound edges, or a very tight introitus may be the result. Moreover, if the episiotomy breaks down only in part, resuture is often unnecessary; it is remarkable what effective healing can be achieved by simple granulation. The patient requires only to keep the area clean by sitting in a bath or bathing the part twice daily and to wear a pad. There is minimal discomfort during this time. When the wound is seen a few weeks later it may be indistinguishable from one healed by first intention.

The puerperium is an admirable time for the surgical treatment of an old third-degree tear. At this time the blood supply is excellent and there will be no tension on the suture-line. Formal repair under general anaesthesia after delivery should be planned for a patient with such a lesion who has become pregnant before repair could be carried out. The principles of operation are those outlined on p. 422.

SUBINVOLUTION

Few diagnoses can have been made so frequently, and at the same time so incorrectly, as that of subinvolution. The process of involution is interfered with seldom, and probably only by infection. Even then, involution may only slightly be retarded, and provided the infection is overcome will be complete shortly. The 'bulky uterus' diagnosed so often during the early puerperium is, in all probability, the normal puerperal uterus perhaps slightly displaced by a full colon or bladder; sometimes, there is not even this excuse for the observation. Ergometrine is then usually prescribed. If indeed there is subinvolution due to mild infection it is questionable if an oxytocic which, if it does anything, will reduce blood flow, is the correct treatment. The multitude of doses of ergometrine prescribed during the puerperium could be withheld in nearly all cases without any disadvantages whatever.

FOOT DROP

Peroneal palsy is an uncommon complication which becomes evident shortly after delivery. It is concerned with injury to the lumbosacral trunk. This structure is formed by the fusion of the 4th and 5th lumbar nerve roots and then passes downwards across the ala of the sacrum to join with the 1st, 2nd and 3rd sacral nerves to form the sciatic nerve. The fibres of the 4th and 5th lumbar nerve are destined to supply, among others, the peroneal muscles in the lower leg. The injury the nerve fibres sustain leads to temporary paralysis of these muscles, and foot drop. The precise nature of the trauma to the lumbosacral trunk is uncertain. It may be concerned with direct injury from the blade of the obstetric forceps in some instances; when the peroneal palsy develops the forceps have often been used. It may in other instances be due to pressure from the foetal head itself; this may be particularly the case if the brim is an unusual shape, leaving the nerve trunk exposed in that situation. Treatment consists in supporting the foot so that it cannot fall below the right-angle, in order to prevent contractures. Thereafter, recovery is usually quick and complete. Physiotherapy will often be helpful.

REFERENCES

BAKER A.A. (1967) *Psychiatric Disorders in Obstetrics.* Oxford, Blackwell Scientific Publications.

BROWSE N. (1969) *Br. med. J.* iv, 676.

DANIEL D.G., CAMPBELL H. & TURNBULL A.C. (1967) *Lancet*, ii, 287.

DANIEL D.G., BLOOM A.L., GIDDINGS J.C., CAMPBELL H. & TURNBULL A.C. (1968) *Br. med. J.* i, 801.

DEWHURST C.J. (1966) *J. Obstet. Gynaec. Br. Commonw.* 73, 53.

EVANS D.S. & CROCKETT F.B. (1969) *Br. med. J.* ii, 802.

EVANS D.S. (1970) *Br. J. Surg.* 57, 726.

FLANC C., KAKKAR V.V. & CLARK M.B. (1969) *Lancet*, i, 477.

FLUTE P.T. (1969) *Br. med. J.* iv, 678.

HOBBS J.T. & DAVIES J.W.L. (1960) *Lancet*, ii, 134.

JEFFCOATE T.N.A., MILLER J., ROOS R.F. & TINDALL V.R. (1968) *Br. med. J.* iii, 19.

KAKKAR V.V., FLANCE C., HOWE C.T., O'SHEA M. & FLUTE P.T. (1969) *Br. med. J.* i, 806, 810.

MAVOR G.E. (1969) *Br. med. J.* iv, 680.

MILLER G.A.H. (1970) *Br. med. J.* ii, 777.

MOIR J.C. (1961) *The Vesico-Vaginal Fistula.* London, Ballière, Tindall & Cassell.

PANETH M. (1970) *Br. med. J.* ii, 778.

REID H.A. & CHAN K.E. (1968) *Lancet*, i, 485.

RICHARDS R.L. (1966) *Br. med. J.* ii, 217.

RUSSELL C. SCOTT (1962) *Vesico-Vaginal Fistulas and Related Matters.* Springfield, Illinois, Thomas.

STALLWORTHY J.A. (1956) *Br. med. J.* i, 393.

CHAPTER 27

MATERNAL INJURIES AND COMPLICATIONS

Serious maternal injury is now rarely seen, and this is a reflection of better antenatal care and the freer use of Caesarean section. Obstetricians are now reluctant to attempt difficult vaginal deliveries, and forceps are seldom used to overcome bony obstruction. In most instances rupture of uterus, extensive lacerations of the birth canal, acute inversion and profound obstetric shock are manifestations of either neglect or mismanagement.

Episiotomy

A deliberate incision of the perineum is most frequently done in primigravida and in hospital practice for a variety of reasons.

INDICATIONS

(i) If the head begins to split the skin of the vestibule an episiotomy should be performed to prevent uncontrolled laceration.

(ii) Delivery face-to-pubes causes gross distension of the vulva and episiotomy may prevent extensive lacerations into the rectum.

(iii) A narrow subpubic arch forces the head backwards towards the rectum and reduces the available pelvic outlet.

(iv) Episiotomy is performed almost as a routine during the course of forceps delivery in the primigravida.

(v) In breech delivery episiotomy aids expulsion of the buttocks, Løvset's man-

oeuvre of the shoulders, reduces compression of the skull, the risk of intracranial haemorrhage, and maternal injury.

(vi) Episiotomy shortens the second stage and may be of value in foetal distress and cord prolapse.

(vii) Caesarean section is probably indicated following the successful repair of a vesicovaginal fistula or colporrhaphy for stress incontinence, but if vaginal delivery is permitted an episiotomy will reduce stretching.

(viii) Compression of the premature foetal skull is reduced by episiotomy.

METHOD

Under local infiltration the perineum is incised with straight, blunt-ended scissors from the posterior mid-point of the vaginal introitus backwards for 2–3 cm either in the mid-line or to one side of the anus. Following delivery of the placenta, the incision is sutured with No. 1 plain catgut (Fig. 27.1). It is important to obtain haemostasis by careful suture of the whole of the vaginal laceration. Pockets beneath sutured tissues must be avoided or haematoma formation and subsequent breakdown will occur.

Extensive lacerations

If lacerations have involved the anal sphincter and anal canal, then suture should be under general anaesthesia. The vagina is sutured first

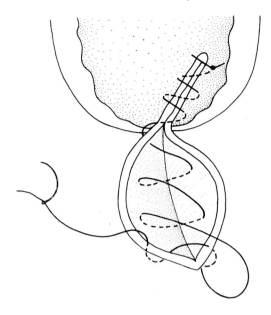

Fig. 27.1. Repair of an episiotomy using one strand of No. 1 plain catgut.

and then the anal mucosa. The torn ends of the anal sphincter are identified, grasped with Allis's tissue forceps and sutured together with No. 2 chromic catgut. The repair is then completed with vertical mattress silkworm or nylon suture, which are removed 5 days later. The bowels are confined for 5 days and then an easy bowel action insured with liquid paraffin by mouth and an olive-oil enema.

Cervical lacerations

Slight tears are very common and often remain unrecognized. More extensive lacerations and deliberate cervical incisions should always be sutured with interrupted catgut.

Lacerations of the cervix may extend upwards into the lower segment, and this is most likely to occur when forceps delivery has been attempted before full cervical dilatation. Exploration under anaesthesia will be wise to ascertain the extent of the damage. The small bowel may prolapse into the vagina. Management will be as for cases of uterine rupture (see below).

Vulval and paravaginal haematomata

The formation of a sizeable haematoma of the vulva (Fig. 27.2) or of the paravaginal tissues is seen often enough for one or other to be suspected in any case in which the recovery of the mother following delivery is slow and bleeding appears still to be in progress. Either may form as a result of imperfect or careless suturing of an episiotomy wound or perineal tear. The paravaginal haematoma, however, may be the result of damage in the upper vagina or in the region of the fornix unrecognized until some hours have gone by; such haematomas are usually not discovered for a time after delivery. The patient's general condition may be giving cause for concern when the discovery may be made as part of a routine investigation into possible reasons for failure of otherwise adequate resuscitative methods to restore the patient.

If blood transfusion and sedation are sufficient to arrest any deterioration in the patient's condition and she then responds well, it will be wise not to undertake surgical exploration of the

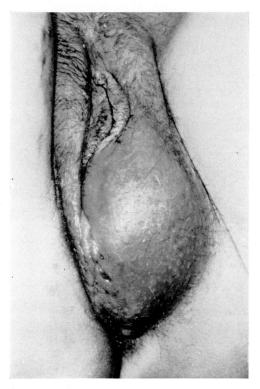

Fig. 27.2. A large vulval haematoma following normal vaginal delivery.

haematoma. It is seldom, if ever, possible to locate a bleeding point within the midst of a large haematoma, and after a fruitless search the operator usually has to resort to the introduction of large mattress stitches (which may cut out anyway) in an attempt to control the bleeding. Meanwhile, resuscitative methods must be continued. Only in the face of continued deterioration of the patient's condition despite adequate resuscitation should any exploration be contemplated; if evacuation of the blood clot and exploration of the area to locate and control bleeding is not quickly successful, consideration must be given to internal iliac artery ligation.

RUPTURE OF THE UTERUS

Rupture of the uterus has always been, and is still, a most serious complication of pregnancy and labour. In common with other serious accidents, it is much less frequent than formerly. This relative infrequency, however, if anything, makes diagnosis more difficult; a further difficulty arises from the changing aetiology of uterine rupture over recent years.

AETIOLOGY

Uterine rupture occurs either spontaneously or following obstetrical intervention of some kind.

Spontaneous rupture may be the end-result of obstructed labour, or may occur at an earlier stage in labour (or even in pregnancy) because of some weakness of the uterine wall. Of the factors weakening the uterine wall, previous Caesarean section is the most common, and by far the most important (Fig. 27.3); less commonly, the injury has been perforation at curettage (Fig. 27.4), the operation of myomectomy or some unusual procedure involving incision of the uterus.

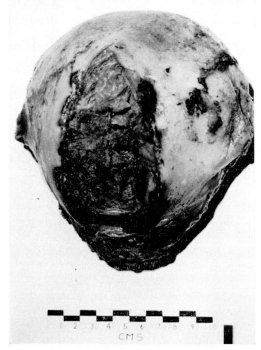

Fig. 27.3. A uterus removed as an emergency procedure following sudden rupture of a classical Caesarean section scar.

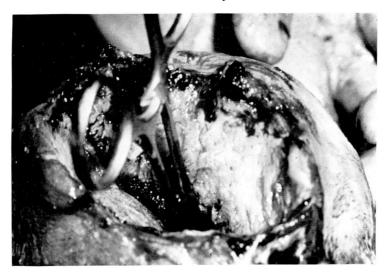

Fig. 27.4. Rupture of the uterus at the fundus through the site of a probable perforation at previous curettage.

In the past, thinning of the uterus due to multiple child-bearing often led to uterine rupture, but this must be less common now, at least in Britain.

The obstetrical management precipitating rupture is usually some intra-uterine manipulation—internal version being the manœuvre most commonly responsible. Other possible precipitating factors are external version (especially under general anaesthesia or in the presence of a uterine scar), the application of forceps before full dilatation of the cervix, or cervical incision, etc. Manual removal of the placenta has sometimes led to rupture, either following great force and ineptitude or when the placenta has burrowed deeply into the muscle, leaving a weakened area. It must not be thought that physical means alone contribute to rupture, however; the unwise use of oxytocics in labour may lead to the same result, unless they are given under strict observation and control (Margulies *et al.* 1966).

The changing aetiology of rupture in recent years had been the reduction in the numbers of cases following obstetrical mismanagement—the neglected transverse lie, the unrecognized hydrocephalic, etc.—and the relative increase in the numbers of cases following minor uterine damage, such as perforation at curettage.

CLINICAL FEATURES

Rupture of a lower-segment Caesarean section scar may occur during pregnancy with few symptoms. The ischaemic scar gradually stretches under the influence of Braxton Hicks's contractions and progressively intra-uterine growth. When eventually the scar gives way, there may be little bleeding and the membranes remain supported by the overlying bladder. The foetus remains *in utero* but can be easily felt through the rupture. Diagnosis may be difficult, and indeed pregnancy may continue for several weeks before a further Caesarean section is performed. Rupture of the lower segment scar is, however, more likely to occur in labour. There will in most cases be extreme local tenderness and pain between uterine contractions. Again, adhesions between the lower segment and the bladder may cause pain and make diagnosis difficult.

If the Caesarean section has been through a classical upper segment incision, then the risk of rupture is over 3%. Rupture may involve the placental site, and there will then be profuse intraperitoneal haemorrhage. Contraction and retraction of the uterus may expel the placenta and the foetus into the abdominal cavity. Labour pains cease; the foetus dies of anoxia; blood in the peritoneal cavity causes severe abdominal pain, and the patient will soon show signs of severe shock (Feeney *et al.* 1956).

Obstructed labour leads to progressive thinning of the lower segment. In the primigravida, secondary uterine inertia usually supervenes, but in the multigravida unrelieved obstruction leads eventually to rupture of the lower segment. Rupture may occur vertically and may involve the uterine vessels; sometimes the lower segment is pinched between the head and symphysis pubis or sacral promontory, and this may cause a transverse laceration. Any form of intra-uterine manipulation will increase the risk of rupture, which is often complicated by infection. Oxytocin given in the presence of obstruction may contribute towards rupture, as already emphasized.

TREATMENT

After rupture has occurred, the patient should be resuscitated with intravenous fluid, electrolytes and blood. The abdomen is opened under general anaesthesia. The foetus and placenta are removed through the uterine opening. If the rupture is small it may be repaired with a continuous catgut ligature and the uterine tubes divided and ligated to prevent further pregnancies (Trivedi *et al.* 1968). A more extensive rupture will be treated by subtotal hysterectomy. Blood and liquor are aspirated from the abdomen. Infection is controlled with antibiotics after taking an intra-uterine swab for culture. Postoperative paralytic ileus is common and should be anticipated by continual gastric aspiration and intravenous fluids until bowel sounds have returned.

PROPHYLAXIS

The risk of rupture of a lower-section Caesarean section scar can be lessened by allowing labour only where easy vaginal delivery seems likely. Labour should not be allowed to continue for more than about 12 hr, and the second stage should be shortened by easy low forceps delivery under pudendal block or skilled general anaesthesia. It is doubtful if, nowadays, labour should ever be permitted after a previous classical section. Any patient who has been delivered

vaginally following a previous Caesarean section operation should have her uterus explored per vaginam as soon as possible to ascertain the soundness of the scar. In the case of the lower-segment procedure, a general anaesthetic may not be necessary if the exploration is carried out as soon as the delivery is complete; exploration of the body of the uterus will, however, call for general anaesthesia to permit thorough examination without discomfort to the patient. It must be emphasized that a deficiency may be found in the scar despite delivery, even spontaneous delivery, per vaginam. If a defect is found the abdomen should be opened and appropriate treatment carried out.

ACUTE INVERSION OF THE UTERUS

This is a complication of the third stage of labour when the uterus becomes partially or completely turned inside out. There must be atonia of the uterine muscle and the inversion is precipitated by heavy pressure on the fundus, attempts at Credé's expression, or cord traction with the placenta still attached to the fundus. Ergometrine given with the delivery of the infant ensures a firmly contracting uterus during the third stage and largely prevents this complication.

As the body of the uterus passes through the cervical ring it drags with it the uterine tubes and ovaries, together with their nerve and blood supply. Further congestion increases the constricting effect of the cervix, and profound shock usually develops rapidly. There is pallor, sweating, tachycardia, hypotension and often a bearing-down feeling. A globular mass is felt in the vagina or protruding through the cervix. This may be mistaken for a fibroid polyp, but in an acute inversion it is not possible to pass a blunt sound into the uterine cavity.

The shock is treated with intravenous blood, fluids and electrolytes until the patient is fit for anaesthesia. Then the placenta, if still attached, is peeled off, and the uterine body returned to its normal position. This can sometimes be obtained by distending the vagina with sterile saline run in under pressure while the vaginal introitus is occluded with the hand. If this fails, it may be possible to replace the uterus slowly by squeezing the lower segment through the cervical ring and then gradually working towards the uterine fundus. Intravenous ergometrine 0·5 mg is then given to increase uterine tone and maintain the reposition (see also p. 407).

OBSTETRIC SHOCK

Shock is a syndrome resulting from depression of many functions, but in which reduction of the effective circulating volume and blood pressure are of basic importance. So-called obstetric or postpartum shock probably does not differ from that seen in other surgical work, but there are many causes of shock which are peculiar to obstetrics.

In many cases it is a combination of factors—especially blood loss, trauma and general anaesthesis—which are responsible.

Blood loss may occur from placenta praevia or accidental antepartum haemorrhage. Following delivery further blood loss from an atonic uterus is superimposed. The patient becomes collapsed and venipuncture is rendered difficult by vasoconstriction. Blood replacement therapy is delayed and the patient soon becomes dangerously ill. Such situations are still witnessed far too frequently, and account for the many avoidable maternal deaths.

Trauma in modern obstetrics should be reduced to a minimum. Difficult forceps, with the head at a high station, should not be attempted. Breech extraction is seldom indicated and Credé's expression of the placenta is a brutal assault, particularly when attempted without anaesthesia. Other causes of trauma which may be held responsible, include manual removal of the placenta, internal version, acute inversion of the uterus and Caesarean section.

Anaesthesia may help to protect the central nervous system from the stimuli of inflicted trauma, but anaesthesia which is too light or too deep and prolonged may in itself contribute towards shock. Epidural, caudal and spinal blocks may reduce blood pressure.

Suprarenal cortical failure may occur in prolonged labour or may complicate shock which has occurred from blood loss and trauma. Haemorrhage and necrosis of the suprarenal cortex may occasionally be seen.

Anaphylaxis may follow incompatible blood transfusion, intravenous oxytocin and blood stream invasion by bacteria. *Clostridium welchii* septicaemia causes rapid haemolysis and profound collapse.

Amniotic fluid embolism may produce hypofibrinogenaemia and severe pulmonary oedema, with respiratory distress, cyanosis and exudation of fluid into the lungs.

The most important measure in treatment is restoration of circulating blood volume. Blood transfusion should be given rapidly under pressure to replace blood lost. Blood volume expanders such as fractionated dextran can be used as blood substitutes in an emergency while awaiting crossmatch, but their use should be limited to 1 l. Vasoconstrictors such as L-noradrenaline are of limited value, and it has been recently suggested that the vasocontraction may increase tissue anoxia and retard recovery. Hydrocortisone 200 mg or more given systemically may relieve suprarenal cortical exhaustion and help to reestablish a normal blood pressure.

REFERENCES

FEENEY K. & BARRY A. (1965) *Br. med. J.* i, 4958.
MARGULIES D. & CRAPANZANO J.T. (1966) *Obstet. Gynec. N.Y.* **27**, 863.
TRIVEDI R.R., PATEL K.C. & SWAMI N.B. (1968) *J. Obstet. Gynaec. Br. Commonw.* **75**, 51.

CHAPTER 28

OBSTETRIC OPERATIONS AND PROCEDURES

The procedures to be dealt with in this chapter are all practical ones. The discussion will, however, be concerned only to a minor extent with *how* they should be carried out. Practical procedures can be learnt only in practice, and descriptions are a poor substitute for seeing and doing them. Rather, will these discussions be devoted to the decision to intervene surgically, the choice of procedure, its advantages and disadvantages, risks, consequences and other matters of this nature. When technical points are relevant to the discussion, however, they will be considered.

INDUCTION OF LABOUR

One of the most common minor procedures in obstetric practice is the induction of labour. For the most part it presents few difficulties, but problems do occasionally arise emphasizing that it should not be undertaken without an adequate reason and should never be regarded as a routine procedure free from risk.

Indications

Labour may require to be induced for reasons which are mainly foetal or mainly maternal; sometimes, the best interests of both are served by getting labour established and accomplishing safe delivery.

In the foetal group the common conditions are:

   (i) Pre-eclampsia.
  (ii) Hypertension.

 (iii) Placental insufficiency which may exist without (i) or (ii).
 (iv) Postmaturity.
  (v) Rhesus incompatibility.
 (vi) Diabetes.
(vii) Repeated unstable lie.

Labour may be induced for predominantly maternal reasons because of:

  (i) Severe pre-eclampsia or hypertension.
 (ii) Gross foetal abnormality.
(iii) A dead foetus.
(iv) Antepartum haemorrhage.

It will be seen that all these are relative indications; whether labour should or should not be induced and, if so, when, are matters concerning which careful consideration may be required in any particular case. None is an absolute indication for induction of labour *per se*, since in the gravest circumstances delivery by Caesarean section may be regarded as preferable. Much skill may be required on behalf of the medical attendant to make a wise decision in many situations involving the 'indications' enumerated above.

Methods of induction

Labour may be induced by methods which are mainly medical, mainly surgical, or both.

MEDICAL INDUCTION

For generations the medical induction of labour consisted of the traditional O.B.E.—castor oil, a hot bath and an enema. The castor oil bottle has, happily, now been transferred from the drug cupboard to the museum; the hot bath, whilst undoubtedly fulfilling a profound need in some patients and being continued for hygienic reasons, probably has little action on the pregnant uterus; the enema alone survives as the sole representative of an earlier regime. It may achieve its purpose on patients who are already on the brink of labour, but it must do so seldom in other circumstances. However, by emptying the lower bowel, and thus avoiding bowel evacuation later, and perhaps by allowing the head to descend more completely on to the cervix, its continuation can be justified.

Oxytocic agents

A far more effective medical means of inducing labour is the use of oxytocics. Opinions have been divided, however, on the efficacy of these preparations and on the best means of using them. Beyond doubt, oxytocics must be given under strict control so that they may be stopped at once if they appear to be inducing too frequent, too powerful or too prolonged uterine contractions. Tetanic contractions can easily be provoked if too much is given quickly, leading to foetal death or even uterine rupture. To be successful, however, large enough doses must be given to make the uterus contract; the dose may require to be increased gradually and, again, this must be under the strictest control. The type of regime advocated by Turnbull & Anderson (1968) appeals most of all. These writers employ three speeds of infusion only, 15, 30 and 60 drops per minute. They point out that if the strength of the infusion is quadrupled with each change, the return from 60 drops per minute to 15 drops per minute when this increase in strength is carried out results in the same amount of oxytocin being given. They suggest commencing with 2 units of oxytocin in 540 ml of 5% dextrose at 15 drops per minute (approximately 4 milliunits per minute). The rate is increased to 30, and then 60, drops at 10-min intervals: if there is no uterine response the strength of the drip is increased to 8 units in 540 ml and later to 32 units in 540 ml. Once the uterus contracts the intervals

between increases in speed are extended to 20 min, until regular adequate contractions are achieved. Turnbull & Anderson's excellent account should be studied for further details.

More precise measurement of the dose of Syntocinon may be obtained by employing an automatic pump (such as a Palmer pump) delivering a dose measured in milliunits per minute. A regime employed in Queen Charlotte's Hospital is to give 2 milliunits per minute for a half hour. The dose is then increased at half-hourly intervals or until labour begins. The maximum dose normally used is 64 milliunits per minute. Increases are not made once contractions commence until it is clear how strong and frequent they are becoming.

Buccal or sublingual oxytocics have been used as alternatives to intravenous infusion in an attempt to induce labour by more simple means with less disturbance for the patient. The type of regime employed is to commence with a buccal tablet of 100 units initially repeating in a half hour and increasing to 200 units in a further half hour. Half-hourly repeats and increases are continued until a response is obtained, or up to a total dose of 4,400 units in some 5 hr. Once a response is obtained, no further increases are made. It seems likely that although this type of regime is effective (Ritchie & Brudenell 1967) better control is available by intravenous methods if these can be made available. Moreover, vigilance requires to be maintained, as a report of a ruptured uterus by Chalmers & Ng (1964) emphasizes.

Repeated injections of oxytocics such as used to be employed at half-hourly intervals do not provide sufficiently precise control, and should be used only when the child is dead, if then.

Whichever method is employed it is important for the patient constantly to be supervised by a midwife or medical attendant. The foetal heart sounds should be listened to frequently and the frequency and strength of uterine contractions recorded. Increases in the strength of the infusion should be employed only when the uterine response is absent or poor and the foetus shows no signs of distress. If strong contractions supervene, the oxytocic must be stopped at least temporarily.

Prostaglandins

In 1968 came the first report of prostaglandins being employed for the induction of labour (Karim *et al.* 1968). These are extremely exciting substances and some consideration of their position in obstetric practice is appropriate.

Prostaglandin was a name given by Euler in 1935 to a smooth-muscle stimulating and vaso-depressor substance found in extracts of human seminal fluid. It is now known that the 'substance' known as a prostaglandin was in fact a family of closely related substances, of which some 13 have been isolated and their chemical structure determined. It is evident also, that their occurrence is in no way confined to semen; they can be found in thymus, pancreas, brain, kidney, menstrual fluid, umbilical cord, liquor amnii, decidua and a number of other tissues as well.

All naturally occurring prostaglandins have 20 carbon atoms. The basic saturated carbon skeleton from which they may be considered to be derived is named prostanoic acid (Fig. 28.1).

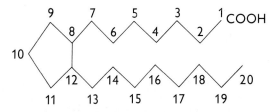

Fig. 28.1. The prostanoic acid nucleus.

Differences occurring in the structure of the 5-carbon atom ring produces four naturally occurring series of prostaglandins called E. F. A and B. The E and F series are of the greatest interest to obstetricians.

In the experimental field the effect of prosta-glandins on uterine muscle strips has been variable, depending upon which prostaglandin has been used and whether the uterus was preg-nant or not. Summarizing the results for sim-plicity, it can be said that the effect of total extract of all 13 prostaglandins on the non-pregnant uterus is mainly inhibitory; the predominant effect of the E series is also inhibitory, whereas $F_{1\alpha}$ and $F_{2\alpha}$ always stimulate non-pregnant isolated muscle strips. The response of the pregnant uterus, however, is different (Embrey 1969). The total effect of seminal extract is stimulatory; E_1 has variable effects but E_2 and $F_{2\alpha}$ always stimulate upper segment strips.

Karim and his colleagues reported the success-ful induction of labour in 10 patients by the infusion of prostaglandin $F_{2\alpha}$ (Karim *et al.* 1968). The preparation was administered con-tinuously by means of an infusion pump at rates of 2·5–5 ng/kg body weight per minute. Uterine contractions, maternal blood pressure and foetal heart rate were all recorded. Karim and his colleagues, in a separate study, noted no significant effect on heart rate, systolic or dia-stolic blood pressure, respiratory rate or E.C.G. pattern in six volunteers infused with con-centrations varying between 1 ng and 2 μg/kg body weight per minute. They later reported further experience with the induction of labour with $F_{2\alpha}$ (Karim *et al.* 1969). Thirty-five women at or near term were given $F_{2\alpha}$ to induce labour, which was successfully achieved in 33. Although $F_{2\alpha}$ was the first prostaglandin used in clinical practice, it appears that E_2 is a more effective preparation. Karim *et al.* (1970) and Beazley *et al.* (1970) both reported on the successful use of prostaglandin E_2 to induce labour near to term.

It remains to be seen what the true place of these preparations will be in obstetric practice. At the time of writing their promise appears immense, although it is not yet possible fully to assess their correct position. The whole subject was recently reviewed at some length by the New York Academy of Medical Sciences (1970) and by Beazley (1971). There appears to be little doubt that prostaglandins $F_{2\alpha}$ and E_2 are effective oxytocic drugs; it remains to be seen if either is superior to Syntocinon. Karim, reporting briefly on a controlled double-blind trial to contrast $F_{2\alpha}$, E_2 and syntocinon, demonstrated E_2 to be the most effective and syntocinon the least effective; the maximum dose of Syntocinon employed, however, was only 8 milliunits per minute which would be regarded as low by many (see p. 429). Beazley & Gillespie (1971), however, found both E_2 and Syntocinon to be equally effective when Syntocinon was given up to 64 milliunits per minute. In midtrimester abortions, however, prostaglandins are far more effective than syntocinon.

SURGICAL INDUCTION

Of the many surgical means of inducing labour which have been employed over the years one only survives in modern obstetric practice—the rupture of the membranes. The forewaters may be ruptured below the foetal head or the hind-waters above it; in either case labour begins within the next 24 hr in many patients and within the succeeding 24 hr in most of the remainder. It seems unlikely that there is much difference in the effectiveness of either variety of membrane rupture, forewater rupture perhaps being slightly the more effective. It is this method which is now generally employed. Hind-water rupture was originally introduced at a time when it was believed that the bag of membranes was a better dilator of the cervix than the head. This belief is not now held, and the principal advantage of hind-water rupture lies in the smaller likelihood of cord prolapse if the head is high; on the other hand, the passage of an instrument, such as a Drew-Smyth catheter which is normally employed, between the membranes and the uterine wall to a point above the head increases the likelihood of uterine or placental injury and, unless the head is high, forewater rupture is preferable.

The disadvantages of membrane rupture are:

(i) the cord may prolapse;
(ii) infection may be introduced;
(iii) labour may not begin for several days.

The risk of cord prolapse may be minimized by employing forewater rupture only when the head is fixed in the brim and hind-water rupture in other circumstances. Alternatively, medical means of induction can first be employed, the membrane rupture being delayed until the uterus is contracting well and the head held against the cervix and pelvic brim.

Infection should seldom be a serious maternal problem but it may give rise to intra-uterine pneumonia, with an increased foetal and maternal mortality and morbidity. The likelihood of significant infection increases with the interval between induction and delivery. Obstetricians nowadays are reluctant to prolong this interval much beyond 48 hr; unless labour is clearly in progress, serious consideration should be given to Caesarean section. For this reason, a combination of oxytocic stimulation and membrane rupture is often employed.

The technique of artificial rupture of the membranes will not be discussed here. Brant (1970) has recently reviewed it. This is, *par excellence*, something to be learnt in practice in the labour ward. The procedure must, however, be regarded as a surgical one and full aseptic precautions employed. Anaesthesia is seldom necessary, although premedication may be given to the increased comfort of the patient.

Under rare circumstances the cervix is found so tightly closed that a finger cannot be introduced through it. It will then be wise to review the indication for induction. If this is a questionable one, a reappraisal of the situation may lead to the decision to postpone induction, for a while at least. If the indication is good, however, induction should be proceeded with, despite the 'unfavourable' cervix. Preliminary infusion with Syntocinon or prostaglandins may then be employed and the membrane rupture delayed until later, as a period of contraction may greatly facilitate the procedure.

INTRA-AMNIOTIC INJECTIONS

Intra-amniotic injections of hypertonic saline or glucose have been used successfully to induce labour, but have been accompanied by such serious infective complications that their continuation cannot be justified.

CHOICE OF METHOD

It has been emphasized already that in the variable circumstances which may prevail when a decision is made to induce labour, some skill and experience will be required to choose the most satisfactory method. General advice only can be given here.

When the head is fixed in the brim, forewater rupture, after the giving of an enema, will probably be the most satisfactory procedure.

This may be followed by an oxytocic infusion if contractions do not start. To proceed with the infusion at once after membrane rupture will probably mean that many infusions will be given unnecessarily, with additional discomfort to the patient and additional extra supervision to the nursing staff. Usually, an interval may be allowed before commencing oxytocics and, during this interval, labour will often begin. The interval before beginning an oxytocic infusion in the absence of contractions may be 6, 12 or 24 hr, depending on the indication for which labour is being induced. When there is some urgency the infusion may be started 3 or 6 hr later, whilst in the most urgent cases the infusion may be employed without delay.

In the presence of a high head, yet a favourable cervix, hind-water rupture may be employed, the case otherwise being managed similarly. If the cervix is very tight and will not admit a finger an oxytocic infusion may be set up first and the patient re-examined later to detect if the cervix is becoming taken up sufficiently to allow for the surgical methods to be used.

If the foetus is dead, surgical methods carry an increased risk of infection and should not be employed.

Rupture of the membranes has one great advantage over other methods—it permits the liquor amnii to be observed to establish if there is evidence of foetal distress. Foetal heart monitoring by a scalp electrode, and foetal blood sampling, may both be employed if required.

FORCEPS DELIVERY

The application of forceps, and the safe delivery of a patient by this means, can be learnt only by practice, first on a model then, under supervision, on individual patients. No description will be given on about how to apply forceps; the account which follows will, however, deal mainly with matters of judgement in forceps delivery—when they should be used and when not, what problems may be encountered and how these may be overcome, etc. During this discussion, however, various technical points will be touched upon.

Indications and conditions

The indications to use forceps are often somewhat loosely said to be:

(i) maternal distress;
(ii) foetal distress;
(iii) delay in the second stage of labour.

When we consider these, however, it is clear that they are not indications for *forceps* delivery, although they may be indications for delivery by the most appropriate means. The decision that delivery is required, precedes that to use forceps to achieve it, and it will help to avoid the wrong use of forceps to consider things in this way. In this sense, the indications for forceps delivery cannot be separated from the conditions which are necessary before they can be applied. These will now be considered.

Conditions necessary for forceps delivery

A conventional list of these conditions is as follows:

(i) the cervix must be fully dilated;
(ii) the presentation must be suitable;
(iii) the position must be suitable;
(iv) the head must be engaged;
(v) the membranes must be ruptured;
(vi) the bladder must be empty;
(vii) there must be no obstruction to delivery at or below the level of the head.

Much more detailed consideration of these considerations will now be undertaken, since doing so many of the problems concerned with forceps delivery can be dealt with. All are excellent rules for the obstetrician in training. Rarely, the expert may consider it wise to break one or more in the best interests of the patient.

CERVIX FULLY DILATED

This is almost, but not quite, an absolute condition. If it is to be ignored, however, the decision to do so must be a deliberate one, once the situation had been fully assessed by an experienced obstetrician.

A tiny rim of cervix remaining undilated will be little barrier to the *application* of forceps for someone experienced in their use. Delivery through this rim, however, may give rise to maternal damage of perhaps considerable extent if the conditions permitting easy delivery are absent. Forceps delivery through an incompletely dilated cervix should be attempted only if the largest diameter of the foetal head has passed through a region of the vaginal vault leaving the rim of cervix, and that alone, as the barrier to delivery (Blakey *et al.* 1958). If the vault is completed dilated in this way forceps may be applied and the head gently drawn down through the rim, which is eased upwards over the head at the same time. Alternatively, the cervix may be cut at 4 o'clock and 8 o'clock to permit the head to be pulled through. Any attempt to carry out this type of manœuvre before the head has passed completely through the vaginal vault is highly likely to lead to serious laceration of the vault and the base of the broad ligament, and the tear produced may involve the uterine vessels or pass upwards into the lower segment of the uterus. For these reasons delivery with forceps before full dilation of the cervix must be regarded as a serious procedure to be undertaken only in exceptional circumstances and if particular conditions apply. Even if the conditions described above are present the vacuum extractor, if available, will be a preferable instrument to use until the head is drawn through the rim of cervix, when forceps may be substituted.

PRESENTATION

The only suitable presentations for forceps delivery, as a rule, are vertex and face. Only under the most unusual circumstances will it ever be otherwise. Exceptionally, a small baby in a large pelvis may descend almost to the pelvic floor as a brow presentation, when the best treatment may be to apply the forceps as the head presents and exert a little traction. Easy delivery is likely either as a brow or by further flexion or extension of the head at the last moment.

POSITION

Forceps may be applied to a vertex presentation with the head in the anterior, lateral or posterior position, but to a face presentation only when it is in the mento-anterior position. Delivery, however, as distinct from application, will occur with the occiput anterior or posterior or the chin anterior. These simple statements will now be amplified.

In a vertex presentation the head will, generally speaking, be delivered more easily as occipito-anterior than occipitoposterior and in most instances rotation of an occipito-posterior position should precede delivery. If the head is very deep in the pelvis as an occipitoposterior, however, delivery in that position will have much to commend it and may be safer than upward displacement, rotation and delivery as an occipito-anterior. With the head at a higher level rotation will almost always be preferable unless there is good reason to believe that the pelvis is predominantly anthropoid in shape.

The occipitolateral position requires rotation to the occipito-anterior one before delivery. Some years ago, manual rotation under general anaesthesia was the preferred method. More recently, rotation with Kielland's forceps has become the more common one, and appears to have some advantages in modern obstetric practice. Local analgesia for forceps delivery is now used widely, and manual rotation is more difficult in these circumstances; Kielland's forceps can, however, be used in some patients, with local analgesia perhaps augmented by self-administered gas and oxygen. Less displacement of the head is needed for forceps rotation, which in many cases can be achieved at the level of arrest or may occur spontaneously on the perineum if the head is drawn downwards to a lower level. The disturbance to the head is also probably less in forceps rotation; a hand grasping the vault for rotation—instead of the face, which is to be preferred—will feel alarming movement at the suture-lines, suggesting that damage can easily be inflicted if too firm a grasp is employed. Thus, Kielland's forceps appears a preferable method of rotation.

Their application will usually be by the wandering method, the anterior blade being manœuvred gently around the face to its position on the anterior parietal bone; occasionally, if the head is very low, direct application of the anterior blade is possible. The classical application of the anterior blade with its cephalic curve forwards, followed by rotation of this blade through 180° after which it is brought downwards into position, should not be employed.

It may be stressed that if the head is in the oblique occipito-anterior position with the occiput pointing to the 2 o'clock or 10 o'clock position, deliberate rotation is unnecessary; the forceps may be applied cephalically or, if this cannot quite be achieved, as close to it as can, and the head drawn down, when spontaneous rotation on the perineum is likely to be observed.

With a face presentation, of course, delivery as a mentoposterior cannot be achieved. Whether delivery can safely be accomplished by forceps with the head in the mento-anterior position is something which can only readily be assessed at the time in a particular patient, and mature judgement and experience will be called for.

ENGAGEMENT OF THE HEAD

Forceps deliveries have for many years been divided into three categories, called high, mid and low forceps.

High forceps, where the biparietal diameter of the head is just at the pelvic brim, is now seldom employed. The kind of case justifying high forceps delivery is that in which some sudden emergency situation for the child—prolapse of the cord for instance—occurs in a multiparous patient, or there is the need to deliver the second of twins from a high level. The problems of high forceps are concerned partly with the greater difficulty of correct application at a high level, but mainly with the large amount of undilated soft tissue below the head. Virtually the whole of the vagina will be undilated, so that in a primigravid patient or one of low parity there may be considerable resistance to delivery from the soft tissues; damage to the foetal head or laceration to the mother, or both, may result. High forceps delivery, therefore, is only for the experienced obstetrician in particular circumstances; one less experienced is likely to do more harm than good. The vacuum extractor, if available, appears more suitable than high forceps in the situations envisaged above.

With mid forceps extraction the largest diameter of the head is between the brim and the ischial spines. Here also, much of the lower vagina will be undilated and manual stretching to facilitate delivery is advisable before the actual extraction proceeds. In considering mid forceps extraction it must be pointed out that it has become customary to describe the station of a head in a pelvis with reference to its lowest point. If the lowest point of a head is at the ischial spinal level the largest diameter is probably just through the pelvic brim provided there is no marked moulding or caput formation (Fig. 12.4). With both these cephalic changes present the largest diameter may be at almost any level (Fig. 12.4). Great care must be taken to ensure that the head is engaged before embarking on forceps delivery. Unless there is an urgent need to interfere, a short wait will often allow the head to descend to a much lower level and the occiput to rotate further forwards. One often seems forceps delivery embarked upon for deep transverse arrest when the head is neither deep nor arrested!

Low forceps describes delivery when the biparietal diameter is at or below the level of the ischial spines. It will seldom cause difficulty.

RUPTURE OF MEMBRANES

Few books or articles on forceps delivery suggest why this requirement must be met. When advance in the second stage is delayed and the membranes are intact, the correct procedure is to rupture them, after which further interference may be unnecessary.

BLADDER EMPTY

For most forceps deliveries this is an excellent rule. It may be, however, that with the head very deep on the perineum, simple 'lift-out' forceps delivery may be accomplished without the need to catheterize the patient, since there may be little urethal bruising with easy voiding of urine afterwards. The risk of introducing infection into the bladder is then minimized.

NO OBSTRUCTION BELOW THE HEAD

This is an absolute rule. The rule should never be pulled past an area of obstruction.

Caesarean section is indicated (see trial of forceps, below).

Varieties of forceps

Since forceps were introduced in obstetric practice many designs have been used, only to be superseded by others, which in their turn were replaced by better ones. Nowadays, several types of forceps are commonly used in this country. With one exception—the Kielland's forceps— each has a pelvic and cephalic curve. Some have axis traction attachments either to the blades themselves or to the shank. It is debatable if any variety (Kielland's excepted) has a special advantage over its rivals. The instrument is asked to do little more than pull the baby from the relatively low position through the pelvic outlet. Axis traction rods, etc. can be completely dispensed with, although no doubt some obstetricians still use them. Indeed, personal preference will generally be the deciding factor between one variety of forceps and another, so that in most situations almost any type will be satisfactory. The very short Wrigley's forceps might, with benefit, be given up. They have an immediate appeal in their small size which may result in an inexperienced operator choosing them unwisely when a larger pair are essential. The use of the Wrigley's forceps to deliver the after-coming head at a breech delivery is an excellent example of this, for unless the head descends well (when it can be delivered in a variety of ways) the instrument will be too short; by the time this is realized dangerous delay will have resulted.

Kielland's forceps have a real value when rotation is necessary, as has already been discussed. Huntingford (1967) has reviewed their place in obstetrics.

Failed forceps

This term was applied some years ago to the situation in which an attempt has been made unsuccessfully to delivery a patient with forceps. Happily, it is a rare circumstance in modern obstetrics. It might be thought that the main reason for failure was unrecognized disproportion. In reality, the two most common causes are examples of fundamental errors of technique— the application of forceps before full dilatation of the cervix, and the failure to recognize that the head is in the occipitoposterio position (Law 1953; Gadd 1954). In either event no progress is achieved when traction is exerted, and the instruments may pull off. Maternal and foetal trauma may be inflicted. These mistakes should not be made, since careful examination will disclose the true state of affairs, and appropriate treatment can be employed. Other possible causes are other malpresentations, such as a brow presentation, unrecognized disproportion, hydrocephalus, etc.

Trial of forceps

The only circumstances when it might be permissible to apply forceps expecting a vaginal delivery and later to remove them and deliver the patient by Caesarean section is when such a trial of forceps is employed as a deliberate manœuvre. It is easier to say that forceps should never be used to deliver a baby when there is no disproportion than it is to decide, in a particular case, if there is disproportion or not. In a busy maternity hospital the situation will occasionally arise when it is not possible in any particular case to be certain if there is mild disproportion or not. In such a circumstance it may be permissible for an experienced obstetrician to apply forceps and to observe progress when reasonable traction is exerted. If advance is maintained, well and good. If not, Caesarean section can be carried out immediately. It will be seen there are obvious advantages to the trial of forceps being conducted in the operating theatre so that there need be no delay if Caesarean section is required. It will be clear, too, that the dividing line here is very narrow. If too great force is exerted the foetus may be damaged and vaginal delivery may result in a stillborn child or one with a cerebral injury. Even if the decision be made to abandon the attempt at vaginal delivery and deliver the patient by Caesarean section, the result may be the same if traction had been exerted too strongly. Trial of forceps, like much else discussed in this chapter, requires skill and mature judgement to be a safe procedure.

VACUUM EXTRACTION

Vacuum extraction, although an old idea, was introduced to obstetrics as a reality by Malmstrom (1954). The instrument has now been used sufficiently long for some assessment to be made of its place in present-day obstetrical practice. The vacuum extractor is a supreme example of the thesis that has pervaded this chapter: that practical procedures can be learnt only in practice. Its wider introduction into obstetrics has undoubtedly been delayed by the fact that it requires an entirely different technique than that of forceps delivery; unless this technique is mastered, poor results will be obtained and the instrument is likely to be blamed rather than the operator.

The vacuum extractor may be used as an alternative to obstetric forceps to deliver a patient whose cervix is fully dilated and on whom forceps would not normally be used. Its second use is to expedite dilatation of the cervix when this apparently ceases and labour is becoming prolonged.

As an alternative to forceps delivery it seems likely that there is little to choose between these methods, given uncomplicated cases and operators skilled in their use. The delivery is probably more comfortable for the patient, since the additional distention of the perineum is less with the vacuum extractor. Local analgesia is all that is required in the majority of instances; indeed, in some multiparous patients no anaesthetic may be required at all and the discomfort of the delivery will be comparable with that of a normal birth. There are circumstances in which the instrument has distinct advantages, some of which have already been indicated in the section on forceps delivery. If the foetal head is high, application of the vacuum extractor may be simpler and safer than is the case with forceps. If the head is occipito-posterior or transverse the application of the cup, followed by traction, may permit good advance and easy rotation on the pelvic floor; this rotation may be assisted by pressure on the knob on the cup, but unless this is gentle, and is accompanied by careful traction strictly at right-angles to the plane of the cup, it may pull off. The instrument is ideally suited for application to the high head of a second twin when delay occurs.

With advantages of this kind it is a little surprising that the extractor has not been more widely received than is the case in this country. The explanation is probably that such a different technique is required that this has not been truly learnt by obstetricians who, after all, need only to take up a pair of forceps to deliver the patients skillfully, easily and safely. The forceps are always available and the vacuum extractor may not be, or perhaps may not be correctly maintained and therefore not in proper working condition. The training of the younger obstetrician in the use of the instrument has therefore been incomplete, and until this gap is filled it is unlikely that forceps extraction will be replaced by vacuum extraction. Chalmers (Chalmers & Fothergill 1960; Chalmers 1964) has been one of the chief protagonists of the vacuum extractor in this country and has obtained excellent results with it.

The use of the vacuum extractor in the first stage of labour when progress has ceased has advantages in very special circumstances. When there is delay in labour—with the cervix more than, say, 6 cm dilated—this delay can sometimes be effectively managed by the vacuum extractor. It is essential, of course, to establish that there is no disproportion before any attempt at extraction is begun. Once the cap has been applied to the head, traction should be exerted gently and intermittently, bringing the head firmly into contact with the undilated portion of the cervix. Initially, little apparent progress may be made, perhaps for 10 or 15 min, but afterwards the cervix will often dilate quite quickly and the remaining rim may be slipped up over the head, which is gently drawn down past it. Delivery may then be completed with the extractor, or forceps may be substituted if there is any difficulty or if the vacuum extraction has already pulled off or been in place too long.

A few technical points will be mentioned. The largest cup which can be applied is always desirable. Traction must be at right-angles to the transverse axis of the cup, or it may pull off. Prolonged application is to be avoided, as it increases the risk of scalp bruising, or sloughing or cephalhaematoma, etc. If there is no progress over 30 min or, at the maximum, 40 min, the procedure should be stopped. Initially, the instrument was introduced in the hope that prolonged, continuous weight traction may assist cervical dilation and permit delivery. Prolonged traction of this kind, however, led to too great trauma of the foetal scalp, and this has been abandoned. It was initially suggested that 6–10 min were essential to build up the necessary vacuum (0·8 kg/cm²) and to fill the cup satisfactorily with the chignon of scalp; it now seems probable that a much shorter time will suffice. Foetal distress, therefore, with the head in the mid-cavity of the pelvis or lower, and the cervix incompletely dilated, may be effectively dealt with by vacuum extraction; the delivery may be accomplished much more quickly than would be possible by resorting to Caesarean section, and with far less trauma to the mother and child than by cervical incision.

The maternal risk of the vacuum extractor seems minimal. The foetal results appear comparable with those of forceps delivery, although Malmstrom believes the instrument to be superior in this respect (Malmstrom & Lange 1964). The special foetal disadvantages of the instrument is scalp trauma. The chignon usually disappears in a few hours. Occasionally, however, superficial necrosis or more widespread sloughing may be observed. These lesions are more common or more extensive with prolonged application than when the instrument has pulled off several times and been reapplied.

CAESAREAN SECTION

This section, like that of forceps delivery, will not be concerned with how to perform the operation but with such aspects as its indications, consequences, difficulties, dangers, timing and variety, etc. Technique will be referred to, however, when special circumstances presenting particular technical problems are discussed.

Indications

With very few exceptions, scarcely ever seen in modern obstetric practice in this country, all the indications for Caesarean section are relative ones. A list of all the conditions which might call for this method of treatment would be very long and quite unhelpful. The indications, however, may be divided into groups, as follows:

(a) IN LABOUR

  (i) Foetal or maternal distress in the first stage of labour.
  (ii) Prolongation of the first stage of labour so as to increase the foetal and maternal risk.
  (iii) Obstructive labour or disproportion becoming evident during labour.

(b) AS AN ELECTIVE PROCEDURE

  (iv) Disproportion or the likelihood of obstructive labour.
  (v) The need to deliver the patient quickly in the presence of some serious pregnancy disorder such as fulminating toxaemia.
  (vi) When vaginal delivery would cause serious risk to the life or health of the mother, child, or both. Placenta praevia would be the main condition in this category. The group includes, however, various conditions which may be adversely affected by vaginal delivery; examples are: previous successful repair for a vesicovaginal fistula, or prolapse, or the existence of a congenital malformation like an ectopic anus.
  (vii) When it is dangerous to allow the uterine contractions of labour because of previous Caesarean section or previous uterine injury or other operation.
  (viii) To minimize the trauma of delivery to the foetus, as in the case of a premature foetus or one affected by placental insufficiency or maternal diabetes.
  (ix) Postmortem, to save the life of the child.

Various points for discussion arise out of this list of general causes.

It has already been stated that indications are relative, and in some circumstances Caesarean section may not be required despite the presence of one or other of the 'indications' mentioned above. A very premature baby, for example, may be so profoundly and quickly affected by foetal distress in labour that it may be decided to withhold Caesarean section as the chances of the child's survival were too slender; maternal distress in labour may be better managed by pain relief such as epidural analgesia might offer; the patient's reaction to a previous Caesarean section may so sway her against its repetition that an attempt at vaginal delivery may be preferred. Many factors must be carefully assessed before deciding on Caesarean section in a particular case.

The pros and cons of some of these decisions have already been discussed in different sections of this book. Several which have not will now be dealt with in greater detail.

PREVIOUS CAESAREAN SECTION

The dictum 'once a Caesarean section always a Caesarean section' had few advocates in Britain in the past. The view has generally prevailed that, provided the first operation was carried out for a non-recurrent cause, and provided the obstetrical situation near to term in the succeeding pregnancy was normal, an attempt, at least, at vaginal delivery was appropriate. In practice, it has even seemed that many obstetricians went further than this aiming at vaginal delivery following Caesarean section even when the foetal head was high at term, or when border-line disproportion had just failed to be overcome on a previous occasion, or in other circumstances in which it could not be truly said that the obstetrical situation was normal. This tendency to resist Caesarean section arose from the wish not to compromise a patient's obstetric future, for by repeating the operation the obstetrician was making it virtually certain that if there should be another pregnancy a third operation would be required.

It is probable that a similar view still prevails, although perhaps to a less extent than formerly. The size of the average family has grown smaller, so that to repeat a Caesarean section will, in many instances, have little effect on the patient's obstetric future, which may only amount to one more pregnancy, if that. In the younger patient there still seems to be a place for attempting to achieve vaginal delivery if the obstetrical situation

in the next pregnancy is normal; if it is not, however, or if the patient is older or is towards the end of her child-bearing life, repeating the operation may be preferable.

The factors to be weighed in the balance are the risk to the mother of repeating the Caesarean section and the risk to her and her child of rupture of the scar if labour is allowed. A realistic mortality rate for relatively uncomplicated Caesarean section is not easy to determine. In the *Confidential Inquiry into Maternal Deaths in England and Wales, 1964–1966*, the calculated fatality rate for the operation was 1·6 per 1,000 Caesarean sections, representing only a slight fall in the figure from 1961–3 (1·8 per 1,000) and 1958–60 (2 per 1,000). This figure is some ten times that for patients delivering per vaginam. However, it almost certainly includes cases with serious complications from which death occurred rather than from the operation. Moreover, the risk to a patient delivered per vaginam following Caesarean section is almost certainly greater than that for maternal mortality as a whole.

The risk of rupture of a classical Caesarean section scar was reported by Dewhurst (1957) to be 2·2% for all cases, 4·7% for those in labour and 8·9% for those delivered vaginally; the figures for the lower segment operation were 0·5%, 0·8% and 1·2%, respectively. Five out of 100 mothers with a ruptured classical scar died and the foetal mortality was 73%; all 55 mothers with a ruptured lower segment scar survived, the foetal mortality rate being 12·5%.

Peel & Chamberlain (1968) and McGarry (1969) review the position further. Peel and Chamberlain make the important observation that the incidence of scar rupture increases in patients allowed to attempt a vaginal delivery after a previous Caesarean section for disproportion; in this group, moreover, the incidence of successful vaginal delivery fell and perinatal mortality rose compared with attempted vaginal delivery following Caesarean section for other indications. Reducing the number of attempted vaginal deliveries after previous Caesarean section in their own hospital corresponded with a fall in perinatal mortality; when 47% of patients were allowed to go into labour following Caesarean section, perinatal mortality was 71 per 1,000, compared with 16 per 1,000 when 33% were permitted to labour. McGarry (1969), however, demonstrates that good results are compatible with vaginal delivery following Caesarean section. He reports on 415 women previously delivered by Caesarean section; 242 (58·3%) were delivered vaginally with a perinatal loss of eight babies (19 per 1,000). The deaths of three of the eight babies, however, were in some measure concerned with delivery vaginally. One scar ruptured in the total of 415 patients.

Other unfavourable factors tending to increase the risk of scar rupture are said to be sepsis following the operation and the implantation of the placenta beneath the scar in a subsequent pregnancy. It seems unlikely that any but gross infection following a Caesarean section would severely affect scar healing. The position of the placenta in the subsequent pregnancy can readily be determined by ultrasound or isotope scanning.

Clearly, there are risks to a patient with a previous Caesarean section whatever is done and, as always, many factors will require to be taken into account when deciding what is best for any individual patient. It is doubtful if vaginal delivery after classical Caesarean section can safely be permitted; if the previous operation has been a lower segment one, the indication non-recurrent, and the subsequent obstetrical situation normal, an attempt at vaginal delivery seems reasonable, at any rate in the younger patients.

Caesarean section in the interests of the foetus

One group in the indication for Caesarean section calling for some comment is that in which the intervention is largely, if not entirely, in the interests of the child. A patient with mild pre-eclampsia, yet with placental insufficiency affecting the foetal well-being *in utero*, is a good example of this kind of problem. If clinical examination, endocrine assay, ultrasonic evidence of retarded growth, etc. indicate a dangerous situation for the foetus at say, 35–36 weeks, what method of delivery should be chosen? The mother is at very little risk from her mild toxaemia but the foetus is in some danger; will vaginal delivery be safe for the foetus or not?

This is the kind of question which is extremely difficult to answer factually, mainly because of the problems of comparing like with like. It has several times been reported that perinatal mortality associated with uncomplicated elective Caesarean section at term exceeds that for normal, vaginal delivery at term (Benson *et al.* 1965). Is it correct, however, to compare uncomplicated elective Caesarean section at term with normal vaginal delivery? Should not the comparison be between elective Caesarean section at term and those patients in whom it is decided to permit vaginal delivery regardless of what happens thereafter? This is the kind of difficulty which has complicated the statistical evidence concerning the foetal risk in Caesarean section. Groups to be compared have been corrected by including this condition and excluding that, but no really satisfactory comparison has emerged. A large series from any centre, for instance, will necessarily go back several years, during which time treatment will certainly have changed—and so will the hospital staff.

It is evident, however, that respiratory distress complications are more common in babies born by Caesarean section than in equally mature babies born vaginally. Here is a definite risk which must be accepted in any patient who is considered for Caesarean section mainly in the interests of a premature baby. This risk still exists, of course, if the premature baby is born per vaginam, and so do other risks. A normal birth occurs in retrospect. When it is over we can say that was a normal confinement. Until it is over, however, there are risks such as anoxia, cord prolapse, infection and others threatening the life of the foetus which will not be factors if delivery is accomplished by operation. All things considered, it seems fair to conclude that faced with many situations in which Caesarean section may be indicated, in the interest of the foetus the risks to the child will probably be smaller if the operation is decided upon.

POSTMORTEM CAESAREAN SECTION

Few obstetricians have been required to perform the procedure, but all may be called on to do so at any time. If the mother has died suddenly there may be little time to weigh the pros and cons, but if maternal death can be foreseen many of the problems concerned can be considered in advance. The chances of a child surviving will decrease the longer the operation is delayed. Cantoni & Rasini (1960) report the case of a live child born 45 min after the mother's death from subarachnoid haemorrhage, the mother's body having been kept oxygenated by ventilation through an endotracheal tube. In general, however, the foetus will die long before this and, if it is to have a reasonable chance of survival, must be delivered as soon as possible after it is certain that the mother is dead.

It may be difficult to be quite certain that death has occurred, and some attempt to revive the mother will generally be appropriate. An attempt to aerate the lungs and carry out external cardiac massage will often be indicated, but if these attempts are unsuccessful after 10 min or so they should be abandoned and the child extracted.

The relatives' permission should be sought, and in a chronic illness can usually be obtained. Even without it, however, there appears to be little likelihood of a successful prosecution of anyone intervening on the infant's behalf (*B.M.J.* 1965).

A classical type of operation is indicated to extract the child with the utmost speed.

TYPE OF OPERATION

It is probably fair to say that the lower-segment Caesarean section should be performed whenever this can safely be done. It will not always be safe, however, and the few indications for classical Caesarean section remain today.

A lower uterine segment containing fibroids may make entry into the uterine cavity extremely difficult, bleeding heavy, and the lower-segment operation very dangerous. The classical Caesarean section should then be employed, placing the incision away from the tumours. Similarly, if the lower segment is covered by adhesions the increased risk involved in the lower-segment approach may make the classical operation preferable. Eastman (1961) reports such a case in which a lower-segment operation was persisted with and the patient died. Classical Caesarean

section is recommended for a patient with carcinoma of the cervix who requires to be delivered by operation before radiotherapy could be carried out. Postmortem, the type of operation should be classical.

Other indications are more debatable. Malpas (1961) suggests that transverse lie should be dealt with in this way; it seems probable, however, that the lower-segment procedure will more often be sufficient if the uterus is relaxed sufficiently by a suitable anaesthetic. Malpas and Eastman advocate classical Caesarean section for central placenta praevia, which is even more debatable still. The bleeding from the lower segment can generally be controlled satisfactorily even though it is necessary to incise the placenta or peel part of it off the uterine wall before extracting the child. Moreover, if very large sinuses bleed heavily they may be directly oversown to control blood loss.

TIMING OF ELECTIVE CAESAREAN SECTION

If elective Caesarean section is to be employed because the foetus *in utero* is in danger of death from placental insufficiency, an estimate of the imminence of that danger will decide the timing of intervention; hormone assay, ultrasonic cephalometry, amnioscopy etc. are the usual means of estimating this foetal risk (see Chapter 11). If the elective Caesarean section is for other reasons—cephalopelvic disproportion, previous Caesarean sections, breech presentation in an older primagravida, etc.—the optimum time for delivery will probably be between 39 and 40 weeks. In such a case it is extremely important to establish the foetal maturity as accurately as possible. If the section is performed at what is thought to be 39 weeks of gestation whereas the real maturity is far less—perhaps only 35 weeks— the child may die. If planned intervention is to be earlier—37–38 weeks in a diabetic or 35–36 weeks in a patient with severe rhesus incompatibility— it is even more important that no mistake in maturity is made. Attention to menstrual history, date of quickening, size of uterus, etc. should establish if doubt exists; if it does, liquor amnii studies (p. 165), ultrasonic biparietal measurement (p. 157) or radiography (p. 157) may be helpful in solving the problem.

X-rays may be helpful also in establishing that the foetal skeleton is normal. Figure 28.2 illustrates an abnormality of a severity likely to influence the decision concerning mode of delivery if no absolute indication for Caesarean section existed. Radiography prior to elective Caesarean section is recommended whenever possible.

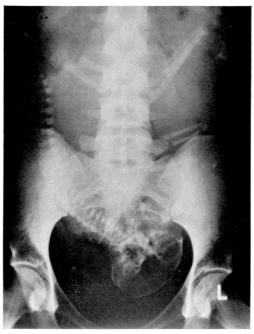

Fig. 28.2. Radiograph in late pregnancy, showing foetal microcephaly.

MORTALITY FROM CAESAREAN SECTION

A Caesarean section is a major operation under any circumstances, and maternal mortality figures emphasize this. The number of deaths associated with Caesarean section in the *Confidential Inquiry into Maternal Mortality, 1964–1966* was 145, a figure which was higher than the two previous reports. The estimated mortality rate for the condition in 1964–6 (1·6 per 1,000 Caesarean sections) was, however, slightly lower than that for the two previous reports (1·8 per 1,000 in 1961–3 and 2 per 1,000 in 1958–60). These are deaths associated with Caesarean section, and not necessarily due to it. Some are undoubtedly due to it, although a precise estimate of this number is very difficult to obtain.

The principal immediate causes of death are: haemorrhage (accounting for 14·5% of section deaths), pre-eclampsia (18·6%—the largest single cause), sepsis and paralytic ileus (17·9%, cardiac failure during and immediately after operation (11%), and toxaemia of pregnancy (4%); 20% of the deaths were from other causes, presumably largely concerned with the patient's general condition and the indication for the operation; 13·8% of deaths were due to anaesthesia (see p. 450). One of the most distressing findings in these figures is that the rate for pulmonary embolism has shown no improvement. Another disturbing finding is that there has been an increase in deaths due to sepsis and paralytic ileus. Emphasis cannot be placed too strongly upon the need to maintain aseptic precautions throughout labour in case Caesarean section be required later. Seventeen of the 20 deaths due to anaesthesia were due to Mendelson's syndrome, the great importance of which is discussed elsewhere (p. 442).

Symphysiotomy is considered on p. 399, external version on p. 364, and foetal destructive procedures on p. 402.

OBSTETRICAL ANAESTHESIA AND ANALGESIA

Reference has been made to various forms of analgesia and anaesthesia, in those sections of this book in which different problems requiring pain relief or anaesthetic assistance are discussed. For completeness, a brief consideration will be undertaken of the problem as a whole.

Nowadays, the obstetrical anaesthetist must be a well-trained specialist in anaesthesia and, therefore, only exceptionally will the obstetrician himself find it necessary or advisable to attempt to give a general anaesthetic. No better illustrations can be obtained of the need for a fully competent anaesthetist to administer an obstetrical anaesthetic than the fatalities referred to in the *Confidential Inquiry into Maternal Deaths in England and Wales, 1964–1966*. Deaths from complications of anaesthesia were higher in that report than in any preceding one; 50 maternal deaths were ascribed to this cause, and 24 of them were considered to have avoidable factors present. The commonest cause of death by far was inhalation of gastric contents (see p. 442).

For this reason, a detailed consideration by an obstetrician for obstetricians of anaesthetic agents, methods and techniques in this increasingly complex field is inappropriate; what is appropriate however, is how various facets of anaesthesia relate to the obstetrician, and what his position and responsibilities are.

INHALATION OF GASTRIC CONTENTS

With this, the most important single cause of death due to obstetrical anaesthesia, the obstetrician must do all he can to minimize its likelihood in patients during labour, any of whom may require a general anaesthetic quickly for some unforeseen complication. Gastric emptying-time during labour is delayed, so that food taken at the beginning of, or even before, labour, may still be in the stomach when a general anaesthetic is required some hours later. Whilst measures to remove gastric contents are possible, they are seldom completely successful and always unpleasant. The passage of a gastric tube to allow removal of stomach contents is upsetting to most patients and may be accompanied by a degree of hypoxia which could be harmful if, for instance, the complication calling for the anaesthetic were foetal distress.

A better approach is to limit the food taken by mouth during labour to that which is likely to be easily digested and passed through into the duodenum, or is sufficiently fluid or semi-fluid to be removed through a gastric tube in an emergency. Drinks may be taken fairly freely, except for glucose, with which care is required. Crawford (1965) suggests that glucose drinks of greater than 5% concentration increase the delay in gastric emptying; they also have more important effect of increasing gastric acidity, for it is not only the inhalation of food which causes

serious complications of general anaesthesia but the inhalation of acid gastric juices also (Mendelson 1946). Such inhalation, generally referred to as Mendelson's syndrome, causes bronchial and bronchiolar spasm with considerable obstruction to ventilation. Cynosis develops with rapid respiration, râles, rhonchi, hypoxia and tachycardia. The inhalation may not be evident immediately, general bronchiolar spasm and dyspnoea developing when the effects of the anaesthetic have passed off. Cynosis, rapid respiration and tachycardia in a patient having just received a general anaesthetic strongly suggest inhalation of gastric contents.

Instructions to be followed for the prevention of inhalation of stomach contents during anaesthesia at Queen Charlotte's Hospital are:

(i) The giving of glucose drinks (including lemonade) is dangerous. From the onset of labour, fluids containing sugar or glucose should be avoided.

(ii) The overloading of the stomach with any fluid is also dangerous. While patients may be allowed to quench their thirst with any beverage they wish, or with water, on no account should the intake of fluids be forced.

(iii) Patients who are in labour should only be given food which will pass through a sieve.

(iv) All patients when established in labour shall be given 15 ml Magnesium Trisilicate Mixture B.P.C., 3-hourly, and a further 15 ml with premedication.

(v) The advisability of passing a stomach tube and of emptying the contents of the stomach before induction of anaesthesia should be considered in every case in which a patient is known to have eaten unsieved food within 24 hr of anaesthesia.

Other possible precautions to reduce the incidence of gastric inhalation—such as rapid intubation with a cuffed tube, utilization of the left lateral position, quick use of the Trendelenburg position, ready availability of suction, etc.—fall within the province of the anaesthetist himself.

LEVEL OF ANAESTHESIA REQUIRED

It is out of place for an obstetrician to tell an anaesthetist what anaesthetic agent to use. He should be able to say, however, what conditions he requires for whatever manipulation he has to perform, and it is the duty of the anaesthetist to provide them if at all possible.

In most instances where a general anaesthetic is called for in obstetrics the operator requires a light general anaesthetic with relaxation of the voluntary muscles but not the uterine muscle. The use of nitrous oxide and oxygen, and a muscle relaxant, will produce these conditions, since the uterine muscle will not be affected by the relaxing agent used. If the mother is kept lightly asleep and well oxygenated the infant should be delivered in good condition and the uterus should contract strongly following an injection of ergometrine after delivery.

There are occasions, however, when relaxation of the uterine muscle is essential to permit the appropriate obstetrical manœuvre to be completed. External version under anaesthesia is such a circumstance, for unless the abdominal muscle and the uterine muscle are relaxed the version may not be successful. The presence of a constriction ring will call for it to be relaxed or incised if delivery is to be achieved, and really deep anaesthesia may be required. Sometimes at Caesarean section, with a baby's head deep in the pelvis, difficulty can be experienced in getting the head out if the uterus remains too irritable; again, some uterine relaxation may be desirable. The great dangers of internal version in the presence of a transverse lie with ruptured membranes have already been stressed, but there are circumstances when this manœuvre may have to be attempted; it will be facilitated if some relaxation of the uterine muscle is obtained. During the third stage of labour, hour-glass uterine contraction below the placenta may cause difficulty in manual removal unless the anaesthetist is able to relax the uterine muscle.

Providing the anaesthetist is informed of the conditions required it should not be difficult for him to provide them, except in rare cases. The problem is to obtain sufficient relaxation to permit delivery or other manipulation and yet to allow the uterus to return to a responsive state so that it can contract immediately, or very soon, after delivery. A skilful anaesthetist can usually achieve this with a minimum of risk by employing halothane, but other techniques are available (see p. 392).

SPINAL ANALGESIA

The disadvantages of spinal analgesia are more pronounced during pregnancy than at other times, and only under exceptional circumstances should this form of treatment be employed. Alterations to the spinal curvature due to the presence of the full-time pregnant uterus increase the difficulty of controlling the level of analgesia in the spinal cord. The anaesthetic agent may pass to a higher level with maternal respiratory difficulty, paralysis or hypotension. Headache can be troublesome in a high percentage of cases.

Epidural and caudal analgesia are discussed on p. 390.

LOCAL ANALGESIA

Local analgesia, as a pudendal block, is employed with considerable benefit in a large proportion of simpler obstetric operations. The technique of pudendal block is easily learnt. The anaesthetic agent should be injected as close to the ischial spines as possible, since the nerve crosses the tip of the spine. An additional nerve supply to the vulval area usually comes from the ilio-inguinal and genitofemoral nerves anteriorly, from the posterior cutaneous nerve of the thigh, and sometimes directly from the sacral plexus. These branches can best be anaesthetized by infiltrating locally towards the symphysis pubis, on each side and across the perineum, and in the lateral vulval tissues.

Dangers are involved in overdosage. If 1% lignocaine or its equivalent is used the maximum volume which can safely be injected is 50 ml, if a vasoconstrictor is added, or 20 ml without one. For $\frac{1}{2}\%$ lignocaine, which is usually adequate, double these amounts may be used. If more is given or the injection is given intravenously in error, convulsions, coma or drowsiness may result and death may ultimately occur. These convulsions should be controlled with thiopentone, and adequate oxygenation and breathing ensured.

RESUSCITATION OF THE NEWBORN

The newborn infant has a tendency towards a respiratory and metabolic acidosis, and this will is slow. Progressive anoxia leads to peripheral circulatory failure with a cold, pale skin, flaccid muscles, feeble heart action, and absent reflex irritability. Irrespective of the degree of asphyxia, it is important to institute methods of resuscitation without delay.

The Apgar scoring system (Apgar 1953) is still an acceptable method of assessing the severity of the asphyxia, and it is usual to make these observations at 1 and 5 min.

Apgar score	0	1	2
Heart rate	Absent	Below 100 per minute	Over 100 per minute
Respiratory effort	Absent	Weak cry. Hypoventilation	Good, strong cry
Muscle tone	Limp	Some flexion of extremities	Active movement. Extremities well flexed
Reflex instability (stimulation with nasal catheter)	No response	Grimace	Cry
Colour	Blue. Pale	Body pink. Extremities blue	Completely pink

be most severe in those infants subjected to anoxia, and particularly the premature infant, who finds it more difficult to compensate by the normal mechanisms of acid-base and fluid balance.

Adequate oxygenation following birth is dependent upon normal expansion of the lungs, and failure will lead to respiratory distress. The underlying causes include immaturity of the lungs, surface tension and airflow obstruction, hyaline membrane formation, aspiration of amniotic fluid, meconium or vernix caseosa, spontaneous pneumothorax, brain damage, traumatic shock, haemorrhagic disease of the newborn, transplacental haemorrhage into the maternal circulation, amniotic infection, twin transfusion syndrome, and abnormalities of the placenta and umbilical cord.

Signs of asphyxia

The infant first becomes blue; the face is swollen; the muscles still have good tone but the heart beat

0–2 points: severely depressed infant.
3–6 points: moderately depressed infant.
7–10 points: Infant in good condition.

APPARATUS FOR RESUSCITATION

This should include a trolley fitted with an adjustable inclined plane and an adjustable water manometer, which permits intermittent flow of oxygen at a maximal predetermined pressure.

A Penlon infant laryngoscope with curved and straight blades and a supply of spare light bulbs.

No. 12 Warne's endotracheal tube.

No. 12 St. Thomas's Hospital endotracheal tube.

No. 3 Leyland red rubber tube.

No. 6 Portsmouth suction tube.

An infant pharyngeal airway.

An infant oxygen funnel mask.

Blease insufflator.

Johnson disposable plastic sterile mucus extractor.

2-ml disposable sterile syringe with No. 17 hypodermic needle.

Ampoules of sterile normal saline.

10-ml ampoule of 5% sodium bicarbonate solution.

Inj. nalorphine hydrobromide (Lethindrone Neonatal) 1 mg in 1 ml.

Inj. phytomenadione or vitamin K (Konakion) 1 mg in 0·5 ml.

Resuscitation

As a routine, the infant is held head downwards immediately after delivery and the upper respiratory passages fully aspirated with a sterile mucus sucker. Oxygen may be given through a funnel mask if respirations are present and the Apgar score is 5 or over. The infant may be stimulated by aspirating the nose or flicking the heels, but digital dilatation of the anal sphincter, back slapping or chest compression is to be condemned.

If the Apgar score is 4 or less then a laryngoscope is passed, the larynx aspirated and an endotracheal tube passed. Oxygen is given at a pressure of 30 cm of water and held for 2 sec. After two such insufflations the pressure is reduced to 15 cm of water and repeated 40 times per minute. When six spontaneous respirations have become established the tube is removed. If the Apgar score is 3 or less and response to oxygen is not immediate then give 5% sterile sodium bicarbonate solution 5 ml by injection into the umbilical vein. This is equivalent to 3 m.equiv. and the dose may be repeated.

If there is cardiac arrest, repeated depression of the sternum at 100 times per minute is alternated with tracheal insufflation 40 times per minute, and this may re-establish an effective circulation, but when this advanced stage of asphyxia has been reached there will be a high incidence of permanent cerebral damage.

Hyperbaric oxygen appears to be of no practical value in the treatment of asphyxia neonatorum. Intragastric oxygen has been used successfully but is often ineffective; it may restrict diaphragmatic movement and may even rupture the stomach. Analeptics are of little value as the therapeutic dosage is close to the convulsive dose

and depression may follow stimulation. Furthermore, they may increase the oxygen requirements of the brain and increase the risk of anoxic damage. Oxygen should be used freely, as retrolental fibroplasia will only develop in the presence of a high arterial oxygen tension over a period of not less than 5 hr.

Hyaline membrane disease appears to develop following anoxia and is most commonly seen in premature infants, infants of diabetic mothers, and those born by Caesarean section.

In these infants there appears to be a deficiency of surfactant, a lipoprotein, which normally forms a monolayer of mutually repellent molecules lining the alveolus and which serves to oppose the adhesive forces keeping the alveolar walls together. The clinical picture is manifested by grunting respiration, increased respiratory rate, intercostal recession, diaphragmatic breathing and recurrent apnoeic attacks. X-ray reveals a typical diffuse reticogranular pattern of collapsed terminal airspaces.

There will be an acidosis, and if blood collected by heel prick shows an alkali reserve of 20 m.equiv./l bicarbonate or less (normal, 25 m.equiv./l) then 5% sodium bicarbonate solution is given. The infant is nursed in an incubator and given intramuscular cloxacillin 25–50 mg twice daily, and streptomycin 5 mg/kg body weight every 12 hr to combat the risk of infection.

Hypoglycaemia is common, and blood sugar estimations should be made with Dextrostix. If necessary, dextrose 10%, sodium bicarbonate 1 m.equiv./ml and heparin 3,000 units in 500 ml is given into the umbilical vein.

A Bennett mechanical respirator may be necessary, and infants liable to apnoeic attacks should be on a special blanket warning device, which rings a bell should respiration cease.

Thick, tenacious mucus and meconium may obstruct the airways and render lung expansion impossible. The trachea is aspirated and intubated. Sterile distilled water 1 ml is passed down the tube and then immediately aspirated with the infant in the head-down position. This may be repeated at hourly intervals.

When lung expansion is incomplete there may follow a vesicular emphysema. Rupture of a bulla may cause a spontaneous pneumothorax with progressive respiratory distress and cyanosis. A plastic catheter is inserted into the pleural space and the risk of infection reduced with an underwater seal.

REFERENCES

AGPAR V. (1953) *Curr. Res. Anesth. Analg.* **36**, 260.

BEAZLEY J.M. & GILLESPIE A. (1971) *Lancet*, **i**, 152.

BEAZLEY J.M. (1971) *Br. J. Hosp. Med.* (in the press).

BEAZLEY J.M., DEWHURST C.J. & GILLESPIE A. (1970) *J. Obstet. Gynaec. Br. Commonw.* **77**, 193.

BENSON R.C., SHUBECK F., CLARK W.M., BERENDES H., WEISS W. & DEUTSCHBERGER J. (1965) *Am. J. Obstet. Gynec.* **91**, 645.

BLAKEY D.H., DEWHURST C.J. & RUSSELL C.S. (1958) *J. Obstet. Gynaec. Br. Commonw.* **65**, 644.

BRANT H.A. (1970) *Br. J. Hosp. Med.* **3**, 116.

CANTONI A. & RASORI C. (1960) *Ann. Obstet. Gynec.* **82**, 31.

CHALMERS J.A. & FOTHERGILL R.J. (1960) *Br. med. J.* **i**, 1684.

CHALMERS J.A. & NG J.L. (1964) *Br. med. J.* **ii**, 1070.

CRAWFORD J.S. (1965) *Principles and Practices of Obstetric Anaesthesia*, 2nd edn. London, Blackwell, p. 209.

DEWHURST C.J. (1957) *J. Obstet. Gynaec. Br. Commonw.* **64**, 113.

EASTMAN N. (1961) *Obstet. Gynaec. Surv.* **16**, 195.

EMBREY M.P. & MORRISON D.L. (1968) *J. Obstet. Gynaec. Br. Commonw.* **75**, 829.

EMBREY M.P. (1969) *J. Obstet. Gynaec. Br. Commonw.* **76**, 783.

GADD R.L. (1954) *Br. med. J.* **i**, 735.

HUNTINGFORD P.J. (1967) *Br. J. Hosp. Med.* **1**, 55.

KARIM S.M.M., TRUSSELL R.R., PATEL R.C. & HILLIER K. (1968) *Br. med. J.* **iv**, 621.

KARIM S.M.M., TRUSSELL R.R., HILLIER K. & PATEL R.C. (1969) *J. Obstet. Gynaec. Br. Commonw.* **76**, 769.

KARIM S.M., TRUSSELL R.R., HILLIER K., PATEL R.C. & TAMUSANGE S. (1970) *J. Obstet. Gynaec. Br. Common.* **77**, 200.

LAW R.G. (1953) *Br. med. J.* **ii**, 955.

Leading Article (1965) *Br. med. J.* **i**, 204.

McGARRY J.A. (1969) *J. Obstet. Gynaec. Br. Commonw.* **76**, 137.

MALMSTROM T. (1954) *Acta obstet. gunec. scand.* **33**, (Supplement IV).

MALMSTROM T. (1957) *Acta obstet. gynec. scand.* **36**, (Supplement III).

MALMSTROM T. & LANGE P. (1964) *Acta obstet. gynec. scand.* **43**, (Supplement I).

MALPAS P. (1960) *Br. J. clin. Pract.* **14**, 879.

MENDELSON C.L. (1944) *Am. J. Obstet. Gynec.* **152**, 191.

New York Academy of Sciences (1970) Conference on prostaglandins.

PEEL J.H. & CHAMBERLAIN G.V.P. (1968) *J. Obstet. Gynaec. Br. Commonw.* **75**, 1282.

Report on Confidential Enquiries into Maternal Deaths in England and Wales, 1964–1966 (1969) London, H.M.S.O., p. 55.

RITCHIE J.M. & BRUDENELL J.M. (1966) *Br. med. J.* **i**, 581.

RITCHIE J.M. & BRUDENELL J.M. (1967) *Br. med. J.* **ii**, 608.

TURNBULL A.C. & ANDERSON A.B.M. (1968) *J. Obstet. Gynaec. Br. Commonw.* **75**, 24; and **75**, 32.

CHAPTER 29

MATERNAL AND PERINATAL MORTALITY

MATERNAL MORTALITY

One measure of the success of our obstetric care might reasonably be thought to be the number of mothers dying as a result of pregnancy, labour and the puerperium. Maternal mortality figures in England and Wales are reported yearly in the *Registrar General's Statistical Review*.

The most recent report available is that for 1969, and it shows the figure of 0·19 per 1,000 total births. This is such a low figure that it is clear that maternal mortality alone cannot be regarded as a satisfactory yardstick against which to judge further improvement or deterioration in our maternity care. A better measure is the perinatal mortality rate, which is the sum of stillbirths and first-week deaths. This, too, is reported in the *Review*; the perinatal mortality rate for 1969 was 23 per 1,000 total births. These are far higher figures than those from maternal mortality, and only when they have been substantially reduced can there be any room for complacency.

Loss of life, whether maternal, foetal or neonatal, should not be the sole criterion imposed, however. All obstetricians of experience know that for any patient whose life is lost there are several who came near to death. And although death is prevented, permanent damage may have been sustained. Morbidity, could it be satisfactorily assessed, might be a better measure still of the personal skill of a doctor or midwife and of the effectiveness of our maternity services. Morbidity is, unhappily, very difficult to assess in the same way as mortality, and no figures—even approximate ones—are available here.

Another approach to evaluating medical, nursing and social service efficiency, has been the publication of the series of triennial reports entitled *Confidential Enquiries into Maternal Deaths in England and Wales*, (1952–4, 1955–7, 1958–60, 1961–3, and 1964–6). These reports have been compiled by a special committee of the Ministry of Health (now Department of Health and Social Security) after the collection and assessment of information supplied by midwives, general practitioners, consultants, medical officers of health and others concerned in the care of maternity patients. These enquiries, carried out as they were with thoroughness and with the cooperation of medical and nursing personnel closely in contact with the patient, provided more information about maternal deaths than simply mortality figures ever could. Moreover, the enquiries permitted the very important assessment to be made as to whether there could be said to be 'avoidable factors' present in each case considered. An examination of maternal mortality through the eyes of this confidential enquiry is therefore appropriate.

Confidential enquiry into maternal deaths

Table 29.1, reproduced from the 1964–6 *Report*, sets the scene for a consideration of maternal and perinatal mortality in England and Wales in the years since 1952, when confidential enquiries commenced. The decline in maternal mortality rates has been accompanied by changes in the chief causes in mortality over this period of time. The table indicates that when the causes of

Table 29.1. Causes of death directly due to pregnancy and childbearing*

	1955–7	1958–60	1961–3	1964–6
Abortion	141	135	139	133
Pulmonary embolism	157	132	129	91
Haemorrhage	138	130	92	68
Toxaemia	171	118	104	67
All other causes	254	227	228	220
Total	861	742	692	579

*Reproduced from the *Report on Confidential Enquiries into Maternal Deaths in England and Wales, 1964–1966*, by kind permission of H.M.S.O.

maternal death directly due to pregnancy and child-bearing are considered, all four major causes have declined in numbers, some to a greater extent than others. In 1955–7 the foremost single cause of death was toxaemia of pregnancy, followed by pulmonary embolism, abortion and haemorrhage, in that order. By 1964–6 toxaemia deaths had been cut by nearly two-thirds, pulmonary embolism deaths by less than a half, and haemorrhage deaths by half; but abortion deaths had scarcely been lowered at all, leaving abortion as the chief single cause of maternal death at the present time. However, the actual cause of death in a case of abortion may be pulmonary embolism, haemorrhage or sepsis; reconsideration of the position if abortion is not given as a specific heading as a cause of death shows that the classification could be as follows:

(1) Haemorrhage, including haemorrhage from abortions, ectopic pregnancy, rupture of the uterus and from Caesarean section   152
(2) Sepsis, including septic abortion, puerperal sepsis and postoperative sepsis   123
(3) Pulmonary embolism, including pulmonary embolism after abortion and ectopic pregnancy   95
(4) Toxaemia   67

Satisfactory though the reduction in numbers of deaths is throughout those years, it is less satisfactory to note no significant change in the percentage of avoidable factors. In 1952–4,

43·1% of deaths directly due to pregnancy and childbirth were considered to have avoidable factors, and in 1964–6 the figure was 44·6%. It should be remembered that the presence of avoidable factors does not necessarily imply that the death could have been prevented; none the less, it might have been. Avoidable factors were less frequent in deaths associated with, but not directly due to, pregnancy and childbearing, 13·1% of the cases examined in 1964–6 being designated avoidable compared with a figure of 16·8% in 1952–4.

Responsibility for error seems to fall on most members of the maternity services. The consultant obstetrician was held entirely responsible in 40 cases in the 1964–6 *Report* the general practitioner in 24, the obstetric registrar or resident in five and the midwife in only one; the anaesthetist was judged entirely responsible in 14 instances. Partial responsibility was attributed more often to the general practitioner (42 times), the midwife (13 times) and the obstetric registrar or resident (14 times). The patient herself, however, was held entirely responsible 128 times and partially so 21 times; in 98 cases this consisted of seeking illegal termination of pregnancy.

It is instructive to look more closely into some of the causes of death dealt with in the *Report*.

Abortion

As we have seen, there has been very little decline in numbers of deaths due to abortion. Illegal interference to bring about interruption of pregnancy was the most significant associated factor, to be found in 98 (73·7%) of 133 abortion deaths. There were, however, 10 maternal deaths from therapeutic abortion; one of these patients was treated by subtotal hysterectomy, five by hysterotomy, two by the introduction of paste into the uterus and two by injection of hypertonic saline into the amniotic cavity. It is worthy of mention that no death was reported from therapeutic termination of an early pregnancy by vaginal evacuation of the uterus.

The precise cause of death is not always apparent, but sepsis or thrombo-embolism is recorded in 69—or a little more than half the total cases; toxaemia is noted in only five. It must be presumed that haemorrhage played a prominent part of the remainder, together with the condition for which the abortion was being procured. Particular emphasis must be laid upon two specific causes of death: air embolism and *Clostridium welchii* infection. Of 45 cases of death from procured abortion in which sepsis and toxaemia were not concerned, 29 were due to air embolism—otherwise an uncommon abnormality; and of 53 cases where sepsis was concerned, the organism was *Clostridium welchii* in 34.

Pulmonary embolism

This condition was the second commonest cause of death in the *Report*, despite the fact that the heading included only cases due to venous thrombosis and excluded those associated with septic emboli and the air emboli due to criminal abortion. In one-quarter of the cases the embolus occurred during pregnancy, in half it followed vaginal delivery, and in a further quarter it followed Caesarean section.

More than half the fatalities appear to have occurred suddenly and unexpectedly, suggesting that they could not have been prevented. However, in a number of the remainder some signs and symptoms—such as phlebothrombosis, superficial thrombophlebitis, chest pain and haemoptysis, etc.—appear to have been ignored, and it is possible that some signs might have been present in the apparently unexpected deaths, if looked for more closely. Moreover, anticoagulant treatment was used less often than was desirable.

The most important aetiological factor was plainly a surgical operation carried out either for delivery or during the puerperium. If puerperal surgery is to be undertaken the greater liability to thrombosis and embolism must be remembered. Obesity, too, appeared to be an important aetiological factor; others were increasing age, especially in primigravid patients, and trauma during delivery. Anaemia was not clearly a factor, although it seems likely that it is important. The association with suppression of lactation by oestrogens had to be examined retrospectively, and it could not be said from the confidential enquiry if it was a significant factor or not.

Haemorrhage

This was the third most frequent cause of maternal death in the 1964–6 *Report*, although, as we have seen, if abortion as a specific cause is omitted, bleeding was the most common single reason for loss of the mother's life. The inclusion of abortion as a cause in the classification, although undoubtedly focusing attention on its importance, tends to minimize that of bleeding, which, despite the facilities readily available for the asking throughout this country, remains far too often the cause of death. This *Report* should be consulted carefully by anyone beginning to doubt the truth of this statement, when it will be seen that precautions to avoid death from haemorrhage are often inadequate, by poor selection of the place of confinement, failure to call for consultant advice, failure to give blood at all or, if it is given, to administer it in sufficient quantities.

Deaths from accidental haemorrhage in particular have not been reduced since the previous *Report*. Blood-coagulation defects are responsible for some of these, and tests to detect such defects are still not employed frequently enough. One effect of inadequate blood transfusion is the failure to prevent acute renal failure—an important cause of death in cases of accidental haemorrhage.

Postpartum haemorrhage deaths, although reduced, still showed avoidable factors in 50% of cases.

Toxaemia of pregnancy

In Britain at the present time an obstetrician in training is unlikely to see more than a handful of cases of eclampsia. To see one, however, is to accept it as a very serious disease indeed, from which the patient may well lose her life. On the other hand, pre-eclampsia is so frequent as to be commonplace; this disorder may be seen so often, and in such a mild form, that it is difficult to accept it as *pre*-eclamptic at all, or to believe that it may be fatal of its own accord. Nevertheless, of 68 cases of death from toxaemia of pregnancy, 40 were attributed to eclampsia and 28 to other toxaemias; in the majority of the latter other conditions were present as an additional cause of death, but in nine cases no such complications were recorded (Table 29.2).

Table 29.2. Deaths caused by toxaemia of pregnancy*

Eclampsia	40
Complicated by	
Intracranial haemorrhage	14
Renal failure	5
Hepatorenal failure	3
Hepatic necrosis	1
Bronchopneumonia	1
Pheochromocytoma	1
Bleeding from a tracheobronchial fistula following treatment of eclampsia	1
No additional complications stated	14
All other toxaemia	28
Complicated by	
Intracranial haemorrhage	5
Renal failure	3
Liver failure	1
Anaesthetic misadventure	3
Haemorrhage during Caesarean section	3
Puerperal sepsis	2
Bronchopneumonia	2
No additional complications stated	9
Total	68

*Reproduced from the *Report on Confidential Enquiries into Maternal Deaths in England and Wales, 1964–1966*, by kind permission of H.M.S.O.

The actual causes of death in the cases considered are set out in Table 29.2 also. Several important associations should be emphasized. It is plain that familiarity still breeds contempt in the common condition of pre-eclamptic toxaemia; patients are still seen too infrequently, are referred for further opinions too late, and are unwisely discharged early from hospital after confinement. Avoidable factors of these and other kinds were present in 56% of cases. Attention is also drawn in the *Report* to possibility of a phaeochromocytoma of the adrenal gland masquerading as toxaemia. Six maternal deaths from this cause were considered, five with signs resembling pre-eclampsia and one eclampsia. Clearly, accurate diagnosis is a necessary pre-

requisite of correct treatment. It will be remembered that pre-eclamptic toxaemia is associated with few, if any, symptoms, and patients are still reluctant to accept advice that hospital admission is required or that the arrangements for confinement should be changed.

Sepsis

Table 29.1 indicating the major causes of maternal death in the various *Reports* since 1952, conceals the fact that sepsis is still a most important cause. The fact is emphasized, however, when abortion, as a specific cause, is omitted. The confidential enquiry considered, in all, 123 deaths due to sepsis, of which 66 occurred after abortion and 29 followed surgical operations. Many readers will show no surprise at the 66 cases following abortion, most of which were illegally procured, and perhaps only a little surprise at the 29 cases following surgical procedures. However, the remaining 28 deaths from sepsis were associated with neither, and in most instances followed spontaneous vaginal delivery. Moreover, even among the deaths from sepsis following Caesarean section, five followed an elective procedure.

It is clear that the risk of maternal death from infection is still present, and attention must still be paid to aseptic techniques if deaths are to be prevented. Undue reliance on antibiotic therapy is unwise, since the acquired resistance in hospital of some strains of organism is well known. Moreover, in many cases the clinical diagnosis of sepsis was not made before death.

Complications of anaesthesia

Deaths from this cause were higher in the 1964–6 *Report* than in any other; moreover, the number considered to have avoidable faults is as high now as it was at the beginning; 50 maternal deaths were ascribed to anaesthesia, 24 having avoidable factors. The predominant cause was inhalation of gastric contents, which was thought to account for 18 deaths out of the 24 with avoidable factors, it was considered likely in one of seven doubtful deaths, and was a probable cause in seven of the 19 deaths assessed as not avoidable. Obstetric anaesthesia is a difficult and potentially dangerous procedure, and requires the skill of an experienced, trained anaesthetist and facilities to deal with any possible complication which may arise; moreover, it requires correct management of the patient during her labour so far as food intake is concerned. The passage of a gastric tube to empty the stomach is an unpleasant procedure for a patient and is never more than partially successful, since solid matter will not be fully removed (see also p. 442).

Other conditions

Several other conditions causing death may be briefly considered.

The highest avoidable factor rate of all was present in cases of uterine rupture—21 out of 30. The rupture of a Caesarean section scar occurred in only three cases, traumatic rupture in 12, and spontaneous rupture in 15. This underlines the changing aetiology of uterine rupture in present-day obstetrics; with better obstetrics being generally practised, the number of ruptured uteri occurring from the classical causes of neglected transverse lie, undiagnosed disproportion, dehiscence of a classical Caesarean section scar, etc., are relatively fewer, and those arising in unusual and less well-defined circumstances relatively commoner. Perforation at curettage (see Fig. 27.4, p. 425) is likely to be more frequent still in the future, as the practice of abortion becomes wider. A cervical tear at the time of an abortion or at delivery may also be responsible, and two cases of rupture following cervical conization in the *Report* emphasize that this too may need to be borne more fully in mind. Despite these newer aetiological factors, however, the well-recognized ones of age and frequency of child-bearing still apply, the chances of dying from rupture of the uterus rising with an increase in age and parity. The association of rupture of uterus with a blood-coagulation defect, presumably due to the release of thromboplastin from traumatized tissue, is one to which attention is rightly drawn.

A total of 30 deaths from amniotic fluid infusion is a surprisingly high figure, emphasizing the importance of this catastrophic complication of labour. Sudden collapse at the time of rupture of the membranes, in association with strong or gigantic uterine contractions, should immediately focus attention upon this possibility. Convulsions or muscle-twitchings, cyanosis and the appearance of blood-stained frothy mucus at the mouth may follow; later, a blood-coagulation defect is highly likely.

Fifty deaths from heart disease makes this condition the most important cause of death associated with, but not directly due to, pregnancy and child-bearing. Rheumatic disease is still clearly the most common variety concerned; congenital malformations accounted for only seven of the total cases. The importance of the increased risk of death with advancing age is again emphasized.

The information to be gained by a careful study of this *Report* should be of immense value to any obstetrician in training or in practice. This brief consideration given here only serves to underline important points. More detailed perusal of the *Report* is strongly recommended.

PERINATAL MORTALITY

Various definitions have been employed to express in numerical terms the numbers of foetuses, newborn babies and older babies who fail to survive. Some years ago the stillbirth rate and neonatal death rate were the chief indices employed in terms of the child of the success of our obstetric management. A stillbirth is defined as any child which has issued forth from its mother after the twenty-eighth week of pregnancy and which does not at any time after being completely expelled from its mother breathe or show any other sign of life; the stillbirth rate is the number of stillbirths occurring per 1,000 total births. A neonatal death is defined as death occurring within the first 4 weeks after birth; the neonatal mortality rate is the number of registered deaths under 1 month of age per 1,000 live births.

As it became more evident that stillbirths and deaths shortly after delivery were due in most instances to similar causes, the concept of perinatal mortality became more popular. The term 'perinatal mortality' refers to the sum of stillbirths and deaths during the first week after birth, and the perinatal mortality rate to this number expressed per 1,000 total births.

However wastage of the viable foetus is measured, a decline in death rate is evident over the last 35 years. The decline has been much slower during the years since 1950 as many, if not most, avoidable deaths are avoided, and we are left with a hard core of conditions—such as congenital malformations and prematurity—which are either impossible or extremely difficult, to overcome. The publication in 1963 of the First Report of the 1958 British Perinatal Mortality Survey provided much more information on perinatal mortality than had been previously available and focused attention more closely on this important problem. A second report in 1969 contained more detailed consideration of some of the aspects of the earlier report. Extensive information such as this cannot easily be condensed into concise form but reference must be made to the main facts determined.

The perinatal mortality rate at the time of the survey was 33·2 per 1,000 total births; the most recent figure available (1969) is 23 per 1,000. The commonest cause of perinatal death was anoxia, accounting for 34·1% of fatalities; in 22·9% the anoxia was intrapartum and in 11·2% antepartum. Cerebral birth trauma was another important cause of death, being present alone or in association with intrapartum asphyxia in 10% of cases. The combination of intrapartum anoxia and/or brain trauma therefore accounted for nearly one-third of the total perinatal deaths, and it is clearly to this group that greatest efforts must be directed in our attempt to reduce perinatal mortality still further.

Congenital malformations were found in 19% of cases. Until more is known of their aetiology it is unlikely that significant reduction in their numbers will be achieved. The disasters of Thalidomide administration and rubella in early pregnancy, however, indicate clearly that every effort must be made to protect the foetus from noxious influences when it is most vulnerable. The numbers of such acquired congenital malformations at least should be capable of reduction. Genetic counselling, too, may prevent the occurrence of some cases where it is thought

a high risk exists. The detection of foetal abnormalities *in utero* by amniocentesis, in which more interest is now being shown, may detect the abnormal child with, for example, an inborn error of metabolism or an autosomal abnormality. Treatment, however, can only be by termination of the pregnancy or by allowing events to take their course, so that in terms of foetal wastage nothing may be gained, although there may be benefits in terms of management of the mother herself. Other important causes of perinatal mortality were hyaline membrane disease, 4·9%; pneumonia, 4·8%; rhesus iso-immunization, 4·3%; intraventricular haemorrhage, 2%; massive pulmonary haemorrhage, 1·8%. No histological lesion was detected in early neonatal deaths in 3%.

So much for an examination of the major causes of perinatal mortality in the First Report of the British Perinatal Mortality Survey. Although this was conducted more than 10 years ago, it is unlikely that significant changes have occurred since. To set out causes in this way, however, is only partly helpful, since varying obstetrical circumstances may be involved in deaths from a particular cause; for instance, anoxic deaths may be due to placental insufficiency or to accidental haemorrhage, placenta praevia, prolapse of the cord, prolonged labour, etc. Moreover, contributory factors may be obscured—prematurity for instance, which is clearly involved in some cases of cerebral injury—anoxia, early neonatal deaths without obvious cause, etc.

It is difficult to overestimate the importance of prematurity as a predisposing factor in perinatal deaths. Prematurity, as a term to be defined, has always presented problems. If it is to be related to gestation, at what point in pregnancy is an infant premature and who is to say what the true duration of pregnancy is? If it is to be in terms of weight, the normal variation in size at term must surely mean that one foetus of 2,500 g is more mature than another of a slightly heavier weight. Whether the duration of pregnancy or a birth weight of 2,500 g or less be employed as an index of prematurity or immaturity, each clearly has an important effect upon perinatal mortality. More than 50% of perinatal deaths occurred in babies of less than 2,500 g birth weight, although only some 6·7% of the total population studied gave birth to babies of such a size. It is important to note that one-third of babies of less than 2,500 g were born after 38 weeks of gestation, emphasizing again the great importance of the small-for-dates baby. When gestation was less than 38 weeks, only 9·4% of patients had been delivered, yet 46·2% of perinatal deaths had already occurred. Postmaturity gave a less striking, but none the less important, association with perinatal deaths.

OBSTETRICAL FACTORS

Several obstetric conditions and circumstances may be examined in terms of perinatal mortality.

Toxaemia of pregnancy showed itself to be an important cause of foetal and neonatal death of course, mortality rising sharply with increasing degrees of toxaemia; when proteinuria was present the mortality was three times the national average. The risk to the baby increased markedly after 40 weeks. Both accidental haemorrhage and placenta praevia were found to be associated with a considerably increased risk to the foetus and newborn. A risk to the foetus greater even than that associated with placenta praevia was found in association with antepartum haemorrhage in which no specific cause was detected; this clearly emphasizes the importance of this group and calls for great caution in discharging from hospital patients with antepartum haemorrhage even if no placenta praevia is discovered.

An increased risk to the child is associated with labour lasting longer than 24 hr, and also with very short labours. Breech delivery was associated with a higher perinatal mortality, even when allowance was made for small, dead, and abnormal babies. Small babies had a high mortality when delivered by the breech, and the mortality rate rose again for babies more than 3,500 g in weight. Irrespective of birth weight, breech delivery in multipara showed a higher foetal mortality than in primipara!

Caesarean section deaths were, for the most part, related to the complication calling for this form of treatment rather than to the operation itself. Deaths from hyaline membrane disease were higher in Caesarean section cases even after a correction for maturity was made. In forceps delivery, the lowest mortality was associated with the procedure being carried out in hospital-booked cases. Very large babies delivered by forceps showed a high mortality, but there was evidence of protection of the premature foetus when forceps were used.

SOCIAL AND GEOGRAPHICAL FACTORS

Increased perinatal mortality was measured in association with increased maternal age over 30 years. A 40 year-old woman had double the normal risk. At ages of less than 20 a somewhat increased risk was evident.

The lowest risk to the child was associated with second confinements. After the first child, which had an above-average risk, the mortality fell with the second confinement, rose slightly through the third and fourth, until the foetal risk in the fifth confinement was approximately that of the first. Thereafter, it rose more sharply.

Social class had an obvious effect, the rate in social class 5 being twice that in social class 1. The effects of age, parity and social class were shown to act independently of each other. A geographical difference in perinatal mortality was evident, the rate being higher in the north and west and lower in the south and the east. The higher rate in the south-west region was, to some extent, associated with an increased percentage of severe congenital malformations.

Some time has been spent discussing the results of the Perinatal Mortality Survey, since it is clearly a valuable document providing important material for study on a national basis. Many smaller studies may show specific differences related to the particular type of the population, the quality of the maternity services, the type of case referred, etc. The main problems, however, are clear: our perinatal mortality will be related directly to the quality of our antenatal supervision, the careful selection of the most appropriate place for confinement, the dietary status of our patients, the early recognition of preventable abnormalities such as anaemia and pre-eclamptic toxaemia, the alert management of labour, the immediate detection of foetal distress, a skilful delivery, and the expertise of

our care of the newborn after birth. Nowhere
can we afford to relax in our efforts to reduce
still further maternal and perinatal mortality.

REFERENCES

Perinatal Mortality. The First Report of the British
    Perinatal Mortality Survey (1963) (edited by N.R.
    Butler & D.G. Bonham). Edinburgh and London,
    Livingstone.
Perinatal Problems. The Second Report of the British
    Perinatal Mortality Survey (1969) (edited by N.R.
    Butler & E.D. Alberman). Edinburgh and London,
    Livingstone.
*Report on Confidential Enquiries into Maternal Deaths in
    England and Wales, 1964–1966*. London, H.M.S.O.

CHAPTER 30

CONTRACEPTION AND STERILIZATION

CONTRACEPTION

Introduction

Contraception is only one aspect of family planning. The latter also includes research into normal reproduction, the investigation and treatment of infertility and habitual abortion, and genetic counselling. In addition, it is concerned with the evaluation of termination of pregnancy as a method of family limitation. An individual may avoid further pregnancy because of illness or for economic and social reasons. Family planning is also important in the context of world and regional over-population, which today constitutes the gravest threat to man's continued existence.

Until the nineteenth century the total world population was less than 1,000 million, and it took a further century to expand by 1,000 million. The next 1,000 million, however, was added in only 30 years, between 1930 and 1960, and if this growth rate continues, by A.D. 2000 world population will reach 7,000 million (Fox 1966). The second half of the present century will have seen a greater increase in world population than in all the previous centuries of man's existence.

In seeking an explanation of this it seems unlikely that human fertility has altered significantly. Advances in community health, however, have produced a fall in death rate, perinatal mortality, and infant mortality. The result is an increased life expectancy which in some developing countries is now similar to that of the Western world.

As an example, the elimination of malaria in Mauritius over a 10-year period in which the birth-rate remained constant resulted in a 40% increase in population (Burnet 1961), and similar trends have been evident in India (Coale & Hoover 1959). If the birth-rate remains steady whilst the death-rate falls, the result is not only a larger but also a younger population, with, consequently a higher proportion of dependants. This is the case in some developing countries, where 40% of the population are aged 15 years or under. As a community develops there occurs a transition from a condition of high birth-rate and high death-rate to one where both birth- and death-rates are low. An intermediate situation of high birth-rate and low death-rate inevitably leads to a crisis of over-population.

Nearly 200 years ago Malthus postulated that population size was limited by disease, war and famine. With decrease in disease the danger of famine increases. For example, between 1964 and 1966, whilst world food production remained static, the world population rose by 70 million. The position in developing countries is aggravated by the fact that the major part of world food production is achieved by those already developed countries in which over-population has not yet reached crisis levels. Novel food sources, e.g. seaweed, seem to be of laboratory rather than of practical importance in the foreseeable future.

When considering the position in the United Kingdom, complacency is soon dispelled by the forecast that in A.D. 2000 the population will exceed the present numbers by 20 million. Even the present population is a third greater than that which is considered optimal by agriculturalists.

The 1967 Family Planning Act provides belated but welcome recognition of the public health importance of contraception. Family size, however, is mainly influenced by social, religious and personal factors. The need for contraception within a community may be obvious to doctors, sociologists and politicians but its adoption by each couple involves a personal decision. Only with the introduction of the pill and the re-introduction of the intra-uterine contraceptive device (I.U.C.D.) have contraceptive methods become available which are not only efficient but also acceptable to a wide range of people.

Previous methods were mainly suited to the middle classes. For an historical review, the reader is referred to Peel & Potts (1969).

Methods available

Most surveys covering the relative popularity of various techniques were made before the pill and the I.U.C.D. achieved their current popularity.

Social class differences become obvious when one considers the method chosen. It is also evident that fewer people from the lower socio-economic groups practise contraception at all, and that when it is attempted by them it is often performed inefficiently. To each couple, therefore, a method must be offered which is appropriate to their intelligence and the emotional and social responses of the group to which they belong. The acceptability of a method may be increased when it is presented as part of a domiciliary service.

Any method exhibits fewer failures when used by people with strong motivation. It has been shown frequently that the failure rate for the same method drops once the chosen family size has been attained. Failure rates are measured by the pregnancy rate per hundred woman years (H.W.Y.). This is the number of accidental pregnancies, whatever their outcome, divided by the number of months exposure and multiplied by 1,2000—the number of months in 100 years.

Failure rate/H.W.Y. =
$$\frac{Total\ accidental\ pregnancies}{Total\ months\ of\ exposure} \times 1{,}200$$

In calculating the total months of exposure, it is usual to deduct 10 for a full term and 4 for an aborted pregnancy.

Contraceptive techniques which are currently in use include:

(1) Coitus interruptus: failure rate about 18/H.W.Y.
(2) The safe period (the rhythm method): failure rate 24/H.W.Y.
(3) Chemical contraceptives, in the form of:
    Cream and jelly
    Pessaries
    Foams and aerosols
(4) The condom or sheath: 14 pregnancies/ H.W.Y.
(5) Diaphragms and various types of cap: 12 pregnancies/H.W.Y.
(6) The I.U.C.D.: 2·5 pregnancies/H.W.Y.
(7) Oral contraceptives: failure rate less than 1/H.W.Y.
    Combined preparations
    Sequential preparations
    Continuous low-dose progestagens
(8) Sterilization
    Of the male
    Of the female

(1) COITUS INTERRUPTUS

Coitus interruptus was found in a 1947 survey to have provided the sole method of birth control for 43% of the recently married British couples who had practised contraception, the percentage rising to 61% in social class 5 (Lewis-Faning 1949). It was still being used by 39% of couples studied by the Population Investigation Committee in 1957, and when one talks to gynaecological patients it becomes evident that the method is still widely employed. Once thought to produce pelvic congestion in women, prostatic hypertrophy in men, and psychological disturbance in both, it is now considered probable that there are no demonstrable ill-effects when both partners have agreed to its use as their preferred method. The efficiency of the technique—as with any form of contraception—is greatest when motivation is strongest, but a failure rate of only 18/ H.W.Y. has been quoted, which is only slightly greater than that with sheath and diaphragm (Loraine & Bell 1968).

(2) THE RHYTHM METHOD

This restricts coitus to a time of physiological sterility, and it is the only method approved by the Catholic Church. It is assumed that during one cycle a single ovum will be shed between the twelfth and sixteenth days counting back from the next expected period, that the ovum is capable of being fertilized for 24 hr after ovulation, and that sperms can fertilize for 48 hr after their deposition in the uterus.

Taking these facts into account for an absolutely predictable 28-day cycle, coitus must not take place on or after the date which falls 18 days before the first day of the next expected period, and must not be resumed until the tenth day before that period is due.

Some recommend the addition of two further days 10 and 19.

The prediction of the date of the next period is vital to the method, and it is essential that a menstrual calendar be kept for a full year beforehand. If the cycle is less than 20 days, or if cycles vary in length by more than 10 days, the method cannot be used. In calculation the earliest possible date of the next period is taken and from this 18 days are subtracted, the date so obtained being the first day on and after which coitus must be avoided. The last day of abstinence is calculated by counting back 11 days from the latest date on which the next period might be expected.

Alternatively, it is possible to use first-morning temperature recording to detect ovulation, though such records are not always easy to interpret.

The method is relatively inefficient. It has been calculated that to achieve a guaranteed 4-year interval between pregnancies only one act of intercourse per cycle can be allowed! More disturbing are suggestions that there may result a higher incidence of ectopic pregnancy because of late fertilization, and of congenital abnormality because of the union of ageing sperm and ovum.

(3) CHEMICAL CONTRACEPTION

Chemical contraceptives in the form of a jelly or cream are an essential adjunct to the use of cap or diaphragm, and are also recommended when the condom is used. Suppositories containing quinine were introduced by Rendell eighty years ago, and Volpar—containing the spermicide phenylmercuric acetate—is still available. They are unsatisfactory, as they take 20 min to melt and achieve poor dispersion. Foam and aerosol preparations are better in this respect, and also hinder sperm transport, but are expensive and have a failure rate which is unacceptable.

(4) THE CONDOM OR SHEATH

This was used in the sixteenth century as a prophylactic against venereal disease, its contraceptive function being recognized subsequently.

In the latter half of the nineteenth century rubber condoms were introduced. This meant that for the first time the condom became relatively inexpensive and freely available. Methods of manufacture improved rapidly, and in England today prepacked, siliconized rubber condoms are still widely used. In 1964 the British Standards Institution published a standard for condoms and rules for quality testing (Peel & Potts 1969). Since 1968 the Population Council has sponsored the manufacture of the even cheaper, thin plastic condom which has a longer storage life. Sales of condoms in Britain exceed 100 million annually, and they are readily accepted among lower social groups. They are freely available without medical supervision, and it is estimated that 50% of couples use them at some time. The condom is especially useful where intercourse occurs infrequently and at irregular intervals. Some couples demand the immediate reassurance which use of the method provides. In cases of trichomonas or monilial vaginitis reinfection may be prevented, whilst a certain degree of protection against the gonococcus is also possible. The method may be suitable when the woman is unwilling or unable to take responsibility for contraception, or may be used to allow her a period of rest from this. The condom must be correctly applied to the erect penis well before ejaculation on all occasions at which intercourse occurs, and it is especially important to ensure that it does not slip off during withdrawal. The coincidental use of a spermicide is strongly advised. The failure rate for the condom is probably about 14/H.W.Y.

(5) OCCLUSIVE DEVICES IN THE FEMALE

Rubber caps and diaphragms became popular from 1880 onwards, following their introduction by Mensinga in Holland. They provided the mainstay of the family planning clinics, whose patients were mainly women, and prior to the introduction of the pill were still being offered to 95% of clinic patients, though providing the method of choice in only one-eighth of couples.

Proper instruction in the method involves a medical examination, which affords an opportunity for breast and pelvic examination and cytology, as well as for fitting. At a second visit the doctor must make certain that the patient knows how to maintain the appliance and can insert and remove it correctly. Use of a diaphragm needs a degree of intelligence and acceptance of the need for self-examination inherent in the technique. Patients must be strongly motivated to use the method. There must be no uterine prolapse or major degree of cystocele, and good vaginal tone is necessary. Patients must be capable of feeling their own cervix. The diaphragm must only be used in conjunction with spermicidal cream or jelly, and optimally should be inserted each night whether or not intercourse is expected to occur and at other times well before coitus takes place. It should remain in place for at least 6 hr after coitus. Patients should be refitted 3 months after the initial visit if coitus is just starting (annually thereafter) following pregnancy or pelvic operations, and when there have been rapid or large alterations in weight.

Types of cap other than the diaphragm are rarely used, cervical caps being suitable only when the cervix is accessible, perfectly healthy, and of a size which will hold the cap. These devices must also be used in conjunction with a spermicidal cream or jelly.

(6) THE I.U.C.D.

Devices described by Grafenberg in 1929 and Ota in 1934 were originally believed to cause a high incidence of pelvic inflammatory disease. Not until 1959 was this fallacy disproved by the results of Oppenheimer in Israel and Ishihama in Japan—who, furthermore, established that the failure rate of the method was only 2·5 per hundred woman years.

Most of the newer devices are made of polyethylene or nylon and take the form of spirals, loops, bows or rings. The most widely used has been the Lippes Loop D (Tietze 1966). Some devices have a tail or stem which can be felt protruding through the cervix, the position of others having to be checked by X-ray or by passing a uterine sound (although one, the Antigon, incorporates a magnet, so that its position can be frequently checked without internal examination).

Insertion of a device is best performed towards the end of a period, as this ensures that an existing pregnancy is not disturbed. Six weeks should elapse after childbirth or abortion and 8 weeks after Caesarean section. If it is considered important to put in the device in the puerperium, it is probably safest to insert it digitally.

Effects of the I.U.C.D.

Myometrial activity which increases at or shortly after insertion has returned to normal after 72 hr. Some authors have even suggested that the uterus subsequently becomes less active than normal.

Tubal activity is prolonged in monkeys where superovulation has been artificially produced, but not in those where ovulation is normal. The effect on tubal motility in women is not fully investigated. Siegler & Hellman (1964) found no alteration in a study of four volunteers. Although the overall reduction in tubal pregnancy among women using the device might suggest accelerated tubal transport, it must not be forgotten that the percentage of tubal pregnancy relative to intrauterine pregnancy actually increases.

Minor histological changes are only seen in the endometrium; they include stromal oedema, increased superficial vascularity and chronic infiltration with plasma cells and lymphocytes. The proliferative phase is prolonged, and this may prevent pregnancy because of the resulting asynchrony between the time of fertilization and the preparedness of the endometrium. No changes occur in endometrial histochemistry. Though endometrial carcinoma has been reported in rats with a device left *in situ* for 2 years, there is no evidence of any such tendency in women. Hysterography in women reveals an increased uterine capacity which could produce rapid expulsion or premature death of the conceptus. Sperm transport is unaltered by the presence of the device.

Following removal of the device fertility is unimpaired, 75% of women conceiving within 6 months and 90% after 1 year (Kleinman 1966).

Complications of the I.U.C.D.

(1) The expulsion rate varies from 2 to 30% according to the device considered. For Lippes Loop D it is 10·4% during the first year of use but only 1·6 and 0·7% in the second and third years respectively (Tietze 1966). Expulsion may occur soon after insertion or subsequently, usually just after a period. As expected, the expulsion rate is higher following reinsertion, though even so two out of five retain a second identical device (Tietze 1967). Expulsion is more common in the young and in patients of low parity. In 20% of cases expulsion is not noticed by the patient (Tietze 1967) and in 15% the device is found to be still in the cervix. The rate of expulsion is lowest for the bow type and highest for the spiral. Including reinsertions, 75% of patients have the device *in situ* at the end of 1 year (Report of International Panel 1968).

(2) Slight vaginal discharge and bleeding are to be expected soon after insertion, and slight intermenstrual loss may occur subsequently. In up to 41% of cases menses become heavier (Tietze 1967). Only if the menorrhagia is severe and persists beyond 3 months is it necessary to remove the device.

(3) Pain on insertion may be acute and accompanied by fainting. In the multipara it is usually not severe, though some discomfort or cramp is noticed by a third of patients. Pain which occurs in a woman who has been free of discomfort may herald expulsion. Patients should be told of this possibility. Removal because of bleeding and pain is least often necessary with

the steel ring, but more often with bow, loop, double coil and spiral, in that order.

(4) Pelvic inflammatory disease, when it occurs, is usually a flare-up of existing disease. An incidence of 2·7% was quoted by Tietze (1966), but in only a sixth was inflammation classed as severe. Antibiotics are given initially. In the one-third where infection persists, it proves necessary to remove the device.

(5) There is no evidence that the devices predispose to carcinoma in women, nor is there a significant alteration in vaginal or cervical smears.

(6) Perforation of the uterus was reported in 0·2% of cases by Tietze (1966) and 1·7 per 1,000 by Burnhill & Birnberg (1967) among 16,338 first insertions performed after confinement. This represents only half the risk of uterine perforation at curettage. However, Ratnam & Yin (1968) reported 8·7 per 1,000 perforations in 8,977 first insertions. Should the device leave the uterus it no longer provides contraception, and also carries a risk to life if intestinal obstruction supervenes. Obstructed cases almost invariably involve closed devices, and if one of these perforates the uterus it must be surgically removed as a matter of urgency.

Contra-indications to use of the I.U.C.D.

(a) Known pelvic inflammatory disease. Optimally, even trichomonas and monilial vaginitis should be eliminated before inserting a device.
(b) Pregnancy
(c) Abnormal uterine bleeding, until this has been fully investigated and treated.
(d) Relative contra-indications: (i) fibromyomata of moderate or large size, (ii) recent hysterotomy or Caesarean section.

The failure rate quoted is from 2 to 2·5/H.W.Y. (London & Anderson 1967; Tietze 1967) (Fig. 30.1). The spiral is most efficient and the double coil less so, whilst the bow is least effective. The rate of failure is highest in the first year of use. If pregnancy occurs with the device still *in situ*, 41% abort compared with 33% where the device has previously been expelled (Kleinman 1966), and an incidence of ectopic gestation of

2·5% has been reported with the device still *in situ* (Tietze 1966).

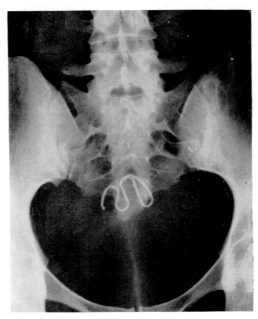

Fig. 30.1. An intra-uterine device *in situ*. The patient is, nevertheless, 16 weeks pregnant.

(7) ORAL CONTRACEPTION IN THE FEMALE

Easy to take, and very effective, the pill is popular among women of all social classes. It was the overwhelming choice among patients of 98·5% of Fellows of the American College surveyed in 1968 and was used by 44% of women aged 20–24 with three or more children in Britain (Inman & Vessey 1968). Usage in Australia and New Zealand is even higher. The position in 1968 was reviewed in WHO Technical Report No. 386 and in a review article by Garcia (1967) with 220 references (see also Borell 1966).

The classical or combined pill contains a progestogen and an oestrogen in combination. The course begins on the fifth day of a cycle (day 1 being the first day of menstruation) and one pill is taken daily for 21 days. For the next 7 days no pill is taken, unless the manufacturer includes 7 placebo pills in the course, when one of these is taken each day. Active pills recommence at the end of 7 days whether or not menstruation has occurred in the interval. The mode of action has been reviewed by Diczfalusy (1968). Inhibition of ovulation via the oestrogen component acting on hypothalamus and pituitary is the most usual feature. Many combined pills have been devised, but all are virtually 100% effective if taken correctly and even when one to five pills were missed Garcia & Pincus (1965) reported a pregnancy rate of only 3/H.W.Y. The total dose of oestrogen and progestogen may be high or low and the relative amounts of each can vary. The main oestrogens (ethinyloestradiol and mestranol) are used, and two main groups of progestogens (17-hydroxyprogesterone derivatives or 19-norsteroid progestogens). The 19-norsteroid derivatives have some oestrogenic effect. The composition of a pill may determine its action as strongly oestrogenic or relatively strongly progestational. If a woman's history suggests that her own hormone balance is oestrogen-dominated (premenstrual tension, fluid retention, heavy menstrual loss, cervical catarrh and erosion) or mainly progestational (full and heavy—but not painful—breasts, acne, light periods) then a pill may be selected to counteract these effects. If one pill causes undesirable side-effects another preparation may prove to be less troublesome.

Before the pill is prescribed

(1) Abnormal cervical and vaginal cytology findings occur more often in pill users than among controls (Attwood 1966; Liu *et al.* 1967). Smears must therefore be taken before the pill is prescribed, and annually thereafter.

(2) By taking a full history and performing a gynaecological examination which includes palpation of the breasts, contra-indications to the pill may become evident.

Contra-indications to the pill

The following are suggested:

(1) History of thrombophlebitis or pulmonary embolism.

(2) Large varicose veins.

(3) Liver disease or previous jaundice.
(4) Hormone-dependent carcinoma, e.g. breast.
(5) Diabetes mellitus.
(6) Large myomata.
(7) Ocular disease and migraine.

Side-effects of the pill

These occur in 5–25% of users, though the incidence varies widely between different studies using the same preparation. Thus with Anovlar various authors have reported excessive weight gain in as few as 1·5% or as many as 54% of patients.

Beneficial side-effects include relief of primary dysmenorrhoea and mittelschmerz, improvement in endometriosis, a lessening of premenstrual tension, decrease in the amount of menstrual loss, and a feeling of well-being. Libido has been said to increase in 50% and to decline in 40%, though Wallach & Garcia (1968) found no alteration at all.

Complications of treatment

(1) Increasing weight—a feature of the early months of treatment, a gain of 3 lb or more is seen in 4–50% of cases. This is less likely with low-dosage preparations and those using 17α-hydroxyprogesterone derivatives.
(2) Breast fullness. This may improve with a more oestrogenic pill. Breast tenderness is seen in 0–27% with various products and may improve a with less oestrogenic preparation.
(3) Headache and migraine.
(4) Alopecia. This has been reported in small groups of patients.
(5) Vaginal discharge and heavier menses— should they occur they may improve with a less oestrogenic preparation.
(6) Gingivitis, rheumatoid effects, and worsening of systemic lupus erythematosus have been reported occasionally.
(7) Various ocular side-effects reported include corneal oedema, which can prove troublesome to wearers of contact lenses.

However, in a study of 184 patients and 361 controls Connell & Kelman (1968) found no serious eye complications.

(8) Metabolic disturbances. Abnormal glucose-tolerance tests have been observed in up to 40% of patients on combined preparations, with an increased incidence in those with a family history of diabetes. These results probably occur from the rise in growth-hormone levels which has been demonstrated. With established diabetes, however, there is no increase in insulin requirements.

Transient changes of little significance were reported in liver-function tests by Mears (1965), but an association with jaundice has been reported by the Swedish Adverse Drug Reaction Committee.

Alteration in P.B.I. shown by Starup & Friis (1968) is not associated with clinically altered thyroid function.

(9) Thrombo-embolic disease. The risk of this occurring was thought by Venning (1963) to be minimal, but it has since been estimated that 1 in 2,000 users will be admitted to hospital annually as a result of this complication, compared with 1 in 20,000 of non-users (Vessey & Doll 1968). An overall mortality due to oral contraceptives of 1·3 per 100,000 in the 20–34 group and 3·4 per 100,000 in the 35–44 group was quoted by Inman & Vessey (1968). It is probable that oestrogen is the prime offender, and the continuous low-dose progestogen pill may prove safer, whilst the sequential pill with its large dose of oestrogen may carry special risks. It must be remembered that even though the above figures suggest that the risk of thrombo-embolism is equal for one pregnancy and 1 year's pill-taking, there are additional risks of childbearing which are avoided in the protected group (Swyer 1966).
(10) Breakthrough bleeding is seen in 7–37% of patients in the first cycle, but declines rapidly after four to six cycles (Venning 1963).

(11) Amenorrhoea is seen in under 4% of cycles, and its incidence is decreased by changing to a tablet containing more oestrogen.

(12) Lactation was reported to be slightly depressed by Pincus (1965), but in a study using Norinyl 1 (norethisterone 1 mg, mestranol 0·5 mg) Kaern (1967) found no change.

Effects of stopping the pill

The rapid reversibility and lack of ill-effects was stressed by Rice-Wray *et al.* (1967). Subsequent fertility does not decline, and may even be temporarily increased (Goldzieher 1964). Hormone levels remain normal. There is no evidence of alteration in the time of menopause—which is, anyway, genetically determined (Loraine & Bell 1968).

In rare cases, ovulation may not occur in the cycles following stopping the pill. If failure continues for 3 months then prednisone 5 mg should be given twice daily for 3 months. In the few patients who still fail to ovulate Clomiphene or human menopausal gonadotrophin may prove necessary.

Other types of pill

Sequential preparations have a higher failure rate than the classical pill, but follow more closely the hormonal changes of the normal menstrual cycle. They may prove helpful in a younger woman who is prepared to accept their decreased efficiency as inhibitors of ovulation (this has been confirmed at laparotomy). It is important to remember that the amount of oestrogen administered during sequential therapy tends to be large compared to that of the low-dosage combined preparations, in which a dose of 50 μg a day is standard.

Continuous administration of progestogens (e.g. chlormadinone acetate) offers protection through not always inhibiting ovulation. Animal work suggests that its action may be to prevent successful implantation by interfering with oestrogen/progesterone balance, or it may produce its effect by altering the quality of cervical mucus, interfering with tubal motility and pre-

venting capacitation of spermatozoa. Though the manufacturers claim a failure rate of 0·6/H.W.Y., an acceptable figure, the failure rate in a preliminary study by the Family Planning Association was ten times as great. An advantage of the method is that by avoiding oestrogen administration the risk of thrombo-embolic disease should be minimal, and laboratory investigation has so far failed to show any alterations in blood-clotting factors in women taking the drug. Continuous progestogen administration demands not only that one tablet be taken daily without fail, but that is should preferably be taken at the same time each day. Omitting to take a single dose cannot subsequently be rectified. Because of its relative inefficiency, this type of pill has now been withdrawn from the British market.

STERILIZATION

In Aberdeen 40 years ago, postpartum tubal ligation was being offered to women aged between 35 and 40 years who had eight or more children. By 1966, Baird could report that in the city 7·2% of all women over 30 years old, and a quarter of the women with five or more children, had been sterilized. Puerperal sterilization accounted for 89% of a series of 902 operations reported by McElin *et al.* (1967), and only 1·9% were performed at the time of therapeutic abortion. This was in contrast to figures from Denmark presented by Hoffmeyer *et al.* (1967), where in 85% of cases the procedure was carried out in connection with abortion, and the series of 1,146 reported by White (1966) from Iowa, where the procedures was an 'interval' operation in 42%. In the United States, Boulware & Ensor (1967) reported a 2·9% incidence of postpartum sterilization in 133 non-Catholic hospitals. Of these, 8% were performed by Caesarean hysterectomy.

Indications

Sterilization may obviously be advised in cases of chronic medical disease, in patients who have had repeated Caesarean section, and for those in whom congenital abnormalities are likely to recur. In general, however, there is no absolute indication for sterilization, and one must consider for each case not only the physical risks to the mother, but also the total burden which she, her husband and the existing family would have to bear in the event of further pregnancy. This involves study of emotional, social and economic facts as well as a full consideration of the efficiency with which available contraceptive methods have been, or are likely to be, utilized. The comments of the patient's general practitioner are very helpful in this regard. The majority of operations are probably performed because of contraceptive failures in multipara. In general, the woman should be aged 30 or more and have at least two living children, though exceptions to both these guides will arise.

No operation should be performed until both husband and wife have been interviewed, have received a full explanation from a named medical practitioner—preferably from the surgeon who will perform the operation—and have given their written consent. During the discussion the question of male sterilization and alternative methods of contraception must be discussed where appropriate. Whilst the essentially irreversible nature of female sterilization must be stressed, it is only right that the (very low) failure rate should be mentioned, though in Britain it is not necessary for any reference to the possibility of failure to appear in the consent form (cf. Woodruff & Pauerstein 1969).

Route, timing and type of operation

Sterilizing operations may be performed at laparotomy, laparoscopy or colpotomy. The route and timing of operation are often dictated by such considerations as the opportunity provided at Caesarean section or termination of pregnancy, or the need for repairing a prolapse. In the presence of fibroids, prolapse, chronic pelvic inflammation and menorrhagia, the appropriate sterilizing operation may be hysterectomy, but an apparently healthy uterus should not normally be sacrificed.

Early puerperal tubal ligation may be simply and satisfactorily performed under local anaesthesia (Bornmann & DeVilliers 1965). The operation is least disturbing when performed with-

in 24 hr of delivery. Some advocate operating on the fourth or fifth day, but this increases the risks of thrombosis and embolism and postoperative pyrexia, whilst at the fifth day there is often histological evidence of acute tubal inflammation. Where operation is not possible within a day of delivery then it is optimal to wait 6 weeks, especially if the laparoscope is available. Each case must, however, be considered separately.

The death-rate from tubal sterilization operations is very low, and series of over 5,000 have been reported with no deaths. In smaller series of over 1,000, White (1966) suggests a figure of between 0·09 and 0·17%. The operation will have the immediate complications of any similar procedure.

Techniques of sterilization

(A) TUBAL SURGERY

Over 100 methods have been described. Tubal ligation or ligation with resection may be employed; the tubes may be crushed with or without ligation; the stumps following ligation (or the fimbrial end of the intact tube as a temporary procedure) have been buried extraperitoneally; the isthmic portion of the tubes and the uterine cornua may be excised together, or the whole of both tubes may be excised. The tubes may be coagulated with diathermy and divided by a vaginal approach (Green-Armytage 1958) or by laparoscopy (Steptoe 1967), though these approaches are not recommended in the puerperium. Finally, it has been suggested that sclerosants could be injected into the tube. Details of many of the techniques are provided by Overstreet (1964) and Dickinson & Gamble (1950).

Five will be mentioned in more detail.

Madlener method

The middle third of the fallopian tube is held up as a loop, the base being first crushed and then ligated with non absorbable material.

Pomeroy technique

The tube is again help up as a loop but the base is *not* crushed and is ligated with fine, absorbable material (o plain catgut), the loop being excised. It is wise to send the excised portions for histological examination. There eventually results quite wide separation of the cut ends, which remain closed. Some authors achieve a similar result by removing a portion of tube between clamps and ligating the stumps separately (Shaw 1960). No attempt is made to bury the stumps.

Irvine technique

The tube is divided some 3 cm from the uterus and each stump ligated with chromic catgut. The free end of the uterine portion of the tube is buried in a cavity formed by dissection in the myometrium of the anterior uterine wall. The cut end of the fimbrial portion of tube is buried extraperitoneally in the broad ligament.

Following tubal sterilization there is a recognized risk of development of hydrosalpinx in 5%, and of tubal pregnancy should the procedure fail. Total bilateral salpingectomy would seem to be the logical method of avoiding these complications.

Injection of sclerosants

This failed in 7·3% of patients traced by Pitkin (1966), who reported on 371 cases treated by intraluminal injection of sodium morrhuate. The method should be abandoned.

Laparoscopic sterilization (see Steptoe 1967)

This should not be used in the puerperium but is eminently suitable for 'interval' operations or following vaginal termination. The tube is picked up under direct vision with the Palmer biopsy forceps and coagulated with diathermy from, and including, the cornu outwards for 3 cm. The devitalized tube is divided and the cut ends once again coagulated.

(B) HYSTERECTOMY

In the U.S.A. the high failure rate of tubal surgery at the time of Caesarean section, together with the high percentage of women so treated who need further gynaecological surgery at a later date, has led to a revival of interest in Caesarean hysterectomy as a method of treatment. It is little used in England. Hysterectomy as a method of sterilization is not infrequently employed in those with gynaecological troubles or in early pregnancy when termination has been agreed. Lewis & Williams (1970) have recently advocated wider use of hysterectomy for this purpose.

Pregnancy following female sterilization procedures

One difficulty of follow-up is illustrated by the paper of Lu & Chun (1967), where only a sixth of patients replied to a questionnaire, and some of the series reported from India, where only a quarter of patients could be contracted. A second problem arises because a long period of time can elapse before failure becomes evident in the form of pregnancy. Follow-up studies should be read critically with these points in mind.

Abdominal pregnancy has been reported even after hysterectomy with conservation of the appendages and, similarly, any tubal operation will have a failure rate. In a review of 29,496 tubal sterilizations, Garb (1957) quoted an overall failure rate of 0·71%. In 7,829 Madlener procedures the rate was double this, and in 5,477 Pomeroy procedures was 0·40%. White (1966) found failures of 1·5 and 0·17% with Madlener and Pomeroy methods, respectively. There had been no failures in 1,056 Irving operations noted by Garb (1957). Similar success with the Irving method was reported by Overstreet (1964). An overall failure rate of 0·84% was noted by Barglow & Eisner (1966) in a 2·7 year follow-up. It has long been known that the failure rate for a given method is increased up to six times when it is performed at the time of hysterotomy or Caesarean section rather than at other times, but the reason for this is not known.

Other effects on patients

Reports suggest that 90% of women are satisfied with the results of the operation and would again choose to have it performed. Those who themselves request sterilization because of muliparity show fewest regrets. Women who were previously emotionally unstable are the most likely to react adversely following the operation (and, one suspects, most likely to reply to follow-up questionnaires).

Psychiatric sequelae were studied by Barglow (1964), who found that among a group of 190 women who had been sterilized (18 by hysterectomy and 172 by tubal ligation) there were 152 (80%) who experienced persistent conscious pregnancy fantasies or symptoms and signs. These persisted even in the 45% of the series judged psychologically healthy for about 1 year. Long-term results were good in 150 of the 152. In 25% of the women who had serious disturbances of personal relationships and psyche pre-operatively there was a temporary acceptance of loss of fertility for 2–3 months, but this was followed by severe pelvic pain, menstrual disturbance and dyspareunia.

It has been estimated that 20% of women who have had tubal ligation will have heavier menses and that 10% of the total will require some form of gynaecological surgery later on. While ligation at Caesarean section is considered the proportion is even higher, and this, together with the increased failure rate of tubal operations performed at this time, have been taken by some surgeons—mainly in the U.S.A.—as indications for Caesarean hysterectomy in such cases.

Sterilization of the male

Whilst vasectomy is increasing in popularity in Britain, the number of operations performed is still small. Large numbers are reported from India, where the campaign for voluntary sterilization has Government backing. The procedure is safe and simple, though at operation the possibility of reduplication of the vas must be borne in mind. Two negative semen tests at 8 and 12 weeks postoperatively are necessary to confirm sterility. Until these are obtained the couple must continue to employ some other adequate method of contraception. Spermatozoa are still formed postoperatively but undergo phagocytosis. A series of 73 patients was followed-up from 1 to 5 years postoperatively by Ferber et al. (1967). The men reported no alteration in their own health and a slight improvement in health of their wives. Coitus occurred more frequently in the majority of couples, and this at an age when sexual activity tends to decline. One important feature of vasectomy is the possibility of successful anatomical repair in from 50 to 90%, which appears to render superfluous methods of temporary male sterilization by intravasal contraceptive devices.

Future developments

(A) THE MALE PILL

The effect upon spermatogenesis of both naturally occurring and synthetic steroid compounds has been studied in animals and in human volunteers, as have compounds such as nitrofurans, thiophenes and *bis*(dichloroacetyl)-diamines. The last has been employed in clinical trials in man and was shown to be effective (MacLeod 1965). Nitrofurans and thiophenes are too toxic to be used and even the *bis*-diamines have unpleasant side-effects if taken with alcohol.

(B) STUDIES OF INFERTILITY IN WOMEN

These have suggested that antibodies to spermatozoa and other fractions of semen can occur (Schwimmer *et al.* 1967), and it may one day become possible to make use of this knowledge as a clinical contraceptive technique.

(C) THE 'MORNING AFTER' PILL

Search for this continues.

(D) PROLONGED CONTRACEPTION

It has been claimed that a single intramuscular injection of 150 mg medroxy-progesterone acetate will provide effective contraception for 3 months. Evaluating studies are in progress.

REFERENCES

ATTWOOD M.E. (1966) *J. Obstet. Gynaec. Br. Commonw.* **73**, 662.
BAIRD D. (1966) *Br. med. J.* i, 850.
BARGLOW P. (1964) *Archs. gen. Psychiat* ii, 571.
BARGLOW P. & EISNER M. (1966) *Am. J. Obstet. Gynec.* **95**, 1083.

BORELL U. (1966) *Acta obstet. gynec. scand.* **45** (Supplement I), 9.

BORNMAN J.J. & DE VILLIERS J.N. (1965) *S. Afr. J. Obstet. Gynaec.* **3**, 50.

BOULWARE T.M. & ENSOR H.C. (1967) *Obstet. Gynec., N.Y.* **29**, 147.

BURNET F.M. (1961) *Eugen. Rev.* **45**, 139.

BURNHILL M.S. & BIRNBERG C.H. (1967) *Am. J. Obstet. Gynec.* **98**, 135.

COALE A.J. & HOOVER E.M. (1959) *Population Growth and Economic Development in Low Income Countries.* London, Oxford University Press.

CONNELL E.B. & KELMAN C.D. (1968) *Obstet. Gynec., N.Y.* **31**, 456.

DICKINSON R.L. & GAMBLE C.J. (1950) *Human Sterilization: Techniques of Permanent Conception Control.* Baltimore, Waverley Press.

DICZFALUSY E. (1968) *Am. J. Obstet. Gynec.* **100**, 136.

FERBER A.S., TIETZE C. & LEWIT S. (1967) *Psychosom. Med.* **29**, 354.

FOX T. (1966) *Lancet,* ii, 175, 1238.

GARB A.E. (1957) *Obstet. Gynec. Survey,* **12**(3), 291.

GARCIA C.R. (1967) *Am. J. med. Sci.* **253**, 718.

GARCIA C.R. (1968) Ed. *Clin. Obstet. Gynec.* **11**, 627.

GARCIA C.R. & PINCUS G. (1965) *Int. J. Fert.* **9**, 95.

GOLDZIEHER J.W. (1964) *Med. Clins. N. Am.* **58**, 529.

GRAFENBERG E. (1929) In *Gebwtenretelung: Vortiäje und Verhandlungen des Ärztekursus Selbstverlag Berlin* (edited by Bendix), p. 50.

GREEN-ARMYTAGE V.B. (1958) In *Operative Surgery,* Vol. 6 (edited by C. Rob & R. Smith). London, Butterworths, p. 107.

HALL H.H. (1966) *Am. J. Obstet. Gynec.* **95**, 879.

HALL R.E. (1966) *Am. J. Obstet. Gynec.* **94**, 65.

HOFFMEYER H., NORGAARD M. & SKALTS V. (1967) *J. Sex. Res.* **3**, 1.

INMAN W.H.W. & VESSEY M.P. (1968) *Br. med. J.* ii, 193.

ISHIHAMA A. (1959) *Yokohama med. J.* **10**, 89.

KAERN T. (1967) *Br. med. J.* iii, 644.

KLEINMAN R.L. (1966) In *Royal Commission Report on Population.* London, PPF.

LEWIS-FANING E. (1949) Cmd. 7695. London, H.M.S.O.

LEWIS A.C.W. & WILLIAMS E.A. (1970) *J. Obstet. Gynaec. Br. Commonw.* **77**, 743.

LIU W., KOEBEL L., SHIPP J. & PRISBY H. (1967) *Obstet. Gynaec., N.Y.* **30**, 228.

LONDON G.D. & ANDERSON G.V. (1967) *Obstet. Gynec., N.Y.* **30**, 851.

LORAINE J.A. & BELL E.T. (1968) *Fertility and Contraception in the Human Female.* Edinburgh, Livingstone.

LU T. & CHUN D. (1967) *J. Obstet. Gynaec. Br. Commonw.* **74**, 875.

McELIN T.W., BUCKINGHAM J.C. & JOHNSON R.E. (1967) *Am. J. Obstet. Gynec.* **97**, 479.

MACLEOD J. (1965) In *Agents affecting Fertility* (edited by C.R. Austin & J.S. Perry). London, Churchill.

MALTHUS T.R. (1798) *An Essay on the Principles of Population.*

MEARS E. (1965) *Handbook on Oral Contraception.* London Churchill.

OPPENHEIMER W. (1959) *Am. J. Obstet. Gynec.* **78**, 446.

OTA T. (1934) *Jap. J. Obstet. Gynec.* **17**, 210.

OVERSTREET E.W. (1964) *Clin. Obstet. Gynec.* **7**, 109.

PEBERDY M. (1964) In *Biological Aspects of Social Problems* (edited by J.E. Meade & A.S. Parkes). Edinburgh, Oliver & Boyd.

PEEL J. & POTTS M. (1969) *Textbook of Contraceptive Practice.* Cambridge University Press.

PINCUS G. (1965) *The Control of Fertility.* New York, Academic Press.

PITKIN R.M. (1966) *Obstet. Gynec., N.Y.* **28**, 680.

Population Council (1964). *2nd International Conference On Intrauterine Contraception.* New York.

RATNAM S.S. & YIN J.C. (1968) *Br. med. J.* i, 612.

RICE-WRAY E., CERVANTES A. & GASTELUM H. (1967) *Int. J. Fertil.* **12**, 312.

SCHWIMMER W.B., USTAY K.A. & BEHRMAN S.J. (1967) *Fertil. Steril.* **18**, 167.

SHAW W. (1970) *Textbook of Operative Gynaecology* (3rd Ed., revised by John Howkins). London, Livingstone, p. 245.

SIEGLER A.M. & HELLMAN L.M. (1964) *Obstet. Gynec., N.Y.* **23**, 173.

STARUP J. & FRIJS T. (1968) *Acta endocr., Copenh.* **56**, 525.

STEPTOE P.C. (1967) *Laparoscopy in Gynaecology.* London, Livingstone.

SWYER G.I.M. (1966) In *Current Medicine and Drugs.* London, Butterworths.

TIETZE C. (1966) *Am. J. Obstet. Gynec.* **96**, 1043.

TIETZE C. (1967) *Proc. Vth World Congress Fertil. Steril.* (Excerpta Medica Int. Conf. Series, Vol. 133).

TIETZE C. (1967) *VIIIth Progress Report Coop. Statist. Program. for Evaluation I.U.D.* (Population Council, Biomedical Division).

TIETZE C. (1968) *Int. J. Fertil.* **13**, 377.

VENNING G.R. (1963) *Proc. Symposium Oral Contraception.* G.D. Searle & Co., p. 43.

VESSEY M.P. & DOLL R. (1968) *Br. med. J.* ii, 199.

WALLACH E.E. & GARCIA C.R. (1968) *J. Am. med. Ass.* **203**, 927.

WHITE C.A. (1966) *Am. J. Obstet. Gynec.* **95**, 31.

WOODRUFF J.D. & PAUERSTEIN C.J. (1969) *The Fallopian Tube.* Baltimore, Williams & Wilkins, p. 351.

WHO (1968) Technical Report Service, No. 386.

CHAPTER 31

PELVIC INFECTION

Despite the availability and ease of administration of many powerful antibiotic drugs, pelvic inflammatory disease is encountered not infrequently in gynaecological practice. Although acute pelvic infection should be more easily treated, chronic inflammatory conditions are still found in patients attending infertility clinics and general out-patient clinics, at which they may complain of troublesome pain and other vague symptoms, including menstrual upsets.

There may be infection of the lower genital tract, including the cervix uteri, the corpus uteri, the uterine tubes, the ovaries and the parametrial tissues. The infection may be acute or chronic and may be due to a number of organisms, including gonococci, gas-forming organisms and tubercle bacilli. There may be an obvious aetiological factor such as a recent abortion or delivery, but in many no source of infection is admitted or found.

ACUTE INFECTION

Puerperal and postabortal infections

After pregnancy, the vascular uterus, and particularly the placental site, provides a good culture medium for infecting organisms, because of the degenerating and vascular tissue present. There is little resistance to the infection which involves the endometrium and then the myometrium. Organisms may then reach the peritoneum and parametrial tissues, with involvement

of the broad ligament, the uterine tubes from the peritoneal aspect and the surface of the ovaries. In abortion, particularly when this has been criminally induced, the instruments or solutions used may not be sterile or, more usually, the cervix or uterus is traumatized. Uterine infection may occur, but the spread to the parametrial tissues is often rapid, with early involvement of the adnexae.

The most common organisms encountered are the *Escherichia coli* and other Gram-negative bacilli, the clostridii, streptococci and staphylococci. They invade rapidly and give rise to a general upset, partly because of bacteraemia and also from toxaemia. This results in 'septic shock' and the death of the patient, if treatment is not commenced immediately and is inadequate.

PATHOLOGY

Acute inflammation is found in the endometrium with hyperaemia and areas of necrosis. Acute salpingitis is of the interstitial type with cellular infiltration of the mesosalpinx and muscularis, while the endosalpinx is only minimally involved. Spread of infection to involve the ovary may lead to oöphoritis or the formation of a tubo-ovarian abscess. Thickening and thrombophlebitis of the veins of the parametrium occurs and involvement of the peritoneum gives rise to the formation of adhesions. Usually, the resultant peritonitis is localized in the pouch of Douglas, but generalized peritonitis may occur, particularly if a tubo-ovarian abscess ruptures (Pedowitz & Bloomfield 1964).

With early antibiotic treatment the systemic upset is less frequently found and usually is of short duration, but chronic changes still develop despite treatment. The abdominal ostium of the tube usually remains open, but adhesions on the peritoneal aspect of the tube may effectively cause its occlusion or involve the ovary, with resultant infertility.

CLINICAL FEATURES

The patient looks ill and is restless, with a marked pyrexia, a rapid pulse and, perhaps, rigors. There is pelvic pain and tenderness especially on movement of the cervix, and perhaps thickening of the parametrium can be felt. There is usually a vaginal discharge, which may be brown or blood-stained and offensive, or may be scanty. Signs of peritonitis are present with rebound tenderness. Bowel sounds are usually present initially, but an ileus may develop later. The uterus may be enlarged and tender.

If there is marked septicaemia and 'septic shock', the blood pressure falls, the pulse becomes imperceptible, the temperature may become subnormal and the patient has a cold, clammy skin. Her urinary output is very low or complete anuria may be found. The first evidence of thrombophlebitis of the pelvic veins may be a pulmonary infarction, although oedema of the lower limbs and tenderness in the iliac fossa may be marked.

The endotoxin may cause peripheral vasomotor collapse in the kidneys, liver, adrenals and lungs—the Schwartzmann reaction.

DIFFERENTIAL DIAGNOSIS

A recent history of abortion or delivery is usually diagnostic, but cannot always be obtained. Acute appendicitis with perforation may produce similar features initially, and if there is doubt about the diagnosis, laparotomy is indicated, but this is only likely early in the disease. Jacobson (1964) has suggested that laparoscopy might be useful in the diagnosis of acute salpingitis.

TREATMENT

If possible, the infecting organism should be identified, but effective antibiotic treatment must be started as early as possible. It is unfortunate that it is very difficult to obtain a culture of the organism except at laparotomy. Vaginal swabs may not reveal any pathogens, and special techniques for anaerobic organisms are not usually employed. It is preferable to use a broad-spectrum bactericidal antibiotic effective against Gram-positive and Gram-negative organisms, ampicillin being the most effective. As there may be a mixed infection, penicillin or kanamycin alone may not be effective. If treatment with large doses of ampicillin is commenced promptly, even anaerobic infections are likely to be overcome. A dose of 500 mg 6-hourly is required for at least 2 weeks, as it is of considerable importance that treatment be continued until all symptoms and signs have disappeared.

Blood loss is replaced and fluid and electrolyte balance is carefully controlled. Oliguria or anuria is more commonly associated with septic abortion, and prompt consultation with a renal physician is required to ensure that treatment by dialysis is given before the condition of the patient deteriorates. If an ileus develops, this is treated by gastrointestinal suction, intravenous fluids and electrolytes.

If it is suspected that products of conception remain within the uterus, these should be removed under antibiotic cover. Once the patient has been resuscitated and has received antibiotics for 12 hr (or, preferably, 24 hr), gentle digital exploration of the uterus should be performed. Ovum or ring forceps can be used, but vigorous curettage is to be avoided because of the danger of uterine perforation, or perhaps, spread of the infection.

If laparotomy has been performed, particularly if damage to the bowel is suspected, no attempt should be made to remove infected organs or tissues in the presence of acute inflammation. If a localized abscess is found, it can be drained by posterior colpotomy into the pouch of Douglas, or by the abdominal route, extraperitoneally, although this is not usually necessary in the early stages.

Gonococcal infection

In gonorrhoea, urethritis and infection of the vulvovaginal glands may occur at the same time as a cervical infection. The latter may resolve more rapidly than infection in the other sites, but spread from the cervix to the uterus occurs rapidly, with involvement of the endometrium. Further spread to the endosalpinx is common with possible exudation into the peritoneal cavity and involvement of the ovaries and peritoneum. Secondary infection would seem to be very likely, and this complicates therapy.

PATHOLOGY

Involvement of the endometrium results in an inflammatory reaction, but this is not usually invasive and after two or three menstrual periods no residual changes may be present. Inflammation in the endosalpinx results in exudation with adhesive occlusion of the tube, particularly at the fimbriated end. A pyosalpinx is formed or the exudation results in the formation of peritoneal adhesions in the pelvis.

The damage to the epithelium may be severe and may lead to subsequent tubal occlusion and infertility. Although prompt treatment may prevent extensive damage, this is not usually possible.

CLINICAL FEATURES

The patient may present while the infection persists in the lower genital tract and organisms can be cultured from the discharge. The discharge precedes the elevation of temperature, and abdominal pain is likely during or immediately after menstruation.

There is bilateral pelvic tenderness and severe pain on movement of the cervix. Swellings or thickening in the appendages may be felt, but examination without anaesthesia is usually too painful to be informative. Despite the pyrexia, the patient is not usually ill, as the systemic upset is minimal.

DIFFERENTIAL DIAGNOSIS

Among the conditions which must be considered are ectopic pregnancy, twisted ovarian cyst, rupture or haemorrhage into a cyst, appendicitis and peritonitis. The history may be helpful and the bilateral nature of the lesion is likely to indicate the diagnosis. If there is doubt and a surgical condition is suspected, laparotomy, or perhaps laparoscopy, will give the diagnosis.

TREATMENT

Antibiotics in large doses are indicated and again prolonged treatment is required. Penicillin intramuscularly in doses of 500,000 units 6-hourly for 10 days is usually sufficient. If the patient is allergic to penicillin, tetracycline 250 mg 6-hourly may be given or intramuscular injections of kanamycin. Ampicillin 500 mg 6-hourly may be more effective if there is secondary infection, and prolonged treatment is necessary.

Peritonitis is managed by rest in a sitting position and attention to the fluid and electrolyte intake and output. Careful follow-up is required to detect any change in the pelvic lesion. Re-infection is a possible explanation for apparent relapse of the condition.

CHRONIC INFECTION

Chronic pelvic infection is an important cause of dysmenorrhoea, dyspareunia, menstrual upsets and infertility. It usually arises because of inadequate or ineffective treatment which may have been commenced too late or not continued for long enough.

The uterus is not usually involved unless chronic infection occurs in retained placental tissue. Chronic inflammatory changes in the myometrium result in the deposition of fibrous tissue among the muscle fibres, and this causes enlargement of the uterus.

Chronic salpingitis and oöphoritis

The main pathological changes encountered are associated with occlusion of the uterine tubes and, in the gonococcal form, destruction of the endosalpinx. Distortion of the tubes with peritubal fixation is also common. If both the fimbrial and isthmic ends of the tube are blocked, a pyosalpinx may form, with thickening and inflammation of the wall. If this subsides and becomes sterile following treatment, a hydrosalpinx may be formed (Fig. 31.1), either with a single cavity or with a number of compartments with trabeculae. The wall is thin and the mucosal cells are flattened by pressure.

CLINICAL FEATURES

A history suggesting previous pelvic infection may be obtained, but this may be concealed by the patient if it were of gonococcal origin. Also, many patients may not associate a puerperal or postabortal pyrexia with later pelvic inflammatory disease. The main complaint is pain,

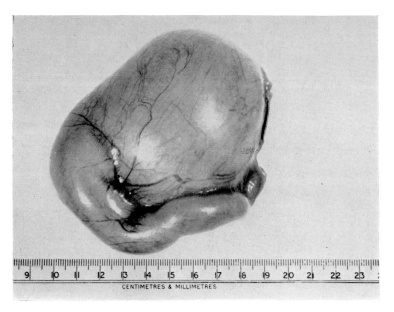

Fig. 31.1. A typical hydrosalpinx.

Extension of the infection from the tube to the ovary results in chronic inflammatory changes or abscess formation, usually with tubal involvement, to form a tubo-ovarian abscess. Occasionally, organisms may penetrate the ovarian stroma, perhaps at ovulation or postoperatively with the formation of an ovarian abscess, in which the tubal involvement is limited to a perisalpingitis (Ledger 1969).

Cystic degeneration of the ovary may result from infection, and the ovary may also become surrounded by dense fibrous adhesions which cause fixation of the pelvic organs and may simulate the changes associated with endometriosis.

sometimes severe, especially with menstruation, but aching or discomfort during or after intercourse may be experienced also. The 'secondary' dysmenorrhoea differs from the type previously experienced and is usually most severe during or immediately before menstruation. Sometimes it is found to persist after menstruation. Backache is a common complaint, although there may be no localization of the discomfort. Rectal symptoms may also be complained of.

Menstrual irregularity, with frequent periods and menorrhagia, is common and is probably related to ovarian involvement in the inflammatory process with the presence of cystic changes. Vaginal discharge from a chronic cervicitis, and frequency of micturition, may also be found. It is surprising that quite a number of patients with chronic inflammatory changes have no symptoms but present with infertility, often having had previous pregnancies or abortions. However, on further enquiry other symptoms may be elicited.

As the symptoms tend to persist for months or even years, it is not surprising that the patient becomes irritable or apprehensive, with bouts of depression. Marital problems may add to her general distress.

It is sometimes possible to detect a mass or bilateral swellings in the lower abdomen, but guarding is likely, and usually this examination is not helpful. On pelvic examination, the uterus is frequently enlarged and fixed in retroversion, and attempts to antevert it are unsuccessful and cause discomfort. Alternatively, it may be displaced by a pelvic mass. Masses of variable size may be detected in both appendages or in the pouch of Douglas, and these are fixed and tender. More usually, thickening of the adnexa is found, and the uterosacral ligaments are prominent, taut and tender.

DIFFERENTIAL DIAGNOSIS

Endometriosis may mimic the features of pelvic inflammatory disease, and laparoscopy or laparotomy is required to determine the diagnosis with certainty. Other causes of pelvic swelling include haemorrhage into—or torsion of—an ovarian cyst, torsion of a pedunculated fibroid and appendix abscess, but these can usually be distinguished by the history and clinical findings.

MANAGEMENT

The treatment of chronic pelvic inflammation is difficult and depends on a number of factors. These include the age and parity of the patient and her aspirations regarding further pregnancies, the causative organisms, the nature of the lesions and their extent in the pelvis, and the response to treatment.

It is good practice to manage pelvic inflammatory disease conservatively by medical measures, but there are indications for surgery, and operation should not be unduly delayed if

these are present. Epstein *et al.* (1962) advocate laparotomy if there is no improvement after 24 hr of treatment.

Medical treatment includes attention to hydration and nutrition, correction of anaemia, analgesics and heat, including short-wave diathermy, and antibiotic therapy. Possibly cauterization, or even amputation, of a grossly infected cervix might be considered as 'conservative' treatment. Antibiotics are not as effective in chronic disease as they are in the acute condition, and there is also the difficulty of obtaining organisms for culture for *in vitro* sensitivity tests. A broad-spectrum, bactericidal agent such as ampicillin 1–2 g daily in divided doses for at least 2 weeks may be of value and is useful as 'cover' when short-wave diathermy or cauterization of the cervix is indicated. More prolonged treatment in the absence of a clinical response is not of value, but may be prescribed if surgery is undertaken. The use of corticosteroids in the management of non-tuberculous inflammatory disease has been described by Hertig (1963), and Campbell (1965) discussed their use along with antibiotics when the parametrium is indurated and fixed. Prednisone 30 mg daily is given initially, with a reduction by 5 mg every 3 days after the temperature has returned to normal. Normally, the course lasts for 3–4 weeks. Surgery is indicated if:

(i) there is no response to intensive therapy and the general health of the patient continues to deteriorate;

(ii) there are repeated and acute exacerbations of chronic inflammatory disease;

(iii) local tenderness persists without improvement;

(iv) masses in the adnexae or pouch of Douglas increase in size or show no diminution;

(v) menstrual disorders continue and cause incapacity.

The laparoscope may be used to determine the nature of the condition and the extent of the disease, but as dense adhesions may be present in long-standing cases, damage to the bowel and other organs is a definite hazard. Laparotomy should be undertaken during antibiotic therapy and, whenever possible, material for bacteriological culture obtained at operation. This is usually sterile, but occasionally organisms, especially anaerobic organisms, may be grown and their sensitivity to antibiotics determined. Blood for transfusion should be held in reserve.

The operation performed depends on the extent of the disease and the age and desire for further pregnancies, but in general as little as possible should be removed. Salpingectomy or salpingo-oöphorectomy may be sufficient, or even bilateral salpingectomy may be indicated. In the premenopausal patient ovarian tissue should be preserved provided it appears to be healthy. If the ovary is involved in an abscess, resection of the infected part may be sufficient provided efficient haemostasis is secured. If there is doubt, it is probably better to remove the ovary because of the likelihood of the recurrence of pelvic symptoms and menstrual disorders.

It is sometimes necessary to remove the uterus, and while this provides the opportunity to drain the pelvis through the vaginal vault, there may be difficulty in effecting haemostasis and there is considerable risk of secondary haemorrhage if the parametrium is extensively involved. It is permissible in certain circumstances to perform a subtotal hysterectomy, provided adequate treatment of the cervix is undertaken and cytological examination of the cervix will be performed at intervals thereafter.

If further pregnancies are desired, the uterus and some portions of a uterine tube and ovary should be preserved, provided this allows the chronically infected tissues which have been causing the symptoms to be removed. The chances of subsequent pregnancy depend on the extent of the destruction of the endosalpinx, the distortion of the tubes by adhesions and the remaining ovarian function, but is is unwise to attempt restorative procedures at the time of operation on patients with the features of chronic inflammation. Salpingostomy and tubal implantation in the uterus may be considered at a later operation. Some form of ventrosuspension operation is beneficial if there have been extensive adhesions in the pouch of Douglas or a tubo-ovarian abscess, in order to prevent fixation of the uterus in retroversion with possible subsequent dyspareunia.

SPECIAL PROBLEMS IN PELVIC INFLAMMATORY DISEASE

(1) TUBO-OVARIAN ABSCESS

A tubo-ovarian abscess may give rise to very few symptoms, or may cause severe abdominal pain and tenderness. Intensive antibiotic therapy is required and when the systemic upset is considered to be controlled, surgical removal or drainage of a persistent abscess is indicated. Drainage is best obtained by means of posterior colpotomy, adhesions being broken down gently and streptokinase–streptodornase in combination being instilled if the pus is thick. Closure of the colpotomy should be prevented until the abscess has subsided. Laparotomy is usually required to prevent recurrence of the abscess, and the removal of the disease organs may be performed 3–6 weeks later under antibiotic cover.

Rupture of a tubo-ovarian abscess results in an acute abdominal emergency. Adhesions to other tissues may predispose to the rupture of the abscess because stretching of the adhesions may cause tearing. Resuscitation is required with early surgery (Mikal et al. 1968), the diagnosis being made by aspiration of purulent material from the pouch of Douglas. At laparotomy removal of the infected organs and drainage of the peritoneal cavity is required and following this intravenous fluids, nasogastric suction and antibiotics are continued for as long as is necessary.

(2) ACUTE INFLAMMATION IN THE PRESENCE OF CHRONIC PELVIC INFLAMMATION

A quiescent chronic pelvic inflammation may flare up, with the development of acute symptoms, including pyrexia and abdominal pain and tenderness. A pelvic abscess may develop but the acute process may be controlled by prompt treatment with antibiotics. Recurrent acute exacerbations are an indication for surgical removal of the diseased tissue and operation should be undertaken when the acute phase has been controlled and during antibiotic therapy.

(3) PELVIC THROMBOPHLEBITIS

As a result of infection, septic thrombophlebitis may develop in the pelvis and cause a persistence in symptoms when improvement is expected. The patient has an intermittent pyrexia and abdominal pain, but otherwise may seem quite well. If antibiotic therapy has been continued without the expected response being obtained, Schulman (1969) suggested that anticoagulant therapy may be beneficial. He gives heparin for 2 or 3 days and if the temperature falls, continues treatment with Warfarin or other oral anti-coagulants for about 3 weeks. If there is no response after 3 days, the anticoagulants are discontinued.

PELVIC TUBERCULOSIS

Tuberculosis of the genital organs is secondary to pulmonary tuberculosis, which is not usually active at the time the pelvic condition is discovered. Spread is initially haematogenous and the disease affects the uterine tube most frequently. Extension from peritonitis or from a tuberculous lymph node is possible, and although spread from the lower genital tract following intercourse with a man with tuberculous epididymitis is reported, it is most unusual. Tubal tuberculosis may spread to the uterus and the peritoneal cavity, with secondary involvement of the ovary.

PATHOLOGY

The changes are similar to those of chronic salpingitis, with the development of a pyosalpinx or interstitial salpingitis. Nodules in the tube may be tuberculous in origin, but salpingitis isthmica nodosa may also occur in the absence of tuberculosis. The medial portion of the tube is most commonly involved, and although the tube is patent on hysterosalpingography, it is rigid and narrowed due to involvement of the endosalpinx and muscular tissue in the wall. The fimbriated end of the tube is everted rather than closed, although pyosalpinx may develop. In miliary tuberculosis, numerous tubercules are present on the peritoneal surface of the tube.

On microscopic examination, the tubercles are typical, with giant cells and endotheliod cells sometimes giving an adenomatous appearance.

Tuberculous peritonitis is now rarely associated with tubal disease but may result in ascites or the formation of adhesions with caseation and subsequent fistula formation. Endometrial tuberculosis has been found in approximately 50% of patients with tubal disease, but the demonstration of endometrial involvement is not always satisfactory. With repeated menstruation, the disease may be minimal in the uterus and curettage may miss an affected area. Similarly, tubal disease cannot be demonstrated in all patients with proven endometrial tuberculosis because of the difficulty of establishing the diagnosis without biopsy or resection of the tubes for examination.

CLINICAL FEATURES

Many patients have no specific complaints and may only be diagnosed after infertility investigations. In others masses are found in the pelvis, although this is now uncommon. Menstrual loss may be scanty or there may be complete amenorrhoea if there is extensive endometrial involvement, but secretory endometrium may be obtained on curettage. Some patients have a persistent vaginal discharge. On further investigation anaemia, an evening pyrexia and weight loss may be detected.

The endometrium obtained at curettage must be examined histologically for the presence of tubercles, but if tuberculosis is suspected tissue must be sent for guinea-pig inoculation. Hysterosalpingography reveals characteristic changes due to thickening and rigidity of the muscularis of the tubal wall with narrowing of the lumen (Fig. 31.2). Laparoscopy or laparotomy may show bilateral tubal enlargement with peritubal adhesions, but the appearance of the tube is not necessarily diagnostic. If any tubal tissue is excised it also should be examined microscopically and bacteriologically.

TREATMENT

After the diagnosis has been made by curettage or biopsy, the patient is given intensive anti-tuberculosis therapy. Many regimens have been

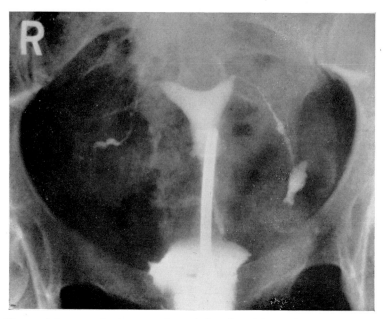

Fig. 31.2. Hysterosalpingogram showing narrowing and distortion of the tubal lumen strongly suggestive of tuberculous salpingitis.

described, but the essentials are to prevent the organism becoming resistant to the drugs used and to continue treatment for sufficient time to prevent recurrence or relapse.

Streptomycin 1 g daily by intramuscular injection, with isoniazid 100 mg orally three times daily and para-aminosalicylic acid 3 g four times daily, should be continued for 3 months until the sensitivity of the organism is determined. Whenever possible, the streptomycin injections are discontinued and outpatient treatment is then possible with isoniazid and PAS. This treatment is required for at least 18 months, and probably 2 years, with curettage being performed after 6 months and at 3- or 6-monthly intervals thereafter. If the infection has not been eradicated or recurs, as demonstrated by the curettings, streptomycin is again required. Investigations such as tubal insufflation or hysterosalpingography and both conservative and radical surgery, should only be undertaken when anti-tuberculous drugs are being given.

The prospects of successful pregnancy are not great if tuberculosis of the tubes has been proved,

although some cases of successful intrauterine pregnancy are reported (Francis 1964). The risk of ectopic pregnancy is considerable and is further increased after salpingostomy and tubal implantation procedures; the patient who seeks a pregnancy should be advised of this. If tubal disease is extensive, removal of the uterus, both tubes and both ovaries is indicated, with intensive chemotherapy for at least 6 months postoperatively.

REFERENCES

CAMPBELL C. (1965) *Penn. med. J.* **68**, 41.
EPSTEIN A.M., BOUTSELIS J.C. & ULLERY J.C. (1962) *Am. J. Surg.* **104**, 555.
FRANCIS W.H.A. (1964) *J. Obstet. Gynaec. Br. Commonw.* **71**, 418.
HERTIG A.J. (1963) *J. int. Coll. Surg.* **40**, 564.
JACOBSON L. (1964) *Acta obstet. gynec. scand.* **43**, 160.
LEDGER W.J. (1969) *Clin. Obstet. Gynec.* **12**, 265.
MIKAL A., SELLMANN A.H. & BEEBE J.L. (1968) *Am. J. Obstet. Gynec.* **100**, 432.
PEDOWITZ P. & BLOOMFIELD R.D. (1964) *Am. J. Obstet. Gynec.* **88**, 721.
SCHULMAN H. (1969) *Clin. Obstet. Gynec.* **12**, 240.

CHAPTER 32

ENDOMETRIOSIS

In endometriosis tissue similar to normal endometrium in structure and function is found in sites other than the lining of the uterine cavity. This tissue, consisting of both glands and stroma, may be in the myometrium of the uterus and has been known as endometriosis interna, but is better referred to as adenomyosis.

If the aberrant tissue is found outside the uterus it is called endometriosis externa, or true endometriosis. It may be in the pelvis, or abdomen, or in more remote sites. Although the two conditions are histologically similar, they are probably of different origin and occur in different types of patient.

ADENOMYOSIS

In this condition, ingrowths of endometrium occur into the myometrium, and glandular and stromal tissue are to be found among the uterine muscle fibres. The lesion is surrounded by muscle, but as it is thought to arise by direct growth from the endometrium, it is likely that a connection exists to the endometrium. It was first described by von Recklinghausen in 1895, and two years later by Cullen.

Aetiology and pathogenesis

The condition is usually found in multiparous women, and it is thought that repeated pregnancies may predispose to the extension of the endometrium into the myometrium. It has been found more commonly in women in the higher socio-economic groups. Vigorous curettage may perhaps lead to damage to the uterine wall, thus allowing access to the endometrium (Ringrose 1962). Cystic glandular hyperplasia of the endometrium may be present in patients with adenomyosis, and it can be postulated from this that hormone imbalance, particularly with oestrogen in excess, may be a contributory aetiological factor (Emge 1958).

Pathology

The uterus is usually enlarged in this condition, but the enlargement is symmetrical. The lesion may be localized or diffuse throughout the uterine wall. Localized lesions are not encapsulated as are fibromyomata, but they may be multiple. The posterior uterine wall is more commonly involved.

If the uterine wall is incised, a number of small, pale areas may be seen with 'blood spots' in their centre. Sometimes, quite large cystic spaces are present in the myometrium, each filled with blood. On histological examination areas of glandular tissue resembling endometrium are found and each is associated with stromal cells with surrounding muscle fibres. The columnar epithelium and the stromal cells of the glandular tissue respond to a variable extent to the cyclical hormonal changes in the menstrual cycle, the major response being to oestrogen. Secretory endometrium may be seen, and also decidual changes in pregnancy, but these are uncommon, because the invading basal layer of the endometrium is less responsive. Menstrual discharge from the adenomyoma may reach the uterine cavity if a patent connection is present, but more often blood collects in the gland 'lumen'.

Clinical features

The condition is found in women near the end of their reproductive lives, and nearly always in multiparous women. The lesions and symptoms may be minimal, but the principal features are menorrhagia, because of interference with the normal uterine haemostatic mechanism, progressive secondary or acquired dysmenorrhoea, and enlargement of the uterus. The uterus may be tender and occasionally irregular, the most usual diagnosis being fibromyomata. Dyspareunia, pelvic discomfort and bladder or bowel irritation may be reported due to adenomyosis, but is sometimes due to coexistent endometriosis, which is reported in 10–20% of patients at operation.

Treatment

If the lesion is localized and further childbearing is desired, an attempt may be made to resect the adenomyoma. More often, however, total hysterectomy is the better operative treatment. The ovaries may be left *in situ* in premenopausal women if there is no associated pelvic endometriosis.

ENDOMETRIOSIS

Aetiology and pathogenesis

Although isolated reports of endometriotic deposits in the pelvis had appeared earlier, Sampson described in some detail perforating chocolate cysts of the ovaries in 1921, and Blair-Bell coined the terms 'endometriosis' and 'endometrioma' in the following year. While numerous theories have been propounded to explain the occurrence of the condition, it seems certain that no one theory will explain all forms of endometriosis. It is not proposed to consider all the theories in detail in this chapter, but merely to mention some of the more plausible of them.

(1) IMPLANTATION THEORY

Sampson (1940) suggested that menstrual blood containing fragments of endometrium might pass along the uterine tubes in a retrograde manner and thus reach the peritoneal cavity. The endometrium would then implant on the peritoneal surface of organs or tissues in the abdomen and pelvis, and in subsequent menstrual cycles it would undergo changes under the influence of ovarian hormones. In support of this theory, it has been possible in animals to produce endometriosis by retrograde menstruation and implantation, and Ridley & Edward (1958) found experimental evidence in women that degenerated endometrium will satisfactorily implant. Ridley (1961) injected menstrual blood into the peritoneal cavities of 15 women, and two subsequently developed endometriosis. Hughesdon (1958) confirmed that retrograde menstruation does occur, and has found evidence of endometriosis in patients who persistently showed this. While retrograde menstruation and implantation explains some peritoneal deposits of endometriosis, it does not explain its occurrence in sites away from the peritoneal cavity.

(2) COELOMIC METAPLASIA THEORY

Ivanoff (1898) and Meyer (1903) independently suggested that endometriosis might result from metaplasia of immature groups of cells which were originally part of the Muellerian epithelial system. The primitive coelomic epithelium gives rise to the epithelial cells lining the Muellerian duct. It is also differentiated into peritoneal and pleural epithelium and the cells on the surface of the ovaries. If these peritoneal or pleural or 'ovarian' cells return to their original embryological function of forming Muellerian epithelium, this could differentiate into ectopic endometrium. It may be that all adult cells derived from the primitive ceolom are capable of reversion and later transformation into Muellerian epithelium, the surrounding cytogenic tissue forming the endometrial stroma. Repeated stimulation by hormones or inflammatory irritation may produce these changes. This theory can explain the occurrence of endometriosis in nearly all the ectopic sites, including the rectovaginal septum and the limbs, because coelomic epithelium may become isolated in unusual sites during development. It is fully described by Novak & de Lima (1948).

(3) LYMPHATIC PERMEATION AND DISSEMINATION

Halban (1924) postulated that endometrium from the uterus reached ectopic sites by means of the lymphatic system. Javert (1949, 1951) has found endometrium in lymph nodes and also in blood vessels. This is not a common mode of spread, but could well explain certain deep-seated areas of endometriosis which have been found.

(4) HAEMATOGENOUS SPREAD

If the endometrium enters a vein as a result of curettage, it may produce emboli which reach the lung, or if there is an anomaly of the circulation the emboli may lodge in other sites. Yeh (1967) reviewed the literature on intrathoracic endometriosis and found eight cases reported of blood-borne 'mestastases'. A lesion which has spread from the pleura to lung tissue would be more readily explained by the coelomic metaplasia theory.

Pathology

The macroscopic appearance of the lesions depends to a large extent on the organ or tissue involved, and the secondary response elicited in the surrounding tissues. They vary in size from very small black 'dots' seen on the peritoneum of the rectovaginal pouch to large cystic masses filled with dark, rather viscous material in the ovaries. If there is haemorrhage from the endometriotic tissue or a cystic lesion ruptures into the peritoneal cavity, peritonitis follows, with a fibrotic reaction around the lesions concerned. Dense adhesions may result from this.

Reabsorption of the fluid content of the blood in the cyst gives rise to the 'chocolate' or tarry material found in these lesions. It is important to appreciate, however, that a chocolate cyst of the ovary may be due to follicular and corpus luteum cyst haemorrhage and to haemorrhage into a cystadenoma after torsion.

Microscopically, endometrial glands, endometrial stroma and, usually, evidence of either recent or old haemorrhage, can be seen. Red cells may be found in the 'lumen' of the glands or haemosiderin pigment may be present in the glands or in macrophages. Because of the pressure within a cyst, the wall may be denuded of epithelium in some areas. During pregnancy the endometrium undergoes a characteristic decidual reaction.

Clinical features

Endometriosis is found during the active reproductive era, although its consequences may still be evident at operation in postmenopausal women. It tends to occur in women between 30 and 45, although it is certainly found in younger women. The patients are usually nulliparous, or have had one or two children some years prior to the onset of symptoms. It is rarely found in Negroes and is more common in women in the higher socioeconomic groups. It would seem that the incidence of the condition is increasing, but in many instances it is detected at operation or autopsy without ever having caused symptoms. The size of the lesion may bear no relation to the severity of the symptoms, the site of the disease and its ability to respond to hormones being of more importance.

Menorrhagia is a common symptom and abdominal pain, backache, secondary dysmenorrhoea and deep dyspareunia are frequently found. The pain may be referred to the rectum if the rectovaginal septum is involved. Patients without symptoms may attend for the investigation of infertility, and be found to have endometriotic deposits.

The pain experienced may be referred to the rectum or perineum, and accompanied by tenesmus. It may also be felt in the lower abdomen, the posterior segment of the pelvis, the vagina and the back. It starts about the time of onset of menstruation, or perhaps 1 or 2 days before. It may continue throughout the period or occur at the end, because the ectopic endometrium does not respond as readily as normal endometrium to the ovarian hormones, and shedding of the endometrium is later than occurs in the uterus. If the lesion is not confined by fibrosis, there may be minimal discomfort. The pain is usually related to the site of the ectopic endometrium.

If ovarian function is altered by bilateral endometriosis, irregular menstruation and menorrhagia may result. Leakage from, or rupture of, an ovarian endometriotic cyst or endometrioma leads to peritonitis, and is an acute abdominal emergency requiring laparotomy.

The patient may have no symptoms but presents for the investigation of infertility. She may have had no pregnancies previously or perhaps one child followed by involuntary infertility.

On examination, hard, fixed nodules of variable size may be detected in the uterosacral ligaments, the pouch of Douglas (rectovaginal cul-de-sac), on the posterior surface of the cervix or the uterine wall. These nodules can be felt on vaginal or more easily on rectal, examination. Other suspicious findings include obliteration of the pouch of Douglas and a fixed retroversion of the uterus. Palpably cystic ovaries, usually bilateral, are found and are usually fixed to surrounding structures. Nodules may be detected in the rectovaginal septum, and a combined vaginal and rectal examination is necessary if endometriosis is suspected.

Speculum examination may reveal a bluish nodule in the posterior fornix if the vaginal wall is involved. Movement of the cervix results in pain and pelvic tenderness is present, particularly during menstruation.

Examination under anaesthesia, and culdoscopy, allow examination of the pelvis, especially the pouch of Douglas, but laparoscopic examination permits visualization of the whole pelvis and aids in determining the most appropriate treatment. Laparotomy may be required if the pelvis contains dense adhesions, and is followed by definitive surgery, if necessary. In certain circumstances, barium enema, intravenous pyelography and cystoscopy may also be indicated if endometriosis of the bowel or urinary tract is suspected.

Differential diagnosis

Depending on the site of the endometriosis, adenomyosis, pelvic inflammatory disease, carcinoma of the colon or rectum and the 'pelvic congestion syndrome' must be considered.

Rupture of an endometriotic cyst results in an acute abdominal emergency. Similar features may be found with a ruptured ectopic pregnancy, haemorrhage into or torsion of an ovarian cyst, or acute sulpingitis.

Sites of endometriosis

(1) OVARIAN ENDOMETRIOSIS

The ovary is the most usual site for endometriosis, and the lesions may be either superficial or deep. The small, superficial, bluish cysts contain altered blood, and from these the escape of small quantities of blood results in the formation of adhesions to the surrounding structures, with subsequent fibrosis. When the adhesions are broken down, the cysts are damaged and 'chocolate' material escapes.

The deeper and larger chocolate cysts have been thought to arise from metaplastic change in follicular or lutein cysts, and also to be downgrowths of ectopic endometrium from surface deposits on the ovary. The features include pelvic pain, backache, dysmenorrhoea, menorrhagia, dyspareuria and infertility. It is often difficult to distinguish the condition from chronic salpingitis.

(2) PELVIC PERITONEAL ENDOMETRIOSIS

There may be a few, or numerous, bluish areas of endometriosis involving the rectovaginal pouch and septum, and the uterosacral ligaments most frequently, as well as the posterior—and sometimes the anterior—layers of the broad ligament and the surface of the uterus. Adhesions may obliterate the rectovaginal pouch, fix the uterus in retroversion and distort the pelvic colon. They cause a variety of symptoms, including dysmenorrhoea, pelvic pain, dyspareunia and bowel discomfort.

(3) BOWEL ENDOMETRIOSIS

The bowel may be involved in endometriosis along with other sites in the pelvis, but sometimes it alone has deposits on its surface. The rectum is involved when there are deposits in the recto-vaginal septum, while peritoneal endometriosis may spread to the bowel. The pelvic colon and rectum are most frequently affected, the lesion being on the peritoneal surface and in the muscular layers, but rarely involving the mucosa. The symptomatology and diagnostic features have been reviewed by Macafee & Hardy Greer (1960) and more recently by Burns (1967). If there is no obstruction, there may be no symptoms, unless there is associated pelvic endometriosis, or perhaps vague abdominal pain at menstruation. If there is obstruction it may be partial or complete, due to fibrosis affecting the wall of the bowel, and this is most commonly seen in the ileal region and the pelvic colon. Although the endometriotic deposits will atrophy and become quiescent after removal of the ovaries or after the menopause, the stenosis due to fibrosis will not disappear and surgical relief may be required. This may entail a colostomy or end-to-end anastomosis. Gray (1966) gives a good account of the management of this problem.

The most important alternative diagnosis is carcinoma of the colon or rectum, and the conditions must be differentiated because of the different management and prognosis. In endometriosis there is a periodicity of symptoms associated with menstruation—diarrhoea, pain in the rectum, blood in the stools, and obstructive symptoms. There may also have been unexplained infertility; there is *no* loss of weight in the presence of symptoms suggestive of carcinoma, and there is dysmenorrhoea. Barium enema may show a long, constant, filling defect, intact bowel mucosa and fixation of the bowel with tenderness and palpation. On sigmoidoscopic examination during or after menstruation, an intact mucosa with reddening and puckering may be seen.

Involvement of the appendix may give rise to symptoms of acute appendicitis at the time of menstruation. While the diagnosis may be incorrect, the management is quite satisfactory, appendicectomy resulting in a complete cure.

It is essential to determine whether there are other endometriotic deposits in the pelvic region before anticipating such a cure, however.

(4) LOWER GENITAL TRACT ENDOMETRIOSIS

Cases of cervical and vaginal endometriosis have been reported (Williams 1960). The lesions are bluish in colour and their cystic consistency is readily palpable. The symptoms include dyspareunia, dysmenorrhoea and minimal metrorrhagia. Perineal deposits may be found in episiotomy scars, but these are not common.

(5) URINARY TRACT ENDOMETRIOSIS

This is well reviewed by Kerr (1966). Bladder endometriosis is very rare but cases have been reported by Laiso & Marcelli (1964), probably as a result of spread from pelvic endometriosis. Blue areas may be seen at cystoscopy if the mucosa is involved, and frequency, dysuria, haematuria and abdominal pain are characteristic.

A ureter is occasionally obstructed by external endometriosis, and Broch (1960) reported five cases of intrinsic obstruction. A diagnosis of carcinoma is likely and can be excluded only by histological examination of the mass after operative removal.

(6) ENDOMETRIOSIS OF THE UMBILICUS

A blue swelling at the umbilicus which bleeds at menstruation is occasionally reported. Steck & Helwig (1965) found 21 lesions out of 82 involving the skin.

(7) ENDOMETRIOSIS IN SCARS

A painful, tender swelling in a laparotomy or Caesarean section scar is highly suggestive of endometriosis. It may follow operation on the uterus or on an abdomen in which there is widespread endometriosis.

(8) OTHER SITES

Spread to the inguinal region by means of the round ligament is reported. A lesion in this region must be distinguished from hernia and lymphadenitis.

Deposits have been found in the limbs when painful swellings have been excised. Haemoptysis may be the first sign of pulmonary endometriosis, probably as a result of blood spread, although spread from the peritoneum to the pleura may be the explanation.

Treatment

This may be radical or conservative, surgical or medical, and depends on the age of the patient, her parity and desire for further family, the site of the lesions and the degree of severity of the symptoms.

If a patient has minimal symptoms but characteristic findings on pelvic examination, no treatment is required, but follow-up examinations every 6 months are advisable because of the possibility of extension of the condition and subsequent complications. If the patient is young and wishes to have children, she should not be observed for too long and if involuntary infertility lasts longer than 1 year, full investigation—including laparoscopy—is indicated. If the patient does not wish further children and is having appreciable pain and other symptoms, more radical surgical treatment is required.

HORMONE THERAPY

As pregnancy frequently has a beneficial effect on endometriotic deposits, causing them ultimately to atrophy and become unresponsive to hormone stimulation, the use of sex hormones to create a pseudopregnancy effect is theoretically sound. Oestrogens in large doses have been used, but most patients are unable to tolerate the doses given and the side-effects are considerable, including severe uterine bleeding.

Progestational agents along with a small amount of oestrogen have been used more recently, the dosage increasing weekly until about ten times the amount required for oral contraception is being administered (Kistner 1958). The preparations which include norethynodrel with ethinyloestradiol, and norethindrone with mestranol given orally, and medroxyprogesterone

by intramuscular injection (Gunnin & Moer 1967) are administered for up to 12 months; the oral preparations are given daily without allowing menstruation to occur. Numerous side-effects have been reported, including breakthrough bleeding, which can usually be controlled by increasing the dose of oestrogen given, heavy bleeding, nausea, breast discomfort, weight gain and psychological upsets (Kistner *et al.* 1965).

The early promise shown by this form of treatment has not been fulfilled in the larger series reported, if success is judged by complete cure. Symptomatic relief may be experienced but many gynaecologists now feel that hormone therapy is a useful pre- or postoperative measure, and only rarely does it replace surgical treatment completely.

Androgen therapy has been used with success, but if the dose is too high the development of virilizing side-effects is distressing. Some women develop these even on low dosage. However, methyltestosterone sublingually in a dose of 5 mg daily for 100 days apparently does not suppress ovulation, and relieves the patient's symptoms without marked virilism.

SURGICAL TREATMENT

The surgical cure of endometriosis requires that all the ovarian tissue or all the endometriotic deposits be removed. The form of treatment employed, therefore, depends on the age of the patient and her desire regarding further pregnancy, as well as the extent of the disease, the symptoms it is causing and the secondary changes which have resulted from it.

In a young woman removal of the ovaries is to be avoided, so local endometriotic deposits are removed and pregnancy is encouraged in the hope that any remaining lesions will undergo atrophy. Of perhaps more importance, a pregnancy may prevent recurrence of the lesions, but, subsequent infertility, and the resultant ovarian changes may interfere with ovulation, causing menstrual upsets. Hormonal pseudopregnancy for 2 or 3 months before operation and for some months afterwards may be beneficial if all the deposits cannot be excised. A full investigation of the patient and her husband is necessary at an early stage if infertility is a major complaint.

This form of conservative treatment consists of the division of pelvic adhesions, mobilization of the appendages and the operative removal of any ovarian endometriomata present. Some form of ventrosuspension of the uterus, after adhesions in the rectovaginal pouch have been divided, is temporarily beneficial, and fertility is likely to be increased by this. Local lesions in the pelvis are excised if possible, or fulgurated with a diathermy pencil. If pain is a prominent feature, presacral neurectomy is sometimes performed, but hormone therapy has, perhaps, superseded this operation. It is necessary to remove endometriomata prior to hormone therapy because of the risk of their rupture, with the development of an acute abdominal emergency.

Radical surgery involves the removal of both ovaries and, usually, the uterus, and its use is confined to women near the menopause who are having distressing symptoms. A more radical approach may be permissible if further pregnancies are definitely not desired. If there is encirclement of the bowel or ureter, treatment must be radical, and even then some form of decompression procedure may be necessary. It may not be technically easy to remove the uterus completely, and in such patients pre-operative hormone therapy possibly has a place for a short time in order to control symptoms and soften the pelvic adhesions.

RADIOTHERAPY

The production of an artificial menopause may be indicated in certain patients in whom operation is contra-indicated, but the number of these is few, and X-ray castration is not likely to be used in any but exceptional cases now.

Malignant change in endometriosis

Malignant change in an endometriotic lesion is very uncommon and when it occurs ovarian endometriosis is invariably involved. There must be both benign and malignant endometriosis present and the malignant tissue must not have invaded the benign tissue to permit this

diagnosis to be made, although late tumours will certainly have invaded the surrounding tissue. Histologically, the tumour is either an adeno-acanthoma or an endometroid carcinoma (adenocarcinoma), the term 'endometroid' being internationally accepted (Scully et al. 1966). Fathalla (1967) reviewed 637 specimens of ovarian endometriosis and found four with malignant features. In a study of 418 primary malignant ovarian tumours, 52 had a histological appearance similar to malignant endometrial changes, and four of these were shown to have a definite endometriotic origin.

Malignant change in adenomyosis is extremely rare, but adenomyosis and adenocarcinoma may coexist in the same uterus.

The possibility of malignant change occurring in endometriosis need not influence the proposed management of a patient. The presence of ovarian malignancy, however, must be considered when an alternative diagnosis is an endometrioma or chocolate cyst of the ovary. Removal of the lesion is the only certain method of establishing this diagnosis.

STROMAL ENDOMETRIOSIS

In tumours designated as stromal endometriosis the cells resemble normal stromal cells of the endometrium and are found in the myometrium. The uterus is enlarged and its cut surface shows protruding worm-like masses of tumour. Extension occurs into the endometrial cavity or into the broad ligaments (Fig. 32.1). The condition has been considered a variant of adenomyosis, but is probably in no way related to either benign or malignant endometriosis or adenomyosis. Gunther (1967) thinks it is an angioplastic sarcoma but that it is of low-grade malignancy.

It is a very uncommon condition, but has been reported in postmenopausal women. Metastases occur which may be fatal, and removal of the ovaries does not appear to cause regression, as would be expected in endometriosis. The main features are menorrhagia and irregular bleeding, and pelvic pain and abdominal swelling may also occur. Treatment consists of total hysterectomy

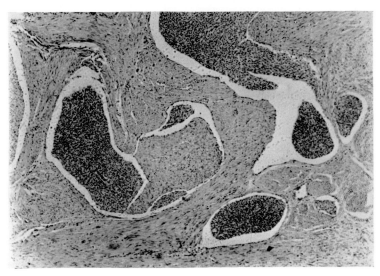

Fig. 32.1. Histological appearances in a case of stromal endometriosis, showing collections of endometrial-like stromal tissue deep in the myometrium. (By courtesy of Drs. Haines and Taylor, and J. & A. Churchill, London.)

with the removal of the ovaries, unless the patient is young and the ovaries are not involved. Radiotherapy may be used if operation is not possible or is incomplete, or if there is a recurrence. Recurrences have been reported by Hunter *et al.* (1956), and therefore the prognosis should be guarded.

REFERENCES

BROCH D.R. (1960) *J. Urol.* **83**, 100

BURNS F.J. (1967) *Dis. Colon Rectum.* **10**, 344

EMGE L.A. (1958) *Am. J. Obstet. Gynac.* **76**, 1059

FATHALLA M.F. (1967) *J. Obstet. Gynaec. Br. Commonw.* **74**, 85.

GRAY L.A. (1966) *Clin. Obstet. Gynec.* **9**, 309.

GUNNING J.E. & MOYER D. (1967) *Fertil. Steril.* **18**, 759.

GUNTHER J. (1967) *Zentbl. Gynäk* **89**, 1857.

HALBAN J. (1924) *Wien. klin. Wschr.* **37**, 1205.

HUGHESDON P.E. (1958) *J. Obstet. Gynaec. Br. Commonw.* **65**, 944.

HUNTER W.C., NOHLGREN J.E. & LANCEFIELD S.M. (1956) *Am. J. Obstet. Gynec.* **72**, 1072.

IVANOFF N.S. (1898) *Mschr. Geburtsh. Gynäk.* **7**, 295.

JAVERT C.T. (1949) *Cander, N.Y.* **2**, 399.

JAVERT C.T. (1951) *Am. J. Obstet. Gynec.* **62**, 477.

KERR W.S. (1966) *Clin. Obst. Gynec.* **9**, 331.

KISTNER R.W. (1958) *Am. J. Obstet. Gynec.* **75**, 264.

KISTNER R.W., GRIFFITHS C.T. & CRAIG J.M. (1965) *Cancer, N.Y.* **18**, 1563.

LAISO E. & MARCELLI G. (1964) *Archo ital. Urol.* **37**, 255.

MACAFEE C.H.G. & HARDY GREER H.L. (1960) *J. Obstet. Gynaec. Br. Commonw.* **67**, 539.

MEYER R. (1903) *Virchows. Arch. path. Anat. Physiol.* **171**, 443.

NOVAK E. & DE LIMA A. (1948) *Am. J. Obstet. Gynec.* **56**, 634.

RIDLEY J.H. (1961) *Am. J. Obstet. Gynec.* **82**, 777.

RIDLEY J.H. & EDWARD J.K. (1958) *Am. J. Obstet. Gynec.* **76**, 783.

RINGROSE C.A.C. (1962) *Can. med. Ass. J.* **83**, 1541.

SAMPSON J.A. (1940) *Am. J. Obstet. Gynec.* **40**, 549.

SCULLY R.E., RICHARDSON G.S. & BARLOW J.F. (1966) *Clin. Obst. Gynec.* **9**, 384.

STECK W.D. & HELWIG E.B. (1965) *J. Am. med. Ass.* **191**, 167.

WILLIAMS G.A. (1960) *Am. J. Obstet. Gynec.* **80**, 734.

YEH T.J. (1967) *J. thorac. cardiovasc. Surg.* **53**, 201.

CHAPTER 33

INFERTILITY AND DYSPAREUNIA

INFERTILITY

In the closing decades of the twentieth century, fertility and infertility are becoming relevant to the overall problem of world population. There is strong pressure to encourage family limitation and to control fertility with modern contraceptive techniques; in many countries a further development is the allowing, or even encouraging, of abortion as a means of controlling the incidence of unwanted pregnancies. Ethical, traditional or modern views of these problems differ enormously, but in the midst of this wider view of the population problem there remains a group of patients who, as individual couples, fail to achieve a pregnancy, and for whom no lengths are too great for them to go in their quest for children of their own. The individual problem of infertility remains, with some recent advance in available methods of treatment and the promise of greater advances ahead.

Infertility refers to the apparent inability of a couple to have children, and in clinical usage is a term to be preferred to sterility, which refers to the absolute inability of a couple to produce children for one or other finite reason. The fertility of any given couple is not absolute and it takes a healthy couple, on average, a year to achieve a pregnancy given normal anatomy, and physiology and sexual function. It is therefore rarely necessary, or wise, to start investigating into reasons why a couple have not achieved success before this time. However, age reduces fertility, and natural anxiety on the part of the patient may make it advisable to institute a

simple examination, at least, with reassurance and good advice at an earlier stage. Infertility is regarded as a primary or secondary problem, depending on whether the difficulty in conception is *ab initio* or follows the birth of previous children.

Factors responsible for infertility

Fertility may be reduced as a result of ignorance, disordered physiology or disease of the genital tract in either partner. Ignorance is not confined to any one group of patients and is seen as often in progessional groups as in any other. Stallworthy (1955) records the incidence of non-consumated marriages as high as 5% in patients attending for infertility. This may be due mainly to a lack of understanding of sexual physiology and therefore a failure to establish normal sexual relationships.

Disordered physiology may be responsible if the patient fails to ovulate or if menstruation is very irregular, making the time of ovulation, which is normally 14 days before the next period, equally erratic. Tubal spasm is believed to play a part in delaying fertility in a small group of patients. There is hystosalpingographic evidence that this is an entity, and some workers claim that anti-spasmodics given before intercourse can lead to success.

Spermatogenesis can be effected by altered thermal control, as seen in undescended testes, in patients with a variocele of the cord, or with the frequent use of restrictive underwear compressing the inguinal region sufficiently to impede venous return from the scrotum. Normal sperm invasion of the cervical canal depends on normal coital function and a healthy receptive cervical mucus. Failure of erection or premature ejaculation will militate against these; in addition, inadequate preparation of the female partner may result in poor cervical mucus output, with resultant poor sperm invasion. The normal production of healthy cervical mucus to bathe the vaginal vault, or the successful penetration of sperms into the cervical canal, are of fundamental importance in this problem.

DISEASE OF THE GENITAL TRACT

Disease in either partner may be responsible for infertility. Thus in the male, congenital absence of the gonads or their failure to descend into the scrotum will result in infertility, as will infections which disorganize the testes or result in blockage of the epididymis or vas deferens. As mentioned earlier, alteration of the thermal regulation of the testes may occur with varicocele of the cord, hernia or hydrocele.

In the female partner also, the essential genital organs may be congenitally absent, as in the many types of intersex (for example, testicular feminization), or imperfectly formed, as in Turner's syndrome. Infections, gonococcal or otherwise, can affect any part of the genital tract and inhibit or prevent fertility. They may act by altering the production of cervical mucus, as in cervicitis, preventing satisfactory imbedding of the ovum, as in endometritis, or most commonly, by the resultant blockage of the fallopian tubes or impairment of their normal function as a result of fibrosis, such tubes being incapable of peristalis and without functioning cilia.

Blockage of the tubes may be cornual, particularly after intrauterine infections following abortion, and in these circumstances the distal portion of the tube may remain healthy. In other patients the fimbrial end of the tube may be blocked and the lumen occluded throughout a varying percentage of its length. The infection may be tuberculous or secondary to abortion, interference or a foreign body, such as an intra-uterine contraceptive device.

Malposition of the uterus—in particular, retroversion—has been blamed for infertility,

but it is only occasionally a factor. Many healthy patients conceive with a normal uterus in the retroverted position. However, this position of the uterus may play a part in reducing fertility when other factors are present. For example, in the patient with a secondary infertility and a relatively capacious vaginal vault and a retroversion, an ejaculate of small volume may fail to find its way into the cervical canal; repeatedly poor postcoital tests prove this. By altering the position of the uterus to anteversion, so that the cervix lies in the posterior fornix, and therefore in the pool of seminal fluid, a good postcoital test can be obtained, and conception may follow in due course. This example may seem remote from reality, but in fact it is just the combination of minor factors which can prevent conception in what appears to be an otherwise healthy couple; and it is by attention to detail that success can be achieved in this work.

Endocrine dysfunction may result in failure of ovulation. This is seen in the hypothalamic-pituitary stress. Dysfunction in other endocrine glands may result in failure to ovulate, as in hyper- and hypothyroidism; similarly, in disordered pituitary or adrenal function, anovulatory cycles commonly occur and successful treatment of these and other endocrine disorders usually results in restoration of menstruation and ovulation. Failure to ovulate may follow endocrine therapy, particularly when the sex steroids are employed. This quite commonly occurs after a patient has been on one of the contraceptive pills for a period of time; the first period after treatment is often delayed by a week or two and, rarely, the patient fails to menstruate or ovulate for some considerable time.

Investigation

This should always be regarded as a joint investigation of husband and wife from the physical and psychological aspects. It should begin with the husband, because examination of him is relatively simple and without physical danger, while the complete investigation of the wife must carry with it a small, but real, risk of complications which attend any minor surgical procedure. Occasionally, for religious or physical reasons, the husband is not able to provide a seminal specimen for analysis; in these circumstances, and in any case as part of the complete investigation, a postcoital test will have to suffice. The latter, as mentioned earlier, tests the sperm invasion of cervical mucus. Before embarking on any special investigation, however, it is necessary to undertake a full history and examination of the patient with regard to her menstrual and sexual function, her past medical history and past obstetric experience. The previous practice of contraception, its methods and timing, and the pattern of normal intercourse in the given couple are all important.

General physical examination of the wife must be performed; general stature, obesity, hirsutism and secondary sex characteristics are noted and detailed clinical examination of the genital tract is undertaken. When these preliminaries are complete, it may be decided that simple reassurance and encouragement are all that are required, depending on the time that the couple have been trying to conceive in which case, an explanation of simple anatomy and physiology, best explained with a simple diagram of the female genital tract, will be most helpful.

If, however, sufficient time and opportunity has passed for conception to occur, had all been normal, detailed investigation should be initiated.

Methods of investigation

SEMEN ANALYSIS AND POSTCOITAL TEST

The first special investigation aims to demonstrate that the husband's semen specimen is capable of fertilizing an ovum. It is undertaken by semen analysis of a masturbation specimen and by a postcoital test. The features of a semen analysis which suggest normality are a pH of 7·5, a volume of 2·5 ml or more, and a count of 60 million per millilitre or more; sperms should be motile and not more than 20% abnormally formed. Thus a specimen of less than 2 ml volume, and certainly a count of less than 40 million per millilitre, is associated with relative infertility, and a volume of less than 1 ml or a count of 20 million per millilitre or less are rarely associated

with fertility. A postcoital test at the time of ovulation gives reassurance that not only are healthy sperms present, but that they are motile and normal in cervical mucus. One poor semen or postcoital test should not be taken as final evidence, but should be repeated.

If the semen test is not normal then the husband should be examined clinically for evidence of disorders. Treatment of varicele or hernia will sometimes effect improvement, and avoidance of restricting underwear, with daily cold bathing of the testes, is not as primitive or unscientific as it sounds, and will lead to improvement if carried out regularly for a few months.

TESTS FOR EVIDENCE OF OVULATION

Anovulatory cycles occur more frequently in the first months and years after the menarche, and in the years before the menopause. They also occur in some patients with irregular cycles, patients whose menstrual patterns react to emotional stress, and in patients soon after childbirth, particularly if the patient is lactating. But at other times it must be uncommon to find evidence of anovulation. Tests which demonstrate the changes which follow ovulation infer that it has occurred, and that it probably occurs in most cycles in that patient. A great deal of information is being obtained by laparoscopic observation at the time of ovulation and in the recovery of the contents of ripe graafian follicles by aspiration after induction of ovulation in some patients. It has even been possible to obtain ova by these means and to effect fertilization in vitro.

Methods available for obtaining evidence of ovulation are as follows: clinical evidence; vaginal smears; basal temperature chart; endometrial biopsy; and direct observation.

The patient may volunteer symptoms which suggest that ovulation has taken place. Pain at the time of ovulation in one or other iliac fossa, associated with slight blood loss, is subjective evidence. These symptoms may vary from being barely susceptible to being severe but of short duration, and of course in many patients no symptoms occur, despite normal ovulation. The subsequent development of primary spasmodic dysmenorrhoea is further evidence of ovulation, as this rarely occurs in patients who have not ovulated.

Cytology of vaginal smears will show the changes in the exfoliated cells which occur during the progestational phase of the cycle and normally only follow ovulation (see p. 27). The advantage of this method is that it is easily repeatable without trauma at different times in any cycle and in subsequent cycles.

Temperature charts

The basal body temperature taken in bed on waking each morning will show a pattern of change at the time of ovulation (Fig. 33.1). Two or three cycles will teach a patient how to recognize the changes for herself, and by con-tinuing with this method she may determine the day of ovulation with reasonable accuracy. Cold, pyrexial illnesses, etc. are common factors which may alter the daily temperature enough to make interpretation difficult on occasions, but the method is relatively accurate, without physical trauma or danger, and can be continued for a long time. It will be seen that the method is of special value in patients who have irregular cycles, when it is not possible to predict the day of ovulation. There is one problem with the method; this is, that patients who are at all sensitive (and most infertility patients seem to be as part of the problem) may find it impossible to carry it out routinely without becoming obsessed with it. The mere recording of temperature as the first waking thought every morning may so

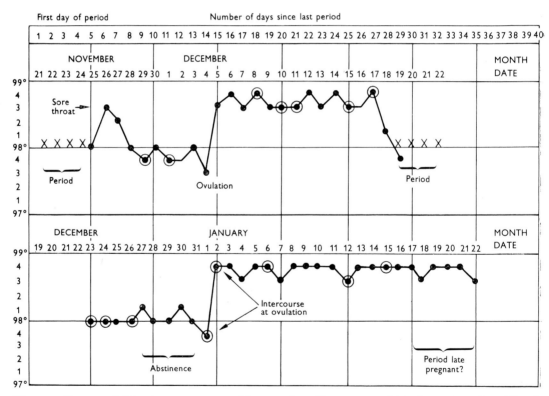

Fig. 33.1. Top: a typical basal temperature record indicating ovulation. At the time of ovulation there is a brief fall in temperature of a few hours' duration, followed by a rise which is maintained until the next period. An ovulatory chart, therefore, has the biphasic pattern shown here. Bottom: an ovulatory temperature chart followed by pregnancy. The rise in temperature is maintained. (By courtesy of John Sherratt & Son and Ortho Pharma-ceuticals Ltd.)

highlight their problem that it becomes an intolerable burden. For the more stoical, and especially those with irregular cycles, it has a definite place.

When considering techniques for the induction of ovulation (see Chapter 34), this method will play an important part in the management of anovulation by clomiphine or gonadotrophic preparations; the rise in temperature will indicate that ovulation has occurred, and if the rise is sustained this confirms that conception has taken place.

Endometrial biopsy

This investigation is useful in that it gives microscopical proof of the changes in the endometrium which follow ovulation, the development of the corpus luteum and its output of progestational steroids. It may also give an indication of any endometrial disorder, such as irregular ripening of the endometrium, or of pathological changes due, for example, to tuberculous infection. It is clearly necessary to take the biopsy as near to the first day of menstruation as possible, and in patients whose periods are very irregular, arrangements must be made to take the biopsy on the first day of the flow to be sure of a correct endometrial sample. The biopsy is taken with a fine endometrial biopsy curette (Sharman), which can usually be passed without anaesthesia with minimal discomfort. Recently, an out-patient suction curette has been shown to be effective (Holt 1970). Having ascertained the position of the uterus on bimanual examination, it is usually easy to pass a uterine sound through the internal os. Having confirmed the direction of the canal and uterine cavity the biopsy curette can then be passed to recover a sample of endometrium sufficient for histological study. Aching menstrual discomfort may attend and follow this procedure. If the patient is left to lie down for a short while and given a mild analgesic this is the most that would be required. When it is not possible to perform this procedure as an out-patient, because the internal os is too tight or the patient uncooperative, the procedure should be carried out under an anaesthetic at the appropriate time (see below).

When there is no evidence of ovulation, then it is advisable to repeat the test in a subsequent cycle, ensuring that the endometrium is immediately premenstrual before anovulation is accepted as a cause of infertility.

Direct observation

By observation at laparotomy or laparoscopy it is possible to see a corpus luteum which has resulted from recent ovulation, or even to see the ruptured follicle on the day of ovulation. Steptoe & Edwards (1970) have carried this observation a step further by inducing ovulation in patients who previously had not ovulated, and on the day of induced ovulation have examined the ovaries and aspirated the contents of any graafian follicles which had developed to maturity; the ova contained have been exposed to seminal fluid *in vitro*. Thus, by direct observation it is possible to detect that ovulation is imminent or has occurred, and in certain special techniques it may be possible to recover an ovum. We must wait a while to find what the practical applications of this work are.

TESTS FOR EVIDENCE OF TUBAL PATENCY

Tubal patency may be tested by various methods, for example:

    (i) Insufflation, using carbon dioxide.
    (ii) Hysterosalpingography.
    (iii) Laparoscopy.

Tubal insufflation

Tubal insufflation—first described by Rubin in 1920—can be performed as an out-patient procedure, providing the patient is cooperative; instrumentation and distension of the tubes can lead to discomfort, but in many patients this is minimal. Air insufflation should never be used, as it may well lead to fatal air embolism. Carbon dioxide is readily absorbed if intravasation should occur, and is therefore safer.

Using a kymograph tracing, insufflation is performed—having ensured a 'gasp-tight' application of the nozzle of the canula in the cervix.

The pressure is slowly increased up to 160 mmHg or higher—even up to 200 mmHg if necessary. A tracing of the pressure and the effect of tubal spasm, peristalis or free-leak through the tubes is seen. It is imperative to ensure that there is no leak in the apparatus or its application to the cervix for good results. Passage of gas through the tubes may be confirmed by auscultation over the abdominal wall in the area of the fimbrial end of the tubes, and the fact that the gas irritates the peritoneal surface of the diaphragm, causing shoulder-tip pain in the next few hours. When there is no evidence of tubal patency, but spasm rather than organic occlusion is suspected, it is possible to give the patient an antispasmodic (e.g. a capsule of amyl nitrite). If the lack of patency is due to spasm, this medication should lead to a picture of subsequent tubal patency.

Insufflation is sometimes inaccurate because of leaks in the apparatus, however careful the operator; and if there is no evidence of patency, then it gives no indication as to the site of blockage. Occasionally, diseased tubes (e.g. in tuberculosis) may give evidence of tubal patency without hint of the disorder; or the impression of patency may be gained as a large hydrosalpinx is distended. The method is the simplest and has the lowest morbidity, but is subject to inaccuracies and errors of interpretation. One, or even two negative insufflations should not be taken as clear evidence of tubal occlusion without further investigation.

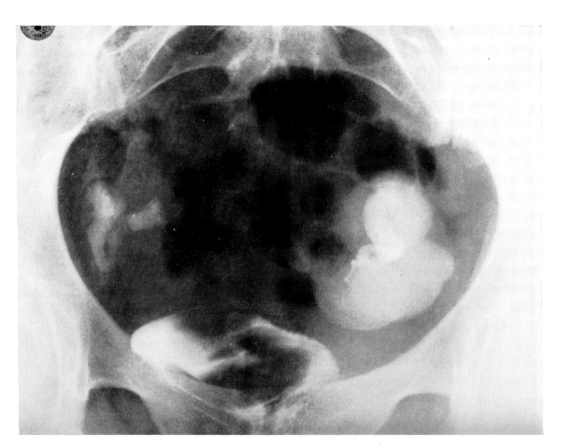

Fig. 33.2. Blocked and diseased tubes demonstrated by salpingogram. On the right of the picture the volume of dye which has collected in the tube suggests a hydrosalpinx to be present.

Hysterosalpingography

This may also be used as an out-patient procedure, but is best performed under light sedation or premedication (Valium 5 mg intravenously or pethidine 100 mg intramuscularly) or even under light general anaesthesia. Using a Labat's syringe (20 ml) and canula a water-soluble radiopaque dye is injected into the uterus using steady pressure. Volvellum forceps on the cervix maintain traction and ensure a water-tight fit. Using X-ray screening, preferably with an image intensifier and a television screen, the dye can be seen to outline the uterus and the tubes with free spill into the peritoneal cavity. Abnormalities of the uterus [fusion faults (Fig. 33.3), submucus fibroids], cervical incompetence, tubal spasm, tubal, cornual or fimbrial occlusion, hydrsalpinx (Fig. 33.2) or tuberculous disease of the tubes and peritubal adhesions leading to loculation of the dye outside the tubes can all be recognized by this method. Nowadays, Water-soluble solutions are used, as the older oily preparations, while they gave better pictures and remained for more than 24 hr for follow-up X-rays, also gave rise to potentially dangerous oil embolism if intravasation into the intra-uterine vessels occurred during injection of the dye. Water-soluble solutions give a less well-defined picture and disperse rapidly, so that any pictures must be taken within 10 or 15 min. However, if intravasation does occur, there appears to be no danger and these solutions are therefore safer, and are now always used.

If tubal occlusion is present it is possible to see the site of blockage. A failure on one occasion of dye to pass into the tubes or to spill should not be taken as certain evidence of permanent occlusion.

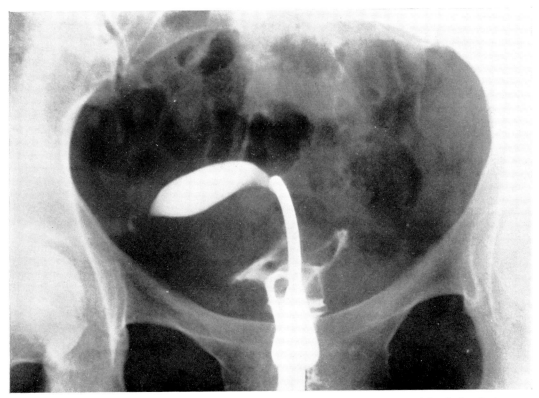

Fig. 33.3. A unicornuate uterus demonstrated by hysterogram. The commencement of the single tube is outlined, but spill is not demonstrated.

Repeat salpingogram or laparoscopy should be performed.

Jeffcoate (1957) found that 37% of 484 negative insufflations were erroneous, while only 15% of 538 salpingograms suggesting occlusion were erroneous. 3·2% of 369 positive insufflations were erroneous, and less than 1% of 380 positive salpingograms were erroneous.

Laparoscopy

This method of direct examination of the intra-abdominal viscera, and especially of the pelvic organs, gained wide popularity on the Continent of Europe, but only in the past 10 years or so has the method become generally accepted in the United Kingdom. This change in practice followed the introduction of the fibro-optic light source and the excellent calibre of modern endoscopic apparatus, making the technique simple and safe and the visual reward of the highest quality. Steptoe's (1967) excellent monograph should be consulted.

Laparoscopy in the study of infertility problems has several advantages. It allows direct inspection of the tubes and ovaries, which is of paramount importance when there is any suspicion of previous inflammatory disease; or in such conditions as the Stein-Levanthal syndrome, the gonads can be examined and, if necessary, an ovarian biopsy taken. If methylene blue solution is injected into the uterine cavity the tubes can be seen to fill and spill, unless there is blockage. If there is evidence of tubo-ovarian disease an accurate assessment can be made of its extent, and an estimate can be made of the chances of improving the prospects for fertility by surgical treatment.

This procedure is more hazardous than other investigations, and the necessary instrumentation runs the same risk of exacerbating any old focus of infection in the tubes and ovaries as do the other methods. No information is derived as to the health and normal development of the uterine cavity, which can only be assessed by hysterography, and if the dye does not pass into the tubes the exact location of the blockage, although presumed to be cornual, cannot be certain. It is the author's belief that the methods of salpingography and laparoscopy are complementary to each other; hysterosalpingography should still be the first method of investigation for tubal patency, proceeding to laparoscopy if for any reason it gives unsatisfactory or inconclusive results. Coltart (1970) has demonstrated the value of laparoscopy as a method of confirming or refuting the findings of salpingography.

Failure of ovulation

Further investigation will be necessary in the patients who do not ovulate as demonstrated by the above investigation, or in patients with amenorrhoea. These are discussed in Chapter 6.

IN SUMMARY

Patients who are infertile are often highly sensitive. Once they consult a specialist for advice, if all is normal in the history and examination and sufficient time has elapsed to allow conception, then investigation should be undertaken. With the exception of the special investigations related to endocrine disorder, the routine tests should be completed within a short space of time efficiently and without pain. There are many ways in which this can be accomplished, but the author believes that the simplest formula is often the best. First, a test to prove the husband's fertility by seminal analysis or a postcoital test. This should be followed by one test under anaesthesia to perform endometrial biopsy and to test tubal patency by hysterosalpingography or, if indicated, laparoscopy. This must be performed in the second half of the cycle to give an informative endometrial sample and the couple must undertake to prevent pregnancy in that cycle by taking precautions, so as not to disturb an early pregnancy in testing after midcycle. In this way, it is rarely necessary to repeat investigations, thus avoiding frustration on the part of the patient.

Treatment

Apart from the induction of ovulation in a patient who is not ovulating, there is little positive treatment in the field of infertility which specifically leads to conception. It is possible to improve the conditions likely to lead to conception, thus hastening the event; examples of this are methods to improve the postcoital test, advice concerning the time of ovulation, and treatment of the wife to allow normal intercourse when this has not been possible. There is a further positive benefit in being able to tell a couple that conception is extremely unlikely because of azoospermia, oligospermia or tubal occlusion in the wife; such information is hard to accept, but for many couples it is better for them to know the truth and build their lives around this knowledge, than to wait in vain year after year for conception which is never to occur. While both partners have the necessary organs and sexual function is normal it is unwise to tell them that pregnancy can *never* occur; it is, however, fair to explain to them how unlikely the chances are, so that they can accept the fact of a childless marriage and develop their interests in other directions or decide to adopt children, depending on their wish.

METHODS OF IMPROVING THE MALE SEMINAL SPECIMEN

The best specimen is produced after an interval of 2 or 3 days' abstinence; a longer or shorter interval gives a less satisfactory specimen, so that if the couple can accept scientific advice to regulate their sexual function, abstinence should occur for 3 days before the day of ovulation; thereafter there are no rules! It is wise to ensure that nothing impedes the normal scrotal temperature by altering the vascularity of the testes. Thus loose underwear, the repair of herniae or varicocele of the cord have all been followed by improved seminal specimens.

While medical measures have had their vogue in animal experiments, there is nothing to suggest that any produce consistent improvement in the semen specimen. In particular, vitamins, thyroid extract and testosterone have all been used, but there is no proof that any is effective; in fact, large doses of testosterone have been shown to depress spermatogenesis. Testosterone may play a small part in increasing libido and ejaculation. Human gonadotrophins have been shown to

be of value as replacement therapy in men who have undergone hypophysectomy, and several successful pregnancies have been reported. However, there seems to be little success following the use of these drugs in the otherwise normal patient with oligospermia. When a patient is found to be azoospermic and yet testicular biopsy shows normal spermatogenesis, obstruction of the vas must be suspect, and if present may be corrected by vaso-epididymostomy.

It is not reasonable to perform any operative treatment for the wife, except operations to allow normal intercourse, until the husband's fertility has been proven.

Methods of helping the wife's fertility are aimed at:

(i) improving the postcoital test;
(ii) inducing ovulation;
(iii) the treatment of tubal occlusion and
(iv) treating incidental problems.

IMPROVING THE POSTCOITAL TEST

If the postcoital test is unsatisfactory despite normal semen analysis, then mechanical factors are often responsible. Either no sperm will be seen, in which case there must be some fault in technique, or the sperms present will be few and barely motile. If there are few sperms, this can be improved by insuring that the semen specimen comes into contact with the cervix by the patient lying with her knees drawn up onto her chest for 15 min after intercourse to be sure that the specimen is retained in the vaginal vault; if this fails, it is possible to teach the patient to collect the semen in a special cervical cap and place this directly onto the cervix. In retroversion the uterus can be anteverted and maintained in the anteverted position with a Hodge pessary; a postcoital test in this circumstance should show a marked improvement. If so, it may be justifiable to perform ventrosuspension or just retain the uterus in the anteverted position with a Hodge pessary for a longer period of time.

If the sperms are not freely motile, it may be that they are rendered less active in transit across the vaginal fornices to the cervical mucus, either because of a capacious vault, or because there is too little cervical mucus bathing the vault in alkaline secretion. The situation can be improved by douching before coitus with a weak alkaline solution (a tsp. of sodium bicarbonate to 300 ml of water) or by improving the cervical mucus by giving oestrogen for a few days before ovulation (Dienoestrol 1 mg daily for 4 days).

If the cervix is unhealthy with cervicitis or erosion, cautery will improve the environment, but care must be taken not to cauterize to excess, and thus produce cervical stenosis or destruction of the mucus-bearing glands in the cervical canal.

By the above measure, it should be possible to obtain a good postcoital test, given a healthy uterus and a normal semen specimen. Rarely, sperm will be present in the cervical mucus in normal density but all will be dead. Evidence has accumulated to show that some patients form antibodies in the cervical mucus which kill sperm on invasion; this has been demonstrated *in vitro* (Parish & Ward 1968), when the sperm attracted to cervical mucus on a slide are seen to perish once contact with the mucus is made.

There is little that can be done to improve this situation, but it is believed that if the sperms are not in contact with the cervical mucus for some time—for example, 3–6 months—by the husband wearing a sheath, then the strength of the antibodies in cervical mucus is reduced, and coitus after this period of time is more likely to be followed by success. Much work is still to be done on this fascinating aspect of infertility, and with greater understanding of the problems involved success from treatment will follow.

Once the seminal specimen has been shown to be normal, the absence of sperm in cervical mucus is usually due to faulty coital technique. It is necessary to ensure that normal intercourse is taking place at the time of ovulation and occasionally, when psychological problems exist, advice to the husband, wife or both, must be arranged to overcome impotence, premature ejaculation, frigidity or vaginismus. Hymenectomy, or Fenton's operation to enlarge the introitus, will be necessary if on initial examination it is seen that for organic reasons full penetration is not possible. If sperm are present, but in reduced numbers, or are non-motile, the various methods outlined above can be considered to improve the sperm invasion of cervical mucus. When the menstrual cycle is irregular, temperature-charting to determine the day of ovulation, if acceptable to the patient, may be of the greatest importance. Some couples cannot order their married life according to scientific principles, and in these circumstances it is unwise to over-investigate or insist on sexual activity by the calendar. These couples must accept that there is likely to be a longer time before conception, which is to be preferred to the distaste and psychological barrier which can build up in some sensible couples when 'under orders' for coitus at a particular time.

INDUCTION OF OVULATION

Treatment for anovulation is dealt with in Chapter 34. There is no place for such treatment except in the proven circumstance of anovulation. Other possible causes of infertility must be excluded. The genital tract should be normal and any other endocrine dysfunction corrected before treatment to induce ovulation is considered.

TREATMENT OF TUBAL OCCLUSION

By far the most important treatment of tubal occlusion lies in its prevention, and it cannot be stressed too strongly or too often that prompt and prolonged treatment of acute salpingo-oöphoritis with appropriate antibiotics is essential to prevent subsequent tubal occlusion.

Once the tubal lumen is occluded, it is rare for pregnancy to occur. It is never wise to tell a patient that pregnancy is impossible while the essential organs are present, albeit chronically diseased, but the chances of a pregnancy occurring cannot be appreciably more than 1%. There are no medical measures which will alter established tubal occlusion.

Surgical treatment

Occlusion may be at the fimbrial or cornual end of the tube, or may result from previous interruption in the lumen by a sterilization procedure. If the block is at the fimbrial end and an hydrosalpinx results, opening the ampullary portion of the tube and suturing the mucosa to the peritoneum will effectively open the tube initially. Hydrotubation is indicated in the immediate postoperative phase by the injection of hydrocortisone and an antibiotic (streptomycin) through the cervix; alternatively, the injection can be given through a fine polythene tube which can be sutured into the new tubal opening and brought out at the abdominal wound to help to reduce the chance of fibrosis and adhesions— and thus reocclusion of the new ostrium—during the healing stage. Unfortunately in such cases, the tubal mucosa is chronically infected, and it is not surprising that in a very high percentage of patients the incidence of subsequent tubal reocclusion is extremely high (more than 90%). Efforts to maintain tubal patency of the new ostium by hydrotubation, or by insufflation with carbon dioxide, have not produced significantly improved results. This is a depressing situation, with poor return for surgical intervention. However, the gynaecologist is often pressed to perform the operation—if only to improve the chances of conception by 1 or 2%—so that the patient can be sure that everything possible has been done. The facts with regard to likely success should be put to the patient pre-operatively, and only on the patient's insistence should the operation be performed.

When the block is cornual there is a much greater possibility that the distal portion of the tube will be relatively, if not entirely, healthy. The healthy segment can then be reimplanted into the cornua and polythene rods sutured in place to splint the tubes in position. This operation dealing with healthy tissue is more likely to be followed by success, and figures of 25–30% have been claimed by some workers. Subsequent pregnancy should be terminated by Caesarean section, for there is a considerable risk of rupture in late pregnancy and labour at the cornua where the tube was implanted.

There is no doubt that in all operative procedures to restore tubal patency, great care must be taken that the tissues are handled gently; haemostasis is effective and postoperative inflammation and fibrosis avoided.

The use of a prosthesis in the fimbrial ends of the tube inserted for a period of 3–6 months for fimbrial occlusion is attractive in principle, but in most surgeon's experience has not effected improved results.

THE TREATMENT OF INCIDENTAL PROBLEMS

Although the specific relationship between obesity and infertility is not known, it is of benefit to such patients to diet and reduce any marked obesity. Other minor endocrine dysfunctions, in particular thyroid dysfunction, should be treated appropriately. There may well be other problems which either reduce fertility or lead to miscarriage if conception occurs. Thus fibroids, particularly if submucus, polypoidal or large, should be removed by myomectomy. When there is acute retroversion fixed by endometriosis, conservative excision or diathermy of the endometriotic areas and ventrosuspension may greatly improve the changes of conception and successful pregnancy.

ARTIFICIAL INSEMINATION

This is rarely justifiable, and in the presence of normal sexual function never indicated. When a husband has a normal seminal specimen on testing, but cannot satisfactorily deposit sperm in the vaginal vault either because of impotence, hypospadias or premature ejaculation, then his sperm can be collected and injected high into the cervical canal at the time of ovulation. There is a specific example of the use of this technique in impotent paraplegics, who, when given Prostigmine, can produce an ejaculate which can be collected and injected in this way.

The problems of artificial insemination using donor semen in patients whose husbands are azoospermic or severely oligospermic is fraught with many difficulties: psychological, ethical and medicolegal. The law relating to such treatment is not clear and this method is therefore not advised, even with the consent of both partners in the marriage.

If artificial insemination is to be considered, it is wise to establish normal fertility on the part of the wife by investigating, as described in this chapter, before the onset of treatment.

There comes a time when all investigations and treatment are complete, when it is necessary to advise a couple that this is so and that there is no advantage to be gained by pursuing further investigations or treatment. Despite this, the obsessive desire for a child often drives a patient from one specialist to another on the flimsiest pretext. If by simple, straightforward reassurance this can be avoided, it is to the advantage of the patient and those who offer counsel.

DYSPAREUNIA

Difficulties with intercourse may arise from physical problems or from a lack of understanding between the partners, or both factors may play a part.

A lack of understanding may arise from ignorance, inexperience, or emotional factors, and it is just as important for a gynaecologist to realize that even in the presence of organic disorders psychological factors may play the greater part, as for a practitioner or a psychiatrist to realize that even with a patient relaxed and in sexual harmony no success will be achieved until physical disorders are successfully treated. Often there is an element of both organic and psychological factors, and only experience will dictate the priorities of treatment.

Women frequently consult a gynaecologist about symptoms for which no organic lesion can be found, and it is part of a gynaecologist's undertaking to sense when this is so and to discern the true problem—which is often a failure to establish or maintain a satisfactory sexual relationship.

Successful intercourse is a composite of many factors: personal harmony, love and respect for the partner, either a desire for pregnancy or a safe acceptable method of contraception—circumstances which allow undisturbed love play and intercourse and complete absence of any guilt or psychological inhibition. Any adverse response in any of these essentials will mar the success of coitus.

Surprisingly, hormone changes have very little effect on libido or sexual response, although androgens are more important in this respect than oestrogens. However, treatment of subnormal response with hormones is rarely rewarding. Sexual interest in the female often continues after the menopause, although there is a wide variation of interest and response at this time. The majority of sexual problems have an emotional or psychological background. Most are capable of resolution by talking to and educating the couple; a few have their origin in psychiatric disorder.

Whatever the difficulty, it is almost always advisable to treat the problem as one in which both husband and wife share the responsibility both for the problem and for overcoming it, and consultation for one partner to the exclusion of the other is rarely as satisfactory or successful as one in which both partners are brought into the management of the situation.

Pain or difficulty with intercourse may well result from anatomical problems, from local disorders, or may be present in the absence of any anatomical or local disorders.

ANATOMICAL FACTORS

Anatomical difficulties arise when there is any narrowing of the introitus or vaginal lumen due to congenital abnormalities such as a rigid hymen, congenital bands or septa, or acquired by narrowing, secondary to surgical insults from episiotomy or prolapse repair. Narrowing may also occur as a result of menopausal atrophy. Dyspareunia may occur on deep penetration if the uterine fundus is retroverted and/or the ovaries are prolapsed in the pouch of Douglas, as either structure may be tender on pressure.

LOCAL DISORDERS

These causes are best related to the problem of difficulty at the introitus, which is often called superficial and relates to difficulties during penetration, or more deeply refers to difficulty or pain after penetration.

Difficulties at the introitus are most likely to be due to infections of the lower vagina or vulva. Thus, trichomonal or fungal infections may present in this way. Atrophic changes after the menopause with secondary infection may be present. Urethral caruncles, kraurosis, vulval ulceration, as in herpes simplex, or swelling, as in bartholinitis, may be the local causative factor.

Difficulties on deep penetration occur due to tenderness around the vaginal fornices. This may be present if there is any inflammatory condition in close proximity, e.g. salpingo-oöphoritis with inflamed tubes and ovaries, especially if adherent in the pouch of Douglas. Occasionally, even with cervicitis, inflamed lymphatics in the parametrium may be responsible for this symptom. Another disorder which leads to areas of tender scarring in the region of the vaginal fornices is endometriosis. The latter condition often gives rise to pain at the time of deep penetration and lower abdominal discomfort for some 24 hr afterwards.

PSYCHOGENIC FACTORS

Dyspareunia in the absence of anatomical or local disorders may be due to ignorance or psychological factors.

Ignorance in either or both partners may lead to failure to establish satisfactory painless intercourse. Premature penetration without sufficient love play to allow vaginal lubrication is an example.

Failure of the female partner to relax due to ignorance or fear may be responsible for vaginismus, spasm of the levator ani and perineal muscles, thus making penetration almost impossible.

Psychogenic factors, often long-standing and deep-rooted, may result in similar spasm of the vaginal muscles, especially the levatores ani and sphincter vaginae (vaginismus). Such spasm may be triggered off initially by local disorders, or by fear of pregnancy, or lack of affection for the partner. These problems can often be difficult to treat, and there is often an element of vaginismus in all patients who complain of dyspareunia. The psychological aspect of the problem must always be borne in mind, as a purely physical approach in the absence of a physical cause may sometimes render subsequent treatment much more difficult.

Treatment

It is essential to approach the problem with understanding and gentleness in order to obtain the patient's respect and confidence. It is essential to arrive at a diagnosis as to the causative factors and to determine what part is played by organic and psychological factors. Once established the treatment is clearly the treatment of the individual cause.

Help ranging from simple instruction with common-sense advice to full psychiatric treatment may be necessary, depending on the level of disturbance, and the need for early, accurate assessment, which leads to knowing how best to advise in this context, cannot be emphasized too greatly. Local disorders will have to be corrected. Thus a rigid hymen may require incision, or digital dilatation under an anaesthetic in hospital. More severe introital difficulties may need the help provided by perineotomy. Simple division of the posterior vaginal wall and perineum in the mid-line is first undertaken. After a little undercutting to free the deeper tissues the incision which was made vertically can be sutured transversely, the upper point of the incision within the vagina being sutured to its lower point on the perineum; two or three further stitches unite the sides of the incision, and sufficient enlargement of the introitus is usually achieved. The wisdom of using vaginal dilators to maintain and dilate the introitus after the initial plastic enlargement will have to be judged in each individual patient; where this can be avoided it should be, but in a few patients it is helpful to encourage them by showing them that dilators can be used and by teaching them to pass them on themselves, thus quickly gaining their confidence and enabling them to change over to normal intercourse in a very short while. When the introitus is narrowed due to atrophy at or after the menopause, the problem is often more troublesome, and any help may require the addition of a small dose of oestrogen to improve the health and tone of the vaginal skin. The problem in this instance is often aggravated by the fact that intercourse takes place less frequently and each episode is a new 'honeymoon' in itself; only with improvement in the health of the vaginal skin, adequate lubrication with a suitable jelly (such as KY jelly) and regular maintenance of dilatation with intercourse or dilators can break the vicious circle of disuse and atrophy. When there is added to this picture a discrepancy in libido, as may so often arise in partners at this stage of their career, then it must be appreciated that very considerable problems will arise, problems which are amongst the most difficult to resolve.

Dyspareunia due to local inflammation and soreness can be corrected by treatment of the specific cause of infection—such as trichomonal, monilial, or bacterial vaginitis—and atrophic changes can be treated by oestrogen preparations as mentioned above.

Treatment of deep dyspareunia will depend on the treatment of the local cause, most likely to be endometriosis or salpingo-oöphoritis, the principle being to remove tender areas and scarring from the region of the vaginal vault by surgery or, where applicable, by medical methods such as progestational steroids for endometriosis, or prolonged antibiotic treatment for pelvic infection. For the milder problems which do not merit interference of this calibre—as in patients with retroversion of the uterus and prolapsed ovaries—an understanding of how the problem has arisen by both partners, the avoidance of very deep penetration, or the use of different coital positions—e.g. prone instead of supine for the female—will often be sufficient to avoid this problem.

While seldom justifiable as an operation itself, when surgery is employed for endometriosis or salpingo-oöphoritis, ventrosuspension as part of the procedure is a wise step to keep the affected organs away from the vaginal fornices during the phase of healing, and for the future.

Where no local cause can be found for dyspareunia, a psychological factor is always present. Emotional factors due to early unsuccessful coitus, clumsiness or selfish action on the part of the husband, lack of real physical attraction and affection or fear of pregnancy, may all play a part. The result is extreme local hyperaesthesia and levator spasm (vaginismus). Such problems can usually be overcome by seeing both partners separately or together, and helping them with

common sense to adjust their approach to help each other. Safe contraceptive advice will bring its own relief and relaxation in this problem. A small group of patients will be left in whom psychological factors play a deeper part, perhaps as part of a psychoneurosis; in these circumstances expert psychiatric advice will be required, and it should be effective before any surgical treatment is undertaken to correct any organic problems.

There is a group of patients who are not able to have intercourse due to: (i) maldevelopment of the vagina or congenital absence of the vagina, septal remnants, or vaginal pits as seen in the testicular feminization syndrome, or (ii) due to severe stenosis of the vagina following over-enthusiastic colporrhaphy operations.

In such problems as testicular feminization syndrome, the vaginal pit will often increase in depth markedly with gentle and repeated attempts at coitus, to allow sufficiently normal relationship to make further interference unnecessary. In patients with vaginal absence the choice will lie between plastic enlargement or creation of a new vagina using Tiersch grafts on a mould after the technique described by McIndoe. The other alternative is to utilize the very much more simple but effective operation described by Williams (1964) (see p. 10), to utilize the labia by building across the introitus to extend the vaginal lumen down to include the introitus; thus lengthening the entrance of the vagina and allowing very satisfactory function. While excellent operations have been devised utilizing lengths of bowel to form an artificial vagina—in particular the operation of Shirodkar in which a lip of sigmoid colon is brought down with its blood supply to make a functioning conduit—these operations have not met with so much favour in the United Kingdom.

REFERENCES

COLTART T.M. (1970) *J. Obstet. Gynaec. Br. Commonw.* **77**, 69.
DOUAYE A. & PALMER R. (1947) *Proceedings of the International Congress of Obstetricians and Gynaecologists.* Dublin, Parkside Press p. 208.

HOLT E.M. (1970) *J. Obstet. Gynaec. Br. Commonw.* **77**, 1043.

JEFFCOATE T.N.A. (1957) *Principles of Gynaecology.* London, Butterworth.

PALMER R. (1920) *Bull. Fed. Soc. Gynec. Obstet.* **203**, 68.

PARISH W.E. & WARD A. (1968) *J. Obstet. Gynaec. Br. Commonw.* **75**, 1089.

RUBIN I.C. (1920) *J. Am. med. Ass.* **75**, 661.

RUBIN I.C. (1932) *Am. J. Obstet. Gynec.* **24**, 561.

STALLWORTHY J.A. (1955) In *British Obstetric and Gynaecological Practice* (edited by E. Holland & A. Bourne). London, Heinemann, p. 663.

STEPTOE P.C. (1967) *Laparoscopy in Gynaecology.* Edinburgh and London, Livingstone.

STEPTOE P.C. & EDWARDS R.G. (1970) *Lancet*, **i**, 683.

WILLIAMS E.A. (1964) *J. Obstet. Gynaec. Br. Commonw.* **71**, 511.

CHAPTER 34

INDUCTION OF OVULATION

It is assumed that before attempts are made to induce ovulation, proper investigation of the anovulatory state, whether primary or secondary, as outlined in Chapters 6 and 33, will have been undertaken. The subject has been fully reviewed recently (Shearman 1969a, b).

Although heterologous gonadotrophins will sometimes induce ovulation (Rydberg 1966), the problem of antihormone production and the increasing availability of human material have caused an eclipse of this therapeutic approach. Radiation to the pituitary and/or ovaries has not been shown to have a success rate greater than would be expected from a placebo effect, and has no place in current therapy.

SURGERY

Where the cause of anovulation lies outside the reproductive axis, surgery may be clearly indicated; sometimes this will be definitive, as in bilateral adrenalectomy followed by steroid substitution in Cushing's syndrome or excision of a virilizing ovarian tumour. In others, hypophysectomy for a pituitary adenoma may resolve the immediate clinical threat, but treatment with gonadotrophins will be necessary to induce ovulation if there is no other contra-indication.

Apart from the obvious need for surgery in the presence of functioning ovarian tumours, a direct surgical assault on the ovaries is only indicated in the presence of polycystic ovaries, and here the place of surgery *versus* medical treatment is controversial.

The published results of bilateral ovarian wedge resection have varied widely. With proper selection of patients, surgery may be expected to effect permanent cure in about 80% of patients (Shearman 1966b) and more or less comparable results may be obtained with clomiphene (see p. 499). At the moment, it seems reasonable to suggest surgery for patients living in remote rural areas—not an uncommon situation in Australia. Otherwise, clomiphene appears to be the treatment of first choice.

CORTICOSTEROIDS

Corticosteroids are indicated unequivocally in patients with adrenal hyperplasia, whether this is diagnosed in infancy or presents after puberty. Ovulation will usually occur and many pregnancies have now been recorded in these women. Urinary 17-oxosteroids in the adult should be maintained between 6 and 10 mg/24 hr. This may usually be accomplished by giving prednisone in a dose of 5–10 mg as a single dose at night. Sometimes the dose may need to be divided two, three or four times daily. Apart from the probability of an increased steroid cover at the time of delivery and a frequent need for Caesarean section due to the sequelae of surgical correction of the abnormal vulva and lower vagina, pregnancy is usually uneventful (Gans & Ser 1959; Mason 1961; Shearman 1962; Swyer & Bonham 1961; Wide & Gemzell 1962).

The non-specific use of corticosteroids rests on less certain ground. Although this use was fairly widespread previously, there now appears to be little justification for the use of corticosteroids in this way when more specific treatments are available.

CLOMIPHENE CITRATE (Clomid)

This compound, 1-(p-(β-diethylaminoethoxy)-phenyl)-1, 2-diphenyl-2-chloroethylene citrate, has recently been shown to exist as two isomers (Greenblatt *et al.* 1967) which have been separated as *cis*- and *trans*-clomiphene. Their formulae are shown in Fig. 34.1. Although preliminary

Jacobson *et al.* (1968) have demonstrated the same response in anovulatory women.

The mechanism of action of clomiphene is not clear. Mahesh & Greenblatt (1964) have produced evidence that oestradiol uptake by the pituitary is blocked, and this is supported by the work of Kobayashi *et al.* (1967) who, in addition, showed that clomiphene reduced the uptake of oestradiol by the anterior hypothalamus.

It is probable that the major stimulus for the ovarian response to clomiphene is mediated via the hypothalamus and pituitary. On the evidence available, it appears that while clomiphene has some direct action on the ovary, its main effects

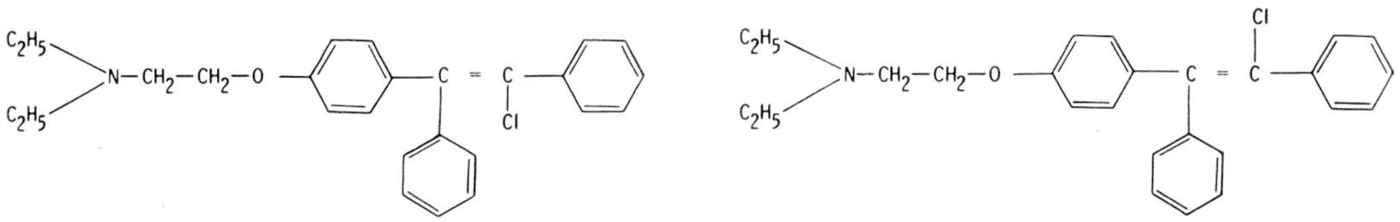

Fig. 34.1. The formulae of *cis*- and *trans*-clomiphene.

data suggest that *cis*-clomiphene is more potent in terms of ovulation induction than *trans*-clomiphene, nearly all published pharmacological data relate to the mixed isomers marketed as Clomid.

In 1961, Greenblatt *et al.* showed that this compound could induce ovulation in some anovulatory females, and this has now been amply confirmed (Jones & Moraes-Ruehsen 1967; Kistner 1965a, b; Kistner 1966; Naville *et al.* 1964; Riley & Evans 1964; Smith *et al.* 1963; Thompson & Mellinger 1965; Vorys *et al.* 1964; Whitelaw *et al.* 1964).

Using 'specific' methods of bioassay for FSH and LH, Roy *et al.* (1963) in a well-documented study of one patient, noted an initial increase in FSH excretion after the start of treatment. This was followed by an increase in excretion of oestrogens and then LH. A peak of LH excretion was followed by a further rise in oestrogen excretion and an increase in urinary pregnanediol. Dickey *et al.* (1965), using similar methods of assay, noted an initial rise in FSH.

Using radio-immunoassay, Odell *et al.* (1967) and Lazarus & Young (1967) noted an increase of plasma LH in men treated with clomiphene.

are mediated by its effect on gonadotrophin release. Certainly, hyperstimulation, seen rarely with excessive dosage of clomiphene, is identical to that seen with the therapeutic use of gonadotrophins.

Selection of patients

There has been some confusion apparent in the literature discussing selection of patients suitable for treatment with clomiphene. The only absolute contra-indication to treatment is the presence of ovarian cysts or tumours. Women with ovarian failure, whether primary or secondary, are not suitable for this or any other form of treatment aimed at inducing ovulation. Since a potentially normal pituitary response is required for the action of clomiphene, patients with panhypopituitarism will not respond to treatment, and should receive gonadotrophins if treatment is indicated. Patients with hypogonadotrophic eunuchoidism do not appear to respond satisfactorily to clomiphene.

For those patients with endometrial hyperplasia where the clinical problem is dominated by infertility, Kistner (1965a) has shown that clomiphene is the treatment of choice. Our own results would support this.

The rate of 'apparent ovulations' in patients with polycystic ovaries following clomiphene treatment is high (Charles *et al.* 1963; Ferriman *et al.* 1967; Kistner 1965a, b; Rabau *et al.* 1967b). Clomiphene, rather than gonadotrophins, is the medical treatment of choice in those patients with polycystic ovaries where pregnancy is desired.

Clomiphene is again the drug of choice in those patients who ovulate two or three times yearly only, and because of this infrequency are infertile. It is also correct initial treatment for patients with persistent anovulatory cycles.

It is not possible to be dogmatic about the best treatment for patients with 'idiopathic' secondary amenorrhoea. Basal oestrogen excretion in these women may be at the postmenopausal level or there may be some evidence of ovarian activity. It has been suggested that clomiphene treatment is more likely to succeed in those patients who show some level of ovarian activity and who have low or normal gonadotrophin excretion (Bell & Loraine 1966; Ferriman *et al.* 1967; Kase *et al.* 1967; Kistner 1965a, b; Kistner 1966; Townsend *et al.* 1966). Much of the data on gonadotrophin levels is, however, based on isolated readings and/or the non-specific 'mouse uterus' assay, so must be accepted with reserve. Vorys *et al.* (1964), after careful pretreatment investigations, could find no correlation between results of treatment and control gonadotrophin levels, except where gonadotrophin excretion was significantly increased.

Low levels of oestrogen excretion appear to be associated with a low success rate, but this does not mean clomiphene should not be used in these patients. We have shown that clomiphene may induce ovulation and pregnancy in these patients (Shearman 1969c), while Spellacy & Cohen (1967) had pregnancies in four of twenty such patients. In a group of women with long-term secondary amenorrhoea after treatment with oral contraceptives where low oestrogen production is found in most patients, we have had six of eleven patients so far treated become pregnant (Shearman 1968b). Where there is associated galactorrhoea the results are even more favourable

(Shearman & Turtle 1969). Although success with gonadotrophins is higher in this group, clomiphene is easier and safer to use. When successful, the stringent precautions that should be adopted when using gonadotrophins have been avoided. It does not seem unreasonable to suggest that these patients should be treated initially with clomiphene, reserving gonadotrophins for those in whom this treatment fails.

Dosage and control

(1) CLOMIPHENE ALONE

When first introduced, clomiphene was frequently administered in doses of 100 mg daily or more for 10–30 days. The possibility of causing the hyperstimulation syndrome with these dose levels is very real (see p. 503). More recently, dosage has been restricted both in amount and duration (Beck *et al.* 1966; Dickey *et al.* 1965; Jones & Moraes-Ruehsen 1967; Kistner 1965a, b; Naville *et al.* 1964; Pildes 1965; Shearman 1966a, b; Wall *et al.* 1965). There appears to be no advantage in prolonged treatment when compared to shorter courses (Ferriman *et al.* 1967), and there may be very considerable disadvantages.

Our own practice now is as follows: in patients with secondary amenorrhoea, after full investigations, including assessment of ovarian responsiveness, treatment is delayed for 2–3 months, as some will begin to ovulate spontaneously during or after these investigations. An initial course of clomiphene is then given in a dose of 50 mg daily for 5 days. Basal body temperature is recorded throughout. If by day 30 menstruation has not occurred and the patient is not pregnant, 100 mg is given for 5 days. If after a further 30 days menstruation has not occurred and the patient is not pregnant, 150 mg is given daily for 5 days. If there is no response to this third course, a fourth at the same dose level is given, and if this too fails, treatment is stopped and human gonadotrophins substituted. If, however, ovulation is induced by any of these courses, clomiphene continues at this dose level, each new course starting on day 5 of the cycle, until the patient conceives or withdraws from treatment. Short anovulatory cycles of 14–20 days are not uncommon on low doses (50 mg daily). If this occurs the dose is increased in subsequent cycles.

Treatment in patients with anovulatory cycles is identical, except that the first course starts most conveniently on day 5 of a spontaneous period.

The patient is seen before each new course of treatment, and ovarian size is assessed by vaginal examination. If enlargement is detected no further treatment is given until complete regression occurs. This usually takes 2–3 more weeks. Providing these precautions are taken and the dosage schedule described here is not exceeded, serious side effects should not occur.

There are difficulties in assessing the response in individual patients. Because of the antioestrogenic effect of clomiphene, serial vaginal smears are even less helpful here than they are in the control of human gonadotrophins. The characteristic thermal shift in basal body temperature seen after ovulation is the most helpful clinical guide, but since clomiphene may cause luteinization of unruptured follicles with progesterone secretion (Jones & Moraes-Ruehsen 1965; Kase *et al.* 1967; Shearman 1966b) such a thermal shift in patients treated with clomiphene does not necessarily reflect ovulation. We have tracked many of our own patients with daily oestrogen and pregnanediol assays, but from the point of view of safety there is not the same necessity to do this when using clomiphene as there is with gonadotrophins.

When ovulation does occur, it is usually 7–12 days after starting a course of treatment (Boutselis *et al.* 1967; Jones & Moraes-Ruehsen 1967; Kase *et al.* 1967; Shearman 1969a).

(2) CLOMIPHENE AND HCG

Kistner (1966) has advocated using HCG after clomiphene therapy in those patients where clomiphene alone does not work. In 20 such patients, apparent ovulation occurred in 38 of 56 treatment cycles. However, only two patients conceived. Cox & Cox (1967) have employed a similar regime for those unresponsive to clomiphene alone.

(3) HMG AND CLOMIPHENE

There is very little published information on this regime. Kistner (1966) succeeded in inducing ovulation in only 5 of 56 treatment cycles with this combination.

Although it is safe to use clomiphene alone without stringent daily control the same cannot yet be said of combinations of clomiphene and gonadotrophins.

Results

Greenblatt & Mahesh (1965) produced apparent ovulation in 77% of 257 patients treated. According to diagnostic classification ovulation occurred in 85% of patients with functional amenorrhoea, 72% with secondary amenorrhoea, 27·8% with primary amenorrhoea, and 85·7% with Stein-Leventhal syndrome. Our own results (Shearman 1969, unpublished) show an overall pregnancy rate of 65%. These results are more favourable than in any published series, but very stringent selection criteria were used.

A wide discrepancy between 'apparent ovulations' and pregnancy rate has been noted by many workers, and there is as yet no satisfactory explanation for this. Since the only absolute proof of ovulation is pregnancy, the term *apparent ovulation* has been used here. The usual criteria employed by most workers have been changes in the basal body temperature and, less frequently, changes in pregnanediol excretion. Both of these are a reflection of increased progesterone secretion, and may be due to factors other than ovulation. Clomiphene is known to be capable of luteinizing both stroma and follicles (Jones & Moraes-Ruehsen 1965; Kase *et al.* 1967; Shearman 1966b). Undoubtedly, this may be a cause of some 'apparent ovulations' without pregnancy, but certainly not all.

We have frequently produced physiological patterns of oestrogen and pregnanediol excretion without conception occurring. This pattern of steroid excretion is so constant in spontaneous cycles and in conceptual cycles after HMG or clomiphene that it is difficult to believe that corpus luteum formation has not occurred. What then, has happened to the ovum? At this stage there is no way of knowing this, but a possibility that cannot be ignored is ovum entrapment. Here, apparent ovulation and corpus luteum formation occur, but the ovum remains within the follicle and the corpus luteum.

Jones & Moraes-Ruehsen (1967) have shown a high incidence of abnormal luteal phases in patients ovulating after clomiphene treatment (19 of 56 patients), and suggest that this may be related to the low conception rate.

The most commonly observed side-effect of clomiphene treatment is the 'heat flash', similar to that described by menopausal patients. About 5–10% of patients treated with current dosage schedules restricted to 5 days will complain of these, and they may persist for several days after the course of treatment. The same patient may not experience these symptoms in all treatment cycles. Occasionally, mild and reversible scalp hair loss may occur (Jones & Moraes-Ruehsen 1967; Kistner 1965a, b), while blurring of vision is seen rarely, and appears to be due to a mydriatic effect (Beck *et al.* 1966). Galactorrhoea may occur very rarely (Leventhal & Scommegna 1963).

Hyperstimulation is much less of a problem with clomiphene than it is with gonadotrophins, but nevertheless may occur. Using the older regime of treatment for 10–30 days, severe hyperstimulation with ascites and hydrothorax has been reported (Southam & Janovski 1962). With the more recent trend to shorter courses of treatment (Beck *et al.* 1966; Dickey *et al.* 1965; Jones & Moraes-Ruehsen 1967; Kistner 1965a, b; Naville *et al.* 1964; Pildes 1965; Shearman 1966a, b; Wall *et al.* 1965) the more serious side-effects relating to ovarian over-stimulation are seen much less frequently, and consist of ovarian enlargement accompanied infrequently by lower abdominal pain. About 5% of patients treated for 4–7 days will have detectable ovarian enlargement (Kistner 1965a, b) but usually this is asymptomatic. In our own series of 86 patients treated with clomiphene for more than 300 cycles slight asymptomatic ovarian enlargement has occurred in seven patients (Shearman 1968a). For reasons that are not clear, this may be unilateral, and the response to the same dose may differ from one treatment cycle to the next.

Multiple pregnancy—usually binovular twins —will occur in about 10% of pregnancies.

HUMAN GONADOTROPHINS

HUMAN CHORIONIC GONADOTROPHIN

This hormone has been discussed more fully in Chapter 3. Biologically, its predominant action is luteinizing and it is the preparation of choice as a luteinizing hormone at the moment.

HUMAN URINARY AND PITUITARY GONADOTROPHINS

Many publications refer to the use of pituitary or urinary FSH, but this is not strictly true. Although apparently biologically pure FSH has been extracted both from urine and the pituitary, this has not yet been used therapeutically. All of the substances used so far have significant LH activity. The amount of LH present, although rarely sufficient by itself to induce ovulation (Gemzell 1965), is a synergistic necessity for the clinical activity of FSH.

It is, therefore, more correct to use the term *human pituitary gonadotrophin* (HPG) for material extracted from the pituitary, and *human menopausal gonadotrophin* (HMG) for extracts of menopausal urine.

It is usual now to express potency in terms of international units (I.U.) of FSH and LH, this international standard being based on the *Second International Reference Preparation of HMG*.

It is desirable that the potency of all human preparations should be expressed in terms of international units of FSH and LH, rather than 'total gonadotrophic' activity.

HPG

Gemzell *et al.* (1958) first showed that HPG would induce follicular maturation, and later demonstrated that when combined with HCG as a luteinizing hormone, ovulation and pregnancy occurred in some women with secondary amenorrhoea (Gemzell 1960, 1961, 1963, 1964, 1965, 1966; Gemzell *et al.* 1959, 1960). These results have been amply confirmed by others, (Apostilakis *et al.* 1962; Bettendorf & Ahrens 1962; Buxton & Herrmann 1961; Crooke *et al.* 1962, 1963; Townsend *et al.* 1966). A limiting factor, however, is the supply of human pituitaries. Most workers using HPG have collected and extracted their own pituitaries, and the slight variation in FSH/LH ratios of materials used clinically does not appear to have affected the outcome. It is probable that some form of national collection supervised by a government agency, as is the practice in Australia, will give the maximum yield of gonadotrophins and other pituitary hormones.

HMG

Preparations of gonadotrophin with predictable potency can be extracted from human menopausal urine (Donini *et al.* 1964a, b) and they are effective in inducing ovulation (Borth *et al.* 1961; Crooke *et al.* 1963; Diczfalusy *et al.* 1964; Furuhjelm *et al.* 1966; Lunenfeld 1963, 1967; Lunenfeld *et al.* 1963; Palmer & Dorangeon 1963; Pasetto & Montanino 1964a; Rabau *et al.* 1967a, b; Rosemberg *et al.* 1963; Shearman 1964, 1966a; Staemmler 1963; Vande Wiele & Turksoy 1965).

The complications of gonadotrophic treatment lie in the very real danger of producing hyperstimulation, and the very high incidence of multiple births.

HYPERSTIMULATION SYNDROME

The most precise classification has come from the Israeli group, (Lunenfeld 1966, 1967; Lunenfeld & Rabau 1967; Rabau *et al.* 1967a, b) and it would help considerably if this categorization could be followed as a standard. This may be summarized as follows:

1. Urinary oestrogens above 150 μg and urinary pregnanediol above 10 mg but no palpable cysts or enlargement of the ovaries.

2. Enlargement of ovaries with or without palpable cyst formation.

3. Enlargement of ovaries, cysts, distension of abdomen, nausea.

4. Enlargement of ovaries, cysts, distension of abdomen, nausea, vomiting and/or diarrhoea.

5. Enlargement of ovaries, cysts, distension of abdomen, nausea, vomiting and/or diarrhoea, plus fluid in abdomen and/or pleura.

6. Same as group 5, plus change in blood volume, viscosity and coagulation time.

The Israeli workers do not consider groups 1 and 2 to be adverse reactions, although clearly they are indicative of excessive stimulation. Groups 3 and 4 are classified as mild adverse reactions requiring hospitalization, and groups 5 and 6 as severe.

Hyperstimulation may result after exposure to heterologous or homologous gonadotrophins. In therapeutic work it is impossible to assess the incidence of grades 1 and 2 hyperstimulation, as the requisite data is lacking in much published literature.

Severe hyperstimulation is a grave complication of treatment given to a previously healthy patient. It usually becomes manifest several days *after* the administration of HCG (Mroueh & Kase 1967; Rabau *et al.* 1967a, b; Vande Wiele & Turksoy 1965). The presenting symptom is frequently 'faintness' with lower abdominal pain or discomfort. Marked ovarian enlargement is followed by the rapid development of ascites and hydrothorax, and, if severe, may be followed by hypovolaemic shock. In extreme cases (Mozes *et al.* 1965) major thrombo-embolic episodes—causing death in one patient and limb amputation in another—may occur apparently due to these sudden changes in fluids, electrolytes and blood viscosity. The presentation as an 'acute abdomen' has resulted in surgical intervention, and indeed, intraperitoneal haemorrhage from rupture of these cysts may require operation (Pasetto & Montanino 1964b). However, if an abdominal disaster such as rupture and/or haemorrhage can be excluded, treatment should be conservative, based on hospitalization, bed-rest and intravenous fluids. Effusions regress and ovaries return to normal size. As in similar situations with varying genesis, continuous monitoring of central venous pressure is invaluable.

No one can yet claim to have developed an infallible system that will prevent all cases of hyperstimulation. Rabau *et al.* (1967b), who have the very considerable experience of treating 134 patients through over 250 cycles, could find no evidence of correlation between the incidence of side-effects and dosage. This is scarcely surprising when the very wide individual responsiveness of patients is considered. There is, however, very suggestive evidence that points to significant factors in the genesis of hyperstimulation.

All workers appear to agree that patients with polycystic ovaries are more likely to develop the hyperstimulation syndrome than others. All efforts should, therefore, be made to exclude this diagnosis before treatment with gonadotrophins is commenced. Also, there appears to be no doubt that—at least in the more severe forms of hyperstimulation (grades 3 to 6)—oestrogen excretion is well above the physiological range *before* HCG is given. But while HMG may load the gun, it takes HCG to pull the trigger.

It is very probable that the only way this potentially serious complication of treatment can be reduced to a minimum is by rigid day-to-day control of dosage, withholding HCG if the response to HMG/HPG is excessive. Using this type of control within the Australian group, no cases of moderate or severe (grades 4, 5 and 6) hyperstimulation have yet occurred.

MULTIPLE BIRTHS

In most published series, multiple ovulation occurs very commonly during treatment with gonadotrophins. Gemzell & Roos (1966), in summarizing their own considerable experience, described multiple births in 23 patients and 20 single deliveries—more than 50% multiple conceptions. Of these 23 patients, 14 had twins and 9 triplets or more. Of 14 pregnancies attained by Vande Wiele and Turksoy, 6 were multiple, including one set of quadruplets (Neuwirth *et al.* 1965a). Rabau *et al.* (1967b) had 12 multiple pregnancies in 33 completed pregnancies, and in a later report (Lunenfeld & Rabau 1967) of 52 completed pregnancies 48·1% were single births, 21·1% twins, 3·9% triplets and 1·9% quadruplets. Gemzell & Roos (1966) show from their own data that there is little quantitative difference in oestrogen and pregnanediol excretion in the

conceptual cycles of twin and single pregnancies, but that pregnanediol excretion is significantly higher in cycles producing triplets or more. Similar findings of steroid levels in single and twin conceptions have been published by Taymor *et al.* (1967).

From their own data, Gemzell & Roos (1966) infer that little can be done to prevent this high incidence of multiple births. Evidence here, however, is not conclusive.

Crooke's group had four multiple pregnancies in 16 patients who conceived, and none of these was more than twins. In Australia, where the three main groups involved in the therapeutic use of gonadotrophins have controlled dosage rigidly and individually (see p. 505), there have been five multiple pregnancies in 24 patients who conceived. There have been four sets of twins and one set of triplets (Adey *et al.* 1967; Cox & Cox 1966; Shearman 1968a; Townsend *et al.* 1966).

Crooke (1966a, 1967) has suggested that repeated injection of HCG are responsible for a high incidence of multiple ovulation. It is not yet possible to be sure whether this is true or not. The three groups working in Australia have used a single 'inducing' injection of HCG varying between 2,000 and 10,000 units, followed if necessary by smaller amounts of 500–1,500 units at 3- or 4-daily intervals throughout the luteal phase. The findings of the New Zealand group suggest that the degree and probably number of follicles matured by HPG/HMG is more important in the question of multiple conceptions than the number of injections of HCG (Seddon *et al.* 1967).

It seems premature to adopt a nihilistic attitude towards the prevention of multiple conceptions. What slender evidence there is, suggests that the total numbers of multiple conceptions (and, more important, the number of multiples greater than twins), may be reduced by rigidly individualized treatment. Although the birth of twins is not a catastrophe, with higher multiples the maternal risk is increased, and foetal wastage from either abortion or prematurity becomes prohibitive. However, it must be accepted at the moment that the rate of multiple conceptions with this treatment is higher than that seen after treatment with clomiphene.

Selection of patients

There are few reasons to use human gonado-trophins as the primary treatment when attempting to induce ovulation. The possibility of over-stimulation is a source of anxiety to the physician and a very real danger for the patient. The stringent precautions necessary to minimize this risk impose a real burden on the patient, will strain the clinical skills of her medical attendant, and place a considerable load on avoidable laboratory facilities.

Undoubtedly, there is an endocrinological elegance in the proper use of gonadotrophins that may be difficult for the investigator to resist. The primary responsibility of the doctor is, however, to his patient, not his own curiosity. Gonadotrophins should, therefore, only be used if chemical induction will not work, or has been tried and failed. Even then their use should be res-tricted to those who have the clinical and labora-tory backing to minimize the risks of this elective treatment.

Since a potentially normal hypothalamic-pituitary axis is essential for chemical induction, gonadotrophins must be used as primary treat-ment in the rare instance of a hypophysectomized patient who wishes to bear, and is capable of bearing, children. Gemzell (1965) has shown the success of this approach. A patient with Shee-han's syndrome would present the same problem.

Greenblatt (1966, 1967) has not found clomi-phene useful in patients with hypogonadotrophic eunuchoidism, and our own experience is similar. Primary treatment in this small group of patients after sexual maturation has been achieved with exogenous steroids, should probably be with gonadotrophins.

It is doubtful if gonadotrophins should be used therapeutically in other patients unless alternative and appropriate methods such as clomiphene citrate have failed.

Gemzell (1967) has summarized the selection of patients for this treatment concisely. 'The ideal subject for treatment with gonadotrophins [is] under 35 with normal, non-functioning ovaries, primary or long-standing secondary amenorrhoea, normally developed sex organs and lack of urinary gonadotrophins as evidence of pituitary failure. She should be fully investigated, show a normal response in an "FSH test", be complaining of infertility, have a normally fertile husband, and show no barriers to conception. Pregnancy should not be contra-indicated on medical grounds and *there should be no preferable alternative methods*.' (Present author's italics.)

Selection of gonadotrophic preparation

All workers agree that HCG is the preparation of choice as a luteinizing hormone. There is no evidence to suggest that preparations of HPG are any better or worse for clinical purposes than HMG, and the choice will usually be dictated by the availability and cost of a particular product.

Again, there is general agreement that some LH content is a necessary component of HPG or HMG. It is probable that the ratio of FSH/LH is important, but there is not yet sufficient evidence to justify dogma, and final judgement must be deferred until there is considerably more information on this point than exists at the moment.

Methods of treatment and control

As stated elsewhere (Shearman 1966a) 'the theory of dosage is disarmingly simple—to secure follicular maturation with either HPG or HMG and then induce ovulation with HCG. In practice it is complex, often difficult and sometimes dangerous'. Individual response is so variable that it must be accepted that there is no such thing as a fixed dosage schedule for all patients. It has also become apparent that the response of the *same* patient to the *same* dose may differ significantly from one cycle to the next. For example, Gemzell (1967) describes one woman who, having aborted seven foetuses after her first treatment, had a single pregnancy after her second without any change of dosage. Crooke *et al.* (1966a) have shown a sevenfold difference in sensitivity between patients. The very small range that there may be 'between a dose that will fail to stimulate follicle ripening at all and one which produces ovarian enlargement or multiple pregnancies' has been clearly shown by Brown's group (Townsend *et al.* 1966).

Method of administration

Following the initial work of Gemzell *et al.* (1958) most groups have administered HPG or HMG intramuscularly each day for about 10 days (Brown 1965; Buxton & Herrmann 1961; Cox 1965; Lunenfeld 1963; Rabau *et al.* 1967a; Rosemberg 1967; Shearman 1964b, 1966a; Taymor *et al.* 1967; Townsend *et al.* 1966; Vande Wiele & Turksoy 1965).

Other methods of administration have involved injection of HMG or HPG four times daily (Jones & Moraes-Ruehsen 1967), in one single dose (Crooke *et al.* 1966b, c), daily for 3 days (Cox *et al.* 1966), or three divided doses on days 1, 4 and 8 (Crooke 1967).

The methods and dosage of HCG administration have varied just as widely. Gemzell (1967) uses 3,000 I.U. daily for 3 days, given after HPG injections have ceased. The Israeli group (Rabau *et al.* 1967a, b) uses three or four injections of 5,000–10,000 I.U. of HCG given daily and overlapping by 2 days the last injections of HMG. Crooke (1967, 1966a, b, c) uses a single dose of either 24,000 I.U. or 12,000 I.U. given 8 days after a single injection of HPG, or on day 10 when HPG is given in three divided doses on days 1, 4 and 8. A similar schedule has been used by Marshall *et al.* (1967).

In Australia and New Zealand it is usual to give a single 'inducing' dose of 2,000–5,000 I.U. HCG after HMG/HPG treatment, followed by smaller injections of 500–1,500 I.U. HCG at 3- or 4-daily intervals throughout the luteal phase if they are needed (Brown 1965; Cox 1965; Seddon *et al.* 1967; Shearman 1966a, c; Townsend *et al.* 1966).

It should be clear from this variability that there is no uniformly satisfactory method of dosage control that will permit the ideal of a uniformly physiological response.

The methods of dosage control used fall into two basic groups:

(1) Dosage controlled by indirect indices of response such as changes in vaginal smears and cervical mucus, with or without retrospective steroid assay.

(2) Dosage controlled by concurrent assay of urinary steroid excretion.

INDIRECT CONTROL

Gemzell (1967) has summarized his long experience using a relatively fixed dosage schedule of HPG with FSH activity 'fairly constant around 100 I.U. per day'. Initially, this was administered daily for 10 days, more recently for 8 days, with a decision then made as to whether to continue HPG injections or not. This decision is based on the presence or absence of ovarian enlargement and a study of serial vaginal smears. HCG is given for 3 days. Assay of urinary steroids was carried out retrospectively.

This relatively fixed dosage schedule causes unphysiological excretion of urinary steroids in the majority of patients; for example, total urinary oestrogens on the last days of HPG/HCG treatment averaged 258 μg/24 hr in patients having single pregnancies (Gemzell 1967; Gemzell & Roos 1966) which is more than twice the mean maximum seen in spontaneous cycles (Brown 1955). The ensuing multiple conception rate of more than 50% (Gemzell & Roos 1966) is far higher than is desirable. Almost all other groups have until now relied on indirect indices of response—change in ovarian size, vaginal smears, cervical mucus, basal body temperature. This may result on the one hand in a low pregnancy rate, or on the other in an unacceptable incidence of hyperstimulation syndrome and multiple births (Buxton & Herrmann 1961; Gemzell & Roos 1966; Mozes *et al.* 1965; Neuwirth *et al.* 1965a, b; Vande Wiele & Turksoy 1965). Taymor *et al.* (1967), using their indirect methods of control and employing retrospective assay of urinary steroids, conclude that 'physicians who do not have a rapid oestrogen method available will have to rely upon the fern test and upon the use of dosage schedules that are less likely to provoke ovarian over-stimulation'.

DIRECT DOSAGE CONTROL BASED ON CONCURRENT STEROID ASSAY

The Birmingham group have done an immense amount of work to determine the optimum method of dosage control (Crooke 1967; Crooke *et al.* 1962, 1963, 1964, 1966a, b, c). The essence of the Birmingham approach is to predetermine individual sensitivity as indicated by urinary oestriol and pregnanediol excretion. Two approaches to dosage method have been employed. The first is to give HPG/HMG in three equally divided doses on days 1, 4 and 8, followed by 24,000 units HCG on day 10. Failure of a positive response (a rise of oestriol of more than 15 μg/24 hr above the control level on day 1, this rise being assessed between the seventh and twentieth day) indicated an increase of HMG/HPG dosage in the next cycle. If, however, the dose is satisfactory and pregnancy does not occur, the same schedule is followed in the next cycle. More recently (Crooke 1967; Crooke et al. 1966b, c), a single dose of HPG/HMG is given every 2 or 3 weeks, increasing each dose by a factor of 50% until a positive oestriol response is obtained. HCG is then given in a dose of 12,000 units 8 days after the HPG. There is no doubt that Crooke's early results are admirable—16 of 18 patients pregnant, only four sets of twins with no higher multiples, and a low incidence of hyperstimulation (Crooke et al. 1966c).

A second apparently satisfactory approach has been developed in Australia following the suggestion of Brown (1963) that each patient be used as her own assay system. FSH and HCG dosage is adjusted according to individual response as indicated by concurrent oestrogen and pregnanediol assay.

The amount of HPG or HMG given is determined by the previous day's oestrogen excretion, administration continuing daily. The dosage used may range widely from between 75 and 400 I.U. of HPG/HMG given daily for 8–10 days, starting with a low dose and increasing if no response is obtained.

The aim is to keep oestrogen excretion in the physiological range. If it more than doubles from day to day, or if total oestrogens reach more than 100 μg/24 hr during HPG/HMG administration, HCG is not given in that treatment cycle. If, however, oestrogen excretion is satisfactory and reaches a level that one knows from assay of normal cycles is compatible with ovulation— usually 50–100 μg of total oestrogen—ovulation is then induced by a single injection of HCG combined with a final injection of FSH, or HCG may be given one or two days after the last

injection of FSH. It has been the practice in this country to use much less HCG (2,000–10,000 I.U.) than is the custom elsewhere. With low doses additional injections of 500–1,500 I.U. of HCG alone may be needed at intervals of 3 or 4 days to maintain luteal function (Brown 1965; Shearman 1966a; Townsend et al. 1966). It is our practice to give the last injection of HCG not more than 11 days after the 'inducing' dose of HCG. In the absence of pregnancy or ovarian enlargement, treatment is recommenced 5 days after the onset of menstrual bleeding. Pregnanediol estimations may be performed in a more leisurely fashion by the method of Klopper et al. (1955) or much more rapidly by a method using gas–liquid chromatography (Cox 1965, 1967).

Using this method of control 24 of 36 patients have conceived (Bettendorf & Ahrens 1962; Cox & Cox 1966; Shearman 1968a). There have been five multiples (one triplets, four twins) and no case of hyperstimulation beyond grade 3. In the writer's personal series (Shearman 1969) there have been 12 pregnancies in 16 treated patients, three sets of twins, one mid-trimester abortion of a singleton foetus and no case of hyperstimulation beyond grade 2.

There can be no doubt that this method of control presents many problems. It is very tedious for the patient, imposes a heavy burden on laboratory facilities and excludes patients who, by reason of geography, cannot reach a suitably equipped laboratory every day. With further experience, and after initial daily assessment of sensitivity, it may ultimately be possible to control treatment by assay of steroids every three or four days. After suitable assessment of sensitivity and with adequate transport provided, we have found it practicable—though tedious— to treat patients up to 300 miles from Sydney.

Crooke (1967) has criticized efforts to control daily dosage on the grounds that 'the response to an effective dose [of HPG/HMG] increases for up to 12 days, indicating that no parameter can be safely used to assess the next day's dose'. His basis for this statement is, however, based on data derived from a study of *HPG/HMG given with HCG*. Our own data, and those of Cox et al. (1966), show clearly that if HMG is given alone the maximum response is reached 4–5 days after injection, unless ovulation is induced by HCG, when there is an immediate drop in oestrogen excretion just as is seen in spontaneous ovulatory cycles. This characteristic pattern has been seen in all conceptual cycles we have studied, whether following spontaneous ovulation or following treatment with HMG or clomiphene.

It should be emphasized that a method of control based on physiological response can only be as good as knowledge of the physiology on which it is based, and can only be satisfactory if the rules of physiology are obeyed. The New Zealand group, although monitoring urinary oestrogens daily, produced six multiple conceptions in their first ten pregnancies (Seddon *et al.* 1967). In these cases oestrogen excretion was more than doubling daily and/or urinary oestrogen exceeded 100 μg daily before HCG was given. Neither of these events occurs in spontaneous ovulatory cycles.

It cannot be stated too often, that induction of ovulation is an elective treatment given to women who are not ill in the usual meaning of the word. Complications of treatment must, therefore, be viewed in a very different light from those— for example—occurring as a result of methotrexate treatment for choriocarcinoma. The problems inherent in this treatment must be explained fully to the patient and her husband and the final decision to embark on treatment should rest with them.

REFERENCES

ADEY D., BROWN J.B., EVANS J.H., TAFT H.P. & JOHNSTONE J.W. (1967) In *Proceedings of Vth World Congress of Gynaecology and Obstetrics.* (edited by C. Wood). Sydney, Butterworths, p. 339.

APOSTILAKIS M., BETTENDORF C. & VOIGT K.D. (1962) *Acta endocr., Copenh.* **41**, 14.

BECK P., GRAYZELL E.F., YOUNG E.S. & KUPPERMAN H.S. (1966) *Obstet. Gynec., N.Y.* **27**, 54.

BELL E.T. & LORAINE J.A. (1966) *Lancet*, i, 626.

BETTENDORF G. & AHRENS D. (1962) *Acta endocr., Copenh.* Supplement 67, p. 133.

BORTH R., LUNENFELD B. & MENZI A. (1961) In *Human Pituitary Gonadotrophins* (edited by A. Albert). Springfield, Thomas, p. 255.

BOUTSELIS J.G., VORYS N. & ULLERY J.C. (1967) *Am. J. Obstet. Gynec.* **97**, 949.

BROWN J.B. (1955) *Lancet*, i, 320.

BROWN J.B. (1963) Personal communication.

BROWN J.B. (1965) In *Recent Advances in Ovarian and Synthetic Steroids and the Control of Ovarian Function* (edited by R.P. Shearman). High Wycombe, Searle, p. 99.

BUXTON C.L. & HERRMANN W. (1961) *Am. J. Obstet. Gynec.* **81**, 584.

CHARLES D., BARR W., BELL E.T., BROWN J.B., FOTHERBY K. & LORAINE J.A. (1963) *Am. J. Obstet. Gynec.* **86**, 913.

COX R.I. (1965) In *Recent Advances in Ovarian and Synthetic Steroids and the Control of Ovarian Function* (edited by R.P. Shearman). High Wycombe, Searle, p. 76.

COX R.I. (1967) In *Proceedings of Vth World Congress of Gynaecology and Obstetrics* (edited by C. Wood). Sydney, Butterworths, p. 343.

COX L.W. & COX R.I. (1967) In *Proceedings of the Vth World Congress of Gynaecology and Obstetrics* (edited by C. Wood). Sydney, Butterworths, p. 343.

COX R.I. & COX L.W. (1966) Personal communication.

COX R.I., COX L.W. & BLACK T.L. (1966) *Lancet*, ii, 888.

CROOKE A.C. (1967) In *Modern Trends in Endocrinology*. Vol. 3 (edited by H. Gardiner-Hill). London, Butterworths, p. 111.

CROOKE A.C., BUTT W.R., MORRIS R. & PALMER R. (1962) *Acta Endocr., Copenh.* Supplement 67, p. 132.

CROOKE A.C., BUTT W.R., PALMER R.F., MORRIS R., EDWARDS R.L. & ANSON C.J. (1963) *J. Obstet. Gynaec. Br. Commonw.* **70**, 604.

CROOKE A.C., BUTT W.R., PALMER R.F., BERTRAND P.V., CARRINGTON S.P., EDWARDS R.L. & ANSON C.J. (1964) *J. Obstet. Gynaec. Br. Commonw.* **72**, 571.

CROOKE A.C., BUTT W.R. & BERTRAND P.V. (1966a) *Acta endocr., Copenh.* Supplement III, p. 1.

CROOKE A.C., BUTT W.R. & BERTRAND P.V. (1966c) *Lancet*, ii, 514.

DICKEY R.P., VORYS N., STEVENS V.C., BESCH P.K., HAMWI G.J. & ULLERY J.C. (1965) *Fert. Steril.* **16**, 485.

DICZFALUSY E., JOHANNISON E., TILLINGER K.G. & BETTENDORF D. (1964) *Acta endocr., Copenh.* Supplement 90, p. 35.

DONINI P., PUZZUOLI D. & MONTEZEMOLO R. (1964a) *Acta endocr., Copenh.* Supplement 45, p. 321.

DONINI P., PUZZUOLI D. & D'ALESSIO I. (1964b) *Acta endocr., Copenh.* **45**, 329.

FERRIMAN D., PURDIE A.W. & CORNS M. (1967) *Br. med. J.* ii, 444.

FURUHJELM M., LUNELL N-O. & ODEBLAD E. (1966) *Acta Obstet. gynec. scand.* **45**, 63.

GANS F. & SER J. (1959) *Acta endocr., Copenh.* **30**, 424.

GEMZELL C.A. (1960) *Ciba Fdn. Colloq. Endocr.* **13**, 191.

GEMZELL C.A. (1961) In *Control of Ovulation* (edited by C.A. Villee). Oxford, Pergamon Press, p. 192.

GEMZELL C.A. (1963) In *Year Book of Obstetrics and Gynecology* (edited by J.P. Greenhill). Chicago Year Book Medical Publishers, p. 331.

GEMZELL C.A. (1964) *Vitams Horm.* **22**, 129.

GEMZELL C.A. (1965) *Recent Prog. Horm. Res.* **321**, 179.

GEMZELL C.A. (1966) In *Ovulation, Stimulation, Suppression, Detection* (edited by R.B. Greenblatt). Philadelphia and Toronto, Lippincott, p. 98.

GEMZELL C.A. (1967) *Clin. Obstet. Gynec.* **10**, 401.

GEMZELL C.A., DICZFALUSY E. & TILLINGER K.G. (1958) *J. clin. Endocr. Metab.* **18**, 1333.

GEMZELL C.A., DICZFALUSY E. & TILLINGER K.G. (1959) *Acta obstet. gynec. scand.* **38**, 465.

GEMZELL C.A., DICZFALUSY E. & TILLINGER K.G. (1960) *Ciba Fdn. Colloq. Endocr.* **13**, 191.

GEMZELL C. & ROOS P. (1966) *Am. J. Obstet. Gynec.* **94**, 490.

GREENBLATT R.B. (1966) *Excerpta medica Int. Congr. Series*, No. 109, p. 6.

GREENBLATT R.B., BARFIELD W.E., JUNGCK E.C. & RAY A.W. (1961) *J. Am. med. Ass.* **178**, 101.

GREENBLATT R.B. & MAHESH V.B. (1965) In *Year Book of Endocrinology* (edited by T.B. Schwartz). Chicago Year Book Medical Publishers, p. 248.

GREENBLATT R.B., MAHESH V.B. & PICO I.R. (1967) In *Proceedings of Vth World Congress of Gynaecology and Obstetrics* (edited by C. Wood). Sydney, Butterworths, p. 301.

JACOBSON A., MARSHALL J.R. & ROSS G.T. (1968) *Am. J. Obstet. Gynec.* **102**, 284.

JONES G.S. & MORAES-RUEHSEN M.D. (1965) *Fert. Steril.* **16**, 461.

JONES G.S. & MORAES-RUEHSEN M.D. (1967) *Am. J. Obstet. Gynec.* **99**, 814.

KASE N., MROUEH A. & OLSON L.E. (1967) *Am. J. Obstet. Gynec.* **98**, 1037.

KISTNER R.W. (1965a) *Am. J. Obstet. Gynec.* **92**, 380.

KISTNER R.W. (1965b) *Obstet. Gynec. Survey*, **20**, 873.

KISTNER R.W. (1966) *Fert. Steril.* **17**, 569.

KLOPPER A.I., MICHIE E.A. & BROWN J.B. (1955) *J. Endocr.* **12**, 209.

KOBAYASHI T., KATO J. & VILLEE C. (1967) In *Proceedings of Vth World Congress of Gynaecology and Obstetrics* (edited by C. Wood. Sydney, Butterworths, p. 351.

LAZARUS L. & YOUNG J.D. (1967) *Proc. Aust. Soc. Med. Res.* **2**, 128.

LEVENTHAL M.L. & SCOMMEGNA A. (1963) *Am. J. Obstet. Gynec.* **87**, 445.

LUNENFELD B. (1963) *J. int. Fed. Gynaec. Obstet.* **1**, 153.

LUNENFELD B. (1966) *Gynéc. Obstét.* **65**, 553.

LUNENFELD B. (1967) In *Recent Research on Gonadotropic Hormones* (edited by E.T. Bell & J.A. Loraine). Edinburgh and London, Livingstone, p. 257.

LUNENFELD B., ESHKOL A., DONINI P., PUZZUOLI D. & SHELSNYAK M.E. (1963) *Harokeach haiv.* **9**, 766.

LUNENFELD B. & RABAU E. (1967) In *Proceedings of Vth World Congress of Gynaecology and Obstetrics* (edited by C. Wood). Sydney, Butterworths, p. 294.

MAHESH V.B. & GREENBLATT R.B. (1964) *Recent. Prog. Horm. Res.* **20**, 341.

MARSHALL J.R., HAMMOND C.B. & JACOBSON A. (1967) In *Proceedings of Vth World Congress of Gynaecology and Obstetrics* (edited by C. Wood). Sydney, Butterworths, p. 356.

MASON A.S. (1961) *Br. med. J.* **i**, 1003.

MOZES M., BOGOKOWSKY H., ANTESI E., LUNENFELD B., RABAU E., SERR D.M., DAVID A. & SALOMY M. (1965) *Lancet*, **ii**, 1213.

MROUEH A. & KASE N. (1967) *Obstet. Gynec., N.Y.* **30**, 346.

NAVILLE A.H., KISTNER R.W., WHEATLEY E.R. & ROCK J. (1964) *Fert. Steril.* **15**, 290.

NEUWIRTH R.S., TODD W.D., TURKSOY R.M. & VANDE WIELE R.L. (1965a) *Am. J. Obstet. Gynec.* **91**, 982.

NEUWIRTH R.S., TURKSOY R.M. & VANDE WIELE R.L. (1965b) *Am. J. Obstet. Gynec.* **91**, 977.

ODELL W.D., ROSS G.T. & PLAYFORD P.L. (1967) *J. clin. Invest.* **46**, 248.

PALMER R. & DORANGEON P. (1963) *Clinique, Paris*, **58**, 239.

PASETTO N. & MONTANINO G. (1964a) *Acta endocr., Copenh.* **47**, 1.

PASETTO N. & MONTANINO G. (1964b) *Minerva ginec.* **16**, 377.

PILDES R.B. (1965) *Am. J. Obstet. Gynec.* **91**, 466.

RABAU E., DAVID A., SERR D.M., MASHIACH S. & LUNENFELD B. (1967a) *Am. J. Obstet. Gynec.* **96**, 92.

RABAU E., SERR D.M., MASHIACH S., INSLER V., SALOMY M. & LUNENFELD B. (1967b) *Br. med. J.* **ii**, 446.

RILEY G.M. & EVANS T.N. (1964) *Am. J. Obstet. Gynec.* **89**, 97.

ROSEMBERG E. (1967) In *Recent Research on Gonadotrophic Hormones* (edited by E.T. Bell & J.A. Loraine). Edinburgh and London, Livingstone, p. 272.

ROSEMBERG E., COLEMAN J., DEMANY M. & GARCIA C.R. (1963) *J. clin. Endocr. Metab.* **23**, 181.

ROY S., GREENBLATT R.B., MAHESH V.B. & JUNGCK E.C. (1963) *Fert. Steril.* **14**, 575.

RYDBERG E. (1966) In *Ovulation* (edited by R.B. Greenblatt). Philadelphia and Toronto, Lippincott, p. 75.

SEDDON R.J., LIGGINS G.C. & IBBERTSON H.K. (1967) In *Proceedings of Vth World Congress of Gynaecology and Obstetrics* (edited by C. Wood). Sydney, Butterworths, p. 363.

SHEARMAN R.P. (1962) *Aust. N.Z. J. Obstet. Gynaec.* **2**, 91.

SHEARMAN R.P. (1964) *Med. Res.* **1**, 115.

SHEARMAN R.P. (1966a) *Australas. Ann. Med.* **15**, 266.

SHEARMAN R.P. (1966b) *Proc. R. Soc. Med.* **59**, 1285.

SHEARMAN R.P. (1966c) In *The Clinical Uses of Human Gonadotrophins*. Proceedings of a Private Scientific Meeting sponsored by G.D. Searle. Royal Society of Medicine, p. 75.

SHEARMAN R.P. (1968a) Unpublished findings.

SHEARMAN R.P. (1968) *Lancet*, **i**, 325.

SHEARMAN R.P. (1969a) *Induction of Ovulation*. Springfield, Thomas, Illinois.

SHEARMAN R.P. (1969b) *Am. J. Obstet. Gynec.* **103**, 444.

SHEARMAN R.P. (1969c) In *Modern Trends in Gynaecology*, Series 4 (edited by R.J. Kellar). London, Butterworths.

SHEARMAN R.P. (1969d) Unpublished findings.

SHEARMAN R.P. & TURTLE J.R. (1969) *Am. J. Obstet. Gynec.* (in press).

SMITH O.W., SMITH G.W. & KISTNER R.W. (1963) *J. Am. med. Ass.* **184**, 878.

SOUTHAM A.L. & JANOVSKI N.A. (1962) *J. Am. med. Ass.* **181**, 443.

SPELLACY W.N. & COHEN W.D. (1967) *Am. J. Obstet. Gynec.* **97**, 943.

STAEMMLER H.J. (1963) *Arch. Gynaek,* **198**, 377.

SWYER G.I.M. & BONHAM D.G. (1961) *Br. med. J.* i, 1005.

TAYMOR M.L., STURGIS S.H., GOLDSTEIN D.P. & LIEBERMAN B. (1967) *Fert. Steril.* **18**, 181.

THOMPSON R.J. & MELLINGER R.C. (1965) *Am. J. Obstet. Gynec.* **92**, 412.

TOWNSEND S.L., BROWN J.B., JOHNSTONE J.W., ADEY F.D., EVANS J.H. & TAFT H.P. (1966) *J. Obstet. Gynaec. Br. Commonw.* **73**, 529.

VANDE WIELE R.L. & TURKSOY R.M. (1965) *J. clin. Endocr. Metab.* **25**, 369.

VORYS N., GANTT C.L., HAMWI G.J., COPELAND W.E. & ULLERY J.C. (1964) *Am. J. Obstet. Gynec.* **88**, 425.

WALL J.A., FRANKLIN R.R., KAUFMAN R.H. & KAPLAN A.L. (1965) *Am. J. Obstet. Gynec.* **93**, 822.

WHITELAW M.J., GRAMS L.R. & STAMM W.J. (1964) *Am. J. Obstet. Gynec.* **90**, 355.

WIDE L. & GEMZELL C. (1962) *Acta endocr., Copenh.* **39**, 539.

CHAPTER 35

DYSFUNCTIONAL UTERINE BLEEDING

Definition

Dysfunctional uterine bleeding has been defined in a wide variety of ways. Probably the most useful and practical at the present state of knowledge is that of Novak *et al.* (1965): 'Dysfunctional uterine bleeding may be defined as abnormal bleeding from the uterus unassociated with tumour, inflammation or pregnancy'; to which may be added 'or any other organic disease of the genital tract'. Dysfunctional uterine bleeding is essentially diagnosed by the exclusion of organic gynaecological disease, and in all probability embraces a whole group of dysfunctional disorders. The term should thus be regarded as describing a group or category of diseases rather than as a specific diagnosis.

The dysfunction may primarily arise in the uterus, ovary, pituitary, in other endocrine organs or in any system of the body. It may also be due to imbalance between these organs or systems. The sole criterion is that it results in uterine bleeding or some disorder of menstruation. A number of authors have limited the term dysfunctional uterine bleeding to include only those states where there is excessive bleeding. As Israel (1967) has pointed out, however, the same endocrine dysfunction may produce either infrequent menstruation or excessive uterine bleeding at different times and the two abnormalities may be intimately related. The term dysfunctional uterine bleeding thus properly includes all the disorders of menstruation, with the exception of amenorrhoea.

The fact that the diagnosis of dysfunctional uterine bleeding is primarily made by excluding organic disease of the genital tract is, in many ways, unsatisfactory. The diagnosis thus depends, as Jeffcoate (1967) noted, 'on the definition of organic lesion and on the care and trouble taken to exclude such a lesion'. Any series of cases of dysfunctional uterine bleeding will inevitably include some cases where organic disease has been overlooked.

Incidence

Dysfunctional uterine bleeding is one of the most frequently encountered conditions in gynaecological practice. It is estimated to account for at least 10% of all new out-patients seen at hospital or privately (Taylor 1965). It may occur at any age between puberty and the well-established menopause. It is said to occur most frequently at the extremes of reproductive life—that is, during adolescence or premenopausally—when menstrual function is either being established or is declining. The true age incidence of dysfunctional uterine bleeding is difficult to determine, as most authors have limited their studies to patients admitted to hospital for curettage. Adolescent girls are rarely admitted to hospital and only when the condition is severe or persistent. All the girls not admitted to hospital, which are the large majority, will be excluded from such series of dysfunctional uterine bleeding. In contrast, virtually all cases of perimenopausal bleeding are admitted to hospital for curettage, even though the abnormality in bleeding may have been trivial or of short duration. Another difficulty in arriving at a true incidence is the great variation in standards that patients adopt in what they regard as abnormal and as necessary to report to a doctor. Gynaecologists also differ very considerably in what they regard as abnormal bleeding. A third difficulty in determining a true incidence is that the diagnosis of dysfunctional uterine bleeding can in fact be made only after uterine curettage. One is therefore obliged to fall back upon series of patients upon whom curettage has been performed, though the limitations and bias of such series should always be borne in mind.

Table 35.1 shows the age incidence of a well-known series of 861 patients with dysfunctional

Table 35.1. Age incidence in patients with dysfunctional uterine bleeding (Sutherland 1949)

Age group	No. of cases	Per cent	Per cent
20 and under	33	3·9	
21–30	194	22·5	56·8
31–40	295	34·3	
41–50	325	37·7	39·3
Over 50	14	1·6	

uterine bleeding studied by Sutherland (1949). It will be noted that only 4% of the patients were adolescents under 20, as compared with 57% in the 20–40 age group and 39% over 40.

Aetiology of dysfunctional uterine bleeding

The causes of dysfunctional uterine bleeding are unknown. It is presumed that most cases of dysfunctional uterine bleeding are due to some abnormality in the process of menstruation and the menstrual cycle and are the result of some dysfunction in the endometrium, ovary, anterior pituitary or hypothalamus. There is probably a second, smaller, category where the abnormal bleeding is secondary to a dysfunction in other endocrine glands, for example the thyroid, or in some other system of the body.

MECHANISM OF MENSTRUATION AND ABNORMAL BLOOD LOSS

Menstruation must be recognized as the only example in mammalian physiology of periodic sloughing from an organ. In normal menstruation the total average blood loss is 60 ml, ranging from 30 to 180 ml. A half to three-quarters of the menstrual discharge is blood, the rest being fragments of endometrial tissue, desquamated vaginal epithelium and mucus. Menstrual blood does not clot readily, and it is suggested that the endometrium normally produces a lytic substance that causes any clots that do form in the uterine cavity to disintegrate. When menstrual loss is excessive, the flow of blood is too great for the amount of lysin available, resulting in the passage of blood clots typical of menorrhagia.

The almost unique feature of menstruating females in all species is the presence of spiral arterioles. In the proliferative phase of the cycle these blood vessels grow upwards from the basal layer of the endometrium to the more superficial layers, where a capillary network develops. During this phase the vessels appear to be in tense contraction. Following ovulation and the formation of the corpus luteum the spiral arterioles are more dilated. There is also a marked increase in the coiling and length of the arterioles. If pregnancy does not occur, the corpus luteum starts to atrophy and there is a decrease in the secretion of progesterone and oestrogen. About 2 days prior to the appearance of menstrual blood, and coinciding with the withdrawal of progesterone and oestrogen, the blood flow through the spiral arterioles decreases. At the same time, the endometrial glands empty of secretion and buckle, and the whole endometrium shrinks, causing the spiral arterioles to become even more coiled and to kink. This is followed by spasmodic contraction of the spiral arterioles, focal necrosis and rupture of their walls, and local extravasation of blood into the endometrium. Numerous venous and capillary lakes appear in the spongiosa, and areas of haemorrhage finally coalesce, to lift off islands of devitalized tissue. Bleeding occurs from the coalesced blood lakes, from the superficial venules which have been torn open, and from the open ends of the remaining parts of the spiral arterioles in the basal layer of the endometrium.

This concept of the process of menstruation, which is based primarily on the changes in the spiral arterioles as propounded by Markee (1950), has been challenged by Okkels (1950), who believes that there is a system of arterio-venous anastomoses in the endometrium which are controlled by nerves terminating in contractile parts of the anastomoses. According to Okkels's theory, just before, and at, menstruation there is a shunting of blood through the arteriovenous anastomoses, creating the lakes which cause the shedding of the endometrium.

The immediate cause of menstruation has been much debated, and has been summarized by Israel (1970). It is probable that the primary cause is the withdrawal of the hormonal stimulus and, in particular, progesterone, which has a direct effect on the spiral arterioles and/or the arteriovenous anastomoses as well as the other structures in the endometrium. It is also believed that at menstruation the degenerating or shed endometrium liberates vasoconstrictor (as well as lytic) substances which cause further con-striction of the spiral arterioles and so accelerate the process of necrosis and shedding of the unshed endometrium. If this is so, it is possible that this vasoconstrictor substance may also cause constriction of the remaining portions of the spiral arterioles in the basal endometrium, and may be a factor in producing haemostasis and in preventing excessive blood loss at menstruation.

The process of menstruation is normally completed in 4–7 days. Repair and resurfacing of the denuded areas of the endometrium com-mence immediately the endometrium is shed, and it is possible that the rate of regeneration and resurfacing of the basal layer may be another factor influencing the amount of blood lost and the duration of menstruation. This in turn may depend upon the secretion of oestrogen by the ovaries. The amount of blood lost in normal menstruation and in cases of dysfunctional bleeding is probably determined by a number of factors, including

(i) the total area of the endometrial cavity;

(ii) the functional state and vascularity of the endometrium, and in particular the functional state of the endometrial blood vessels;

(iii) the amount of haemorrhage into the endometrium and the precise nature and rate of the shedding process;

(iv) the number, size and patency of the blood vessels in the denuded basal endometrium;

(v) the clotting and lytic factors in the en-dometrium and menstrual blood;

(vi) the rate of regeneration of the endometrium.

The changes in the spiral arterioles and other blood vessels of the endometrium in dysfunctional uterine bleeding have received scant attention. Salvatore (1958) studied the changes in the spiral arterioles and in the endometrium in 100 cases of dysfunctional uterine bleeding. Nineteen of the patients had normal endometrium, and of these 13 (68·5%) had normal arterioles and 6 (31·5%) showed some abnormal changes. The remaining 81 patients had some variety of en-dometrial hyperplasia, and in these patients 16 (19·7%) had normal arterioles and 65 (80·3%) showed abnormal changes. In the 71 patients with abnormal spiral arterioles, the abnormalities found were: perivascular fibrosis (48%), sub-endothelial hyaline degeneration (33%), hyper-plasia and hypertrophy of the smooth muscle (23%), and elastosis (4%) (Fig. 35.1). Though there was no strict relation between the changes in the endometrium and those in the spiral arterioles, Salvatore (1958) concluded that 'alterations of the spiral arterioles of the en-dometrium constitute an important local factor in haemorrhage. Altered arterioles probably react to oestrogen deprivation differently from the way normal arterioles react and interfere in the bleeding mechanism, making more difficult (1) the scaling of the endometrium, (2) re-epithelialization of the scaled surfaces, and (3) the vascular contractions and constriction that make up the haemostatic mechanism. This results in the prolongation and increase in endometrial bleeding'.

How much uterine bleeding comes from the spiral arterioles and how much from the venous sinuses is not known. Sippe (1962) has described

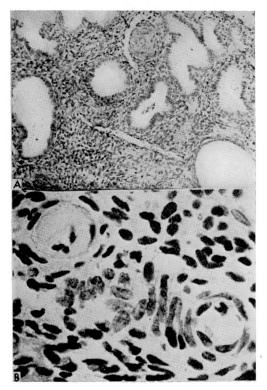

Fig. 35.1. Spiral arterioles. Cystic glandular hyperplasia of endometrium. (A) Hypertrophy and hyperplasia of muscular tunics of spiral arterioles (× 360). (B) Hyaline degeneration of spiral arteriole and normal spiral arteriole (× 920) (Salvatore 1958).

the occurrence of large, thin-walled, venous sinuses in the superficial layers of the endometrium, particularly in endometrial hyperplasia. There was, however, no correlation between the number and size of the sinuses and the intensity of the hyperplastic process. Sippe considers that the rupture of the sinuses is responsible for the uterine haemorrhage in endometrial hyperplasia and some other types of dysfunctional uterine bleeding.

The structural changes in the spiral arterioles and the venous sinuses of the endometrium which have been described may be an important part of the pathogenesis in at least some cases of dysfunctional uterine bleeding. It is nevertheless probable that in the majority of cases the cause of the abnormal bleeding is some disturbance in the functioning of the spiral arterioles and other vascular structures in the endometrium, and possibly of the other factors which normally control menstrual blood loss. This dysfunction of the spiral arterioles and other blood vessels is probably a direct result of the changes in oestrogen and progesterone secretion, though it is possible that other factors—for example, thyroid hormone—may have a direct effect on the blood vessels.

CAUSES OF DYSFUNCTIONAL UTERINE BLEEDING

The present concept is that in the majority of cases of dysfunctional uterine bleeding the essential defect is in the secretion of oestrogen and progesterone by the ovary. The oestrogen or progesterone may be deficient or excessive in amount or may not be secreted in the necessary cyclical sequence. This dysfunction of the ovary may be primary or secondary to inadequate or inappropriate stimulation by the pituitary. This may result in irregularity of the menstrual cycle, excessive menstrual blood loss or acyclical uterine bleeding.

In cases of pubertal dysfunctional uterine bleeding it is believed that the primary fault lies in the pituitary, which fails to secrete gonadotrophins in the correct cyclical sequence. In premenopausal bleeding, in contrast, it is believed that the fault lies primarily in the ovary, which fails to respond to gonadotrophins. In both cases there is a failure of ovulation and anovulatory bleeding.

In the child-bearing period of life it is believed that ovulation is normal but that the fault lies in the corpus luteum, which fails to complete its normal cycle of luteinization and atrophy.

A classification of dysfunctional uterine bleeding which is based on the presumed dysfunction of the ovary and which is useful in practice has been put forward by Vorys & Neri (1968) (see Table 35.2).

(1) *Ovulatory dysfunctional uterine bleeding*

Disorders of menstruation, associated with normal ovulation, more commonly result in the

Table 35.2. Classification of dysfunctional uterine bleeding according to aetiology and common symptoms (after Vorys & Neri 1968)

(1) *Ovulatory*	(a) Long proliferative or secretory phases	Oligomenorrhoea
	(b) Short proliferative or secretory phases	Polymenorrhoea
(2) *Corpus luteum abnormality*	(a) Insufficiency	Premenstrual spotting Menorrhagia Polymenorrhoea
	(b) Prolonged	Menorrhagia Oligomenorrhoea
(3) *Anovulatory*	(a) Cyclical	Oligomenorrhoea Menorrhagia
	(b) Acyclical	Metrorrhagia

disturbance of the cycle than excess menstrual loss.

(*a*) *Ovulatory oligomenorrhoea* is usually due to a prolonged proliferative phase. It most commonly occurs in adolescence and may be a normal feature of the menarche. It may, however, be a forerunner of the Stein-Leventhal or polycystic ovary syndrome. Ovulatory oligomenorrhoea also occurs—but less commonly—in older women, when it may precede the menopause. To what extent the oligomenorrhoea is due to a primary unresponsiveness of the ovary with a slow development of a follicle or is secondary to pituitary dysfunction is not known. The secretory phases of these menstrual cycles are usually normal.

(*b*) *Ovulatory polymenorrhoea* is commonly due to a shortening of the proliferative phase— particularly in adolescence, when it is thought to be due to hypersensitivity of the ovary. Ovulation is normal and there is no abnormality in the amount of menstrual blood loss. Polymenorrhoea with a shortened secretory phase may occur in older women and may progress to oligomenorrhoea and amenorrhoea of ovarian failure. It is due to premature degeneration of the corpus luteum and is really a form of corpus luteum insufficiency.

(2) *Dysfunctional bleeding with corpus luteum abnormalities*

This is said to occur most commonly in the adult reproductive years.

(*a*) *Corpus luteum insufficiency* is due to failure in the development of the corpus luteum, with a decreased secretion of progesterone and oestrogen in the second half of the cycle. Endometrial biopsy at the time of menstruation may show 'irregular ripening' of the endometrium (Traut & Kuder 1935). The condition is typically associated with hypermenorrhoea and premenstrual spotting. Early involution of the corpus luteum may also occur and may result in a shortening of the menstrual cycle and polymenorrhoea.

(*b*) *Corpus luteum prolonged activity.* In some cycles the corpus luteum may fail to involute at the correct time and the secretory activity may be abnormally prolonged. In a group of cases of dysfunctional uterine bleeding, McKelvey & Samuels (1947) have demonstrated an 'irregular shedding of the endometrium' associated with the secretion of pregnanediol persisting throughout the bleeding period. This abnormality is comparatively rare and may be associated with the development of a corpus luteum cyst. It results in prolonged and excessive menstruation, and possibly in oligomenorrhoea due to the prolonged cycles.

(3) *Anovulatory dysfunctional uterine bleeding*

Failure of ovulation is the most common abnormality of the menstrual cycle. It may result in

(a) normal regular cycles with apparently normal periods;

(b) regular cycles with excessive loss—anovulatory hypermenorrhoea;

(c) irregular menstruation in which periods of amenorrhoea are followed by excessive loss — metropathia haemorrhagica — or completely acyclical bleeding.

Anovular menstruation occurs at both extremes of reproductive life—namely, at the menarche and preceding the menopause. It is the rule rather than the exception at these times, and should be regarded as normal provided there is no abnormal uterine bleeding.

There are three main types of anovulatory uterine bleeding. In the first there is a progressive rise of oestrogen secretion to comparatively high levels of 100 μg or more per day, which is then followed by a sudden fall in secretion due to feedback inhibition of the pituitary and of FSH secretion. With the fall in oestrogen secretion the endometrium which is proliferative does not undergo the generalized ischaemic process as normally occurs at menstruation. The shedding of the endometrium is, in consequence, often irregular, incomplete and prolonged, resulting in excessive blood loss. The cycles in these cases are nevertheless regular or only slightly irregular.

The second type is the classical form of dysfunctional uterine bleeding—metropathia haemorrhagica. In this type there is a slowly increasing secretion of oestrogen but no secondary feedback inhibition of the pituitary and consequent fall in oestrogen secretion. The cycle is therefore prolonged, resulting in a period of amenorrhoea, and the prolonged stimulation of the endometrium by oestrogen causes a hyperplasia of the endometrium. The hyperplasia continues until such time as there is a fall in oestrogen secretion or until particular areas of the endometrium outgrow their blood supply and slough. The blood loss from the hyperplastic endometrium may be considerable, and may occasionally exsanguinate the patient. The hyperplastic endometrium may be shed and a normal menstrual cycle may follow, though the episodes of metropathia haemorrhagica tend to recur. Sometimes, the endometrium may not be completely shed, and this results in continuous or acyclical bleeding. This type of anovulatory

bleeding is often associated with the formation of multiple follicular cysts of the ovary. The Graafian follicles presumably fail to rupture, and continue to produce oestrogen until such time as the granulosa and theca cells degenerate. A third type of anovulatory abnormality is when the oestrogen secretion does not increase but 'teeters' about a critical threshold below which the endometrium cannot be maintained and therefore bleeds. This results in so-called 'threshold bleeding', which is often completely irregular and acyclical and in which no periodic loss can be distinguished.

Oestrogen, progesterone and gonadotrophin estimation in dysfunctional uterine bleeding

The measurement of oestrogens, progestogens and gonadotrophins is time-consuming and difficult. Methods for the measurement of these substances in blood, which require a high degree of sensitivity and specificity, have only recently been developed. Most of the knowledge we have is based on the urinary excretion or metabolites, usually over a 24 hr period. The main excretion products of oestrogen are oestriol, oestrone and oestradiol, and the main excretion product of progesterone is pregnanediol. Pregnanediol is also a major metabolite of the adrenocortical steroids.

In order to make a satisfactory assessment of endocrine function, it is necessary to make serial estimations of a relatively large number of hormones and their metabolites over several cycles. Loraine & Bell (1966 and 1967) have reviewed the literature and also summarized their own extensive researches at the Medical Research Council Clinical Endocrinology Research Unit at Edinburgh. They found a considerable variation in the hormone excretion in normal menstrual cycles from one individual to another. The hormone excretion in a composite normal menstrual cycle is shown in Fig. 35.2.

The major features in women with dysfunctional uterine bleeding and oligomenorrhoea were the extreme variability in the hormone excretion patterns and the not infrequent finding of very high readings, sometimes up to and above

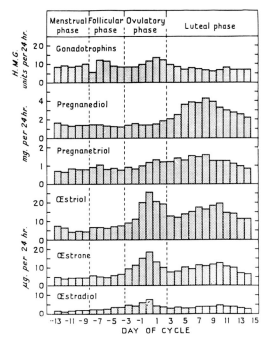

Fig. 35.2. Mean hormone excretion during the normal menstrual cycle (15 cycles) (Loraine & Bell 1963).

100 μg of total oestrogens per 24 hr. Brown *et al.* (1959) were unable to establish any correlation between oestrogen output, endometrial histology and pattern of uterine bleeding. In one patient with endometrial hyperplasia, however, studied by Loraine & Bell (1967) (Fig. 35.3), cessation of bleeding was associated with rising oestrogen levels, while bleeding recommenced when oestrogen readings fell.

The variability of both the endocrinological and clinical picture in patients with dysfunctional uterine bleeding is illustrated in Fig. 35.4. This patient had unequivocal cystic glandular hyperplasia at endometrial biopsy some weeks prior to the study. However, during the period of investigation the patient had three normal ovulatory cycles. This variability in successive cycles constitutes one of the greatest difficulties in the study of dysfunctional uterine bleeding.

Goldzieher (1970), in reviewing the relation between dysfunctional bleeding and oestrogen and progesterone excretion, comments that 'functional abnormalities of the endometrium are associated more with a lack of cyclical variation in the oestrogen levels than with abnormal levels of production and excretion. However, serial daily urinary excretion studies have failed to show an invariable correlation between a drop in oestrogen production and the onset of uterine bleeding. Even on the basis of the meagre evidence available it must be concluded that the initiation of bleeding is a more complex phenomenon than is generally supposed'. Goldzieher also discussed the relation between oestrogen excretion, the functional state of the endometrium and vaginal cytology: 'The vaginal epithelium is the most sensitive indicator of oestrogen action in the body; thus alone or in conjunction with the endometrium it can serve as a valuable index of oestrogenic activity. It must be remembered, however, that the effect of oestrogen as seen in the vaginal smear represents not only the effect on the most oestrogen sensitive tissue of the body but it also reflects the integrated effect of a slow response: in the menopausal woman, for example, an injection of oestrogen begins to show effects on the vaginal epithelium after an interval of several days and persists for a week or more. Thus, the poor correlation between vaginal and endometrial response on the one hand and urinary oestrogen levels on the other hand may be more apparent than real.' On the basis it would seem that vaginal cytology may well provide a better guide to the functional state of the endometrium than measurements of oestrogen or progesterone secretion.

Other possible causes for dysfunctional uterine bleeding

The causes of dysfunctional uterine bleeding will remain a mystery as long as we are uncertain of the precise mechanism of menstruation and uterine bleeding. Inasmuch as the two ovarian steroids oestrogen and progesterone are the principal factors controlling the growth of the endometrium, it is logical to look upon abnormalities in their production and utilization and abnormalities in the function of the pituitary which controls their production as the main causes for dysfunctional uterine bleeding. This does not, however, exclude other factors. Three

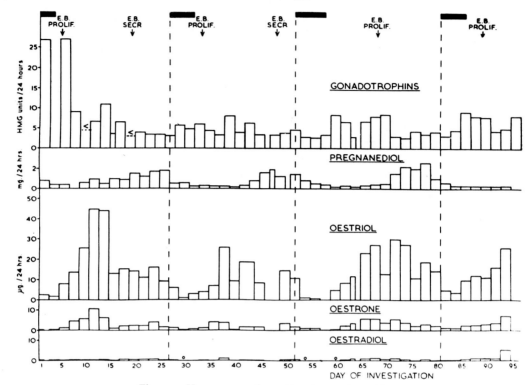

Fig. 35.3. Hormone excretion pattern in a patient with
cystic glandular hyperplasia. (Loraine & Bell 1966).

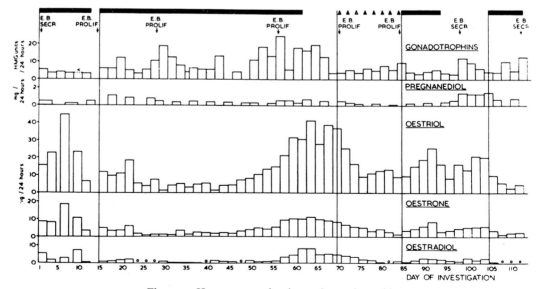

Fig. 35.4. Hormone excretion in another patient with
cystic glandula hyperplasia (Loraine & Bell 1966).

abnormalities which from time to time are said to cause dysfunctional bleeding are (1) thyroid disease, (2) haematological bleeding disorders, and (3) iron-deficiency anaemia.

(1) THYROID DISEASE

The relationship between thyroid function and menstruation has not been defined, but it would appear that the lack of thyroid hormone prevents ovulation by interference with the production of LH by the anterior pituitary gland, whereas excessive amounts of thyroid hormone depress ovarian function (Scheenberg 1970). Whether this latter is a direct action upon the ovary or is mediated via the pituitary has not been settled.

In 50 women with myxoedema studied by Scott & Mussey (1964), 23 had menstrual disorders characterized by excessive bleeding, 22 had normal menses, five had hypomenorrhoea and only two patients had amenorrhoea (two patients showed two patterns). In 10 women with myxoedema, Goldsmith *et al.* (1952) reported that eight had menstrual abnormalities. Five had severe metrorrhagia, two had menorrhagia and one had amenorrhoea; in six of the eight there was no evidence of ovulation. Abnormal menstruation in hypothyroid patients responds promptly to therapy, and frequently to doses insufficient to correct completely all other stigmata of hypothyroidism.

In hyperthyroid patients the usual menstrual disorder is amenorrhoea or oligomenorrhoea, though menorrhagia does occur. Goldsmith *et al.* (1952) studied 18 patients with thyrotoxicosis. Fourteen had a moderate to marked decrease in flow and three had amenorrhoea. Benson & Dailey (1955) studied 241 patients with hyperthyroidism and found an almost linear relationship between the decrease in flow and the severity of the thyrotoxicosis. Successful treatment of the thyrotoxicosis relieved the menstrual disorders promptly. The hypomenorrhoea of hyperthyroidism occurs without marked ovarian or endometrial abnormalities, as evidenced by normal ovulation and the production of a secretory endometrium. It would therefore appear that there is no significant change in the pituitary or ovarian function in thyrotoxicosis. The excess thyroid hormone may have a direct effect on the endometrial blood vessels.

(2) HAEMATOLOGICAL DISORDERS

Abnormal uterine bleeding is characteristic of several, but not all, of the hereditary bleeding disorders (Simpson & Christakos 1969). Excessive menstrual bleeding is common in thrombocytopoenic purpura and in Minot-von Willebrand syndrome, and may be the first sign of these diseases. This may be due to the diminution in platelets and increasing capillary fragility normally seen in the luteal phase of the cycle. Quick (1966), in an excellent paper, discusses the relation between menorrhagia and coagulation and bleeding disorders. He states 'Because normal menstruation is observed in afibrinogenaemia, severe hypothrombinaemia, marked reduction of factor VII and hyperheparinaemia, it can be concluded that the control and termination of the cyclic uterine bleeding depends upon a mechanism other than the clotting of blood. Menorrhagia is associated with lack of bloodclotting factors V, VII and X and is common in platelet deficiency as well as in the Minot-von Willebrand syndrome.' In investigating patients with menorrhagia who are suspected of having some bleeding or coagulation disorder, it is important to ask for epistaxis and early bruising in childhood and to inspect the arms and legs for ecchymoses. The initial investigations should include haemoglobin estimation, blood smear, platelet count, prothrombin time, bleeding time and torniquet test. By means of a careful history and laboratory studies it is usually possible to determine whether menorrhagia is due to a failure in systemic haemostasis, and to institute appropriate therapy. In treating excessive menstruation and in preparing patients for operation, fresh frozen plasma or, in the case of thrombocytopenic purpura, fresh, platelet-rich plasma, is very useful in producing haemostasis.

(3) ANAEMIA AND IRON DEFICIENCY

Though anaemia is common in dysfunctional uterine bleeding, the precise relationship between anaemia and abnormal menstruation is difficult to establish. Many gynaecologists regard the blood haemoglobin level as a measure of the amount of menstrual blood loss. It is maintained that if uterine bleeding is excessive it will produce anaemia, and that a patient with a normal haemoglobin concentration cannot have excessive blood loss. There may be some general truth in these widely held beliefs, but they would seem to ignore the fact that men and women, such as blood donors, can lose relatively large amounts of blood over long periods without any persisting effect on the haemoglobin levels. Fowler & Barer (1942) thus found that women blood donors can lose on an average 555 ml or 2·2 g haemoglobin in addition to the normal blood loss, and that the haemoglobin will return to normal in an average of 52 days (range 43–73 days). As the frequency of blood withdrawal (for the same overall blood loss) did not affect the rate of blood regeneration, this would mean that a woman can lose on average an additional 300 ml of blood per period without any persisting effect on the haemoglobin levels. It would therefore appear that at least some women can lose excessive amounts of blood at menstruation (up to 300 ml) and maintain a normal haemoglobin. The development of anaemia probably depends upon a number of factors, such as the iron intake and the efficiency of the erythropoietic system, as well as upon the amount of menstrual blood loss.

Some investigators maintain that iron deficiency and anaemia are causative factors in dysfunctional uterine bleeding (Taymor 1964). Others hold that anaemia may cause a reduction in menstrual blood loss. Jacobs & Butler (1965) measured the blood loss in 17 normal women and in 15 women with iron-deficiency anaemia. In 13 of the women the measurement was repeated after the anaemia had been fully treated and the haemoglobin level had returned to normal. The mean blood loss per period in the normal women was 13·7 ± 5·8 ml, as compared with 85·5 ± 14·9 ml in the women with untreated anaemia; a sixfold difference which was statistically significant.

When the blood loss was measured after the anaemia had been fully treated, many of the anaemic women had a considerable increase in menstrual flow, the mean blood loss per period

after treatment being 157·7 ± 28·0 ml, or approximately double. The increase in blood loss following treatment was observed to be greatest in those women whose initial blood loss was above average. There was one exception. A woman who had an alarming haemorrhage was treated with an intravenous infusion of 2,250 mg of iron, which resulted in complete remission of her anaemia. After treatment the blood loss in this patient was very much less, though still excessive. Jacobs & Butler (1965) arrive at the important conclusion that in the majority of their cases the development of iron-deficiency anaemia initiated a compensatory mechanism which tends to reduce the menstrual blood loss, and that the menstrual blood loss after treatment represents the original flow or the menstrual blood loss the patient would have in the absence of anaemia. In dysfunctional uterine bleeding with excessive blood loss, the development of anaemia would appear to cause a relative reduction in the menstrual blood loss in the majority of cases. Their one patient who improved on treatment, however, is interesting, and suggests that there may be a few cases where iron deficiency may perhaps be an aetiological factor in the dysfunctional uterine bleeding.

PATHOLOGY

Endometrium

Dysfunctional uterine bleeding may be associated with almost any type of endometrium, even apparently normal endometrium. This does not mean that the histological examination of the endometrium is of little or no value. As Fluhmann (1956) has emphasized, 'the bleeding, after all that is said about the many causes of this serious complication, is from the endometrium and a microscopic examination most often points the way to the final method of treatment'.

The endometrial findings in two well-known series of dysfunctional uterine bleeding (Sutherland 1949; Kistner 1964a) are shown in Table 35.3. The agreement in the relative percentages of the different types of abnormality, and the percentage of normal endometria, is striking.

Table 35.3. Histology of endometrium in dysfunctional uterine bleeding

Diagnosis	Sutherland (1949)		Kistner (1964a)	
	No.	Per cent	No.	Per cent
Normal	547	63·5	230	57·5
Hyperplasia	265	30·8	123	30·8
Irregular ripening	26	3·0	—	—
Chronic menstrual	—	—	31	7·8
Irregular shedding	13	1·5	9	2·2
Atrophy	10	1·2	7	1·7
Total	861	100	400	100

The incidence of abnormal endometrial findings probably represents that found in routine gynaecological practice. It does not, however, necessarily indicate the true incidence of abnormalities of the endometrium, as the incidence of abnormality will depend greatly upon the time when the endometrial biopsy was performed, both in relation to the cycle and to the episode of bleeding.

In Sutherland's (1949) series 'the patients were admitted to hospital from the waiting list and no attempt was made in any case to obtain endometrium at any time in the cycle'. In many cases, therefore, it may well have been that the curettage was performed in the first half of the cycle when no abnormality would be detected or, alternatively, that the curettage was performed *after* the menstrual abnormality had in fact corrected itself. This is one of the chief difficulties in determining the significance of endometrial findings in cases of dysfunctional uterine bleeding. If endometrium abnormalities are to be detected, curettage must be performed in the second half of the cycle, preferably immediately before menstruation, or else during the period of actual bleeding. The performance of curettage in cases of dysfunctional uterine bleeding in the first half of the cycle is useless unless it is done solely with the purpose of excluding organic disease, though even then tuberculous endometritis may well be missed. A positive effort should be made to perform uterine curettage or endometrial biopsy 4 or 5 days before the expected onset of menstruation. In cases of irregular or acyclical bleeding the value of curettage at the time of bleeding must not be underestimated, as not only may haemorrhage be arrested but endometrial hyperplasia and other abnormalities such as 'irregular shedding of the endometrium' may frequently be diagnosed in this way.

The endometrial abnormalities in dysfunctional uterine bleeding are of three main types:

(1) *Ovulatory*

    (a) Irregular ripening of the endometrium.
    (b) Irregular shedding of the endometrium.

(2) *Anovulatory*

    (a) Proliferative endometrium.
    (b) Endometrial hyperplasia.

(3) *Atrophic*

(1) OVULATORY ENDOMETRIUM

(a) Irregular ripening of the endometrium

This condition was first described by Traut & Kuder (1935), and an example is shown in Fig. 35.5. On histological examination of the endometrium obtained in the second half of the cycle, there is a mixture of both proliferative and secretory phases, with considerable areas that are definitely non-secretory and others which are as definitely secretory. Traut & Kuder (1935) stress that the changes must be found in the peripheral or superficial zone of the endometrium, as it is well-recognized that the basal layers of the glands adjacent to the myometrium are almost completely unresponsive to the secretory stimulus of the ovary. They also stress that it is important to exclude myomata and polypi, as the endometrium is frequently refractory in the vicinity of submucous fibroids and polyps. In a series of 100 cases of dysfunctional uterine bleeding, Traut & Kuder (1935) found 21 cases of irregular ripening of the endometrium. Fourteen of the cases presented with bleeding commencing in the middle of the cycle. All responded to curettage without recurrence. It is suggested that there is either a functional defect of the corpus luteum or an irregular response of

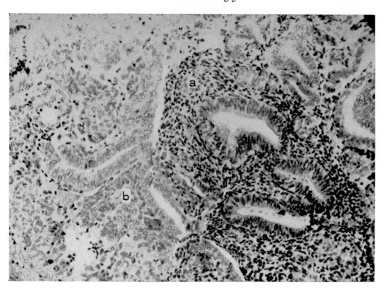

Fig. 35.5. Irregular ripening of endometrium. (a) Glands and stroma in proliferative phase. (b) Early secretory glands and stroma (× 85) (Traut & Kuder 1935).

the endometrium to the normal hormonal influence. Sutherland (1949) has commented that this condition has received relatively little attention, and that routine premenstrual biopsy would probably reveal a higher incidence than the 2·6% he found.

(b) Irregular shedding of the endometrium

Irregular shedding of the endometrium was first described by Driessen (1914) and was also discussed by Traut & Kuder (1935). They summarized their findings as follows: 'The history of the patient and the histological findings point definitely to maldeciduation of the endometrium with prolonged and exhausting secretory activity in the glandular elements of those fragments of the spongiosa which remain attached to the basalis, while the stroma becomes shrunken and most often its cells have changed from large round nucleated forms to the spindle shape which is characteristic of the proliferative phase of the cycle'. (See Fig. 35.6.) They found 11 cases in their series of 100 patients with dysfunctional uterine bleeding. The women all gave a history of having had normal menstrual periods until

they came under observation because of a prolonged or profuse menses or of recurrent bleeding immediately following what was supposed to have been a normal menstrual period. The duration of the bleeding was from 10 to 43 days, though curettage, when performed, caused prompt cessation of the bleeding. McKelvey & Samuels (1947) describe 34 cases in which the endometrium had the same characteristics and was associated with prolonged and profuse menstrual bleeding. They emphasized that the endometrium must be taken on the fifth day of the bleeding or a day or two later. If the endometrium is taken earlier, or at the end of the bleeding, accurate diagnosis is difficult. They also studied the pregnanediol excretion in six patients through 6 days of bleeding, after which curettage was performed to establish the diagnosis. In five of the six cases pregnanediol was excreted throughout the periods. Holmstrom & McLennan (1947) showed that an identical microscopic picture to that of irregular shedding of the endometrium could be produced in normal patients by the administration of progesterone either immediately before or during menstruation. It has been suggested that the condition is due to

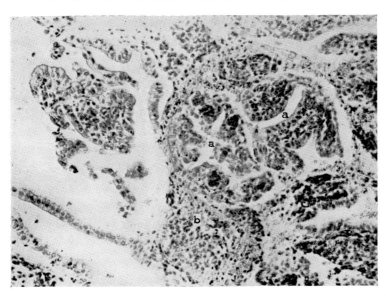

Fig. 35.6. Irregular shedding of endometrium. (a) Collapsed 'star-shaped' glands with secretory epithelium. (b) Shrunken, inactive endometrium (× 85) (Traut & Kuder 1935).

retarded regression of the corpus luteum, which is 'dead but will not lie down' (Kistner 1964b). The incidence of irregular shedding in series of cases of dysfunctional uterine bleeding varies from 3·7 to 25% (Sutherland 1949). Sutherland (1949) commented that a much higher incidence will probably be found if curettage is done more frequently at the time of bleeding.

(2) ANOVULATORY ENDOMETRIUM

(a) Proliferative endometrium

Anovulatory cycles are common in adolescence and before the menopause. Though the mechanism is not known, the menstrual bleeding associated with the shedding of proliferative endometrium is frequently excessive and prolonged. The finding of proliferative endometrium in the second half of the cycle should always be regarded as abnormal in dysfunctional uterine bleeding.

(b) Endometrial hyperplasia

This is the classical and most common abnormality of the endometrium in dysfunctional uterine bleeding, and is associated with metropathia haemorrhagica or completely acyclical bleeding. The hyperplasia varies from slight exaggeration of the proliferative phase to marked overgrowth simulating adenocarcinoma of the endometrium. The overgrowth affects both the stroma and the glands, which increase in number and size, producing the typical 'Swiss cheese' endometrium. There is also abnormal vasculization with numerous large, thick-walled blood vessels and markedly dilated veins or sinuses just under the endometrial surface (Fig. 35.7). As Schroeder (1954) repeatedly emphasized, endometrial specimens obtained during bleeding show infarction and thrombosis of the blood vessels, with areas of necrosis and sloughing of the superficial layers of the endometrium. With the increased vascularity, and often grossly abnormal endometrium, it is not difficult to visualize that endometrial hyperplasia is associated with bleeding, which is frequently very heavy.

The incidence of endometrial hyperplasia in dysfunctional uterine bleeding has been quoted as high as 90%. Sutherland (1949), however, in an analysis of 4,850 cases from 31 papers, found an incidence of 39·4%, which is in reasonable

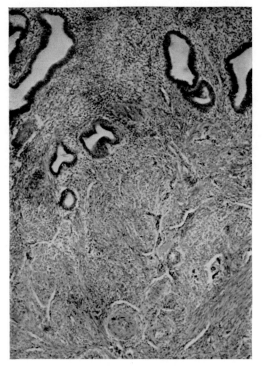

Fig. 35.7. Glandular endometrial hyperplasia showing dilated glands with 'Swiss cheese' appearance and blood vessels.

agreement with the figure of 30·8% which he found in his own series.

Discussion of the significance of endometrial hyperplasia, particularly in relation to the subsequent development of endometrial carcinoma, has occupied a large place in gynaecological literature. The subject has been reviewed by Kistner (1964c) with particular reference to the effect of new progestational agents.

(3) ATROPHY OF THE ENDOMETRIUM

There is considerable variation in the histological criteria for the diagnosis of this condition and in the incidence in different series, which ranges from 1·9 to 21·9% (Sutherland 1949). It is probably the least common abnormality in any age group, though there seems little doubt that dysfunctional uterine bleeding can occur with a completely atrophic endometrium.

Ovary

The findings in the ovary in dysfunctional uterine bleeding vary with the age of the patient and the endometrial changes. In pubertal girls the ovaries may contain follicular cysts which may be up to 3 cm in diameter, but there are usually no recent or old corpora lutea. In women of childbearing age with dysfunctional menorrhagia the ovaries usually appear normal, though there may occasionally be a persistent corpus luteum or corpus luteum cyst. The ovaries of premenopausal women, in contrast, frequently contain multiple cysts of various types, and these are particularly associated with endometrial hyperplasia.

Other associated findings

In this chapter on dysfunctional uterine bleeding, pathological findings have been excluded by definition. It is nevertheless important to have some idea of the proportion of pathological conditions which may be overlooked. The series of 861 cases of Sutherland (1949) was derived from 1,000 cases of abnormal uterine bleeding in which careful pelvic examination under general anaesthesia failed to reveal any recognizable pathological lesion which might explain the haemorrhage. The pathological findings in the remaining 139 cases, or 13·9% of the total cases, are shown in Table 35.4. The main pathological conditions—polyps, tuberculous endometritis and malignant disease—accounted for ap-

Table 35.4. Organic lesions of the uterus in abnormal uterine bleeding without clinical abnormality (Sutherland 1949)

Condition	No. of cases	Per cent of Organic lesions	Per cent of total series
Chronic endometritis	110	79	11
Uterine polyps	11	7·9	1
Tuberculous endometritis	10	7·2	1
Malignant disease	8	5·6	1
Total all cases	1,000	100	14

proximately 1% each of the total cases. Jacobs *et al.* (1957) reported 20 incorrect diagnoses in 112 cases of 'dysfunctional uterine bleeding', including six pelvic inflammatory disease, four fibroids, four incomplete abortions, three threatened abortions and one polyp, one sub-involution and one case of precocious puberty.

CLINICAL FEATURES OF DYSFUNCTIONAL UTERINE BLEEDING

Dysfunctional bleeding from the uterus may be abnormal in amount or duration, in its regularity or frequency, and its relation to menstruation. There is no specific pattern of bleeding which is characteristically dysfunctional and no specific pattern which is associated with organic disease. The incidence of pathological diseases and the prognosis varies both with age and the type of bleeding. In dealing with cases of abnormal uterine bleeding it is useful to consider the patients under three age groups and three types of bleeding.

The age groups are: (a) under 20—Adolescent uterine bleeding; (b) 20–40—uterine bleeding of adult reproductive years; (c) over 40—peri-menopausal bleeding. And the types of bleeding are: (i) regular or cyclical bleeding; (ii) irregular or acyclical bleeding; (iii) intermenstrual bleeding.

It must be stressed, however, that these groupings are generalizations, and should be regarded as guidelines only. What is said of an adolescent of 19 may equally apply to a woman of 21, and what is said of a 'perimenopausal' patient of 41 may well apply to the adult reproductive patient of 39. The distinction between regular and irregular bleeding is, similarly, often only one of degree.

Adolescent uterine bleeding

Uterine bleeding in adolescent girls (under the age of 20) is almost always dysfunctional in origin. The pathological findings in a group of 200 girls aged 20 or under investigated by Sutherland (1953) is shown in Table 35.5. No

Table 35.5. Histology of endometrium in pubertal uterine bleeding (Sutherland 1953)

Diagnosis	No.	Per cent
Normal endometrium	147	73·5
Hyperplasia	31	15·5
Chronic endometritis	10	5
Atrophy	4	2
Tuberculosis	8	4
Total cases	200	100

cases of malignancy were found, but there were eight cases of unsuspected tuberculous endometritis.

It is estimated that as many as the first 30 to 40 cycles after menarche may be anovulatory. Distinction must be made between (a) transitory oligomenorrhoea or some transitory irregularity of the cycles which may be regarded as physiological and a normal part of puberty, and (b) persisting oligomenorrhoea and polymenorrhoea or excessive blood loss. Menorrhagia or metrorrhagia can be severe in adolescents and accounts for about 4% of cases of dysfunctional uterine bleeding seen by gynaecologists.

Southam & Richart (1966) have published a valuable series of 291 patients with dysfunctional uterine bleeding and 247 with oligomenorrhoea presenting as adolescents, with a follow-up extending to 20 or more years.

Of 291 girls with dysfunctional uterine bleeding, the symptoms started with the menarche in 103 cases. The remaining 188 cases either had normal periods or oligomenorrhoea initially. The rate of continuing abnormality over 13 years of follow-up is shown in Fig. 35.8. Approximately 40% had returned to normal over the first 2 years, when the rate of recovery was greatest, but, surprisingly, recovery could take up to 10 years. At this time only 30% of patients had a continuing abnormality. The prognosis appears to be better in those patients whose symptoms started later after a period of normal menstruation, as compared with those whose symptoms started at the menarche.

Of the 291 patients with pubertal dysfunctional uterine bleeding, 177 had one or more curettages, 43 required blood transfusions and nine had

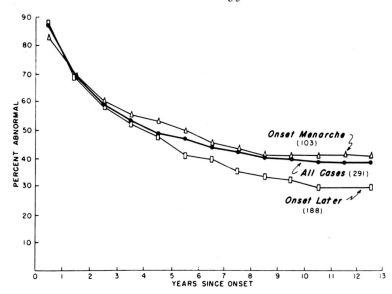

Fig. 35.8. Adolescent dysfunctional uterine bleeding. Rate of continued abnormality (Southam & Richart 1966).

hysterectomies. Four of the nine hysterectomies were done for endometrial carcinoma at the ages of 23, 29, 30 and 33 years, respectively. Southam & Richart (1966) also observed that patients with dysfunctional bleeding had poor obstetrical histories. Out of 97 pregnancies, only 36 women gave birth to 58 term infants, of whom three were anencephalics.

In the series of 247 adolescents presenting with oligomenorrhoea there was a marked difference in prognosis between those where the oligomenorrhoea started at menarche as compared with those of later onset (Fig. 35.9). In oligomenorrhoea commencing at the menarche, 30% had returned to normal in 1 year and 60% at 10 years. In oligomenorrhoea of later onset 60% had returned to normal in 1 year and 80% in 10 years. In all patients presenting with oligomenorrhoea, 71 were known to have married, 45 were known to have become pregnant, and 29 out of 36 patients whose obstetrical history was known delivered successfully. There was therefore no marked infertility, and there was surprisingly no apparent difference in fertility between those who had resumed regular periods and those who continued to have oligomenorrhoea.

These figures probably overstate the seriousness of dysfunctional uterine bleeding and oligomenorrhoea in adolescence, as this series is based on cases seen at a special gynaecological endocrine clinic, most of whom were referred because of recurrent or persistent abnormality. It nevertheless clearly shows that patients with dysfunctional uterine bleeding may not return to normal for up to 10 years, and that the overall prognosis for recovery is good.

Dysfunctional uterine bleeding in adult reproductive years

Abnormal uterine bleeding between the ages of 20–40 is most commonly due to benign tumour, pelvic inflammatory disease or some complication of pregnancy. A diagnosis of dysfunctional uterine bleeding should therefore not be made until organic disease has been excluded. It is sometimes said that dysfunctional uterine bleeding is uncommon in this age group. However, this is not borne out in the published series. Over 50% of Sutherland's (1949) patients were between the ages of 20 and 40. Dysfunctional uterine bleeding is frequent in the puerperium,

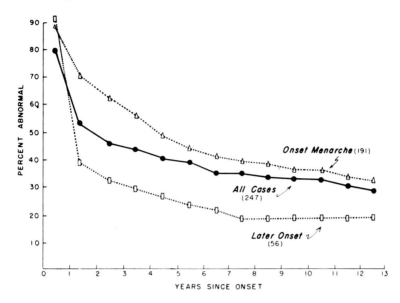

Fig. 35.9. Adolescent oligomenorrhoea. Rate of continued abnormality (Southam & Richart 1966).

and occurs in parous women more often than in nulliparae. The bleeding is most frequently ovulatory in type, and probably—due to some defect in the corpus luteum—results in irregular ripening or irregular shedding of the endometrium. Anovulatory bleeding and endometrial hyperplasia does, however, occur, and was present in 21% of Sutherland's (1949) patients of childbearing age with dysfunctional bleeding.

The prognosis in ovulatory dysfunctional uterine bleeding is good. Most of such cases either undergo spontaneous cure or remit after curettage or hormone therapy. The prognosis is, however, less favourable in patients with anovulatory bleeding and endometrial hyperplasia, which tends to recur.

Perimenopausal dysfunctional uterine bleeding

Abnormal uterine bleeding in women over the age of 40 is commonly due to organic disease. Carcinoma of the endometrium and of the cervix occurs with increasing frequency with increasing age, and constitutes an important and serious cause of uterine bleeding in this age group. It is therefore essential to take every step to exclude carcinoma in all cases of perimenopausal bleeding. This period of life nevertheless has a high incidence of dysfunctional uterine bleeding associated with the alteration in ovarian or pituitary function preceding the menopause. The bleeding tends to be acyclical, and approximately 50% of cases are associated with endometrial hyperplasia. The prognosis and management of such cases depends on the significance attached to endometrial hyperplasia.

Some gynaecologists believe that endometrial hyperplasia is precancerous. Kistner (1964c), however, has reviewed the evidence and maintains that there is only meagre evidence that cystic hyperplasia is causally related to carcinoma of the endometrium, though in predisposed women adenomatous endometrial hyperplasia or anaplasia may progress to carcinoma *in situ* and eventually invasive carcinoma of the endometrium.

Cystic and atypical hyperplasia may also develop postmenopausally and accounts for a significant proportion of cases of postmenopausal bleeding (McBride 1954). Though this may strictly be regarded as dysfunctional uterine bleeding, postmenopausal bleeding is usually considered in a separate category due to the high incidence of gynaecological carcinoma in these cases.

REGULAR OR CYCLICAL BLEEDING

Regular or cyclical uterine bleeding is frequently dysfunctional in origin, and if due to organic disease is rarely associated with malignancy. Cyclical dysfunctional bleeding is more commonly ovulatory, and the prognosis is, accordingly, good. Regular uterine bleeding is therefore usually considered relatively favourably, and uterine curettage may be deferred in younger women with menorrhagia of short duration in the absence of obvious organic disease.

IRREGULAR OR ACYCLICAL BLEEDING

Irregular or acyclical uterine bleeding is more often associated with organic disease and may be due to carcinoma of the cervix, endometrium or elsewhere in the genital tract.

Acyclical dysfunctional uterine bleeding is frequently associated with endometrial hyperplasia, which is more difficult to treat and is associated with the suspicion of carcinoma. Acyclical or irregular uterine bleeding is therefore regarded less favourably and uterine curettage must be performed in every case.

INTERMENSTRUAL BLEEDING

Intermenstrual bleeding with normal regular periods falls into a separate category. If regular and occurring midcycle, it is often physiological, and is due to the fall in oestrogen secretion following the oestrogen surge associated with ovulation. It usually lasts only 2–3 days, but may occasionally linger until the next period. It is said to occur in 20% of women with mittelschmerz (Diddle 1948) and in 60% of ovulatory women if the midcycle mucus is examined for erythrocytes (Kurzor et al. 1953). Intermenstrual bleeding is, however, common with endometrial polyps, submucous fibromyomata and cervical carcinoma. It is therefore essential to regard all cases of intermenstrual bleeding as abnormal until proved otherwise.

DIAGNOSIS

The steps taken to diagnose dysfunctional uterine bleeding are the traditional history, examination and special investigations. It should be stressed that it is not sufficient simply to make a diagnosis of 'dysfunctional uterine bleeding', but that every effort should be made to diagnose the nature of the underlying defect. This positive approach will bring far more rewards than the simple exclusion of organic disease.

History

The history should include a detailed menstrual history and an assessment of the blood loss and general condition of the patient. The presence or absence of associated menstrual symptoms and of symptoms of endocrine or other organic disease may provide an important guide to the diagnosis. It is also important to elicit the patient's background, home and marital circumstances and any history of emotional stress or psychiatric abnormality.

Examination

Pelvic examination must be performed and the cervix visualized as a matter of principle *in every patient* complaining of any abnormality of menstruation. In adolescents and young unmarried women with intact hymen this principle may be transgressed, depending upon the duration of the abnormality, the age of the patient and the circumstances. If the abnormality persists more than 3 months, a pelvic examination per rectum, as well as an abdominal examination, must be performed, as a minimum, to exclude palpable uterine or ovarian enlargement and obvious organic disease. A general examination is essential to assess the general condition of the patient and to exclude systemic endocrine and other diseases.

Special investigations

These include:

(1) Curettage of the uterus and endometrial biopsy.

(2) Basal body-temperature charts, vaginal and cervical smears, and examination of the cervical mucus.

(3) Oestrogen and progesterone estimations.

(4) Other endocrine investigations.

(5) Haematological investigations.

(6) Other gynaecological investigations.

(1) UTERINE CURETTAGE AND ENDO-METRIAL BIOPSY

(a) Uterine curettage

Curettage of the uterus is the most important measure in the management of patients with abnormal uterine bleeding. It is, however, a procedure which should be performed with purpose, thought and care, not 'unadvisedly, lightly or wantonly'. The objects of curettage are:

(a) to exclude any lesion in the uterus such as incomplete abortion or endometrial polyp or carcinoma;

(b) to obtain endometrium for histological examination, to determine the functional state of the endometrium, and to exclude disease such as tuberculous endometritis;

(c) for any possible therapeutic effect.

The precise indications for curettage are difficult to specify. In general it may be said 'the older the patient the more irregular the haemorrhage and the longer its duration the greater the indication for curettage.' Most gynaecologists are agreed that

(a) *in adolescence* (*under 20*) curettage should be deferred unless the bleeding is severe or fails to respond to other measures;

(b) *in reproductive years* (*20–40*) it may be postponed for a limited period (not more than 3 months) provided there is no suspicion of organic disease and no abnormality on examination;

(c) *in the perimenopause* (*over 40*) it is mandatory and must be performed without delay in every patient.

The timing of the curettage is crucial in determining the functional state of the en-dometrium. Curettage must be performed in the second half of the cycle and preferably 5–6 days before menstruation. Only at this stage can failure of ovulation, the response of the endometrium to progesterone and oestrogen, and tuberculous endometritis be diagnosed.

A much neglected procedure, particularly in patients with prolonged periods, is curettage *at the time of the bleeding.* Apart from arresting haemorrhage, it is of value diagnostically. 'Irregular shedding' of the endometrium, in particular, can only be diagnosed when curettage is performed on the fourth or fifth day of bleeding.

(b) Endometrial biopsy

Most gynaecologists are agreed that formal dilatation and curettage under general anaesthesia is essential in virtually all cases of abnormal uterine bleeding to exclude organic disease. Endometrial biopsy, by means of Sharman's or Novak's curette, can be carried out as an office procedure, and some gynaecologists, such as Abell (1968), believe that endometrial specimens so obtained are of great value in the investigation and management of dysfunctional uterine bleeding. The procedure may be of advantage if it is desired to obtain repeat biopsies to assess the endometrial changes in different cycles or the effect of treatment. There is, however, a sharp division among gynaecologists as to the safety of the procedure and the degree of discomfort to the patient. Some feel that these disadvantages, together with the fact that organic conditions may be missed, make its use unwarranted. Others feel that it is a quick, easy, safe procedure that can be performed in the office or clinic without hazarding or hurting the patient. The use of endometrial biopsy will depend upon the inclination and skills of the particular gynaecologist and the use he will make of the information obtained from the biopsy.

(2) (a) BASAL BODY-TEMPERATURE CHARTS
(b) VAGINAL AND CERVICAL SMEARS
(c) EXAMINATION OF CERVICAL MUCUS

These three simple investigations may provide useful information on the endocrine state of the genital tract, the occurrence of ovulation and the function of the corpus luteum.

(a) Basal body-temperature charts

When combined with menstrual calendar, daily basal body-temperature charts may be of considerable value in the diagnosis and management of dysfunctional uterine bleeding (Palmer 1959). Besides providing a precise record of the amount and pattern of the bleeding, which in many cases resolves spontaneously, basal body-temperature charts provide evidence of the absence or presence of ovulation and the function of the corpus luteum as measured by the thermogenic effect.

(b) Vaginal and cervical smears

Examination of the vaginal smear may provide most useful information on the 'endocrine status' of the genital tract, the occurrence of ovulation and the effect of sex hormone therapy (Wied 1968). To be of value, however, serial smears must be taken at intervals throughout the cycle, and the findings—including the various indices of maturation, such as the karyopyknotic index, the occurrence and degree of the 'progesterone effect' and the presence of navicular cells—must be related to the time of the menstrual cycle. Cervical smears must, of course, be taken in all cases, to exclude cervical carcinoma.

(c) Examination of the cervical mucus

The examination of the cervical mucus and the presence of ferning in the dried specimen may provide useful evidence of oestrogenic activity. If serial vaginal smears are being taken for exfoliative cytology a specimen of cervical mucus is easily obtained at the same examination. The finding of ferning in the first half of the cycle which subsequently disappears is good evidence of ovulation and of a normally functioning corpus luteum.

(3) OESTROGEN AND PROGESTERONE ESTIMATION

The estimation of the secretion of oestrogen and progesterone and metabolites in the urine and,

more particularly, the estimation of their levels in the blood is difficult, time-consuming and often difficult to interpret. They have in general been found of little value in dysfunctional uterine bleeding, except under special circumstances such as suspected feminizing tumour of the ovary.

(4) OTHER ENDOCRINE INVESTIGATIONS

Tests of thyroid and adrenal function are indicated in all cases where there is clinical suspicion of associated endocrine disease. Tests of pituitary function and X-ray of the skull may be indicated in cases of oligomenorrhoea, particularly when this is of sudden onset and has occurred for no apparent reason.

(5) HAEMATOLOGICAL INVESTIGATIONS

All cases of dysfunctional uterine bleeding must have a haemoglobin estimation and appropriate investigation of anaemia if present. Patients with persistent and unexplained dysfunctional uterine bleeding should have a blood smear, platelet count, bleeding and tourniquet test to exclude idiopathic thrombocytopenic purpura or other haematological cause for the bleeding.

(6) OTHER GYNAECOLOGICAL INVESTIGATIONS

It is sometimes very difficult to exclude an organic gynaecological lesion, particularly when it is not readily accessible to pelvic examination or uterine curettage. In all cases of presumed dysfunctional uterine bleeding which fail to resolve or to respond to treatment it is important to question the diagnosis. The patient must be re-examined and a repeat curettage performed. Two other gynaecological procedures, hysterosalpingography and laparoscopy may be of great value in certain circumstances. Hysterosalpingography is invaluable in diagnosing uterine polypi—particularly small, single fibroid polyps—and also malformations of the uterus, which may be easily overlooked on curettage. Laparoscopy is useful in the diagnosis of endometriosis, pelvic inflammation and unsuspected ovarian tumours, and should be performed in all obscure cases of uterine bleeding, particularly when this is accompanied by pain.

MANAGEMENT OF DYSFUNCTIONAL UTERINE BLEEDING

Three principles should be borne in mind:

(1) it is essential to take all appropriate steps to exclude organic disease, if necessary by repeated examination and special investigations;
(2) it is desirable to make a positive diagnosis of the endocrinopathy or functional defect underlying the dysfunctional bleeding;
(3) treatment should be individualized according to:
  (a) age, parity, emotional and social background of patient;
  (b) the severity, pattern and duration of the bleeding and the general disturbance of the patient;
  (c) the nature of the underlying defect, the prognosis and the likelihood of organic disease.

Three main measures are available in the treatment of dysfunctional uterine bleeding: uterine curettage, hormone therapy and hysterectomy; a general strategy of management is set out in Table 35.6. Before discussing these methods of treatment, it is first necessary to consider general measures conventionally employed.

(1) General measures

If the patient is exsanguinated and shows signs of shock, blood transfusion may, on rare occasions be necessary. It is usually advised, if bleeding is heavy, that the patient should rest in bed and be given sedation. Mental and physical rest is also advised, with active exercise between bleeding episodes. Attention to diet, carbohydrate restriction in obese patients, generous and well-balanced diet in undernourished patients and vitamins for all patients is recommended. Immediate investigation and treatment of anaemia is essential, as apart from improving the condition of the patient it may occasionally be an aetiological factor in the bleeding. This also applies to any other generalized endocrine or systemic disease which may be suspected. One of the most important steps is explanation and reassurance of the patient, and the investigation and treatment of any emotional or psychological disturbance, particularly in adolescents. The most useful general measure of all, however, is to ask the patient to keep a detailed menstrual calendar with a precise record of the amount of blood loss for 2 or 3 months. Most episodes of dysfunctional uterine bleeding will resolve spon-

Table 35.6. Strategy of management of dysfunctional uterine bleeding

Age	Dilatation and curettage	Hormone therapy	Hysterectomy
20 and under	*Only* if bleeding persists or is severe	*Whenever indicated*, e.g. excessive bleeding	*Never* (or almost never)
20–40	*Always*, but may be deferred (up to 3 months) if bleeding moderate, regular, and there is no suspicion of organic disease	*First resort* after dilatation and curettage	*Seldom*, only if bleeding is persistent or severe after dilatation and curettage and hormone therapy
40 and over	*Mandatory* in all cases	*Only after dilatation and curettage*, in absence of organic disease	*First resort* if bleeding is persistent after dilatation and curettage and hormone therapy

taneously and no specific treatment will be required. In those cases which persist, the menstrual calendar provides a precise and accurate record on which to base treatment.

(2) Uterine curettage

The possible therapeutic effect of uterine curettage in dysfunctional uterine bleeding has been much discussed. It seems to be generally agreed that during episodes of profuse bleeding curettage may have a useful therapeutic effect in arresting haemorrhage, probably by removing the necrotic areas of endometrium. Israel (1967) states 'it is not only the best therapeutic measure to arrest bleeding but it is also the most informative diagnostically'.

In less severe cases, and in the intervals between bleeding, the therapeutic value of curettage is a much more open question. Jeffcoate (1967) states 'any therapeutic value the operation may have is incidental.' Israel (1967b), on the other hand, claims, quoting his own experience and that of four other authors, that 'when curettage is employed as the sole treatment for prolonged dysfunctional uterine bleeding a cure rate of between 40% to 60%, depending upon the presence or absence of hyperplasia, is thereby attained'. It is possible to argue, as many gynaecologists have done, that this proportion of cases would have reverted to normal spontaneously. With the difficulty of obtaining suitably matched cases and carrying out a properly controlled series, it is probable that we shall never know the answer to this question. It is, however, largely an academic problem, as curettage is essential to exclude organic disease and to establish the diagnosis of dysfunctional uterine bleeding.

(3) Hormone therapy

(a) OESTROGENS

With the advent of potent progestational agents, oestrogens are now not often used by themselves in the treatment of dysfunctional uterine bleeding. This is because on discontinuing treatment they produce an oestrogen-withdrawal bleeding which is itself often prolonged or excessive. There is also the very small, but proven, increase in incidence of thrombo-embolic disease in patients given oestrogens (Inman *et al.* 1970). The incidence of thrombo-embolus, and the associated mortality, appears to be related to the dose of oestrogen. When considered as a group, women taking oral contraceptives containing 100 μg of ethinyloestradiol were found to have treble the mortality of women taking oral contraceptives containing 50 μg of ethinyloestradiol. If oestrogens are to be used in the treatment of dysfunctional uterine bleeding it will be necessary to show that the benefits outweigh the risks. Assuming that they receive oestrogens according to a regime similar to that for oral contraceptives, it will not be justifiable, on present evidence, to exceed 0·05 mg ethinyloestradiol or 1 mg stilboestrol daily. The specific instances which were previously regarded as indications for oestrogen therapy in dysfunctional uterine bleeding were:

(i) bleeding at ovulation;
(ii) polymenorrhoea due to shortened proliferative phase;
(iii) to arrest haemorrhage.

Oestrogens are very effective in controlling severe bleeding, but must be given in large doses. In view of the risk of thrombo-embolus, however, and the fact that other means of arresting haemorrhage are available, this method of treatment will presumably have to be abandoned.

(b) PROGESTOGENS

The introduction of potent, orally active progestogens has revolutionized the hormonal treatment of dysfunctional uterine bleeding. Unlike oestrogens, the different synthetic progestational agents have different effects, so that correct selection of the progestogen is important. Most of the progestogens are in part metabolized to oestrogens, but some are more oestrogenic than others. Others, particularly those derived from 19-nortestosterone, have an androgenic effect and appear to be more effective in controlling dysfunctional uterine bleeding. Most of the compounds are only available in formulations for oral contraception, when they are combined with various dosages of ethinyloestradiol or its 3-methylether, mestranol, as shown in Table 35.7.

Table 35.7. Progestational agents: 19-nortestosterone derivatives (formulation per tablet)

Trade name (manufacturer)	Progestogen (mg)	Oestrogen (μg)
SH 420 (Schering)	Norethisterone acetate, 10	None
Norlutin-A (Parke-Davis)	Norethisterone, 5	None
Primolut-N (Schering)	Norethisterone, 5	None
Orgametril (Organon)	Lynoestrenol, 5	None
Gestanin (Organon)	Allyloestrenol, 5	None
Anovlar-21 (Schering)	Norethisterone acetate, 4	EO*, 50
Gynovlar-21 (Schering)	Norethisterone acetate, 3	EO, 50
Norlestrin (Parke-Davis)	Norethisterone acetate, 2·5	EO, 50
Minovlar (Schering)	Norethisterone acetate, 1	EO, 50
Orlest (Parke-Davis)	Norethisterone acetate, 1	EO, 50
Norinyl-2 (Syntex)	Norethisterone, 2	3-M, EO†, 100
Orthonovin (Ortho)	Norethisterone, 2	3-M, EO, 100
Norinyl-1 (Syntex)	Norethisterone, 1	3-M, EO, 50
Orthonovum 1/80 (Ortho)	Norethisterone, 1	3-M, EO, 80
Metrulen (Searle)	Ethynodiol acetate, 2	3-M, EO, 100
Ovulen (Searle)	Ethynodiol acetate, 1	3-M, EO, 100
Ovral (Wyeth)	Norgestrol, 0·5	EO, 50
Enavid (Searle)	Norethynodrel, 9·85	3-M, EO, 150
Enavid (Searle)	Norethynodrel, 4·925	3-M, EO, 75
Conovid-E (Searle)	Norethynodrel, 2·5	3-M, EO, 100
Previson (Roussel)	Norethynodrel, 2·5	3-M, EO, 100
Noracyclin (Ciba)	Lynoestrenol 5·0	3-M, EO, 150
Lyndiol (Organon)	Lynoestrenol, 5·0	3-M, EO, 150
Lyndiol-2·5 (Organon)	Lynoestrenol, 2·5	3-M, EO, 75

*EO = Ethinyloestradiol.
† 3-M, EO = 3-Methyl-Ether-ethinyloestradiol (mestranol).

Progestational agents are used in three ways in the treatment of dysfunctional uterine bleeding:

(1) to arrest haemorrhage;
(2) cyclically throughout menstrual cycle (fifth to twenty-fifth days);
(3) cyclically in second half of cycle (twentieth to twenty-fifth day).

(1) The use of progestogens to arrest haemorrhage

The most generally accepted regime for the arrest of haemorrhage is to give a 19-nortestosterone derivative such as norethisterone without added oestrogen—for example, Norlutin-A (Parke-Davis) Primulot-N (Schering)—20–30 mg daily for 3 days or until the bleeding stops, which it usually does within 24–48 hr.

The patient should be warned that a withdrawal bleeding will occur 2–4 days after cessation of treatment, but that this will stop of its own accord after 4 days or so. Kistner (1969a) recommends that cyclical progestogen therapy should be commenced on the fourth or fifth day of the withdrawal flow. If endometrial biopsy has shown endometrium of a simple proliferative nature, cyclical progestogen therapy should be continued for at least 3 months. If the biopsy has shown endometrial hyperplasia or anaplasia, however, Kistner deems it advisable to continue cyclical therapy for 9 months to 1 year and then to perform repeat uterine curettage. Other authors prefer to arrest the haemorrhage and then await events, and to institute cyclical progestogen therapy only if there is further abnormal bleeding.

(2) Cyclical progestogen therapy in dysfunctional uterine bleeding throughout menstrual cycle

(a) Ovulatory bleeding

In ovulatory bleeding with polymenorrhoea and menorrhagia, normal cycles may be produced by giving 19-nortestosterone derivatives with oestrogens from the fifth to the twenty-fifth day of the cycle, according to the usual regime adopted for contraception (Table 35.8). This treatment is continued for three cycles. On

Table 35.8. Progestational therapy: dysfunctional uterine bleeding

	Dosage
(1) *To arrest haemorrhage* Norethisterone acetate (SH-420, Schering) Norethisterone (Norlutin-A, Parke-Davis; Primolut-N, Schering) Lynoestrenol (orgametril, Organon)	20–30 mg daily for 3 days
(2) *To control cycles** Anovlar Gynovlar Norlestrin Minovlar Orlest Conovid-E Previson Lyndiol 2·5	1 tablet from fifth to twenty-fifth day of cycle or for 21 days every 28 days
(3) *For premenstrual spotting* As for (2) above	One tablet twentieth to twenty-fifth day of cycle

* The compounds listed are those combined oral contraceptives available in the United Kingdom which have been reported to have a below average association with thrombo-embolic disease (Inman *et al.* 1970).

discontinuing treatment normal menstruation is said to be resumed in the majority of cases due to the 'rebound phenomenon with restoration of a normally balanced pituitary-ovarian-endometrial axis'.

As many types of ovulatory bleeding are thought to be due to a defective corpus luteum, it might be supposed that cyclical progestogen therapy in the second half of the cycle would produce normal menstruation. Klopper (1962) and Kistner (1969b), however, found that if treatment is given only during the 7–10 days before the next expected period benefit is unlikely to occur. To control menstrual bleeding it is necessary to give progestogen from the fifth to the twenty-fifth day and to inhibit ovulation. According to Klopper (1962) the main action of the 19-nortestosterone derivatives is to suppress the pituitary and ovarian function, and the endogenous production of ovarian steroids.

(b) Anovulatory bleeding

Anovulatory bleeding may be acyclical and is sometimes excessive, and measures such as dilatation and curettage or progestational therapy may be required to arrest the haemorrhage, as previously discussed. In adolescents and younger women of child-bearing age every endeavour should be made to find the cause of anovulation and to institute appropriate treatment. If no cause is found the excessive bleeding may be controlled by cyclical progestogen therapy for 2–3 months. In cases of endometrial hyperplasia, Kistner (1969a) recommends that cyclical progestogen therapy should be continued for 9 months to 1 year, when repeat curettage should be performed. Steiner et al. (1965) treated 23 patients with cystic and adenomatous hyperplasia and eight patients with carcinoma in situ of the endometrium with progestational agents. Repeat histological examination of the endometrium showed glandular atrophy and stromal decidua in every case, though one-third of the patients showed residual hyperplasia with 'drug effect'. None of the women, all of whom were menopausal or postmenopausal, developed endometrial carcinoma at the time or subsequently. Prolonged progestational therapy causes regression of benign cystic, adenomatous and atypical endometrial hyperplasia and may obviate the need for hysterectomy, particularly in the younger patient. Many gynaecologists nevertheless prefer abdominal hysterectomy, particularly in the premenopausal patient, because of the very small risk of progression to invasive carcinoma.

(3) Cyclical progestogen therapy in dysfunctional uterine bleeding in second half of cycle

Administration of progestogens in the second half of the cycle has found relatively little place in the treatment of dysfunctional uterine bleeding. One specific indication is of premenstrual staining which may be associated with 'irregular ripening' or a 'progestationally immature' endometrium. In these cases 19-nortestosterone derivatives, with or without oestrogen, should be given from the twentieth to the twenty-fifth day and repeated for three or more cycles. This treatment has the advantage of not suppressing ovulation. For those women who wish to avoid pregnancy, it will be necessary to revert to the standard contraceptive regime, with progestogen from the fifth to the twenty-fifth day of the cycle. If premenstrual staining continues while the patient is on treatment, an unrecognized organic cause should be suspected.

(c) ANDROGEN THERAPY

Androgens have been used extensively in the treatment of dysfunctional uterine bleeding in the past and are an effective form of treatment. Because of the fear of masculinization, most gynaecologists now prefer to use one of the new progestogens. Some gynaecologists, such as Israel (1967c), however, still feel there is a place for androgens in the treatment of dysfunctional uterine bleeding, particularly in the premenopausal women. Israel gives methyltestosterone 10 mg daily either for 7 days preceding menstruation in cyclical menorrhagia or in 15-day courses with 10-day rest periods in acyclical bleeding. He claims that this is highly effective and does not evoke even temporary masculinization.

(d) CLOMIPHENE

Clomiphene is an anti-oestrogenic compound which either directly or indirectly through the pituitary or hypothalamus stimulates the ovary to ovulate and to produce large quantities of oestrogen. It produces ovulation in 70% of anovulatory patients and has been used to stimulate ovulation in infertile patients, including those with oligomenorrhoea and with dysfunctional uterine bleeding. It has been used to treat anovulatory dysfunctional uterine bleeding and endometrial hyperplasia (Charles et al. 1964; Kistner 1968). The use of clomiphene is, however, not without side-effects and complications such as hot flushes and over-stimulation of the ovaries, with massive enlargement and ascites. If given by chance in an ovulatory cycle, it may produce polyovulation and multiple pregnancies. Clomiphene, therefore, should be reserved for the induction of ovulation in anovulatory infertility where pregnancy is desired, and should not be used in dysfunctional uterine bleeding (Bishop 1970).

(4) Surgery and radiotherapy

(a) UTERINE CURETTAGE

This is primarily a diagnostic procedure, though it may have a therapeutic effect, as previously discussed.

(b) WEDGE RESECTION OF THE OVARY

Wedge resection of the ovaries has been widely used in the treatment of patients with polycystic ovary or Stein-Leventhal syndrome with dysfunctional uterine bleeding. Goldzieher (1968) has reviewed the published series and found that an average of 80% of patients with polycystic ovary syndrome are reported to resume normal ovulatory menstrual function after wedge resection. The condition nevertheless does tend to recur, and the operation is now usually reserved until the patient wishes to have children, no treatment being given in the interval. Goldzieher, however, feels that treatment should be started as soon as the syndrome develops, particularly if this is associated with dysfunctional uterine bleeding, on the grounds that:

  (a) the bleeding may be severe;
  (b) endometrial hyperplasia is frequently found in association with polycystic ovary syndrome and there are at least 46 documented cases which were left untreated and developed endometrial carcinoma;
  (c) the underlying adrenal and/or ovarian production of androgens in untreated cases will cause obesity and hirsutes, which does not readily regress and may be responsible for the capsular fibrosis of the ovaries.

He advocates cyclical progestogen and oestrogen therapy from the time of the diagnosis 'until wedge resection or other alternative treatment becomes appropriate'. This treatment will control the bleeding and help counteract the effect of the androgen secretion.

Excellent results have recently been obtained in cases of Stein-Leventhal syndrome with clomiphene and human pituitary gonadotrophin particularly with regard to induction of ovulation and pregnancy (Kistner 1968).

The rightful place of wedge resection in the treatment of dysfunctional uterine bleeding associated with Stein-Leventhal syndrome is difficult to determine. It has recently been suggested, that, for the reasons given above and because wedge resection does reduce the abnormal androgen production, the operation should be performed whenever there is a persisting menstrual abnormality, even before the patient is desirous of having children. Clomiphene may then be given if necessary to induce ovulation at a later date when pregnancy is desired. Wedge resection would seem to be particularly indicated in cases of polycystic ovary syndrome associated with endometrial hyperplasia. Should a follicular cyst be found in such cases, puncture or rupture of the cyst will frequently terminate the bleeding episode.

(c) HYSTERECTOMY

The place of hysterectomy in the treatment of dysfunctional uterine bleeding depends upon the age of the patient. *In girls* and younger women of child-bearing age it should be a last resort. The need to preserve reproductive function and to avoid a psychologically mutilating operation is paramount. The possibility of remission of symptoms for up to 10 years from the onset of the dysfunctional bleeding (Southam & Richart 1966) more than justifies an ultraconservative approach. *In women in their thirties* it should be performed with reluctance, and only after full investigation and failure of hormone treatment. It may be considered in women who have completed their family, and much will depend on the wishes of the patient and her psychological attitude. *In older women over 40* hysterectomy should be considered in all cases of persistent or recurrent bleeding, particularly after a repeat curettage. In this age group the uterus is of less importance psychologically and, provided there is no contra-indication, hysterectomy is the treatment of choice in all cases where bleeding is persistent or severe. Though spontaneous cure may occur with the menopause, the possibility of a malignant or other organic lesion which may have been overlooked or may develop in the future fully justifies the operation in cases of persistent bleeding.

(d) RADIOTHERAPY

This probably has a small place in the treatment of dysfunctional uterine bleeding in women over 40 who are unfit for operation. Its advantages are that

(i) it is free of immediate risk;
(ii) it causes little disturbance to the patient;
(iii) it is effective in producing amenorrhoea in 95% to 99% of cases.

Its disadvantages are

(i) operation is not completely avoided, because it is essential to perform a dilatation and curettage in all cases to exclude malignancy;
(ii) the method is not without side-effects and complications. Doll & Smith (1968) in the long-term follow-up of 2,068 patients with metropathia haemorrhagica and other benign gynaecological disease treated by various forms of radiation over 20 years found that there was a fourfold increase in leukaemia in these patients, and an excess of cancer of the various organs in the heavily radiated areas.
(iii) the procedure leaves a damaged organ which may develop haematometra, pyometra or carcinoma. Corscaden *et al.* (1946) and Turnbull (1956) report an incidence of carcinoma of the cervix and endometrium of 1·5% in patients treated with radium or X-rays for benign uterine bleeding;
(iv) it does not permit organic disease to be definitely excluded;
(v) ovarian function is always suppressed, and menopausal symptoms are common;
(vi) in women under 40 amenorrhoea may not be permanent and menstruation, and ovulation may recommence after 1–2 years.

In most cases the disadvantages associated with radiotherapy heavily outweigh the advantages. Where radiotherapy is decided upon, external irradiation to the ovaries is now considered preferable to radium insertion, because the dose of radiation to the various pelvic tissues can be more closely controlled and because of the lower incidence and serious side-effects, such as radiation cystitis and proctitis, and of complications such as radium burns.

A safe and effective treatment is to irradiate the whole pelvis using two or four back and front fields with a calculated central dose of 1,200–1,500 r. This should be given in divided doses of 200 to 250 r for 5 days, which will avoid any general disturbance to the patient or skin reaction.

REFERENCES

ABELL M.A. (1968) In *Textbook of Gynaecologic Endocrinology* (edited by J.J. Gold). New York, Hoeber.

BENSON R.C. & DAILEY M.E. (1955) *Surgery Gynec. Obstet.* **100**, 19.

BISHOP P.M.F. (1970) *Br. med. Bull.* **26**, 22.

BROWN J.B., KELLAR R. & MATTHEW G.D. (1959) *J. Obstet. Gynaec. Br. Commonw.* **66**, 177.

CHARLES D., BARR W. & McEWAN H.P. (1964) *J. Obstet. Gynaec. Br. Commonw.* **71**, 66.

CORSCADEN J.A., FERTIG J.W. & GUSBERG S.B. (1946) *Am. J. Obstet. Gynec.* **51**, 1.

DIDDLE A.W. (1948) *Am. J. Obstet. Gynec.* **56**, 537.

DOLL R. & SMITH P.G. (1968) *Br. J. Radiol.* **41**, 362.

DRIESSEN L.F. (1914) *Zentbl. Gynäk.* **38**, 618.

FLUHMANN C.F. (1956) *The Management of Menstrual Disorders*, 5th edn. Philadelphia, Saunders.

FOWLER W.M. & BARER P.A. (1942) *J. Am. med. Ass.* **118**, 421.

GOLDSMITH R.E., STURGIS S.H., LERMAN J. & STANBURY J.B. (1952) *J. clin. Endocr. Metab.* **12**, 846.

GOLDZIEHER J.W. (1968) In *Progress in Infertility* (edited by S.J. Behrman & R.W. Kistner). Boston, Little, Brown, p. 351.

GOLDZIEHER J.W. (1970) In *Progress in Gynecology*, Vol. 5 (edited by S.H. Sturgis & M.L. Taymor). New York, Grune & Stratton.

HOLMSTROM E.G. & McCLENNAN C.E. (1947) *Am. J. Obstet. Gynec.* **53**, 727.

INMAN W.H.W., VESSEY M.P., WESTERHOLM B. & ENGELUND A. (1970) *Br. med. J.* **i**, 203.

ISRAEL S.L. (1970) *Menstruation in Scientific Foundations of Obstetrics and Gynaecology* (edited by E.E. Phillip *et al.*). London, Heinemann.

ISRAEL S.L. (1967) *Menstrual Disorders and Sterility*, 5th edn. New York, Hoeber.

Jacobs A. & Butler E.B. (1965) *Lancet*, **ii**, 407.
Jacobs W.M., Leazar M.A. & Lindley J.E. (1957) *Obstet. Gynec., N.Y.* **10**, 274.
Jeffcoate T.N.A. (1967) *Principles of Gynaecology*, 3rd edn. London, Butterworths.
Kistner R.W. (1964) *Gynecology. Principles and Practice.* Chicago, Year Book Medical Publishers.
Kistner R.W. (1968) In *Progress in Infertility* (edited by S.J. & R.W. Kistner). London, Churchill.
Kistner R.W. (1969) *Progestins in Obstetrics and Gynaecology.* Chicago, Year Book Medical Publishers.
Klopper A. (1962) *Proc. R. Soc. Med.* **55**, 865.
Kurzor R., Wilson L. & Birnberg C.H. (1953) *Fert. Steril.* **4**, 479.
Loraine J.A. & Bell E.T. (1966) *Hormone Assays and their Clinical Application*, 2nd edn. London, Churchill, p. 478.
Loraine J.A. & Bell E.T. (1967) *Obstet. Gynec. Survey*, **22**, 467.
Markee J.E. (1950) In *Progress in Gynecology*, Vol. 2 (edited by J.V. Meigs & S.H. Sturgis). New York, Grune & Stratton.
McBride J.M. (1954) *J. Obstet. Gynaec. Br. Commonw.* **61**, 691.
McKelvey J.L. & Samuels L.T. (1947) *Am. J. Obstet. Gynec.* **53**, 627.
Novak E.R., Jones G.S. & Jones H.W. (1965) *Novak's Textbook of Gynecology*, 7th edn. Baltimore, Williams & Wilkins, p. 625.
Okkels H. (1950) In *Menstruation and Its Disorders* (edited by E.T. Engle). Springfield, Thomas.

Palmer A. (1959) *Clin. Obstet. Gynec.* **2**, 153.
Quick A.J. (1966) *Obstet. Gynec., N.Y.* **28**, 37.
Salvatore C.A. (1958) *J. int. Coll. Surg.* **29**, 599.
Scheenberg N.G. (1970) In *Menstrual Disorders and Sterility*, 5th edn. New York, Hoeber, p. 274.
Schröder R. (1954) *Am. J. Obstet. Gynec.* **68**, 294.
Scott J.C. & Mussey E. (1964) *Am. J. Obstet. Gynec.* **90**, 161.
Simpson J.L. & Christakos A.C. (1969) *Obstet. Gynec. Survey*, **24**, 580.
Sippe G. (1962) *J. Obstet. Gynaec. Br. Commonw.* **69**, 1015.
Southam A.L. & Richart R.M. (1966) *Am. J. Obstet. Gynec.* **94**, 637.
Steiner G.J., Kistner R.W. & Craig J.M. (1965) *Metabolism*, **14**, 356.
Sutherland A.M. (1949) *Glasg. med. J.* **30**, 303.
Sutherland A.M. (1953) *Glasg. med. J.* **34**, 496.
Taylor E.S. (1965) *Essentials of Gynecology*, 3rd edn. Philadelphia, Lea & Ferbiger, p. 429.
Taylor M.L., Sturgis S.H. & Yohia C. (1964) *J. Am. med. Ass.* **187**, 323.
Traut H.F. & Kuder A. (1935) *Surgery Gynec. Obstet.* **61**, 145.
Turnbull A.C. (1956) *J. Obstet. Gynaec. Br. Commonw.* **63**, 179.
Vorys N. & Neri A.S. (1968) In *Textbook of Gynaecologic Endocrinology* (edited by J.J. Gold). New York, Hoeber.
Wied G.L. (1968) In *Textbook of Gynecologic Endocrinology* (edited by J.J. Gold). New York, Hoeber.

CHAPTER 36

THE MENOPAUSE AND CLIMACTERIC

The words menopause and climacteric are often used synonymously, although the meaning is not the same. The term menopause refers specifically to the final cessation of menstruation, whilst the word climacteric refers to the time during which the body is passing from the reproductive to the postreproductive periods of life and is becoming adjusted to a different hormonal and emotional environment. The menopause is related to the climacteric as the menarche is to adolescence.

THE MENOPAUSE

Menstrual periods finally cease in most women between the ages of 45 and 50 years. The periods may stop between 40 and 45 years or continue for a few years until 52 or 53 and may still be regarded as within normal limits. If the menopause occurs before the age of 40 years, however, it should be regarded as premature and may call for investigation to a limited or more extensive degree depending on the circumstances. Continued menstruation to the age of 54 or 55 must also be considered potentially abnormal and an indication for treatment even though the periods are still comparatively regular. Despite much speculation, no close relationship has been shown between the age of the menarche and that of the menopause. Fluhmann (1956) has reviewed scattered earlier literature on the age of menopause which is less extensive than that devoted to the menarche; it seems possible that over many years the average age of the menopause has

become later, just as the average age of the menarche has become earlier, suggesting a similar environmental or nutritional cause.

It seems likely that menstruation finally ceases when the ovary runs out of eggs. Marchant (1969) suggests that the number of ova are reduced from 200,000 about the age of 25 years to less than 10,000 between 40 and 45 years. Many follicles undoubtedly commence maturation and never achieve it in every cycle, thus relentlessly reducing the ovarian store until none remain to respond to gonadotrophic stimulation.

The cessation of menstruation is, in most cases, a gradual process, the periods becoming less frequent and the amount of loss smaller. Considerable variation occurs, however; many more cycles are anovulatory and the pattern may be established of a longer interval between periods and a greater duration of loss (see metropathia haemorrhagica, p. 516).

THE CLIMACTERIC

The changes which occur during the climacteric include general ones throughout the body as a whole, such as arthritic, bony and vascular changes, physical changes in the genital organs themselves and emotional alterations.

CHANGES IN THE GENITAL ORGANS

All the pelvic tissues undergo atrophic changes during the climacteric years. With the gradual disappearance of ova, and fibrosis of old follicles and corpora lutea, the ovaries become more sclerotic, until they have a whitish, somewhat wrinkled appearance and a fibrous consistency on palpation; histologically, arterial obliterative changes, fibrosis and traces of old corpora albicantia are to be seen. The fallopian tubes become similarly atrophic and appear thinner and shorter.

Atrophy of the corpus uteri and cervix takes place also, the former often to the greater extent, with a return to the 1:2 ratio of corpus/cervix encountered in childhood. Endometrial thinning is common, the glands becoming simple and fewer in number and the stroma more fibrous. Glands sometimes persist in cystic but inactive form, however, for many years (Fig. 36.1).

the amount of hair and subcutaneous fat, the tissues slowly become more flattened and shrunken, and the characteristic features less prominent.

ENDOCRINE CHANGES

Decline in oestrogen production is the principal cause of the physical changes in the genital organs during the climacteric era. The whole subject of postmenopausal urinary excretion of oestrogens, gonadotrophins and adrenal steroids has recently been reviewed by Procopé (1968). Total oestrogen excretion after the menopause has been reported to vary between 5·5 μg/24 hr (Brown & Matthew 1962) to 28·1 μg/24 hr

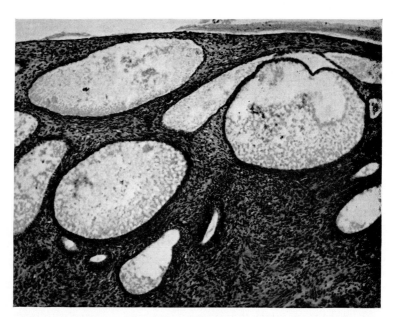

Fig. 36.1. Cystic inactive endometrium sometimes seen in the postmenopausal patient.

The vagina becomes less rugose, narrower and drier as time goes by, the walls taking on a smooth, shiny appearance. The epithelium is reduced to only a few layers of cells, without the maturation of superficial layers seen during reproductive life. Lactogenic bacteria disappear, the vaginal secretion is reduced and the reaction becomes alkaline. The vulva demonstrates diminution in

(Furuhjelm 1966). Furuhjelm's figures were obtained by employing the technique of Furhujelm & Waller (1958); the remaining modern authors have employed Brown's (1955) method, when the highest total oestrogen excretion reported has been 17·1 μg/24 hr.

Continued oestrogen reduction at a low level has continued, however, into old age, although its source is not known with certainty. It seems unlikely that the sclerotic ovaries of the elderly are the source of much oestrogen. It is more likely that some, perhaps most, is adrenal in origin. Bulbrook & Greenwood (1957) reported similar urinary oestrogen levels in patients whose ovaries had been removed and other patients who had undergone a spontaneous menopause, providing support for an extra-ovarian site of production. Even after oöphorectomy and adrenalectomy, however, some excretion of oestrogens in the urine continues, although the source of this is more mysterious still.

Progesterone production probably declines to some extent once corpus luteum formation becomes less frequent. Certainly, after the menopause reduced excretion of pregnanediol in the urine is reported.

As oestrogen production declines, there is a rise in gonadotrophin production as the pituitary is released from oestrogenic inhibition. Earlier workers (Loraine & Brown 1956), using essentially imprecise biological methods of assay, found extracts of postmenopausal urine to be approximately 20 times as potent as extracts from women within the reproductive era for total gonadotrophic activity. Whilst there is undoubtedly greatly increased gonadotrophic excretion in the postmenopausal period of life, it is not easy to express this in modern terms; in the laboratories at the Chelsea Hospital for Women values of 0·2–2 mg (second IRP–HMG) per 24 hr are recorded from normal premenopausal women and value two to ten times higher than this after the menopause; modern techniques of immuno-assay should determine the levels more precisely still. The marked rise in gonadotrophic excretion after the menopause is not continued for the rest of the patient's life, since excretion declines again after some 10 years or so.

Plotz & Friedlander (1967) suggests that there is no similar increase in the production of the other trophic hormones stimulating the thyroid, growth hormone and adrenal. 17-oxosteroids and 17-oxogenic steroids appear to be less directly influenced by the climacteric *per se*. 17-oxosteroid levels in urine are maximal about the age of 20–30 years, after which there is a steady decline to old age. The excretion of 17 oxogenic steroids is reported to be similar by Borth *et al.* (1957), although Lavell *et al.* (1957) showed that levels attained around the age of 25 years were thereafter maintained.

Clinical features

Most women experience symptoms of some kind related to the climacteric. For the most part, however, such symptoms are comparatively minor or, if more troublesome, are brief in duration. Less commonly, the years of readjustment prove troublesome ones, and the symptoms present are many, varied and difficult to treat. These symptoms are broadly vasomotor and emotional in nature.

The vasomotor disturbances (or hot flushes) consist of feelings of warmth over the body, especially in the region of the face, neck and upper chest. At the same time there is reddening of the effected area. Later, marked sweating may lead to a feeling of cold and shivering. The frequency of hot flushes is subject to great variation. Many women experience perhaps two or three daily for a few weeks only; others may have almost as many hourly, when they can cause considerable distress. Flushes occurring at night often give the greatest concern, since the patient can be awakened, sometimes several times, bathed in perspiration, and her rest is much interrupted. Hot flushes appear sometime after the actual menopause in most patients. They persist for weeks or months, gradually disappearing either following treatment or spontaneously. Exceptionally, they continue for longer, especially if treatment with oestrogens has been undertaken for too long at too high a dose level and resumed as soon as any further flushes are experienced. It is probable that in some cases the degree of distress the patient suffers is greater than the actual physical disturbance caused by the flushes. She, being aware of their origin, may be acutely embarrassed by them and may imagine that others will readily notice the flushing, will realize their implication and will know that she is 'in the change'.

The cause of the hot flushes is not known. It may be concerned with oestrogen deprivation, although this seems unlikely since other classes of individuals with oestrogen lack, such as prepubertal girls and patients with secondary amenorrhoea, do not experience them. A more likely explanation is that they are concerned with gonadotrophic excess. Objections also apply to this possibility, however, since not all patients with high gonadotrophic excretion suffer the symptoms, which can, in any event, be controlled by oestrogen dosages unlikely significantly to reduce gonadotrophic levels.

The emotional problems of the climacteric may present as many and varied physical symptoms, but their causation is concerned with 'change of life' and all that is believed to imply. To some women (and men) growing older is a concept which they find most unwelcome. Whether a woman accepts what is inevitable realistically or resists it strongly will depend on her own character and personality, the circumstances of her home, the attitudes of her husband and children and the habits of her friends in the community. A well-adjusted person, happily married, with a considerate family will probably act calmly to the change which is taking place and may require a minimum of medical advice and therapy. A patient with family and financial worries, one previously liable to neurotic symptoms, an older woman trying hard to hold a younger husband (or obtain one) and other women in similar difficult circumstances may react more violently and may require help.

Common symptoms at this time are headache, dizziness, sleeplessness, depression, apathy and irritability; pain in various sites may be a prominent complaint. Loss of libido may be a feature, although some women achieve greater enjoyment from intercourse after the possibility of a further pregnancy is removed. It is likely that the degree of satisfaction obtained from coitus in the past will influence the reaction here. In rare cases the climacteric may be attended by more profound disorders, such as involutional melancholia; very rarely, a marked increase in sexual desire amounting to nymphomania may be encountered.

OTHER CHANGES

The symptoms arising from the genital atrophy discussed above are not usually marked during climacteric years, although they may be more in evidence as the patient grows older still. Genital prolapse commonly becomes more troublesome at this time. Although the damage sustained formerly at childbirth is initially responsible for prolapse, the genital atrophy of the climacteric may cause sufficient additional weakness in the pelvic supports to make any degree of prolapse much worse, and bring the patient to the gynaecologist. Increasing weight may be an additional factor.

Menopausal irregularity and excessive menstrual loss are, of course, common at this time (see Chapter 35).

Osteoporosis begins in many bones during this period, and continues thereafter. The risk of coronary thrombosis, which is normally low in premenopausal women, rises about the time of the climacteric to become almost equal to that in men.

Treatment

The management of the climacteric problems will necessarily take several forms. Hot flushes, if infrequent and not greatly distressing to the patient, should initially be approached by explanation. Any consultation at this time is a good opportunity to outline what is really happening during the climacteric, in contrast to what many women mistakenly believe to be the case. A sympathetic doctor who is prepared to spend a little time talking and listening to his patient can do a lot to inculcate correct attitudes for the period of time ahead. Treatment for hot flushes should aim to reduce them and the disturbance they cause whilst allowing them to decline completely, which they will most certainly do over a few weeks or months. In many patients explanation alone may be sufficient; sometimes, mild sedative treatment may be needed as well. In other patients the use of oestrogens in diminishing doses is certainly indicated. Ethinyloestradiol 0·01 mg may be given daily and gradually reduced over a period of 1–2 months. Flushes should be reduced, but not eliminated, by this therapy, so adjustment of dosage may be required. If too high a dosage is given for too long, withdrawal bleeding may be caused or flushes may return to some extent as soon as the dosage is reduced, which may tempt the patient to take more tablets.

In some circumstances, oestrogens are not indicated. This may be so if there has been endometrial hyperplasia or endometriosis. Androgens in small doses may be helpful here, but if too much is used, or they are given for too long, voice changes or hirsutes may result.

For predominantly emotional symptoms psychotherapy should be employed. This does not necessarily involve a psychiatrist, but will certainly call for time, sympathy and encouragement from the family doctor and the gynaecologist. Careful general and local examination is essential to exclude associated disease and a cervical smear test must be taken. Reassurance of the absence of significant disease may in itself be very helpful.

Tranquillizing drugs can be useful, but only if they are combined with the approach outlined above.

Premenstrual tension

This name has been given to a group of somewhat ill-defined symptoms which occur during the week or so preceding menstruation. There is still speculation as to its aetiology and, to a less extent, its management.

Many women are aware of the imminence of their menstrual period, either by the occurrence of such local symptoms as pelvic heaviness and vague pelvic pain or more general ones of breast tenderness, weight gain, etc. Most do not find such manifestations unduly disturbing unless they become very pronounced. Premenstrual tension, as a clinical condition calling for medical attention, implies greater disturbance still. The symptoms of pelvic pain and breast discomfort may become much more marked and may be accompanied by less well-defined sensations, such as apprehension, irritability 'nervous tension', restlessness and insomnia. Headache, backache and aches and pains elsewhere may appear or become accentuated. Weight gain during this time is common and may exceed the gain of 2 or 3 lb which not uncommonly occurs during the premenstrual week. Symptoms are almost always relieved by the menstrual flow. In marked cases, however, this relief may be short-lived and the patient may describe the reappearance of symptoms after a few days, with gradual increasing intensity until the next period begins. The symptoms of premenstrual tension are not confined to the immediate premenopausal period of life but are more common at that time, a fact of possible aetiological significance.

The aetiology of premenstrual tension has been described to excess of oestrogens alone, or of oestrogen and progesterone, giving rise to sodium and water retention. It is believed by many, that psychogenic factors figure prominently in most cases of premenstrual tension. It is doubtful if they are ever the sole factor concerned but are chiefly responsible for turning the minor physiological changes of the premenstrual week into disturbing symptoms.

Management is best approached by attention to psychological factors, and the correction, by diuretics, of water retention. The thiazide group of drugs should give a satisfactory diuresis within a short period of time. The selected drug need be given only for the week or so during which symptoms arise and, for such a short period, electrolyte imbalance is unlikely to be precipitated. The psychotherapeutic approach should include enquiry into the patient's family and social background, financial or sexual worries and other possible related factors. If the premenstrual tension is not severe a sympathetic consideration of the patient's problems, together with the diuretic therapy outlined above, should be sufficient. In more severe cases the assistance of a consultant psychiatrist may be required and more intensive psychotherapy applied. The use of a tranquillizer may then be helpful. Hormone therapy is not indicated in most cases, but in refractory ones the use of a progestogen to inhibit ovulation may coincide with improvement; whether such a therapy can be regarded as specifically the reason for the relief of symptoms is less certain.

Long-term oestrogen replacement

Several of the physical changes, and the symptoms of the postmenopausal years, have been shown to be concerned with the decline in oestrogen production. The atrophic changes in the genital organs are certainly caused by oestrogen lack;

hot flushes are directly or indirectly concerned and are relieved by oestrogen therapy. Some of the symptoms labelled, in general terms, emotional—such as headaches, palpitations and dizziness—may be due, in part at least, to vasomotor instability, of which the hot flushes are the clearest sign. The osteoporosis and increased tendency to atherosclerosis are mianly due to oestrogen deficiency.

With so much evidently due to oestrogen deprivation, the suggestion has been made in recent years that oestrogen replacement therapy be used more frequently, and for longer, in some, or even all, women after the menopause. This practice has been more common in America than in Britain. Two reviews by Overstreet (1966) and Rogers (1969) deal with much of the evidence for and against this kind of regime.

To use oestrogens more often in women deprived of them would seem to have obvious advantages in some circumstances. In the present context it seems logical to employ them in patients having a spontaneous premature menopause or in others unlucky enough to undergo bilateral oöphorectomy at a youthful age. The frequency and severity of atherosclerosis in such women is raised. Rogers believes that they should be given oestrogens, and reports that the progress of atherosclerosis is delayed. It is less certain that the onset of atherosclerosis and its progress is likely to be influenced by oestrogens given after the menopause which occurs at the normal age. The widespread use of oestrogens for this reason has little to commend it, but their use in certain patients prone to such vascular disorders and demonstrating marked oestrogen lack might be indicated. Similar considerations apply to osteoporosis. The role of oestrogens here is still in some doubt, although the balance of evidence suggests that oestrogen deficiency is certainly an important, but not the only, factor. Overstreet (1966) suggests that only about 25% of untreated postmenopausal women ever develop significant osteoporosis; even this figure seems high. Clearly, oestrogen therapy for this reason is likely to be indicated only if obvious manifestations are present, when the drug might be employed in consultation with a colleague in the appropriate speciality.

In the management of flushes it has been stressed that the purpose of treatment is to diminish them and to reduce the distress caused by them, not to eliminate them completely. The period of vasomotor instability must be allowed to pass with as much relief as possible. Long-term therapy is not indicated here unless flushes are unusually protracted. The emotional disorders described are unlikely to be directly helped by oestrogens. Marked atrophic genital changes giving rise to symptoms are clearly an indication for oestrogen therapy, but in many instances short-term therapy and local application may be better than long-term replacement.

The dosage used has varied but is usually low, to avoid, or at any rate minimize, the risk of withdrawal haemorrhage. Overstreet believes Premarin 0·3 mg daily may be sufficient (but he would, if necessary, give much more). He suggests that small doses, sufficient to control the vasomotor or atrophic signs and symptoms, should be the aim. Rogers suggests the simple regime of stilboestrol 0·1–0·5 mg daily for 21 days followed by 7 days without treatment. Clearly, the risk in therapy of this kind is withdrawal haemorrhage, which, if it appears, may or may not be due to oestrogens. It is not clear from many reports on the subject if withdrawal haemorrhage occurs frequently or seldom, and if—and how—it is investigated to ensure that there is no malignancy. MacBride (1967) makes the surprising comment that this symptom was observed in *only* 60% of his small series of patients who still retained the uterus! Lack of experience in Britain with this type of treatment does not permit detailed comment at present, but it would seem that more than scientific considerations apply here. The philosophy of one culture group is not necessarily the same as that of another, and these differences appear to be important so far as concepts such as long-term oestrogen therapy are concerned. It appears doubtful if this kind of treatment has more than a very small place in gynaecological practice in this country at the present time.

REFERENCES

BORTH R., LINDER A. & RIONDEL A. (1957) *Acta endocr., Copenh.* **25**, 33.

Brown J.B. & Matthew G.D. (1962) *Rec. Prog. Horm. Res.* **18**, 337.

Brown J.B. (1955) *Biochem. J.* **60**, 185.

Bulbrook R.D. & Greenwood F.D. (1957) *Br. med. J.* i, 662.

Fluhmann C.F. (1956) *The Management of Menstrual Disorders.* Philadelphia and London, Saunders, p. 307.

Furuhjelm M. (1966) *Acta obstet. gynec. scand.* **45**, 352.

Furuhjelm M. & Waller R. (1958) *Acta endocr., Copenh.* **27**, 482.

Levell M.J., Mitchell J.L., Paine C.G. & Jordan A. (1957) *J. clin. Path.* **10**, 72.

Loraine J.A. & Brown J.B. (1956) *J. clin. Endocr. Metab.* **16**, 1180.

Marchant D.J. (1969) *Clin. Obstet. Gynec.* **12**, 705.

McBride W.G. (1967) *Postgrad. med. J.* (Supplement to December issue, p. 55).

Overstreet E.W. (1966) *Am. J. Obstet. Gynec.* **95**, 354.

Plolz E.J. & Friedlander R.L. (1967) *Clin. Obstet. Gynec.* **10**, 466.

Procopé B. (1968) *Acta endocr., Copenh.* (Supplement), 135.

Rogers J. (1969) *New Engl. J. Med.* **280**, 364.

CHAPTER 37

PROLAPSE AND STRESS INCONTINENCE
OF URINE

A major part of the gynaecologist's activity is concerned with the problems of prolapse and stress incontinence. Although the closeness of the relationship between prolapse and stress incontinence has been held in question (Jeffcoate 1961), this is a minority view, and from a practical point of view operative treatment for stress incontinence is most commonly combined with some procedure to rectify prolapse, and vice versa.

Prolapse can be interpreted, in its common form in the parous woman, as an exaggerated local manifestation of the ageing process. The arthritis, diminished muscle and mental power of old age may be regarded as similar manifestations. There is, however, the difference from the examples quoted that prolapse does not *always* present in advanced old age. In parous women prolapse *may* present any time after childbirth, but it most commonly causes the patient to come to the gynaecologist at, or shortly after, the menopause. 'Cure' in the commonly accepted sense is not the essential aim, but rather correction of any distressing symptoms without producing undesirable side-effects.

The term 'prolapse' in gynaecological connotation classically refers to prolapse of the uterine cervix. A numerical staging is sometimes employed:

Stage I: descent of the cervix to the introitus

Stage II: descent of the cervix, but not the whole uterus, through the introitus

Stage III: descent of the cervix *and* the whole uterus through the introitus.

In stage III, on palpating the prolapse the fingers can be made to meet above the uterine fundus outside the introitus. If the cervix or uterus has been removed prolapse may, of course, still occur, and in this situation the vaginal vault is the point of assessment.

Uterine descent is rarely an isolated phenomenon, being accompanied by prolapse of anterior and/or posterior vaginal walls in most cases. If the lower anterior vaginal wall lying in relation to the urethra descends, it is referred to as *urethrocele*; if the higher portion in relation to the bladder, as *cystocele*. Posteriorly, descent of the upper third of the vaginal wall which lies in contact with the pouch of Douglas is referred to as *enterocele* or *pouch of Douglas hernia*, and of the lower portion as *rectocele*.

AETIOLOGY AND
PREDISPOSING FACTORS

Prolapse is a consequence of failure of the uterine supports. This may be due to congenital weakness, but only a very small proportion of patients develop prolapse without the occurrence of pregnancy. True 'congenital' prolapse may be associated with spina bifida—overt or occult.

The effects of pregnancy and parturition are complex. The hormonal changes lead to softening of the ligaments and other supporting tissue. As the uterus enlarges and rises from the pelvis, stretching and distortion as compared to the non-pregnant state inevitably takes place. If the labour is long there will be more pressure of the foetal presenting part on the back of the symphysis, with bruising and, possibly, permanent damage. This type of effect will, of course, particularly tend to be operative if the second stage is prolonged. The stretching of the cervix in the first stage must produce changes. It is probable that the greatest damage is done if 'bearing down' occurs before full cervical dilatation, in which case the cervical supporting ligaments are subjected to the full strain of all the effort the mother can muster. Laceration of the cervix and of the lower genital tract in the second stage, with disruption of the pelvic floor musculature at delivery, all may play a part. In the third stage of labour (and after) injudicious downward pressure on the uterus in misguided attempts to deliver the placenta or control bleeding may do much harm. Inadequate repair of injuries or episiotomies have been claimed to be a factor, but this is doubtful. In this connection it is relevant that prolapse is virtually never found in association with a 'complete' or third-degree perineal tear. This is almost certainly because the unfortunate woman comes to utilize her levatores ani to try to get some degree of faecal continence. The development of levator tone and strength presumably prevents the occurrence of prolapse. In Victorian times it was claimed that too early ambulatory activity in the puerperium was important, but it is now generally accepted that this is of little relevance. There is no evidence that the modern trend to early ambulation has led to more prolapse, nor that primitive peoples, denied the benefit of obstetric care and puerperal rest, have a high incidence.

After congenital weakness and childbearing, the menopause is the most generally relevant factor in prolapse. It appears that with the withdrawal of the influence of the ovarian hormones on the pelvic tissues which are sensitive to them, the ligaments become atrophic and prolapse develops. Ultimately, a tendency to prolapse, produced by one or more of the factors mentioned, may develop into frank prolapse when chronically raised intra-abdominal pressure develops from a variety of causes, the most important being obesity and chronic bronchitis.

The main mechanical feature of uterine prolapse is stretching of the supporting ligaments. The transverse cervical and uterosacrals are the prime ones, but in addition the round and broad ligaments which have little or no supportive strength are also inevitably stretched. Divarication of the pelvic floor muscles is also usually a factor, as may be perineal muscular deficiency. Stretching of the vaginal walls and the tissues deep to them is another usual component. As the uterus descends, its body comes into the axial position, *not* the retroverted position as is sometimes stated. The pull of the broad ligament when descent occurs is such that both anteverted and retroverted uteri move into the axial position as they descend.

Elongation of the supravaginal cervix is a usual feature of significant uterine descent (Fig. 37.1); it is apparently a consequence of the tension on the supporting ligaments at the side of their uterine insertion. This anatomical feature is of particular relevance in relation to the Manchester repair technique.

For the uninitiated exploring the literature it is important to appreciate that different writers and operators have described different structures in the composition of the female pelvic supporting tissue, or given different names to imaginary structures. Ball (1966) reviews some of this controversy concerning tissues with labels such as 'pubovaginal fascia', 'subvesical fascia', 'fascia endopelvina', 'mesovaginal fascia', 'uterovesical ligaments', 'musculofascial hammock', bladder pillars', etc. He points out that many surgeons who claim to be suturing such fascias are in fact stitching the bladder, and he denies their existence as anatomical entities. Uhlenhuth & Nolley (1957) put a similar point of view in a paper entitled 'Vaginal fascia, a myth?'.

SYMPTOMS

Gross prolapse may be present without any symptoms. On the other hand, there may be a lot of discomfort from relatively minor degrees. One explanation put forward for this paradox is that the symptoms in the early stages are often related to abnormal tension on the nerves in the

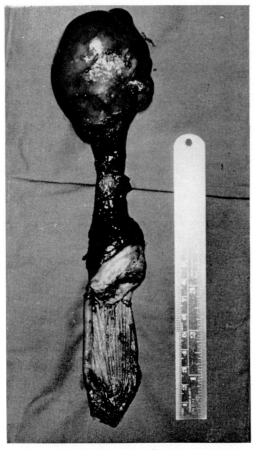

Fig. 37.1. Specimen removed at operation to repair prolapse in an 80 year-old woman. A vaginal hysterectomy was performed. Instead of the short uterine length usual at this age, the uterus is greatly elongated, this particularly involving the uterine isthmic region.

tissues being stretched by the prolapse, particularly the uterosacral ligaments. As the stretching increases, these nerve fibres, which are inelastic, become disrupted and cease to be a source of stimuli.

NON-URINARY SYMPTOMS

A sensation of an uncomfortable swelling at the introital region, referred to with uncanny frequency in patients' histories as 'something coming down', is the classic and commonest symptom. Sometimes there is also a 'dragging'

sensation. If ulceration of the protruding cervix has occurred there will be discharge, probably purulent, possibly blood-stained. Backache may occur, but evaluation is difficult. It is situated in the mid-line of the lumbosacral region, mediated through the nerve fibres previously referred to running in the uterosacral tissues. If backache is due to prolapse *it is only present when the patient is on her feet, gets worse as the day goes on, and is relieved by lying down.* Many women with prolapse have backache which does not have these characteristics, and it is almost certainly *not due to the prolapse.* If atypical backache is the main symptom, then operation is not indicated. If there are other reasons for operating then it should be made clear to the patient that there is no guarantee that her backache will be relieved.

There may be bowel symptoms if a large rectocele is present. In particular, the patient may be unable to empty her rectum unless she applies pressure on the bulging rectocele.

URINARY SYMPTOMS

(1) *Frequency*

Frequency of micturition is extremely common. It may be caused by urinary infection, or mechanical irritation because of the prolapse, or related to large volumes of residual urine. On the other hand, it may be a protective phenomenon aimed at minimizing the embarrassment of concomitant stress incontinence. It is essential that intrinsic urinary tract causes be excluded prior to performing a repair operation.

(2) *Urgency and urgency incontinence*

The desire to micturate develops with disconcerting speed and intensity to such an extent that the patient has to drop what she is doing and seek the refuge of the toilet. If she cannot do this quickly enough incontinence is the consequence.

Urgency is to be regarded as a disorder of the function of the detrusor muscle rather than a mechanical disturbance of the urethrovesical anatomy as is the case with stress incontinence. For this reason it is even more important in these patients to seek any possible intrinsic irritative lesion of the bladder. These symptoms are often associated with frequency, particularly if there is some form of cystitis. They may also be associated with stress incontinence, and such cases present a peculiarly difficult problem. It may be that in these cases a small quantity of urine gets into the upper urethra, with a sudden increase in the intra-abdominal pressure. If there is increased irritability this triggers off a detrusor contraction which would not otherwise occur (Beck *et al.* 1966; Warrell 1969). McLeod & Howkins (1964) and Beck *et al.* (1966) claim that some patients with urgency are relieved by repair operation. It is probable that in these cases elevation of the bladder neck corrects this type of detrusor stimulation from urine in the upper urethra. In general, however, *urgency is unlikely to be cured by anterior colporrhaphy in the absence of cystourethrocele.*

(3) *Retention*

If there is a large cystocele but a well-supported urethra, the patient may find she is unable to void urine when the prolapse is down. If she rests and the prolapse goes back, or if she manually replaces the cystocele, bladder emptying becomes possible. Occasionally, this situation may be associated with overflow incontinence. It is one which obviously predisposes to the occurrence of urinary infections.

(4) *Stress incontinence*

This is the urinary symptom which presents most problems in relation to prolapse. The term was first introduced by Sir Eardley Holland in 1922 to describe the occurrence of incontinence of urine on sudden elevation of the intra-abdominal pressure—as on coughing or sneezing.

Reference has been made to the controversy as to the precise relationship of stress incontinence and prolapse. The fact is agreed, however, that in a high proportion of cases of stress incontinence associated with prolapse, a repair operation with special attention to supporting the urethra and urethrovesical junction will lead to relief of the symptom.

In relation to the matter of stress incontinence it is important, if it is not volunteered as a symptom, to ask a specific question about it. Many women regard it as part of 'woman's lot' and hesitate to mention it even when it is causing them great inconvenience. Yet it is one of the most distressing symptoms in gynaecology, and its relief is one of the gynaecologist's greatest contributions. To assess its severity it is important to get from the patient a statement as to its *approximate frequency in terms of time*—hours, days or weeks. 'Occasional' is useless; it may mean once in a year, which is often not sufficient to justify surgery, or it may mean several times a day. In relation to this point it is interesting that in a study of 1,327 young nulliparae, Nemir & Middleton (1954) found that 52·4% had experienced some degree of stress incontinence. Stress incontinence must therefore be considered as a *relative* rather than an *absolute* phenomenon.

The severity of stress incontinence can also be related to the volume of urine in the bladder at the time stress incontinence is demonstrable (Low 1967; Beck *et al.* 1968). In severe cases incontinence is present when there is only a small volume of urine or introduced fluid in the bladder.

EXAMINATION

Examination to detect prolapse and determine its extent requires modifications of the techniques used for other gynaecological examinations. Fortunately, demonstration of prolapse is of importance *only* if the patient has symptoms which could be due to this or if hysterectomy is being contemplated for some other condition, so these modifications need only be employed in selected patients.

The vulva and introitus are first inspected and any obvious prolapse or perineal deficiency noted. Then the patient is asked to cough, and the situation reassessed. This is repeated when two fingers have been inserted to the vagina, and the posterior vaginal wall and perineum retracted. At the same time as observing any degree of cysto-urethrocele, any stress incontinence is noted. Stress incontinence may be absent initially but become evident when the perineum is retracted. True stress incontinence should cease to be evident when the anterior vaginal wall is elevated by pressure of the tips of the examining fingers in the region of the bladder neck (Bonney's test or sign).

While it is the preference of many gynaecologists to perform routine examination with the patient in the dorsal position utilizing a bivalve type of speculum for cervical exposure, to demonstrate a prolapse completely and assess its components the use of a Sims's speculum in the left lateral position is desirable. The degree of anterior wall descent on straining can be defined and the uterine descent also assessed. Where doubt exists, a gentle attempt may be made to apply a tenaculum forceps to the cervix; in most cases this produces little discomfort and traction may be exerted to determine the precise degree of descent. Of course, if the patient resents application of the forceps to the cervix, the procedure must be abandoned. The degree of posterior wall prolapse can be assessed by asking the patient to strain while the speculum is slowly removed. It is difficult on clinical examination to prove with certainty the presence of an enterocele. Theoretically, by asking the patient to cough while one examining finger is in the rectum and another in the vagina, it should be possible to detect an impulse in the hernial sac. However, it usually requires a degree of prior conviction to allow persuasion that such an impulse is palpable! Reference is sometimes made to 'high rectocele', but any herniation of the upper vaginal wall almost certainly betokens enterocele, regardless of whether an impulse has been elicited or not.

It is important to appreciate when examining a patient with regard to probable prolapse that *any* woman who has had a baby will inevitably show *some* deficiency of the perineum and some laxity of anterior and posterior vaginal walls. Categorizing a particular degree as constituting prolapse is highly subjective.

If the cervix has been protruding from the introitus when the patient has been on her feet it is very difficult to get a satisfactory cervical smear. All the cells which would be removed by the spatula have already been rubbed off by friction on underclothing. This situation, even if the protruding cervix is not evident at examina-

tion on the couch, can be surmised by the dull, matt appearance of the cervical epithelium compared with the moist, glistening appearance of the normal cervix with its thin coating of mucus.

It may be difficult to decide whether the whole uterus is outside the introitus; passing a uterine sound will give the answer. It is often found that the uterus is very much longer than normal, due to elongation of the supravaginal portion of the cervix uteri, the site of attachment of the supporting ligaments (Fig. 37.1).

A bimanual examination must never be omitted no matter how obvious the diagnosis may be on inspection. Just occasionally, prolapse is caused by the weight of a pelvic mass; to miss such a cause is a major blunder. A general medical examination including neurological assessment is, of course, important.

Specialized investigations have little place in relation to prolapse, but where there are urinary symptoms, special urinary tract investigations are, of course, often indicated. Bacteriological examination of the urine should be performed, together with checking of the volume of residual urine, bladder capacity, cystoscopy, blood urea and, sometimes, intravenous pyelography. Cystometry is helpful in some cases. Normally, the pressure rise from 'empty' to 'full' is less than 10 cm of water; if it is over 15 cm the bladder is abnormally irritable, probably due to inflammatory effects (Warrell 1969). Cysto-urethrography may be considered, but it is a procedure which is more relevant to research investigation than clinical assessment. It may, however, be worth performing to help define the anatomical situation precisely in cases where one operative procedure for stress incontinence has failed and a secondary operation such as a fascial sling is being contemplated. The same applies to cystometry. Where urological problems exist it is always wise to bear in mind that these may have a neurological basis and carry out an appropriate examination.

PRE-OPERATIVE EVALUATION

If operation is contemplated, critical assessment must be made. The first question concerning which the gynaecologist must satisfy himself before considering operating on a patient with prolapse, is that of *whether the patient has symptoms*. This becomes increasingly important in these days of 'well-woman' examination facilities; in the course of such examinations many women are ill-advisedly informed of minor gynaecological abnormalities such as prolapse which carry no risk to life. Only in most exceptional circumstances would it be justifiable to operate on a woman with symptomless prolapse, for example if prolonged protrusion of the cervix was causing chronic cervical ulceration or if there was evidence that the prolapse was producing hydro-ureter and hydronephrosis with renal damage (Te Linde 1966).

If the answer to this is in the affirmative, he must then decide *whether her symptoms are referable to her prolapse*. A woman informed of a prolapse of which she has not been aware may attribute a multitude of unrelated symptoms. Those which may reasonably be attributed to prolapse have been detailed. Any other symptoms of which a woman with prolapse complains should be regarded as unrelated and unlikely to be cured by any operation for the prolapse.

It must next be decided *whether the symptoms are sufficient to justify operation*. In coming to a decision about this it is helpful to explain frankly to the patient that any prolapse present carries no risk to life; it is purely a matter of her own comfort and convenience. If operation is decided against, this decision can be reviewed at any time, and should the prolapse increase in degree the operation is not going to be technically more difficult or less likely to be successful. The only circumstance in which any element of positive persuasion is indicated is when the patient has obviously got distressing symptomatology, such as severe stress incontinence, yet is hesitant about having an operation. It should then be explained that the operation mortality is negligible and the complication rate low, while, presuming proper selection, the relief rate is high.

The general condition must obviously be taken into consideration. However, the patient who is able to be active enough to get prolapse symptoms is almost always fit for operation, given proper care for any disease she may have. Exceptions

to this generalization are few. More commonly, a decision having been made about operation, it is appropriate to take measures to correct general abnormalities which predispose to the occurrence of prolapse, such as obesity or chronic bronchitis. If such factors are present, optimum relief must always be obtained before operation. Furthermore, the patient should be made aware that the prospects for long-term success of the procedure will be much greater if recurrence of obesity or bronchitis does not occur. If there has been a recent pregnancy, operation should be delayed for at least 6, and preferably 9, months. Local factors such as ulceration may also need attention, and any urinary infection treated.

A most important point to be decided before operation is whether coitus is taking place. In a woman still in the reproductive life it should always be assumed that it may be attempted in the future. After the menopause, if coitus has ceased it may influence the choice of procedure. If there is a large or recurrent prolapse, or the tissues are of poor quality, then it may be considered wise to narrow the vagina deliberately, and thus obtain a better repair. It is important to emphasize to the patient that in the ordinary course of events a repair operation should not preclude subsequent coitus, and to explain that if it should prove difficult postoperatively this can be put to rights readily by giving oestrogens and/or dilating the vagina.

A clear decision should be taken at the time of the pre-operative assessment, in the light of the coital situation and all other factors, precisely what type of repair operation should be performed. This plan should be adhered to unless major unexpected problems arise in the course of the operation. Whether or not a posterior repair is performed, for example, is not a matter which should be left to the aesthetic whims of the operator on the day in question.

NON-OPERATIVE THERAPY

Gross prolapse cannot be cured by measures other than surgery. When there is a minor degree of prolapse, however, a number of conservative measures may at least alleviate some of the symptomatology temporarily. The main procedures which are relevant are (a) physiotherapy to the pelvic floor; (b) the use of mechanical pessaries; and (c) measures to improve general condition, such as dieting. It might be claimed that rest is another effective form of conservative therapy. All prolapses, however, are naturally relieved by rest, and patients recognize this instinctively. The whole aim of treatment of prolapse is to keep the patient symptom-free and active with *the avoidance of enforced rest*. It seems inappropriate in this light to regard 'rest' as an acceptable therapy. An exception is the special circumstance of an ulcerated procidentia, when a period of rest is extremely helpful in allowing the ulceration to heal and make the condition amenable to surgery. Administration of small doses of oestrogens to postmenopausal women with this complication may accelerate healing.

(a) *Physiotherapy and electrical techniques*

Various forms of pelvic floor exercises are widely practiced in the puerperal phase. It is presumed that they are effective in reducing the incidence of prolapse, and they certainly can do little harm. When prolapse has already developed it is debatable whether any benefit will result, but if the patient is anxious to avoid operation it may be worth trying. It is difficult for a patient to know when she is contracting her levators, and an instrument which helps in this respect is Kegel's perineometer (Kegel 1948, 1956). This is a rubber or plastic phallic device with a basal flange which fits into the introitus. From the cavity of this a tube runs to a pressure gauge. The patient can then read off pressure achieved each time she does her exercises.

Electrical stimulation has been utilized in various ways to try to relieve stress incontinence. Intermittent faradism may be applied to the levators, but unless in unusual situations, this is probably not superior to voluntary exercising. Implantation techniques have been experimented with increasingly in relation to various forms of incontinence, and Caldwell and his colleagues (1968) report on 31 cases in which a radio-frequency transformer was used to pass electrical energy to an implanted electronic unit from which leads conveyed the impulses to the selected excitation points. They used 4-V pulses, lasting 1–4 msec, repeated 20 times per second. The electrodes were sited at points 5 cm deep, one each side of the perineum 5 cm posterior to the pubic symphysis and 1·5 cm from the midline. These points were found on perineal approach for testing, but the definitive electrodes were passed down to them from an abdominal incision made to insert the electronic receptor unit. Twenty-three out of 31 cases were regarded as successes; most of the failures were due to technical problems.

Alexander & Rowan (1968), Hill *et al.* (1968), de Soldenhoff & McDonnell (1969) and Paterson & Harrison (1970) have described electrode-bearing pessaries which have been of some value in relief of stress incontinence.

(b) *Mechanical pessaries*

A generation ago, mechanical pessary therapy for prolapse was one of the gynaecologist's main activities. The frequency with which pessaries are used, however, has diminished remarkably in the last few decades. The reasons for this are several. It has come to be appreciated that the chronic irritative effect of the pessaries upon the vaginal epithelium, which often produces ulceration, can proceed to the development of carcinoma (Russell 1961). This, of course, is particularly liable to occur if the pessary is neglected. There has been a great advance in the safety of surgery and anaesthesia, and it has come to be appreciated that advanced years—a common feature of prolapse patients—is not at all a necessary contraindication to surgery. Providing careful preoperative assessment and care is applied, old ladies withstand repair operations extremely well to day. It is, in fact, very unusual to encounter a patient who is sufficiently active to be symptomatically troubled by prolapse yet is not fit to undergo operation. Fell (1963), for example, recorded operations for prolapse on 44 women over 70 years of age; 18 had vaginal hysterectomy and repair and 15 had Manchester-type repairs. The mortality was nil, the complication rate low, and the results very gratifying. No patient was refused operation on account of age, and this is now widespread policy.

There are, however, a number of circumstances in which it is still appropriate to consider the use of a pessary—usually on a temporary basis. If there is likely to be delay in operation due to hospital waiting-lists or other factors, then it may be considered appropriate to insert a ring pessary. Prolapse in early pregnancy and the immediate postpartum phase are other indications for the use of a pessary. Pessaries may also be employed to assess whether the patient's symptoms are in fact due to the prolapse; all prolapse symptoms except stress incontinence should be relieved effectively by pessary control. Once a time for surgery is fixed it is important to remove the pessary a few weeks in advance, in order that any ulceration will heal.

Modern pessaries are superior to earlier types. Polythene ring pessaries of a semi-rigid nature can become mouldable when heated in tap water. Non-toxic polyvinyl chloride (PVC) ring pessaries are also available, and possess the elasticity of rubber but are much less irritant than the old-fashioned rubber pessaries. No special toilet procedures are required when the pessaries are *in situ*, but they should be removed and cleaned every 3–6 months. At this time the posterior fornix should be inspected carefully for any sign of ulceration. If this is present, the pessary should not be reinserted.

(c) Measures to improve the general condition

The two common general conditions relevant to the problem of prolapse are obesity and chronic bronchitis. These are not only major predisposing factors to prolapse but, as has been mentioned, the presence of one or both militates strongly against successful operative cure. Any benefit to prolapse already present by correcting them is probably insignificant, but the symptoms may be less troublesome, sometimes to such an extent that the patient no longer desires operation. Both obesity, a consequence of over-eating, and chronic bronchitis, frequently secondary to over-smoking, are often beyond the capacity of medical therapy to cure. To ask a woman who has a high calorific intake of sweetmeats and smokes heavily to desist immediately from both these weaknesses of the flesh, is to ask the impossible. It must rest

with the clinician's acumen to decide when maximal benefit has been achieved and operation should be undertaken.

Conservative measures which may be helpful in relation to urgency and urgency incontinence are referred to below (p. 565).

OPERATIVE TREATMENT

Many and varied are the operative manœuvres which have been utilized to try to correct prolapse and its attendant symptoms. No attempt will be made to catalogue these, for which texts in operative gynaecology should be studied (Howkins 1968; McLeod & Howkins 1964). Instead, attention is directed to the main principles common to most successful procedures. These involve (i) excision of redundant or bulging skin over the vaginal walls and of any pouch of Douglas hernial sac; (ii) supporting the tissue deep to the areas of excision by deep suture; (iii) narrowing the vagina may also be done as a deliberate policy particularly in elderly widows by means of a perineorrhaphy but both of the first two procedures may have this unintentional effect; (iv) amputation or excision of such uterine tissue as may be considered desirable; and (v) supporting the vaginal vault utilizing the 'ligamentum transversale colli' (transverse cervical, cardinal or Mackenrodt's ligament) and the uterosacral ligaments.

It is the last of these procedures which is the cornerstone of any sound operation for uterine prolapse. Much disputation has taken place as to whether vaginal hysterectomy or a cervical amputation procedure, as in the Manchester operation (Fothergill 1914), is preferable. Most of this has been irrelevant, however, as the important feature is not the uterine tissue excised but the efficiency with which the vaginal vault is supported by shortening the transverse cervical and uterosacral ligaments. Whether this is done by plicating the ligaments or suturing the divided, shortened ligaments anterior to the cervix or to the vaginal vault, the end-result is that precisely the same structures are carrying the support of the vaginal vault. *Vaginal hysterectomy* per se *does nothing to cure prolapse; it is the concomitant suturing to support the vaginal vault which is important.*

In the majority of cases, whether to perform a Manchester-type repair or a vaginal hysterectomy with repair is a matter which can, and should, be left to the preference of the individual surgeon concerned. There are, however, a number of circumstances in which specific factors weigh in favour of one or other procedure. For example, if the patient is over 40 and has no desire or expectation of further children but is experiencing menstrual disturbance attributable to dysfunctional uterine haemorrhage or small fibroids, then there is obviously much to be said in favour of vaginal hysterectomy as part of the repair procedure. If, on the other hand, the individual has a strong psychological aversion to hysterectomy, then it is wrong that the operator should let his own personal operative preference be overriding, if it be for vaginal hysterectomy. It is, of course, obvious that if subsequent pregnancy is desired, vaginal hysterectomy should be avoided. But the classical Manchester procedure is not suitable either in such circumstances and some modification is usually appropriate (see below, p. 556).

Whatever procedure is performed to support the vaginal vault, this is combined with such measures as may be necessary to deal with (a) *anterior vaginal wall prolapse and/or stress incontinence*; (b) *enterocele* (or herniation of the pouch of Douglas); (c) *rectocele*. Only in a small proportion of cases is it appropriate to perform one of these ancillary procedures in isolation, but an example is when there is stress incontinence but no vault prolapse. The methods employed are not significantly affected by whether the main procedure has been a vaginal hysterectomy or a Manchester operation.

(a) ANTERIOR COLPORRHAPHY

It is virtually always desirable to perform an anterior colporrhaphy whenever a vaginal vault-supporting procedure is performed, *even if there is no anterior wall prolapse evident*. The reason for this is that although stress incontinence may not have been present prior to operation, the adjustment in anatomical relationships produced by the repair of vault prolapse may result in the development of stress incontinence *as a consequence of the operation*. Obviously some sort of anterior wall procedure will always be indicated if there *is* pre-operative stress incontinence.

A triangle of vaginal skin is excised, apex towards the urethra. After lateral dissection to free bladder, bladder neck and urethra, supporting stitches are introduced, with particular emphasis to the region between the urethral meatus and the urethrovesical junction. Where stress incontinence has been a problem, more attention is paid to the extent and tightness of this suturing. These will have the effect of (i) compressing the urethra; (ii) lengthening the urethra—as measured by how far a balloon catheter can be drawn down (this is strictly a measure of corrected urethral funnelling); and (iii) increasing the urethrovesical angle*. All of these changes will tend to help towards achievement of urinary continence in the face of suddenly increased intra-abdominal pressure—the factor productive of stress incontinence. Different surgeons use different tissues for this purpose. Some (e.g. Kelly & Dumm 1914 and Kennedy 1937) place plicatory stitches in the so-called pubocervical or vesical fascia, while others utilize the pubococcygeus muscle, approximating it in the midline beneath the urethrovesical junction (Pacey 1949), or join the divided muscle beneath the urethra (Ingelman-Sundberg 1947).

(b) REPAIR OF ENTEROCELE

A common cause of failure of a repair operation to relieve the patient's sensation of 'something coming down' is failure to deal with, or deal *adequately* with, a hernia of the pouch of Douglas or enterocele. Again, practice should be the same whether a Manchester type of repair or vaginal hysterectomy and repair has been performed; in *every case* the pouch of Douglas should be explored for any redundant peritoneum. If present this should be excised, the pouch closed,

---

* Urethrovesical angle refers to the angle between the bladder and the urethra as demonstrated by laterally projected X-rays when bladder and urethra are occupied by contrast media (Roberts 1952; Jeffcoate & Roberts 1952).

and supporting stitches inserted to approximate the uterosacral ligaments in the mid-line to prevent further herniation.

A particular problem arises when enterocele develops after vaginal hysterectomy, as it is much more prone to do than after a Manchester repair. (It may also develop after abdominal hysterectomy done for some condition quite unconnected with prolapse.) An attempt may be made to repair the enterocele vaginally. After dissecting redundant vaginal wall and peritoneal tissue the problem is to secure support for the vault of the vagina. It is usually difficult, or impossible, to define strong uterosacral ligaments, but advantage must be taken of whatever tissue can be defined. Prospects of success are greatly enhanced in this difficult situation if the age and marital situation make it possible to narrow the vagina to one-finger capacity.

If this technique fails or is considered inappropriate, then an abdominal approach may be tried. Various techniques of vault suspension have been described, including the use of external, oblique aponeurosis strips, cut as for the Aldridge operation, passed through the broad ligaments along the course of the round ligaments and attached to the vaginal vault (Howkins 1968). At the same time, the hernial sac is obliterated and the uterosacral tissue shortened and attached to the vaginal vault to give additional support.

(c) POSTERIOR COLPOPERINEORRHAPHY

The most controversial of the additional procedures which may be performed is posterior colpoperineorrhaphy, a procedure basically designed to correct posterior vaginal wall prolapse (rectocele) together with any perineal deficiency. Triangles of vaginal and perineal skin are excised, their bases at the introitus. The levatores ani are stitched together anterior to the rectum before approximating the lateral edges of the excision. If the patient is elderly and coitus has ceased there is much to be said for this procedure, which automatically brings about narrowing of the vagina and will thereby reduce the possibility of recurrence of prolapse. If intercourse is taking place, avoiding interference with this is much

more important than other considerations. Formerly, a colpoperineorrhaphy was performed rather as an after-thought to almost every repair, but thanks to the appreciation that it frequently interferes with subsequent coitus (Francis & Jeffcoate 1961), it has been dispensed with as a routine by many surgeons. This trend has also been accelerated by the appreciation that rectoceles and perineal deficiency rarely cause symptoms *per se*. Furthermore, the postoperative convalescence is much less uncomfortable when the perineum is left intact; there are more sensory nerve fibres in this area than in any other which may be involved in a vaginal repair.

The question of a sterilizing procedure should always be considered at the time of any repair operation. No pressure should be brought to bear on the patient in this regard but, rather, she should be made aware that it is usually possible to combine it with the repair without extra risk or longer hospital stay, and if she is confident that she has completed her family it may be advantageous. In such circumstances if the operator favours vaginal hysterectomy and this is practicable it is, of course, the obvious procedure. If this should not be the case then tubal ligation may be performed at the same time as the Manchester operation, through either anterior or posterior fornix, according to choice.

A number of procedures are now of little more than historic interest in most centres. These include colpocleisis (vaginal obliteration); Le Fort's operation (suturing the anterior and post-vaginal walls together in the mid-line, leaving a channel down each side); the interposition operation of Watkins and Wertheim (stitching the anteverted uterus under the bladder base); ventrofixation or hysteropexy (attachment of the uterus to the anterior abdominal wall); and the Spalding-Richardson operation (amputation of the cervix followed by supravaginal hysterectomy with preservation of the cervical isthmus).

Various operations have been used in the past to support the prolapsed uterus from above. Most of these have fallen into disuse with appreciation that vaginal procedures devised on a basis of knowledge of the main supporting function of the uterosacral and transverse cervical ligaments are highly effective. There are, however, a very few cases in which abdominal support may be considered, and procedures of this type have been described by Arthure & Savage (1957) and Shirodkar (1967). Shirodkar devised a sling operation* for use when the utero-sacral tissues are of poor quality. A strip of Mersilene tape is passed round the rectum, attached to the posterior aspect of the uterus close to the insertion of the uterosacral ligaments or, if subsequent childbearing is not desired, round the front of the uterus. Posteriorly, the tape is attached to the anterior of the anterior longitudinal lumbosacral ligament; on the left side it is also attached to the psoas muscle to avoid pressure on the rectum.

Operations for prolapse in the young woman

In patients who are past the child-bearing age, the decision to operate and the choice of operation present little difficulty. The situation is very different in the younger age group, however, when the woman may specifically want more children or, alternatively, the gynaecologist knows that some future change in her social situation may cause her to desire another child. The standard operations—vaginal hysterectomy and repair or the Manchester type of repair—are absolute and relative barriers respectively to further conception. In these circumstances very careful thought has to be given to the best course. Formerly, it was general policy to defer repair operations until the child-bearing era was past, but this is now generally accepted as being unreasonably harsh on many patients. If operation is denied to a woman of 25 years who happens to have stress incontinence associated with pro-lapse, she is likely to have to endure many years of misery, as the non-operative measures available are most unlikely to produce relief. Accordingly, search has been made for modifications of tech-

nique which will preserve fertility and make miscarriage due to cervical incompetence un-likely.

The simplest modification is to perform a Manchester type of operation but restrict the amount of cervix amputated. This will reduce the risk of subsequent cervical incompetence should a pregnancy occur. Such an approach will not, however, affect the matter of infertility said to be a consequence of covering the cervical stump with vaginal epithelium inimical to the ascent of the spermatozoa.

Three other procedures are worth considering. (a) The Hunter operation (Hunter 1938); (b) the 'fore-quarter' operation (Currie 1953); and (c) Shirodkar's (1967) 'extended Man-chester' operation. All these procedures adopt the basic principle of the Manchester repair, in utilizing shortening of the transverse cervical or cardinal ligaments as the mainstay of the repair.

(a) The Hunter operation

This operation devised by one of the Manchester school, involves no interference with the cervical canal whatever. Two circumferential incisions are made round the cervix. One is close to the external os and the other is at a higher level (usually approximately 2–3 cm higher). The vaginal epithelium between these is removed, and by upward dissection in the lateral position the transverse cervical ligaments can be ap-proached and sutured together anterior to the cervix, affecting elevation. The raw epithelial edges are then approximated by radially placed interrupted sutures. Anterior colporrhaphy is performed if necessary, which it usually is.

(b) The 'fore-quarter' operation

This treatment involves the excision of a wedge of tissue from the anterior segment of the cervix. From this exposure access to the cardinal liga-ments is obtained. The canal is then recon-stituted and the transverse cervical ligaments approximated anteriorly as in the other pro-cedures. Again, no cervical length is lost and it is therefore unlikely that cervical incompetence would be a subsequent problem (Figs. 37·2–37·6).

---

* It is important to appreciate that the term 'sling operation' is used in two entirely distinct ways in relation to prolapse and stress incontinence. There is one group of sling procedures in which the sling passes beneath the urethrovesical junction, and the aim is to control stress incontinence which is present without prolapse. The second group of procedures is designed to support the uterus or vaginal vault from within the abdomen.

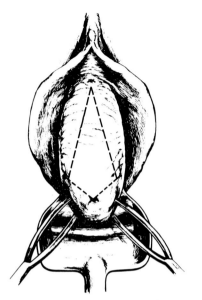

Fig. 37.2. Incision for 'fore-quarter repair operation'.

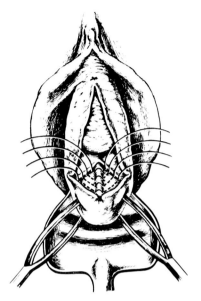

Fig. 37.4. The cervix is reconstituted.

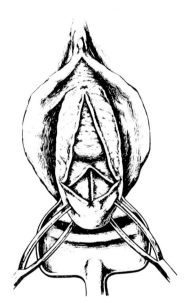

Fig. 37.3. After bladder dissection a wedge has been removed from the cervix, excising its 'fore-quarter'.

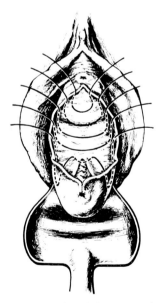

Fig. 37.5. Deep supporting stitches are now inserted; the one proximal to the cervix is passed out laterally to take the transverse cervical ligaments which are pulled anterior to the cervix by it, thereby elevating the cervix and drawing it backwards.

558   CHAPTER 37

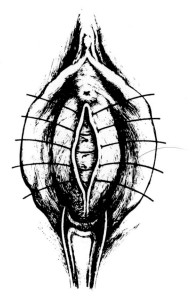

Fig. 37.6. The vaginal wall is closed in the usual manner.

(c) The Shirodkar 'extended Manchester' operation

This operation involves dissecting the anterior flaps lateral to the uterus and exposing the attachment of the transverse cervical ligaments. The incision is extended posteriorly round the cervix and any enterocele dissected free. The pouch of Douglas is opened and the uterosacral ligaments divided close to the cervix and mobilized from the peritoneum and the transverse cervical ligament. (This usually involves sharp dissection.) These are ultimately crossed anterior to the cervix. The posterior vaginal wall incision is then closed and the divided uterosacral ligaments brought through to the anterior position and stitched together on to the front of the cervix, adjusting the tension appropriately to maintain the cervix at its proper height. The basis of this procedure is very similar to the Hunter technique, except that the elevating sling is composed of utero-sacral, rather than transverse, cervical tissue.

OTHER OPERATIONS FOR STRESS INCONTINENCE

In a variable proportion of cases of stress incontinence vaginal repair fails to effect cure, and other procedures must be sought. This should not be more than a very small number, however, provided good case-selection has been followed by skilled surgery. Just occasionally, there are cases in which it seems that a vaginal repair would be futile. To meet such infrequent contingencies three main approaches have been developed; (a) sling operations; (b) vesico-urethropexy procedures; and (c) vesico-urethrolysis.

(a) Sling operations

A bewildering variety of sling operations have been described. The method of Aldridge (1942, 1946), however, is probably that which has been most widely employed, and the principles of other procedures are similar. In the Aldridge technique a combined abdomino-vaginal approach is employed. Through a transverse suprapubic incision, strips of fascia approximately 2 cm broad are fashioned from the external oblique aponeurosis. The medial attachment of the strips is preserved and they are then passed retropubically down either side of the urethra. Through a vaginal incision the strips are picked up and sutured together under the region of the urethrovesical junction. The great problem of the operation is to achieve the perfect tension of this strip. Micturition must be able to take place unimpeded, but whenever the patient strains suddenly, which will inevitably be associated with tightening of the abdominal muscles, the strip is drawn up just sufficiently to prevent stress incontinence. The end result of the operation is thus a dynamic one with a built-in protection to urethral leakage at the very time it is suddenly needed. In this respect it is, of all the operations, *theoretically* the ideal one for stress incontinence. *In practice* it is not used as the elective, first-choice procedure in most cases, because the technical difficulties of getting a good result are much greater than in the vaginal repair operations. The bladder neck may be damaged at the operation; if the sling is too tight it may sever the urethra or lead to chronic urinary retention; if too loose the stress incontinence persists. The natural tendency is to make the sling too tight. If a finger can just be admitted at operation between the sling and the urethra, the tension when the patient is awake and contracting her abdominal muscles should just be about correct.

After such operations patients have to be re-educated in bladder emptying. If they employ Valsalva stress in the usual way the sling mechanism is activated and the urethra occluded. They must learn to sit in a relaxed way on the toilet and allow the detrusor to effect bladder emptying unassisted by raising of the abdominal pressure. Sometimes, patients find they have to adopt bizarre positions to secure bladder evacuation. Not uncommonly, emptying is most easily achieved in a semi-standing position.

Other procedures involve the use of different fascias—autologous, homologous and heterologous—or synthetic material to form the sling and modified techniques of placement.

(b) Vesico-urethropexy

The best known procedure in this category is that described by Marshall et al. (1949). The cave of Retzuis is approached through an abdominal incision and the bladder neck stitched to the posterior aspect of the symphysis pubis and lower rectus muscle, thus affecting elevation. The result lacks the same degree of dynamic efficiency of the Aldridge sling type of procedure but it can be done at the conclusion of an abdominal hysterectomy in a case where stress incontinence is a problem. It does not demand as high a degree of personal judgement on the part of the operator as does the sling technique.

(c) Urethrovesicolysis

For the 'frozen-bladder syndrome' referred to on page 565 where scarring and fibrosis around the bladder prevent the usual automatic adjustment to sudden Valsalva pressure, Mulvany (1957, 1958) has described a procedure of 'vesicourethrolysis' which should be particularly appropriate. Some degree of freeing of the bladder neck is a feature of almost all repair operations, but in his technique it is the mainstay. The difficulty is to ensure that adhesions do not re-form; to help in this regard adjacent vascularized tissue can be drawn into the region of the urethrovesical junction.

Individual surgeons have their own strong preferences for operations in one particular category, and providing good results are achieved there is no reason why such preferences should not be followed. Given good primary vaginal surgery, however, opportunities for acquiring experience in these techniques should be infrequent in the average gynaecological surgeon's practice. A young gynaecologist who may never have had more than isolated experience of such operations in his training will, if faced with a problem case requiring this type of approach, be well advised to seek the help of a senior colleague. Only when he has had the opportunity of working with an expert on a number of occasions would he be prudent to embark on a sling procedure on his own. There is, in fact, a great deal to be said for referring such cases to centres where a special interest in female urinary incontinence has been developed. Such centres will have efficient facilities for good-quality investigation by the more complex techniques, in addition to surgeons with special experience.

OPERATIVE COMPLICATIONS

At the time of operation, damage to related structures—urethra, bladder, ureters or rectum—may occur, and if recognized should be dealt with immediately. If not recognized, the injury may later be the cause of abscess and fistula development. Haemorrhage may be a problem at operation, immediately afterwards ('reactionary') or secondarily at the time of slough separation. The injection of a sympathomimetic solution such as adrenalin $1 : 1,000$, 3 ml in 60 ml of $\frac{1}{2}\%$ procaine will help to reduce the operative blood loss, and also facilitates tissue plane dissection. The problem of bleeding from large vessels is, however, unaffected by this, and meticulous attention to details of haemostasis is, of course, an essential requirement. Particular difficulties tend to arise with large venous channels alongside the bladder neck. It is usually difficult, or impossible, to deal with specific bleeding points in this region and attempts may merely lead to worse tearing and increased haemorrhage. Fortunately, the effect of deep levator stitches inserted transversely to support the bladder neck is usually to control such bleeding. Keeping the lateral dissection to the minimum necessary is also important. If significant bleeding occurs in the immediate postoperative phase it is desirable to re-anaesthetize the patient and explore the operation site; merely packing the vagina without exploration is rarely satisfactory.

Postoperative hypotensive collapse in the absence of haemorrhage is an occasional complication. It is, of course, important to be quite sure that concealed blood loss is not taking place. Factors to be considered are the effect of (a) anaesthetic agents; (b) drugs which the patient is (or has been) taking; and (c) the depression of the patient's legs from the lithotomy position— if this is the cause, re-elevation of the feet in relation to the head is followed by rapid correction of the collapse.

In the early postoperative phase, retention of urine is the commonest complication. Different policies are adopted with regard to this—indwelling catheters, intermittent catheterization and suprapubic aspiration. Policy is, to some extent, governed by the individual situation (e.g. the continuous availability of skilled staff for catheterization 'on demand'), but as a consequence of the widespread appreciation of the higher incidence of urinary infection when an indwelling catheter is used, many gynaecologists now avoid this unless in particular circumstances. If an indwelling catheter is used, then it is wise to administer a urinary antiseptic such as sulphamethoxypyridazine 0·5 g daily. Hawkins (1962) found that short-acting sulphonamides were of little value, but that a long-acting preparation reduced the incidence of infection by one-third. Regular checks should be made on the sterility of urine specimens obtained. Pre-operative catheterization can also be avoided with complete safety prior to vaginal procedures.

Donald *et al.* (1962) point out that urinary infection accounts for more than all the other complications put together. Paterson *et al.* (1960) found that using an indwelling catheter for 48 hr after repair operations there was an appalling 92·5% incidence of urinary infection. With intermittent catheterization this dropped to 70%, while the instillation of 60 ml of

chlorhexidine diacetate solution (1 in 5,000) after catheterization reduced the incidence to 13·5%. This regime with the use of solid rather than rubber catheters and dry hands is the one now followed in our unit. Pre-operative catheterization is not done, and postoperatively it is performed only for specific indications. This involves about 50% patients being catheterized (Donald *et al.* 1962). Barr & Paterson (1962) studied the effect of these postoperative infections on symptomatic results of operation. They concluded that they contributed significantly to urinary symptoms present at follow-up.

Reference has been made elsewhere to the fact that *repair operation may result in stress incontinence in women who did not suffer from it previously.* Enquiry about this should be a routine feature of every postoperative check consultation.

Incidentally, it is becoming widely accepted that just as indwelling catheters after repair operation are unnecessary, so also are vaginal packs (Donald *et al.* 1962; Cope 1962).

Pelvic infection is not uncommon, probably related to the fact that absolute sterility of the vagina and perineal areas is hard to achieve. It is commoner when there have been problems of haemostasis, and some degree of haematoma formation is the usual nidus of infection. While prophylactic antibiotic cover may be given, this is not generally favoured, and antibiotics are usually reserved for administration when infection develops, being prescribed as far as possible following sensitivity testing. If pyrexia fails to settle with appropriate antibiotics then a pelvic collection of pus is likely, and drainage is usually best effected by digital opening of the suture line near the vaginal vault.

Thrombo-embolic complications represent a major problem. Patients with prolapse often have varicose veins, with the concomitant phlebothrombotic tendency; pelvic operations of all sorts are predisposing factors, but this is particularly so when the lithotomy position has to be employed. Important points in prophylaxis include careful positioning of the legs, which should lie *inside* the lithotomy poles so that there is no pressure on the calves; early deep breathing and leg exercises, together with early ambulation;

the consideration of prophylactic anticoagulants in bad-risk cases or the use of medium-molecular-weight dextrans to cover operation. Chalmers *et al.* (1960) reported on the use of phenindione prophylactically in 1,877 obstetrical and gynaecological cases, and went so far as to recommend that anticoagulants should be used routinely in gynaecological cases.

Cervical stenosis after a Manchester-type procedure can result in haematometra and pyometra. If dilatation is not effective hysterectomy may be required.

Dyspareunia has been referred to. This, or apareunia, is a complication which is obviously of major importance, yet embarrassment frequently causes patients to refrain from mentioning it; many in fact regard it as a necessary consequence of the operation. *It is in the circumstances the duty of the gynaecologist to enquire specifically about the problem at postoperative consultations*; if coitus has been practised up to the time of operation the patient should not be discharged from gynaecological care until it has been re-established. Usually, the use of graduated glass vaginal dilators will overcome the problem, along with oestrogen therapy where appropriate, but occasionally it may be necessary to carry out dilatation under anaesthesia.

PROBLEMS RELATED TO SUBSEQUENT PREGNANCY

A major problem, though not perhaps strictly a complication, is the possible subsequent occurrence of pregnancy after repair operation. The consequence of this may be to undo the benefits of the procedure if it has been successful. However, given proper management the risks of this are not great and it is wrong to imagine that pregnancy is contra-indicated in women who have had repair operations. This is not the only problem in relation to pregnancy. The common complications can be listed as:

(1) infertility;
(2) cervical incompetence;
(3) cervical rigidity or stenosis;
(4) recurrence of the prolapse or stress incontinence after a pregnancy.

(1) *Infertility*

Women who have prolapse operations may be infertile for a variety of reasons. Firstly, it may be the case, particularly if a posterior repair has been performed, that intercourse is difficult or impossible (Francis & Jeffcoate 1961). Secondly, even if full insemination occurs the spermatozoa may find the vaginal epithelium, which is stitched over the cervical stump in the Manchester procedure, inimical to their ascent to the uterus and tubes. Thirdly, infection following the repair operation may have produced tubal or peritubal adhesions which interfere with sperm and ovum transport or fertilization.

(2) *Cervical incompetence*

Amputation of the cervix being an integral part of the Manchester procedure, it is obviously possible that the amputation level may be such that the sphincteric mechanisms at internal os level which control the retention of the foetus in the uterus may be disturbed. This, of course, is likely in subsequent pregnancies to result in second trimester abortion or premature labour early in the third trimester. The classical cervical incompetence presentation, with unexpected rupture of the membranes followed by an almost painless abortion or labour, may occur, but sometimes after membrane rupture has occurred, completion of the cervical dilatation may be interfered with by scarring from the operation and paradoxically completion of the uterine-emptying process is delayed and may necessitate intervention.

Unlike cervical incompetence due to other causes such as over-zealous cervical dilatation, it is extremely difficult to deal with such cases by procedures such as the Shirodkar suturing technique, as the relevant tissue is not damaged but absent.

(3) *Cervical rigidity*

As mentioned above, the cervical scarring may interfere with cervical dilatation. While this may present after early rupture of the membranes, it more commonly occurs when the pregnancy has continued to near term. The cervix fails to dilate and Caesarean section has to be under-taken. Alternatively, and more seriously, tearing may take place along a line of scar tissue and serious haemorrhage ensues from torn vessels.

(4) *Recurrence of prolapse or stress incontinence*

The aetiology of prolapse and stress incontinence is widely accepted as being closely related to pregnancy and labour. There is some debate as to the relative importance of pregnancy and labour in relation to the aetiology of stress incontinence, though a majority view seems to be that labour is a major factor. This problem is increased by virtue of the fact that a repeat surgical attempt to cure prolapse or stress incontinence which has recurred following a pregnancy is technically more difficult and much less likely to be successful than a primary procedure. Prolapse and stress incontinence are rarely seen in women who have had all their deliveries by elective Caesarean section.

It follows from these observations that if a patient is pregnant after a previous repair opera-tion careful consideration must be given to the question of whether or not vaginal delivery should be attempted or elective Caesarean section per-formed. No rules can be laid down, but there are some guiding general principles which apply.

The most distressing and most difficult symptom to relieve at repair operations is stress incontinence. If stress incontinence was a major indication for the operation and it has been successfully relieved, this would be a major consideration. In such circumstances most gynaecologists favour elective Caesarean section. If on the other hand the repair operation has been unsatisfactory in its results, then there would be little or nothing to be said against allowing an attempt at vaginal delivery. Other factors which may weigh are whether or not the patient desires that this should be her last pregnancy and it is intended to perform tubal ligation; whether or not the cervix has been amputated, and the degree of scarring which appears to have resulted therefrom.

If labour is allowed, special precautions are indicated. If in the first stage cervical dilatation is slow it must be suspected that this is due to cervical rigidity from scarring. If this suspicion arises it is prudent to resort immediately to section. Allowing labour to continue may result in serious lacerations. If cervical dilatation pro-ceeds uneventfully, then everything possible should be done to make the second stage of labour as atraumatic as possible. A prompt and generous episiotomy, combined if necessary with the application of forceps, will help to relieve the amount of pressure of the foetal head upon the region of the urethrovesical junction.

After every pregnancy subsequent to a repair it is appropriate to give serious consideration to the advisability of a sterilizing procedure. The fact that one delivery has been achieved without interference with the efficacy of the repair does not mean that this will be so with subsequent pregnancies.

SPECIAL PROBLEMS OF URINARY CONTINENCE

MECHANISMS OF URINARY CONTINENCE

In considering the problem of stress incontinence it is relevant to consider the anatomy and physiology of urinary continence in the normal female. Not, of course, that one can necessarily restore precisely the same mechanisms in a repairative procedure, but knowledge of the normal may point to the types of approach most likely to give consistent results. It is important to bear in mind the possibility that the prime mechanism may be valvular rather than sphinc-teric in relation to protection from stress in-continence.

BLADDER AND URETHRAL ANATOMY

Unfortunately, there has been much disputation about what appears to be simple anatomical fact, quite apart from controversy concerning physiol-ogy. The main smooth muscle of the viscus which produces the contraction leading to evacuation, the detrusor muscle (Latin, *detrudere*, to thrust away) is arranged as a meshwork with some degree of layering. On the urine surface of the bladder, fibres are arranged longitudinally and are continuous with the inner layer of the urethra. The middle circular layer does not extend to the urethra, while the outer longitudinal layer is continuous with the outer circular layer of the urethra (Tanagho & Smith 1966).

The female urethra is a tubular structure 3–5·5 cm in length and 7–10 mm in diameter. There is an intra-abdominal portion above the urogenital diaphragm and an extra-abdominal segment below it. It is the upper part which is concerned in the maintenance of continence (Ball 1966).

The outer circular fibres of the urethra have been described as constituting a sphincter (Denny-Brown 1936) but this does not represent a separate mass of muscle as, for example, the pyloric sphincter. Ball (1967) deals with the situation outspokenly: 'Many concepts in medicine die after a reasonable terminal illness, but the sphincters of the female urethra have an extraordinary capacity for survival . . . they have only existed in the imagination of medical artists instructed by urologists and gynaecologists to draw them since it seemed the least painful way to explain the mechanism of urinary control'. There are a few circular striated muscle fibres at the distal end of the sphincter which may be regarded as constituting an external sphincter, but these are of little physiological importance.

Fibres of the levator ani are inserted into the paraurethral tissue and are almost certainly relevant in urinary control by increasing the urethral compression on contraction. The normal urethra has an inherent elasticity which is probably an important factor (Ball 1967).

NERVOUS CONTROL OF THE BLADDER AND URETHRA

Parasympathetic autonomic fibres from S. 2, 3 and 4 pass to the vesical plexus, and probably also to the urethra, and are the main motor supply. Sympathetic fibres (T. 11, 12 and L. 1, 2) pass to the bladder via the hypogastric plexus but their function is uncertain. The few external sphincteric striated fibres are innervated by the pudendal nerve. Afferent impulses pass via the pelvic splanchnic nerves. Sympathetic afferents are probably concerned with visceral pain. The operation at spinal level of reflexes through these autonomic pathways can be influenced by higher centres in different ways—passive or active inhibition or facilitation.

BLADDER AND URETHRAL PHYSIOLOGY

Accepting the idea that emerges of the detrusor and urethral muscle constituting one muscular unit with common innervation, the problem arises of how the bladder contracts to empty and the urethra dilates to allow emptying as part of the same movement. Hodgkinson & Morgan (1969) in a careful review concluded that, to varying degrees, detrusor contraction and Valsalva stress pressures were responsible for initiating micturition, but once flow was established the Valsalva component tended to decrease. They could not, however, despite careful study, define the precise voiding mechanism. Lapides (1958) has suggested that the effect of bladder plus urethral contraction is to convert the urethra, which is normally a tube with walls tending to lie in apposition, into a funnel-shaped structure, terminating at the external meatus (Fig. 37.7). This implies that the normal mechanism of urethral continence is a passive one.

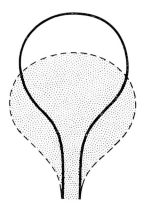

Fig. 37.7. Diagrammatic representation (after Lapides) of bladder and urethra at rest (solid line) and during detrusor contraction (broken line). The effect of contraction of the combined bladder and urethral musculature is to shorten the effective urethra and cause a funnelling which terminates at the external urethral meatus. The effect of this is that the total pressure is projected on the external meatus and urine tends to pass out.

When the bladder is at rest, the pressure within it is close to that of the pressure in the peritoneal cavity. On coughing or sneezing the intraperitoneal pressure is raised, and this is transmitted directly to the bladder. Enhörning (1961) measured cough pressure in urethra and bladder simultaneously and observed that cough pressure was transferred to the urethra as well as the bladder. Furthermore, this transfer was more effective in women who did not have stress incontinence. He therefore postulated that any surge of urine under pressure from the bladder upon coughing was met by a counter-pressure generated directly in the urethra by the cough. This counter-pressure would prevent the advance of the wave.

Enhörning & Westin (1963) and Warrell *et al.* (1963), working quite independently, later confirmed that on sudden straining the pressure in the upper urethra in the continent patient exceeded that in the bladder. If stress incontinence was present this did not occur. In normal subjects the intravesical pressure ranges from 10 to 60 cm H_2O, while that in the upper urethra is from 50 to 135. Enhörning & Hinman (1964) define the *closure pressure* as the difference between the highest intra-urethral pressure and the bladder pressure. In patients with stress incontinence this figure is reduced (Ball 1967; Toews 1967). Beck *et al.* (1968) refer to this situation as 'pressure equalization stress incontinence'.

The urethrovesical angle concept (Roberts 1952; Jeffcoate & Roberts 1952) suggests that a flap-valve type of effect operates to prevent incontinence on sudden Valsalva stress when the urethra is set at an appropriate angle to the bladder (Fig. 37.8). This is a two-dimensional concept. Lapides *et al*.'s (1960) explanation of urethral funnelling as the important feature in stress

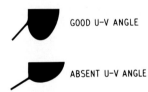

GOOD U–V ANGLE

ABSENT U–V ANGLE

Fig. 37.8. Diagrammatic representation of the urethrovesical junction as seen on lateral, contrast cysto-urethrography. Above there is a good angle and the patient was continent. Below there is a poor or absent angle and the patient had stress incontinence.

incontinence can be regarded as the same idea in three-dimensional terms.

Many of the bitter debates on this subject have been between workers with data on different parameters which in fact have inferred the same type of process. Some of the arguments on the importance of urethral compression, urethral lengthening and increasing the urethrovesical angle were conducted on the assumption that they were rival and exclusive theories of urinary continence. In fact, *the evidence from all these different measurements points to the fact that the urethral continence mechanism is a passive one.* The adherents of each of these 'theories' used to claim support of their validity on the basis that operations designed to increase the particular parameters they measured and championed, relieved established stress incontinence. In fact, any operation designed to increase the urethrovesical angle will *inevitably* tend to lengthen the urethra and increase the degree of its compression. Operations aimed at increasing each of the other two parameters mentioned will also increase all three.

The clinical facts are in favour of this idea of a mechanical, valvular effect. No active smooth muscle-type sphincter could meet the demands placed on the urethral mechanism by the sudden increase in intravesical pressure as occurs with sneezing and coughing. The fact that operative procedures which ignore the vesical and urethral muscular tissues are effective in relieving stress incontinence, makes this notion much easier to accept. By the same token, the idea that when standing continence is aided by the contraction of the levator muscles (an essential to the maintenance of the erect posture) fits with clinical experience that operations designed to strengthen the levatores—for example, the Pacey operation (Pacey 1949)—successfully relieve stress incontinence.

The evidence can be summarized by saying that the mechanism of protection of urinary continence against stress is a passive phenomenon, and that contributory factors include:

(a) the natural tone of the urethra;
(b) the pressure effect on the urethra of external structures, particularly the levatores

ani which automatically contract with Valsalva stress and therefore give counter-pressure at the moment it is needed;

(c) the urethrovesical angle;
(d) the shape of the internal urethra, with its lack of 'funnelling';
(e) the length of the urethra;
(f) the direct influence of intra-abdominal pressure on the proximal segment of the urethra which normally lies above the levatores ani (the so-called 'intra-abdominal urethra').

MECHANISMS OF STRESS INCONTINENCE

The common type of stress incontinence occurs in parous women. Furthermore, they frequently have anterior vaginal wall prolapse (Warrell 1969). The symptom may occur for the first time in pregnancy (Francis 1960), but some women do develop stress incontinence after delivery for the first time (Beck & Hsu 1965) and it is hard to escape the conclusion that it is a consequence in these circumstances.

It is probable that the underlying cause of stress incontinence is a deficiency of some (or all) of the factors mentioned which tend to maintain continence. Whenever urethral compression forces are diminished the urethrovesical angle will probably be reduced, and the urethral shortening or funnelling will also tend to be present. Weak levator tone or levator separation will tend to aggravate this situation.

As Warrell (1969) puts the problem after, considering reported data on pressure measurements: 'Perhaps the question which should be asked is "Under what circumstances does transmitted intra-abdominal pressure operate as a force opening the internal urethral meatus rather than as a force closing the urethra?" '. This is, of course, particularly liable to happen if the urethrovesical junction drops downwards, as is the case if there is prolapse *of that portion of the anterior vaginal wall which is directly opposed to the junction* (Hodgkinson 1963). This fits with the loss of the urethrovesical angle concept and the 'funnelling' concept of Lapides with loss of urethral length (Lapides *et al.* 1960). Jeffcoate's (1961) claim that anterior vaginal wall prolapse is not concerned,

probably relates more particularly to women with cystoceles. If there is a large cystocele but the urethra and urethrovesical angle are well supported, there is little tendency to stress incontinence.

Ball (1966) describes *posterior cystocele*, prolapse of the bladder lying behind the inter-ureteric bar, which is not conducive to stress incontinence. Herniation arising lower (or more anteriorly) he refers to as an *anterior cystocele* (or cysto-urethrocele), and this *does* tend to be associated with stress incontinence.

A particular group of patients (who are unrelieved by the usual operative procedures), are those who have stress incontinence associated with severe scarring around the bladder neck region. This fixes the tissues—'frozen bladder syndrome' (Ball *et al.* 1966). The automatic adjustments which appear to be a direct mechanical consequence of the forces from sudden increase in the abdominal pressure do not occur and incontinence is manifest.

URGENCY INCONTINENCE WITHOUT ORGANIC LESION

Urgency is usually a symptom of bladder inflammation, and treatment to correct this is the appropriate course. A difficult problem is presented by the patient with urgency or urgency incontinence, usually combined with frequency, and in whom no organic lesion is discovered. It may be said that such patients are strictly the responsibility of the urologist, but in practice very many of them present to the gynaecologist. Jeffcoate & Francis (1966) in a review of 300 cases of urgency incontinence record that 131 were referred as having stress incontinence. Fifty-four of the 300 were shown to have organic disease of genito-urinary or nervous systems. In the remainder the cause was assessed as basically psychological or environmental. Precipitating factors included marital troubles, widowhood, accidents or illnesses to close relatives, together with postoperative retention and cystitis. With relief of any specific factor, plus conservative educational policies and anticholinergic medication 166 were cured after one year and 54 considerably improved.

As indicated, a repair operation is unlikely to be helpful unless stress incontinence and prolapse are present also. General measures may give relief, however, in a high proportion of cases at least temporarily. This is probably because in many cases the basic problem is merely faulty bladder habit.

The underlying dysfunction may be one of poor cortical processing of the stimuli resulting from bladder distention. This can be helped by a regime of 'bladder drill'. This starts with filling the bladder to capacity at the time of cystoscopy. Instead of draining it at completion the fluid is left in, and on recovering consciousness the patient voids what is usually a very much larger volume of fluid than she has done for a long period. The psychological influence of discovering that her bladder can accommodate this quantity may not be irrelevant. The patient is kept in hospital and a regime of voiding 'by the clock', regardless of whether or not she desires to micturate, is initiated. Starting ½-hourly, the time of emptying is increased by ½-hr increments daily to 3 or 4 hr. Even if 2 hr is the longest that can be achieved, this is usually a great improvement on the previous situation. The success of this regime is often helped by prescribing a mild sedative or tranquillizer together with a preparation such as propantheline bromide (Pro-Banthine) 15 mg t.d.s. plus 30 mg at night, which counteracts bladder spasm.

Some authorities recommend urethral dilatation but the rationale of this is unclear, unless it be that some factor causing irritation in the proximal urethra is relieved by the stretching.

It cannot be too strongly emphasized that *full* genito-urinary tract investigation must be performed before embarking on the type of regime outlined above. If this is not done, from time to time patients with serious and treatable pathology of the urinary tract, such as tuberculosis, may be denied specific therapy.

RESULTS OF OPERATION

The results of operations for repair of prolapse and relief of stress incontinence like any other procedure depend on the skill of the surgeon. However, to a very much greater degree they depend on the selection of cases. This is particularly important in relation to stress incontinence. The time of any follow-up assessment is very important; both prolapse and stress incontinence have a tendency to recur with passage of the years.

In Hawksworth & Roux's (1958) published figures for 1,000 patients who had vaginal hysterectomy and repair performed, the mortality was 0·1%. Of 54 patients with stress incontinence 51 were cured at 1 year. There was a 6% incidence of enterocele in Hawksworth and Roux's initial series, but with modification of their technique this was virtually eliminated. Krige (1962) reviewed 2,973 repairs with vaginal hysterectomy and graded 2·6% (including three deaths) as failures.

Bailey (1954, 1956) suggests that only 50% patients with severe stress incontinence will be cured by vaginal repair. This figure is reached after critical follow-up over 6 years. Beck *et al.* (1968) record a cure rate of 62·2% and a failure rate of 20·4%, figures very similar to Jeffcoate's (1961), Cullen & Welch's (1961), Green's (1962) and Low's (1967). Beck and his colleagues (1965) recorded pressures achieved within the urethra and bladder at the time of operation. They found that where the differential achieved 1–2 cm from the bladder neck exceeded 30 mmHg, the chances of ultimate success were higher. Taking all cases and assuming good selection and operative technique, probably about 80–85% success at primary operation can be regarded as an average expectation *at initial follow-up* (Hodgkinson 1965; Howkins 1968). If the follow-up interval after operation is long then, of course, lower success rates are recorded, for the degenerative ravages of time must be expected to lead to recurrence in a proportion of cases. The fact that recurrence occurs after 10 years, often in association with new aetiological factors like obesity or bronchitis, should not be regarded as a fault of the initial operation. The results for stress incontinence are subject also to considerable variation in relation to the number of the procedures which are primary ones. With large numbers of cases having secondary procedures after failure of primary operation, the results which can be expected are, inevitably, less satisfactory.

Examples of what can be achieved in relation to secondary sling procedures in expert hands are Moir's (1968) and Low's (1969) figures. Using a modified Aldridge sling procedure which he called the 'gauge-hammock operation', Moir obtained cure or substantial improvement in 59 of 75 cases; improvement, but still occasional stress incontinence, in eight cases, and failure in four. Low, using a combined procedure with plication of the bladder neck and the introduction of a sling derived from fascia lata, reported resolution of *demonstrable* stress incontinence in 41 of 43 patients. Of these 41, four occasionally experienced incontinence and 14 had persisting frequency and urgency.

Warrell & Russell (1965) grouped together cases of 'complicated' incontinence, of which 81 had had previous surgery and 125 had insufficient prolapse present to account for the incontinence. Of those previously operated upon, 52 had anatomical faults, of which scarring and devitalization were the major ones. They freed the urethra and bladder after the style of Mulvany. Where necessary, and possible, they inserted tissue with intact blood supply from surrounding structures to try to prevent fresh adhesion formation. Forty-two of these 52 were cured. Of the 29 without anatomical abnormality cystitis was the commonest feature; 17 of these 29 were cured by conservative management. Of the 125 patients who had *not* had an operation before, mechanical 'sphincter' weakness was diagnosed in 25, bladder or urethral inflammation in 38, a combination of these in 42 and abnormal bladder action not due to local inflammation in 20 including six cases in which no cause was found. All 25 with anatomical 'sphincter' abnormalities were cured by vaginal surgery, 22 of the 38 with inflammation were cured by medical treatment. Of the 42 'combined' cases, all were given initial medical treatment and seven were cured to an extent that they did not wish surgery. Twenty-nine of the remainder had urethroplasty and 24 were cured. They emphasized that relief of chronic bronchitis, and weight reduction, play an important part in management.

It is wise not to become too involved in the intense arguments which rage on the best operative technique. The grounds for assessing success are too imprecise to justify strong claims. There is also the not irrelevant fact that some surgeons are preferentially satisfied with their own handiwork. Hodgkinson (1965), after a comprehensive review of the literature on the subject for the preceding decade, concluded that the variables largely invalidated statistical accuracy. He emphasizes that case-selection is of the greatest importance. Those who report a high success rate are very probably applying less stringent standards than those with a low rate. It cannot be too strongly emphasized that *results are much more related to the selection of cases than to the operation.*

REFERENCES

ALDRIDGE A.H. (1942) *Am. J. Obstet. Gynec.* **44**, 398.
ALDRIDGE A.H. (1946) *Am. J. Obstet. Gynec.* **51**, 299.
ALEXANDER S. & ROWAN D. (1968) *Lancet*, i, 728.
ARTHURE H.G.E. & SAVAGE D. (1957) *J. Obstet. Gynaec. Br. Commonw.* **64**, 355.
BAILEY K.V. (1954) *J. Obstet. Gynaec. Br. Commonw.* **61**, 291.
Ibid, Part II (1956) *J. Obstet. Gynaec. Br. Commonw.* **63**, 663.
BALL T.L. (1966) *Clin. Obstet. Gynec.* **9**, 1062.
BALL T.L. (1967) In *Advances in Obstetrics and Gynaecology*, Vol. 1 (edited by S.L. Marcus & C.C. Marcus). Baltimore, Williams & Wilkins, p. 542.
BALL T.L., KNAPP R.C., NATHANSON B. & LAGASSE L.D. (1966) *Am. J. Obstet. Gynec.* **94**, 997.
BARR W. & PATERSON M.L. (1962) *J. Obstet. Gynaec. Br. Commonw.* **69**, 110.
BECK R.P. & HSU N. (1965) *Am. J. Obstet. Gynec.* **91**, 820.
BECK R.P., HSU N. & MAUGHAN G.B. (1965) *Am. J. Obstet. Gynec.* **91**, 314.
BECK R.P., THOMAS E.A. & MAUGHAN G.B. (1966) *Am. J. Obstet. Gynec.* **94**, 483.
BECK R.P., THOMAS E.A. & MAUGHAN G.B. (1968) *Am. J. Obstet. Gynec.* **100**, 483.
CALDWELL K.P.S., COOK P.J., FLACK F.C. & JAMES E.D. (1968) *J. Obstet. Gynaec. Br. Commonw.* **75**, 777.
CHALMERS D.G., MARKS J., BOTTOMLEY J.E. & LLOYD O. (1960) *Lancet*, ii, 220.
COPE E. (1962) *J. Obstet. Gynaec. Br. Commonw.* **69**, 857.
CULLEN P.K. & WELCH J.S. (1961) *Surgery Gynec. Obstet.* **113**, 85.
CURRIE D.W. (1953) *Trans. N. Engl. obstet. gynaec. Soc.* 56.
DENNY-BROWN D.E. (1936) *New Engl. J. Med.* **215**, 647.
DONALD I., BARR W. & McGARRY J. (1962) *J. Obstet. Gynaec. Br. Commonw.* **69**, 837.
ENHÖRNING G. (1961) *Acta chir. scand.* Supplement 276, p. 1.

ENHÖRNING G. & HINMAN F. (1964) *Surgery Gynaec. Obstet.* **118**, 507.

ENHÖRNING G. & WESTIN B. (1963) *Acta obstet. gynec. scand.* **42**, 328.

FELL M.R. (1963) *Lancet*, **i**, 799.

FOTHERGILL W.E. (1914) *J. Obstet. Gynaec. Br. Commonw.* **26**, 29.

FRANCIS W.J.A. (1960) *J. Obstet. Gynaec. Br. Commonw.* **67**, 899.

FRANCIS W.J.A. & JEFFCOATE T.N.A. (1961) *J. Obstet. Gynaec. Br. Commonw.* **68**, 1.

GREEN T.H. (1962) *Am. J. Obstet. Gynec.* **83**, 632.

HAWKINS D.F. (1962) *J. Obstet. Gynaec. Br. Commonw.* **69**, 585.

HAWKSWORTH W. & ROUX J.P. (1958) *J. Obstet. Gynaec. Br. Commonw.* **65**, 214.

HILL D.W., MABLE S.E.R., WALLACE D.M. & DEWHURST C.J. (1968) *Lancet*, **ii**, 112.

HODGKINSON C.P. (1963) *Clin. Obstet. Gynec.* **6**, 154.

HODGKINSON C.P. (1965) *Surgery Gynec. Obstet.* **120**, 595.

HODGKINSON C.P. & MORGAN J.E. (1969) *Am. J. Obstet. Gynec.* **103**, 755.

HOWKINS J. (1968) *Shaw's Textbook of Operative Gynaecology*, 3rd edn. Edinburgh and London, Livingstone.

HUNTER J.W.A. (1938) *Br. med. J.* **ii**, 991.

INGELMAN-SUNDBERG A. (1947) *Gynaecologia*, **123**, 242.

JEFFCOATE T.N.A. (1961) *Jl R. Coll. Surg. Edinb.* **7**, 28.

JEFFCOATE T.N.A. & FRANCIS W.J.A. (1966) *Am. J. Obstet. Gynec.* **94**, 604.

JEFFCOATE T.N.A. & ROBERTS H. (1952) *J. Obstet. Gynaec. Br. Commonw.* **59**, 685.

KEGEL A.H. (1948) *Am. J. Obstet. Gynec.* **56**, 238.

KEGAL A.H. (1956) *Obstet. Gynec., N.Y.* **8**, 545.

KELLY H.L. & DUMM W.M. (1914) *Surgery Gynec. Obstet.* **18**, 444.

KENNEDY W.T. (1937) *Am. J. Obstet. Gynec.* **34**, 576.

KRIGE C.F. (1962) *J. Obstet. Gynaec. Br. Commonw.* **69**, 570.

LAPIDES J. (1958) *J. Urol.* **80**, 341.

LAPIDES J., AJEMIAN E.P., STEWART B.H., BREAKEY B.A. & LICHTWARDT J.R. (1960) *J. Urol.* **84**, 86.

LOW J.A. (1967) *Am. J. Obstet. Gynec.* **97**, 308.

LOW J.A. (1969) *Am. J. Obstet. Gynec.* **105**, 149.

MARSHALL V.F., MARCHETTI A.A. & KRANTZ K.E. (1949) *Surgery Gynec. Obstet.* **88**, 509.

McLEOD D.H. & HOWKINS J. (1964) *Bonney's Gynaecological Surgery*, 7th edn. London, Cassell.

MOIR J.C. (1968) *J. Obstet. Gynaec. Br. Commonw.* **75**, 1.

MULVANY J.H. (1957) *J. Obstet. Gynaec. Br. Commonw.* **64**, 531.

MULVANY J.H. (1958) *Surgery Gynec. Obstet.* **107**, 511.

NEMIR A. & MIDDLETON R.P. (1954) *Am. J. Obstet. Gynec.* **68**, 1166.

PACEY K. (1949) *J. Obstet. Gynaec. Br. Commonw.* **56**, 1.

PATERSON M.L., BARR W. & MACDONALD S. (1960) *J. Obstet. Gynaec. Br. Commonw.* **67**, 394.

PATERSON P.J. & HARRISON N.W. (1970) *J. Obstet. Gynaec. Br. Commonw.* **77**, 732.

ROBERTS H. (1952) *Br. J. Radiol.* **25**, 253.

RUSSELL J.K. (1961) *Br. med. J.* **ii**, 1595.

SHIRODKAR V.N. (1967) In *Advances in Obstetrics and Gynaecology*, Vol. 1 (edited by S.L. Marcus & C.C. Marcus). Baltimore, Williams & Wilkins Co., p. 567.

SOLDENHOFF R. DE & McDONNELL H. (1969) *Br. med. J.* **iv**, 230.

TANAGHO E.A. & SMITH R.D. (1966) *Br. J. Urol.* **38**, 54.

TE LINDE R.W. (1966) *Am. J. Obstet. Gynec.* **94**, 444.

TOEWS H.A. (1967) *Obstet. Gynec., N.Y.* **29**, 613.

UHLENHUTH E. & NOLLEY G.W. (1957) *Obstet. Gynec., N.Y.* **10**, 349.

WARRELL D.W. (1969) In *Modern Trends in Gynaecology*, Vol. 4 (edited by R.J. Kellar). London, Butterworths, p. 186.

WARRELL D.W. & RUSSELL C.S. (1965) *J. Obstet. Gynaec. Br. Commonw.* **72**, 564.

WARRELL D.W., WATSON B.W. & SHELLEY T. (1963) *J. Obstet. Gynaec. Br. Commonw.* **70**, 959.

CHAPTER 38

BENIGN AND PREMALIGNANT LESIONS OF THE VULVA, VAGINA AND CERVIX

LESIONS OF THE VULVA

A number of vulval lesions may be encountered in everyday gynaecological practice. These often cause distressing symptoms quite out of proportion to their apparent severity. Many present with symptoms of vulval irritation, and will be discussed under that heading.

Vulval irritation

Vulval irritation, often described as pruritus vulvae, is a most upsetting symptom. It may be encountered in children, as already described on p. 19; it may be met during reproductive life; but it is most troublesome when it occurs in the elderly. Vulval irritation may arise from a variety of causes, some of which are set out below.

(1) *Irritation from a vaginal discharge.* This is particularly the case with discharges caused by *Trichomonas vaginalis* or *Candida albicans*.

(2) *Application of irritating substances to the vulval skin.* Antiseptics, detergents and the like are apt to set up severe irritation of the vulva in susceptible patients. It seems probable that some patients are prone to develop vulval soreness from comparatively mild vulval irritants, which would not affect others. The failure to take a bath for one or two nights may be sufficient to provoke vulval irritation in such an individual. Other minor insults to which a vulval reaction may arise are imperfectly rinsed underclothing containing irritating soapflakes, or small quantities of household antiseptic lotions added to bath water.

(3) *Local vulval skin disorders.* These may be vulval manifestations of generalized skin disorders such as psoriasis or lichen sclerosus; or they may be specific vulval lesions—for example, leucoplakia vulvae and kraurosis vulvae.

(4) *Diabetic vulvitis.* This is an angry, red vulvitis seen in uncontrolled diabetic patients. To some extent, it is probably due to vulval irritation from heavily sugar-laden urine, but an associated *Candida albicans* infestation is a frequent finding.

(5) *Psychological causes.* Vulval irritation is sometimes a manifestation of a stress disorder in gynaecology. In these cases the patient may display features of such psychological disturbance—sexual conflicts earlier in life, sexual frustration, fear of cancer, longing for love and affection, and many other features of this kind. Much time may need to be spent with a patient to reveal the true cause of her complaint and to relieve it.

(6) *Various ulcerative conditions.* These include granuloma venereum, lymphogranuloma inguinale and Behçets syndrome.

(7) *Condylomata accuminata.* These are viral papillomata, which may be sparse or widespread on the vulva and around the vaginal introitus. They can be extremely irritating. Each 'wart' shows a central core of collective tissue with a papillomatous, heaped-up area of squamous epithelium on its surface.

(8) *Malignant lesions.* These may be present as vulval irritations, especially if carcinoma of the vulva has developed upon pre-existing leucoplakia.

History and examination

History-taking must always explore fully the onset, severity, duration, etc. of the symptom. The possibility of irritation from a local substance must be remembered and enquiry about recent creams, lotions, etc. applied to the vulva must be undertaken; specific questioning about additions to the bath water is advised. Sexual contact should be thought of as a possible cause; questioning about this aspect will be unnecessary if the patient is a married woman, and must be delicately approached if she is not. History-taking must also explore the possibility of a deep-seated psychological conflict at the root of the trouble.

The examination of the patient complaining of a vulval irritation will require to be very careful and thorough. A general examination is necessary to locate a possible skin lesion elsewhere on the body surface. A careful vaginal examination is necessary too, to exclude or confirm vaginitis or vaginal discharge as a causative factor.

Treatment

Treatment will depend upon the cause. The various causes and treatments of vaginal discharge are dealt with under specific headings later in the chapter.

Irritation from chemical substances such as antiseptics usually responds very quickly to cessation of the offending practice; a local application of a bland ointment such as Eucerin or zinc and castor oil for a short time will give relief and allow the skin to return to normal. In all cases the patient must be instructed to wash and dry very carefully; only plain water, or water with a good soap, should be used. Drying must be with a soft towel. If, for any reason, a bland ointment is not well tolerated, a little dusting powder may be applied; this tends to 'cake' if too much is used, however, and is generally less satisfactory than a simple ointment.

A generalized skin disorder with vulval manifestations will require treatment appropriate to the affection present. A dermatologist may be consulted. Cockerell & Knox (1962) have reviewed this subject.

Diabetic vulvitis usually responds well to effective control of the diabetes, and if an associated *Candida* infestation is present nystatin pessaries or similar therapy will be helpful.

Psychological causes will require careful psychotherapy; several visits may be required before progress is made. A sympathetic and skilful psychiatrist can be invaluable under such circumstances. It must, of course, be established that a local lesion does not exist. If scratching has led to much vulval excoriation a simple bland ointment such as zinc and castor oil will be helpful.

Condylomata acuminata (Fig. 40.1, p. 590) may well respond to applications of podophyllin. The 25% suspension in liquid paraffin is the most satisfactory to apply; if the solution in spirit is used, considerable pain and excoriation may be produced. If the lesions do not respond to podophyllin they can easily be removed under general anaesthesia with a pair of scissors. Each wart is snipped off at a very superficial level; there is little bleeding, which stops easily with pressure, and healing is rapid.

The remaining conditions will now be considered more fully under separate headings.

Vulval ulceration

GRANULOMA VENEREUM

This condition is found mainly, but not exclusively, in Negresses. It is common in the Southern parts of the United States of America, in the Caribbean and in different parts of Africa. Venereal infection is the common method of spread.

The condition arises as a papule, nodule or vesicle; there is ulceration quite quickly, the ulcer having a clearly defined margin and reddened floor. Later, heaped-up granulation tissue spreads over the edges of the ulcer and a chronic, indurated lesion results. The vulva may be massively involved in this way. Lymph glands may be palpable in the inguinal regions if there has been much secondary infection, but they are not common.

Granuloma venereum is probably caused by a small bacterium, *Donovania granulomatis*. This organism is found inside mononuclear cells in affected areas. The diagnosis may be established for certain by demonstrating the Donovan bodies within these large, mononuclear cells. These cells, however, lie beneath the ulcer base, and unless a small portion of tissue is obtained with a knife or biopsy forceps, they may be missed.

Antibiotics are now generally employed for treatment. Stewart (1967) recommends streptomycin, tetracycline, oxytretacycline and chloramphenicol, in that order. These lesions may predispose to cancer.

LYMPHOGRANULOMA INGUINALE

This is a virus disorder common in the same general areas as those in which granuloma venereum is endemic. Again, it is usually acquired by sexual intercourse. There is an early primary ulcer of the vulval area, which may heal spontaneously. Stewart reports that it is seldom seen in women, but may be evident in the male. Inguinal glands become swollen a few weeks later; they tend to be dark in colour and rubbery to feel. Destructive vulval lesions appear later. They may cause destruction of large areas of the fouchette, or fenestration of the labia, or urethal destruction. Rectal stricture and proctitis may be found.

Diagnosis can be difficult of confirmation unless the Frei test is strongly positive. Treatment is with sulphonamides or tetracyclines. Treatment for 10–14 days or more may be necessary and may be required on more than one occasion, the drugs being alternated.

It is rare for gynaecologists in Britain to acquire first-hand knowledge of these conditions, so diagnosis may be difficult. Our understanding of them is somewhat hampered, too, by their confusing nomenclature and by the fact that both are common in the same areas of the world (see Chapter 40).

VULVAL AND ORAL ULCERATION WITH OCULAR INFLAMMATION

Behçet's syndrome

This name is attached to the association of vulval and oral ulcers with acute inflammatory lesions in the eye. Close examination of this triad of symptoms, however, reveals that various separate diseases may be present with these features. The main condition in this group are Behçets syndrome, erythema multiforme and ocular pemphigus (Dewhurst 1955).

The term Behçet's syndrome (Behçet 1937) is applied to aphthous ulcers of the mouth in association with similar aphthous lesions of the vulva (Fig. 38.1). The ulcers themselves are small, round or oval lesions; they may have a reddened border and a sloughing base, and are often both tender and painful. They may occur singly or in groups. Healing is usually rapid.

Occasionally, a lesion may be larger and deeper, and healing is considerably delayed. In such a lesion a degree of induration may be evident and secondary infection in the ulcer will give rise to enlargement of the lymph glands. The ocular changes may be conjunctivitis or corneal ulceration, or even more extensive lesions such as iritis with hypopyon or panophthalmitis.

Behçet's syndrome in its more severe generalized form has other important associations. Smith et al. (1967) report retinal vascular changes; Hall et al. (1968) describe neurological manifestations; Cunliffe & Menon (1969) report the association of pulmonary embolism, and Hills (1969) the occurrence of aortic aneurysms. Other generalized complications have been described. Despite much speculation, the aetiology remains unknown.

Erythema multiforme, by contrast, is a condition mainly characterized by a maculopapular rash, which can be vesicular or bullous in type. It occurs on extensor surfaces of the limbs, on the palms and soles, and occasionally on the face and trunk. If the bullous lesions occur in the mouth and on the vulva (Fig. 38.2) they may easily be abraded and become ulcerated. A more severe form of the disease is sometimes associated with widespread oral sloughing, when the patient may also develop purulent conjunctivitis, urethritis and vaginitis. This more generalized form is known as the Stevens-Johnson syndrome.

Ocular pemphigus tends to affect an older age group, and the affected patient is usually postmenopausal. Here, the characteristic changes are in the eye. There is catarrhal inflammation

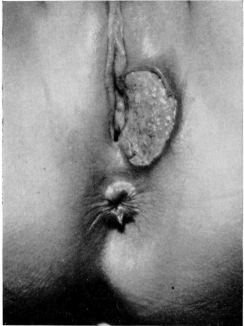

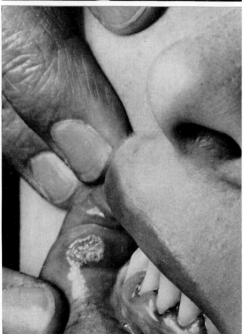

Fig. 38.1. Aphthous ulceration of the mouth and vulva (Behçet's syndrome). The vulval ulcer was very large and slow to heal. (By courtesy of the editor of *Journal of Obstetrics and Gynaecology of the British Commonwealth.*)

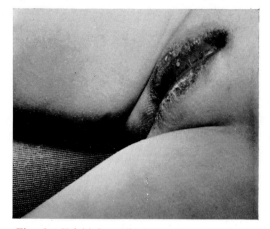

Fig. 38.2. Vulvitis in a child with erythema multiforme.

of the eye, followed later by much scar-tissue formation. Adhesions become marked and the globe may be fixed, leading to corneal ulceration and perforation. Vesicles and superficial erosions occur in the mouth and vulva. Again, these heal with much scarring, and vaginal stenosis may result.

Treatment for Behçet's syndrome has been employed in a variety of ways. Cortisone acetate 50–70 mg daily was used with success by Phillips & Scott (1955). Prednisolone 5 mg daily by mouth was used successfully by the author in a recent case. Aureomycin cream has also been used with benefit. Hill (1967) suggests that corticosteroids suppress troublesome general symptoms, but there is no evidence that they affect the underlying process. It seems clear that our understanding of the cause of this condition is most incomplete, and until we know more about it treatment will remain empirical.

OTHER VULVAL ULCERATIONS

Vulval ulceration can arise in other circumstances. Vulval herpes infection proved by virology has been described on several occasions (Hutfield & Longson 1968). In this condition, the vulva is affected by a vesicular eruption and generalized erythema (Fig. 38.3). Vesicles may rupture, to form ulcers. If there is secondary infection there may be large, tender, inguinal

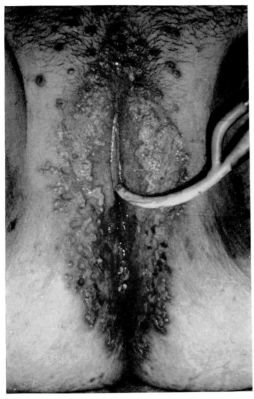

Fig. 38.3. Vulval herpes.

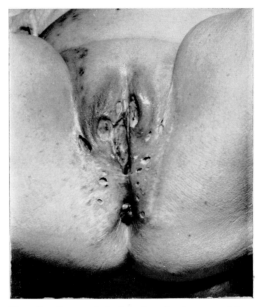

Fig. 38.4. Acute vulval ulceration of unknown aetiology. It responded well to local therapy.

glands palpable. Viral studies on vesicular fluid should confirm the diagnosis. Treatment is with bland local application and, if there is secondary infection, antibiotics. Considerable care and attention to the vulva may be required. Rarely, vulval vaccinia may be encountered.

Non-specific vulval ulcerations may follow damage to the vulval skin from scratching, antiseptic applications, etc. (Fig. 38.4); again, local applications of bland ointments or cortisone preparations will be helpful. Antibiotics are less likely to be required. Acute ulcers of this kind have been described by various names in the past (ulcus vulvae acutum, etc.). Despite speculation, the real aetiology is not known.

Tuberculous vulval ulceration is very uncommon in Britain, although it may be seen more often elsewhere. Such ulcers may have a hard, infiltrated margin, and the resemblance to cancer can be very close. A biopsy will be required in

these circumstances to establish the diagnosis. Treatment should be given with streptomycin, isoniazid and PAS once the presence or absence of tuberculous elsewhere in the genital tract or in some other system has been established.

Syphilitic ulcerations must be remembered. The primary chancre appears initially as a firm nodule which then develops superficial ulceration; occasionally, primary ulcers are multiple; they are often oedematous. The secondary lesions are condylomata lata. They are slightly raised, flat-topped outgrowths which may run together to cover a wide area. Tertiary gummatous ulcers are very uncommon.

Malignant ulcers are considered in Chapter 40.

It will be evident from this account of vulval ulceration that considerable care must be taken to establish the diagnosis in any such case. In some instances, local external examination will not be sufficient to permit a confident diagnosis. Then viral studies, a search for Donovan bodies, a Frei test, biopsy, or all these measures together may be called for. A biopsy will usually be wise at an early stage if the diagnosis is not clearly apparent.

Chronic vulval dystrophies

Few subjects can be less confusing than chronic vulval dystrophies. Many names have been applied to conditions with similar appearances—leucoplakia, in hypertrophic and atrophic form; lichen sclerosus; kraurosis vulvae; intra-epithelial carcinoma; Bowen's disease; erythroplasia; Paget's disease. This variety of names suggests our real ignorance of the processes involved, and it must be our aim to reduce them to a smaller, more intelligible, number.

The group of chronic vulval dystrophies have a number of points in common. They occur predominantly, but not exclusively, after the menopause; they are associated with white patches on the vulval skin; they are associated with evidence of atrophy in other parts of the vulval skin; they affect the area of the clitoris, labia minora and majora but do not extend into the vagina itself, although they may pass backwards to the anal region; cracking and fissuring are common; carcinoma is closely associated with some.

The commonest term to be applied to cases of this kind has been leucoplakia.

LEUCOPLAKIA

Earlier descriptions of leucoplakia refer to it as occurring in two stages, in which the hypertrophic stage was believed to precede the atrophic one. Hypertrophic leucoplakia demonstrated the following hystological appearances (Fig. 40.3, p. 593). The epithelium was affected by (1) hyperkeratosis; (ii) thickening of the epidermis; (iii) enlargement, downgrowth and bizarre forking of the rete pegs; and (iv) thickening and increased activity of the Malphigian layer.

In the dermis the changes were (i) disappearance of elastic fibres; (ii) round-cell infiltration; and (iii) oedema and hyaline change.

The activity of the cells of the Malphigian layer was marked. Although this layer was thickened and the pegs dipped down deeply into the dermis, normal stratification was evident in the superficial aspects.

The atrophic stage in the disease, which was believed to follow the hypertrophic stage, was characterized by (i) hyperkeratosis; (ii) atrophy of the epithelium with flattening of the rete pegs and Malphigian layer; and (iii) dermal changes similar to those described in the hypertrophic form.

This so-called atrophic stage is identical in appearance with the condition of lichen sclerosus —or to give it its full title, lichen sclerosus et atrophicus.

LICHEN SCLEROSUS

Lichen sclerosus may appear at almost any point on the body surface, but it has a particular tendency to affect the vulval regions. Its early lesions show discrete, ivory-white, flat-topped papules, but these later coalesce to form larger plugs. The disease runs a rather prolonged course, during which considerable atrophy of affected areas may occur. Shrinkage of the labia minora along with flattening of the skin folds here and around the clitoris are evident. The entire vulval and perianal region shows a patchy or diffuse, atrophic, white appearance similar to that usually referred to in general terms as leucoplakia.

This condition is, in one respect, an exception to the others described in this section in that it may be evident in childhood (Fig. 38.5), (see also p. 21).

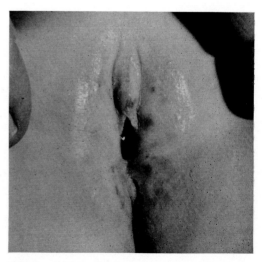

Fig. 38.5. Lichen sclerosus of the vulva in a 5 year-old child.

The evidence now strongly supports the view that the so-called atrophic stage of leucoplakia is lichen sclerosus. This term will therefore be reserved for the atrophic disorder just described, and the term leucoplakia will be reserved for the hypertrophic form. Lichen sclerosus may later progress to leucoplakia, however (Wallace & Whimster 1951; Vickers & Sneddon 1957; Stening & Elliott 1959).

KRAUROSIS VULVAE

This is a less distinct entity in which the predominant feature is atrophy of all the vulval tissues with extreme shrinkage and contraction, especially around the vaginal introitus. The histological appearances associated with it are variable, but quite often they resemble those of lichen sclerosus. The term kraurosis, if used at all, is best restricted to those cases in which atrophy and contraction of the introitus are very marked.

This view of the distinctions drawn here between these various conditions is not held by Jeffcoate & Woodcock (1961), who consider that there is no evidence to support the view that lichen sclerosus and leucoplakia are separate disease entities. Their view of the malignancy risk involved, however, is similar to that outlined below.

RISK OF MALIGNANCY

Jeffcoate and Woodcock hold the view that when great epithelial activity, increase in the Malphigian layer, and bizarre downgrowth of the rete pegs exist—and in those cases only—we are dealing with a condition possessing an increased cancer risk. The risk in this type of case, which we have labelled here leucoplakia, is suggested by Jeffcoate & Woodcock to be approximately 10%. It seems probable that in lichen sclerosus and kraurosis no direct cancer risk exists, although there may be an indirect one concerned with the progression from lichen sclerosus to leucoplakia. Wallace & Whimster (1951), for instance, describe 20 cases of lichen sclerosus of the vulva with atrophy of the rete pegs and flattening of the Maphigian layer, five of whom later showed a change to intense epithelial activity with down-dipping rete pegs; two of these five later developed carcinomatous change. Nonetheless, it is a fact that the hyperplastic type of vulval condition called here leucoplakia is the dangerous one which may call for prophylactic surgical removal of the vulva (see below). Although lichen sclerosus is not directly prone to malignant change, however, it may be so indirectly via the leucoplakic stage.

MORE ADVANCED LESIONS

There are other cases in which intra-epithelial carcinoma can be said already to exist. Here, too, various names have been employed—Queyrat's erythroplasia; Bowen's disease; Paget's disease; carcinoma *in situ*. In essence, however, there is the type of epithelial activity seen in carcinoma of the cervix—hyperactivity with numerous mitotic figures evident in the Malphigian layer, but without the normal stratification through the more superficial layers of the epithelium. Cellular pleomorphism and mitoses are evident at all levels of the epithelium (Fig. 40.4, p. 595). Corps ronds and epithelial pearl formation may be seen. No downgrowths through the basement membrane are present. It would seem wise to limit the term carcinoma *in situ* to this type of change, eliminating erythroplasia and Bowen's disease completely in this context. It seems possible, however, that Paget's disease does have more distinctive features, being a much more chronic condition which may remain limited to a localized area of the vulva for years. Here, the characteristic Paget cells will be evident—large, pale cells identical with those seen in the same disease in the nipple. There is some evidence that Paget's disease of the vulval skin may be associated with an underlying similar disorder of the apocrine glands.

Attempting some form of summary of this complex situation, it appears that the vulval dystrophies and associated conditions may be reduced to:

(a) An atrophic type of lesion here described as lichen sclerosus. This condition may be chronic and non-progressive, but may at some point develop into leucoplakia.

(b) Leucoplakia. This is a hyperplastic condition with similar dermal changes to those of lichen sclerosus, but with marked Malphigian activity. This is evident as increased thickness of this layer and down-dipping and bizarre-shaping of rete pegs; the stratification of superficial layers of squamous epithelium is retained, however. The condition has a premalignant tendency. Some 10% or so of cases may develop carcinoma if untreated.

(c) In addition, the vulva may be affected by extreme atrophy and shrinkage of tissues, especially around the vaginal introitus. Various histological appearances may be associated with this atrophy. The condition may be labelled kraurosis, but this term, if used at all, must be strictly limited to cases where shrinkage of tissue is very marked indeed.

More serious conditions are:

(d) Carcinoma *in situ*, where histological changes similar to those of carcinoma *in situ* of the cervix are evident. Invasion sooner or later—probably sooner—is likely.

(e) Paget's disease. This is uncommon, and is a form of carcinoma *in situ* which may be associated with a similar change in apocrine glands. It is a very slowly developing condition which may remain unchanged for many years, although it may later spread very rapidly.

CLINICAL FEATURES

There are similarities between the features of the various chronic vulval dystrophies and *in situ* malignant lesions which make precise diagnosis difficult without biopsy. Atrophy of the tissue in parts of the vulva is likely with all; the presence of white patches as distinct areas or over the whole of the vulval area are a common feature. There are differences, however, which may help to suggest which of the conditions under review we are likely to be dealing with.

The presence of lesions elsewhere on the body surface may indicate the diagnosis of lichen sclerosus. The vulva affected by this condition usually shows considerable atrophy, with flattening of skin folds; the whitened areas are free from induration; spread of the condition backwards to encroach upon the anal area, should suggest a diagnosis of lichen sclerosus.

Leucoplakia may be almost indistinguishable from lichen sclerosus by ordinary clinical methods, and biopsy will be necessary to establish the degree of activity of the epithelium. Raised, irregular, whitish areas with increased cornification and, if not induration, firmness to the touch, cannot be assumed to be free from leucoplakic activity. This heaping-up of keratin can give distinctly raised white patches which may lie adjacent to shallower, reddened areas where it appears the keratin has been rubbed off by some local irritant action. Cracking and fissuring, aggravated by scratching, may be evident in this condition, and in lichen sclerosus also. It must be remembered, too, that one part of the vulva may demonstrate atrophic changes of lichen sclerosus and another hyperplastic epithelial activity; this makes it unwise to rely solely on clinical observation in suspicious cases.

Extreme atrophy and shrinkage of the vulval area, especially in the region of the introitus, may be termed kraurosis vulvae, although 'vulval atrophy' seems an adequate term. The vaginal introitus may be greatly narrowed and examination well-nigh impossible. Sometimes, the labia minora adhere together (Fig. 38.6), as in the very young child (see labial adhesions, p. 22).

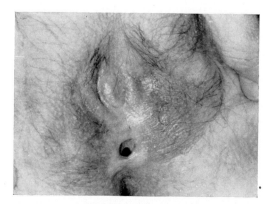

Fig. 38.6. Sealed labia in an old lady. The labia minora are adherent to each other, reducing the vaginal introitus to a tiny opening.

The clinical features of carcinoma *in situ* are far from distinct. Again, firm or indurated areas must be regarded with suspicion. Absence of keratin from some lesions affected by carcinoma *in situ* leads to a dull, reddened appearance of the affected skin. The presence of Paget's disease tends to give similar clinical appearances, with slightly raised reddened areas alternating with whitish patches where hyperkeratosis is marked (Fig. 38.7).

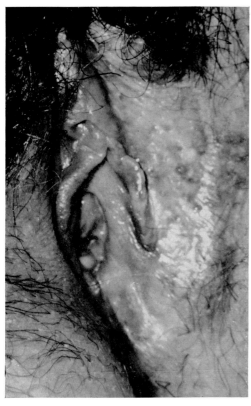

Fig. 38.7. Paget's disease of the vulva. The anterior portion of the labium majorum on the patient's left shows thinning and reddening of the vulval skin alternating with whitish areas. The histological appearances are those of Paget's disease.

TREATMENT

Management of the postmenopausal patient with a chronic vulval lesion of the variety under discussion will initially involve a careful decision as to whether biopsy is indicated or not. Any suggestion that the disorder may be leucoplakia, as defined here, will call for biopsy of suspicious areas; those more indurated, raised or reddened may be chosen. If a localized area alone is affected and is sufficiently limited to allow excision biopsy, this will be preferable. If, however, there is clinical evidence to support lichen sclerosus alone as the lesion present, biopsy may be withheld at the time until the effect of local treatment has been observed. In other circumstances early biopsy will be the best course, conservative treatment being employed later if a premalignant lesion can be excluded.

Treatment of lichen sclerosus can be conducted, for a time at least, without the need for prophylactic surgery. Attention to general health and to vulval hygiene are both important. Correction of anaemia, insistence on a correct diet, weight reduction where appropriate, etc. may not seem likely to influence the course of the disease significantly, but it is probable, nonetheless, that they have a general beneficial effect. So, too, does attention to the patient's emotional outlook. On many occasions one has noted more troublesome symptoms from a vulval lesion during a period of anxiety and overwork. This aspect of the case must receive attention.

Local vulval hygienic measures are even more important. The skin must be treated with great delicacy. Washing and drying must be gentle, a good soap and a soft towel only being used; underclothes must be washed in a non-irritant soap and rinsing must be very thorough, as in the case of more acute vulvitis already dealt with. Lichen sclerosus in postmenopausal patients responds well to local steroid therapy with a betamethazone, or similar preparations. They may be used for some months at a time, but it is better that they be stopped once there is sufficient local improvement and kept in reserve for some future exacerbation. Meanwhile, the hygenic measures discussed above must be continued; if any ointment is required a simple, bland one such as zinc and castor oil may be helpful. Patients with lichen sclerosus may be kept in comfort for years in this way. There will be periods of increased irritation and itching but, once controlled as above, a remission may last for many months. Biopsy must be kept in mind if any obvious change in the vulval appearance takes place.

Leucoplakia is premalignant, as already indicated, and if it is established that significant hyperplasia is present in the vulval skin, and that malignancy must be considered a risk, prophylactic simple vulvectomy is indicated. It may not be easy in all cases to decide if the epithelial activity present is sufficiently marked and disordered to call for this measure. Careful consultation with the pathologist can be very helpful here.

The progress of the disorder, after the type of conservative approach just described for lichen sclerosus, may be helpful in deciding if further observation is safe or if operation is desirable at once.

If the changes observed in the vulval biopsy are even more marked, and fall within the category of carcinoma *in situ*, vulvectomy without gland dissection is certainly indicated. Moreover, whenever surgery is performed a careful follow-up is important, since recurrences in the new vulval skin are not unlikely. After surgery, considerable care of the vulval area should be continued in an attempt to minimize these recurrences. There is further consideration of these subjects in Chapter 40.

Other vulval lesions

BARTHOLIN CYSTS AND ABSCESSES

Bartholin cysts are common gynaecological lesions. They arise as a result of an obstruction to the duct of Bartholin's gland on one or other side, resulting in a cystic swelling deep to the posterior part of the labium. The gland secretion, normally discharged from the orifice of the duct just external to the hymen in the 5 o'clock and 7 o'clock positions, is retained and the cyst forms. Such cysts are not usually of large size, and do not usually exceed 5 or 6 cm in diameter (Fig. 38.8).

The presence of the cyst itself may be the most disturbing feature for the patient. When she becomes aware of its presence, she may worry that she has a serious lesion, although few symp-

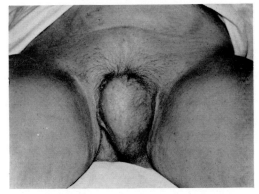

Fig. 38.8. A very large Bartholin's cyst.

toms *per se* arise from uncomplicated Bartholin cysts.

Bartholin abscess formation, however, is another matter. A swelling becomes very painful and tender. It is red and angry and clearly infected. The patient may have difficulty in walking, or even sitting, without considerable discomfort. It is probable that one of various organisms such as *Escherichia coli*, streptococci, staphylococci and gonococci will be the infecting agent. It used to be said that the gonococcus was especially common, but this is certainly not true in Britain today; however, it might apply elsewhere. Recurrent infections in Bartholin's glands may well be seen. Following the bursting or incision of an abscess, there is rapid relief of symptoms and the infection subsides. It may, however, return within weeks or months, and unless definitive treatment is undertaken a patient may suffer several such episodes a year.

Bartholin cysts and abscesses are best dealt with by marsupialization. An incision is made some 2·5 cm in length over the vaginal aspect of the swelling along the line of the labium minus. The cyst fluid is drained out and the lining is sutured to the skin by four or five interrupted cat-gut stitches. If there is no infection the procedure can be done in the out-patient department under local anaesthesia, or under general anaesthesia as a day case. If infection is present, then greater care is required to unite the skin and the more fragile cyst lining. With this treatment, the ostium of the gland is preserved, and its function also. Recurrences after marsupialization are uncommon (Blakey *et al.* 1966). Kelly (1969) has recently reviewed these lesions. Other minor cysts and swellings are dealt with in Chapter 40.

FEMALE CIRCUMCISION

Occasionally, the effects of female circumcision are encountered in patients living in, or visiting, Great Britain. A brief account of this seems appropriate.

Mutilating procedures which are collectively called female circumcision have been practised for hundreds, perhaps thousands, of years. It seems probable that the practice reaches back so far into the past that no-one can say when it began. The ritual is most common in the continent of Africa in general, and in the upper reaches of the River Nile in particular, although it is occasionally practised elsewhere. Laycock

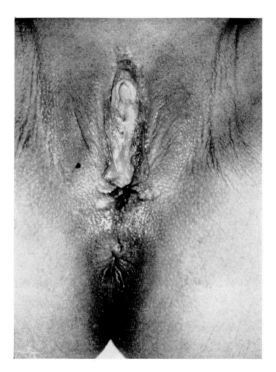

Fig. 38.9. The results of infibulation in childhood. The labia minora have been stitched together, obscurring the vagina.

(1950) distinguishes two main types of procedure —excision and infibulation. In excision it may be the clitoris alone which is excised, or parts of the labia minora as well. During healing, especially if extensive procedures have been employed, considerable scarring may result. Infibulation—the fastening with a fibula or clasp—aims at occluding the introitus completely by fastening the labia minora together (Fig. 38.9); this may be done with some form of suture material or they may be transfixed with thorns.

As may be imagined, numerous complications have occurred as a result of this practice—deep scar tissue, haemorrhage and infection being the principal ones. Extensions of incisions into the rectum or urethra have also occurred.

VAGINAL LESIONS

Infections

Pyogenic infection of the vagina is uncommon during the child-bearing years because of the protection afforded by the acid vaginal reaction. The action of the oestrogens on the vaginal epithelium is to cause growth, maturation and exfoliation of the squamous cells. The surface cells are rich in glycogen and this is acted upon by the lactogenic bacilli present in the vagina to produce lactic acid; the pH of the vagina during reproductive life is about 4 or 5. There is a constant small amount of vaginal discharge present under normal circumstances, and this is composed of the desquamated superficial cells of the vaginal epithelium and cervical mucoid discharge. The secretion from Bartholin's gland, which occurs most markedly at the times of intercourse, contributes also.

During childhood there is little oestrogen to act upon the vagina. The epithelium is thin and easily abraded and the pH of the vagina is alkaline. After the menopause, a similar situation prevails.

Vaginitis during childhood is not uncommon, and is considered on p. 19. After the menopause, the vaginal skin may also become easily abraded, and infection (atrophic or 'senile' vaginitis) is common. Vaginal infections during reproductive life are rare and are confined to infestations with *Trichomonas vaginalis* and *Candida albicans*, and to those infections associated with irritation from a foreign body, such as a neglected tampon.

Trichomonas vaginalis VAGINITIS

The *Trichomonas vaginalis* organism is a flagellated, unicellular organism some 20 μm in length. It has four flagellae anteriorly and a terminal membranous stylus. The organism is similar in size to a pus cell, but may sometimes be slightly larger.

It seems probable that infection is spread by sexual intercourse, since the organism is clearly harboured by the male, though it probably produces few symptoms under normal circumstances. The organism may be found in the vagina of patients without symptoms, and it seems probable that its simple presence is not sufficient alone to allow it to establish itself and cause trouble. Possibly the reduction in the pH of the vagina shortly after menstruation allows the infection to arise and symptoms of vaginal discharge and vulval itching to follow.

The discharge associated with *Trichomonas* infestations is fluid, greenish in colour and slightly frothy in appearance. The quantity of discharge varies, but in acute cases it is usually profuse. On inspection the vaginal walls show tiny punctate 'strawberry' spots and these, together with the typical appearance of the discharge, often permits the diagnosis to be made confidently on inspection alone. For confirmation a drop of discharge is taken, mixed with a drop of saline on a slide and examined at once under the microscope. The motile organisms are clearly visible when viewed in this way.

Treatment is simple. Metronidazole (Flagyl) may be given by mouth in doses of 200 mg three times daily for 7–10 days. Most cases respond well to this treatment, but relapses are common. They may follow further intercourse with the infected partner or may perhaps follow the continued presence of the *Trichomonas* in the various vulval glands, Skene's ducts, etc. The male partner should be treated with the same dose whenever there has been a recurrence, and it may be wise to treat him on the first occasion.

Candida albicans VAGINITIS

This infection is due to the presence of the yeast-like fungus *Candida albicans*. It is evident in a specimen of discharge stained by Gram's stain as long filaments (mycelia) or as spores. Culture will confirm the diagnosis in doubtful cases. This organism thrives in the presence of carbohydrate, and is common in diabetics and during pregnancy when sugar-containing urine may be passed. It is generally held in check by the presence of other vaginal organisms, but if antibiotic treatment has been given and these organisms destroyed, the *Candida* may thrive.

The discharge produced is thick, white and cheesey in appearance, and tends to stick to the walls of the vagina. The vagina itself is extremely sore and examination may be very painful. Great itching is complained of.

Infection responds well to antifungal pessaries such as nystatin—one or two pessaries being inserted into the vagina nightly for 2 weeks. Painting with 1% aqueous solution of gentian violet, which was formally used, is seldom needed now. Recurrences may arise and are usually associated with the basic underlying conditions—such as glycosuria—or with antibiotic therapy; sometimes, general ill-health in the patient tends to predispose to infection in this way.

ATROPHIC VAGINITIS

The very thin vaginal epithelium of the postmenopausal woman is easily injured and infected, as already indicated. Non-specific organisms of low virulence are usually responsible. The walls of the vagina appear red and angry and tiny bleeding spots may be visible. A thin, purulent discharge may be evident. Examination is often difficult, in view of the pain experienced. Unless it can be established for certain that no other lesion is present—particularly cancer of the cervix, if the discharge is slightly blood-stained—examination under anaesthesia will be wise. Vaginal and vulval soreness are the symptoms usually experienced. Sometimes, the patient has a sensation of 'something coming down,' and may believe she has a prolapse.

Oestrogen therapy applied locally has a rapid effect. Oestrogen pessaries inserted high into the vagina for 2 weeks are usually all that is required. If preferred, oestrogens may be given by mouth, but local application appears preferable. If there is early recurrence, which is uncommon, consideration should be given to long-term, low-dose, oestrogen therapy.

The discharge associated with the retention of a tampon or other foreign body in the vagina is usually foul-smelling and blood-stained. Removal of the offending article is all that is necessary.

Other vaginal lesions

VAGINAL CYSTS

Vaginal cysts are usually remnants of the lower portion of the Wolffian duct. The duct runs alongside the vagina at an early stage of development and then usually retrogresses totally. If a portion persists, a vaginal cyst may result.

These cysts are thin-walled structures and may lie at almost any point in the vagina, although they are somewhat more common in the upper portion. They seldom achieve any appreciable size and rarely give rise to important symptoms. Discovery is usually accidental during a vaginal examination to take a cervical smear or for some other symptom.

It seems probable that most, if not all, vaginal cysts can be ignored, as the patient is unaware of their presence and they are causing no trouble. Very rarely, those in the upper vagina burrow fairly deeply into the broad ligament, and then attempted removal may lead to a deep, bloody and dangerous dissection, during which the bladder or ureter or both may be injured. Left alone, they do not harm.

VAGINAL ADENOSIS

Vaginal adenosis is a far more serious condition. The normal squamous epithelium covering the vagina is replaced by columnar, gland-bearing epithelium. One unpleasant feature of the condition is the excessive mucus secretion, which causes quite profuse vaginal discharge. Examination shows that much of the vagina, and perhaps even the cervix too, contains cysts varying in

size from a pin-head to several millimeters in diameter. Sometimes larger aggregations cause heaped up masses of glandular tissue (Fig. 38.10).

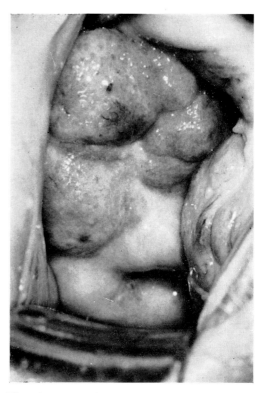

Fig. 38.10. Vaginal adenosis. This patient has large aggregations of cysts throughout the vagina and was very disturbed by the profuse vaginal discharge.

A very striking feature is the large amount of mucus poured out from these various lesions. Stabler (1961) described several patients greatly troubled by this type of profuse discharge.

The histological picture is that of closely packed glands similar to those seen in the cervical canal; they lie close to the surface, most of which is denuded by its squamous epithelium. The stroma surrounding the glandular area may show oedema or chronic inflammatory change and fibrosis. Treatment for this condition can be quite difficult. Excision is likely to be an extensive procedure, and, indeed, in the more marked cases will involve the removal of almost all the vaginal epithelium. Such a surgical undertaking is of course possible and may be followed by skin grafting of the area, but will clearly require very careful consideration before it is decided upon (Stabler 1967). A recent personal case appeared to improve on the contraceptive pill and another improved significantly after the menopause. Malignancy developing in these areas has been reported (Sandberg *et al.* 1968).

VAGINITIS EMPHYSEMATOSA

This is an unusual condition in which gas-filled cysts lie beneath the epithelium of the vagina. The lesions are smooth, tense, discrete, grey cysts. They may be very small or a centimeter or two in diameter. They tend to occur in groups, forming a firm, palpable mass. If a cyst is pricked a tiny plop may be heard, but no fluid escapes. Most recorded cases have been in patients who were pregnant and who experienced few, or no, symptoms from the lesion. Microscopic examination from the excised areas shows sub-epidermal, air-filled spaces, sometimes lined by endothelial cells and sometimes by squamous epithelium. Treatment appears unnecessary, since few symptoms can be attributed to the lesion. Rowland & Inman (1968) have recently reviewed the condition.

LESIONS OF THE CERVIX

Cervicitis, cervical erosion, ectropion

These are all terms which are employed from time to time in clinical gynaecological practice without any real attempt at precise diagnosis. The cervical situation usually so described is that in which the red vascular columnar epithelium of the endocervix is clearly visible around the external os; there may be variable amounts of cervical mucus evident, and sometimes greenish mucoid pus as well. In many cases, the whole cervix appears enlarged. These terms are usually employed without special care and attention because this whole subject is far from clearly elucidated. Some attempt at clarification will be made.

CERVICAL EPITHELIUM

The cervix is covered by two types of epithelium. The vaginal portion is covered, on its external aspect, by stratified squamous epithelium up to the external os. Within the cervical canal the epithelium is thrown into very complex folds and lined by tall, columnar, mucus-secreting cells.

The junction of the squamous and columnar portions may show a sudden change from one variety to the other, or there may be a broader transitional zone present.

The cervical os in the nulliparous patient is small and circular and no columnar epithelium is visible. In the parous patient the os is more slit-like following the almost inevitable trauma of delivery. A small portion of the columnar epithelium lining the canal is often visible on one or other or, less often, both cervical lips.

The canal itself is lined by deep, cervical glands. Whether these are true glands or not appears questionable; their gland-like appearance may be due to the extremely complex infolding of mucosa which is certainly evident within the canal. In any event, deep, crypt-like spaces occur which are effectively glandular, since mucus production is continuous from the tall, columnar cells of the epithelium.

Ectropion is strictly an eversion of the cervical lips permitting the endocervical epithelium to be seen on inspection. If bilateral minor lacerations have occurred to the cervix, giving it a longer than usual slit-like os, the anterior and posterior lips may fall somewhat apart, so allowing the epithelium within the canal to assume a partially external situation and to be clearly visible. Of itself, this cannot be regarded as abnormal. If associated with the production of excessive cervical mucus, however, causing troublesome symptoms, treatment as indicated below may be required.

A cervical erosion is, in some respects, similar, inasmuch as columnar epithelium is again visible on the ectocervix. Here, however, it seems probable that damage has occurred to the squamous epithelium of the vaginal portion of the cervix and the columnar epithelium has grown over the area, extending itself at the expense of the squamous variety. The extent of this erosion may be variable. If minor, it is unimportant and like ectopian can be ignored apart from the taking of a cervical smear if one has not been done recently. If more extensive, but unassociated with symptoms, it can probably again be ignored. If a vaginal discharge is complained of, however, and the pouring out of mucus from the cervix is clearly excessive, treatment is again necessary (see below).

Cervicitis is less easy to define. If there is considerable mucus production in either ec-tropion or erosion, it is probable that cervicitis is present to some extent. This does not imply predominantly an effective condition with virulent organisms present. It implies rather that there is a general increase in the glandular mucus-producing elements in the cervix, and that super-ficial minor infection is probably present in those areas. Certainly, the mucus seen on such a cervix is often yellowish and unpleasant, and seems likely to be due, in part at least, to a minor infective element.

A big cervix with a large area of columnar mucus producing epithelium visible is commonly seen in patients attending postnatal clinics. The impression given is that involution in the cervical glands is not quite complete. Some of the hypertrophy and hyperplasia which occurred as a result of pregnancy may remain and may in itself be the underlying change in some large cervices with profuse mucoid discharge. Other local irritants such as contraceptive caps, etc. may excite a similar reaction.

Sometimes, a cervix of this type, recognized at the postnatal clinic, may later be seen to be smaller, with less or no columnar epithelium visible; there may, however, be small cysts visible in the cervical substance, the domes protruding slightly above the surface. These are Nabothian follicles, formed, it is believed, by growth of the squamous epithelium over the mouths of the cervical glands formerly present in that area, trapping mucus within the follicles. This is a common finding in patients with no symptoms whatsoever.

The to and fro growth of columnar and squamous epithelium in the region of the external os is obviously a distinct entity. In cervices re-moved with the uterus at hysterectomy, or in

portions of cervix removed at biopsy, another type of epithelial change may be evident. Here, squamous epithelium is seen partially replacing columnar epithelium within the glands of the endocervix. This is epidermidization, and is not, of itself, a significant finding, although in cervices showing dysplasia or carcinoma *in situ* the glandular portions of the squamous epithelium may be similarly affected.

CLINICAL FEATURES

In clinical terms, the importance of these cervical changes is concerned with the symptoms they produce. An excessive vaginal discharge is the most common symptom; this may disturb the patient simply by its presence; or it may so soil her clothing that she must either change frequently or wear a pad constantly; or she may be con-cerned about the unpleasant odour which she believes is offensive to other people; the dis-charge may, of course, cause considerable vulval soreness.

When the discharge is thick, yellow and offensive, it seems probable that a true, if super-ficial, infection is present in association with the excessive mucus produced. Intermenstrual bleed-ing, small in amount and usually following local cervical irritation or trauma such as that occurring at intercourse, may be an additional symptom.

It is questionable how often, if at all, lower abdominal pain can be said to arise from these cervical changes. Patients sometimes make this complaint in association with vaginal discharge, but this cannot be taken as clear evidence of cause and effect. Bladder symptoms of frequency and urgency are also sometimes attributed to cervitis. Here, too, it is questionable if a direct relationship exists on more than a few occasions. Such symptoms are more likely to be due to other causes distinct from cervicitis.

Examination of a patient with symptoms just described must of course be conducted with the possibility of a cervical cause in mind. The size, appearance and feel of the cervix are all important. The cervix with 'erosion', 'ectropion' or 'cer-vicitis' present usually feels soft; occasionally, a slightly granular sensation is appreciated by the palpating finger. Some bleeding is not uncommon on the more vascular cervices when they are touched or scraped.

The principal differential diagnosis is carcinoma of the cervix, and this must always be kept firmly in mind. A cervical smear is essential. Probing of the cervix with a fine probe is often an excellent means of detecting an early clinical cancer; a fine probe, gently pressed against the area of normal (if misplaced) columnar epithelium, will not penetrate the surface but it will sink with ease for a short distance into a malignant area. If there is clinical doubt a biopsy is important, even if a negative smear has been obtained. Coppleston (see p. 626) has urged the wider use of colposcopy in such cases.

Treatment should be reserved for those patients in whom cervical epithelial changes are associated with symptoms. Since, in most cases, the symptoms are due to excessive mucus production, destruction by cauterization or cryo-surgery of the mucus-producing areas is required. This should be done by radial strokes of the cautery at a superficial level. It may be undertaken as an outpatient procedure without anaesthesia. Healing is usually complete within a few weeks. If the cervical changes are extensive it will be wiser to carry out the cautery under general anaesthesia, and to follow it by cervical dilation to ensure that stenosis of the cervix does not result. It is rare for more elaborate cervical operations to be required. The association of considerable cervical damage at previous confinement with the changes described above may, however, suggest that a cervical plastic repair procedure, with excision of some of the glandular areas and reconstruction of the cervix to something approaching its normal appearance, may be contemplated if simpler measures have failed to relieve symptoms. Such trachylorrhaphy operations are more difficult and less successful than may be imagined, and they are rarely indicated. Other vulval, vaginal and cervical lesions are considered in Chapter 40.

REFERENCES

BLAKEY D.H., DEWHURST C.J. & TIPTON R.H. (1966) *J. Obstet. Gynaec. Br. Commonw.* **73**, 1008.

CUNLIFFE W.J. & MENON I.S. (1969) *Lancet*, i, 1239.

DEWHURST C.J. (1955) *J. Obstet. Gynaec. Br. Commonw.* **62**, 563.

FOWLER T.J., HUMPSTON D.J., NUSSEY A.M. & SMALL M. (1968) *Br. med. J.* ii, 473.

HILLS E.A. (1967) *Br. med. J.* iv, 152.

HUTFIELD D.C. & LONGSON M. (1968) *J. Obstet. Gynaec. Br. Commonw.* **75**, 768.

JEFFCOATE T.N.A. & WOODCOCK A.S. (1961) *Br. med. J.* ii, 127.

KELLY J. (1969) *Br. J. Hosp. Med.* **3**, 1696.

SANDBERG E.C., DANIELSON R.W., CAUWET R.W. & BONAR B.E. (1965) *Am. J. Obstet. Gynec.* **93**, 209.

SMITH R.B.W., PRIOR I.A.M. & STURMAN D. (1967) *Br. med. J.* ii, 220.

STABLER F. (1961) *J. Obstet. Gynaec. Br. Commonw.* **68**, 857.

STABLER F. (1967) *J. Obstet. Br. Commonw.* **74**, 493.

STENING M. & ELLIOT P.G. (1959) *J. Obstet. Gynaec. Br. Commonw.* **66**, 897.

STEWART D.B. (1967) In *Obsetrics & Gynaecology in the Tropics* (edited by J.B. Lawson & D.B. Stewart). London, Edward Arnold, p. 432.

VICKERS H.R. & SNEDDON I.B. (1957) *Modern Trends in Geriatrics*. London, Butterworths.

WALLACE H.J. & WHIMSTER I.W. (1951) *Br. J. Derm.* **63**, 241.

CHAPTER 39

TUMOURS OF THE FEMALE GENITAL TRACT

The female genital tract is the site of a large number of tumours of considerable diversity but many of them are extremely rare and even those regarded as common are not seen sufficiently often to become commonplace to postgraduate students of medicine. The tumour occurring with the greatest frequency is undoubtedly the benign fibromyoma or uterine fibroid, a tumour so familiar that ignorance regarding its aetiology, apart from a nod in the direction of hormones, is accepted somewhat complacently. Simple cervical and endometrial polyps are also frequently found, but, as they cause only minor symptoms and are easily removed by minor operations, they attract little attention. Benign tumours of the ovary are fairly often seen and of these the benign teratoma or dermoid cyst, the mucinous and the serous cystadenomata are those which are usually found. The term mucinous cyst has been adopted universally instead of pseudomucinous, now that the nature of the cyst content is known. But pseudomyxoma peritonei remains the name for that rare form of spread to the peritoneum resulting in the accumulation of the glutinous material within the abdominal cavity. Most interest and research is reserved for the malignant tumours, and of these the most important are carcinoma of the cervix, adenocarcinoma of the corpus uteri and ovarian carcinoma, as these are the commonest, and therefore responsible for many unpleasant deaths in women (see Table 39.1).

Certain changes in respect of incidence and mortality rates are to be observed. There is a general increase in all cases of cancer, more for

Table 39.1. New cases of malignant disease in women of all ages: rates per 100,000 women, 1964 (adapted from the *Registrar General's Review, 1962–1964*).

Leukaemia		5·3
Ovary		14·6
Lung		15·5
Stomach		18·1
Uterus		17·5
Cervix		21·8
Large bowel	23·7	37·4
Rectum	13·7	
Breast		65·8

Table 39.2. Malignant disease, all new cases, England and Wales (adapted from the *Registrar General's Review, 1962–1964*).

	1962	1963	1964
Stomach	4,170	4,300	4,406
Large bowel	5,142	5,454	5,777
Lung	3,003	3,371	3,781
Breast	14,697	15,880	16,031
Cervix	4,377	4,731	5,301
Uterus	3,140	3,208	3,434
Ovary	3,162	3,424	3,547
Leukaemia	1,237	1,248	1,303

men than for women; growing points for women are lung and carcinoma of the large bowel (see Table 39.2). Within the genital tract, changing incidences have been observed in uterine cancer. Earlier in the century it was commonly held that carcinoma of the cervix was seen eight times as frequently as carcinoma of the endometrium.

This ratio has changed considerably, so that many reports give a 3 to 2 ratio in favour of the cervix, whilst in the United Kingdom the incidence is nearly equal. The reasons for this are not clear, but it has been suggested that there is a decrease in the incidence of carcinoma of the cervix due to changed economic circumstances; that there is an increase in carcinoma of the corpus uteri due to increased longevity in the population at large, and that there is an improved diagnosis in carcinoma of the corpus uteri, which previously may well have been reported as carcinoma of the cervix.

The aetiology of malignant disease remains as obscure as ever, despite recurrent prophecies that the solution is imminent. Too often, aetiological factors have been proclaimed without proper relation to controls or statistical analysis, and often more work has to be done to refute claims than was done to state them. Carcinoma of the cervix has remained a happy hunting ground for this sort of activity and so far, despite an enormous literature, the only indisputable facts are that coitus and child bearing predispose a woman to this condition! In the case of carcinoma of the corpus uteri, a number of factors have been invoked to try to formulate an endocrine basis, but whilst there are many reports of much interest both as regards oestrogen stimulating and progesterone inhibiting the condition, the knowledge remains of limited value in the management of the majority of patients.

The histogenesis of ovarian tumours has always been an extremely confused area because of the great diversity of tumours which may occur in this one gland. There is a welcome tendency to simplify the approach to this problem, in that the cells of the ovary itself are considered to be capable of giving rise to all the various types of primary tumour. The predilection for a number of tumours to metastasize to the ovary has long been known, and this sometimes gives rise to difficulties in diagnosis. The similarity in appearance of some ovarian tumours to uterine adenocarcinoma has aroused interest in recent years, and has given rise to the use of the term endometrioid carcinoma; this is considered to arise from endometrioisis of the ovary, but proof of this is only rarely forthcoming. Some authorities

regard endometrioid carcinoma in a rather special light, believing it to carry a better prognosis than most other types of ovarian cancer, but this is not generally agreed. The group of tumours showing endocrine activity have attracted a degree of interest in inverse proportion to their frequency, for they form only a small proportion of all ovarian tumours. Increasing knowledge has destroyed the original concept that these tumours could be divided neatly into feminizing, masculinizing or inert categories; it is now recognized that the hormone stimulus produced may be very variable, even to the extent of both masculinizing and feminizing effects being produced by the same tumour, and also that tumours such as mucinous cystadenomata may, on occasion, be associated with some hormone activity.

Treatment of malignant disease of the genital tract has undergone various changes over the years, but no startling changes in cure rates have been evident, except as a result of very early diagnosis. Prior to the discovery of radium and X-rays, surgery offered the only hope of treatment. At first, surgery was directed towards the removal of the primary tumour and its immediate surroundings. As knowledge of the spread of cancer grew and surgical technique developed, more extensive operations were developed, such as those described by Wertheim, Schauta and Bassett.

An abdominal approach to gynaecological surgery was inevitable in the United Kingdom as the early gynaecologists were general surgeons who turned to pelvic surgery; amongst these, Victor Bonney was pre-eminent. Vaginal surgery had always been more popular on the Continent of Europe, and this approach was encouraged in the more radical operations by the very slow development of anaesthesiology. Since the Second World War anaesthetic standards have improved considerably, and with this improvement has come a resurgence of the radical abdominal hysterectomy. Radiotherapy in its infancy seemed to hold out the promise of a cure for cancer, but whilst it is invaluable in cancer therapy, that promise has not been entirely fulfilled. Since those early days when the pioneers subjected their patients and themselves to dangerously high doses of radium and its emanations, standards and techniques have improved dramatically and now the regulations governing the use of radioactive sources are so strict that treatment can only be carried out in well-organized units. The hope has always been that more powerful machines delivering even greater doses would show greatly improved results. Such marked improvement in results has not been forthcoming; some improvement has obviously been obtained, but in the main the value of sophisticated machinery has been to increase the flexibility of treatment and reduce the discomfort and morbidity for the patient. Today, radiotherapy remains the mainstay of treatment in cancer of the cervix and the vagina, it can be a useful adjunct to surgery in cancer of the corpus uteri and the ovary, but has little place in cancer of the vulva.

Chemotherapy was the next bright star to arise on the scene of cancer therapy, but with a few notable exceptions—such as choriocarcinoma of the uterus—the results to date have been disappointing. A number of different agents have been employed with varying degrees of toxicity, and the choice of which to use has been empirical and subject to the whims of the therapist. A more logical method of choice has been suggested by Limburg (1969) who has devised a method of *in vitro* testing of chemical agents on tissue cultures of the tumour. To date, ovarian carcinoma has been the main field of action for the use of this form of treatment, and the present situation is that chemotherapy tends to be reserved for late stages of the disease and for recurrences when surgery and radiotherapy have failed; the most that can be expected is some prolongation of life in some cases, although in a few, dramatic results may be achieved, even to the extent of encouraging 'second look'operations.

Hormone therapy with high doses of progestogens has been successfully used in some cases of carcinoma of the corpus uteri; soft-tissue secondary masses, particularly in the lungs, have been shown to resolve and some workers have shown that local application to the primary tumour has achieved reversal to normal endometrium in some cases. Naturally, there has been much speculation on the possible long-term effects of prolonged oral contraception, but whilst it is recognized that the pill alters the characteristics of the cervical smear, so far there has only been unconfirmed rumour that carcinoma *in situ* or invasive carcinoma is more common in users of the pill than in other women. On the other hand, it is postulated that by preventing endometrial hyperplasia the pill might in fact protect women from developing cancer of the endometrium.

Early diagnosis and the detection of premalignant conditions has been the most exciting development in recent years. Once again, however, early promise has not been fulfilled; despite the enthusiasm generated over cervical cytology, cancer of the cervix is still far from being eradicated. However, discovery of premalignant and micro-invasive conditions has highlighted the value of early detection and, together with the more widespread acceptance of criteria for staging, latterly through the activities of F.I.G.O., it is realized that the results of treatment in early stages of cancer can be very gratifying (see Table 39.3). It is a sad comment on the failure of society to make full use of the facilities available, that so many of the cases of cancer when first treated are at such a late stage. Whilst the value of cervical cytology in detecting carcinoma *in situ* and early invasive carcinoma is generally accepted, attempts

Table 39.3. Results of treatment in the early stages of invasive malignant disease

Organ	Stage	Treatment	5-year survival rate (%)	Authors
Cervix	I	Surgery	82·9	Kelso & Funnell (1967)
		Radiotherapy	83	McLennan *et al.* (1967)
Corpus	I	Surgery	83	McGarrity & Scott (1968)
Ovary	Ia	Surgery	84	Munnell (1968)
Vulva	Node-free	Surgery	72·9	Gopelrud & Keetal (1968)

at more widespread screening with 'do-it-yourself' kits have remained largely in the realm of research, and only in British Columbia have money, enthusiasm and organization been applied in an attempt to screen a whole population, but even here 25% of the population remain unscreened— and this may be the most important 25%. The value of such efforts is not universally accepted, for Green (1966) feels that the impact on mortality rates is not yet conclusive, and Ashley (1966) suggests that not all cases of cancer of the cervix are preceded by an *in situ* stage. The results of cytology have stimulated other methods of screening such as the enzyme test described by Bonham & Gibbs (1962), but to date these do not carry the simplicity, ease and accuracy of cytology. Attempts to uncover the early stages of other genital tract malignancies are rendered more difficult because they are in less accessible sites than the cervix. Some successes have been recorded with intra-uterine aspiration for carcinoma of the corpus, and with cul-de-sac puncture for carcinoma of the ovary, but it is difficult to see how these can become routine in busy gynaecological clinics let alone be applied to mass screening methods. At present, the main hope must be that increasing education of doctors and the public alike will lead to early diagnosis, so that the benefits of treatment can be applied as soon as possible in the development of the disease.

REFERENCES

Ashley D.J.B. (1966) *J. Obstet. Gynaec. Br. Commonw.* **73**, 372.

Bonham D.G. & Gibbs D.F. (1962) *Br. med. J.* ii, 823.

Green H. (1966) *Am. J. Obstet. Gynec.* **94**, 1009.

Kelso J.W. & Funnell J.W. (1967) *J. Okla. St. med. Ass.* **60**, 503.

Limburg H.G. (1969) *Proc. R. Soc. Med.* **62**, 361.

McGarrity K.A. & Scott G.C. (1968) *J. Obstet. Gynaec. Br. Commonw.* **75**, 14.

McLennan C.E., McLennan M.T. & Bagshawe M.A. (1967) *Am. J. Obstet. Gynec.* **98**, 675.

Munnell E.W. (1968) *Am. J. Obstet. Gynec.* **100**, 790.

CHAPTER 40

TUMOURS OF THE VULVA AND VAGINA

TUMOURS OF THE VULVA

Forming part of the body integument, the vulva can be afflicted by any pathology known to arise in skin and its related structures. Not all of these lesions will be new growths but many will give rise to swelling or ulcers which must be considered in differential diagnosis and others may be precursors to tumour formation. The number of conditions to be considered is inevitably large but the number causing symptoms or being of significance is small.

Benign tumours of epidermal origin

As elsewhere in the skin, these tumours are fairly common on the vulva but they are, on the whole, unremarkable. To the clinician there is no distinction to be made between *sebaceous* and *epidermal cysts*, but Knox & Freeman (1965) consider that more than 90% of cutaneous cysts are epidermal. Epidermal cysts have a lining of stratified squamous epithelium and are filled with keratin. Sebaceous cysts have foamy, plump, sebaceous-type cells in their stratified squamous epithelium and have a sebum and keratin content which is often foul-smelling. Both types of cysts are clinically similar, being firm and dome-shaped with a central punctum. If the cysts discharge or become infected they may cause symptoms, otherwise they require removal only for cosmetic reasons.

Seborrhoeic keratoses vary in size, from being miniscule to several millimetres in diameter, and in appearance from macules to polypoidal projections. They are light brown and rather greasy, are often multiple and occur in older women.

Achrocordons are seen in young and, in particular, pregnant, women; they are in effect fibro-epithelial polyps or squamous papillomata. *Pigmented naevi* arise as localized accumulations of melanocytes in the basal layer and develop into collections of naevus cells in the dermis, forming intradermal naevi. They appear as macular, brown pigmented spots which become papular or polypoidal as they develop intradermally. They are removed for aesthetic reasons or if it is thought that they might become malignant. Warning of malignancy is denoted by increase in intensity or extent of pigmentation, increasing size, ulceration and bleeding or discharge. If the naevus is easily traumatized by clothing, as is usual on the vulva, then it is also best removed. Removal must be adequate with a generous margin of normal skin and underlying tissue. Histological examination is essential.

Benign proliferation of sebaceous glands appearing as small, yellow papules in *Fordyce's disease*, or singly as *sebaceous adenoma*, are rare, and are usually diagnosed only on histological examination if excised.

VIRAL WARTS

These are the most important members of this group, in that they are common and give rise to symptoms. They occur most often in the child-bearing years and are common during pregnancy, when their growth is luxuriant and profuse.

There is often associated vulvovaginal infection with discharge, when *Trichomonas vaginalis*, *Candida albicans* or the gonococcus may be found. Whilst warts may occur in the absence of these conditions, they are almost certainly venereal in transmission. The lesions are small, discrete, papillary processes which are nearly always multiple and tend to spread and to coalesce to form larger papillary growths. The fresh warts are pinkish-white, whilst older ones become brown, like the surrounding skin.

The larger, flatter, lesions on the perineum and perianal skin are moist, and are designated condyloma accuminata (Fig. 40.1). The basic

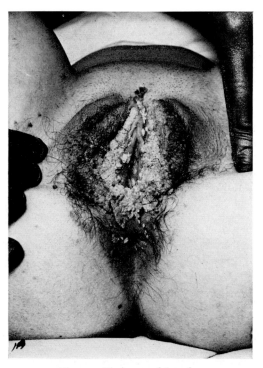

Fig. 40.1. Viral warts of the vulva.

histology is common to all types, with thickened epithelium thrown into folds around connective-tissue stalks. There is acanthosis with little hyperkeratosis and a variable amount of inflammatory reaction in the dermis. Mitotic figures may occur and their appearance is aggravated after the unsuccessful use of podophyllin.

Malignant change in condyloma accuminata has been reported on rare occasions. The warts are seen mainly on the skin of the labia majora, the perineum and perianal skin; the vagina may be involved in severe cases, more particularly in pregnancy, but the anal canal less commonly. The associated vaginitis is likely to cause more acute symptoms than the warts, but they may themselves give rise to pruritis or soreness and, if large and necrotic, to foul-smelling discharge.

Treatment will depend on the size and extent of the lesions. Any associated infection should first be treated, and this may result in the disappearance of the warts. Specific treatment is the application of a 20% solution of podophyllin in tincture of benzoin to the wart surface alone, carefully avoiding the surrounding skin. The warts blanch and then slough off in 3–4 days. Repeated applications are usually required for larger lesions and for fresh outcrops. Large and more extensive lesions are best removed by the diathermy loop, and any residual warts then touched with podophyllin. Some cases are very resistant and despite energetic treatment will persist for a number of years before finally disappearing. In pregnancy, when the lesions tend to be extensive and the tissues vascular, it is wiser to confine treatment to any associated infection and leave definitive treatment of the warts until after delivery, when they may in any case disappear spontaneously.

SWEAT-GLAND TUMOURS

Sweat glands on the vulva are of two main types: (a) small coil, or eccrine, which occur in practically every part of the skin and secrete clear fluid; they are not related to hair follicles, and (b) large coil, or apocrine, which occur at special sites: the axillae, breasts and genital region. The ducts open into the lower wall of a hair follicle. The secretion is fluid, contains part of the cell substance and has an odour. They begin to secrete at puberty and show some cyclical activity related to ovarian function.

Hidradenomata develop from the apocrine sweat glands. Mostly they are small, symptomless tumours less than 1 cm diameter and occurring on the labium majus. If they ulcerate they may cause bleeding and suggest malignancy. They are almost universally benign, and their rather bizarre microscopical appearance is characteristic.

Benign mesodermal tumours

These tumours are rare and basically symptomless. They seldom require treatment, but where indicated simple excision suffices. They may on occasion reach large size.

Fibroma

This is usually a pedunculated, firm, solid mass and is the commonest of this rare group.

Lipoma

This is a soft, round, lobulated swelling of variable size which may also become pedunculated.

Neurofibroma

This is more common than is usually realized, and is often mistaken for a fibro-epithelial polyp or small fibroma. Neurofibromata are small, fleshy papules or polyps, which may be single or multiple.

Leiomyoma

In contrast to the extreme frequency of this tumour in the uterus, its presence in the vulva is very rare.

Microscopically, all these mesodermal tumours are the same as their counterparts elsewhere in the body.

GRANULAR-CELL MYOBLASTOMA

As its name implies this is an oddity. It is a very rare tumour which occurs in other parts of the body also, notably the tongue. Kaufman & Gardner (1965) in a review of the histogenesis favour the view put forward by Fisher & Wecksler (1962), that these tumours arise in the nerve sheath-cell rather than in muscle cells, histiocytes or fibroblasts, which earlier observers postulated. This makes the terminology incorrect, but as a curiosity the name is likely to persist. The tumour is a small, solid nodule tending to infiltrate locally and thus to recur unless widely excised. Microscopically, the characteristic feature is of irregularly arranged bundles of large, pink-staining, round and polyhedral cells with indistinct cell borders (Fig. 40.2). Numerous

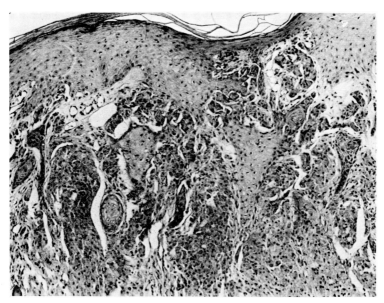

Fig. 40.2. Granular-cell myoblastoma. Marked epithelial hyperplasia with groups of 'myoblastoma' cells in the subepithelial connective tissue.

eosionophylic granules in the cytoplasm have given rise to the term granular-cell myoblastoma.

HAEMANGIOMA

There are a number of tumours arising from blood vessels, and these may be seen on the vulva, as elsewhere.

(1) *Strawberry haemangioma* is the typical red blotch which, in this area, is of no significance.

(2) *Cavernous haemangioma.* If small, this is of no importance, but occasionally the lesion is large and widespread. Because of the extreme vascularity, treatment is best avoided, but may become obligatory in the event of ulceration and bleeding. The method of treatment will be dictated by the age of the patient and the extent of the lesion. Smaller swellings may be dealt with by cryotherapy using a carbon dioxide stick. In some cases the injection of sclerosants will help. External irradiation with X-rays can be valuable in extensive lesions, but is not suitable for children and young women. Surgical excision is possible in less extensive lesions, but in larger ones can be fraught with considerable risk of severe bleeding.

(3) *Senile haemangioma.* Presenting as small, soft, bright-red papules, these are not so uncommon in the elderly. They are symptomless and unimportant.

(4) *Angiokeratoma.* This is a warty type of haemangioma with papillary formation and hyperkeratosis; it is very rare and is usually excised for diagnostic purposes.

(5) *Granuloma pyogenicum* is a dull-brown papule or papilloma with a scab formed after ulceration of the thinned, overlying epidermis and this, again, tends to be excised for diagnosis.

LYMPHANGIOMA

Even more uncommon than the various types of haemangioma, lymphangioma may present in simple form as a diffuse, soft, compressible, grey-pink nodule, or in more extensive cavernous form.

Carcinoma of the vulva

Incidence

As stated in Chapter 39, carcinoma of the vulva is a rare condition. Most gynaecologists see but one or two cases yearly, and for information about the condition it is necessary to study the reports of surgeons such as Taussig (1940), Green (1958) and Way (1954), who have collected relatively large series of cases.

Age

The majority of cases occur in women aged between 50 and 70 years. Seldom are the young or very old afflicted; Way (1951) in a series of 314 cases reported only 18 in women under 40 and only two in women over 80 years.

AETIOLOGY

Embryologically, the skin of the vulva is analogous to that of the scrotum, and it is of interest to note the occurrence of mule-spinners' cancer in females as well as males in the days when carcinogenic oils came into contact with the skin of the area. Of more significance is the recognition of certain changes in the vulval skin which may be precancerous. Leucoplakia vulvae has long been recognized as of importance in this respect. In the past any condition of the vulval skin presenting with pruritus and showing macroscopical skin changes, particularly if white patches were evident, tended to be designated as leucoplakia, regarded as precancerous and treated by vulvectomy. Such surgical treatment was regarded as both a cure for the symptoms and a prophylactic measure against the development of cancer. The fact that associated leucoplakia was found in well over half the patients suffering from carcinoma of the vulva, seemed to justify this approach. A more careful classification of the various changes found in the vulval skin, the use of skin biopsy to aid diagnosis, and the advent of topical cortisone preparations, have all led to a much more conservative policy in the management of what Jeffcoate *et al.* (1961) have preferred to name the chronic vulval dystrophies.

In his consideration of the subject he concluded that between 2·5 and 3% of cases so designated will have early invasive or intradermal carcinoma when first seen; 4–8% of the remainder will show microscopical signs of disorderly activity in the epidermis (Fig. 40.3), and the risk of invasive carcinoma developing in these is but one case in ten. Wallace & Whimster (1961)

of opinion as to nomenclature, and the conditions variously described are:

  (i) Bowen's disease.
 (ii) Erythroplasia of Queyrat.
(iii) Intra-epidermal carcinoma or carcinoma *in situ.*
 (iv) Paget's disease of the vulva.

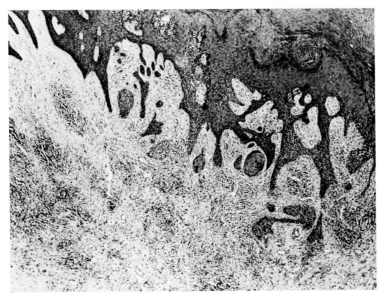

Fig. 40.3. Leucoplakia showing markedly atypical epithelium and early invasion.

preferred to differentiate the various conditions affecting the vulval skin, and described in particular four conditions:

  (i) Leucoplakia, which may be premalignant.
 (ii) Lichen sclerosus.
(iii) Primary atrophy. Both (ii) and (iii) may develop leucoplakic change and thus be premalignant.
 (iv) Senile atrophy, which does not lead to malignant change.

In addition to these conditions which may sometimes lead to malignancy there are others, less common, which are more clearly premalignant and which do not warrant conservative treatment. Once again, there is some different

These conditions are described elsewhere (Chapter 38) and here it is only necessary to indicate those features which should guide the clinician to regard a particular lesion with suspicion and to take preventative or early curative action. It must be admitted that the problem is not easy to solve even with the information obtained at biopsy, because tissue may be removed which shows a relatively benign appearance whereas, close by, a more sinister pathology may exist. For this reason many surgeons still adopt a radical approach to all such lesions. Such an approach leads to an increased number of mutilating operations which are not always successful, in that recurrences are common. Kaufman & Gardner (1965) have had some success with a method reported by Collins (1965) for selecting the appropriate area for biopsy. The vulva is painted with 1% toluidine blue and then washed with 1% acetic acid. In areas of invasive or *in situ* carcinoma the blue stain is retained but normal epithelium is washed clean. False-positive results may occur with areas of superficial ulceration. Clearly, cases which do not respond to adequate conservative treatment must undergo surgery, if only for the relief of symptoms. There are a number of cases where symptoms are more or less controlled but in which physical signs persist or deteriorate, and in these, repeated biopsy is necessary; the presence of cracks and fissures in the skin or of raised, indurated areas are such signs. The microscopical appearances which give rise to disquiet are an hyperactive-looking epithelium with long rete pegs and basal-cell activity which becomes disorderly, pleomorphic and atypical (see Fig. 40.3). There can be a range of appearances, from a clear-cut hypertrophic leucoplakia to those of intra-epidermal carcinoma and, of course, to microscopical evidence of invasion of the corium. The more disorderly and atypical the epithelium, the more likely is it to be premalignant and to warrant vulvectomy.

The various forms of intra-epidermal carcinoma have been described in some detail by Kaufman & Gardner (1965), but distinction is not clear. Difficulties arise because the macroscopic and microscopic appearances can be very similar. Haines & Taylor (1962) prefer to consider Bowen's disease as occurring, as originally described, on the skin elsewhere than the vulva, and to recognize only the other three lesions. Certainly, it seems difficult to distinguish between Bowen's disease and erythroplasia of the vulva. Willis (1953) goes further and considers that all the conditions are different stages of the same disease process. Paget's disease of the vulva does seem to present a very different histological picture in most cases (although Paget-type cells have been observed in cases described as Bowen's disease), but it is associated with an underlying apocrine carcinoma only in about 30% of cases, in contradistinction to Paget's disease of the breast. Macroscopical appearances in these various conditions are varied and the correct

diagnosis is seldom made without microscopical examination. Most patients present with pruritus vulvae and are found to have a dull or bright red, raised area with a well-defined margin [Fig. 40.4(a)]; the surface of the patch is either moist or dry and scaly. There may be associated leucoplakia or lichen sclerosus. Kaufman & Gardner (1965) are inclined to recognize distinctive clinical features with subtle histological differences. The main features of intra-epidermal carcinoma are thickening of the Malphigian layer which may contain vacuolated round cells or 'corps ronds', broad rete pegs tending to coalesce and loss of stratification, with irregular mitotic figures throughout the epidermis but no invasion of the dermis [Fig. 40.4(b)]. In Paget's disease, however, the normal stratification is maintained; the rete pegs tend to be enlarged and longer or broader; the characteristic feature being the presence of large, rounded or oval cells with pale, vacuolated cytoplasm, devoid of prickles; the latter are the Paget cells.

A microscopical picture compatible with an intra-epidermal carcinoma is sufficient to warrant a complete vulvectomy. Where disorderly activity of the epidermis is a feature a similar course should be followed. In all other types of chronic vulval dystrophy conservative therapy necessitates constant supervision to exclude, or diagnose as soon as possible, any changes for the worse, but the results of prospective surveys confirm the safety of this course. Hunt (1940) followed the progress of 96 cases of lichen sclerosus, of whom only four developed carcinoma; similarly, Jeffcoate & Woodcock (1961) found only four cases of carcinoma developing in 98 cases of chronic vulval dystrophy. Furthermore, Langley (1951) followed 122 cases treated by vulvectomy and noted a recurrence in 59%, with the development of only one carcinoma.

In a small proportion of cases syphylis seems to be associated, in that cancer of the vulva develops in an earlier age group in patients so afflicted, and in Green's (1958) series the association was noted in Negresses in whom otherwise the incidence of vulval carcinoma is low.

Two tropical diseases are reputed to be premalignant: granuloma venereum (Donovanosis) and lymphogranuloma inguinale. May & Cole

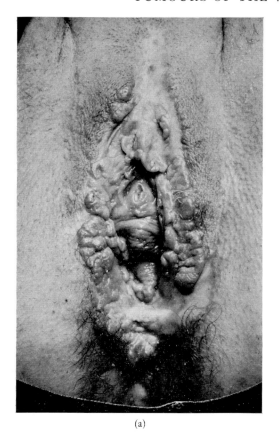

(a)

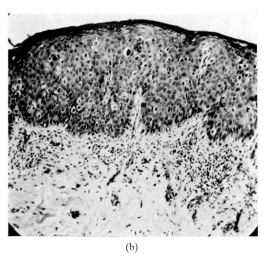

(b)

Fig. 40.4. Carcinoma *in situ*. (a) Macroscopic. This patient had vulval warts treated ineffectually with podophyllin many years before. (b) Microscopic.

(1969) in a group of 52 West Indian patients with carcinoma of the vulva found 65% to have evidence of either one or both of these infections; in these patients the mean age incidence of 36 years was 20 years younger than those patients developing cancer without such prior infection. Lunin (1949) had similar results in a group of Negresses. Cancer of the vulva appears to occur in women with other primary growths rather more frequently than do other genital-tract cancers; Taussig (1940) found this in 6·4% of his cases.

SYMPTOMS

The patient presents, most commonly, complaining of a lump, which is often painful, in contradistinction to most cancers of the genital tract. Pruritus will be the leading symptom if leucoplakia coexists with the cancer. Bleeding, discharge and urinary symptoms are all less common manifestations. Surprisingly, there is often considerable delay before the patient seeks advice, so that the lump may be quite large when first seen.

SIGNS

On examination there may be evidence of leucoplakia or one of the other precursors. The growth is either an hypertrophic lesion of varying size (Fig. 40.5) or, more commonly, a typical epitheliomatous ulcer; less often, the nodular infiltrating type of tumour is seen (Fig. 40.6).

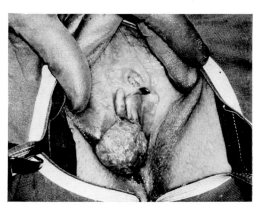

Fig. 40.5. Hypertrophic carcinoma of the vulva.

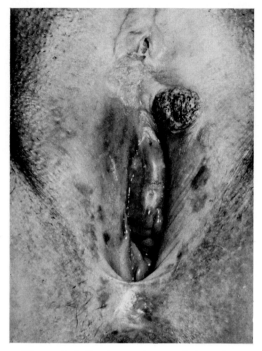

Fig. 40.6. Infiltrative carcinoma of the vulva.

Only in very early lesions, developing in association with one of the premalignant conditions, will diagnosis be difficult. Small lesions may be confused with rodent ulcer or hidradenoma, and areas of hyperkeratosis may present difficulties, but the diagnosis can be established by biopsy and microscopic examination.

PATHOLOGY

The growth is a well-differentiated squamous-cell carcinoma; anaplastic forms are less common. In a good proportion of cases the associated epithelium will show the atypical changes discussed in the aetiology of the condition.

Commonly, the tumour is found in the anterior half of the vulva and affects mainly the skin of the labia majora. Spread of the tumour occurs directly to other parts of the vulva, and the clitoris is often involved, but cancer originating in the clitoris is rare. In neglected cases the urethra, vagina, perineum or perivulval skin may be infiltrated. Multicentric origin accounts for the so-called 'kiss' cancer.

Metastasis is mainly by lymphatic channels. Knowledge of the lymphatic drainage of the vulva has been clarified by the studies of Way (1948), Green (1958), Parry-Jones (1960) and Reiffenstuhl (1964), amongst others. There are five groups of nodes arranged in two layers, a superficial and a deep layer:

Superficial (i) Medial and lateral inguinal.
              (ii) Medial and lateral femoral.
Deep   (i) Inguinal.
              (ii) Femoral.
              (iii) External iliac.

The superficial inguinal nodes are arranged in a lateral chain on a line below the inguinal ligament and a medial group lying inferior to the superficial inguinal ring. The deep inguinal nodes, when present, lie in the inguinal canal. The superficial femoral nodes are clustered in two groups on either side of the saphenous vein as it enters the femoral vein at the fossa ovalis [Fig. 40.7(a)]. The deep femoral nodes lie in the femoral canal and are usually represented by a single node only—the node of Cloquet, which lies more on the abdominal side of the opening with only its lower pole in the proximal part of the canal [Fig. 40.7(b)]. The external iliac nodes are disposed in three groups, the most important lying medial and inferior to the external iliac vein, another situated lateral to the artery, and the anterior group—when present—is in the sulcus between artery and vein.

The lymphatic vessels of the vulva are numerous and interconnecting, they run upwards and laterally to the superficial and deep nodes but do not cross the labiocrural fold. The lymphatics from the perineum, however, may travel in the fold alongside the vulva, as do those from the skin lateral to the vulva. The vessels travel through the mons veneris to reach their destination, and those from the clitoris and urethra run upwards and medially to enter the pelvic cavity between the origins of the abdominis rectus muscles and then turn laterally on the superior ramus of the pubic bone, on the inner surface of which may be found an intermediary lymph node which interconnects with the node of Cloquet. The superficial and deep nodes intercommunicate and all drain into the node of

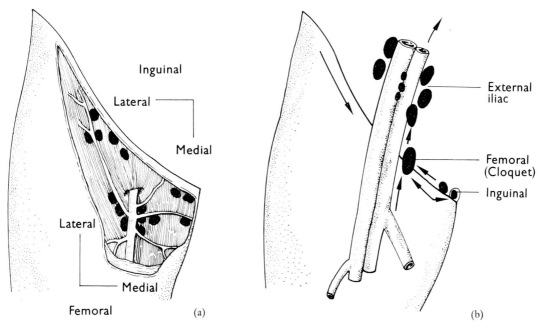

Fig. 40.7. Vulval lymph drainage. (a) Superficial nodes. (b) Deep nodes.

Cloquet, which thus assumes great importance as being the recipient of all the lymphatic drainage of the vulva. Then the flow is upwards through the external iliac, common iliac and paraaortic nodes, finally reaching the thoracic duct.

Lymphatic drainage from tumours of the vulva may be to the ipsilateral or contralateral nodes or to those of both sides; the more medial the tumour the more likely is the spread to be bilateral, but it is important to realize that it can occur in any case.

It is clear that there are no clinical means of determining whether or not the nodes are involved by growth. Palpation is notoriously unreliable and in Way's (1951) series in only just over half of those patients where the nodes were palpable were they involved by growth, whereas in just over one-third they were involved but impalpable. There is little correlation between node involvement and length of history, tumour size and macroscopical appearance, but if the lesion is anaplastic the chance of node involvement is somewhat higher than in well-differentiated tumours. This means that bilateral lymphaden-

ectomy is always necessary in any but palliative procedures.

The incidence of lymph node involvement is about 50–60% of cases.

TREATMENT

In contradistinction to malignant disease of the cervix uteri, radiotherapy is disappointing in its application to the vulval skin, which reacts unfavourably with necrosis and ulceration; furthermore, stimulation of a premalignant epithelium may encourage further malignant change. Therefore, surgical treatment is preferred, and in order to avoid a major and mutilating skin removal, electrocoagulation has been tried. Bervan (1949) has reported on 286 cases so treated in conjunction with teleradium to the lymph nodes and, in some cases, their excision. The relative 5 year survival rate was 38·1%, which is an improvement on limited surgical excision accompanied by superficial lymph node dissection—this procedure can be expected to give a 25% survival rate only. Both these methods may be of value in palliative treatment on recurrences or in those unfit for major surgery. Modern treatment follows the recommendations of Taussig (1940), Way (1960) and Green *et al.* (1958), who advocate a radical vulvectomy with bilateral superficial and deep ilio-inguinal lymphadenectomy as the ideal. The procedure is relatively simple to perform but is attended by a high mortality when, as is so often the case, the patient is elderly. Way (1966) reporting his late results on 69 cases followed for 15 years, gave a figure of 19% for patients who die in hospital after operation, but this includes all the cases at the beginning of his series, when resuscitation and postoperative care were less advanced than now. With modern aids to surgery a lower operative mortality of between 5 and 10% can be hoped for, and there is some evidence that staged operation might be less hazardous in terms of primary mortality than one-step procedures. Nevertheless, by present standards this remains a high mortality for a surgical procedure if compared with figures for other major operations such as Wertheim's hysterectomy and major bowel resections. The main causes of death are pulmonary embolism, sepsis and haemorrhage; loss of serum from the large, raw area is less of a problem today than in the early days of such major surgery.

There are two major problems connected with this operation, of which the first is whether or not to attempt closure of the radical vulvectomy wound. If the extent of the excision follows the advice of Way (1954) this is virtually impossible unless some form of plastic skin cover is essayed. On the whole, the use of flaps and skin grafts has been disappointing, because of the difficulty in avoiding haematoma formation and serous discharge under the grafts. McGregor (1966) described a method of delayed grafting with careful attention to detail which in 26 patients was rewarded by 96% take of the graft and healed wounds within 10–14 days of grafting. The majority of surgeons, however, try to reduce the raw area by approximation of as much skin to vagina as possible. Parry-Jones (1960) as a result of his studies claims that it is not necessary to incise the skin wide of the groin crease, but, unfortunately, the situation of the growth often demands a wider excision; on the opposite side, if there is no tumour, the advice to cut along the fold may be followed and closure is easier. The incision posteriorly passes across the perineum just anterior to the anus; if the latter is involved by growth, excision of anus and anal canal, with formation of a terminal colostomy, will be necessary. Similarly, extension to the urethra will require excision of the lower one half to two-thirds of this structure.

The second problem is the extent of the lymph node dissection to be undertaken. Ideally, this should extend as far up as the division of the common iliac vessels on each side, and in young, fit women this should always be performed. In the elderly or unfit patient such an extensive dissection above the inguinal ligament increases the primary mortality of the operation, and probably is unjustified. Way (1960), in an attempt to decide in which cases to extend and in which to limit the operation, removes the gland of Cloquet and makes a fresh smear; if malignant cells are found he proceeds, and if not he goes no further. Way believes the node involvement to be sequential from below upwards, but Green (1958) believes that 'skipping' can occur; the latter is common in other tumours. Probably, however, the gland of Cloquet is always involved in cases where growth has extended above the inguinal ligament, as it is the node to which all the lymphatics of the vulva drain.

Treatment should be chosen to suit the needs of the individual patient, and whilst the aim should be towards the method which gives the best results as regards survival, this must always be tempered by consideration of morbidity and mortality rates. In the young, fit patient with operable disease, a radical vulvectomy with bilateral ilio-inguinal lymphadenectomy in one stage is the method of choice. If the patient is unfit for such a major procedure then a staged procedure can be adopted. There is a theoretical dispute about the order in which the stages should be performed. The advantages of first removing the primary growth are:

(i) The psychological benefit to the patient of knowing that the growth has been removed.

(ii) The removal, in some cases of a large, ulcerated and infected tumour.

(iii) The prevention of further metastasis from the primary lesion.

The disadvantage is that delayed healing of the large raw area or the supervention of sepsis might postpone the completion of the subsequent lymphadenectomy, and it has been argued that it is therefore, better to undertake the lymph node dissection first in one or two stages. Unfortunately, breakdown of the groin wounds is also common and this may delay removal of the primary growth, which most surgeons would consider to be a more serious drawback. Whether the lymphadenectomy should be performed in one or two stages, again will depend on the patient's fitness for the procedures. Most patients and their surgeons prefer to limit the number of stages as far as possible. In more advanced cases, particularly in the very aged, the extent of the surgical attack should be more limited, but not at the expense of the vulvectomy. The latter should always aim at a radical removal of the vulva to avoid local recurrence, which is always the danger following inadequate surgery, is distressing to the patient, and may prove very difficult to treat. In such cases lymphadenectomy, to include the superficial inguinal nodes and superficial and deep femoral nodes—including the gland of Cloquet, which can usually be removed without seriously disrupting the integrity of the abdominal wall or destroying the inguinal ligament—is desirable. Where the nodes are obviously involved and fixed, their removal may not be feasible because of attachment to the vessels, but it is surprising how often there is a layer of cleaveage allowing the node mass to be removed without damage to the vessel.

The management of patients with recurrent disease can be difficult because there is fungating infected growth on the vulva, in the groins or in all areas. If a local, wide excision which encompasses the tumour on the vulva can be achieved this is obviously to be performed, otherwise fulguration of the mass is all that can be offered. Recurrence in the groins presents a rather hopeless problem, but fortunately relief often comes with death from haemorrhage following erosion of the femoral vessels.

RESULTS OF TREATMENT

Operability rates for this condition are generally high, about 80–90% of cases seen being deemed fit for major surgery despite their relatively advanced age. Operative mortality rates have decreased with improved techniques of anaesthesia and resuscitation from near 20% to somewhere between 2 and 5%. Survival rates improve markedly with more radical operations. Involvement of lymph nodes more than doubled operative mortality in Way's (1960) series, and is generally reported to reduce 5 year survival rates to 45–50% as against 70–80% where nodes are found to be free of growth.

The results of non-radical vulvectomy are poor. Way (1951) reported 87 cases, with a 24% 5 year survival and Green (1958) 78, also with a 24% 5 year survival. Radiotherapy gives similar results: Paterson (1950) reporting 100 cases with a 24% 5 year survival. Fulguration and some additional irradiation slightly improves the situation, Berven (1941) describing 177 cases with a 36·7% 5 year survival.

Increasing the radicality of the vulvectomy, together with superficial node dissection, improves the results further. Lees (1961) quoted 11 cases with a 55% 5 year survival and Goplerud (1968) 31 cases with a 45% 5 year survival. The most impressive results follow radical vulvectomy and bilateral superficial, and deep ilio-femoral-inguinal lymphadenectomy—Taussig (1940) describes 41 cases with a 58% 5 year survival; Green (1958) 65 with a 61% 5 year survival; and Way (1966) reports 69 cases with a 61% 5 year survival.

Rare malignant tumours of the vulva

For most gynaecologists, the rarer malignant tumours are of academic interest, for their frequency is low compared with epithelioma, itself a rare tumour (see Table 40.1).

Basal-cell carcinoma

This condition represents about 2–4% of all vulval malignancies, and presents a typical appearance of a rodent ulcer. A nodule appears, breaks down, and forms an ulcer with a rolled,

Table 40.1.

	Rutledge (1965) Cases	Brunschwig (1967) Cases
Squamous-cell carcinoma	153	155
Carcinoma *in situ*	29	12
Basal-cell carcinoma	2	5
Bartholin's gland carcinoma	14	2
Sarcoma	5	2
Melanoma	19	14
Adenocarcinoma		5
Paget's disease	7	4
Unknown pathology		3
Urethra (10 year survey)	25	
Total	254	202

beaded edge. The lesion is invasive locally and then only slowly. Care in the histological examination is required to exclude coexistent invasive squamous carcinoma. Treatment of rodent ulcer is wide local excision.

Melanoma

Here, as elsewhere, this may be either benign or malignant, and the latter accounts for about 4% of vulval malignancies. It presents as a soft, fungating, protuberant mass of black or purplish colour, but early lesions are small and nodular [Figs. 40.8(a) and (b)]. Metastasis is to the regional lymph nodes and by the bloodstream. The only hope of cure is by radical surgery in cases diagnosed early. Prophylaxis by wide excision of benign pigmented naevi is recommended, because in this area they are inevitably traumatized.

Carcinoma of Bartholin's gland

This is very rare, unilateral and an adenocarcinoma in most cases, although squamous carcinoma can arise from the duct. The appearances are similar to epithelioma when ulceration occurs; beforehand there is a hard, indurated swelling in the region of the gland. Treatment is as for carcinoma of the vulva.

Sarcoma

This can be fibrosarcoma or leiomyosarcoma. Differentiation from malignant melanoma or undifferentiated squamous carcinoma can be difficult.

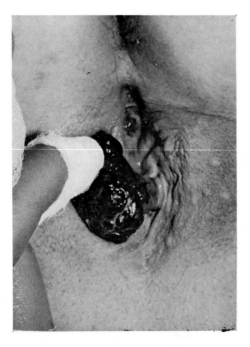

(a)

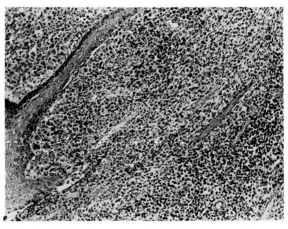

(b)

Fig. 40.8. Melanoma. (a) Macroscopic. (b) Microscopic. Broad sheets of cells containing pigment.

Carcinoma of the urethra

This condition may rarely present to the gynaecologist in the guise of a vulval carcinoma. The latter is far more likely to involve the urethra by direct spread than is a primary urethral tumour to arise. The histology is usually squamous cell, but may be adenocarcinoma arising from the paraurethral glands. Apart from the swelling, the patient experiences haematuria and dysuria. If the lesion is in the distal urethra metastasis may be solely to the inguinal nodes, and then the radical operation for vulval carcinoma will be suitable, but more extensive lesions will also metastasize to the pelvic nodes, and then radiotherapy by needling—and subsequent external irradiation—will be more appropriate.

Secondary metastases

Metastases may spread to the vulva from primary growths of the corpus or cervix uteri, vagina, anal canal, ovary or kidney, and also from chorioncarcinoma.

Other vulval swellings

Developmental abnormalities

These are seldom the cause of vulval tumour formation, but *hypertrophy of the clitoris* occurs when a female foetus is subjected to masculinizing influences, as in the congenital adrenogenital syndrome. Asymmetry of the labia minora may be regarded as abnormal by the patient or a parent and may be aggravated by trauma: amongst certain African primitives this is regarded as aesthetically pleasing, hence the 'Hottentot apron'. Small cysts arising from the terminal end of the Wolffian (Gartner's) duct may be found around the hymen or clitoris, but seldom cause trouble unless they become infected. Cysts of the *canal of Nuck* may appear in the upper part of the labium majus and must be distinguished from inguinal hernia by the lack of cough impulse and from vulval varices by irreducibility. Such cysts usually require excision because of their prominent position. As the milk line runs through the vulva, *supernumerary nipples* or mammary tissues can occur there.

Trauma

Accidental trauma is uncommon, as the vulva is a relatively well protected area, and it is usually children who suffer. *Haematoma* and contusion may result from falling astride a hard object or from criminal assault, and can be diagnosed without difficulty. More common, are injuries arising from obstetric or surgical trauma. Haematomata may follow disruption of perineal or vaginal vessels by a tear or episiotomy, or by repair operations; in the latter case the collection is usually subvaginal and extends upwards, but in the former it tends to collect in the ischiorectal fossa and bulge into the perineum. The amount of blood may be quite large, with extensive bruising; considerable pain may be occasioned with reflex inhibition of micturition or defaecation. Such collections are best extirpated and the resultant cavity packed with gauze; small haematomata may be left to resolve. Epidermal *inclusion cysts* may result from enclosure of skin deep to the surface of repair procedures, and are therefore lined with stratified squamous epithelium and contain a thin, yellow fluid; they are usually symptomless. *Fibro-epithelial polyps* result from malocclusion of suture lines, and only cause trouble if they become irritated by trauma or inflammation.

Oedema of the vulva

Here, as elsewhere, there are many causes of oedema. As part of a generalized process it may be due to pre-eclampsia, cardiac or renal failure, or as a form of angioneurotic oedema. Local factors may be inflammatory or traumatic, or more commonly the obstruction of lymphatic or venous drainage; thus vulval oedema may be a sign of intrapelvic tumours, usually malignant, or pelvic sepsis, usually postoperative. Ablation of lymphatics by radical operations for cancer of the vulva and cervix may be followed temporarily by oedema.

Genital prolapse and tumours arising in the uterus, cervix or vagina may present at the vulva but should cause no difficulty in diagnosis.

BARTHOLIN'S CYST

Bartholin's glands lie, one on each side, deep to the posterior third of the labium majus, superficial to the deep perineal compartment. It is a compound racemose gland with tall, mucus-secreting cells. The collecting ducts open into the vagina just distal to the hymen at 5 o'clock and 7 o'clock on the circumference. The secretion is produced (as a result of erotic stimuli) to lubricate the introitus and to facilitate sexual intercourse. The duct may become obstructed marsupialization, the cyst being incised freely and the lining wall on each side being sutured to the adjacent skin [Fig. 40.9(b)]. The cyst soon shrinks and the gland secretion is enabled to drain. Abscesses may be treated similarly, except that in very acute cases the lining wall may be too necrotic, then the incision should be cruciate, with saucerization of the cavity to encourage healing from the depths by granulation. Occasionally, the gland itself becomes infected and can be felt as a tender, indurated swelling; in such cases excision of the gland itself is indicated. This

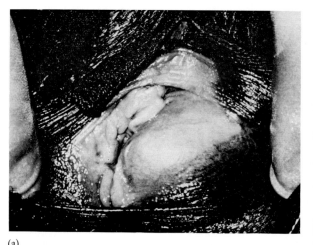

(a)

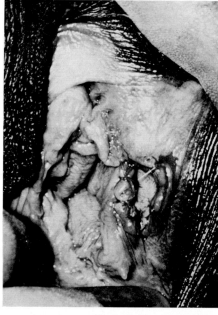

(b)

Fig. 40.9. (a) A Bartholin cyst. (b) Bartholin cyst marsupialized.

as a result of infection or of trauma associated with parturition and then becomes distended, to form a Bartholin's cyst [Fig. 40.9(a)]. The wall of the cyst is lined by transitional epithelium. Small cysts are often symptomless, larger ones are noticed by the patient but even then no complaint may be aroused until infection supervenes and an abscess is formed. Because of its situation, such an abscess is very painful and is often relieved by spontaneous rupture; an event which tends to be followed by recurrent abscess formation. Treatment of Bartholin's cysts is by

operation can be a difficult and bloody procedure, leaving a deep cavity oozing blood and requiring obliteration by suturing in layers, preferably with drainage. Bruising of the perineum and dehiscence of the wound is a common complication of excision.

SKENE'S DUCT CYSTS

Cysts around the urethra arise in Skene's ducts or in the suburethral glands. In the case of the latter, abscesses are likely to form, and this is currently believed to be the cause of suburethral diverticulitis. Tancer (1965) believes this to be a condition commonly overlooked by both gynaecologist and urologist. The symptoms which tend to be recurrent are dysuria and increased frequency of micturition, together with superficial dyspareunia; pyuria and haematuria may also be present. Examination may reveal a tender, suburethral swelling which, on compression, discharges pus through the urethral meatus, or tenderness alone may be elicited. Urethroscopy should reveal the opening of the sac. In addition, Tancer (1965) recommends the procedure of urethrography, using a Hyman or double-balloon catheter to isolate the urethra and allow positive pressure-instillation of dye. Ideally, excision of the sac and urethral repair is performed, but the tissues may be too friable and then partial excision, closure of the urethral defect and obliteration of the cavity may be all that is possible.

URETHRAL CARUNCLE

There is some debate as to whether a caruncle is a true entity or whether it should more properly be regarded as partial prolapse of the posterior urethral membrane. Most gynaecologists, however, designate any reddened area involving the posterior margin of the urethral orifice as a caruncle, and consider urethral prolapse as the diagnosis when the whole circumference of the urethral membrane is seen to prolapse (Fig. 40.10). The latter condition is fairly easy to recognize and can occur in any age group, even young children, and may follow straining or an acute urinary infection. On occasion, however, the prolapse is infarcted due to thrombosis in the underlying suburethral venous plexus, and the appearance is then of a small, black or plum-coloured swelling which may at first sight look malignant. Urethral prolapse may initially be quite painful and be associated with some blood-staining, but the condition produces few symptoms in the chronic phase. Excision and suture at the muco cutaneous junction with fine, plain catgut is all that is necessary.

Caruncles are described as being of three types. The *angiomatous* type could well be a localized

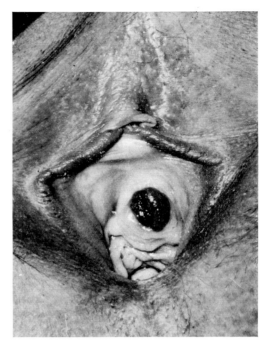

Fig. 40.10. Urethra. Prolapse of musosa.

prolapse of the posterior urethral wall. There is a red or cherry-red swelling, varying in size from a match-head to a pea. The caruncle is covered by stratified squamous or transitional epithelium, which has deep crypts due to infolding. On section, these crypts appear as epithelial islands deep in the stroma, which may simulate malignant invasion. In the stroma are numerous, submucous capillaries are distended with red-blood cells, and when the epithelial islands are infrequent (as may be the case in the angiomatous variety) the appearance is similar to urethral prolapse.

The *polypoid* type presents as a cherry-red blob on a stalk arising from the posterior urethral margin. Microscopically, the epithelial islands are more prominent and rest in a loose stroma. The *granulomatous* variety (Fig. 40.11) is more likely to be associated with infection and appears as a red, granular area around the posterior urethral margin, and in severe cases the urethral margin may be deficient. Jeffcoate (1962) believes many of these to be due to a chronic *Trichomonas* infestation. The surface epithelium is often missing, the stroma shows extreme vascularity,

TUMOURS OF THE VAGINA

Benign tumours

Any benign tumour of structures associated with stratified squamous epithelium may be found in the vagina, and so cases of papilloma, fibroma, fibromyoma and neurofibroma have been reported. Most papillomatous lesions of the vagina are due to malocclusion following natural or surgical repair after trauma. Warts occur occasionally and are usually due to secondary spread from the vulva. The commonest benign tumours found in the vagina are cystic lesions. The commonest of these is a simple cyst widely thought to be a mesonephric (Gartner's) duct cyst, but according to Evans & Paine (1965) the majority have a paramesonephric (Muellerian) origin.

Both ducts develop in the urogenital ridges, which lie longitudinally on the posterior wall of the embryonic peritoneal cavity. The mesonephric ducts appear first and run down to open into the cloacal cavity. The paramesonephric ducts develop later as invaginations of the coelom, lateral to the proximal end of each mesonephric duct. The fusion of the distal parts of these form the uterus and vagina. It is fairly well accepted that an upgrowth of stratified squamous epithelium from the dorsal wall of the urogenital sinus replaces the columnar epithelium of the paramesonephric ducts. Evans and Paine believe that remnants of the Muellerian epithelium may persist to form paramesonephric duct cysts or tumours. Such cysts have a lining of cervical or tube-like epithelium. They are all situated in the subepithelial connective tissue of the vaginal wall, and do not penetrate its muscular coat. The cysts are generally symptomless and are found during examination; they are usually single and most often are found in the upper vagina near the fornices. Treatment is seldom necessary, but if excision is required care must be taken of the bladder and ureters.

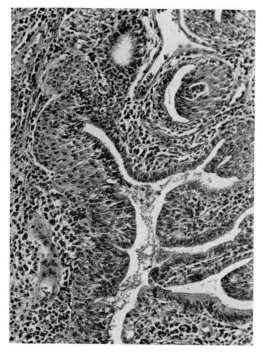

Fig. 40.11. Urethral caruncle showing granulomatous pattern with included paraurethral glands.

and leucocytic infiltration is more marked than in the other varieties.

Caruncles are often symptomless and are most frequently found in postmenopausal women. When giving rise to symptoms, pain or discomfort, and occasional blood-staining, are the most common. Exquisite tenderness is sometimes present, and superficial dyspareunia may be the result. The granulomatous variety is likely to cause the most soreness. Treatment is only indicated in the presence of symptoms, and diathermy excision of the caruncle and the area of the urethra from which it arises is the best method. Although the lesion is benign, it has a tendency to recur. In granulomatous varieties infection should be diligently sought and treated; oestrogens may be of value to improve the resistance of the tissues. Excision may still be required even in this type, and if the urethra is deficient as a result of ulceration or previous surgery a simple plastic elongation of the urethra may be required.

ADENOSIS VAGINAE

This condition, first described by Bonney & Glendenning (1910) as adenomatosis, consists of multiple mucus-secreting glands or cysts in the vagina. The cysts may rupture, with subsequent ulceration and secondary infection, but more usually leucorrhoea is the symptom. Contact bleeding and dyspareunia may be occasioned. On examination the appearance is of multiple small cysts or a granular, red, swollen area which bleeds on touching. Adenoma and adenocarcinoma have been described. Cysts are best left alone, but the other lesions require excision biopsy for a diagnosis.

MESONEPHRIC (GARTNER'S) DUCT CYSTS

These are sausage-shaped with a lining layer of cubical epithelium on a well-defined basement membrane, and surrounded by a wall of smooth muscle. They lie along the course of the duct, anterolaterally in the vaginal wall. They are usually solitary and symptomless, and do not require treatment. Those in the lower vagina need to be distinguished from bladder diverticula.

Cancer of the vagina

It is fortunate that the vagina is an uncommon site in the genital tract for malignant disease, because the prognosis is poor. Most series are small, as the condition forms only 1–2% of all genital tract malignancies, as shown by Way (1951) and McGarrity (1967). The tumour may be primary or secondary in the vagina. The secondary metastases may be from the uterus (either body or cervix), from the vulva and, occasionally, the ovary; also, from kidney, bladder or urethra, from rectum or large bowel and, of course, from chorionic carcinoma. With tumours arising in proximity to the cervix or vulva it may be difficult to decide which is the primary site. The corpus uteri has a special relationship in regard to secondary metastasis in the vagina. The commonest form is the recurrence at the vault of the vagina subsequent to surgical removal of the primary growth; less often, the metastasis forms at the lower end of the vagina, is usually, but not always, suburethral in position, and is often present before the primary is treated.

There are no common aetiological factors, but the occasional case has been reported as developing in the traumatic ulcer created by a long-retained ring pessary, and also as arising in endometriosis of the rectovaginal septum. It is important to realize that carcinoma *in situ* may be found in the vagina as well as the cervix, and occasionally the epithelial change is noted throughout the length of the canal; this accounts for the rare case of squamous carcinoma developing in the vagina after hysterectomy for carcinoma *in situ* of the cervix.

The histology is that of a squamous-cell carcinoma in the majority of cases, but a few adenocarcinomas are found and these are thought to arise either from the epithelium of Gartner's duct or possibly from aberrant Muellerian glandular epithelium. In a few cases, malignant melanoma has been observed. Macroscopically, the tumour appears in one of three forms: (i) infiltrative; (ii) proliferative; (iii) ulcerative.

Most of the tumours occur in the upper half of the vagina and are more often on the posterior vaginal wall than the anterior. Direct spread occurs within the vaginal wall, but despite the proximity of bladder and rectum these organs are involved only in late stages of the disease and then fistula formation may occur. Despite their late involvement, however, it is the very close

Table 40.2. Staging of carcinoma of the vagina (F.I.G.O., 1965)

Pre-invasive carcinoma of the vagina
Stage 0: Carcinoma *in situ*; intra-epithelial carcinoma

Invasive carcinoma of the vagina
Stage I: The carcinoma is limited to the vaginal wall

Stage II: The carcinoma has involved the subvaginal tissues but has not extended on to the pelvic wall

Stage III: The carcinoma has extended on to the pelvic wall

Stage IV: The carcinoma has extended beyond the true pelvis or has involved the mucosa of the bladder or rectum. (A bullous oedema, as such, does not permit allotment of a case to Stage IV)

relationship of these organs which renders treatment difficult and probably accounts for the poor results. Lymphatic spread is to the deep pelvic nodes from the upper two-thirds of the vagina and to the inguinal nodes from the lower third.

The recommended staging of cancer of the vagina by F.I.G.O. is shown in Table 40.2.

CLINICAL FEATURES

The presenting symptom is either bleeding or watery discharge, and as the disease, like cancer of the vulva, occurs in the late age group with a mean somewhere around 65 years, such an occurrence in a postmenopausal woman should alarm her sufficiently to report her symptoms. Although Corscaden (1967) reports a combined patient–physician delay of approximately 11 months, McGarrity (1967) found most cases to be relatively early as regards clinical staging (see Table 40.3).

Table 40.3. Primary carcinoma of the vagina: staging (From McGarrity (1967), by courtesy of the Editor of *Australian and New Zealand Journal of Obstetrics and Gynaecology*)

Stage	% cases
o	1
I	43
II	39
III	6
IV	11

TREATMENT

Treatment presents great problems, largely because the condition is too rare to allow any individual to gain sufficient experience to determine the best form of therapy. Added to this the desire to avoid damaging the bladder and rectum, inclines surgeons and radiotherapists to an approach which is less than radical and therefore likely to be inadequate. Lesions involving the upper third of the vagina are suitable for treatment by the methods available for carcinoma of the cervix; that is:

(i) *Surgery.* Radical abdominal hysterectomy and pelvic lymphadenectomy including removal of the upper three-quarters or even the whole vagina.
(ii) *Radiotherapy.* Intracavitary radium using specially adapted applicators and followed by external radiotherapy.

(iii) *A combination of surgery and radiotherapy.* This is probably the wisest approach, unless the condition is too advanced for surgical removal.

Involvement, or suspected involvement, of bladder or rectum, which may only be determined at operation, will require anterior of posterior exenteration, and in a few cases total exenteration.

Tumours of the lower third of the vagina can either be treated by radium needling or included in a radical vulvectomy and inguinal lymphadenectomy, depending on the extent and situation of the disease. Supplementary external radiotherapy to the pelvic lymph nodes will be necessary, as spread to them may occur. Middle third tumours present the greatest problem, and are probably best treated by radiotherapy. External radiotherapy delivered by supervoltage machines is probably the best and is suitable for all types in this situation. Intracavitary radium can be applied to suitably sized tumours, mainly of the infiltrating or ulcerative type; supplementary external radiation to the pelvic nodes will be required. Radium needling, providing good access is available and the tumour is not too large, is a further possibility; again, supplementary external radiation will be necessary.

McGarrity (1967) noted clinical involvement of lymph nodes in 20% of patients, and in 25% of surgically removed nodes there was histological evidence of metastases.

If surgery is contemplated for middle third tumours, nothing less than some form of exenteration is essential. The reported results to date are poor, as in the case of carcinoma of the ovary,

Table 40.4. Results of treatment of carcinoma of the vagina (From McGarrity (1967), by courtesy of the Editor of *Australian and New Zealand Journal of Obstetrics and Gynaecology*)

Author	No. of cases	5-year survival rate (%)
Livingstone (1950)	970	12
Bivens (1953)	81	12
F.I.G.O. Annual Report, Vol. 13	1,199	33·5
McGarrity (1967)	90	33·8

and do not exceed a 5 year survival rate much over 30% (Table 40.4).

REFERENCES

BERVEN E. (1949) *Br. J. Radiol.* **22**, 498.

BIVENS M.D. (1953) *Am. J. Obstet. Gynec.* **65**, 390.

BONNEY V. & GLENDINNING B. (1910) *Proc. R. Soc. Med.* **4**, 18.

BRUNSCHWIG A. & BROCKUNIER A. Jnr. (1967) *Obstet. Gynec., N.Y.* **29**, 362.

COLLINS C. (1965) *Am. J. Obstet. Gynec.* **91**, 818.

CORSCADEN J.A. (1962) *Gynaecologic Cancer.* Baltimore, Williams and Wilkins.

EVANS D.M. & PAINE C.G. (1965) *Clin. Obstet. Gynec.* **8**, 997.

FISHER E.R. & WEEKSTER H. (1962) *Cancer, N.Y.* **15**, 936.

GOPLERUD D.R. & KEETEL W.C. (1968) *Am. J. Obstet. Gynec.* **100**, 550.

GREEN T.H. Jnr., ULFELDER H. & MEIGS J.V. (1958) *Am. J. Obstet. Gynec.* **75**, 834.

HAINES M. & TAYLOR C.W. (1962) *Gynaecological Pathology.* London, Churchill.

HAY D.M. & COLE F.M. (1969) *J. Obstet. Gynaec. Br. Commonw.* **76**, 821.

HUNT E. (1940) *Diseases Affecting the Vulva.* London, Kimpton.

JEFFCOATE T.N.A. (1962) *Principles of Gynaecology.* London, Butterworths.

JEFFCOATE T.N.A. & WOODCOCK A.S. (1961) *Br. med. J.* ii, 127.

KAUFFMAN R.H. & GARDNER H.L. (1965) *Clin. Obstet. Gynec.* **8**, 1035.

KNOX J.M. & FREEMAN R.G. (1965) *Clin. Obstet. Gynec.* **8**, 925.

LANGLEY I.I., HERTIG A.T. & SMITH G. VAN S. (1951) *Am. J. Obstet. Gynec.* **62**, 127.

LEES D.H. (1961) *J. Obstet. Gynaec. Br. Commonw.* **68**, 730.

LIVINGSTONE R.G. (1950) *Primary Carcinoma of the Vagina.* Springfield, Thomas.

LUNIN A.B. (1949) *Am. J. Obstet. Gynec.* **57**, 742.

MCGARRITY K.A. (1967) *Aust. N. Z. J. Obstet. Gynaec.* **7**, 170.

MCGREGOR I.A. (1966) *J. Obstet. Gynaec. Br. Commonw.* **73**, 599.

PATERSON R., TOD M. & RUSSELL M. (1950) *The Results of Radium and X-ray Therapy in Malignant Disease.* Edinburgh, E. and S. Livingstone.

PARRY-JONES E. (1960) *J. Obstet. Gynaec. Br. Commonw.* **67**, 919.

REIFFENSTUHL G. (1964) *The Lymphatics of the Female Genital Organs.* Philadelphia and Montreal, J.B. Lippincott.

RUTLEDGE F.N. (1965) *Clin. Obstet. Gynec.* **8**, 1051.

TANCER M.L. (1965) *Clin. Obstet. Gynec.* **8**, 982.

TAUSSIG F.J. (1940) *Am. J. Obstet. Gynec.* **40**, 764.

WALLACE H.J. & WHIMSTER I.W. (1961) *Br. med. J.* ii, 453.

WAY S. (1948) *Ann. R. Coll. Surg.* **3**, 187.

WAY S. (1951) *Malignant Disease of the Female Genital Tract.* London, Churchill.

WAY S. (1954) *Br. med. J.* ii, 780.

WAY S. (1960) *Am. J. Obstet. Gynec.* **79**, 692.

WAY S. (1966) *J. Obstet. Gynaec. Br. Commonw.* **73**, 594.

WILLIS R.A. (1953) *Pathology of Tumours*, 2nd edn. London, Butterworths.

CHAPTER 41

BENIGN TUMOURS OF THE UTERUS

UTERINE POLYPS

Polyps are common tumours in the uterus, and may occur in either the cervix or the corpus. They are of various types and are usually benign, apart from polypoidal masses found in carcinoma or sarcoma of the endometrium. Rarely, malignant change can occur in a benign polyp. The following are seen:

(1) *Corpus* Adenomatous or endometrial polyps
Fibroid polyps (Fig. 41.1)
Adenofibromatous polyps
Adenomyomatous polyps
Placental polyps
(2) *Cervix* Mucous polyps (Fig. 41.2)
Fibro-epithelial polyps

Adenomatous or endometrial polyps are the commonest occurring in the corpus uteri, they are usually multiple and may form part of an hyperplastic endometrium. Postmenopausally they are single or only a few in number. There is a tendency to recur, but this must sometimes be due to failure to remove them all at operation. A relationship with subsequent development of carcinoma of the endometrium has been noted by Armenia (1967), but in no sense are they to be regarded as premalignant.

PATHOLOGY

They are small, red or pinkish-white tumours projecting from endometrial surface; only occasionally do they have a long stalk allowing them to present through the cervix, or even at the vulva. Microscopically the adenomatous polyp is com-

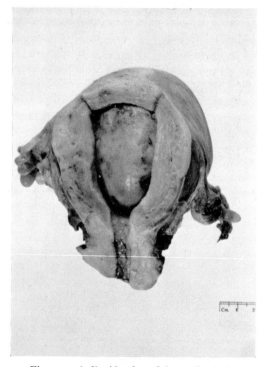

Fig. 41.1. A fibroid polyp of the uterine body.

posed of endometrial stroma and glands covered by a single layer of columnar epithelium. There is a variable response of the glands to the ovarian hormones. Atypical changes and squamous metaplasia may cause difficulty in diagnosis from malignancy, but attention to the usual criteria for malignancy should avoid this hazard. Malignancy may rarely occur. Adenofibromatous

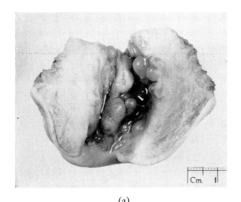

(a)

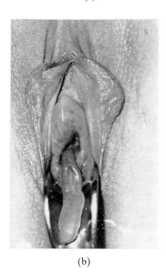

(b)

Fig. 41.2. (a) Mucous polypi within the canal of an amputated cervix. (b) A single, long endocervical polyp.

polyps occur more commonly postmenopausally and are differentiated by the presence of a fibrous stroma. Fibromyomatous and adenomyomatous polyps show the characteristic microscopical features to be expected.

Placental polyps are due to organization of small pieces of retained placental tissue, they are unusual but are of significance on two counts; they may cause severe haemorrhage on avulsion and they must be carefully distinguished from chorion carcinoma.

CLINICAL FEATURES

If part of an endometrial hyperplasia (Fig. 41.3), the symptoms are those associated with dysfunctional uterine bleeding usually with increased menstrual loss. In particular, however, polyps are associated with intermenstrual bleeding or postmenopausal bleeding in the older woman. If extruded from the cervix there may be discharge, intermenstrual bleeding or even post coital bleeding, and sometimes the patient herself discovers the polyp in the vagina.

TREATMENT

They are easily removed by small sponge forceps and by curettage; the former are the more useful and should always be introduced after dilatation

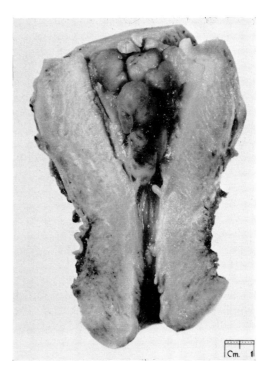

Fig. 41.3. Pronounced endometrial hyperplasia.

of the cervix before inserting the curette, as the latter on its own may miss the polyp. Careful histological examination of all polyps is necessary to exclude malignant change.

Cervical polyps

These are called mucous polyps, because of their histological appearance. It has been suggested that they may be distention cysts of the cervical racemose glands which have become extruded. Macroscopically they are single or multiple, small, cherry-red swellings appearing at the cervix and usually arising within the canal. Microscopically the polyp consists of cervical mucous glands, sometimes distended, in a vascular bed of fine fibrous tissue and covered usually by columnar, but sometimes by squamous, epithelium. Inflammation and ulceration of the apex is common.

Their main symptom is mucous discharge, which may be blood-stained. Intermenstrual bleeding and postcoital bleeding are also occasioned when the polyps are more vascular or if there is degeneration or inflammation of the apex. They are easily removed by avulsion, scissors or curettage; the canal should be dilated and explored for the presence of further unseen polyps and the stalk carefully removed and its base cauterized, or recurrence is likely. Uterine curettage is also advisable, as there are often associated endometrial polyps. Larger polyps may have quite a large artery in the stalk. For the above reasons it is wiser to remove cervical polyps under anaesthesia rather than in the outpatient department.

UTERINE FIBROIDS

Fibromyoma—more correctly leiomyoma and, by general usage, fibroid—is not only the commonest tumour found in the uterus, or even in the female genital tract, but in the human body. It is estimated that 20% of all women have one or more present in the uterus at death; the vast majority of these have been symptomless and often are small to the point of insignificance. The aetiology is quite unknown, but inevitably the female sex hormones have been incriminated. Experimental production of myomata has been conspicuously unsuccessful and the tumours produced by oestrogen stimulation do not persist when the hormone is withdrawn, tend to be more fibrous than myomatous, and do not occur solely in the uterus. The theory that the tumours arise from smooth-muscle cells is supported by the tissue-culture experiments of Millar & Ludovici (1955). It has been noted that myomata in women receiving hormone treatment (usually oral contraceptives) have, in some cases, enlarged quite rapidly. Whilst it is accepted that tumours are commonest in women who have not borne children, this is not always the case; there is an obvious racial factor in women of Negro origin, many of whom develop myomata when young and despite having had children. The association with nulliparity is common to endometriosis and carcinoma of the corpus uteri, in association with either of which myomata may be found. In European women fibroids tend to cause symptoms around the age of 30 and are then more frequently observed until the menopause, when they cease to cause trouble because they no longer grow and, indeed, undergo atrophy along with the uterus. Jeffcoate (1962), however, states that they do sometimes grow after the menopause.

Pathology

Macroscopically the appearance is of a firm, round tumour in the uterine wall, which itself may be thickened and hypertrophied (Fig. 41.4). When

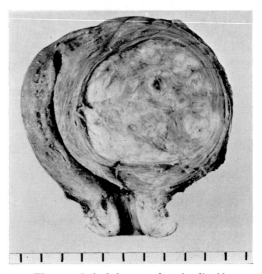

Fig. 41.4. A single intramural uterine fibroid.

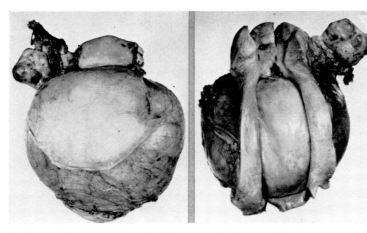

Fig. 41.5. A single, large cervical submucous fibroid: the anterior surface is seen on the left and the posterior wall of the canal has been opened (right) to display the tumour.

within the wall of the uterus, fibroids are described as being intramural, if projecting from the peritoneal surface of the uterus as subserous, if between the layers of the broad ligaments as intraligamentary, and if projecting into the cavity as submucous. Submucous fibroids may become polypoidal and subserous ones pedunculated. Pedunculated fibroids may become adherent to other structures, particularly the omentum, gain a secondary blood supply, and lose their uterine attachment; they are then called parasitic. The tumours may arise either in the body of the uterus—which is the commoner—or in the cervix (Fig. 41.5); infrequently, they spring from the round ligaments. They may be single or multiple, and large numbers have been reported. Their size varies from microscopic to huge, when they may fill the whole abdomen. Characteristically, they are firm in consistency but as a result of degeneration may be soft and cystic, or rock-hard due to calcification. A single fibroid can cause symmetrical enlargement of the uterus, whereas multiple fibroids transform the organ into an irregular mass. On cutting into a uterus containing fibroids it is immediately apparent that the tumour is enclosed in a false capsule of compressed uterine muscle, thus allowing it to be easily enucleated; this is in contradistinction to an adenomyoma (Fig. 41.6). As the myometrium retracts, the fibroid stands proud above the cut

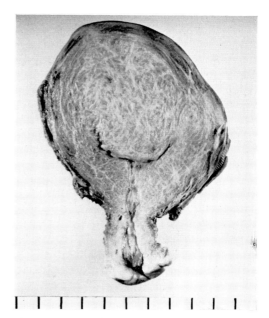

Fig. 41.6. A fundal adenomyoma. Note lack of false capsule (compare Fig. 41.4).

surface. The tumour itself is white with a characteristic whorled appearance. On microscopical examination the tumours when small are mainly composed of smooth-muscle cells, but as they become larger fibrous tissue is more abundant and degenerative changes become more frequent. The muscle cells are arranged in bundles in the classically whorled pattern. The proportion of muscle cells to fibrous tissue is very variable; a preponderance of the former gives a superficial resemblance to sarcoma and of the latter to fibroma. The blood supply enters from the periphery and the tumours are relatively avascular, encouraging the degenerative changes which are common in all but the smaller tumours. The degenerative changes which may occur are as follows.

Hyaline

This is present to some degree in most tumours. There is a tendency to liquefaction of larger areas of hyaline change and this leads on to cystic degeneration.

Cystic

Usually this occurs irregularly and gives a sponge-like appearance and soft consistency to the tumour, but there may be formation of a cystic cavity (Fig. 41.7).

Calcification

This is seen more in pedunculated fibroids with poor blood supply, and also with postmenopausal atrophy. The fibroid becomes rock-hard, shows up on X-ray and represents what used to be called a 'womb-stone'.

Infection

Infection occurs in minor degree when fibroids become adherent to bowel or pyosalpinges; abscess formation is uncommon but may occur, particularly in submucous fibroids or in fibroid polyps in the puerperium. Sometimes a fibroid polyp sloughs off as a result of infection.

Necrosis

This may occur in any tumour, particularly following other degenerations and may be either microscopical or macroscopical, when a putty-like area is seen, usually in the centre of the tumour.

Necrobiosis or red degeneration

This occurs commonly in pregnancy and near the menopause, but can occur at any time. It is similar to the process of infarction. Necrosis occurs either in diffuse or focal distribution; there is thrombosis of the peripheral vessels, loss of the fibromyomatous pattern with absence of nuclei, and distended thin-walled vessels are

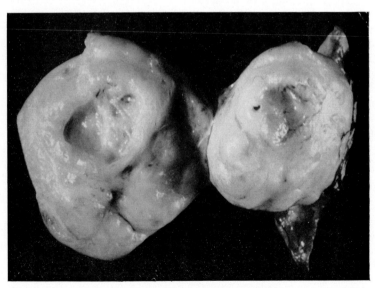

Fig. 41.7. Cystic degeneration with a fibroid.

engorged with red blood cells. If the fibroid is freshly sectioned its colour is the appearance of raw beef, but it soon turns to a dull red on exposure; later, the colour may turn a greenish yellow. Later still, central necrosis—and even cyst formation—may occur.

Sarcomatous degeneration

This is of very infrequent occurrence. Typically there is a soft homogeneous area in the fibroid, and this may extend into the adjacent myometrium at one area on the circumference. In a gross case diagnosis is easy, but real difficulty may be encountered with what are known as cellular myomata, where there is lack of distinctive fibrous tissue and a preponderance of muscle cells.

Clinical features

The symptoms of fibroids are extremely variable, but often they are symptomless even when of considerable size. It is extremely rare for fibroids to cause symptoms after the menopause, as they usually undergo atrophy along with the uterus. Such atrophy occasionally allows an abdominal mass to drop back into the pelvis and cause increased frequency of micturition or acute retention of urine, but in general it is unwise to diagnose as being a fibroid a tumour which causes symptoms after the menopause.

Abdominal swelling is a common method of presentation and may be noticed by the patient herself or by her doctor at a routine examination. The swelling is due to the mass itself appearing in the abdomen. The patient might first notice it by feeling the mass move if it is pedunculated. Slow increase in girth is often ignored as being due to menopausal obesity.

Pressure effects may be produced on the pelvic veins or on the inferior vena cava. Oedema and varicose veins in the leg will result and will be either unilateral or bilateral depending on which vessel is subjected to pressure. Haemorrhoids may similarly occur. A large tumour filling the abdomen may embarrass respiration and cause dyspnoea. Pressure on the bladder may cause increased frequency of micturition, and

on occasion appears to cause stress incontinence of urine. Cervical fibroids or fundal fibroids in a retroverted uterus may so displace the cervix as to cause retention of urine in the same manner as an impacted retroverted gravid uterus. Constipation is not caused by fibroids.

Disturbance of uterine function is one of the commonest symptoms. Increased menstrual loss is very common and the reason is not always obvious unless the uterine cavity is enlarged by submucous fibroids; often, quite large tumours may be present without any increase in size of the cavity. If heavy periods occur in these women it may be due to the generally increased vascularity of the uterus. But in cases where heavy periods are associated with only small fibroids the conclusion drawn is that the condition is one of dysfunctional uterine bleeding, either coincidental or associated, in that some unspecified hormonal disturbance is responsible for both. Intermenstrual bleeding may occur as a result of a fibroid polyp with ulceration of the apex. Infertility has a relationship with fibroids rather like endometriosis. Infertility, either voluntary or involuntary, is likely to be followed in time by the development of uterine fibroids, whereas once fibroids have developed fertility is likely to be decreased or in abeyance. Whilst uterine distortion or mechanical obstruction of the fallopian tubes by fibroids is an understandable cause for infertility, this may also be present when the uterine cavity and fallopian tubes are apparently normal and undisturbed by the tumours; occasionally, pregnancy occurs in a uterus grossly distorted by fibroids. At operation about 10% of patients with uterine fibroids are found to have associated hydrosalpinges, the latter probably precede, and cause, the tumour formation by producing infertility. Once pregnancy has occurred then abortion may follow; this is thought to be more likely if implantation occurs in relation to a submucous fibroid; most pregnancies, however, continue undisturbed. During pregnancy, fibroids may increase in size as the uterus enlarges, but not to any great extent and, in fact, due to a marked oedema in the connective tissue, they soften and flatten out and may become more difficult to distinguish. In the puerperium they undergo involution and usually become smaller than before pregnancy started.

Pain may result from the presence of uterine fibroids. This may be a simple congestive dysmenorrhoea resulting from the increased vascularity in the pelvis or it may be more constant and in the form of backache when the fibroids are of moderate size in a retroverted uterus. Torsion of a pedunculated fibroid will result in a pain of an acute or subacute nature demanding fairly urgent treatment. Less severe, but still unpleasant, pain is associated with red degeneration, which occurs most commonly during pregnancy or near the menopause, but which can occur at any time. A fibroid polyp may be associated with some degree of uterine colic as the uterus tries to expel it through the cervix. Infection and sarcomatous degeneration also cause pain but are, of course, rare complications.

The physical signs associated with uterine fibroids are also extremely variable and can simulate conditions as dissimilar as pregnancy and malignant disease. Much depends on the size, number, situation and type and, further on, the presence of degenerative changes. Fibroids are so common that they may occur coincidentally with other pelvic pathology and may thus obscure a more important lesion such as an ovarian tumour or carcinoma of the endometrium. The differential diagnosis must include all those conditions which might be mistaken for a pelvic tumour, as well as other pelvic tumours. Fortunately, in the majority of cases the diagnosis is relatively simple, and perhaps the most distinctive feature is that of consistency: 'fibroids feel like fibroids'. The tumours are rounded, smooth swellings of characteristic firm consistency. Mostly intramural, they distort the shape of the uterus, but if single can cause symmetrical enlargement. If it can be certain that they are situated in the uterus, there is little difficulty, unless there is cystic degeneration of a single fibroid, which can then simulate pregnancy; the reverse mistake is more important to avoid, as a laparotomy for fibroids which reveals a pregnant uterus is an unfortunate error. Pedunculated fibroids may be thought to be ovarian tumours, either cystic or solid, and if calcified may be mistaken for ovarian fibromas; sometimes, it is possible to feel the pedicle of attachment to the uterus. Small fibroid polypi cause no uterine enlargement, and may only be assumed to be present from the history or be found at curettage. Sometimes, the polyp is seen extruding through the cervical canal, but occasionally this sighting may be intermittent and only during menstruation. The difference between myoma and adenomyoma may not be appreciated until attempted removal reveals the lack of capsule, but in general the latter are firmer tumours and there is severe dysmenorrhoea. The main differential diagnosis is from ovarian tumours where, as a rule, the uterus can be detected as separate from the swelling and where menstrual disorders are not so common; but if the ovarian tumour is adherent to the uterus then difficulty may ensue, and it is not unusual for the correct diagnosis to be reached only at laparotomy. Ascites is uncommon, but may result from peritoneal irritation by a freely mobile, firm, pedunculated tumour.

Treatment

Conservative treatment undoubtedly has a place in the management of uterine fibroids. Where the tumours are small, the diagnosis is certain and there are no symptoms, patients may be reassured but must be kept under regular supervision to detect any subsequent enlargement. During pregnancy any attempt to remove the tumours may be attended by severe haemorrhage, which will be difficult to control, and so conservative management is the rule. Near the menopause larger, symptomless, fibroids may also be left untreated, in the anticipation of atrophy subsequent to cessation of the periods, but the patient must be kept under regular supervision. The advent of symptoms or increase in size of the tumours demands surgical intervention, in case the diagnosis is incorrect or malignant degeneration has supervened.

In cases where, apart from the finding of a few small fibroids, the diagnosis would be dysfunctional uterine bleeding, then a diagnostic curettage may be all that is required; if the abnormal bleeding persists, hormone therapy with progestogens may be instituted, but the fibroids must be carefully observed in case they are stimulated to grow.

Where fibroids are causing symptoms, where the diagnosis is in doubt, or where they are larger than a size corresponding to a 16 week pregnancy, then surgical treatment is indicated. Two main forms of operation are possible: myomectomy or hysterectomy. Both are usually performed abdominally, but occasionally the vaginal route is preferred. Hysterectomy is the better procedure, because the fibroids cannot recur and the symptoms can be relieved with certainty. The operation is easier to perform, there is less blood loss, and less postoperative morbidity. Obviously it is only indicated where the age of the patient and parity are such as to render further pregnancy unlikely or undesirable. For younger patients myomectomy is indicated, as it is possible for successful pregnancy to occur after this operation. It must be understood, of course, that recurrence of the fibroids is a distinct possibility, either from seedling fibroids overlooked at the time of operation or because the stimulus to regrowth is maintained. In performing myomectomy the surgeon must be careful to avoid damaging the fallopian tubes in their course through the myometrium. Incisions on the posterior uterine wall are to be avoided as far as possible because of the increased risk of adhesions involving the intestines. Those interested in the techniques of myomectomy should read Bonney (1946), whose treatise remains a classic textbook, also Louros (1966), who has described an ingenious and effective way of occluding the cavity left by myomectomy. The operation is often followed by a slightly stormy convalescence associated with abdominal pain and raised temperature; this is seldom due to infection and usually results from oozing of blood into either the myomectomy cavity in the uterus or into the peritoneal cavity. Intestinal obstruction is the most serious complication, resulting from the small bowel becoming adherent to the uterine scar. Rupture of a myomectomy scar in a subsequent pregnancy or labour is excessively rare, but has been described. The uterus which is often still quite enlarged after the operation tends to shrink to normal size within 2–3 months.

In the Negro races, in whom removal of the uterus is considered a serious mutilation and permission for hysterectomy is not often granted, even where multiple fibroids are associated with gross pelvic sepsis and where there is no possible hope of subsequent pregnancy, a modified subtotal hysterectomy which leaves a modicum of functioning endometrium may be the most acceptable procedure.

UTERINE FIBROIDS AND PREGNANCY

During pregnancy myomata tend to become soft as a result of intestitial oedema and as there is little hypertrophy of the muscle tissue of the tumour as compared with the normal uterine muscle, there is a tendency for the intramural myomata to flatten out and become indistinct during the course of the pregnancy. Subserous tumours, on the other hand, may be readily palpated as the uterus enlarges, and on occasion may be mistaken for foetal parts. Certain accidents and degenerations are more common in fibroids during pregnancy, and of these red degeneration is the most common, as this is the main time when this occurs. There is subacute abdominal pain which may be severe enough to require opiates for relief, tenderness over the fibroid and, at times, signs of peritoneal irritation with rigidity and guarding in the area. Constitutional effects are slight, but there may be initial vomiting and both temperature and pulse will be minimally raised. In the non-pregnant there is an associated leucocytosis, but in pregnancy, this will not signify, in view of the physiological leucocytosis of pregnancy. The differential diagnosis from acute appendicitis may be difficult if the fibroid is situated in the right iliac fossa but usually there is a more constitutional effect in this condition, with a rapid thready pulse raised out of proportion to the body temperature, which is only slightly raised or may even be subnormal. Pyelonephritis may also have to be considered in the diagnosis, but here the temperature is high and there is less tachycardia; there is also symptomatic and bacteriological evidence of urinary tract infection. The treatment of red degeneration in fibroids is conservative; bed-rest, reassurance and analgesics to relieve pain will result in subsidence of symptoms and signs within about 10 days.

Torsion of pedunculated fibroids may occur during pregnancy, but is more likely to occur in the early puerperium, when there is rapid uterine involution and more mobility of intra-abdominal contents associated with laxity of the abdominal wall. Symptoms and signs of an acute or subacute abdomen follow, but guarding and rigidity will be absent due to the lax abdominal muscles. Diagnosis is seldom difficult and laparotomy with myomectomy should be performed. Infection in fibroids may also occur postpartum or, more commonly, after an abortion; fibroid polypi and submucous fibroids are more likely to be infected, the former may be cured spontaneously by sloughing and being passed per vaginam.

The fibroids may influence the course of pregnancy and labour. In early pregnancy abortion may result, this is thought to be more likely if implantation occurs over a submucous fibroid. Inconsistency of uterine size in relation to period of gestation may cause difficulty in estimation of the expected date of delivery. Cervical fibroids, or those situated in the lower half of the corpus, may cause non-engagement of the head, instability of the foetal lie, or persistent abnormal lie or presentation. During labour, fibroids seldom interfere with uterine action, but if multiple and intramural they may do so by causing incoordinate action and, as a result, prolonged labour. Pregnancy in association with a cervical fibroid is a very rare finding, and will inevitably result in obstructed labour, the latter may also result where the tumour is in the lower segment of the uterus, but here it is more usual for the fibroid to be pulled up and out of the way as the lower segment is taken up during the course of the labour.

Obstructed labour must be relieved by Caesarean section, but the temptation to undertake Caesarean myomectomy should be resisted unless the fibroid is actually in the line of the incision; uncontrollable haemorrhage may be the reward of such intervention. Caesarean hysterectomy is a safer procedure if it is deemed that removal of the uterus is both desirable and inevitable. Postpartum haemorrhage is a more common complication, the presence of the fibroids interfering with proper contraction of the uterus. In the puerperium, retarded involution may be real or simulated, and retroversion may be produced particularly by posterior wall fibroids. The ultimate effect of pregnancy on fibroids is variable, they may become much smaller or they may remain unchanged; they do not increase in size.

REFERENCES

ARMENIA C.S. (1967) *Obstet. Gynec., N.Y.* **30**, 524.

BONNEY V. (1946) *The Technical Minutiae of Extended Myomectomy and Ovarian Cystectomy.* London, Cassell.

JEFFCOATE T.N.A. (1962) *Principles of Gynaecology.* London, Butterworths.

LOUROS N.C. (1966) *Three Gynaecological Surgical Techniques.* Springfield, Thomas.

MILLAR N.F. & LUDOVICI P.P. (1955) *Am. J. Obstet. Gynec.* **70**, 720.

CHAPTER 42

MALIGNANT DISEASE OF THE CERVIX

CANCER OF THE CERVIX

After the breast, the cervix is the most notorious site for cancer in women and it is the most feared of all malignant tumours of the female genital tract. It is what women understand as cancer of the womb; it has been the commonest malignant tumour in the genital tract; Lewis (1964) calculated that one woman in every 100 would die from it; and its terminal phases can be painful and distressing in the extreme. Yet, by reason of accessibility, cervical cancer is one of the most easily diagnosed and can now be detected in the very earliest stages of the disease, when the chance of cure is high. Despite this, and the fact that the symptoms produced are relatively dramatic, there is often unfortunate delay by patient and physician before treatment is sought. In the early stages 80–90% of patients, or more, can be cured, but the overall cure rate of all cases seen is around 40%; the means of early detection are available now, it seems that only the will to apply those means is lacking. Although cancer of the cervix commands such dread attention, it is by no means as dangerous as cancer of the ovary, which is inaccessible, tends to be diagnosed later, and thus has an overall cure rate of only some 25%. More women die each year from cancer of the ovary than from cancer of the cervix (see Table 42.1).

The maximum age incidence is around 48 years, but the condition can occur at any age, having been described in children and women of advanced age. It is more common in multiparous than nulliparous women, but the latter are not

Table 42.1. Deaths from cancer of ovary and cervix (adapted from the *Registrar General's Report, 1967*)

Year	Cervix	Ovary
1958	2,866	2,702
1962	2,511	3,032
1967	2,449	3,274

immune. Women of Jewish origin are relatively immune to cancer of the cervix.

Pathological types

Squamous-cell lesions comprise the great majority of carcinomas of the cervix. Some 95% are generally regarded as falling into this category, the remaining 5% being adenocarcinomas which usually arise in the endocervix. It is interesting, too, that when carcinoma of the cervix arises in the very young patient—under 20 years of age— it is almost always of the adenocarcinoma variety.

Aetiology

Myself when young did eagerly frequent
Doctor and Saint, and heard great argument
About it and about : but evermore
Came out by the same door as in I went

Omar Khayyám's comment could well apply to the aetiology of carcinoma of the cervix. A considerable number of factors have been considered, promulgated, relegated and generally debated upon by their protagonists and antagonists over the years. At the present time certain aspects seem to emerge from the welter of reports on the subject. Few, if any, would dispute that to remain a virgin renders a woman as free from the risk of contracting cancer of the cervix as is humanly possible. The researches of Gagnon (1950) and Towne (1955) underline this, by showing the extreme rarity of this disease in nuns. The strange suggestion that such a natural act as coitus must be involved in the aetiology has lead to investigation in some detail, and the present consensus of opinion highlights certain associated features relating to intercourse.

Age at first coitus

Boyd & Doll (1964) in a statistical analysis satisfied themselves that first coitus in adolescence is a common feature in women who develop cancer of the cervix. Terris & Oalmann (1960) found that just over half the patients with cancer of the cervix had first intercourse before the age of 17 years, compared with one-quarter the number of the controls. Rotkin (1967) had similar findings and further substantiated the relationship of first marriage at an early age and the development of this cancer.

Promiscuity

Increased promiscuity is underlined by the findings of Moghissi et al. (1968) that cancer of the cervix was four times as common in a group of female prisoners, one-third of whom were known prostitutes, than in controls. Similar results have been found in association with venereal infections such as syphilis, gonorrhoea and *Trichomonas vaginalis* infections, where women with these conditions are found to have a higher incidence of cancer. Boyd & Doll (1964) and Aitken-Swan & Baird (1965) found some evidence for the protective element in obstructive methods of contraception, but on the whole the evidence is somewhat inconclusive.

Circumcision

Circumcision of male partners has long been held to be a protective factor because of the in-

frequency of the disease in Jewesses, and of some inconclusive evidence on the carcinogenetic role of smegma. A number of authors have contradicted this thesis, amongst them Abou-Daoud (1967), who found no difference in incidence of the disease between Lebanese Christians and Moslems despite their different circumcision status.

Social status

It is generally agreed that the condition is more common in the lower socio-economic groups, and many reasons have been given—such as poor hygiene, promiscuity, poverty and poor medical care.

Race

All observers are agreed that Jewesses are a very low risk group and a diversity of reasons has been suggested, of which the most likely seems to be heredity; but factors such as circumcision of the male, reduced intercourse during pregnancy and the postpartum period, and the strong ethnic ties to solidarity of family life, as against the more permissive sexual habits of other groups, have all been cited.

Carcinogens

As in the aetiology of most cancers, the possibility of carcinogenetic factors has been considered. The possibility of virus infection has recently been resuscitated by Rawls et al. (1968), who have found a higher incidence of infection with herpes simplex virus (type 2) in patients with carcinoma of the cervix than in controls. Coppelson (1969), in an extensive review of the subject, ingeniously proposes that carcinoma of the cervix develops from atypical squamous metaplasia found in adolescence and first pregnancy and that the cells of this abnormal epithelium, by phagocytosis of spermatozoa and incorporation of the sperm DNA into their nuclei, may undergo genetic mutation to become carcinogenetic cells.

If it is true that promiscuity, unguarded intercourse, first intercourse and first pregnancy at an early age, are major factors in the development of carcinoma of the cervix, then the present-day permissive society should show a marked increase in the incidence of the disease in the next decades.

Carcinoma *in situ*

The lesion now recognized as carcinoma *in situ*, or stage o carcinoma of the cervix, was originally described by Schauenstein (1908), but interest in it has largely stemmed from the researches of Rubin (1910) and Schiller (1927) in particular. Papanicolau & Traut (1941, 1943), who demonstrated the ability to recognize abnormal cells in appropriately stained smears of vaginal secretion, gave a considerable impetus to research into the condition because they provided a means of diagnosing it in what appeared to be, by ordinary clinical examination, a normal cervix. A more successful yield was obtained by scraping the cervix with a wooden spatula, the smear being taken from the squamocolumnar junction, which is in most cases the site of origin of the condition Ayre (1951). The aspirations and smears when suitably stained show abnormal cells which may be shed from the surface of a variety of abnormal lesions such as basal-cell hyperplasia, carcinoma *in situ*, and micro-invasive carcinoma of the cervix, all of which can be confirmed only by microscopical examination of material obtained by cervical biopsy. Such cells can also be obtained from early invasive lesions which are clinically obvious, but frank epitheliomatous ulcers may give a negative result, as the surface of the ulcer is composed of granulation tissue and the malignant cells are in the deeper layers. The lesions which may be found on histological examination have been clearly described by Govan *et al.* (1966), in a paper which also reiterates the fact that diagnosis of these lesions is not always easy. Errors may be due to insufficient biopsy material, inadequate staining, examination of an insufficient number of sections, or lack of experience in the observer. The lesions to be considered are listed by Govan as:

Bland lesions
  (1) Squamous hyperplasia
      (a) Reactive hyperplasia
      (b) Basal-cell hyperactivity

  (2) Reserve cell proliferation
  (3) Metaplasia
      (a) Incomplete
      (b) Complete

Malign lesions
  (1) Dysplasia
      (a) Mild
      (b) Severe (Fig. 42.1)
  (2) Carcinoma *in situ* (Fig. 42.2)
  (3) Micro invasive carcinoma (Fig. 42.3)

The malign lesions are characterized by disorder in the arrangement, morphology and activity of the epithelial cells. The most important feature of carcinoma *in situ* is complete loss of stratification, which of course allows the abnormal cells to be exfoliated and thus to be collected by the cervical smear. However, errors in taking the smear are not uncommon, there are times when even an experienced gynaecologist can have difficulty, and, unless the smear is fixed immediately in 95% ethyl alcohol solution or 5–10% Carbowax, difficulty may arise in interpretation due to artefacts in the cells caused by drying. Furthermore, inflammatory changes in the cervix and vagina, often due to *Trichomonas vaginalis*, and changes induced by pregnancy or by exogenous hormone administration, particularly oral contraceptives (Fig. 42.4), may complicate the picture. Despite this, cervical smears are generally accepted as being successful in detecting malign lesions in 98% of cases. The false-positive rate varies with the experience of the cytologist, and can be expected to fall from about 10% initially to well under 1% with increasing experience. Assessment of false-negative results is, naturally, more difficult, but Anderson (1956) reported 14 patients in 12,920 women screened who, having negative reports, subsequently developed cancer, an incidence of 0.11% known false-negatives. Tuncer *et al.* (1967) reviewed 100 patients with invasive carcinoma of the cervix; in less than half had a smear been taken, and in 48 patients in whom one had been taken, there were seven negative reports, of which six on review were found to show cancer cells. The incidence of unsuspected malign lesions detected by cytology varies with the type of populations screened, being high in high-risk

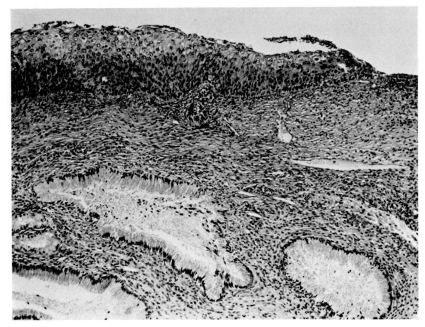

Fig. 42.1. Cervical dysplasia.

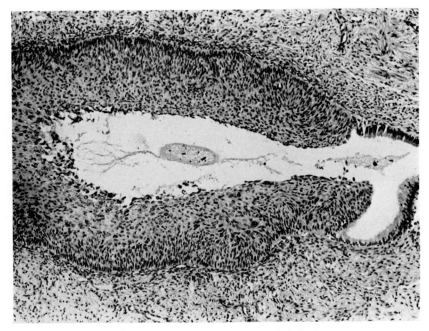

Fig. 42.2. Carcinoma *in situ* in a cervical gland.

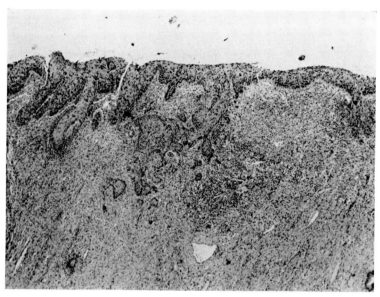

Fig. 42.3. Carcinoma *in situ* with micro-invasion.

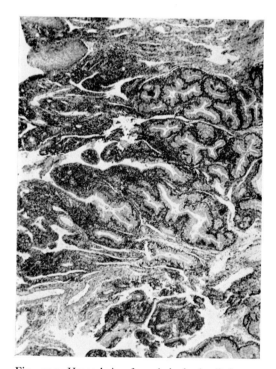

Fig. 42.4. Hyperplasia of cervical glands. Patient on treatment with oral contraceptives.

groups such as prostitutes and the clientele of venereal disease clinics. Interpretation of the stained smear is reported in different ways by different cytologists or pathologists, the standard result being expressed as one of five grades:

Grade I: Normal smears.
Grade II: Slightly atypical cells (as occurs in metaplasia and infection).
Grade III: More marked dysplasia.
Grade IV: Marked dysplasia with a few suspicious malignant cells.
Grade V: Very marked dysplasia with abundant malignant cells showing nuclear changes and basal dyskaryosis.

Grades I and II are regarded as benign or negative, grade III as suspicious, and grades IV and V as malignant or positive.

When faced with a positive or suspicious smear, the clinician must act warily; most important, he must ensure that his patient is made to understand clearly the implications. Too often a patient is referred to hospital in an aura of suspense, fully convinced that she has cancer.

Evidence of inflammation requires treatment of that inflammation and then repetition of the smear. Doubtful or suspicious smears require repetition. Positive smears must be repeated to avoid clerical and observer errors. If two positive smears are obtained then histological confirmation must be from cervical biopsy. At the present time this means cone biopsy. A cone biopsy must include most of the ectocervix, together with a cone reaching to an apex just below the internal os or approximately 2 cm in the non-pregnant patient and rather less, approximately 1 cm, in the pregnant. Less than this may miss endocervical lesions, more may lead to subsequent cervical incompetence and to abortion when the patient becomes pregnant.

The cone should be cut with the cold knife to avoid obscuring the histology by diathermy burning, and is best done after injecting around the cervix a solution of 1 in 250,000 phenylephrine in order to reduce bleeding. It is customary to mark the cone at 12 o'clock on the cervical circumference with a suture to help the pathologist orientate the lesion. The report should describe the lesion and, where possible, state whether it has been circumscribed or not. The report is limited to the tissue sent to the pathologist, and if the cone is inadequate the report may be inconclusive. Considerable reaction follows in the cervix and paracervical tissues, usually with some local sepsis; this does not give rise to any systemic reaction, but is sufficient to cause trouble if further surgery is contemplated. Such surgery should be performed within 48 hr or be deferred until 6 weeks later; that is, before or after the inflammatory reaction. The septic reaction is the cause of the secondary haemorrhage which is a common complication of the operation and which occurs about 10 days afterwards. Late complications of cone biopsy are cervical incompetence, caused by extending the excision to the region of the internal os; and cervical stenosis, due to an excessive fibrous tissue reaction. This stenosis may result in cervical dystocia in any subsequent pregnancy. There are those who feel that cone biopsy is a crude and excessively traumatic diagnostic weapon and prefer to use biopsy at selected sites. The use of Schiller's iodine may indicate the points from which biopsy should be taken, areas containing malignant cells fail to stain brown due to lack of glycogen; toluidine blue may similarly be used. These methods may be particularly valuable in the vagina, where on occasion the *in situ* lesion may spread. Schiller's test and toluidine blue are not sufficiently reliable, however, and colposcopy and colpomicroscopy are more selective and reliable tools, but are usually practised only by a few enthusiasts.

If some method of selecting the correct site for biopsy is not available then the use of cone biopsy is inevitable.

There will be few gynaecologists who, given the facilities, would not now take routine smears on all their obstetric and gynaecological patients and who would not recommend routine cytology for all women over the age of 20. There have now been enough reports to show that the prevalence of carcinoma *in situ* in a freshly screened symptomless population is about 2 to 4 per 1,000 and of microinvasive carcinoma about 1 to 2 per 1,000; cancer of the corpus uteri, ovary and fallopian tube are detected rarely and with insufficient accuracy. Fidler *et al.* (1968) report that in a population already screened, invasive carcinoma of the cervix develops at a rate of approximately 4·5 per 100,000, whereas the rate in the unscreened population is about 29 per 100,000. They also find that the incidence of clinical invasive carcinoma has steadily fallen from 28·4 per 100,000 in 1955 to 13·6 per 100,000 women in 1966. The inference is that a total population screening programme would remove preclinical cancer and, assuming that this condition always precedes invasive cancer, that the latter would ultimately be eradicated. However, even with the enthusiasm and drive of the British Colombia experiment, it had taken 8 years to reach the position where 75% of the female population over 20 years had been screened, and it was felt that the remaining 25% probably contained a number of high-risk women. It is generally recognized that women in the higher socioeconomic classes tend to take advantage of positive health and screening programmes to a greater extent than their less fortunate sisters in whom the diseases it is wished to detect are likely to be more prevalent. Green (1966) is not convinced that such population screening programmes have been shown to reduce the mortality from cancer of the cervix, and believes that the incidence rates fluctuate quite markedly over the years. It seems that crude mortality rates have not been influenced greatly, but Fidler et al. (1968) argue that the true picture will not emerge for 15–20 years. All are agreed that the detection of micro-invasive cancer is a major advance, for the survival rates of treatment in this stage of the disease are nearly 100%. Even so, screening programmes remain inadequate because of financial stringency, lack of trained technical staff and apathy in profession and lay public alike.

Corscaden (1962) emphasizes the point that really early diagnosis and prompt treatment is possible now and can prevent the ravages of carcinoma of the cervix, but Ashley (1966), in postulating two distinct varieties of cancer of the cervix, sounds a more cautious note and believes that those cases preceded by in situ lesions are of a more favourable, slowly developing type, nearly always diagnosed at an early favourable stage, and that the other type—occurring in an older age group—has no precursor stage, develops rapidly and has a poor prognosis.

In the early days of cytology, carcinoma in situ was regarded as an inevitable precursor of invasive disease, and treatment, believed to be prophylactic, tended to be radical, usually by hysterectomy, sometimes even a Wertheim's or, in some cases, by radiotherapy. A progression from normal epithelium to basal-cell hyperplasia, carcinoma in situ and, finally, to micro-invasive and then clinically detectable cancer, is believed to occur. Basal-cell hyperplasia is considered to be frequently reversible to normal, and carcinoma in situ probably also reversible, because some cases have been observed to regress and disappear, but as diagnosis incurs operative interference with the lesion, it is not known how often this happens spontaneously. Because diagnostic procedures are often curative, it is not known how many cases of carcinoma in situ become invasive and how many regress spontaneously. That the former occurs, is known from the reports of many observers amongst whom Te Linde et al. (1957) found 17 cases of pre-

invasive cancer in biopsies which had been taken in patients who subsequently were found to have invasive cancer; Kottmeier (1953) followed 59 untreated cases of pre-invasive cancer over 10 years and found that 8 or 13% became invasive; Younge (1952) followed 41 cases, and 14 became invasive; and Petersen (1956) followed 127 patients and found that 4% had become invasive in 1 year, 11% in 3 years, 22% in 5 years, and 33% in 9 years.

Boyes et al. (1962) believe that the average duration of pre-invasive lesions before becoming invasive is about 12 years, which fits in with a maximum age incidence for invasive cancer of 48 years of age and of pre-invasive cancer of 38 years.

It is assumed that at least 30% of pre-invasive lesions become invasive, but this implies that many such lesions regress or remain unchanged. Further, recurrences have been found in the vagina even after hysterectomy either as new lesions or because they were missed at the time of the original diagnosis; pre-invasive lesions have been described throughout the length of the vagina, and even extending on to the vulva. This means that whether the patient receives minor or major surgery as treatment, interminable follow-up with smears is necessary. As a result, the present tendency is towards more conservative management, particularly in younger women, and Green (1966) has even suggested this in certain patients with micro-invasive lesions.

Whilst individual gynaecologists vary in their attitude towards the abnormal findings that may be made as a result of cytology, in general the present procedure after obtaining two positive smears would be to perform a cone biopsy. Abnormal lesions, including carcinoma in situ, shown to be completely cleared by the biopsy, should be followed by routine smears at 3-monthly, then two 6-monthly intervals, and subsequently at yearly intervals, assuming that the smears remain negative. If it is considered by the pathologist that the excision has not cleared the lesion, and it is a case of carcinoma in situ, it is safe to wait 3 months and repeat the smear. If the smear is negative then further close follow-up, using smears, is indicated. If the smear is positive, or if it becomes positive subsequently, then the choice rests between a further biopsy or hysterectomy with removal of a cuff of vagina. Which of these steps is taken will depend on the age, parity and wishes of the patient. Green (1966) claims that it is better to wait until 6 months, as the smear may by then have become negative. Micro-invasive lesions of the cervix which have been removed *in toto* by the cone biopsy can, in the opinion of Green, be treated conservatively, and in essence this is logical if the lesion has in fact been cleared, and indeed will be desirable in some young patients. Most gynaecologists would prefer to perform an extended hysterectomy with removal of a cuff of vagina in older patients whenever micro-invasive lesions are found.

Finally, if micro-invasion is found but has patently not been completely excised in the cone biopsy then further surgery must be undertaken. Extending the hysterectomy is mainly to enable the surgeon to remove a cuff of vagina, a procedure often more simply done by vaginal hysterectomy —which does not require dissection of the lower end of the ureter. The cuff is removed because the *in situ* change may be present here as well, and the extent of the lesion may not reliably be demarcated by Schiller's iodine staining.

More difficulty arises in the management of positive smears found in the pregnant patient. Smears are commonly taken at the first antenatal visit, because of the large number of defaulters at the postnatal clinics. If the smear is positive, the question of a biopsy arises. When the cervix is healthy and there are no suspicious symptoms such as bleeding, then a further smear is taken after the lying-in period, and if still positive a cone biopsy is taken from the cervix. If suspicious lesions exist, or suspicious symptoms are present, then a modified cone is taken, despite the risk of haemorrhage, abortion, or cervical dystocia due to fibrosis. Further intervention would only be indicated if micro-invasion were found to be present and the age and parity of the patient allowed. Such intervention would be an extended hysterectomy with a cuff of vagina where the patient was agreeable, but if the pregnancy were very precious then a more limited attack confined to the cervix might be first essayed, but extending the extent of the cervical excision

increases the risk of abortion. It is in the pregnant patient with a positive smear that colposcopy can be very valuable, in that a much more limited biopsy, confined to the area of epithelial abnormality, can be taken; or in some cases with suspicious smears, a colposcopic examination alone will obviate the need for any interference at all.

Clinical features

In carcinoma *in situ* and micro-invasive lesions of the cervix, there are usually no symptoms, and these conditions are mostly detected only by screening methods. Once the disease has become clinically detectable abnormal bleeding is the most likely symptom. Frequently this followed minor trauma to the cervix, as during coitus, micturition or defaecation. As the same symptoms may occur with *in situ* or micro-invasive lesions, all cases of postcoital bleeding should have a cervical biopsy taken, even in the face of a negative smear report. In premenopausal women the bleeding in carcinoma of the cervix will be mainly intermenstrual and slight in amount, but it can take the form of heavy or prolonged periods, and in neglected cases the loss can be profuse. In postmenopausal women the bleeding is more likely to concern the patient and the physician. In women not practising coitus there may be insufficient disturbance of the tumour to cause bleeding. It is noteworthy that the disease can reach a late stage of development before bleeding occurs. Corscaden (1962) reports on 252 patients with inoperable cancer of the cervix (stages III and IV), one-third of whom had bled for less than 2 months when first seen and five of whom had suffered no bleeding. Any abnormal bleeding, therefore, in any woman warrants a careful digital and per speculum examination of the pelvic organs, together with such further investigation as may be indicated.

Vaginal discharge presents much less frequently and occurs at a later stage of development than bleeding, because it indicates ulceration and infection of the tumour. The discharge may be serosanquinous or purulent, and is often offensive; rarely, it may be the only symptom.

Disturbances of micturition or defaecation are not characteristic of this condition in the early stages.

Pain is a phenomenon found only in the terminal phase of the disease. It is of two main types, (i) visceral, due to the presence of a large infective mass of growth and characterized by a dull, aching pain in the pelvis, or (ii) somatic, due to involvement of the lumbosacral nerve plexus, when the pain is severe and in the distribution of the sciatic nerve.

In late and neglected cases uraemia due to obstruction of the ureters by paracervical spread will usually kill the patient before malignant cachexia supervenes. Involvement of bladder or rectum will give rise to urinary or bowel symptoms, such as frequency and urgency of micturition or diarrhoea and tenesmus. Fistula formation will be associated with incontinence of urine or faeces.

On examining the patient it will be found, in the majority of cases, that the outward appearance is normal and there is no loss of weight. If bleeding has been severe the patient may be anaemic, but this is not the rule. Examination of the abdomen is usually unrevealing. Examination of the external genitalia shows no abnormality either. The demands of cytology have made it usual these days to pass a speculum so as to inspect the vagina and cervix and take a smear before proceeding to digital examination. In cases where the history is highly suggestive of carcinoma of the cervix it is wiser to perform an initial gentle digital examination so as to avoid troublesome and distressing bleeding which may occur in the more advanced cases. On inspection per speculum the cervix may appear normal in carcinoma *in situ*, subclinical or endocervical carcinoma. In more advanced cases a vascular erosion may be present or a more obvious roughened, red, papillary area asymmetrically disposed on the surface of the cervix. Extension of the abnormal area onto the vagina is highly suspicious. The presence of obvious ulceration or of a cauliflower-type mass springing from the cervix is practically diagnostic. On occasion the lesion is nodular in type, and the cervix will then appear irregular and nodular, but may have an unbroken surface.

Digital examination of the cervix in very early cases may not be informative, but where the surface epithelium is broken there is likely to be brisk bleeding as a result of the examination, and this will be aggravated when the smear is taken. Early lesions feel rough and granular, more advanced lesions show friability of the surface with induration of the base. Friability may be obvious on palpation, but in cases of doubt the probe test can be applied; the probe will sink into the substance of a growth, whereas a healthy cervix resists its passage. Extension of the growth into the fornices and down the vagina may be realized more readily by touch than by sight. Where extensions to the paracervical tissues have occurred the mobility of the cervix will be limited. Bimanual examination of the body of the uterus and the adnexae will usually be unremarkable, unless a pyometra is present, when some enlargement may be detected.

Rectal examination should now be performed to determine the degree of involvement of paracervical tissues, by this means the cardinal and uterosacral ligaments can be palpated throughout their course from cervix to pelvic attachment; induration indicates direct extension of growth or inflammatory reaction, and whilst it is often not possible to distinguish these clinically, for the purposes of staging it must be reported as extension of growth. Isolated lymph-node masses may be palpated on the pelvic side-wall in advanced cases.

Management

Once a presumptive or definite diagnosis of carcinoma of the cervix has been made on clinical grounds, confirmation by histological examination must follow. In addition, a full assessment of the extent of the lesion and of the patient's general condition must be made before the method of treatment can be decided. In advanced cases pieces of growth may fall free into the vagina during digital examination, and these should be sent for microscopy, but in most cases surgical biopsy is required. In early cases staging of the extent of the disease may be achieved when the patient is first examined, but often, in order to avoid unnecessary bleeding and discomfort, this procedure must await examination under anaesthesia.

On admission to hospital, in addition to a routine assessment of the patient's general fitness for operation, certain particular investigations are necessary. The haemoglobin concentration and the red and white blood cell count should be determined, as anaemia must be corrected before either radiotherapy or major surgery. Intravenous pyelography and estimation of the blood urea will give information on kidney function. Parametrial extension of the growth may involve the lower ureter and cause obstruction with resultant hydronephrosis which will influence management. Before major surgery involving dissection of the ureters, the presence of ureterorenal abnormalities must be excluded, or if present their nature carefully observed. Chest X-ray is also routine, and if other sites of possible extrapelvic metastasis are indicated by symptoms or clinical signs, then the necessary investigations—such as X-ray of long bones, or the spine and, where available, liver-scanning procedures—should be performed. Examination under anaesthesia now follows, to stage the extent of the growth and to decide the method of treatment. Staging is performed by digital examination of the pelvic organs. First, a vaginal examination will discover the nature of the tumour—whether ulcerative, proliferative or nodular and the extent to which the cervix is involved; the extent to which the vagina is involved should next be determined, as this is often more readily appreciated by palpation than by direct vision. Bimanual palpation of the uterus and adnexae reveals the degree to which the uterus is tethered by the parametria, and also any uterine enlargement or adnexal swellings; uterine enlargement may be due to pyometra or uterine fibroids, and adnexal swellings are more likely to be inflammatory than neoplastic. Extension into the parametria, i.e. the cardinal and uterosacral ligaments, is not readily appreciated on vaginal examination as these structures lie above the lateral vaginal fornices which limit the extent of digital examination; rectal examination is obligatory and allows palpation of the ligaments throughout their whole length and thickness, and also the detection of isolated

lymph node metastases on the pelvic side-walls. A useful method, often employed, is simultaneous rectal and vaginal examination with the index finger in the vagina and the middle finger in the rectum. Unless really hard, induration of the parametrial tissues cannot be distinguished for certain as being neoplastic rather than inflammatory. Carcinoma of the cervix is staged from stage 0 to stage IV, and Table 42.2. shows the definition of the different clinical stages.

Table 42.2. Staging of carcinoma of the cervix uteri (adapted from F.I.G.O., 1965)

Pre-invasive carcinoma of the cervix
  Stage 0: Carcinoma *in situ*; intra-epithelial carcinoma. (*Note*: Cases of stage 0 should not be included in any therapeutic statistics).

Invasive carcinoma of the cervix
  Stage I: Carcinoma strictly confined to the cervix (extension to the corpus should be disregarded).

  Stage Ia: Cases of preclinical carcinoma and of so-called 'early stromal invasion'.

  Stage Ib: All other cases of stage I.

  Stage II: The carcinoma extends beyond the cervix but has not extended on to the pelvic wall.
    The carcinoma involves the vagina, but not the lower third.
    Subgrouping of stage II cases into IIa (no parametrial involvement) and IIb (parametrial involvement) is recommended.
    Every institution reporting cases of stage II should, as well, give information on the number of cases allotted to stage III.

  Stage III: The carcinoma has extended on to the pelvic wall. On rectal examination there is no cancer-free space between the tumour and the pelvic wall.
    The tumour involves the lower third of the vagina.

  Stage IV: The carcinoma has extended beyond the true pelvis or has involved the mucosa of the bladder or rectum. (A bullous oedema, as such, does not permit allotment of a case to stage IV.)

Dilatation and curettage is the next procedure. A uterine sound is passed and the direction and length of the cavity is measured. Where there is extensive destruction of the cervix this can be a very difficult and hazardous procedure, for the internal os may be difficult to find and perforation is liable to occur because of the friable and necrotic tissues; the use of fine probes may help, but they perforate more easily and so require to be used with extra caution. In cases of failure a second attempt may be more successful after external irradiation or intravaginal radium has caused the growth to shrink. In some cases, dilatation of the cervix releases a pyometra, which must then be drained by a rubber tube sutured to the cervix. Careful curettage of the endocervix and uterine cavity may help to delineate extension of the tumour upwards into the uterus.

Schiller's iodine test

The Schiller test is the application of a solution of iodine made up as follows: iodine 1 g, potassium iodide 2 g, water 300 ml.

Normal cells containing glycogen stain brown; malignant cells are unstained, but so are areas with loss of epithelium as in prolapse ulcers, erosions and atrophy, as well as endocervical epithelium. It may help to indicate areas suitable for biopsy, particularly in early invasive or preinvasive cases. By no means in general usage, it is an adjunctive diagnostic tool which can be valuable—as long as its limitations are recognized.

Colposcopy

The colposcope, devised by Hinselmann (1925), is even less commonly used than the iodine test, but undoubtedly it is much more accurate and useful. It is a binocular illuminated optical instrument introduced into the vagina and giving a magnification of 12 diameters. It requires experience to operate it correctly and is thought to be time-consuming, and as a result tends to be used only be enthusiasts; it is much more popular in Europe than in the U.K. and America. Coppleson & Reid (1967) have had extensive experience with the instrument and claim that, when used in conjunction with cytology, it increases their diagnostic accuracy to 98%, as against 93% for cytology alone. The main value seems to be in indicating the site and type of biopsy and as a research tool.

Certainly, as used by Coppleson and his colleagues the instrument is easy to use as a routine procedure in the operating theatre and, in conjunction with cytology, allows a much more accurate diagnosis and greater discrimination in deciding treatment.

Colpomicroscopy

The colpomicroscope is basically a development of the colposcope, giving a magnification up to 200 diameters, and the cervical epithelium stained with haematoxylin can be examined. This also requires expertise and expenditure of time, and is not in general usage. Antoine & Grunberger (1956), who developed the instrument, have produced an atlas showing the results that can be obtained.

Biopsy of the cervix

Ideally, a generous biopsy of obvious malignant tissue—together with an equally generous piece of underlying normal cervical tissue—should be taken for histological examination; this is even more important in very early or suspicious cases, as it is necessary for the pathologist to be able to say whether penetration of the normal tissues has occurred, and to what extent. In gross cases, adequate portions of malignant tissue suffice, and, indeed, it may be impossible to find any remnant of normal cervix; often in such cases the material is best removed with a curette. If the degree of vaginal wall extension is uncertain, then biopsies should be taken from the suspicious areas. Bleeding from the biopsy site can be controlled by suture, diathermy coagulation or packing the vaginal cavity.

Cystoscopy

Examination of the bladder should now be performed, although evidence of involvement of the bladder is seldom seen unless it is clear on clinical assessment that such involvement is probable. The evidence to be sought is bullous oedema, indicating spread to the underlying bladder muscle; direct invasion of the bladder mucosa will be found in less than 2% of cases (Fig. 42.5).

Rectal involvement by carcinoma of the cervix is rare and is only likely in very advanced cases or where the pouch of Douglas has been obliterated

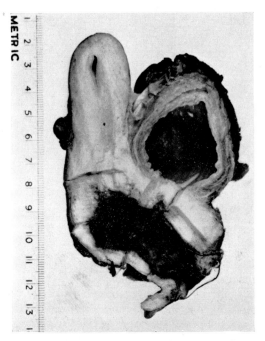

Fig. 42.5. Direct invasion of the bladder by carcinoma of the cervix.

by endometriotic or inflammatory adhesions; such involvement will be readily apparent to the examining finger and will rarely require endoscopic examination.

In advanced cases assessment of operability is important; suitable cases will have mobility of the malignant mass in the pelvis and absence of firm attachment to the pelvic side-wall. Naturally, the final judgement in such cases often has to await the findings at exploratory laparotomy. Where radiotherapy is indicated either as definitive or as pre-operative treatment, and the diagnosis is certain, then the first radium application can be made at the same time as the assessment under anaesthesia. In cases where histological confirmation is required, measurement of the vaginal vault and length of the uterine cavity will enable the correct size of radium applicators to be prepared for subsequent insertion.

Treatment

The question of treatment of carcinoma of the cervix has aroused much debate and argument,

and there are still divisions of opinion as to which method is to be preferred. Unfortunately, this has led to rigid attitudes being adopted which are not always in the best interests of the individual patient. Historically, apart from ancient remedies involving local applications more remarkable for their nature than for their efficacy, surgery was the only treatment available. In 1870, Marian Sims was expelled from the very hospital he had founded for trying to admit and treat cases of carcinoma of the cervix, then considered to be contagious. In the last quarter of the nineteenth century simple hysterectomy and removal of the growth was shown to be inadequate, and more ambitious surgery, compatible with the ideas of Halstead as related to cancer of the breast, was attempted. At the beginning of the century Wertheim (1905) developed the procedure now known by his name, and usually meant to infer a radical abdominal hysterectomy; the operation as described by him (1925) fell somewhat short of the measures later adopted by Bonney (1941) and others of the twentieth-century school of gynaecologists. Improvements in anaesthesia, antisepsis and resuscitation have enabled surgeons to carry out more radical procedures, even to the extent of exenteration as practised by Brunschwig (1948). Where Wertheim removed only palpably enlarged lymph nodes, his successors have striven to remove all the lymphatics and nodes possible. Whilst Wertheim was promoting the abdominal approach, Schauta (1904) was developing the radical vaginal hysterectomy now associated with his name and developed by Amreich (1941), Navratil (1954), Bastiaanse (1955) and Mitra (1954). This operation allows removal of the uterus and adnexae, and is, if anything, a more radical excision of the paracervical tissues than the Wertheim, but it does not allow removal of the pelvic lymph nodes (a deficiency Mitra resolved by combining it with extraperitoneal lymphadenectomy). As the early surgeons were developing their skills, a rival form of treatment appeared. In 1895 Roentgen discovered X-rays, and in 1898 the Curies discovered radium; the physical properties, and physiological and pathological effects, of both were soon appreciated, and their application in the treatment of cancer rapidly followed. In the early days of surgery and radiotherapy patients suffered high mortality rates and often appalling injuries, but the improving survival rates justified their continued usage.

There now developed an unfortunate era of competition between surgeons and radiotherapists which to this day has not completely subsided. Most agree that for carcinoma of the cervix the basic treatment must be radiotherapy and that surgery must be reserved for carefully selected cases. Even where operability rates can be increased by the use of pre-operative radiotherapy, there still remains a group of patients in whom the disease is too far advanced, or who are too infirm to withstand radical surgical procedures. It must be conceded that the surgical technique required is of a high order, and that greater proficiency comes only with constant practice, thus surgery can compete only when it is performed by experienced surgeons in selected cases. Nevertheless, the radical operation needs to be kept alive for those cases unsuitable for radiotherapy, to enable surgeons to progress to the even more radical procedures occasionally required for recurrent lesions, and because it is more suitable for young women in whom the ovaries can be conserved. If features of the present liberal attitude—such as early age of marriage, more frequent broken marriages, promiscuity and unguarded intercourse—persist, then perhaps cancer of the cervix will occur in earlier age groups than is now the case. Certainly cytology, even if it does not entirely prevent the occurrence of invasive cancer, should bring the latter to light in the earliest stages. Thus there would be the need for more frequent use of surgery.

Patients should be treated individually rather than collectively, and their treatment should be selected from all the methods available in whatever single method or combination of methods best suits their particular problem.

RADIOTHERAPY

When considering radiotherapy there are a variety of methods from which to choose; some are detailed below.

(1) Intracavitary radium supplemented by external deep X-ray therapy remains the method of choice. The means of application are varied, and the differences depend basically on the time–dose ratio. A large source can only be applied for short periods of time without danger to normal tissues, and therefore repeated applications must be made, as in the Stockholm technique. A small source can be left in for a longer time and a continuous single application becomes possible, as in the Paris technique. The Manchester technique lies somewhere between the two. The difference also extends to the apparatus in which the radium source is applied—boxes, cylinders or ovoids, for example. Important also, is the method by which the radium source is kept in the correct position, for any shift after the original siting will alter the maximum impact of the radiation and may result in trauma to normal tissues. Various techniques use different types of colpostat, such as the Fletcher (1962) or Fordyce, reported by Corscaden (1959). Radiodiagnostic methods are employed after the sources have been positioned, in order to ensure that errors have not occurred due to shifting. Scintillation counters are used also, to ascertain that dangerous doses are not being received by bladder and rectum. In an effort to allow even more accurate placing of the sources—and, in addition, to protect staff—after-loading techniques are being employed whereby the applicators are positioned and small test sources are introduced from which the appropriate calculations are made, then the definitive dose of radium can be inserted in a special radium ward or treatment room. A sophistication of this method is the cathetron, where the patient is placed in a heavily screened cell, the applicators are put in place and then a very high dosage source is introduced from a storage machine for a very short time (O'Connell *et al.* 1967).

(2) External irradiation. This can be administered by means of high-voltage machines of varied powers, radium or cobalt-60 bombs, betatrons, neutrons and protrons. The hope is always expressed that the more powerful the machine the better will be the results; this is not always the case, and much will depend on the experience of the radiotherapist. The main advantages accrue from a higher depth-dose combined with a lower skin-dose, and for the

same tumour-dose there is a lower volume-dose; the biological effect on the cell, however, remains the same. In order still further to reduce skin-dosage, rotational methods can be applied whereby either the patient rotates around the source, or vice versa; by this means individual ports of entry are eliminated in favour of a circumferential attack. External irradiation is mainly employed as an adjunct to intracavitary radium, but, with the more powerful machines available, some centres have delivered the whole dose of radiation by this means.

(3) Interstitial irradiation using radium needles, cobalt or colloidal gold, have been tried in a few centres but the method had not been very popular in the case of the cervix, as the application to the paracervical tissues has to be made blind, and most authorities prefer its usage in more superficial growths where needles can be inserted and arranged under direct vision.

(4) Transvaginal roentgen rays have been superseded by external irradiation, as being more accurate and less unpleasant for the patient.

In the definitive treatment of carcinoma of the cervix by radiotherapy, the local tumour and its immediate paracervical spread is attacked with intra-uterine and intravaginal radium, whilst lymph nodes on the pelvic side-wall, and their immediate lymphatic tributaries, are dealt with mainly by external irradiation.

A dispute between surgeons and radiotherapists has long centred on the question of who best could deal with the lymph-node metastases. Surgeons have demonstrated the effect that operation can achieve in cases where the lymph nodes are involved by growth (see Table 42.3).

Radiotherapy suffers from the disadvantage that the incidence of definite node involvement in

successfully treated cases cannot easily be demonstrated. Rutledge (1962) demonstrated what radiotherapy can achieve in involved lymph nodes by performing lymphadenectomy after such treatment and comparing his results with the incidence of involved nodes collated by Navratil (1954) from several series (see Table 42.4). Other workers have demonstrated similar

Table 42.4. Effect of radiotherapy on pelvic lymph nodes (percentage nodes involved by growth)

	Surgery alone *	Surgery preceded by radiotherapy †
Stage I	11·2	3·3
Stage II	23·1	11·9
Stage III	43·5	19·0

* Navratil (1954)
† Rutledge (1962)

results. Moreover, the results obtained by radiotherapy when the expected incidence of lymph node involvement is considered, together with the findings at pre- and postoperative lymphangiography, confirm the opinion that radiotherapy can destroy malignant disease in the pelvic lymph nodes, but does not, of course, do so in all cases.

The incidence of new primary growths in the treated area and of subsequent sarcomatous change in the uterus after radiotherapy is so small as to have no bearing on the argument. There has always been a feeling that certain types of cancer must be more suitably treated by radiotherapy and others by surgery, and that, if they could by some means be separated and the appropriate type of treatment applied, then the overall results would be improved. Efforts in this direction have been made by Glucksman & Spear (1945), Graham & Graham (1960), and others, by methods involving histology and cytology. Although some success in prediction has resulted, the overall results in treatment have not been markedly improved, and these methods so far remain in the hands of dedicated enthusiasts and have not become generally used. Unfortunately, it seems to be broadly true that the cases that do well with surgery do equally well with radiotherapy, and that the final results of any

Table 42.3. Results of surgical treatment in cases with lymph-node involvement

Author	5 year survival rate (%)
Bonney (1941)	21
Schlink (1960)	29
Currie (1962)	42
Brunschwig & Daniel (1962)	32
Stallworthy (1964)	27

treatment depend more on the special characteristics of the tumour, the resistance of the host tissues and, most important, the stage at which the disease is detected, than on the particular method of treatment employed.

COMPLICATIONS OF RADIOTHERAPY

Radium and external irradiation affect normal tissue cells in a similar manner, but to a lesser degree than malignant cells. Varying degrees of inflammatory reaction result, ranging from mild erythema to necrotic slough as a result of tissue death. The therapist must aim at the maximum lethal dose to the tumour concomitant with a safe dose to nearby normal tissues. The structures most at risk during treatment of carcinoma of the cervix are the skin, bladder and lower intestinal tract.

Skin

The use of multiple ports of entry, rotational methods and, in particular, high-voltage therapy, have resulted in the virtual elimination of severe skin burns, so that initial erythema and subsequent pigmentation are the main changes occurring in the skin as a result of external irradiation.

Urinary tract

The bladder is the most likely part of the urinary tract to be injured. Increased frequency of micturition, urgency and dysuria due to a simple acute cystitis are almost inevitable during treatment, as the radium applied to the cervix reacts upon that part of the bladder in contact with the cervix. This cystitis is only transient and subsides without treatment—provided there is no associated urinary tract infection, aggravated or produced by catheterization. With overdosage, the clinical features may be prolonged and there may be haematuria due to haemorrhagic cystitis when there is a more acute inflammation of the mucosa.

This inflammatory reaction is likely to be followed by an area of atrophy of the bladder mucosa with telangiectasia and the possibility of more severe bleeding from a ruptured dilated vessel, which may require fulgurization. A more serious injury is the formation of an ulcer, usually found on the postero-inferior region of the bladder close to the cervix. The ulcer has clear-cut outlines and is covered with a tough, yellow slough which is firmly adherent and in time becomes encrusted with deposits of urinary salts. Such ulcers are very chronic and may persist for 2 or 3 years before healing spontaneously; at any time, however, perforation with the formation of a vesicovaginal fistula may occur. Such ulcers are late injuries and may arise some months to a year or more after treatment, and may produce only mild urinary symptoms. The distinction from a malignant ulcer due to persistence or recurrence of the growth may be difficult, but such a degree of bladder involvement is rare without evidence of recrudescence of growth elsewhere in the pelvis. Vesicovaginal fistula due to radiotherapy usually follows some 3–8 months after treatment, but cases have been reported at much later intervals; as with the ulcers, the possibility of the lesion being due to recrudescence of growth must be considered, and in fact with modern methods of treatment the latter is much the most likely cause. Treatment of radiation-induced fistulae is rendered difficult because of the avascularity of the tissues, and the best method is by colpocleisis, although more extensive procedures utilizing fresh tissues from other areas in order to introduce a new blood supply have been successfully used; such methods involve the use of grafts from the labium majus, the gracilis muscle or the greater omentum. The ureters are seldom, if ever, damaged as a result of radiotherapy but they may become obstructed by fibrosis consequent on treatment, particularly if the parametrial tissues are heavily infiltrated by growth; such obstruction can lead to hydronephrosis and loss of kidney function. As a result of modern techniques, accuracy of dosage calculations and the use of dosimeters, severe injuries to the urinary tract are now uncommon from radiotherapy.

Bladder contraction may occur after extensive external irradiation, but is more likely to do so when such treatment is followed by radical surgery; the blood supply of the bladder, already diminished by the irradiation, is further endangered by the surgery, which also interrupts the nerve supply. The affect on the bladder is aggravated by prolonged catheterization and concomitant infection, and a contracted bladder of low capacity results. The extreme frequency and urgency of mucturition produced will necessitate some form of urinary deviation.

Intestinal tract

The intestinal epithelium is very susceptible to injury by radium and X-rays. Radiation sickness is common, due to an enterocolitis, and is associated with diarrhoea, nausea and a feeling of prostration. Mucus discharge is common also, but bleeding is not. Spontaneous recovery is usual but occasionally treatment must temporarily be interrupted. With more severe injury there is an acute enteritis with bleeding from the haemorrhagic mucosa; such bleeding may continue for months or years following treatment. Ulcer formation as seen in the bladder also occurs and, similarly, is a late reaction; the commonest sites are first the rectosigmoid and then the anterior wall of the rectum. The symptoms are discharge of mucus and blood, the treatment is palliative. Fistula formation is uncommon.

Following exterior irradiation with high-voltage therapy, particularly if used as the sole form of treatment, a plastic peritonitis may result. Extensive adhesions are formed between the loops of small bowel, and obstruction may occur. More extensive damage leads to intestinal necrosis and fatal peritonitis.

Fractured neck of the femur due to avascular necrosis has been reported following deep X-ray therapy, but is uncommon now that the possibility is recognized.

Leucopenia is usual following radiotherapy, and requires repeated blood counts to observe the degree to which the white cell count falls; this is seldom to the degree induced by chemotherapy.

Unsuspected pelvic inflammatory disease may flare up as a result of radiotherapy (more usually intracavitary applications), and if the condition cannot be controlled by antibiotics surgery may be required either to remove the infected organs before radiotherapy can recommence or as definitive treatment for the carcinoma. Pyometra must be drained prior to radium insertion.

COMBINED METHODS

As both methods of treatment give more or less similar results (Table 42.5), there are those who feel that a combination of the two will give even better results, and Schlink (1960), Welch *et al.* (1961) and Stallworthy (1964) have shown what can be achieved by these methods (Table 42.6). It has yet to be shown that the method improves the overall results in all cases seen, and does not merely render more cases operable. There is no doubt that in stages two and three pre-operative radium will reduce the size of the tumour mass and resolve some paracervical induration, particularly if it be inflammatory in nature. Some dispute exists as to whether such preliminary radiotherapy should consist of a full or partial tumour dose. Many surgeons prefer one-half to two-thirds of the full dose, but Schlink (1960) and Stallworthy (1964) have favoured the use of a full dose. The decision will rest on what the operator is trying to achieve by the radium, if it be merely to clean up inflammation, reduce tumour mass and increase operability, it will not be necessary to give a full dose. If the radium is intended to destroy the tumour, then a full dose is required, and the need for subsequent surgery must be in doubt.

Table 42.5. Results of treatment in cancer of cervix

Author		Surgery		Radiotherapy	
		Cases	5 year survival rate (%)	Cases	5 year survival rate (%)
Masabuchi *et al.* (1969)	Stage I	296	90·5	152	88·2
	Stage II	266	74·5	450	68·7
Blaikley *et al.* (1969)	Stage I	47	63·8	183	63·3
	Stage II	19	47·3	368	44·0

Table 42.6. Results of treatment in cancer of cervix; surgery preceded by radiotherapy.

	Schlink (1960)		Welch *et al.* (1961)		Stallworthy (1964)	
	Cases	5 year survival rate (%)	Cases	5 year survival rate (%)	Cases	5 year survival rate (%)
Stage I	61	72·1	52	90·4		
Stage II	113	60·2	77	71·6		
Stage III	46	43·5	13	66·7		
All			149	77·9	244	71

SURGERY

As with radiotherapy, there are a variety of surgical procedures by which the various stages of cancer of the cervix may be treated. These range from simple conization of the cervix for micro-invasive carcinoma, as advocated in some cases by Green (1966), through hysterectomy (abdominal or vaginal), extended hysterectomy, Schauta's or Wertheim's radical hysterectomy, to some form of exenteration procedure. It is not known for certain to what extent dangerous lymphatic embolism occurs in the early stages of invasive carcinoma, but it is probably that the lymph nodes can deal with occasional malignant cells, just as the showers of cells which reach the blood stream must be destroyed.

In 67 stage Ia cases Kovacic *et al.* (1968) found no cases of node involvement, whereas in 700 stage I cases Kolstad (1968) found nodes involved in 20%, a rather higher figure than usually reported.

Nor is it known how important it is to remove extensively the paracervical tissues in cases where there is no clinical spread to this area, but by the extent of this excision the surgeon reckons his radicality. The investigations of Hill (1960) and Stallworthy (1964) tend to show that the para-

Table 42.7. Persistence of malignant cells in operation specimens after preliminary radiotherapy

Author	Uterus	Parametrium	Lymph nodes
Hill (1960)	43%	8%	22%
Stallworthy (1964)		3·4%	24%

cervical tissues are less important than the nodes themselves (Table 42.7).

Where there is obvious parametrial involvement there can be no doubt as to the need to extend the dissection well clear of the growth, but in the earlier stages it is desirable to strike a balance between what is necessary in the interests of a cure and what is dangerous to the patient's well-being by reason of undue extension of the surgical excision. Certainly there is no need routinely to sacrifice healthy ovaries, for extension to them of the malignant process does not occur in any but advanced tumours, and there is no evidence that cancer of the cervix is an endocrine-dependent tumour. The more extensive the surgery, and the greater the dose of pre-operative radium, the more likely is injury to ureter or bladder, and the greater the chance of increased morbidity due to haemorrhage and sepsis, and the higher the operative mortality.

Micro-invasive carcinoma is the earliest form of the disease, and as Green (1966) has shown this can be removed by the diagnostic cone biopsy, but most surgeons would prefer a more extensive removal such as a total hysterectomy incorporating a cuff of vagina, or even an extended hysterectomy. There does not seem to be any necessity for lymphadenectomy at this early stage, and if indicated the ovaries may be conserved. With overt invasion nothing less than the Wertheim procedure is really adequate if the best results from surgery are to be obtained. In stage I cases there would seem to be little logic in the use of preliminary radiotherapy which will increase the number of surgical procedures to be borne by the patient and also the morbidity of the more radical operation without offering any striking advantage

Table 42.8. Cooperative study of cancer of the cervix uteri (13th vol., 1964);
5 year survival rates (%)

Country	Stage I	Stage II	Stage III	Stage IV	All stages
Japan	86	65	37	14	59
Scandinavia	77	56	30	11	53
U.S.A.	76	53	34	9	52
Australia	73	48	18	0	48
U.K.	68	43	24	7	41

in results. In such cases, should the lymph nodes be found to be involved, postoperative external irradiation should be given.

In more advanced stages there is a better case for the use of radiotherapy in conjunction with surgery, because the operability rate will be increased and growth which might otherwise have been in the line of dissection may be destroyed. Again, postoperative external irradiation will be necessary. Amongst the very advanced cases, or those in which other treatment has failed, there remain some where extraradical surgery in the form of exenteration will be feasible.

The consensus of opinion throughout the world favours radiotherapy as the definitive treatment of choice for cancer of the cervix in all stages, but in most countries there are centres where surgical treatment is preferred. Balancing the best results of surgery against the best results of radiotherapy there seems to be little to choose between them, but by no means all centres can reproduce similar results. There is in fact a distressingly uneven span of results from different countries which is difficult to explain (Table 42.8).

COMPLICATIONS OF SURGERY

The complications of any major surgical procedure—such as shock, haemorrhage and sepsis—are possible, but less common under present-day conditions; however, such complications do contribute to the much higher mortality following exenteration procedures. Pulmonary embolism remains a dread complication and is more prone to occur if patients become anaemic, develop sepsis or suffer complications such as paralytic ileus which interfere with early ambulation.

The complication uppermost in the surgeon's mind in relation to the Wertheim operation is

ureteric fistula, and it has even been stated that only those surgeons with a high fistula rate were doing a sufficiently radical operation. Experienced surgeons have shown that a low fistula rate is possible with a radical clearance and good survival rates (Table 42.9).

Table 42.9. Incidence of ureteric fistula in series of surgically treated cases with good survival rates

Author	No. of fistulae (%)	5 year survival rate (%)
Currie (1957)	2·3	79
Schlink (1960)	1·4	59
Stallworthy (1964)	0·7	71

Ureteric fistula may result from direct trauma, when urinary incontinence will follow immediately or soon after operation, but more usually it is due to avascular neurosis, and the leakage may then occur any time from 6 weeks to 6 months postoperatively.

The blood supply of the ureter within the pelvis is contributed to by the common iliac, internal iliac, uterine, inferior and superior vesical arteries; these vessels feed an arterial plexus which runs longitudinally over the surface of the ureter. If during the dissection the ureter is stripped from pelvic brim to bladder angle, this longitudinal plexus is the sole source of blood supply. Too close stripping of the ureter, or rough handling, will endanger the longitudinal plexus, and a fistula may follow, usually about 3–4 cm from the bladder angle. Different surgeons have different ideas as to how the blood supply to the ureter may best be preserved. Gentle handling, the avoidance of instruments and tapes to hold the ureter and of stripping the ureter too free of its surrounding loose connective tissue are fairly obvious measures. The lower end of the ureter must be dissected free as it runs across the field of dissection of the parametria, and it is only here that it may be involved in growth; that part of the ureter lying on the posterior leaf of the broad ligament need not be disturbed, as growth will seldom be found in this area, and indeed if it is, the case is not suitable for surgical treatment. Stallworthy & Bourne (1966) make a point of leaving the ureter attached to a loose areolar mesentery containing vessels arising from the pelvic floor and, like many others, of preserving the superior vesical artery. Novak (1963) ligates but does not divide the uterine artery until the ureter has been dissected in its terminal part; this avoids dissection of the lateral side of the ureter which contains the contribution from the superior vesical artery. He also advocates an intraperitoneal course for the terminal ureter in order to avoid kinking, but care must be taken not to constrict it during reperitonization of the pelvic floor. Collections of blood, serous or septic exudates will be followed by an increase of the usual fibrous tissue reaction in the pelvis, this will further endanger the blood supply of the ureter; such collections are less likely to accumulate if the pelvic cavity is drained adequately after operation.

Pre-operative radiotherapy diminishes blood supply by causing endarteritis and fibrosis and is likely to increase the risks of fistula formation, but Currie (1963), reporting a fistula rate of 2% and a relative 5-year survival rate of 75%, and Stallworthy (1966), with a 0·6% fistula rate and a 5 year survival rate of 73%, have both shown that this risk can be overcome by the experienced surgeon.

Fraser (1966) investigated the late results on the renal tract of 46 Wertheim operations, and showed that 50% had severe urinary symptoms on questioning and a similar incidence of abnormally high-residual urine volumes on investigation. Kobayashi & Matsuzawa (1967) have described a method of preserving the nervi erigentes which allows rapid return of bladder function postoperatively and does not reduce the radicality of the operation. This should also help to reduce the incidence of stress incontinence,

which can be a very trying symptom for patients undergoing radical surgery for cancer of the cervix and which is even more prevalent after the vaginal method than the abdominal. Some degree of hydronephrosis and hydroureter is common after such surgery, but it is usually transient and if it recurs is most likely to be due to recurrence of growth.

Injury to the bladder can occur during the operation, but immediate repair is nearly always successful; vesical fistulae are not very common and are more likely to follow surgery combined with radiotherapy; the same is true of rectal fistulae.

Deep-vein thrombosis is more common after major pelvic procedures and may, of course, lead to pulmonary embolism. Oedema of the legs may also follow this event, or may be due to the interruption of lymphatic drainage; it is usually transient if due to the latter, and its reappearance is again most often due to recurrence of growth.

Lymphocyst

This is an interesting complication with a wide range of incidence in different series. Rutledge (1962) recorded a 31% incidence in 100 consecutive stage III cases of cancer of the cervix where lymphadenectomy had followed a full course of radiotherapy, and 24% for all stages of the disease similarly treated. Most reports do not mention the occurrence, probably because the majority of lymphocysts are symptomless and therefore overlooked. The lymphocyst is a collection of fluid on the pelvic side-wall, the larger ones being palpable in the iliac fossa. They are thought to follow extensive excision of the nodes and lymphatics and to be more prevalent after preliminary radiotherapy. The commoner type of cyst is soft and flaccid and is discovered soon after operation, and may require aspiration. The other type more likely to be associated with symptoms is of a more chronic nature and has a thick capsule rendering it smooth, hard and fixed; there is thus a tendency to regard it as a recurrence. Pressure symptoms may be caused by the larger cysts which may abut on the ureter, bladder, rectosigmoid or blood vessels; infection in the

cyst will aggravate the symptoms. If the lymphocyst requires treatment then marsupialization
suffices.

Treatment of terminal carcinoma

The terminal management of the patient with
inoperable cancer of the genital tract depends,
naturally enough, on the site of the primary
tumour, the symptoms engendered and the
general condition of the patient. The question
of whether the patient should be told the nature of
her condition and the inevitability of its outcome
receives sharply divided answers both from the
medical profession and the public; there are those
who believe the patient should always be told and
those who would never tell her, but such a didactic
approach ignores the extreme variability of the
human condition. It seems wiser for the physician
to try and decide which approach would best suit
his particular patient, even though this can be a
very difficult decision. It is essential not to
abandon the patient even though no further practical treatment can be offered, for it is important
that those with a terminal illness should feel that
they are still under care.

RELIEF OF PAIN

Contrary to expectation, severe pain is not a
feature of most malignant disease of the genital
tract, even in its terminal phases. Metastases in
bone can be very painful but they seldom occur
secondary to genital tract disease, endometrial
cancer being the most likely, and if they do can
usually be relieved by external irradiation. Visceral
pain associated with intra-abdominal and intrapelvic masses is not, as a rule, severe and can be
relieved by the use of analgesic drugs in adequate
amounts and, where necessary, increasing potency.
The most severe pain is experienced when the
lumbosacral nerve roots are invaded by cancer
of the cervix; in such cases where death is close
at hand, morphia, heroin and cocaine must be
given in increasing doses. Where, however, the
physical condition of the patient is still strong
and the expectation of life is to be reckoned in
months a different approach is required. Interruption of the sensory nerve pathways can be

achieved by intrathecal injection of alcohol or
phenol.

A more permanent affect is achieved by
chordotomy, but fortunately this is seldom required.

EXENTERATION PROCEDURES

Brunschwig (1948) has been the main exponent
of the exenteration procedure as a means of
salvaging patients with the late stages of the
disease. There are three variations of the operation—anterior, when, in conjunction with a
radical hysterectomy and lymphadenectomy, the
bladder is removed; posterior, when the rectum
is removed; and total, when both organs are
removed, a true pelvic clearance. The operation
may be performed as the initial procedure, but
more usually there has been prior ineffectual
radiotherapy or surgery. As a rule the total
exenteration is the most effective, desperate cases
need desperate measures and it is wiser to operate
in as radical a fashion as possible or not at all.
But the removal of the bladder may become
necessary during a Wertheim operation if
difficulty is encountered in separating the bladder
from the cervix because of unexpected extension
of the growth. In some cases after radiotherapy,
separation from the bladder is technically possible
and then it is tempting to save the organ, leaving
the patient with only a terminal colostomy.
Unfortunately, the blood supply of the bladder
will have been impaired by the radiotherapy and
the subsequent major surgery, usually requiring
ligation of the internal iliac arteries, will cause
further interference with the blood supply, so
that a small-capacity bladder results; the latter
is further contributed to by the need for prolonged catheterization for retention following
disruption of the nerve supply. The distress
caused by such a bladder often necessitates a
secondary operation to deviate the urinary flow
and this will now be technically difficult, whereas
it would have been relatively simple at the
initial procedure. The decision when to perform
an exenteration is difficult and is mainly to be
considered when useful expectation of life is to
be achieved, and not merely for short-term
palliation which can be achieved by simpler

procedures. The indications are limited, therefore, to patients who have a mobile ceutral pelvic mass which is giving rise to pain and toxic effects from necrosis and infection. Such pain is visceral, and is not to be confused with somatic pain due to involvement of the lumbosacral plexus, which

deviation are preferable to a 'wet' colostomy discharging both urine and faeces, and it is sensible to operate with a urological and gynaecological team to undertake the appropriate parts of the procedure. The results that can be achieved are shown in Table 42.10.

Table 42.10. Results of extenteration operations

Surgeon	No. of cases	Mortality (%)	Survivals for 0–5 years (%)	5 year survival rate (%)
Rutledge (1962)	50	24	32	
Brunschwig & Daniel (1962)	592	17	27	17

is severe in nature and of sciatic nerve distribution, and which will not be relieved by exenteration. The other indication is the otherwise fit patient with a central mobile mass in whom prospect of a cure can be anticipated. Haemorrhage and fistula formation or incipient fistula formation are not in themselves indications, for they can be dealt with by simpler diversionary procedures. An operation with a mortality rate of 15–25% and a high incidence of distressing complications is not to be undertaken without due consideration.

Having decided the indication the surgeon must then determine the feasibility of the operation. First must be excluded extrapelvic metastases, fortunately seen in about 17% of cases only, and this requires X-ray of the chest and of any other sites which might be suspect by virtue of symptoms, such as skeletal pain; where available, a liver scan is also helpful.

The mobility of the mass and the absence of fixed side-wall masses can best be determined by examination under anaesthesia, but the final decision remains to be taken at laparotomy. The procedure will have to be abandoned if unexpected intra-abdominal metastases are discovered or if separation at the pelvic side-wall cannot be achieved; the dissection must start, therefore, on the side-wall. Sacrifice of the external iliac vein is acceptable, but not the artery, as the internal iliac artery will have to be tied in most cases and the viability of the leg will then be in jeopardy. A terminal colostomy and an ileal loop urinary

Apart from the more usual complications, the main problems following the operation are intestinal and urinary fistulae and intestinal obstruction; once these serious complications arise the patient is usually doomed to weeks of intensive care in hospital, repeated operations, and ultimate demise.

Cancer of the cervix in pregnancy

This combination is a rare finding, the incidence varies between 1 in 5,000 to 1 in 20,000 pregnancies, according to the class of population sampled. Blaikley et al. (1969) at the Chelsea Hospital for Women report an incidence of 0·4% in 1,970 cases. The incidence of carcinoma in situ is also variably reported, but McLaren (1961) reported an incidence of 1·8 per 1,000 cases in a survey of 5,000 pregnant women. In most respects carcinoma of the cervix in the pregnant uterus behaves as in the non-pregnant but, naturally, it is much more vascular and occurs in a younger age group. The main problem arises in treatment because of the presence of the pregnancy. Now that cervical cytology is a routine examination in pregnancy, overt cases are diagnosed early in the pregnancy, and in fact the more common problem is that of the positive smear in the absence of clinically detectable cancer. However, whether or not cytology has already been performed, any bleeding or blood-stained discharge at any time in pregnancy requires inspection of the cervix and cytological examination. Diagnostic features of overt cancer, apart from the increased vascularity, are similar to those found in the non-pregnant cervix. Pregnancy somewhat alters the cytological pattern of the smear, with an increase in parabasal cells and increased dyskariosis of superficial cells, there may also be changes associated with coincidental infection, but none of these should embarrass the experienced cytologist. If a positive smear is reported and confirmed by a second smear a dilemma faces the obstetrician. Should the patient be further investigated, or should such procedures be deferred until some months later when the pregnancy is completed? If definite malignant cells are seen in the smear and there has been bleeding, or there is any clinically detectable abnormality of the cervix, then a modified cone biopsy should be performed. In the absence of physical signs or symptoms it is not unreasonable to wait until after delivery before performing the cone biopsy. This approach is a compromise, because a micro-invasive tumour can be present in an apparently healthy looking cervix and may not cause symptoms. However, cone biopsy does carry slightly more risks in the pregnant patient. Increased vascularity predisposes to haemorrhage, but this has not, in practice, been a major problem; more important is the fact that in fear of this event an inadequate biopsy may be taken. The risk of causing an abortion cannot be denied, but appears to be minimal. Subsequent cervical dystocia consequent upon excessive fibrotic reaction in the cervix is a practical disadvantage in some cases. If colposcopy is available then punch biopsy can be used for suspicious areas, in preference to the rather cruder method of cone biopsy.

Once invasive cancer has been diagnosed the management depends largely upon the stage of pregnancy. Naturally the patient's wishes with regard to the sanctity of the child must influence the decision, but this apart the pregnancy will usually be sacrificed in the interests of the mother. In the first 3 months the choice lies between radical hysterectomy and radiotherapy. As the patients are usually young, surgery and conservation of ovarian function is to be preferred. The operation is in fact facilitated by the oedema-tous tissues, which separate easily; increased vascularity is overcome by epidural or hypotensive anaesthesia. Radiotherapy involves the prior use of external irradiation; initially the foetus dies and will then abort spontaneously whilst the pelvic side-walls are being irradiated. A few days after abortion is complete intracavitary radium can be applied. From the twelfth week until the child is viable, the same choice of treatment exists but it is considered preferable to evacuate the uterus abdominally rather than vaginally for fear of severe trauma to the diseased cervix and the risks of disseminating the growth. When the child is viable, Caesarean section naturally precedes treatment; if surgery is preferred it is better to defer the radical procedure for a few days to allow the extreme vascularity of the full-term pelvic organs to subside. For this reason many prefer radiotherapy, which can be started fairly soon in the puerperium without the necessity for reopening the abdomen. A more difficult decision has to be made when the foetus is not quite viable but would become so if allowed a few more weeks of intra-uterine life. The wishes of the patient, her circumstances and her parity will be of great importance, but if the pregnancy is allowed to be continued it is difficult to suppress the desire to start some treatment. Where the foetal head is still not engaged in the pelvis, a carefully calculated dose of intravaginal radium may be applied, but if the calculation is incorrect the risk of producing a microcephalic idiot is high, and failing this the risks of temporary alopecia are also high (Corscaden 1962).

The results of treatment are difficult to assess as most series are small and varied methods of treatment have been adopted, but in general they compare well with results of treatment in the non-pregnant. Too often the disease has reached a late stage before being diagnosed, and this is particularly true in late pregnancy and post-partum. Cervical cytology should stop this late diagnosis.

REFERENCES

Abou-Daoud K.T. (1967) *Cancer, Philad.* **20**, 1706.
Aitken-Swan J. & Baird D. (1965) *Br. J. Cancer.* **19**, 217.
Amreich J. (1930) *Gynakol Operationslehre.* Berlin.

ANDERSON A.F. (1956) *J. Obstet. Gynaec. Br. Commonw.* **63**, 439.

ANTOINE T. & GRUNEBERGER V. (1956) *Atlas der Kolpomiscroskopie.* Stuttgart, G. Thieme.

ASHLEY D.J.B. (1966) *J. Obstet. Gynaec. Br. Commonw.* **73**, 372.

AYRE J.E. (1947) *Am. J. Obstet. Gynec.* **54**, 609.

BASTIAANSE M.A. VAN B. (1955) *14th British Congress of Obstetrics and Gynaecology.*

BLAIKLEY J.B., LEDERMAN M. & POLLARD W. (1969) *J. Obstet. Gynaec. Br. Commonw.* **76**, 729.

BONNEY V. (1941) *J. Obstet. Gynaec. Br. Commonw.* **48**, 421

BOYD J.T. & DOLL R. (1964) *Br. J. Cancer,* **18**, 419.

BOYES D.A., FIDLER H.K. & LOCK D.R. (1962) *Br. med. J.* i, 203.

BRUNSCHWIG A. & DANIEL W.W. (1962) *Ann. Surg.* **151**, 571.

COPPLESON J.V.M. & REID B.L. (1967) *Preclinical Carcinoma of the Cervix Uteri,* Oxford, Pergamon Press.

COPPLESON M. (1969) *Br. J. Hosp. Med.* **2**, 961.

CORSCADEN J.A. (1959) *Clin. Obstet. Gynec.* **2**, 1136.

CORSCADEN J.A. (editor) (1962) *Gynecologic Cancer.* Baltimore, Williams and Wilkins.

CURRIE D.W. (1963) *Proc. R. Soc. Med.* **56**, 878.

FIDLER H.K., BOYES D.A. & WORTH A.J. (1968) *J. Obstet. Gynaec. Br. Commonw.* **75**, 392.

FLETCHER G.H., STOVELL M. & SAMPIERE V. (1962) *Carcinoma of the Uterine Cervix, Endometrium and Ovary.* Chicago, Year Book Medical Publishers.

FORDYCE R.G. (1962) In *Gynecologic Cancer* (edited by J.A. Corscaden). Baltimore, Williams and Wilkins.

FRASER A.C. (1966) *J. Obstet. Gynaec. Br. Commonw.* **73**, 1002.

GAGNON F. (1950) *Am. J. Obstet. Gynec.* **60**, 516.

GRAHAM J.B. & GRAHAM R.M. (1960) *Cancer, N.Y.* **13**, 5.

GLUCKSMAN A. & SPEAR F.G. (1945) *Br. J. Radiol.* **18**, 313.

GOVAN A.D.T., HAINES R.M., LANGLEY F.A., TAYLOR C.W. & WOODCOCK A.S. (1966) *J. Obstet. Gynaec. Br. Commonw.* **73**, 883.

GREEN H. (1966) *Am. J. Obstet. Gynec.* **94**, 1009.

HILL A.M. (1960) *J. Obstet. Gynaec. Br. Commonw.* **67**, 717.

HINSELMANN M. (1925) *Münch. med. Wschr.* **77**, 1733.

KOBAYASHI T. & MATSUZAWA M. (1967) *Fifth World Congress of Gynaecology and Obstetrics.* Sydney, Butterworths.

KOLSTAD P. (1968) *Aust. N.Z. J. Obstet. Gynaec.* **8**, 107.

KOTTMEIER H.L. (1953) *Carcinoma of the Female Genitalia.* Baltimore, Williams and Wilkins.

KOVACIC J., LAVRIC V. & PESTEVSEK R. (1967) *Ginek. i opstet.* **4**, 345.

LEWIS T.L.T. (1964) *Progress in Clinical Obstetrics and Gynaecology.* London, Churchill.

McLAREN H.C. (1961) *Proc. R. Soc. Med.* **54**, 712.

MITRA S. (1954) In *Surgical Treatment of Carcinoma of the Cervix* (edited by J. V. Meigs). New York, Grune and Stratton.

MOGHISSI K.S., MACK H.C. & PORZAK J.P. (1968) *Am. J. Obstet. Gynec.* **100**, 607.

NAVRATIL E. (1954) In *Surgical Treatment of Carcinoma of the Cervix* (edited by J. V. Meigs). New York, Grune and Stratton.

NOVAK F. (1963) *Proc. R. Soc. Med.* **56**, 881.

O'CONNELL D., JOSLIN C.A., HOWARD N., RAMSEY N.W. & LIVERSAGE W.E. (1967) *Br. J. Radiol.* **40**, 882.

PAPANICOLAOU G.N. & TRAUT H.F. (1941) *Am. J. Obstet. Gynec.* **42**, 193.

PAPANICOLAOU G.N. & TRAUT H.F. (1943) *Diagnosis of Uterine Cancer by the Vaginal Smear.* New York, The Commonwealth Fund.

PETERSEN O. (1955) *Acta radiol.* Supplement 127.

RAWLS W.E., TOMPKINS W.A.F., FIGUERON M.E. & MELNICK J.L. (1968) *Science,* **16**, 1255.

ROTKIN I.D. (1967) *Cancer Res.* **27**, 603.

RUBIN I.C. (1910) *Am. J. Obstet. Gynec.* **62**, 668.

RUTLEDGE F.N. (1962) *Cancer of the Uterine Cervix, Endometrium and Ovary.* Chicago, Year Book Medical Publishers.

SCHAUENSTEIN W. (1908) *Arch. Gynaek.* **85**, 576.

SCHAUTA F. (1904) *Mschr. Oeburtsh Gynak.* **19**, 475.

SCHILLER W. (1927) *Vitchows Arch. path. Anat. Physiol.* **263**, 279.

SCHLINK H.H. (1960) *J. Obstet. Gynaec. Br. Commonw.* **67**, 402.

STALLWORTHY J. (1964) *Ann. R. Coll. Surg.* **34**, 161.

STALLWORTHY J. & BOURNE G. (1966) *Recent Advances in Obstetrics and Gynecology.* London, Churchill.

TE LINDE R.W., GALVIN G.A. & JONES H.W. Jnr. (1957) *Am. J. Obstet. Gynec.* **74**, 792.

TERRISS M. & OALMANN M.C. (1960) *J. Am. med. Ass.* **174**, 1847.

TOWNE J. (1955) *Am. J. Obstet. Gynec.* **60**, 606.

TUNCER M., GRAHAM R. & GRAHAM J. (1967) *N.Y. St. J. Med.* **67**, 2317.

WELCH J.S., PRATT J.H. & SYMMONDS R.E. (1961) *Am. J. Obstet. Gynec.* **81**, 978.

WERTHEIM A. (1905) *Br. med. J.* ii, 689.

YOUNGE P.A. (1952) *Proc. natn. Cancer. Conf.* **1**, 668.

CHAPTER 43

MALIGNANT DISEASE OF THE UTERINE BODY

Malignant disease of the uterus presents some difficulties of classification in the rarer conditions. In the cervix the commonest tumour is squamous-cell carcinoma and in a few cases adenocarcinoma is found; whereas in the corpus, adenocarcinoma is the commonest tumour and squamous-cell carcinoma is rare. Because these tumours differ so markedly in nearly every respect, it is customary to consider the cervix and the corpus uteri under quite separate headings. Other malignant tumours occurring are found mainly in the corpus, and are rare.

CARCINOMA OF THE CORPUS UTERI

Although carcinoma of the corpus occurs in the same organ as carcinoma of the cervix, it differs considerably as regards aetiology, pathology, prognosis and treatment; the symptoms in the two conditions are, however, very similar.

Aetiology

Whilst the main interest in carcinoma of the cervix centres around coitus as being of prime aetiological importance, in carcinoma of the endometrium the condition is more common in virgins and nulliparous women. However, a number of additional factors have been noted in relation to the development of the condition.

(1) *Age*. An older age group is found than in carcinoma of the cervix, and the maximum incidence is about 61 years, with three-quarters of the patients being over 50 and very few under 40 years old (see Table 43.1). At the maximum age incidence, carcinoma of the corpus is more frequently observed than carcinoma of the cervix, but before and after this the cervical lesion is more prevalent.

(2) *Parity*. Whilst it is generally agreed that nulliparity or relative infertility is a common feature and occurs much more frequently for example than in the case of carcinoma of the cervix, it is as well to remember that from 40 to 60% of women with carcinoma of the corpus will have had one or more children (Speert 1948; Roberts 1961).

(3) *Obesity*. Unfortunately for the surgeon, big, overweight women are commonly afflicted, and this is as true for the younger as for the older woman (Dockerty *et al.* 1951).

(4) *Menstrual abnormalities*. These are reported in the histories of both young and older women who have developed carcinoma of the corpus. According to Corscaden (1962), who discusses the matter fully, in about half the cases there is a history of menorrhagia.

(5) *Age at menopause*. A fairly high proportion of cases are reported to have reached the menopause after the age of 50–35% according to Randall *et al.* (1951). Roberts (1961) reported that 73% of his cases were aged between 51 and 55 years when periods ceased, but he also observed that one-quarter were premenopausal.

(6) *Radium menopause*. Although it has been calculated by Palmer & Spratt (1956), amongst others, that women undergoing a radium meno-

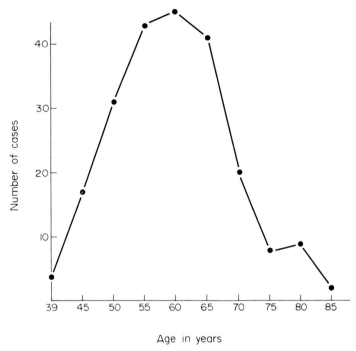

Table 43.1. Age distribution: carcinoma of the corpus uteri.

pause are three times more likely to develop carcinoma of the corpus than expected, Corscaden (1962) argues that this is due not so much to the radium as to the fact that the menopause has been induced for heavy bleeding, and thus in a selected population who are more prone to develop the condition.

(7) *Diabetes*. The relationship of diabetes mellitus to carcinoma of the endometrium remains obscure. Much of the difficulty lies in the criteria for diagnosis, and this probably accounts for the extreme variation in the reported incidence of diabetes in various series, from 1·3% Roberts (1961) to 29% Way (1954). Those with access to large diabetic populations do not report a high incidence of cancer of the uterus, Joslin (1952) reports an incidence of only 2·6% in over 10,000 cases of diabetes, whilst referrals of cases with postmenopausal bleeding from the large diabetic clinic at King's College Hospital are unusual; still less, is there a high incidence of carcinoma of the endometrium. Dunn *et al.* (1968) attempted to evaluate factors which might influence glucose tolerance, such as age, parity, obesity, hypertension, family history of diabetes and anterior pituitary function. They compared 55 patients with endometrial carcinoma against 114 control patients, and concluded that abnormal carbohydrate metabolism and hypertension were no more common in the carcinoma group than in the controls, but that obesity and diminished parity were.

(8) *Hypertension*. As mentioned above, hypertension tends to be prevalent in this age group, and is not significantly more common in association with this type of cancer.

(9) *Uterine myomata*. These are common and are seen in association with endometrial cancer quite frequently, but probably no more frequently than might be expected in women of this age group.

(10) *Oestrogens*. It is interesting to speculate on the relationship of ovarian hormones in the development of this tumour. Many gynaecologists have seen women who after prolonged exogenous oestrogen therapy for menopausal symptoms

have developed an endometrial carcinoma. Such cases are few in number considering the large number of women who must be taking oestrogens. It has been shown by Meissner *et al.* (1957) that cancer of the uterus can be induced in certain strains of rabbit by exogenous oestrogen administration. The relationship between menstrual abnormality and the development of endometrial carcinoma has already been noted, and considerable interest has been aroused in the relationship between endometrial hyperplasia and the development of the tumour. There are those who see a progression from normal endometrium, through endometrial hyperplasia, to atypical endometrial hyperplasia (regarded by some as carcinoma *in situ* of the endometrium), and finally to adenocarcinoma. Whilst this indubitably occurs in some cases, such progression is not necessarily always the case; in the postmenopausal patients, for example, the hyperplasia itself should give rise to warning bleeding. Te Linde *et al.* (1953) reported three small groups of cases; the first group had gross atypical hyperplasia where distinction from carcinoma was in doubt, on hysterectomy 11 of 13 cases showed carcinoma to be present; the second group had similar changes but were treated conservatively, and months to years later developed cancer; the third group had normal endometrium shown prior to the finding of cancer. In some cases of cholanthine-induced cancer of the uterus in animals there is a preliminary stage of endometrial hyperplasia. It is well recognized that oestrogens administered exogenously can give rise to endometrial hyperplasia, and a suggestion is that in certain circumstances such hyperplasia, can eventually pass on to cancer formation. Twombly *et al.* (1961) have suggested that there is a relationship between obesity and oestrogen stimulation in that oestrogens are stored in fat, and therefore obese patients are likely to accumulate oestrogens and the endometrium will thus be subjected to more prolonged stimulation. Turning to the role of endogenous oestrogen stimulation in the formation of endometrial cancer, there is some evidence for this taking place. Feminizing tumours, particularly those with a predominance of theca cells, have been found in association with en-

dometrial carcinoma in a varying proportion of cases; according to Novak & Woodruff (1947) the frequency is as high as 15–27% of cases when the ovarian tumour occurs in postmenopausal women. Unfortunately, the opportunity to examine the endometrium has not always been seized, and as a result the true incidence is unknown. Dinnerstein & O'Leary (1968) record 102 women with feminizing tumours in whom the endometrium was examined in only 64 cases, and of these 30 showed cystic glandular hyperplasia and three adenocarcinoma. In younger women carcinoma of the endometrium has been reported in relation with the Stein-Leventhal syndrome in a small number of cases, the theory being that anovulation leads to unopposed oestrogenic stimulation and subsequent endometrial hyperplasia which, unchecked, may progress to adenocarcinoma. Finally, co-existing hyperplasia is often seen in the endometrium adjacent to adenocarcinoma, but this is by no means always the case.

(11) *Endometrial polyps.* A relationship between endometrial polyps and endometrial cancer has been postulated from time to time. Armenia (1967) reviewed 959 cases of benign endometrial polyps and concluded that the risk of endometrial carcinoma developing in such patients was nine times that expected.

(12) *Foreign bodies.* Contrary to expectations, there is no evidence to date to suggest that intrauterine contraceptive devices are conducive to the development of malignancy.

(13) *Progesterone.* The beneficial results of treatment with large doses of progestational steroids in some cases of endometrial carcinoma with metastasis support, at least, the contention that carcinoma of the endometrium may be an endocrine-dependent tumour. Way (1954) has suggested that the primary fault may lie in the pars anterior of the pituitary gland, and that this would account for such features as the menstrual irregularity, the endometrial hyperplasia, the late menopause, the obesity, the relative infertility, and, in his series, the high incidence of abnormal carbohydrate metabolism. Others, like Corscaden (1962) and Novak & Woodruff (1967), are concerned to underline the significance of abnormal oestrogen levels.

Pathology

The tumour is nearly always an adenocarcinoma of polypoid or nodular type which spreads around the endometrium or projects into the cavity (Fig. 43.1). The lesion may be diffuse or localized, and in the latter case may in be the form of a single, large polyp. In the early stages the growth is usually confined to the fundus, but as it spreads it may come to involve the whole endometrium

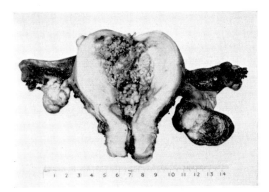

Fig. 43.1. Uterus. Proliferative adenocarcinoma of body.

and spread into the cervical canal. The uterine wall may become very thin and friable, and this will be more so if pyometra due to cervical stenosis is present; the latter is usually the result of infection rather than obstruction by the tumour itself. Associated lesions are fibroids commonly and granulosa–theca cell ovarian tumours rarely. The uterus will be enlarged in just over one-half of cases examined postoperatively, but such enlargement may not easily be detected on clinical examination. Microscopically the tumour is an adenocarcinoma, and rarely is the diagnosis in doubt, but difficulties do arise in the case of atypical hyperplasia. All grades of abnormality may be seen, from benign cystic glandular hyperplasia, through grossly atypical hyperplasia where an experienced pathologist may have difficulty in deciding whether the lesion is benign or malignant, to obvious cancer; occasionally, the whole gamut of such changes may be observed in the same specimen. The pathologist is at a disadvantage in that he has to make his decision on inspection of fragmented curettings and is not given a specimen containing an ade-

quate amount of subjacent normal tissue for comparison as is usual with biopsy specimens, and the final diagnosis is sometimes not reached until the uterus has been removed. As a result the diagnosis rests on the glandular pattern and the cell structure, and the relationship of the cells to the basement membrane. The main difficulty arises where pattern and structure suggest malignancy but the basement membrane remains intact; for such cases there are those who employ the terminology carcinoma *in situ*, but many authorities, amongst them Haines & Taylor (1962), dislike this concept as applied to the endometrium, and prefer to classify such lesions as grossly atypical (Fig. 43.2).

The main problem for the clinician is the management of such cases, and in most, hysterectomy is recommended for fear of cancer subsequently developing. That such a fear is reasonably justified, is shown by the reports of Hertig *et al.* (1949) and Te Linde (1953), amongst others, all of whom show clear evidence of cases of adenomatous hyperplasia preceding, or being noticed before, the development of endometrial carcinoma in a large proportion of cases. The difficulty arises when the degree of hyperplasia is equivocal, and the patient is reluctant to agree to hysterectomy, or is not suitable for operation by reason of concomitant disease. When the hyperplasia is found in the postmenopausal patient conservative treatment is less likely to be adopted in the more grossly atypical cases, particularly if there are associated factors such as obesity and nulliparity; but in milder degrees of hyperplasia conservative management is permissible unless postmenopausal bleeding recurs. Hyperplasia thought to have been induced by exogenous oestrogen therapy can be reversed if the patient is weaned off the oestrogens, but if this is not possible then hysterectomy should be performed. In cases of obvious carcinoma the histological picture varies from one of good differentiation, as in the adenoma malignum where the malignancy is confined to the endometrium, to poorly differentiated patterns, where the use of Broders's index is applicable.

Spread of the tumour is direct in the endometrium itself and, to a lesser degree into the myometrium; the latter, in contradistinction to

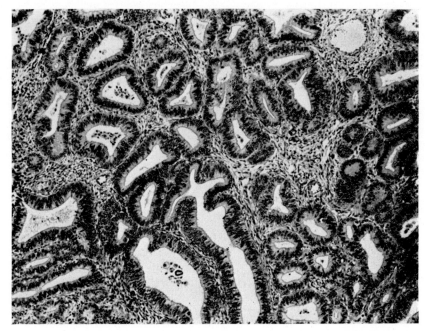

Fig. 43.2. Endometrium showing atypical hyperplasia with a crowded abnormal gland pattern.

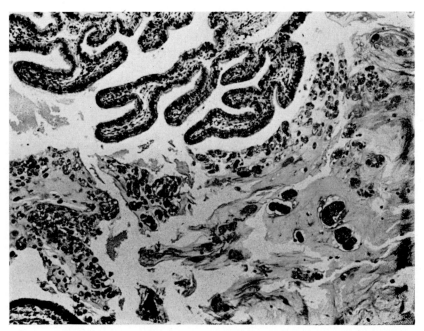

Fig. 43.3. Tumour emboli in the tube from a case of carcinoma of the body of the uterus.

the cervix and paracervical tissues, is fairly resistant to the invasion of tumour, presumably because of the close, interlacing network of muscle fibres, so that penetration to the serosa

Table 43.2. Staging of carcinoma of the corpus uteri (F.I.G.O. 1965)

Stage 0: Histological findings suspicious of malignancy but not proven

Stage I: The carcinoma is confined to the corpus

Stage II: The carcinoma has involved the corpus and the cervix

Stage III: The carcinoma has extended outside the uterus but not outside the true pelvis

Stage IV: The carcinoma has extended outside the true pelvis or has obviously involved the mucosa of the bladder or rectum

Note : In rare cases it may be difficult to decide whether the carcinoma actually is a carcinoma of the endocervix or a carcinoma of the corpus and endocervix. If a clear decision cannot be made at the fractional curettage, an adenocarcinoma should be allotted to carcinoma of the corpus and an epidermal carcinoma to carcinoma of the cervix

Histological gradings to be added to the above (F.I.G.O., 1968)

G.1.: Carcinoma, well defined

G.2.: Carcinoma showing various degrees of differentiation

G.3.: Carcinoma, low differentiation or anaplastic

is unusual; staging is indicated in Table 43.2. If there is penetration to the outer half of the thickness of the myometrium the prognosis is worse, and this is an indication for postoperative external irradiation. Lymphatic spread occurs mainly via the pathway of the ovarian vessels to the para-aortic lymph nodes, and in view of the results obtained by treatment which makes no attempt to include them, would appear to be uncommon. However, it is a means by which the ovaries may be involved; the ovaries may also be involved (as may the peritoneum of the pouch of Douglas) by transtubal embolism (Fig. 43.3). Ovarian secondaries are found in about 5–7% of cases. Rarely, metastasis to the inguinal lymph nodes is occasioned via the lymphatics accompanying the round ligament. There has been considerable discussion about the

frequency of involvement of the pelvic lymph nodes, and varying figures have been quoted (Table 43.3). Winterton (1954) and Rickford

Table. 43.3. Frequency of involvement of lymph nodes

	Cases	Glands invaded (%)
Javert (1954)	50	20
Schwarz & Brunschwig (1957)	96	13
Liu & Meigs (1955)	47	23
Lees (1969)	76	17

(1968), who have carried out routine Wertheim hysterectomies on all cases, show how small is the number of patients in whom involvement of pelvic lymph nodes occur (Table 43.4). Whilst it

Table 43.4. Involvement of pelvic lymph nodes

Winterton (1954)	85 cases treated
Glands sectioned	28
Glands invaded	2 = 7·1%
Rickford (1967)	50 cases treated
Glands invaded	5 = 10%
Stage I glands	
invaded	2 = 5·5%

is true that the results of these surgeons are good and the mortality low, routine use of such a major procedure seems unjustified, and a measure of selection preferable.

Clinical features

As for carcinoma of the cervix, the symptom is abnormal bleeding; this is mainly postmenopausal, as that is when the majority of cases occur; the bleeding may simulate a period or be no more than a show, and there may be long intervals between each episode of bleeding. Occasionally, the first symptom in a postmenopausal women is a persistent, watery discharge coming from the uterus. In premenopausal women the bleeding is usually intermenstrual, but may only be manifested as prolonged or heavy menstruation. Mild uterine colic may be present, but is a symptom more often elicited than volunteered. Evidence of extra-uterine metastasis in lungs, spine or long bones occurs late in the disease and has practically always been preceded by abnormal bleeding.

On examination it will be found that many of the patients are obese. Examination of the abdomen and pelvis is usually unremarkable—as often, enlargement of the uterus, if present, is not clinically apparent. In the postmenopausal patient it may appear to be of normal size for a woman in the menstrual era, rather than small and atrophic. Pyometra, if present, will of course enlarge the uterus, but this may not be detected clinically, as the uterine wall will be thin and soft and the patient is usually obese. Rarely, a secondary metastasis at the lower end of the vagina presents as a red or plum-coloured swelling, whose surface may be broken and bleeding or be intact and smooth. It is usually situated on the anterior vaginal wall suburethrally. Very rarely, metastasis causing enlargement of inguinal lymph nodes may be detected.

The diagnosis must always be made by histological examination of uterine curettings. Dilatation and curettage must always be performed with extreme care, because the uterine wall may be soft and thin and be easily perforated. Associated pyometra is best drained through a rubber tube sown into the uterus and left for 2–3 days. Fractional curettage—where the surgeon curettes first the endocervical canal then dilates the cervix and then curettes first fundus and then lower uterine walls—is reputed by some to indicate the extent of the lesion, but not all are agreed as to its accuracy; too often, growth exudes from the cervix during dilatation, and it is difficult not to catch a tumour in the lower uterus on withdrawing the curette from the fundus. European surgeons favour the use of hysterography to delineate the tumour, but the method has not found favour in Britain because of the theoretical fear of disseminating the growth.

Cervical cytology has stimulated attempts towards early diagnosis of this lesion but difficulty of access, particularly in the senile uterus with a relatively stenosed cervix, renders this less simple than taking a cervical smear. Posterior fornix smears or aspirates will detect a few cases, but too many false-negatives render the method insufficiently reliable. Attempts at smearing the uterine cavity and suction aspiration of the cavity have proved more successful, but remain too complicated to become routine in the same way as has the cervical smear. In most cases, therefore, it is necessary for the patient to present with symptoms before being able to make a diagnosis, always a relatively late stage of any cancer.

Treatment

In cancer of the corpus uteri there is little dispute about the basic method of treatment, which is surgical. Simple total hysterectomy and bilateral salpingo-oöphorectomy will give a 5 year survival rate in approximately 60% of patients treated, but there will be a number of recurrences in the vault of the vagina. These are almost certainly due to spill of viable cancer cells into the freshly cut edge of the vagina at operation. Such implantation is known to occur in carcinoma of the colon. Retrograde lymphatic spread is an unsatisfactory explanation because:

(i) Deposits have not been demonstrated in the upper vagina in operation specimens.
(ii) Retrograde spread occurs mainly where the ascending lymphatic channels are blocked.
(iii) The lymphatic drainage of the corpus uteri and the vagina is quite different.

Because of the fairly high rate of vault recurrences, it was suggested by Dobbie (1953) that these could be prevented by postoperative insertion of radium into the vagina in a tubular applicator, and by so doing she reduced the incidence of such recurrences.

The results of radiotherapy in this condition have never been as satisfactory as those of surgery, perhaps because of the difficulties of application. The uterine cavity is often distorted and enlarged, the wall of the uterus thin, and radium sources can only be introduced with real danger of perforating the uterus; furthermore, it cannot be certain that all areas of the growth are equally irradiated. Nevertheless, Heyman's intracavitary packing with multiple small sources is a method of treating patients considered to be unfit for surgery. The results obtained at the Radium hemmet are shown to be inferior to those obtained by surgery, and although a properly controlled trial comparing the methods has not been carried out, most authorities prefer to treat carcinoma of the corpus uteri surgically.

The use of radium in conjunction with surgery is now widespread, and the method favoured is pre-operative intracavitary and vault radium, applied usually by the Stockholm or Manchester technique. There is no firm decision regarding the correct dosage, but most prefer only one application, believing this to be sufficient to inactivate any superficial cells which might be shed at operation. Two applications are more certain to achieve this, and in a number of cases after such doses there is no residual tumour in the extirpated uterus; it does mean, however, that the patient has to undergo three small operations, if one includes the diagnostic dilatation and curettage before her major procedure.

It has been suggested that the results would be improved by performing the Wertheim operation, and the results of this approach have been shown by Winterton (1954), who obtained a 5 year survival rate of 82% in 57 cases operated upon (93% of all cases seen, in which the survival rate was 76%). Although the results are good, the incidence of lymph-node involvement is too low to warrant routine use of the operation in patients who are often less suited to it than those suffering from carcinoma of the cervix. The patient with carcinoma of the corpus is in an older age group, is obese, and, if she is nulliparous, the uterus is less mobile and the vagina smaller, all of which render the operation more difficult and more dangerous if carried out by the relatively inexperienced. Here there is a case to be made for individual treatment for individual patients.

The standard method of treatment adopted by most surgeons is a preliminary application of intracavitary radium, followed 1 week later by total hysterectomy and bilateral salpingo-oöphorectomy. Although the radium is relied upon to prevent vault recurrence, some method of occluding the cervix is attempted, usually by means of suturing the anterior and posterior lips of the cervix together. This is a rather ineffectual way of trying to contain cancer cells. Percival (1952) has described a special clamp which can be applied to the cervix prior to operation which occludes the cervix completely and is removed with the operation specimen. Certain points of techniques are observed during the hysterectomy: first, a preliminary exploration of the abdomen should be carried out, particularly to discover whether or not the para-aortic lymph nodes are involved. Secondly, before handling the uterus the ampullary ends of the fallopian tubes are ligated to prevent spill of tumour cells during the operation. Finally, the round ligaments are divided as near to the internal inguinal ring as possible in case there is spread along the lymphatic channel communicating with the inquinal lymph nodes by the same route as is taken by the round ligament. If the diagnosis is suspected before the diagnostic curettage, radium can be applied at the same time if the patient is postmenopausal, because even if the diagnosis is not sustained on microscopical examination of the curettings no harm will have been done. In the premenopausal patient, of course, radium application must be deferred until diagnosis has been histologically confirmed. Unfortunately, a number of cases are not diagnosed until the curettings have been examined under the microscope, and so the intracavitary radium application has to be carried out after the initial diagnostic curettage.

In early cases with a well-differentiated tumour and a small uterus the radium application can be dispensed with, providing that satisfactory measures are taken to prevent the spill of viable cancer cells into the cut edge of the vagina. This can be achieved by fashioning a cuff of vagina, and inserting into it a swab soaked in perchloride of mercury tightly packed against the cervix and sewn in by approximating the edges of the vaginal cuff. The operation then performed is an extended hysterectomy. This involves dissecting out the lower ureter, achieved by dividing the uterine vessels as they cross the ureteric tunnel, and then removing the uterus tubes and ovaries, together with the vaginal cuff and a reasonable amount of paracervical tissue; the latter is facilitated by the preliminary fashioning of the vaginal cuff. The uterus can then be opened and the extent of the tumour confirmed. If the lesion is extensive and involves the cervix or that part of the uterine cavity just above the internal os, then metastasis to the pelvic lymph nodes is more likely and these can be dissected out and removed, so that the final operation is a Wertheim hysterectomy after the fashion originally described by Bonney (1947). If the lesion is confined to the fundus then the lymph-node dissection need not be performed. The advantage of the extended hysterectomy is that preliminary radiotherapy is not required and a more extensive removal of the peritoneum of the pouch of Douglas is performed; it is probable that transtubal spread of tumour cells to this area occurs in the same way as it may do to the ovaries.

A similar approach can be carried out in those patients who have a uterus enlarged by multiple fibroids which cause considerable distortion of the uterine cavity and where intracavitary radium might be more difficult and less effective. Where, however, the cavity of the uterus is uniformly enlarged the walls are likely to be soft and thin, in such cases it is possible for the uterus to be torn during the operative manipulations, with resultant spill of tumour into the peritoneal cavity. Preliminary intracavitary radium applied in two doses will have the effect of destroying much of the tumour, shrinking the size of the cavity and making such disruption of the uterus during operation much less likely. Where the lesion is considered to be involving the lower uterus and cervix, a Wertheim procedure preceded by intracavitary radium in two doses is required.

RADIOTHERAPY

Pre-operative radiotherapy has already been mentioned; definitive radiotherapy by packing the uterine cavity with Heyman's capsules is indicated in the few cases where the patient is considered unfit for surgery. On the whole, operability rates for this condition are high

Table 43.5. Operability rates for cancer of the corpus uteri

Author	Operability (%)
Winterton (1954)	93
McGarrity & Scott (1968)	88
Lees (1969)	88

(Table 43.5). Supplemental postoperative external irradiation of the pelvis tends to be given in a rather empirical fashion, being recommended if the tumour extends through 50% or more of the thickness of the uterine wall as judged at microscopical examination, if the ovaries are involved, or if the growth extends down towards the cervix.

Recurrent disease

Recurrent disease may occur
 (i) At the vault of the vagina.
 (ii) In the lower third of the vagina.
 (iii) As a mass within the pelvic cavity usually on the side wall and probably arising from lymph node involvement.
 (iv) As distant metastases in lungs or bone.

Recurrences at the vault of the vagina can be excised, but are probably better treated by intravaginal or external radiotherapy. Metastasis at the lower end of the vagina can be satisfactorily treated by radium needling. Tumour masses in the pelvis are best treated by external radiotherapy as only occasionally, when they are solitary and mobile, will they be amenable to surgical removal. Metastases in the lungs, spine and long bones can be treated with radiotherapy but have also in some cases responded dramatically to hormone therapy.

HORMONE THERAPY

Kelly & Baker (1961) reported on the effect o high-dosage progestogen therapy in advanced cases of endometrial cancer. Other reports have been forthcoming which support their results (Kennedy 1968). The dosage recommended is at least twice weekly intramuscular injections of 0·5–1 g of hydroxyprogesterone caproate, or 100–300 mg of medroxyprogesterone by mouth daily; the treatment can be continued for an unlimited time, and, if nothing else, induces a sense of well-being in the patient. It is most valuable where the growth is slow-growing, well-differentiated and, in particular, where there are pulmonary metastases; resolution of the latter has been achieved in a number of cases. Assessment of the effect locally in slowly growing tumours is more difficult, but some prolongation of life is claimed. Some recent reports have shown that a few well-differentiated tumours can be made to regress by the installation of a solution of the progestogen into the uterine cavity. For the present, hormone therapy remains a useful adjunct when conventional methods have failed. Clomiphene has been used by Wall *et al.* (1964) to convert adenocarcinoma of the endometrium back to a secretory, and then to an atrophic, endometrial pattern in two out of ten cases; such reports are more interesting with regard to the possible oestrogenic stimulus to adenocarcinoma formation in the uterus than as methods of treatment.

SARCOMA OF THE UTERUS

Sarcoma of the uterus is rare, but tends to be more malignant than most other varieties of uterine tumour. The corpus is more commonly affected than the cervix uteri. There are a number of different types of lesion, and not a little disagreement amongst pathologists over classification. All recognize the leiomyosarcoma which may arise from either normal myometrium or as a malignant degeneration of a leiomyofibroma or fibroid. Leiomyosarcomata are the commonest type of this rare condition, and comprise about 50% of most series, Aaro *et al.* (1966) recording 105 such tumours out of a series of 177 uterine sarcomata. The less common types arise from the endometrial stroma, and various types have been described:

 (i) Stromal sarcoma.
 (ii) Fibromyxosarcoma.
 (iii) Carcinosarcoma.
 (iv) Mesodermal mixed tumours.

A further confusion arises in the case of stromal endometriosis, which may show varying degrees of differentiation and of clinical behaviour, being at times definitely malignant and therefore indistinguishable from endometrial sarcoma, and indeed there are some, such as Novak (1956) and Koss *et al.* (1965), who prefer to consider stromal endometriosis as endometrial sarcoma. Mixed mesodermal-cell tumours are found in the cervix and vagina as well as the corpus uteri; in the cervix and vagina they have been known in the past as sarcoma botyroides, from their polypoidal or grape-like appearance. They are stromal sarcomata (Fig. 43.4) in which mesodermal elements such as bone, cartilage and striped muscle are found. The tumours are thought to arise from Muellerian tissue, the Muellerian mesoderm providing the mesodermal elements of the tumour. If carcinoma is found concomitant to the sarcoma, the term carcinosarcoma is used, although Haines & Taylor (1962) dislike the nomenclature and consider such tumours to be examples of mixed mesodermal tumours, or if there be two separate tumours with adjoining intermingled edges, to regard this as a 'collision' of the two tumours. In addition, there are described certain vascular tumours, haemangiosarcoma and haemangiopericytoma, the latter like stromal endometriosis falling into the category of tumours of doubtful or low grade malignancy. Lymphosarcoma of the uterus has also been described, Aaro *et al.*

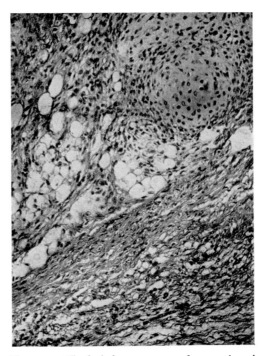

Fig. 43.4. Histological appearances of a mesodermal mixed tumour of the uterus.

Table 43.6. Types of uterine sarcoma

Leiomyosarcoma
  (1) Arising in leimyofibroma
  (2) Arising in myometrium
Endometrial sarcoma
  (1) Stromal sarcoma, to include some or all cases of stromal endometriosis
  (2) Mixed mesodermal-cell tumour, to include:
      Sarcoma botyroides
      Osteosarcoma
      Chondrosarcoma
      Rhabdomyosarcoma
      Fibromyxosarcoma
      Carcinosarcoma
Vascular
  Angiosarcoma
  Haemangiopericytoma: some cases
Lymphosarcoma

(1966) reporting three cases in their series. In summary the following types of uterine sarcoma must be considered (see Table 43.6 also).

LEIOMYOSARCOMA

These tumours are the commonest single group amongst all the sarcomata of the uterus. They may arise either from the myometrium or from a leiomyofibroma or fibroid. The incidence of the latter is very rare and is difficult to estimate, much depends on whether one considers the number of fibroids sectioned or the number of patients with fibroids. Difficulties in diagnosis from cellular fibroids, mixed mesodermal tumours and vascular tumours further complicate the issue, but probably less than 1 in 300 patients with uterine fibroids will be found to have sarcomatous degeneration present. Rarely, cases are recorded of the recurrence in the pelvis of apparently benign fibroids following hysterectomy and also of metastasis, usually to the lungs. A further oddity is the so-called intravenous leiomyomatosis, where cords of tumour spread through the uterus and into the broad ligament; such intravenous extensions are postulated to originate in the muscle wall of the vein; pulmonary metastases have also been recorded in some of these cases. These rarities are further examples of histologically benign tumours behaving in a low-grade, malignant fashion.

Pathology

The general appearance is one of degeneration occurring within a fibroid with a softened,

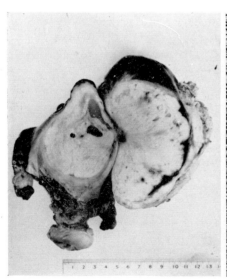

(a)

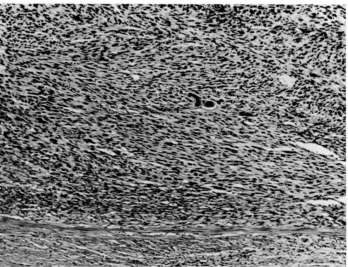

(b)

Fig. 43.5. Uterine leiomyosarcoma. (a) Gross appearances. (b) Histology.

necrotic, haemorrhagic area. When arising from the myometrium, the appearance may be of a more diffuse, nodular, polypoidal tumour [Fig. 43.5(a)]. The histological picture is very similar to cellular myoma, and indeed the distinction between the latter and sarcoma may be very close, but there is scanty stroma, pleomorphism, cellular atypia, giant-cell formation, and most important, mitotic activity [Fig. 43.5(b)]; in short, the usual criteria for the diagnosis of malignancy are to be sought, but in the very low-grade tumours a very thorough search may be required.

Clinical features

Most patients are in the age group 40–60 years, and about two-thirds are postmenopausal. The commonest symptoms are abnormal bleeding and abdominal pain; less common are the findings of a mass by the patient or of cough due to pulmonary metastases. The finding of a uterine mass is by far the commonest physical sign.

Treatment

As lymphatic spread is uncommon, total hysterectomy and bilateral salpingo-oöphorectomy is indicated. Radiotherapy is not very effective and should be reserved to follow incomplete surgery or for cases of recurrence which cannot be treated surgically. Chemotherapy may offer some palliation in a few cases.

ENDOMETRIAL SARCOMA

These usually arise from the upper part of the corpus uteri in the form of large, fleshy polyps; usually, demarcation from the myometrium is clear-cut, particularly with mixed mesodermal tumours, but at times infiltration is seen. The surface may be smooth and glistening, or ulcerated. The tumour is soft and brain-like when cut. Histological examination reveals closely packed fusiform cells with large nuclei and numerous mitoses. In mixed mesodermal tumours the appearances vary with the presence of the various heterotopic tissues, but myxomatous tissue, cartilage and striated muscle

are frequent findings, the last may require an extensive search and special staining techniques.

Clinical features

The majority of patients are, as those with carcinoma of the corpus uteri, 50–70 years old; an older age group than with leiomyosarcoma. A small number of mixed mesodermal tumours of the cervix and vagina occur in young children in the first decade of life, and these are the so-called sarcoma botyroides. Again, abnormal bleeding and abdominal pain are predominant symptoms and a uterine or cervical mass the commonest physical sign.

Treatment

Again, total hysterectomy and bilateral salpingo-oöphorectomy is the main hope, and in this group more help of a palliative nature can be expected from radiotherapy and chemotherapy.

Prognosis

Much depends on the degree of malignancy and the all-important factor of early diagnosis in reaching a prognosis. Most series are too small to be reliable indices of the value of treatment. Aaro et al. (1966) reported 25 of 60 patients with leiomyosarcoma and 17 of 53 patients, with endometrial sarcoma to have survived 5 years after definitive treatment. They also noted that in 6.5% of leiomyosarcoma and 26% of endometrial sarcoma the uterus had been subjected to radium or radiotherapy at some time before. Other reports of this association with previous radiotherapy have been noted but it is not a universal finding, and in view of the rarity of the condition it is not easy to decide how significant is the relationship.

CARCINOMA OF THE FALLOPIAN TUBE

The tube may, of course, be secondarily involved by ovarian carcinoma, and this is more common than primary malignant disease of the

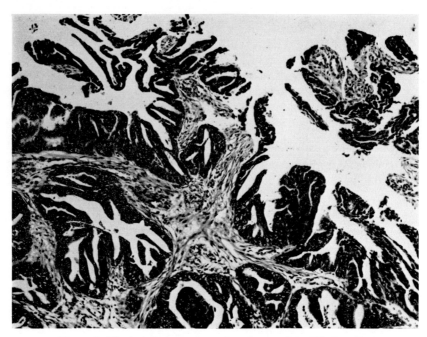

Fig. 43.6. Histological appearances of carcinoma of the fallopian tube.

tube, which is excessively rare, with an incidence amongst genital tract cancer of about 0·3%. It occurs in women between 40 and 60 years old, with a maximum age incidence of around 50 years. Approximately 50% of patients are nulliparous.

PATHOLOGY

The tumour is variable in size, but usually large by the time it is diagnosed. It is mostly unilateral, but bilateral disease is reported in a few cases in the various series reported. The tumour is a papillary adenocarcinoma, and some attempt at alveolar formation is common in most tumours. Necrosis and inflammatory change is also common (Fig. 43.6).

CLINICAL FEATURES

The condition is seldom diagnosed preoperatively, most cases being mistaken for ovarian tumours. Most tumours are diagnosed late, for the same reasons as apply to ovarian cancer. Three-quarters of the patients have a clear or sanguinous vaginal discharge, one-third have abdominal pain and two-thirds have a palpable mass; few cases have all three.

TREATMENT

Surgery, in the form of total hysterectomy and bilateral salpingo-oöphorectomy, is the most usual treatment. As the disease is usually found at a late stage, subsequent external irradiation, with chemotherapy as an adjunctive or alternative, is also given. Hanton *et al.* (1966) report a 44% 5 year survival rate in 27 cases, but this is higher than most series, which give salvage rates between 5 and 25% at 5 years. As with other tumours, all depends on the stage at which the disease is discovered.

REFERENCES

AARO L.A., SYMMONDS R.E. & DOCKERTY M.B. (1966) *Am. J. Obstet. Gynec.* **94**, 101.
ARMENIA C.S. (1967) *Obstet. Gynec., N.Y.* **30**, 524.

BONNEY V. (1947) *Gynaecological Surgery*. London, Cassell.

CORSCADEN J.A. (1962) *Gynecologic Cancer*. Baltimore, Williams and Wilkins.

DINNERSTEIN A.S. & O'LEARY J.A. (1968) *Obstet. Gynec., N.Y.* **31**, 654.

DOBBIE B.M.W. (1953) *J. Obstet. Gynaec. Br. Commonw.* **60**, 702.

DOCKERTY M.B., LOVELADY S.B. & FOUST G.T. Jr. (1951) *Am. J. Obstet. Gynec.* **61**, 966.

DUNN L.J., MARCHANT J.A., BRADBURY J.T. & STONE D.B. (1968) *Archs. intern. Med.* **121**, 246.

HAINES M. & TAYLOR C.W. (1962) *Gynaecologic Pathology*. London, Churchill.

HANTON E.M., MALKASIAN G.D. Jr. & DAHLIN D.C. (1966) *Am. J. Obstet. Gynec.* **94**, 832.

HERTIG A.T., SOMMERS S.C. & BENGLOFF H. (1949) *Cancer, N.Y.* **2**, 957.

HEYMAN J. (1947) *J. Am. med. Ass.* **135**, 412.

JOSLIN E.P. (1952) *Treatment of Diabetes Mellitus* 9th edn. London, Henry Kimpton.

KELLEY R.M. & BAKER W.H. (1961) *New Engl. J. Med.* **264**, 216.

KENNEDY B.J. (1968) *Surgery Gynec. Obstet.* **127**, 103.

KOSS L.G., SPIRO R.H. & BRUNSCHWIG A. (1965) *Surgery Gynec. Obstet.* **121**, 531.

MEISSNER A., SOMMERS S.C. & SHERMAN G. (1957) *Cancer, N.Y.* **10**, 505.

NOVAK E. (1956) *Obstet. Gynec. Survey* **72**, 1072.

NOVAK E.R. & WOODRUFF J.D. (1967) *Gynecologic and Obstetric Pathology*. Philadelphia and London, Saunders.

PALMER J.P. & SPRATT D.W. (1956) *Am. J. Obstet. Gynec.* **72**, 497.

PERCIVAL R. (1952) *Lancet*, ii, 810.

RANDALL J.H., MIRICK D.F. & WIEBEN E.E. (1951) *Am. J. Obstet. Gynec.* **61**, 596.

RICKFORD R.B.K. (1967) *Fifth World Congress of Gynaecology and Obstetrics*. Sydney, Butterworths.

ROBERTS D.W.T. (1961) *J. Obstet. Gynaec. Br. Commonw.* **68**, 132.

SPEERT H. (1948) *Cancer, N.Y.* **1**, 584.

TE LINDE R.W., JONES H.W. & GALVIN G.A. (1953) *Am. J. Obstet. Gynec.* **66**, 953.

TWOMBLY G.H., SCHEINER S. & LEVITZ M. (1961) *Am. J. Obstet. Gynec.* **82**, 424.

WALL J.A., FRANKLIN R.R. & KAUFMAN R.H. (1964) *Am. J. Obstet. Gynec.* **88**, 1072.

WAY S. (1954) *J. Obstet. Gynaec. Br. Commonw.* **61**, 46.

WINTERTON W.R. (1954) *Proc. R. Soc. Med.* **47**, 895.

CHAPTER 44

TUMOURS OF THE OVARY

Ovarian tumours present a number of problems with regard to aetiology, classification, diagnosis and treatment. No organ in the body produces such a multiplicity or diversity of tumours. The picture is further confused by the cystic changes which may develop as a result of the physiological activity of the ovary; these cysts of the follicular system need to be differentiated from true neoplasms and this can be difficult, and indeed is not always possible until they are removed.

The clinical picture associated with these follicular cysts will be discussed later in the chapter.

NEW GROWTHS OF THE OVARY

Many different forms of ovarian new growth have been described, and the study of their pathological features and their histogenesis is a fascinating one. In clinical practice, however, one seldom knows the nature of an ovarian tumour until the abdomen is opened and not always then. We become aware of them clinically as pelvic swellings—large or small, with or without symptoms. Since this is how they present to the clinician this is how we will consider them here—first clinically, then in relation to certain features in their pathology, and finally in their histogenesis.

Clinical features

Neoplasms of the ovary may be found accidentally at a routine examination; in younger women this may be at an antenatal clinic, or nowadays in association with routine cervical cytology examinations, and they are then often benign cystic teratomata (dermoid cysts).

They may also present as a result of accidents occurring to the cysts. These accidents give rise to acute or subacute abdominal symptoms. They are as follows.

(1) *Torsion*

The cyst is nearly always benign, of moderate size and the pedicle long. The reason for torsion occurring is not known but it is probably quite accidental. There may be a number of twists on the pedicle and consequent infarction of the ovary, cyst and related tube will occur. There is acute or subacute pain in the lower abdomen and pelvis on the appropriate side, perhaps with associated vomiting. The patient is mildly shocked with a rapid pulse. The lower abdomen is tender with guarding and rigidity. Pelvic examination reveals an acutely tender swelling in one fornix separate from the uterus. The diagnosis is relatively obvious. Laparotomy is indicated and the tumour mass must be excised; seldom will it be possible to conserve any of the affected ovarian tissue.'

(2) *Rupture*

This may occur with cysts of any size; in small to medium-size cysts it is the whole cyst that bursts but with larger cysts it is usually a loculus. The acuteness of the symptoms will depend on the amount and character of the contents disgorged into the peritoneal cavity. The contents of a chocolate or dermoid cyst are extremely irritant and may cause acute collapse, whereas rupture of a simple serous cyst or the loculus of a mucinous cyst will only cause momentary pain or discomfort. The physical signs will vary from those of an acute abdomen to mild tenderness in association with a mass originating in the pelvis.

(3) Haemorrhage

Haemorrhage occurring into a cyst or part of a cyst is associated with pain, mild, but sometimes more severe, in character. It seldom causes acute symptoms and usually only serves to draw attention to the tumour.

(4) Infection

This is not a common complication of ovarian tumours and is more likely to occur with chocolate cysts which become adherent to the large bowel. Again, subacute or acute symptoms will be engendered, with the general reactions to infection of pyrexia and a raised pulse rate; due to the peritoneal irritation, there will be localizing signs in the abdomen of tenderness, rigidity and guarding. Should the cyst rupture with dispersal of pus into the body cavity, then the result may be devastating with pelvic or general peritonitis supervening. Most malignant tumours have loculi containing purulent contents, but these are seldom sufficient to give rise to any particular sign or symptom.

(5) Malignant change

Malignant tumours of the ovary draw attention to their presence by virtue of their size or by causing pain. But early malignant change in a benign ovarian tumour seldom causes new and dramatic symptoms.

In the absence of such accidents described above, ovarian tumours will usually present with abdominal enlargement or, occasionally, with pressure signs. They are usually slow growing and symptomless, and hence tend to be of large size before being detected. The patient may notice abdominal enlargement, but often, in middle-aged women, this is ignored and attributed to menopausal obesity. Sometimes the patient notices the tumour herself. Pressure on pelvic veins or the inferior vena cava may cause unilateral or bilateral lower-limb oedema and varicosities. or haemorrhoids. Pressure on the bladder may give rise to increased frequency or urgency of micturition. Rarely, the tumour becomes impacted in the pelvis, with the production of acute retention of urine by mechanisms similar to that of the impacted retroverted gravid uterus. Even in the terminal stages of malignant ovarian disease constipation is not a symptom. Large tumours, by filling the abdomen and raising the diaphragm, may cause dyspnoea. Excessively large tumours, of a size seldom seen except in underdeveloped countries, by interfering with absorption and digestive processes may be associated with extreme cachexia, so that a diagnosis of malignancy is automatically but erroneously entertained. These very large tumours are always benign. Malignant ovarian tumours have caused symptoms and destroyed the patient before reaching such a size. Malignant ovarian tumours are nearly always found in patients of normal general appearance; it is only in the terminal phases of the disease that cachexia supervenes. These tumours are distressingly silent in their development and do not give rise to symptoms until they spread outside the ovarian capsule and are thus in an advanced stage which renders cure much less likely. If abdominal enlargement is the first symptom then it is due either to the tumour, which to have reached noticeable size is almost certain to have involved nearby structures, or to ascites, the development of which is an almost certain indication of malignancy. The other symptom is pain, and this pain which, unfortunately for diagnostic purposes, is seldom of an acute nature, is due to the involvement of other structures by spread beyond the ovary.

The only benign ovarian tumour conspicuously accompanied by ascites is the ovarian fibroma, and then the finding of hard, mobile masses in an abdomen full of free fluid encourages a mistaken diagnosis of malignancy. The added finding of hydrothorax, usually right-sided, provides the clinical picture known as Meigs's syndrome;

this, however, is not confined to the benign fibroma, but may also occur with other benign or malignant tumours.

The more bizarre tumours which are of considerable interest to gynaecologists and pathologists alike are rare and they can either be diagnosed only under the microscope or, more rarely, they present with such outstanding clinical features that they require no great diagnostic skill. Masculinizing tumours such as the arrhenoblastoma cause, first, defeminization, with amenorrhoea and atrophy of the breasts and then masculinization, with acne, hirsutism, deepening of the voice and enlargement of the clitoris. Feminizing tumours such as the granulosa-cell tumour cause varying clinical pictures according to their age of onset. In prepubertal girls precocious puberty occurs, and in postmenopausal women postmenopausal bleeding due to oestrogenic stimulation of the atrophic endometrium. In women in menstrual life the abnormal oestrogenic stimulus often induces cystic glandular hyperplasia of the endometrium and the clinical picture of metropathia haemorrhagia. A noteworthy incidence of carcinoma of the corpus uteri has been found in association with the feminizing tumours. In some cases of dysgerminoma, where there is no hormone activity, pseudohermaphroditism is found. However, recent reports have indicated that the separation into masculinizing or feminizing tumours, depending on the clinical picture, is not always so simple. The rarest among these rarities is the ovarian struma, where active thyroid tissue causes symptoms of thyrotoxicosis.

The physical signs are usually not difficult to elicit. Where the tumour is benign and intrapelvic it should be relatively easy to distinguish an adnexal swelling distinct from the uterus. Benign tumours other than endometriomata are usually smooth and mobile. The main differential diagnosis will be presented by tubo-ovarian or tubal inflammatory lesions, but these are more likely to be bilateral, fixed and have associated symptoms. Broad-ligament cysts are unilateral, fixed and deflect the uterus to one side. Pedunculated fibroids have a characteristic consistency, unless subject to degenerative changes, and it is sometimes possible to feel the pedicle. The differentiation between early neoplasms and follicular cysts can be difficult, but this is a problem which is uncommon in clinical gynaecology; the difficulty can be resolved by observation over a period of time to see if the cyst enlarges or disappears, or, if necessary, by direct inspection. The cyst can be visualized by culdoscopy, culdotomy, laparoscopy or laparotomy.

Ovarian cysts rising into the abdomen are also fairly easy to diagnose, they tend to be situated more to one or other side of the abdomen and to have their lower pole in the pelvis. Their borders are discrete and their surface and consistency varies with their nature. The uterus can, as a rule, be palpated separate from the tumour. The tumours themselves are, of course, dull to percussion. However, certain difficulties in diagnosis do arise, and being fairly well known will only be mentioned briefly.

(1) A full bladder can be eliminated by the patient voiding urine or being catheterized.

(2) Abdominal distension with flatus is characterized by resonance.

(3) Faeces collected in the intestines can give rise to a large mass, but is rarely seen these days as a diagnostic problem.

(4) Free fluid is evidenced by dulness in the flanks, shifting dulness and, possibly, a fluid thrill. It must be remembered that it may be present in association with an ovarian tumour. Encysted ascites, as found in tuberculous peritonitis, will create greater difficulties, but the patient usually will present with general systemic signs and symptoms; these latter may be mistaken for malignant cachexia.

(5) Fibroids may give rise to problems, particularly if they are the seat of degenerative change, cystic degeneration being the most confusing.

(6) Pregnancy, especially if accompanied by a false history, can mislead even the most experienced observers.

(7) Much less common differential diagnoses are large hydrosalpinges (particularly tuberculous), hydronephrosis, enlarged spleen, accessory lobes of the liver, mesenteric cysts, pancreatic and pseudopancreatic cysts. Lesions of the pelvic colon such as endometrioma and diverticulitis and, more rarely, carcinoma, may

on occasion cause difficulty. A mobile pelvic caecum can at times be the cause of error.

(8) Obesity can cause great difficulty and percussion is of great value here, but sometimes examination under anesthesia is necessary to exclude the presence of a soft, flaccid cyst in an obese abdomen. Ultrasound may also be valuable in this situation.

(9) Pseudocyesis is a rarity, but a distended abdomen which the patient cannot relax is not uncommon.

Malignant tumours tend to present fairly well marked characteristics. Ascites is common. Fixity is usual. Nodular deposits in the pouch of Douglas are often found. Cachexia occurs in late cases only. Moderate abdominal pain and discomfort accompany the abdominal enlargement. Disturbances of menstruation do not occur unless the tumour is hormone-producing, but in postmenopausal women there may be slight bleeding. The possibility of malignant tumours being secondary metastases must be entertained and signs or symptoms referable to the breast, stomach, or large bowel must be sought. Krukenberg tumours, which are rare, will not present the more usual features of malignant ovarian tumours, being bilateral, smooth, encapsulated, lobulated tumours of moderate size (Fig. 44.1). Hormone-secreting tumours may be quite small and yet still produce their rather dramatic systemic effects; recourse to more extensive investigations such as gynaecography, culdoscopy, laparoscopy, and even laparotomy, may be necessary.

When all is said and done the final diagnosis of ovarian tumour often is not made until the abdomen has been opened. At this moment the diagnosis of malignancy is often clear-cut due to spread through the capsule and widespread metastasis to pelvic peritoneum, outer surface of large bowel, omentum and parietal peritoneum. A search for a primary site in stomach or large bowel should be made, and also for metastasis to the para-aortic lymph nodes and to the liver. In less advanced cases malignancy will be suggested by deposits in the pouch of Douglas or by the macroscopic appearance of the tumour when examined after removal. Hard, solid areas or soft, mushy proliferative masses are suggestive, as are loculi containing purulent-looking material. Proliferative processes sprouting through the capsule give cause for concern. However, there are times when it is not possible to make a definite diagnosis at laparotomy. In patients in the older age groups where conservation of ovarian function is not important no problem arises, as the uterus and both ovaries may be removed. In the very young it is best to remove the affected ovary and retain the uterus and other normal-looking ovary, from which a full slice biopsy should be taken. If the patient survives she retains her reproductive powers, whereas if she is destined to die from her condition the result is unlikely to have been influenced by conserving a normal ovary. Great difficulty may arise with bilateral tumours or with suspicious-looking unilateral tumours in women in their late thirties, where castration may pro-

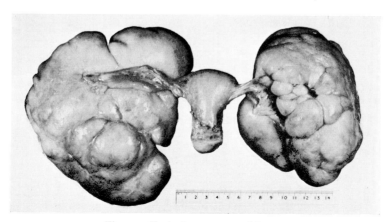

Fig. 44.1. Krukenberg tumours of the ovary.

duce severe menopausal symptoms and considerable psychological trauma. It is in these cases that the frozen-section technique may be of some value. The difficulty here, however, is that of deciding from which area to take the biopsy and the very pleomorphic nature of these tumours. If the tumour is wholly maligant there will be little difficulty, but in benign tumours in which there is malignant change the diagnosis could be missed; this is quite apart from the difficulties of interpretation.

Treatment

Treatment of benign ovarian tumours is relatively simple, providing that the diagnosis is clear. Where age and parity demand conservation of ovarian function then enucleation or excision of the cyst, or cysts, is all that is required, and it is usually possible to conserve some healthy ovarian tissue. At times one ovary is so heavily involved that it must be removed *in toto*, and this is usually so in the larger cysts; providing the whole or part of the remaining ovary can be conserved this is acceptable. In the older age groups where the patient is premenopausal it is customary to remove both ovaries and the uterus.

The management of ovarian malignant disease is at present in a state of flux, in which the prominent attitude is one of despair engendered by the universally agreed poor results of any form of therapy. These poor results are generally acknowledged to be due to the late stage at which most tumours are discovered. The markedly

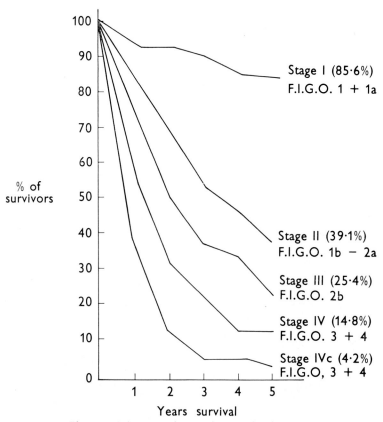

Fig. 44.2. Primary carcinoma of ovary. Graph showing cumulative relative survival rates by stages—R.A.C.O.G. and F.I.G.O. (From McGarrity & Scott 1967).

improved results of treatment undertaken in less advanced stages of the disease is obvious (Fig. 44.2). To correlate results from different centres it is preferable that F.I.G.O. staging be employed (Tables 44.1 and 44.2). Because of this, the present emphasis is directed towards early diagnosis and prophylaxis. With regard to the latter the question of conservation of ovaries at hysterectomy must be considered. The incidence of subsequent tumour formation in such ovaries is estimated to be between 1 in 300 and 1 in 3,000 (Jeffcoate 1962), although Terz et al. (1967) found that 8·8% of 624 patients undergoing laparotomy for benign conditions subsequently presented with ovarian carcinoma. Obviously, prophylactic removal at the initial operation would save a small number of women from developing ovarian cancer. The disadvantages to the remaining great majority would be a sudden and severe onset of menopausal symptoms and an increased incidence of coronary thrombosis. In favour of routine removal of normal ovaries it has been claimed that the ovaries atrophy within 2 years of hysterectomy. Clinical experience and the researches of Richards (1951) and Bancroft Livingston (1954) do not confirm this. Most surgeons have an arbitrary approach to the problem, either removing the ovaries routinely at hysterectomy or removing them in women over 45 years old. However, women vary considerably in their appearance and attitude, and many are still young for their years in this age group. There is little doubt that normal functioning ovaries are better value to a woman than synthetic hormones. Once the menopause has been reached there should be no question of conservation.

Early diagnosis presents a more difficult problem, because the ovary is not a surface organ. Routine examinations associated with cervical cytology will uncover a few cases. Graham & Graham (1967) have shown that early lesions can be discovered by aspiration of the posterior fornix before clinical signs become evident, but this is hardly to be considered a routine screening procedure. If a simple enzyme or similar screening test could reliably indicate those patients most likely to have a cancerous lesion somewhere in the body then such methods could be applied more selectively.

Table 44.1. Clinical staging of tumours of the ovary (F.I.G.O., 1965)

Stage I: Growth limited to ovaries
Stage Ia: Growth limited to one ovary no ascites
Stage Ib: Growth limited to both ovaries: no ascites
Stage Ic: Growth limited to one or both ovaries: ascites plus malignant cells in fluid

Stage II: Growth involving one or both ovaries with pelvic extension
Stage IIa: Extension and metastasis to the uterus and tubes only
Stage IIb: Extension to other pelvic tissues

Stage III: Growth involving one or both ovaries with widespread intraperitoneal metastasis to the abdomen (the omentum, small intestine and its mesentery)

Stage IV: Growth involving one or both ovaries with distant metastasis outside the peritoneal cavity

Special category: Unexplored cases which are thought to be ovarian cancer (surgery, explorative or therapeutic not having been performed)

Note: The presence of ascites does not influence the staging for stages II, III and IV.

Table 44.2. Histological classification of tumours of the ovary (F.I.G.O., 1965)

I. Serous cystomas
   A. Serous benign cystadenoma
   B. Serous cystadenoma with proliferative activity of the epithelial cells and nuclear abnormalities, but with no infiltrative growth (low potential malignancy)
   C. Serous cystadenocarcinoma

II. Mucinous cystomas
   A. Mucinous benign cystadenoma
   B. Mucinous cystadenoma (low potential malignancy)
   C. Mucinous cystadenocarcinoma

III. Endometrioid tumours (similar to adenocarcinoma in the endometrium)
   A. Endometrioid cysts
   B. Endometrioid cysts (low potential malignancy)
   C. Endometrioid adenocarcinoma

IV. Concomitant carcinomata. Unclassified carcinomata (tumours which cannot be allotted to one of the groups I, II or III)

Treatment of ovarian cancer is undergoing a more aggressive approach at the present time. Where the disease is confined to one or both ovaries total hysterectomy and bilateral salpingo-oöphorectomy will give as good a result as any treatment, and supplementary radiotherapy does not appear to enhance the results. There is a definite improvement in survival rates, however, if such radiotherapy is employed in the later stages of the disease where complete removal is doubtful or impossible; in these cases the surgeon removes as much cancerous tissue as possible, including the uterus and both adnexae. It has also been suggested that removal of the greater omentum reduces the chance of recurrent ascites, and certainly the procedure does not considerably enlarge the operation, but whether it is worth-while is not yet proven. In those more advanced cases where complete removal of the growth seems at first to be impossible it can be achieved in some cases by performing a retrograde hysterectomy and excising the pelvic peritoneum with the enclosed tumour mass en bloc, for the tumour seldom spreads through the peritoneum. This procedure has been described by Hudson (1968) and Dellepiane (1967). So far no results are forthcoming. Most surgeons presented with the surgically hopeless case prefer to excise as much of the tumour as is possible and then refer the patient for radiotherapy. In some cases the

results of therapy are so encouraging that a second-look operation is justified, and the uterus and adnexae can then be easily removed.

Chemotherapy has, of course, produced its most resounding successes in tumours of the genital tract in the treatment of choriocarcinoma. Its only other place of value to date, if one excludes the remarkable but transient results achieved by Trussell (1963), is an ovarian cancer, and here the value is limited. Usually, chemotherapy is utilized in the treatment of inoperable cases, and often after radiotherapy has proved to be of no avail. From time to time good results are reported and second-look operations have been possible. Till recently the decision as to which of many therapeutic agents to employ has been resolved by the personal whim of the physician, the desire to evaluate a new drug, or trial and error. Heckmann & Limburg (1967) have described a method of assessing drug sensitivity of *in vitro* cell cultures grown from biopsy material which may make chemotherapy more logical, if not more effective. It may be that preliminary radiotherapy diminishes the value of subsequent chemotherapy by reducing the blood supply to

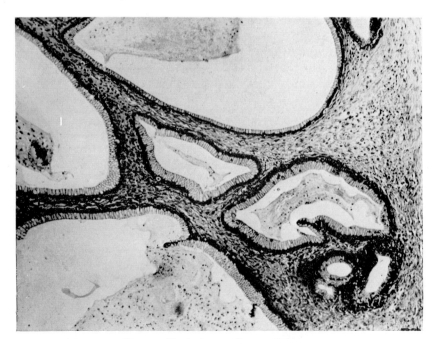

Fig. 44.3. Mucinous cystadenoma of the ovary.

the tumour. In considering the use of either radiotherapy or chemotherapy it is important to weigh the toxic consequences of the treatment against the quality of any prolongation of life that is obtained. In the absence of any response to either form of therapy the patient will succumb, usually quite rapidly, to malignant cachexia, but there may be an intervening stage when the patient's discomfort can be temporarily relieved by abdominal paracentesis to remove accumulated ascites; in most cases this will have to be repeated at increasingly frequent intervals, and soon becomes less effective due to loculation of the collected fluid by adhesions.

Pathological features

MUCINOUS CYSTADENOMATA

These tend to be large, unilateral cysts, sometimes of enormous size. They are multilocular with smooth outer and inner surface. The fluid content is mucinous, of variable consistency but characteristically jelly-like. The loculi are lined by a single layer of tall mucus-secreting columnar cells with darkly staining nuclei, and are of variable size (Fig. 44.3). Papillary processes are rarely seen and are very suggestive of malignancy. Malignant degeneration is in the form of adenocarcinoma, and probably occurs in 5–10% of cases. Pseudomyxoma peritonei is a rare complication due to spontaneous perforation of the cyst and implantation of cells of low malignancy on the peritoneum; these continue to secrete mucin, necessitating repeated removal. Mucocoele of the appendix may also be a cause of this condition. The patient usually dies from malignant cachexia after several laparotomies to remove the collected mucin; unfortunately, treatment seems to be of little avail.

SEROUS CYSTADENOMA

Serous cystadenoma is usually a smaller cyst than the mucinous variety and is bilateral in approximately 50% of cases. The cyst is most often unilocular, with a smooth outer surface [Fig. 44.4(a)], the interior, however, nearly always contains papilliferous processes [Fig. 44.4(b)]. The fluid content is a thin, serous fluid. The papillae may be few in number and just cause a localized roughened area or fill the whole cyst so that it appears solid, with all gradations between. The papillae may sprout through the capsule, in which case ascites may be present, and although this is very suggestive of malignancy, such tumours may be histologically benign. The lining cells are cubical or columnar and may be ciliated; they often resemble the epithelium of the fallopian tube. Small deposits of calcium, known as psammoma bodies, are often seen in the stroma. Occasionally, a cyst may show both mucinous and serous-type epithelium, suggesting a common histogenesis. Considerable interest is aroused by the papilliferous group, in that all gradations may be seen—from a well-differentiated benign pattern to an obviously malignant one with anaplasia. In this group of tumours there is an intermediary pattern which the pathologist may have difficulty in assigning to a benign or malignant state, and from the clinician's point of view there is the group which, histologically, is benign but which implants on surrounding structures and recurs locally; such cases tend to run a protracted course with recurrent operations and a final outcome of definite malignant change.

DERMOID CYSTS

These lesions do not, as a rule, present problems of diagnosis or treatment. They are the commonest cysts found in young women, occurring in 53 of 147 patients below 18 years of age in a 35-year survey by Moore et al. (1967), but they may be discovered at any time in a woman's life. Malkasian et al. (1967), in a review of 581 cases over an 18-year period, found the mean age of discovery to be 42·6 years, and it is interesting to note that 28·6% of the patients were postmenopausal. Dermoid cysts tend to be found at routine examinations, being, in general, symptomless. Acute accidents such as torsion and rupture may occur, particularly in pregnancy. In around 10% of cases there are cysts in both ovaries. The cysts are heavy and for some reason often come to lie in the uterovesical pouch of peritoneum; they are seldom larger than 12 cm diameter. The surface

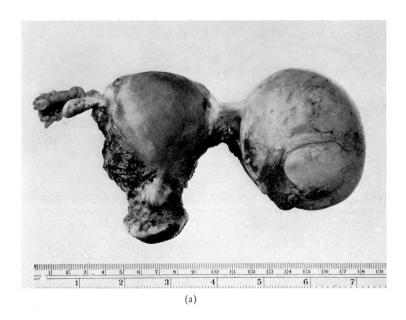

(a)

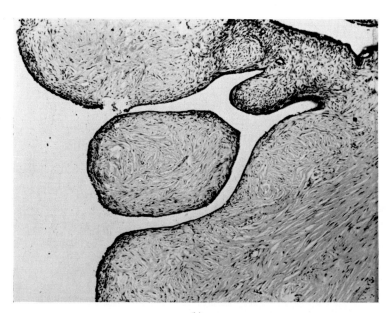

(b)

Fig. 44.4. Serous cystadenoma of ovary. (a) Macroscopic, and (b) microscopic appearances.

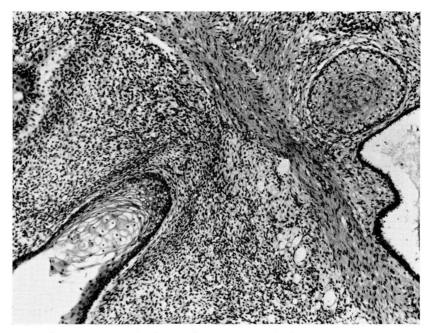

Fig. 44.5. A malignant teratoma showing cartilage, squamous epithelium and undifferentiated mesenchyme.

is smooth and the consistency doughy, with one or more hard areas, and the wall of the cyst is opaque and yellow. The contents are yellow, greasy and the consistency of thin porridge; a variable amount of hair is present. In most cysts there is a single loculus into which projects a raised area or mamilla from which the hairs arise and in which may be embedded dentigerous structures.

Histologically, the main constituent is skin, with its associated structures, hair, sebaceous and sweat glands. From the squamous epithelium epidermoid cancer can arise, but this is rare. A great variety of tissues may be found, such as alimentary or respiratory epithelium, neural tissue, cartilage, bone and thyroid tissue; preponderance of the latter is thought to engender the rare struma ovarii. Whilst solid teratomata may be benign, they are more usually malignant, showing a variety of immature or embryonic tissues on histological examination (Fig. 44.5); extremely rarely, imperfect embryo formation is attempted (fetus in fetu). Primary chorio-carcinoma, carcinoid and melanoma have been described in the ovary, and some believe that

their origin is initially in an ovarian teratoma. The teeth in a dermoid cyst may, of course, be observed pre-operatively on X-rays of the pelvis. Benign cysts can be enucleated intact from the ovary in most cases; the contralateral ovary should be carefully inspected, even to the extent of bisection if doubt exists, to exclude the presence of small cysts.

FIBROMA

These tumours occur infrequently and present as large, hard, mobile, lobulated tumours with a white, glistening surface, they are bilateral in about 10% of cases. They often produce ascites, and thus present an important diagnostic problem; hard masses in the abdomen associated with ascites suggest malignancy, and patients not subjected to laparotomy may be abandoned as hopelessly incurable until their continued well-being suggests a reappraisal of the diagnosis. Well known is the syndrome of ovarian fibroma, ascites and pleural effusion (usually right-sided), and Meigs (1954) indicated the benign and curable nature of the former syndrome now commonly known by his name, and differentiated it from the other types of malignant ovarian tumour also associated with ascites and hydrothorax with a very different prognosis. Small fibropapillary nodules are often found on the surface of the ovary; if they contain gland-like structures they are regarded as adenofibromata, the latter may, of course, be large and similar in appearance to fibromata. Novak & Woodruff (1967) suggests that many fibromata may in fact be Brenner tumours in which the epithelial elements are largely overshadowed by the immense fibrous tissue growth and thus may be overlooked by the pathologist. Other solid tumours of the ovary— such as fibromyoma, haemangioma, lymphangioma, adenomatoid and neutral tumours—are pathological rarities which have no distinguishing clinical pattern.

SPECIAL TUMOURS

In turning to the so-called special tumours of the ovary, it is to be stressed that they are rare, and have generated much interest because of their possible histogenesis and, in some cases, their associated endocrine effects. Whilst it is convenient to consider (i) feminizing tumours, (ii) masculinizing tumours, and (iii) inert tumours as the three basic patterns, according to the observed endocrine effect, this is too simple to cover all types of tumour described. Assuming an origin from the ovarian mesenchyme, and allowing that this cell is totipotential, then mixed patterns can be expected, and indeed have been described.

The *feminizing tumours* are the granulosa- and theca-cell tumours, and are the commonest of the special ovarian tumours; of the two, the granulosa cell is found more often. Whilst it is customary to describe the two as separate entities, it is more common to find elements of both, to greater or lesser degree, in any one tumour. Granulosa-cell tumour occurs in any age group, is usually unilateral, and varies in size from a small nodule to a large tumour. It is round, lobulated, its consistency is solid with cystic areas and its colour mainly yellow, with red or blue areas due to the cysts containing

blood-stained fluid. The histological picture is variable but the cells, which are usually in sheets, are very similar to those of the membrana granulosa in the ripening follicle. The cells are grouped around spaces of varying size, suggesting primordial follicles (Fig. 44.6). Variations in connective tissue, usually inconspicuous, may break the cells up into patterns described as cylindromatous and gyriform, as opposed to the more usual diffuse arrangement. The theca-cell tumour is usually unilateral, of moderate size, and is a firm, solid tumour with a bright yellow colour. The cells are plump spindles resembling the follicle theca cells, arranged in intertwining bundles (Fig. 44.7). Both granulosa- and theca-cell tumours may show evidence of lutenization in some of the constituent cells.

Clinically, the classical picture has been related to the influence of the oestrogen produced by the cells. This, in girls before the menstrual era, induces precocious puberty; in women during it, cystic glandular hyperplasia with resultant menstrual disturbance; in those beyond it postmenopausal bleeding can be expected. However, granulosa-cell tumour is quite frequently malignant; 25 out of 47 cases in a series reported by Dinnerstein & O'Leary (1968) as against two out of 46 theca-cell tumours; in these cases a mass with or without ascites was the method of presentation in 53%, abdominal pain in 29% and bleeding per vaginam in only 18%; of the 64 endometrial examples out of 102 cases, 30 showed cystic glandular hyperplasia and three adenocarcinoma. Clearly, a marked endocrine response is not always to be found in these tumours. It is generally held that the granulosa-cell tumour has a lower level of malignancy than other ovarian tumours, but this is perhaps dependent on the stage of diagnosis and the fact that recurrences of the tumour may arise at extremely long intervals after the original treatment, 10–20 years in some cases. Several workers have reported a high incidence of endometrial carcinoma in association with feminizing tumours, in particular the thecoma; the figures are variable but are of interest in relation to the possible dependency of the uterine cancer on oestrogen, and also in that they point to the theca cells being the source of that hormone.

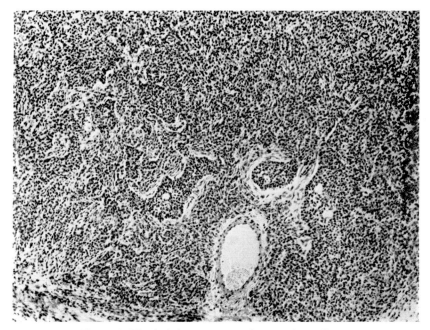

Fig. 44.6. Histological appearances of a granulosa-cell tumour.

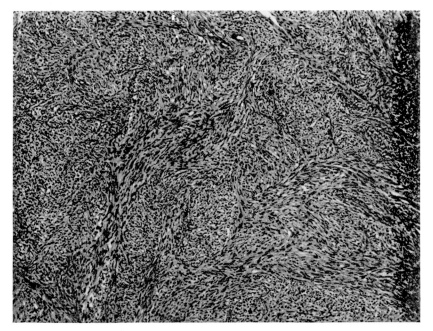

Fig. 44.7. A theca-cell tumour.

Masculinizing tumours

The best known is the arrhenoblastoma, in which tubular structures resembling those found in the testis are seen in varying degrees of differentiation. Three main varieties are described:

(1) Highly differentiated, resembling testicular adenoma (Fig. 44.8).

(2) Intermediate (the commonest), showing strands of cells with imperfect tubule formation.

(3) The undifferentiated, showing a sarcomatous appearance.

In all three, intestitial or Leydig-like cells are to be found in greater or less degree and are responsible for a corresponding degree of virilizing effect. This shows itself first as defeminization, with the menstrual periods becoming less frequent and finally developing into secondary amenorrhoea, atrophy of the breasts; and then masculinization is shown, with hirsutes, enlargement of the clitoris and deepening of the voice. The tumour occurs most often in young women and is unilateral. It is seldom large, is smooth and solid, with a greyish-pink or yellow

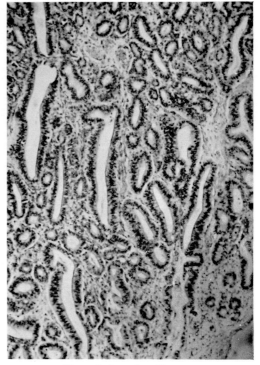

Fig. 44.8. An arrhenoblastoma.

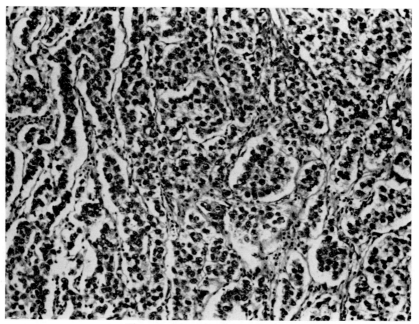

Fig. 44.9. An ovarian dysgerminoma.

substance; cystic degeneration occurs frequently. At least a quarter of the tumours are malignant. Where microscopical features characteristic of both granulosa-cell tumour and arrhenoblastoma are found in the same tumour, the designation gynandroblastoma has been used. In the less well-differentiated tumours the appearances of one may mimic the other and lead to difficulties of interpretation, it is in such cases that the term gonadal stroma tumour is best applied.

A number of tumours associated with masculinizing effect are composed of cells with a high lipoid content and this has resulted in a confusing array of names such as lipoid-cell tumour, virilizing lipoid tumour, adrenal-like tumour, masculinovoblastoma, hilar-cell tumour, and Leydig-cell tumour. There is equal confusion regarding the identity and histogenesis of such tumours, those who favour adrenal rests and hilar cell activity, such as Novak & Woodruff (1967), prefer to consider adrenal tumours as arising from such rests and the Leydig-cell or hilar tumours as arising from hilar cells, and to credit these cells with the ability to manufacture a variety of steroids because of the associated finding of endometrial hyperplasia and virilization. The alternative explanation is simpler and more in line with present tendencies regarding histogenesis of ovarian tumours; that both hilar-cell and adrenal-like tumours arise from the ovarian stroma cell, thus bringing all these special tumours under the umbrella name of gonadal stromal tumour, with either masculinizing, or feminizing, or even mixed, effects. The tumours themselves are usually unilateral, small and yellow in colour.

Dysgerminoma

This is rare in the group of special tumours and morphologically is similar to seminoma of the testis with large, polyhedral cells arranged in cords or nests separated by fibrous tissue (Fig. 44.9). About 10% of tumours show a mixed pattern with teratomatous elements. The tumours are considered by most authorities to arise from the germ cell. Although originally thought to be commonly associated with developmental abnormalities of the genital tract, par-

ticularly pseudohermaphroditism, recent studies have not confirmed this. Asodourian & Taylor (1969) observed no such association in 117 cases. The tumour is bilateral in 5–10% of cases, is of moderate size (about 15 cm diameter), is round or lobulated, solid and rubbery in consistency, pinkish-grey in colour and shows haemorrhagic and necrotic areas. It is found most commonly in the age group 20–30 years. The main presenting symptoms are a mass, with or without pain. Prognosis is generally good, providing the tumour is encapsulated, limited to one ovary, and in the pure form. Conservative surgery is therefore applicable in the younger women where these criteria apply. As the tumour is very radiosensitive, late stages and recurrences are best treated by this means.

Brenner tumour

This, again, is mainly of interest from the point of view of histogenesis. It presents nests of epithelial cells [Fig. 44.10(a)] similar in appearance to Walthard's cell rests which are surrounded by a dense fibrous tissue stroma. When cystic degeneration [Fig. 44.10(b)] occurs in the islands, leaving central debris, the appearance is suggestive of a Graffian follicle, and this gave rise to Brenner's original nomenclature of oöphoroma folliculare. A more interesting feature of the epithelial islands with cystic degeneration is the presence of cells resembling those seen in mucinous cystadenoma; conversely, Brenner tumours have been noted in the wall of some mucinous cysts. Furthermore, the fibrous tissue element of the Brenner tumour is comparable to that in the fibroma of the ovary and if, as may be the case, the epithelial elements are sparse, a wrong diagnosis may be made. The tumour of variable size, is hard and round or lobulated, and macroscopically resembles a fibroma. It is unilateral and basically benign in behaviour.

It will be appreciated that in most cases the definitive diagnosis is not made in this group of tumours until after operation, and when all the available evidence, clinical and pathological has been collated. Since some of these tumours are malignant and may occur in young women, a

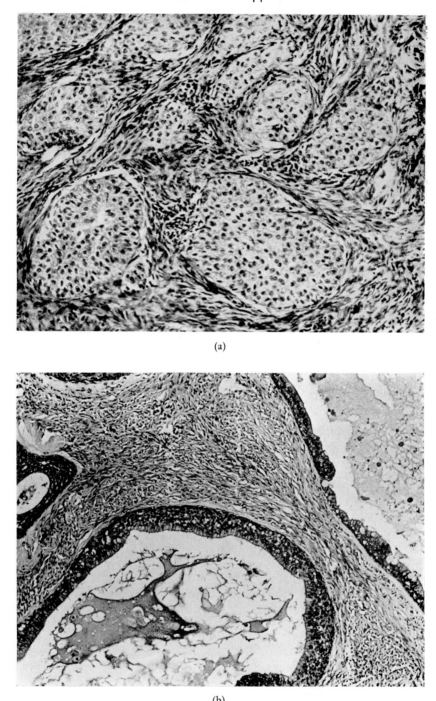

(a)

(b)

Fig. 44.10. Brenner tumour. (a) Nests of cells surrounded by fibrous septa. (b) Cystic change, showing loculi lined by mucinous epithelium.

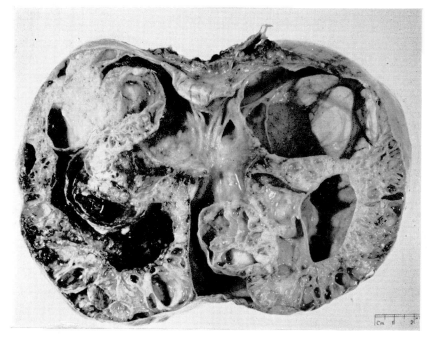

(a)

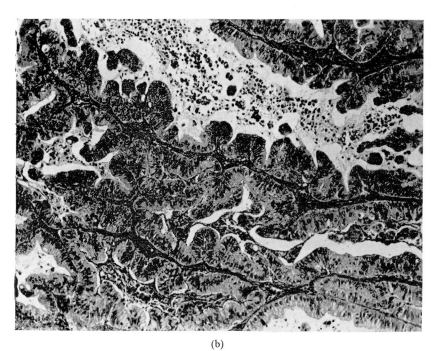

(b)

Fig. 44.11. Mucinous cystadenocarcinoma. (a) Gross appearances. (b) Microscopic appearances.

problem arises for the surgeon who is faced at operation with what he suspects is a tumour belonging to this group. In general, the prognosis is favourable where the tumour is unilateral and encapsulated (as in most ovarian cancer) and so conservative surgery is adequate providing a careful observation is made of the other ovary, including full-thickness biopsy, and that careful follow-up of the patient's condition is observed. For older women more radical surgery is employed, with removal of both the ovaries and the uterus. The principles, in fact, do not differ from those to be observed with ovarian tumours in general.

MALIGNANT OVARIAN TUMOURS

Apart from the borderline cases, seen most commonly in the papilliferous cysts, malignant ovarian tumours present little difficulty in diagnosis. The most frequently occurring are the cystadenocarcinomata, with the serous group in preponderance (Figs. 44.11, 44.12).

The special group of tumours, as has been noted, are rare. Distinction must be made, if possible, between primary and secondary tumours; the latter are metastatic from endometrial cancer, from adenocarcinoma of the stomach and large bowel, and from the breast. Carcinoma of the tube involves the ovary by direct extension, but is so rare as to be unworthy of note in this context. Secondary cancer of the ovary is mostly bilateral; the growth may reach the ovary by blood or lymphatic emboli or by direct implantation onto the surface. Usually, the pattern of the primary tumour can be recognized, but in anaplastic tumours it may not be possible to confirm whether the tumour is primary or secondary, unless the primary site can be determined. A special form of secondary tumour of the ovary which has attracted much attention, but which is rare, is the Krukenberg tumour. Most often this is secondary to a tumour in the stomach but on occasion the large bowel, and sometimes the breast, is the primary. As a rule, the primary is small and may be unrecognized, whilst the ovarian lesion presents first as bilateral fairly large, solid, lobulated, mobile tumours. In outward appearance they resemble fibroma or

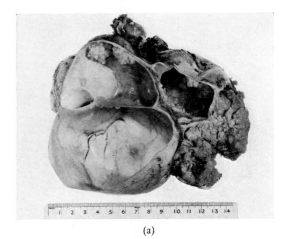

(a)

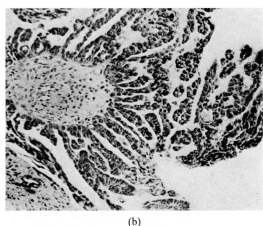

(b)

Fig. 44.12. Serous cystadenocarcinoma. (a) Gross appearances. (b) Microscopic appearances.

thecoma of the ovary, but the characteristic microscopical finding of signet-ring cells containing mucin enables the diagnosis to be made. Interest has been aroused as to the method of spread; at present vascular spread seems to be more accepted than transcoelomic or retrograde lymphatic spread.

Primary carcinoma of the ovary is either solid, or cystic, or a mixture of the two. Most primary tumours are probably malignant *ab initio*, but malignant change in a benign cyst does occur in a small number of cases, the proportion is difficult to assess, but is thought not to be very high. Such malignant change can occur in:

(1) Mucinous cystadenoma.
(2) Serous cystadenoma.
(3) Dermoid cysts (usually squamous-cell carcinoma).
(4) Endometrial cysts.

Apart from borderline cases, the histological appearance of mucinous and serous papilliferous cystadenocarcinoma is fairly typical. Solid ovarian tumours are less common than the cystic type, they present a variety of microscopical pictures which are given descriptive names such as adenocarcinoma, papillary carcinoma, medullary, schirrous, alveolar, and plexiform carcinoma, most of which are probably better defined as undifferentiated carcinoma. There has been much interest in the so-called endometroid carcinoma in recent years; these tumours are thought to arise in areas of endometriosis (a difficult point to prove in most cases) and present a pattern similar to endometrial adenocarcinoma. They are reputed to be of a lower degree of malignancy than other types of ovarian cancer and to be only locally invasive. Many authorities dislike the term, which has, however, been accepted in the F.I.G.O. classification (1965). Gray & Barnes (1967) had difficulty in distinguishing the tumour in a group of 142 ovarian malignancies which were compared with 240 endometrial adenocarcinomata, and they concluded that the prognosis was better only if the stage of the disease was early. McGarrity & Scott (1967) also found a low salvage rate in endometrioid tumours.

Some dispute remains regarding certain rare histological appearances in ovarian cancer. Clear-cell carcinoma, or hypernephroma, and mesonephroma are described by some as clear-cut entities, but Haines & Taylor (1962) accord with Willis (1953) in the view that these patterns are variants of undifferentiated cancer or of mucinous cystadenocarcinoma.

The spread of the malignant process in carcinoma of the ovary is direct, by lymphatic channels, and by the blood stream. Direct spread is to the peritoneum, mainly of the pelvis, particularly the pouch of Douglas, to the uterus, contralateral ovary, and to the omentum. Bowel may also be involved by becoming adherent to the tumour. The disease may be widespread throughout the abdominal cavity, and peritoneal involvement is commonly associated with ascites. Both ovaries are grossly involved in over 50% of cases, probably as bilateral primary tumours. Lymphatic spread to tube, uterus and contralateral ovary may occur. The para-aortic lymph nodes are the main drainage-channel for the ovaries but they are seldom obviously involved, as the patient succumbs to her disease before symptoms of such involvement develop. In terminal cases more distant nodes may be involved, in particular the supraclavicular nodes. Blood stream spread may give rise to distant metastases, but this is uncommon apart from lung involvement; bone metastases is rare. Local spread is pre-emptive.

Histogenesis

A logical classification of ovarian tumours, is at present, impossible. The histogenesis of most tumours remains in doubt; more than one variety of tumour may be found in the one ovary; the histology may be extremely confusing, and in the so-called 'special tumours' the endocrine effects can be very variable; these effects have been described in association with the commoner tumours.

There seems now to be a move towards accepting a simpler and more inclusive theory of histogenesis, based on the idea that all ovarian tumours other than secondary ones can arise from the constituent cells of the ovary, thus avoiding the need to invoke rests and remnants. Moreover, there is a growing realization that, just as the normal ovary produces several steroids, so may the tumours, and therefore a rather rigid concept of feminizing and masculinizing tumours has given way to the idea that the gonadal stroma forming such tumours is capable of a varied endocrine influence; and this in turn seems to be leading to a less definite distinction between the special tumours and the avoidance of some of the more bizarre terms. It is believed that in the adult ovary, the stromal and epithelial cells are capable of considerable differentiation, and this is supported by experimentally produced tumours such as the granulosa-cell tumours produced by light irradiation of mice (Furth & Butterworth 1936) and the ovarian transplantation experiments of Biskind & Biskind (1949). Serous cystadenomata are thought to be derived from the surface coelomic epithelium; alternatively, they may develop from germinal inclusion cysts. Adenofibroma would then have a similar development, but the ovarian cortical stroma would provide the abundance of fibrous tissue.

Two lines of thought exist regarding the histogenesis of mucinous cystadenomata. One of these postulates that the coelomic epithelium can differentiate into the tall, columnar cells found in the tumour which bear a strong resemblance to endocervical cells, whilst the cells of the serous cystadenoma resemble those of the fallopian tube. The Muellerian epithelium does, of course, form both cervix and tube during embryological development. The other view is that the epithelium of mucinous cysts is comparable to the intestinal mucosa and that these tumours represent an overgrowth of this tissue in a dermoid cyst, such as occurs with thyroid tissue in struma ovarii. The fact that pseudomyxoma peritonei may result from either mucinous cysts or from mucocoele of the appendix, lends some support to this argument, but although the coexistence of mucinous and dermoid cysts in the same ovary is well recognized, it is not as common a finding as would be expected if this explanation were correct.

The place of the Brenner tumour in relation to mucinous cystadenoma has to be considered also. The two tumours are discovered in coexistence, which has led to the belief that there is a common aetiology from the germinal epithelium; indeed, many have accepted the view that the Brenner tumour arises from Walthard rests, which themselves are thought to be examples of serosal metaplasia, but which are more commonly seen in the fallopian tube than the ovary. Endocrine effects have been observed in relation to Brenner tumours, and to a lesser extent with mucinous cystadenomata; these are mainly oestrogenic, in the form of endometrial hyperplasia (Farrar *et al.* 1960), but occasionally andro-genic. The hormone production is considered to result from the conversion of the mesenchymal cells of the stroma to theca lutein cells. Fibromata are generally considered to arise from the ovarian stroma, but some are thought to be undiagnosed Brenner tumours where the epithelial elements have been overlooked (Novak & Woodruff 1967) others to be indistinguishable from theca-cell tumours (Haines & Taylor 1962). Teratomata are thought to originate in some way from the germ cells, because of their predilection for the gonads, but the evidence is only by inference.

The special tumours have attracted considerable attention, from pathologists and clinicians alike, because of their bizarre microscopy and their endocrine effects. They are, however, rare compared with the tumours already considered. In the past a somewhat simple classification according to endocrine effects was accepted—feminizing tumours (granulosa- and theca-cell tumours); masculinizing tumours (arrhenoblastomata); and inert (dysgerminomata).

To this classification was appended a number of even rarer tumours, adrenal rest tumours, hilus or leydig tumours.

The discovery of mixed tumours, gynandroblastoma, together with the finding that endocrine effects vary with similar histological varieties and may occur with supposedly non-functioning tumours, has undermined this approach. Closer study has indicated that all these special tumours are closely related and are probably derived from the gonadal mesenchyme, which in embryological development can give rise to either ovarian or testicular cells and which therefore can develop through all the phases of gonadal development of either sex. This theory allows for the presence of granulosa, theca, Leydig, or Sertoli cells in the ovary, or of combinations of them. In this way, granulosa-cell tumour, theca-cell tumour, fibroma, arrhenoblastoma and the functioning stromal element of some Brenner tumours can be seen to have a common ancestry, and gynandroblastoma is explained. Some dispute still exists regarding lipoid-cell tumours. These are mainly masculinizing tumours and their main component is a polyhedral lipoid-containing cell resembling those of the suprarenal cortex, ovarian hilar cells or testicular Leydig cells; it is tempting to infer that all these variations can arise from the ovarian mesenchyme, thus bringing them in to line with the other tumours discussed, but there are those who prefer an origin from ovarian hilar cells or adrenal rests. Dysgerminoma is considered to arise from the germ cells, and is indistinguishable from seminoma of the testis, although some postulate an origin from teratoma along with choriocarcinoma. Haines & Taylor (1962) stress that, where possible, tumours should be assigned the names associated with their obvious morphology, but that in those cases where doubt exists the label gonadal stromal tumour be applied.

Most ovarian malignant disease arises on the basis of serous and mucinous cystadenoma. The malignancy is estimated as being secondary to a benign cyst in about 5–10% of cases, but it is impossible to assess the true figure. Some carcinomata are composed of undifferentiated cells and cannot be allotted to either group. Many different patterns may be found, and are named accordingly, such as medullary, schirrous, alveolar and plexiform, but they are all undifferentiated carcinoma. Two particular types are thought by some to have a different origin: the clear-cell carcinoma and the mesonephroma. The former has been regarded as originating from renal rests, hence the name, hypernephroma of the ovary, and the latter from mesonephric rests. Novak *et al.* (1968) regard them both as variants of mesonephroma, but Haines & Taylor (1962) follow Willis (1953) in believing both to be variants of either serous or undifferentiated carcinoma. Carcinoma arising from endometriosis is recorded, but few cases show the clear-cut graduation from benign to malignant change which is required for diagnosis. Carcinoma resembling endometrial carcinoma in the body of the uterus is now generally recognized, and has been accorded the nomenclature of endometrioid carcinoma of the ovary.

OTHER OVARIAN SWELLINGS

FOLLICULAR CYSTS

This is what is known as a 'cystic ovary'; such a cyst is seldom more than 5 cm in diameter, but on rare occasions can be large and palpable per abdomen; the latter may be the case with the cysts produced by overdosage with clomiphene or human pituitary gonadotrophin. The cysts may arise in either the follicular or the luteal phase, and haemorrhage into them resulting in a small haematoma is not uncommon. The altered blood may then produce a macroscopical appearance identical with endometriosis. Most follicular cysts, which are extremely common, are symptomless, but the following clinical pictures may arise.

(1) Pain in one or other iliac fossa associated with rupture or haemorrhage. This may be minimal or quite severe, and if associated with slight menstrual disturbance may call ectopic pregnancy into the differential diagnosis.

(2) Attacks of recurring pain in either iliac fossa with repeated cyst formation may quite seriously incapacitate the patient.

(3) Persistence of the corpus luteum will be associated with delayed menstruation and a suggestion of early pregnancy, either intra-uterine or ectopic.

(4) In patients receiving human pituitary gonadotrophin or clomiphene larger cysts may develop quite rapidly and be associated with symptoms of acute or subacute abdominal pain (see Chapter 34).

Most of these aberrations of follicular development can be suppressed by anovular therapy induced by cyclical hormone administration, but the last group of cysts require more careful control of the stimulatory agents.

The majority of follicular cysts disperse spontaneously and require no treatment. They may rupture during bimanual examination of the pelvic organs, and this event is usually quite painless, but on occasions the patient may experience some discomfort.

Metropathia haemorrhagica and uterine fibroids are often associated with small follicular cysts in the ovaries. In hydatidiform mole and chorion carcinoma the theca lutein cysts may reach quite large size, due to the stimulation by the chorionic gonadotrophic hormone; occasionally, such large cysts are seen in association with normal pregnancy.

Enlargement of the ovaries with small, multiple cysts occurs in association with the Stein–Levanthal complex, but here diagnosis is initially suggested by associated symptoms.

The important group of endometriomatous ovarian cysts is discussed in Chapter 32.

OVARIAN TUMOURS IN PREGNANCY

Fortunately, most ovarian tumours found in pregnant women, who necessarily are in the younger age groups, are benign. In societies well organized from a medical viewpoint, women attend first for antenatal care in early pregnancy, and pelvic tumours should be detected before the pregnancy is too advanced. Where attendance for antenatal care is less good, tumours are brought to light as a result of accidents occurring to them, or perhaps not until labour is in progress. When an ovarian cyst is found in early pregnancy the diagnosis is usually easy, but a pedunculated fibroid may cause difficulty. The commonest type of tumour is the dermoid cyst but any other types may occur, including, in a small proportion of cases, malignant tumours. Corpus luteum cysts and luteomas of pregnancy rarely occur, but are worth considering as they may spontaneously regress as pregnancy advances. Any of the accidents occurring to ovarian tumours in the non-pregnant may, of course, happen in the pregnant woman; malignant degeneration of a simple tumour is probably the least likely event. Torsion occurs most commonly during pregnancy and in the puerperium, when involution of the uterus and lax abdominal muscles allow greater freedom of movement to the cyst. Haemorrhage into the cyst and rupture are more likely during labour, and infection during the puerperium. Torsion is, however, the commonest complication.

In early pregnancy the presence of a tumour may cause the uterus to appear higher in the abdomen than expected. In late pregnancy if the cyst is impacted in the pelvis a malpresentation or non-engaged presenting part will result, and in the unlikely event of its not being discovered obstructed labour may ultimately develop; such events are rare in the extreme.

TREATMENT

Ovarian tumours discovered in the first and second trimesters of pregnancy should be removed. The optimum time for removal is between the fourteenth and eighteenth week, when the risk of early abortion is over and the uterus not too large to limit access. This time also is recommended to avoid possible disturbance of the corpus luteum of pregnancy. Since the observations of Frankell (1903) many other animal experiments indicate the importance of the corpus luteum in early pregnancy before the formation of the placenta, but is has been shown by Melinkoff (1950) amongst others that this is not so important in the human. When the tumour is first discovered in late pregnancy it is better to defer operation until the puerperium. In the rare cases of obstructed labour operation must be undertaken as an emergency, and usually the uterus must be emptied by Caesarean section before the tumour can be removed from the pelvis. Ramoso-Jalbuena et al. (1967) in 119,903 pregnancies recorded 97 ovarian tumours, an incidence of 1 in 1,236 pregnancies; 4% or 1 in 30,000, were malignant. There were 43% of dermoid cysts and 21% of serous cystadenomata. Complications to the cyst were noted in 66% of cases, torsion being the commonest and occurring most often at 7–8 weeks' gestation.

REFERENCES

ASODOURIAN L.A. & TAYLOR H.B. (1969) *Obstet. Gynec. N.Y.* 33, 370.

BANCROFT-LIVINGSTON G. (1954) *J. Obstet. Gynaec. Br. Commonw.* 61, 628.

BISKIND G.R. & BISKIND M.S. (1949) *Am. J. clin. Path.* 19, 501.

DELLEPIANE G. (1967) *Fifth World Congress of Gynaecology and Obstetrics.* Sydney, Butterworths.

DINNERSTEIN A.S. & O'LEARY J.A. (1968) *Obstet. Gynec., N.Y.* 31, 654.

FARRAR H.K., ELESH R. & LIBRETTI J. (1960) *Obstet. Gynec. Survey,* 15, 1.

FRANKEL L. (1903) *Arch. Gynaek.* 68, 438.

FURTH J. & BUTTERWORTH J.S. (1936) *Am. J. Cancer,* 28, 66.

GRAHAM J.B. & GRAHAM R.M. (1967) *J. Obstet. Gynaec. Br. Commonw.* 74, 371.

GRAY L.A. & BARNES M.L. (1967) *Obstet. Gynec., N.Y.* 29, 694.

HAINES M. & TAYLOR C.W. (1962) *Gynaecological Pathology.* London, Churchill.

HECKMANN U. & LIMBURG H. (1967) *Fifth World Congress of Gynaecology and Obstetrics.* Sydney, Australia.

HUDSON C.N. (1968) *J. Obstet. Gynaec. Br. Commonw.* **75,** 1155.

JEFFCOATE T.N.A. (1962) *Principles of Gynaecology.* London, Butterworths.

McGARRITY K.A. & SCOTT G.C. (1967) *Fifth World Congress of Gynaecology and Obstetrics.* Sydney, Butterworths.

MALKASIAN G.D. Jnr., DOCKERTY M.B. & SYMMONDS R.E. (1967) *Obstet. Gynec., N.Y.* **29,** 725.

MEIGS J.V. (1954) *Am. J. Obstet. Gynec.* **67,** 962.

MEIGS J.V. (1954) *Obstet. Gynec., N.Y.* **3,** 471.

MELINKOFF E. (1950) *Am. J. Obstet. Gynec.* **60,** 437.

MOORE J.G., SCHIFRIN B.S. & EREZ S. (1967) *Am. J Obstet. Gynec.* **99,** 913.

NOVAK E., WOODRUFF J.D. & NOVAK E.R. (1954) *Am. J. Obstet. Gynec.* **68,** 1222.

NOVAK E.R. & WOODRUFF J.D. (1967) *Gynecologic and Obstetric Pathology.* Philadelphia and London, Saunders.

RAMOSO-JALBUENA ALMIRANTE & SOTTO (1967) *J. Philipp. med. Ass.* **43,** 242.

RICHARDS N.A. (1951) *Proc. R. Soc. Med.* **44,** 496.

TERZ J.J., BARBER H.R.K. & BRUNSCHWIG A. (1967) *Am. J. Surg.* **113,** 511.

TRUSSEL R.T. (1963) in *Modern Trends in Gynaecology* (edited by R.J. Kellar). London, Butterworth, p. 52.

WILLIS R.A. (1953) *Pathology of Tumours.* London, Butterworths.

CHAPTER 45

GENERAL SURGICAL PROCEDURES.
URINARY TRACT INJURIES

Surgical technique has been given little consideration in this book, since we believe that practical matters should, in general, be learned in practice, and by reference to specialized treatises where necessary. There will, however, be some technical considerations in this section, because the procedures prescribed are likely to be less familiar to the gynaecologist, and it is felt some discussion of them is appropriate.

THE GYNAECOLOGIST
AS GENERAL SURGEON

It is obviously desirable that a surgeon who embarks on a surgical procedure should be competent to deal with any complication he may meet during its performance. The gynaecologist should therefore open the abdomen only if he feels able to deal with the more common general surgical conditions which may be mistaken for gynaecological lesions, and with general surgical problems which may arise as a result of gynaecological procedures. For this reason the basic general surgical principles of resection and repair of bowel should be understood by the gynaecologist, and he should in his training have practical experience of them. The more exotic aspects of general abdominal surgery will be beyond the gynaecologist's ability, but fortunately these will only rarely be met with.

The better the gynaecologist is as a diagnostician the less often will he be faced with the unexpected general surgical problem and the less experienced, therefore, will he be in dealing with it. By using modern diagnostic techniques, especially radiology and laparoscopy, as well as the traditional examination under anaesthesia, errors should be kept to a minimum. In doubtful cases, referral for a general surgical opinion is a wise step. If doubt still exists an invitation should be extended to an agreeable surgical colleague to attend the operation and assist, or be assisted by, the gynaecologist, according to the operative findings. In such cases the pre-operative preparation of the patient should be aimed at covering all eventualities, and if, for example, colonic surgery seems a possibility, the bowel should be prepared with antibiotics accordingly. In the busy general hospital of today it is rare for a surgical list not to be going on at the same time as the gynaecological list, or at least for a general surgeon to be available in the hospital. In this situation it is in the best interests of the patient for the gynaecologist to summon experienced general surgical assistance rather than embark on a procedure, such as resection for a neoplasm of the colon, in which his technique may perforce have become rusty. Rusty or not, however, the technique must be capable of being carried out, since in an emergency the situation may arise when no general surgical assistance is available.

BOWEL RESECTION AND
ANASTOMOSIS

Small bowel

Resection of small bowel will most often be required in gynaecological operations as a result of the bowel becoming involved in pelvic inflammatory or endometriomatous masses. Since resection always carries some risk, it should be avoided where possible, and so every effort should be made to free the bowel. If this cannot be done, or if it is damaged beyond simple repair of minor perforations, resection will have to be carried out. The level of resection should always be well to each side of the affected area. At the levels selected for resection a hole is made in an avascular area of the mesentery. The mesentery is then divided between these two points in the line of a shallow V, the apex of which points to the root of the mesentery (Fig. 45.1). The vessels in the mesentery are clamped and divided seriatim, and are then tied off. A crushing clamp is now applied to each end of the segment of bowel to be resected, exactly opposite the line of division of the mesentery. After applying light, non-crushing clamps to the healthy bowel on either side, the bowel is divided close to the crushing clamps, every effort being made to mop up any leakage of intestinal contents. After removing the resected bowel the anastomosis is carried out. End-to-end anastomosis is the procedure of choice and can almost invariably be carried out, unless there is much disparity between the size of the bowel above and below the resected portion. The non-crushing clamps are approximated so that the open ends of the bowel lie in apposition. The anastomosis is effected by two layers of sutures (Figs. 45.2 and 45.3). The first layer is made up of a continuous suture through all layers of the bowel wall, beginning at the anti-mesenteric border and continuing round the entire circumference. The individual sutures should be placed close together and locked at intervals to prevent a concertina effect. The mucosa should be inverted as far as possible. No. oo chromic catgut is suitable suture material, and can also be used for the outer layer of sutures which complete the anastomosis. This outer layer should be of interrupted sutures, which should not penetrate the lumen. They bury and reinforce the inner suture line. Special attention should be paid to reinforcing the suture line at the point where it meets the mesentery, for here there is a small area of bowel uncovered by serosa and so prone to leakage. The final step consists in closing the gap in the mesentery with a few interrupted stitches, which should be placed so as to avoid blood vessels running close to the cut edges. Before returning the anastomosed bowel to the abdomen it should be inspected and palpated carefully to confirm that a good lumen has been left at the site of junction and that haemostasis has been secured. Drainage of the peritoneal cavity is not required.

Large bowel

The only portion of the large bowel which the gynaecologist is likely to have to resect is the pelvic colon. This will usually be because of the discovery during the course of a gynaecological laparotomy of a localized lesion, most commonly an annular carcinoma. Occasionally, the pelvic colon may be involved in ovarian or uterine neoplasma, and will need resection along with the other affected pelvic organs. Unless the bowel is obstructed, resection and end-to-end anastomosis can be carried out in the same way as for the small bowel (Figs. 45.4, 45.5 and 45.6), except that a non-absorbable material such as Mersaline should be used for the outer suture line, and great care should be taken to avoid soiling the peritoneal cavity with large bowel contents. Where the resection is done for malignant disease a much wider resection should be performed, with a deep V of mesentery extending to the point where the sigmoid arteries arise from the inferior mesenteric artery. The marginal artery ensures a good blood supply to the bowel throughout much of the length of the colon, and providing the cut edges bleed freely at the time of resection the blood supply will be adequate for good healing.

The problem is complicated when the colon is obstructed at the site of the lesion. In this situation the simplest solution is to bring out a loop of transverse colon through a separate upper abdominal incision and then close the abdomen, leaving the lesion *in situ*. The loop colostomy thus formed can be opened subsequently to relieve the obstruction (Figs. 45.7 and 45.8). If the patient's general condition is poor, or the gynaecologist very inexperienced in bowel surgery, performing a transverse colostomy is

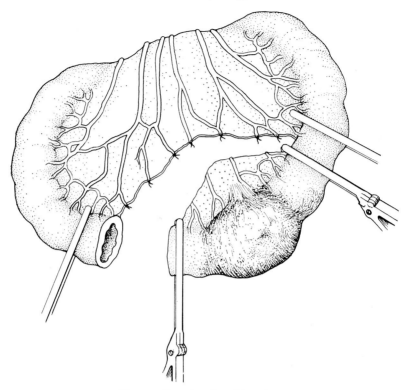

Fig. 45.1. Resection of small bowel.

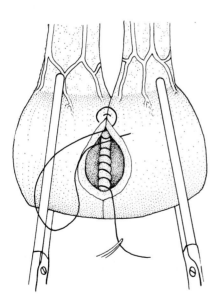

Fig. 45.2. Anastomosis of small bowel: inner suture line.

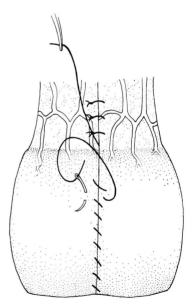

Fig. 45.3. Anastomosis of small bowel: outer suture line.

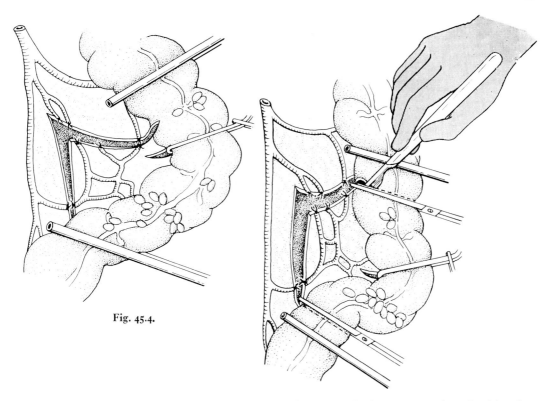

Fig. 45.4.

Fig. 45.4 and Fig. 45.5. Resection of pelvic colon.

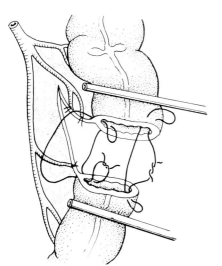

Fig. 45.6. Anastomosis of pelvic colon.

safe and quick. It does have the disadvantage that the definitive operation is postponed for 2 or 3 weeks, and a third operation will be needed to close the colostomy thereafter. Two alternative solutions are available and either may be used, depending on the degree of obstruction. If the colon is only partially obstructed or, if complete obstruction has been present for only a short time, the disparity in size between the colon above and below the obstruction will not be great. Resection and end-to-end anastomosis will then be possible as described above. It should only be done in this situation, however, if the strain can be taken off the suture-line by means of a defunctioning transverse colostomy or a caecostomy. The latter has much to commend it, and is performed through a small McBurney incision in the right iliac fossa. The caecum is carefully sutured to the incision and then incised to allow the insertion of a small Foley catheter

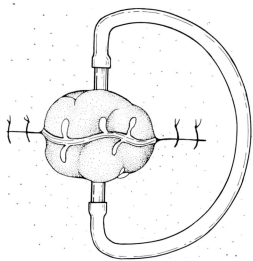

Fig. 45.7. Loop colostomy before opening.

(Fig. 45.9). The bag on the catheter is blown up and serves to minimize leakage, whilst at the same time the catheter acts as a valve through which flatus and fluid bowel contents can escape. Once the anastomosis has healed the catheter is withdrawn, and the small fistula will then close spontaneously. The second alternative solution to carcinoma of the pelvic colon complicated by obstruction is the time-hallowed Paul Mikulicz operation (Fig. 45.10). In this procedure the obstructed loop of pelvic colon containing the lesion is exteriorized through an oblique incision in the left iliac fossa. The abdomen is then closed and thereafter the exteriorised loop cut off leaving a 'double-barrelled' colostomy which can be closed in the usual way at a subsequent operation when the effects of the obstruction have disappeared.

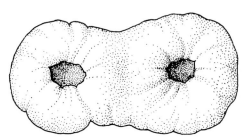

Fig. 45.8. Loop colostomy: end result.

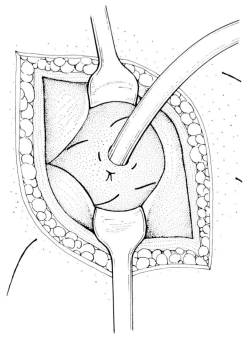

Fig. 45.9. Caecostomy using Foley catheter.

Appendicitis

Acute appendicitis will often feature in the differential diagnosis of an acute admission to the gynaecological ward. In young women with lower abdominal pain of sudden onset the distinction between acute appendicitis, acute salpingitis, ectopic pregnancy, urinary tract infection and even incomplete abortion may be difficult to make on clinical grounds. The central abdominal site of the pain at its onset and its later localization to the right iliac fossa—together with anorexia, vomiting, and the absence of menstrual or urinary disturbance—point to appendicitis. If careful clinical assessment cannot exclude a gynaecological cause for the pain, the patient should be examined under anaesthesia and a laparoscopy performed. If this shows the pelvic organs to be normal the appendix can then be removed through an incision in the right iliac fossa. This is a preferable procedure to performing a mid-line lower abdominal laparotomy and then finding that the patient's symptoms are

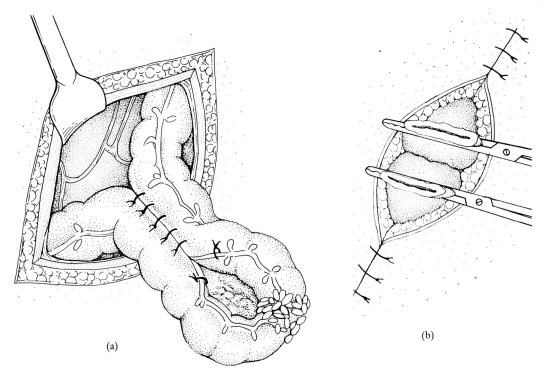

(a)

(b)

Fig. 45.10. (a) Paul Mikulicz operation. Exteriorizing the loop. (b) Paul Mikulicz operation. Loop excised. The clamps are removed, leaving a double-barrelled colostomy.

due to an inflamed retrocaecal appendix. Removal of the appendix in this situation may be difficult from the mid-line approach.

ROUTINE APPENDICECTOMY DURING
GYNAECOLOGICAL OPERATIONS

Some gynaecologists make a practice of removing the appendix as a routine when performing a laparotomy for a gynaecological condition. If this is done, however, there is a risk of post-operative complications relating to the appendicectomy—mainly the spread of infection from the appendix stump to the pelvic peritoneum and any traumatized tissue or haematoma that may result from the gynaecological operation especially hysterectomy. In young women with a history of pain in the right lower abdomen the appendix should be removed even if the pain seems likely to have arisen from the gynaecological

condition for which the operation is performed. In most patients subjected to gynaecological abdominal surgery, however, there will be no such history, and the slight risk of added post-operative complications outweighs the small risk that the patient will subsequently get acute appendicitis.

Inversion appendicectomy

If removal of the appendix is thought necessary the technique of inversion is recommended. In this procedure the appendix is cleaned by ligation and division of its mesentery, and the removal of any attached fatty tissue. Using a blunt-ended probe, and starting at the tip of the organ, the appendix is inverted into the caecum. When inversion is complete the appendix lies 'inside out' in the lumen of the caecum and its site is marked only by a dimple in the caecal wall. This is closed with a single catgut suture and the procedure is complete. The appendix sloughs off and is 'digested', in the course of its passage round the colon, with the bowel contents. The advantage of this method is that the risk of infection is minimized, since the bowel lumen is never opened. Apart from this the pleasure of turning a long appendix inside out, especially in the presence of an astonished general surgical audience, makes the procedure one which should be in every gynaecologist's armamentarium. (A little quiet practice is advisable before a public demonstration is attempted, for a fibrosed appendix may be very difficult to invert!)

Diverticulitis

Modern general surgical opinion favours immediate resection and end-to-end anastomosis in many cases of acute diverticulitis. The gynaecologist faced with a previously undiagnosed acute diverticulitis of the pelvic colon should seek expert general surgical assistance if possible, for these resections are sometimes difficult and call for considerable surgical skill. The main problem is likely to be mobilization of the inflamed segment of bowel. Once this has been achieved resection and end-to-end anastomosis can be performed in the usual way. A simple defunctioning caecostomy as described above should be combined with the procedure. If it is felt that immediate resection is likely to prove too difficult an operation, the gynaecologist should be content with closing the abdomen and treating the acute attack with antibiotics. If perforation of the bowel has occurred an attempt should be made to close the perforation. A large, rubber-tube drain should be led through a separate stab incision in the iliac fossa, down to the site of the perforation. Where a localized pericolic abscess has formed it should be drained in the same way. A defunctioning colostomy is not usually indicated unless it seems likely that continuing leakage of bowel contents will occur.

Excision of the rectum

The fifth edition of Berkely and Bonney's famous textbook *Gynaecological Surgery* devotes a whole chapter to the various methods of excising the rectum when a carcinoma of that part of the bowel had been mistaken for a tumour of the uterus. Nowadays the gynaecologist should never have to carry out excision of the rectum except during the course of an exenteration operation for advanced pelvic cancer. The indications and technique for this very extensive surgical procedure are beyond the scope of this present work. In the unlikely event of a carcinoma of the rectum being discovered during the course of a gynaecological laparotomy the services of a competent rectal surgeon should be sought at once. If such an individual is not immediately available the wisest course is to close the abdomen and refer the patient for surgical treatment at a later date. A pelvic colostomy should not be performed unless the lesion is causing obstruction.

Benign conditions of the rectum and anal canal

PROLAPSE OF THE RECTUM

The gynaecologist's help is sometimes sought in this condition when it occurs in elderly women in association with vaginal prolapse. A successful repair operation with excision of any enterocoele sac which may be present may improve the rectal prolapse and facilitate such surgical measures that may be necessary to complete the cure.

HAEMORRHOIDS

Parous women commonly suffer from piles, to a greater or lesser degree, especially in association with vaginal prolapse. As with rectal prolapse, a successful posterior vaginal wall repair may improve matters, but further surgical treatment by injection or dissection and ligature will usually be required. The temptation to combine the posterior repair with a haemorrhoidectomy should usually be resisted, since the discomfort to the patient in the postoperative period after such a combined assault is very considerable.

ANAL FISSURE

This lesion is very commonly seen in gynaecological patients, especially shortly after delivery.

It is most commonly situated in the mid-line posteriorly and gives rise to severe pain, especially on defaecation. Recent fissures will usually heal with soothing local ointments and the avoidance of constipation, but longer-standing fissures become indurated and require surgical treatment. If this condition is met with during the course of gynaecological operation it should be dealt with by stretching of the internal anal sphincter. This is effected by slowly inserting first one, then two, and then three or four fingers into the anal canal. Very long-standing fissures, which usually are accompanied by a 'sentinal' pile, require excision, and this is best done as a separate surgical procedure and not combined with the gynaecological operation.

URINARY TRACT LESIONS IN GYNAECOLOGY

It is a sad fact that, apart from the bladder and urethral conditions incidental to vaginal prolapse, urinary tract lesions met with by the gynaecologist are most often of his own making. Because of the close proximity between the lower ends of the ureters and the bladder to the uterus and vagina, gynaecological operations may from time to time result in damage to these parts of the urinary tract. In only about one-third of cases of ureteric damage will the injury be recognized at the time of operation, although a much higher proportion of bladder injuries will be noticed at once. The practising gynaecologist should be able to carry out any necessary immediate reparative surgery. When ureteric damage is only recognized in the postoperative period the advice and assistance of a urologist may be prudently sought. Vesicovaginal fistula, the product in this instance of unrecognized or badly repaired bladder damage, is best regarded as a specialized gynaecological problem, to be dealt with by a gynaecologist with special experience in this field.

Injuries to the bladder

Apart from penetration of the anterior vaginal and bladder walls by protruding sharp objects in 'falling astride', accidents the bladder is most commonly injured during the course of abdominal hysterectomy or vaginal repair. In carrying out abdominal hysterectomy great care must be taken when dissecting the bladder off the anterior aspect of the cervix and upper vagina. Once the uterovesical fold of peritoneum has been incised the plane of cleavage between bladder and uterus should be sought in the mid-line; the bladder can then be stripped down by gentle finger or gauze dissection. Although the separation is usually easy it may be attended by troublesome bleeding from the paravesical plexus of veins. This bleeding must be carefully controlled, as the dissection proceeds by means of diathermy forceps or fine ligatures. Difficulty in separating off the bladder is especially likely to occur when the patient has had a previous Caesarean section or Manchester operation. Sharp dissection with scissors may then be needed, and in this case every effort should be made to keep close to the anterior aspect of the uterus.

Even in seemingly uncomplicated cases, injury to the bladder may occur, the characteristic appearance of bladder mucosa announcing the sad fact that the organ has been breached. It is usually best in this situation to complete the removal of the uterus before turning attention to the repair of the bladder. Once the uterus has been removed the extent of the bladder damage should be defined, the edges of the hole being picked up with fine tissue forceps. As with the repair of holes in the bowel, a two-layer closure should be aimed at. The first layer is made up of a continuous suture of fine (oo) chromic catgut through the bladder mucosa alone. This suture line is now buried by a second suture line of interrupted, fine, chromic catgut sutures. As well as closing the opening the two suture lines should ensure haemostasis, which is a prerequisite for good healing. The suture line should be rendered extraperitoneal by closure of the pelvic peritoneum in the usual fashion. A fine plastic or rubber-tube drain may be led down extraperitoneally to the site of injury being brought out to the surface through a small separate suprapubic stab wound. Such a drain is only needed if the injury has been extensive or persistent oozing makes haematoma formation seem likely.

Efficient closed-catheter drainage of the bladder is essential for a minimum of 10 days; particular care must be taken to ensure that blockage of the catheter does not occur. A No. 14 Foley catheter with a 5 ml bag is suitable, and the nursing staff should be instructed to record the volume of urine drained every hour for the first 48 hr and every 4 hr for the next 5 days. A broad-spectrum antibiotic should be given to reduce the chance of infection at the site of injury. In most cases healing will occur uneventfully, and the patient's bladder function will thereafter be unimpaired.

Injury to the bladder may occur during vaginal repair operations and, as with abdominal hysterectomy, is most likely during the dissection of the bladder off the anterior aspect of the cervix. Once the vaginal epithelium has been removed or reflected laterally the extent to which the bladder is attached to the cervix is usually apparent, a well-marked fold denoting the point of reflexion. In case of doubt, and especially when there has been a previous repair operation or Caesarean section, a bladder sound passed per urethram will accurately delineate the bladder margins. When the bladder is adherent sharp dissection may be preferable to finger or gauze dissection, but if the scissors are used they must be kept close to the anterior wall of the uterus. It is well to remember the old maxim that it is better to leave a small portion of the uterine wall on the bladder than vice versa!

When the bladder is opened during the course of a vaginal operation similar steps should be taken to close the opening. The more restricted approach to the lesion may make the procedure more difficult but, with care and patience, satisfactory closure should always be possible. Since the opening is likely to be closer to the bladder neck, care must be taken to avoid the ureteric orifices when inserting the bladder sutures. If it seems likely that the Foley catheter bag will impinge on the suture line a simple No. 14 plastic catheter may be used, but care must be taken to secure it in position by strips of adhesive plaster. Suprapubic drainage of the damaged bladder is not usually necessary nowadays, but may be employed if it seems likely that urethral catheter drainage will be inefficient.

Injuries to the ureter

It has been said that no one can assume the title of gynaecologist until they have inadvertently cut a ureter at operation. Most modern aspirants strive to avoid this distinction, however, and with good reason for the accident is usually, but not always, the result of poor operative technique. Abdominal gynaecological operations are more likely to cause ureteric damage than vaginal operations. Feeney (1969) analysed 29 cases, of which 24 were the result of abdominal and five the result of vaginal procedures. The commonest types of injury by far are crushing, division and ligation, in various combinations.

SITE OF INJURY

The ureter may be injured at one of three sites.

(a) At, or adjacent to, the pelvic brim

The ureter is most often damaged at this site during ligation and division of the infundibulo pelvic ligament, and care must always be taken when carrying out this step to palpate the bundle before applying the clamp. The ureter adheres to the deep surface of the parietal peritoneum and may be drawn up with it. Lateral extension of the peritoneal incision during a presacral neurectomy may easily involve the ureter.

(b) At, or adjacent to, the crossing of the uterine artery

This is not a common site for injury to the ureter, but it must always be remembered that the normal anatomical relationships may not apply in the presence of fibroids arising from the lower part of the uterus, especially when these extend laterally into the broad ligament. The only safe course of action in this circumstance is positively to identify the ureter, if necessary tracing it down from the pelvic brim, before applying the uterine artery clamp. Endometriosis and chronic pelvic inflammatory disease may also distort normal anatomical relationships and impair the normal mobility of the ureter.

(c) At, or adjacent to, the entry into the bladder

This is by far the commonest site of injury in abdominal procedures, and is the invariable site in vaginal operations. A clamp placed alongside the cervix to include the cervical branch of the uterine artery and the main attachment of the lateral cervical ligament is usually responsible for the ureteric damage. Placing the clamp too far laterally or failing to displace the bladder sufficiently off the anterior aspect of the cervix are the commonest faults, although the hurried application of a clamp to arrest haemorrhage may be responsible. The temptation to 'grab' a bundle of tissue in the region of the lateral vaginal fornix to stop what may be an alarming haemorrhage should always be resisted. Firm pressure with a pack will always control the situation until the site of the bleeding can be accurately identified.

TIME AND RECOGNITION OF THE INJURY

Unfortunately, in only one-quarter of all cases is the ureteric injury recognized at the time of the initial operation. In the remainder, recognition comes during the postoperative period, usually in the first few days, depending upon the nature of the injury. Where the ureter has been completely obstructed the patient develops severe continuous pain in the affected kidney and usually a high, swinging temperature. If both ureters are damaged anuria results. This condition should be noted within the first 12 hr of operation, but its recognition has sometimes been inexplicably delayed, with disastrous results to the patient.

Incomplete occlusion of the ureter will be associated with lesser symptoms; where the ureter has been cut and not ligated leakage of urine through the vaginal vault or abdominal wound will occur. The leak may not become immediately manifest, being preceded by a local collection of urine in the pelvis, with an inevitable abscess formation.

DIAGNOSIS

Immediate recognition that a ureter has been damaged during the course of an operation will save the patient much discomfort, and in most cases the need for a further operation. If it is suspected that the ureter may have been clamped or divided a very careful appraisal of the situation should be made, the course of the ureter being carefully traced by palpation or, if necessary, by exposure. Where it seems likely that a particular 'bundle' contains the ureter, whether divided or not, the ligature or clamp should be carefully removed. When this is done free bleeding will occur from any cut vessels, which can then be picked up separately with artery forceps. The cut end of a ureter which is said to 'pout' may not be easily visible, but palpation will detect its characteristic cord-like feel. Postoperative diagnosis will be made on the clinical features, which, as mentioned above, include loin pain and swelling, high temperature and rigors, and ultimately a leak of urine through the abdominal or vaginal incisions. The intravenous pyelogram is a very valuable aid to diagnosis and will show poor or absent function in the affected kidney or a leak of urine into the pelvis if the ureter is not completely occluded.

TREATMENT

Every endeavour should be made to restore the situation so that the ureter drains into the bladder again. If the ureter is clamped or ligated without being cut, prompt removal of the clamp or ligature will usually be followed by complete recovery without leakage. Diagnosis of ureteric occlusion within 72 hr of operation calls for an immediate attempt to relieve the occlusion. Later, diagnosis associated with free drainage of urine through the abdominal incision or vagina is best managed by postponing operation for 3 months. By the end of this time local inflammation should have settled down and the definitive surgery can more easily be carried out. Of the possible operative approaches to the problem of the damaged ureter, cutaneous ureterostomy, simple ligation and nephrectomy should not normally be considered by the gynaecologist.

Implantation of the ureter into the bladder

This is the procedure of choice and can be carried out in the majority of cases, especially if full use is made of the freedom with which the bladder can be mobilized and of the Boari technique. The operative considerations apply to both immediate and delayed operations on the damaged ureter. When the ureter is of sufficient length to lie without tension on the bladder wall, a simple method of implantation is employed. The end of the ureter is cut obliquely and an incision is made in the bladder wall close to the site of the original ureteric opening. The incision is placed in the line in which the ureter is to lie and penetrates completely through the bladder wall only at its distal end. At this point the ureteric end should be sutured with very fine (ooo) catgut to the exposed bladder mucosa so as to give, as far as possible, a suture line from the bladder mucosa to ureteric mucosa (Fig. 45.11). The remainder of the incision in the

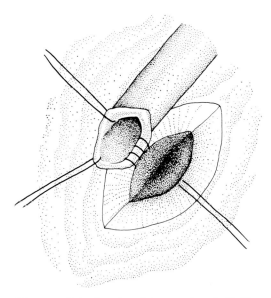

Fig. 45.11. Reimplantation of the ureter into the bladder.

bladder wall is closed round the ureter, so as to give a short, intramural course to the new ureterovesical junction. The site of implantation should be made extraperitoneal by repairing the pelvic peritoneum as necessary. An extraperitoneal drain is employed and the bladder is drained with a urethral catheter for at least 10 days.

Boari's operation

When the ureter is too short even after mobilization of the bladder, a rectangular flap of bladder is outlined (see Fig. 45.12) and cut in such a way as to leave its base hinged in the region of the trigone. The ureter is split and anchored to the bladder flap, which is then sutured so as to form a tube. Fine catgut sutures (ooo) are employed for this purpose. The bladder is closed but must be efficiently drained by a urethral catheter for 10–14 days. The site of anastomosis is drained extraperitoneally as before. This drain should be left *in situ* until all leakage of urine through it has ceased.

Uretero-ureteric anastomosis

End-to-end anastomosis of the ureter is not difficult, but the results are not good, stricture formation being common. Where the ureter is damaged at a considerable distance from the bladder it may, however, be employed as an alternative to nephrectomy or more elaborate techniques of ureteric replacement by a segment of bowel. The cut ends of the ureter are trimmed obliquely and sutured together with fine catgut sutures. The site of anastomosis should be drained extraperitoneally.

Ileal conduits

The use of an isolated segment of ileum, either to replace the lower end of a ureter or to act as an alternative receptacle to the bladder, is part of the specialized field of urology, and will normally only be performed by gynaecologists employing exenteration with removal of the bladder as a means of treatment of advanced carcinoma of the cervix. It is worth noting that the use of an ileal bladder is now considered preferable to ureterocolic anastomosis, which used to be favoured.

Vesicovaginal fistulae

The historical importance of the vesicovaginal fistula to modern gynaecology is immense, and is based on the pioneer work of J. Marian Sims. The efforts made by Sims to deal with this most

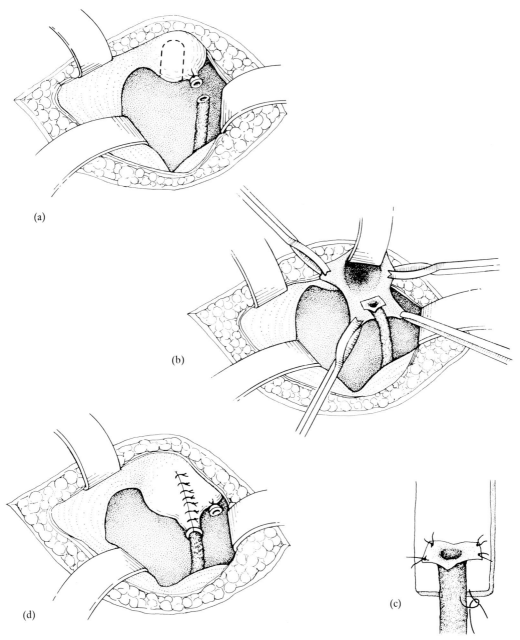

Fig. 45.12. The Boari operation. (a) Bladder flap fashioned. (b) Bladder flap and ureter approximated. (c) Cut end of ureter split and sutured to the bladder flap. (d) Bladder flap closed.

debilitating of gynaecological lesions laid the foundations of vaginal surgery as it is practised today. Sim's achievements—in the middle of the nineteenth century and before the advent of anaesthesia and antisepsis—were the result of a single-minded dedication and determination which has rarely been seen in medicine before or since. Today's vesico-vaginal fistulae result from obstetric, gynaecological or radiotherapeutic trauma of one sort or another. The problem of management is too complex a subject to be considered in the present context. The reader is referred to the classic monographs of Moir (1967) and Russell (1962).

REFERENCES

FEENEY J.K. (1969) Lecture to gynaecological travellers in Dublin.

MOIR J.C. (1967) *The Vesicovaginal Fistula*, 2nd edn. London, Baillière, Tindall & Cassell.
RUSSELL C.S. (1962) *Vesicovaginal Fistulas and Related Matters*. Springfield, Thomas.

Textbooks of
Operative General Surgery

FARQUHARSON E.L. (1969) *Textbook of Operative Surgery*. Edinburgh and London, Livingstone.
McNAIR T.J. (editor) (1967) *Hamilton Bailey's Emergency Surgery*. Bristol, John Wright.

INDEX

Ligaments
  broad 124–5
  pelvic 125
  round 123–4
  uteroscral 124
Lippes Loop D 458
Liquor amnii 440
  abnormalities 378–82
  volume 379
Lochial flow, in puerperium 203
Long-acting thyroid stimulator
  (LATS) 328, 330
Lorain-Lévi syndrome 56
Lovset manoeuvre, in breech delivery
  368
Luteal phase deficiency 208
Luteinizing hormone *see* LH
Luteinizing hormone release factor
  see LRF
Lutembachers syndrome 289
Luteolysis 35
Lymphadenectomy 599, 630, 633
  pelvic 606
Lymphangiography 630
Lymphangioma 664
Lymphatic permeation 477
Lymphocyst 635–6
Lymphogranuloma inguinale 570,
  594–5
Lymphosarcoma 649

McIndoe/Read technique 10, 11
Madlener method, of sterilization
  463, 464
Magnesium sulphate, in eclampsia
  275, 277, 278
Male intersex 13
  cryptorchid hypospadiac 46, 50–
  1, 58–9
Male pill 465
Malformations, congenital 13–14, 18,
  321, 452
Malignant tumours, of vulva 599–
  601
Malnutrition, foetal 153, 155–6
Manchester procedure 554, 555, 556
  in prolapse 560, 561
Mannitol
  in abortion kidney 224
  in urinary suppression 275
Manual rotation, and forceps delivery
  356, 401
Masculine differentiation 45
Masculinizing tumour 78–9, 664,
  666–7, 672
Maternal
  disease, as cause of abortion 209
  factors, causing abortion 207
  injuries, and complications 422–7
  mortality 231–2, 319

Maternal-foetal glucose 315–16
Mauriceau-Smellie-Vertical method,
  of delivery 368
Meclozinehydrochloride (Ancolan)
  349
Medroxy-progesterone acetate, and
  contraception 465
Melanocyte-stimulating hormone
  (MSH), in pregnancy 127, 151
Melatonin 34
Membrane rupture
  in forceps delivery 434
  to induce labour 431–2
Menarche 23, 55
  age of 28
  delayed 61
Mendelson's syndrome 441, 442
Menopause 69, 539
  age of 640
  and uterine prolapse 547
  in triple X female 47
  premature 63, 64, 67, 69, 71
Menstrual bleeding 10–12
  abnormalities 640
  excessive 30
Menstruation 37, 123
  and FSH 38–41
  cessation of *see* Menopause
  delay in 57
  disorders of 511
  failure 9
  following delivery 203
  in adrenal hyperplasia 79–80
  mechanism of 512–14
  normal 55
  onset of 28
  physiology of 22–8, 30
  spontaneous 58
Mental disorders 340, 341
Mentoposterior position 358, 359
Mentovertical presentation 183, 184
Mesonephric duct 2, 5, *see also*
  Wolffian duct
Mestranol, treatment in Turner's
  syndrome 60
Metabolism, iron 132–3
Metholrexate
  in abdominal pregnancy 231
  in chorionic carcinoma 243–4, 245
Metronidozole (Flagyl) 21, 580
Metropathia haemorrhagica 516, 673
Minot-von-Willebrand syndrome
  519
Molar metastases 239–40
Mole
  hydatidiform 232, 234, 235–7, 237–
  42, 269, 673
  invasive 234, 235, 241
  metastasizing 241
  transitional 234, 235

Monilia albicans 123, 318
Montgomery's tubercles, in pregnancy
  127
Morphia, and abortion 214
Mortality
  maternal 231–2, 319, 447–51
  perinatal 451–4
'Mouse uterus' test 68
Muellerian ducts 44, 45, 113, 219,
  476, 604, 649
  anomalies of 216, 218–19
  inhibition 49, 50
  involvement 2–5
Multiple births 504
Multiple pregnancy 375–8
  abortion in 219
  diagnosis of 375–6
  by X-ray 141
  labour in 376–7
Mumps
  effects in pregnancy 335
  effects on foetus 101
Myasthenia gravis, and effects of
  pregnancy 339
Myoblastoma, granular cell 591–2
Myomectomy 359, 424
  of uterine fibroids 615
Myometrial contraction 170

Nalidixic acid, treatment of acute
  pyelonephritis 309
Necrosis 275
  avascular 632
  renal cortical 254
Neonatal
  death 319, 320
  disorders 18–19
  hypoglycaemia 320
Neoplasia, trophoblastic 233–7
  aetiology 35–6
  classification 234–5
  geographical distribution 235–7
Nephrectomy 14, 686
Nephritis 266, 268, 282
Nephrotic syndrome 266, 268, 287,
  see also Renal disease
Nerve supply, to uterus in pregnancy
  116
Nervous disorders, in pregnancy
  338–41
Neurotic reactions, in puerperium
  419
Nitrofurantoin treatment, of pyelonephritis 309
Norethisterone 30, 71, 221
Norethynodrel (Enavid) 30
Nystatin 21

Obesity
  and amenorrhoea 84